The Fourth Monkey

An Untold History of the Lyme Disease Epidemic

PJ Langhoff

The Fourth Monkey
An Untold History of the Lyme Disease Epidemic

Published by Allegory Press, LLC, Hustisford, WI 53034
Printed in the United States of America, First Standard Edition

Library of Congress Control Number: 2012902131
ISBN: 978-0-9833765-1-4

For more information please contact the author at:
PJ Langhoff c/o Allegory Press LLC
PO Box 444, Hustisford, WI 53034
books@allegorypress.com

PJ Langhoff's books are available in large-print, audio, hand-held, and E-book formats. Please see the publisher's web site for more information on available formats for each book.

Patient Stories From the Front Lines (Book 1 – "It's All In Your Head" Series)
Around the World in 80 Lyme Patient Stories (Book 2)
The Baker's Dozen & the Lunatic Fringe: Has Junk Science Shifted the Lyme Disease Paradigm? (Book 3)
God Science: The Secret World of Rampant Genetics, Hidden Illness, and Biotech Profiteering (Book 4)
The Singing Forest, A Journey Through Lyme Disease
Right Behind You, Spiritual Helpers from Beyond the Earth Plane
Jordan and the Naughty Camels (English and Spanish versions)

Available at: www.AllegoryPress.com, www.Amazon.com, and other retailers.

PJ Langhoff is available for private research projects in the medical and legal arenas.

Front Cover and title page art: H Lucas. Front and back cover and book designs: PJ Langhoff.
Back Cover Images: "Tools of Technology" top row: Three Mile Island, Middletown, Pennsylvania, CDC image; Crop dusting the fields, 1952 Dick Robbins/CDC; Inside a coal mine, circa late 1940s, CDC image.
Row two: Protozoan *Acanthamoeba* species, 2009 Janice Haney Carr/CDC; Soil bacteria *Bacillus cereus*, 2010 Pete Seidel/CDC; Fungus *Beauveria bassiana*, 1961 Lucille K. Georg/CDC.
Bottom row: Soil or water spirochetes leptospira species, 1998 Janice Haney Carr/CDC; Deer tick or black-legged tick *Ixodes scapularis*, Jim Gathany/CDC; and Soil bacteria *Pseudomonas aeruginosa*, Janice Haney Carr/CDC.

The Fourth Monkey

An Untold History of the Lyme Disease Epidemic

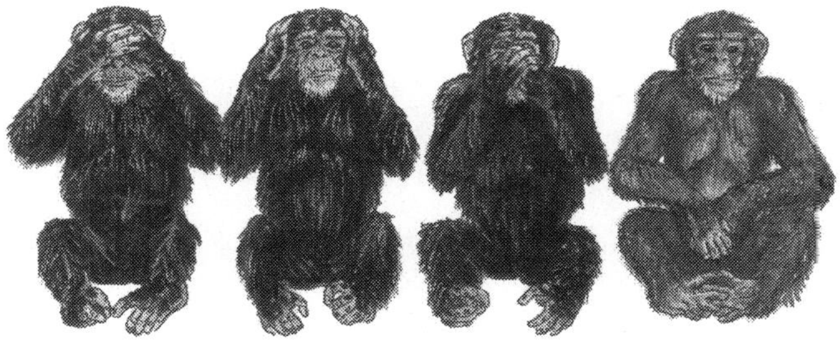

In Japanese culture, the three wise monkeys or mystic apes (Mizaru, Kikazaru, and Iwazaru) represent a pictorial metaphor. They embody the principals "hear no evil, speak no evil," and "see no evil." There is however a little known fourth monkey named Shizaru who symbolizes the principal of "do no evil."

In medicine, the Hippocratic Oath is a pledge that has historically been uttered by new physicians and other healthcare professionals as a rite of passage in many countries. Individuals under oath swear to practice medicine using the highest ethical standards. Although the oath's verbiage varies by country, the heart of the oath includes the words "never do harm to anyone." It is an oath that is well heeded by those who place the value of human life above all else. In the scientific arena common sense and sound moral judgment to "do no harm" should prevail above matters of political and private interests. While there are many who work diligently at all levels of industry and government to protect the interests of public health, it is because of those who do not and have not, that this book has come to be written.

Public health reports often state that Lyme disease does not kill its patients. In the real world however, patients and their families live with this disease undetected, misdiagnosed, untreated, or under treated; and they can attest that it can, it does, and it has, killed. This book is dedicated also to the heroic physicians and researchers boldly blazing new pathways to better diagnostic and treatment options despite stern opposition in the medical and scientific arenas. And to the millions who walked before us, and those who have become infected with agents that should never have, and probably never would have entered their bodies had someone spoken up decades ago.

In memory of Jean Kreilkamp, who left us to battle Lyme in her stead.
And so we shall, and we shall win.

Special thanks to the Jean Kreilkamp family; to H. Lucas, S. Langhoff, Nancy Mackay, Walter Lehman, Susan Green, Dr. Rudolph Scrimenti; the staff at Hustisford Library, Hustisford, Wisconsin; Judy O'Brien and Joanne Humphrey; and Amy Vanderboom, Jørgen Eilenberg (University of Copenhagen) and Niels Bohse Hendriksen (Aarhus University) Denmark.

To our Creator, I am your humble servant, always.

Disclaimer

This book is a representation of ideas and hypotheses based upon extensive research over an eight-year period. The information was gathered from hundreds of sources, and has helped formulate the opinions and hypotheses of the author, which are expressed herein. Note that the author is a Lyme patient and a student of science and medicine; therefore accuracy and opinions are affected by same. The reader is warned not to take any thoughts, information, or hypotheses with anything but casual observation for educational purposes. Some ideas expressed in this book may be the result of conclusions drawn from published literature where the content thereof may or may not have been accurate. Inasmuch as the author relied upon scientific papers and texts for some information gathering, the author and publisher do not warrant that anything contained in this book in any of its forms is necessarily factual, or that it has been scientifically or otherwise verified. Readers are encouraged to do their own research to prove or disprove the author's observations or hypotheses; even in the presence of what may seem to be compelling or irrefutable evidence.

While there are many good and properly motivated individuals in the scientific, biotech, public health, and government communities; the trends toward the denial of epidemics; and the individuals, agencies, or industries whose actions, products, or services grant favor toward industry or profits above the welfare of human health are those addressed in this book. Scientific, medical, or public health organizations including the ADA, AEC, AMA, CDC, EPA, FAO, FDA, IAEA, IDSA, ILADS, UN, WHO, etc. have memberships which include highly respected individuals. Absolutely no criticisms are made about a specific organization or its membership in whole or in part. References to "IDSA," "IDSA guidelines," or "ILADS" or "ILADS guidelines" refer simply to Lyme disease medical guidelines or the individuals responsible for writing them in any edition.

Please note that with respect to references made to the "military" or any military branch; or government department, agency, or its affiliates or subcontractors, such references pertain only to individuals who performed research or experiments involving agriculture, microbes, biowarfare or agricultural "weapons," medicines, or other industrial processes or products discussed as related to the story in this book. When any public health, government, or independent agency, division, or publicly or privately held company, institution, university, non-profit, laboratory, medical organization, or corporation from any country is referenced; such reference pertains only to the individual(s) from the named entity who are or were involved in the specific topic of discussion. No other inferences or connections are made or should be assumed. All individuals and entities named in the book are to be considered innocent of any wrongdoing or inappropriate intent unless and until found guilty in a proper court of law. There are no allegations made or intended as to right or wrong actions by any parties, even if made or seemingly implied. Some information was not cited directly, because it was used only transiently to uncover additional resources. The author thanks these unnamed sources. For more information about biowarfare, Lyme and related topics, please see *God Science: The Secret World of Rampant Genetics, Hidden Illness, and Biotech Profiteering*, also available from Allegory Press, LLC.

Readers are advised that the author is not a healthcare professional, scientist, nor someone with formal training in medicine. The author cannot and is not providing medical advice or recommendations for the prevention, diagnosis, or treatment of any medical condition. **Do not rely upon any information or ideas in this book as medical advice. Always seek the advice of a qualified medical practitioner before undertaking any therapy or change in therapy.**

This book is a collection of ideas presented solely for informational purposes and independent study. There is no guarantee of accuracy made or implied in any portion of this book in any of its formats. Although this book is based on historical facts, events, and evidence; the story told within this book and the timeline of events have been assembled based on the author's hypotheses as to the origins of one or more animal and human epidemic diseases. The story in this book is not necessarily accurate and should be understood solely as the author's opinion and hypotheses.

Note: There is a lot of technical information in this book. Please do not get hung up on the names of various microbes. Simply read over them and in time many will become familiar. It is unnecessary to memorize the names of microbes. It is however, important to see their names since they play a role in the formation of mutant organisms which may cause human diseases.

TABLE OF CONTENTS

First, Do No Harm.

Introduction

I chuckled slightly when I saw the photograph of a headstone with the epitaph "I told you I was sick." That is the story of my life and the lives of hundreds of thousands of people who live in all parts of the world, who live with a mysterious illness called Lyme disease. Many of these people will have been told their illness is "something else." Others will be told their symptoms are too perplexing for their doctors to diagnose so they must be imaging them and their problem is "all in their heads." I am one of these people and I have heard it all more times than I have heard acknowledgement that maybe the symptoms I have been dealing with are real. And while many Lyme patients look "great" on paper with respect to routine laboratory tests, when the right kinds of tests are ordered, voilà, suddenly we don't look quite so normal.

I would not learn about Lyme disease until I was bitten for the second time by a hard-shelled, black-legged *Ixodes scapularis* or deer tick in 1992. The first time was in 1969 when I was just a kid. But three decades later, a new tick bite, and a month after grueling symptoms arrived, one of my physicians declared "there is no Lyme disease in Wisconsin." In retrospect the huge bull's-eye rash which covered my entire back should have been a red flag for any astute doctor. Had I known right away what it was, I would not have listened to my doctors for as long as I did. After all, this strange new infection was wreaking absolute havoc upon my health.

Out of frustration I went to the local library. There I was fortunate enough to locate a small blurb and a photograph of a bull's-eye rash in an encyclopedia. As I read the description of symptoms, I felt as if I was reading my own story. That day I felt certain I had found the source of my illness: Lyme disease. It would be a dozen and a half more years however before I would find a single physician willing to listen with an open mind to my ills, and who would diagnose it properly so I could begin some kind of meaningful treatments and the delay was most unfortunate.

At the start of the journey, my first doctor dismissed my rash and symptoms. He suggested that I get a colonoscopy since I was having gut issues. The request seemed odd since I had a skin rash, but I complied. The test showed nothing out of the ordinary. When my body produced a second series of raised red rashes, I visited a Milwaukee Dermatologist for a second opinion.

The new physician appeared sincere as he looked at my rashes. They had assumed the form of thirty to thirty-five red "footballs" that peppered my trunk. After donning an antiquated light reflector, he frowned, raised his eyebrows, and told me "not to worry" about them, they would go away. The bull's-eye rash had disappeared two weeks earlier and was replaced by an unsightly mess that probably would have been difficult for any doctor to diagnose. After some time the physician handed me a bottle of pink goop that reminded me of calamine lotion, and sent me on my way.

Despite many different kinds of treatments and the passage of decades, when cultured properly my blood still yields tiny, live spirochetes that have been proven in the laboratory to be the spirochetes of Lyme disease. Despite this some doctors will still tell me I can't possibly have Lyme because I was treated with antibiotics. Others will say I must have "something else." When asked, they do not offer any helpful information to identify what that something else might be. However they might venture a guess at a diagnosis since many Lyme symptoms are attributable to depression, perimenopause, or even stress. This doesn't change the fact that spirochetes are alive inside my body.

Like many others who have the misfortune not to be diagnosed correctly during the acute phase of infection, I remain infected and rejected by mainstream infectious disease physicians. Most physicians willing to treat "chronic" Lyme disease do not accept insurance. If they do, insurance companies will usually not cover the treatments. It is because of the difficulty obtaining an accurate diagnosis, treatment, and acknowledgement in the medical arena that I vowed years ago to get to the bottom of why Lyme patients seem to get the raw end of the stick. I also wanted to learn why patients today are discouraged from talking about or even having Lyme disease, when none of us chose to become infected with it in the first place.

After spending an exhausting number of years reading and deciphering a room full of research materials, I pieced together what was previously a most puzzling history of Lyme disease, biowarfare weapons, and infectious diseases. I published my theories April 2011 in the book *God Science: The Secret World of Rampant Genetics, Hidden Illness, and Biotech Profiteering.* It was a difficult process since I am one person, but I believe it to be the beginning of what I hope will be the truth about Lyme disease and other illnesses. The book covers a century and a half of history, and there is an audio version. The objective of this current book then is to more simply tell the story of modern Lyme and Lyme-like illnesses. These revelations are needed since many patients have waited decades for curative solutions which never arrive. It is time to hear the story of some of the most powerful "biowarfare weapons" ever engineered, and what those tools may mean to the history of insect-borne diseases.

While the history of Lyme disease may prove to have had humble beginnings, aspects of Lyme history seem to have been locked securely away by powerful individuals in the upper echelon of public health, with no hope of seeing daylight. It seems also that if there are secrets, there are strong motivations behind them. Why are government scientists babysat by government employees during public interviews? Why aren't doctors "allowed" to diagnose Lyme disease? Who is afraid of the truth coming out? What is the truth about Lyme disease, and why is it the Pandora's box of the scientific and medical communities?

While human disease epidemics have occurred throughout world history, it is only within the last century or so that the world's public health agencies have come into existence. These institutions are valuable commodities in times of infectious disease outbreaks, and are charged with guarding public health and safety. But when epidemics rapidly overshadow any agency's ability to stifle public panic, roles quickly change and can be overridden by a lack of common sense or compromised moral ethics. If globally useful and highly valuable tools are found to not only be inherently flawed, but also responsible for outbreaks of animal and human diseases; what are public health agencies to do, shut down entire industries? Are the public to be informed when an industrial accident of global proportion occurs? Who is left to clean up the mess if the best of scientific intentions should fail, and how do we prevent similar future events?

In the realm of diseases possibly caused by the biowarfare tools of the past century and a half, the threat of costly mistakes and liabilities easily provides the temptation of silencing any accidents caused by these new technologies at any cost. The potential loss of valuable agricultural, military, industrial, and medical inventions leads us through a murky underworld of tainted research, hidden agendas, patent profits, and disinformation campaigns meant to prolong the useful life of products that may in effect be "junk science." When the value of currency and profits supersedes public health objectives, the results are unspoken secrets, stifled knowledge, ruined careers, and countless victims of epidemic diseases with "no known cause," or cure. In such a world there seems to be an arcanum of scientists "in the know" who are sworn to secrecy, and who will only reveal as much as is absolutely necessary, and only when pressed to do so with brute force.

I will say simply, may important truths finally be told. For without such revelations we can in no measure take steps toward understanding the devastating infection called Lyme disease. And neither may we have any hope for establishing meaningful treatment therapies for the thousands of patients around the world who are so needlessly suffering in silence. ❑

A Moving Target

If studying insect pathology or bacterial genomics at 1:30 in the morning does not sound exciting to you when you feel healthy, imagine how tedious it must be when you do not feel at all well. And yet this is how I spent the past decade of my life – studying bizarre medical topics at all hours of the night and day. Born in the Midwestern United States of European parentage; I have been functionally ill most of my life, from what in modern times is called Lyme disease. I recall a tick bite in 1992, but I found my first bull's-eye rash in 1969 on my arm. The lack of explanation for my lifetime of ill health and an equal lack of meaningful treatment therapies and acknowledgement in the medical and public health communities has unfortunately necessitated that someone put on their thinking cap to find answers. Many people have attempted to do this for a long time, myself included. Since I was unable to find anyone who might shed light on the numerous questions I had about this thing called Lyme, I thought what the heck maybe I should try to figure it out for myself.

There are literally millions of people at the present time around the world who suffer from "unexplained" illnesses; or those with names that were unfamiliar to the ear only a few decades ago. Many who are ill are wondering from where these illnesses and "syndromes" have originated, and also why. Unfortunately even in this highly technical world, we cannot always find answers quickly enough, especially where illnesses are concerned. Therefore extreme measures must be undertaken in order to solve what are in fact, extreme problems. For myself, this meant dedicating a decade to the study of infectious diseases.

Since 1969 when I first discovered a bull's-eye rash on my left wrist after my family moved from Illinois to Pennsylvania and back again, my life could never again be considered normal. I struggled throughout elementary school with weird "viruses" and illnesses which resembled the "flu"; upper respiratory infections, debilitating fatigue, and unusual "growing pains." I became a sleepwalker; I experienced night terrors, and had a pervasive feeling of apathy. My rail-thin body and digestive problems contributed to a semi-permanent brain fog throughout my school days. Most of the time I struggled to retain facts learned the day before, or even to make sense of classes each day. It was as if there was a mental road block on learning facts and figures that I could not bypass no matter how hard I tried. Anorexia visited my twenties and it was difficult eating even one meal a day. For years I battled restlessness, extreme irritability, menstrual problems, migraines, and sleeplessness; and was clueless that I might have untreated infections.

By 1994 me, my first husband, and our two small children moved from a Chicago, Illinois suburb to a southeast suburb of Milwaukee, Wisconsin. After living there for only a few months I was bitten by a black-legged deer tick that I removed from my left shoulder blade. I had never seen a tick before that day, and I was completely ignorant about tickborne diseases. That summer truly marked the turning point in my life where nothing would ever again be the same. It was also the first time I realized that physicians in my state were clueless about an infection called Lyme disease.

Ten months of debilitating illness followed, which included but was not limited to gastrointestinal problems, soaring fevers, migraines, intractable fatigue, dizziness, hyperirritability, gallbladder attacks, insomnia, weakness, numbness, and vertigo. A huge bull's-eye rash on my back erupted on my shoulder and spread across my entire back. Two weeks later a new eruption of multiple red rashes would also appear. Despite this nothing provoked more than the bored curiosity of doctors, nor contributed to a diagnosis of any infectious disease. I also suffered random anxiety attacks, usually while driving on the highway. I would realize later on that my brain was having difficulty processing the motion of the vehicle, and the sights and sounds of daily life that were absorbed by my other senses.

By 1994, two years after my acute infection, I managed to convince a Rheumatologist to treat me with antibiotics in case I had Lyme, but only after I pleaded several times. I took this approach because previous doctors were not helpful with any diagnosis, I had terrible joint pain, and I was feeling extremely ill. After all I had seen a picture of a bull's-eye rash in a library book. I assumed that I was infected with Lyme disease, even if doctors refused to test me for it. Unfortunately none of the other extensive tests I had undergone were able to validate the infection, but then doctors weren't looking for tickborne diseases. If they had, the available tests would probably not have detected any since they were not specific, and are notoriously inaccurate.

Hospital staff inserting IVs into my dehydrated body told me I had a "virus." Doctors told me I was working too hard. What I found extremely odd at this point was that medical experts were dodging and sometimes flatly refusing to discuss this curious illness. One physician actually closed his office door and frankly told me that he was "not allowed" to diagnose Lyme disease even if I had it. The Rheumatologist I begged did reluctantly prescribe an oral regimen of doxycycline and penicillin for about a month, followed by a sulfa medication, which I was unable to take more than once or twice before I became allergic or reactive to it. My Lyme symptoms never entirely resolved despite intermittent antibiotics over decades. The enormous passage of time between onset and treatment during acute infection allowed the organism to disseminate throughout my body. I was now what you might call bacterial "toast."

In 2000 I was once again bitten by a tick of unknown species, this time on my scalp. The event occurred during a camping trip at Pardeeville, Wisconsin a few hours north of my home. Curiously the town was a short distance from Fort McCoy, a military base where Yale University scientists had been studying Lyme disease prevalence a few years before my 1994 tick bite. This was the same year that multiple doctors wrongly informed me there was "no Lyme disease in Wisconsin."[1]

By 2003 I could no longer work outside the home and I was unofficially medically disabled. As it would happen, I did not receive disability benefits until the government officially declared me disabled two years later. This was not because I lacked a disability, but was due to the paperwork and the lengthy processes involved with filing. Delays are not uncommon for patients when applying for disability. One disability agent told me, "It doesn't matter that you have been diagnosed with Lyme disease, I need to know what is making you so ill." That was stunning to hear because Lyme disease had disabled me; and because the ignorance surrounding this illness is so prevalent. An attorney advised me to move on with my life and to accept the agency's disability "onset" date even though it came two years late. But how do you move forward when doctors and public health experts ignore that an illness exists? The answer is that you can't do it very well without a lot of effort. Losing one's livelihood is no small matter when there is a dependent family and a debilitating illness that keeps you largely homebound.

In December 2004 through an "alternative" practitioner, I found one of only three Wisconsin doctors known to be somewhat knowledgeable about treating Lyme disease. I was finally diagnosed with Lyme after being ill since 1969 with a host of symptoms, and having been re-bitten by ticks at least twice. By 2004 my left side was horribly dysfunctional and at times partially paralyzed. I had already suffered facial paralysis (Bell's Palsy) in 2000 for nine weeks, which left permanently damaged nerves on the left side of my face. By 2005 I could no longer lift my left arm above my head, I was using a cane to walk, I had fatigue so badly I could not walk around or drive; I had intermittent cardiac issues and a host of neurological and arthritic symptoms. I was quite literally in very bad shape and rapidly going downhill in physical and cognitive health.

A Lyme treating physician delivered the bad news that I might need a pacemaker. Before this happened he offered high-dose intravenous antibiotics. It never dawned on me that this might be risky. I was so grateful anyone was willing to treat my symptoms that I simply said "do whatever you need to, I can't live like this." We made the one hundred mile round trip every day for the first week. After that I received a home infusion pump and a few hours of instruction on how to self-infuse. Talk about a crash course in medicine. Although still disabled by Lyme, I continued as my body would allow, to take antibiotics, herbals, and to use alternative therapies to try to regain my health and function. As I sit writing this book I have lost most of my hair and have somewhat better, but precarious health. Despite the years of difficulty and an uncertain future, I retained both my sense of humor and my desire to tell "the story" of Lyme.

I now work with a Naturopath and other "alternative" practitioners using treatments designed to restore my gut function so that I can continue treatments. I want to get well, but my liver function is dicey, my body is in metabolic tilt, I have parasites, and no idea how we will surmount the remaining infections since I can no longer take antibiotics and many nutritional supplements.

Between emergency room visits and routine office visits over decades, I have seen more than one hundred physicians in four states. Only one by 2004 was willing to test me for, and to diagnose my symptoms of Lyme disease. Typically if Lyme infected patients are not diagnosed immediately during acute infection, then they must wait an average of two years and see up to twenty treating physicians before their infections are properly diagnosed and finally treated. This delay in timing is devastating during tickborne infections; some of which are life-threatening, and all of which are debilitating.

This is a taste of what life is like for the so-called "chronic" Lyme patients who are left misdiagnosed, undiagnosed, and/or untreated for years. It is a very different experience than that of patients who are diagnosed and treated for a classic ECM-rash illness at onset of infection. In the latter experience, those lucky enough to take antibiotics "long enough" have an easier time "curing" Lyme and any co-infections present. The longer a patient is forced to wait, the more likely the infections can multiply and disseminate throughout the body. There they remain hidden from the immune system among organs, tissues, and intracellular spaces. This makes detection and treatment far more difficult and requires a multi-tiered approach for a substantially longer period to restore optimal health, because short-term antibiotics are simply not enough.

There is another side to today's Lyme disease that many people refuse to discuss. These are the psychiatric aspects that come from the disease, called neuropsychiatric Lyme. Psychiatric symptoms caused by brain infections can become extremely intense and frightening. The kind of depression that can accompany Lyme disease occurs on many levels and is unlike anything one might think is associated with feeling "down." This depression seems to be caused by the extreme alterations in body chemistry that come about from depressed immunity, crashing hormones, and imbalanced brain neurotransmitters.

Lyme symptoms are intensified by nutritional deficiencies in vitamins, minerals, and amino acids important for health and vitality which can affect brain and mood function. Some patients have tragically committed suicide as a result of such severe pain and biochemical changes that there probably seemed to be no where else to go but to leave their bodies. What some people don't know or fail to comprehend is that during this level of brain dysfunction, the severely suffering individual is not the normal rational person they would be. Something in the brain fails to "think" before acting, and there comes a sudden disconnect like a shortage in an electrical system. The result can bring about a spontaneous anomaly of behavior that never would have occurred had the patient's brain not been infected with disease. This can be as subtle as irritability or impatience; to extremes in rage, or worse.

Patients can go from crying to laughing to introversion in a moment, as if a light switch is turned on or off in the brain. One can have momentary lapses of function or thought in a mini-seizure. Patients can also suffer mild or severe memory loss, word-finding difficulties, obsessive compulsive or attention deficit disorders, paranoia, dementia, or delusional thinking. Symptom flares may rapidly arise or be present in a chronic form.

Lyme symptoms mimic many illnesses, hence the name "the new great imitator" that is ascribed to the agent of Lyme disease, *Borrelia burgdorferi* ("Bb"). Due to the complex presentation of symptoms from a systemic Bb infection, patients are often misdiagnosed. Lyme-infected patients have heard well-meaning doctors diagnose Lupus, Fibromyalgia, Rheumatoid Arthritis, Chronic Fatigue, Multiple Sclerosis, Amyotrophic Lateral Sclerosis (ALS), Parkinson's, Multiple Chemical Sensitivities, and other illnesses. These may include those with psychiatric presentations (i.e. ADD, ADHD, depression, anxiety, schizophrenia).

Some patients describe random anxiety attacks in the middle of crowded stores or movie theatres. Some have ventured out in their car only to suddenly fail to recognize where they were driving, or remember where they had been. Some have observed road signs or words on a printed page which suddenly disappeared from view. Due to cognitive problems, children may be called by the names of their pets, and vice versa. Visual problems may cause strange flashes of light which appear like beautiful sparklers. Many Lyme patients suffer through multiple prescription lenses for eyesight quality which comes and goes like the weather.

Tinnitus, migraine headaches, and feelings of "invisible insects" that are biting or stinging are common. The pains come from the sharp, knife-like jabs of misfiring nerves. The tingling, numbness, burning and shooting pains, and intense itching, or skin that is too painful to touch are other symptoms described by Lyme patients. Nerve pain can be mild to absolutely debilitating. Unfortunately many Lyme patients spend a considerable portion of their lives home-bound. Travelling is difficult for many reasons, nonetheleast of which are the vibrations upon the nervous system and joints. Jarring motions can also set off extreme panic attacks, as can overexposures to lights, sounds, temperature extremes, or the vibrations of moving vehicles.

Many Lyme patients find it easier to travel at night, probably because the autonomic nervous system and brain are not overwhelmed by the rapid processing of movement, sound, and imagery that accompanies daily life. The infected brain simply can no longer keep up with routine brain functions. The "fight or flight" autonomic nervous system becomes like a cat whose tail gets stepped on, on a daily basis. The patient responds to everything around them with stress hormones and panic attacks. Over time, he or she "learns" to be afraid of everything around them because everything around them appears stressful.

The slightest irritation can set a Lyme patient on edge, and even the calmest tempered person can become overtly hostile. One of the most important things that family members can do for Lyme patients is to understand that they may not look sick, but they are sick, and they don't really want to have to keep explaining what is wrong day after day. With Lyme, symptoms are widely varied each day, and they are a given, period. Yes I'm still sick. No I'm not cured yet. Yes I have a right to park in the handicapped zone. Although I can drive a car today and walk today, in five minutes I may not be able to do it very well. If you follow me around long enough you will see that I have to stop and rest every hundred feet or so from terrible fatigue, joint pain, or neurological issues. On the worst days, two minutes after I get to the store I may not even remember why I came.

Lyme disease is an extremely isolating illness. A person who is Lyme infected can feel incredibly lonely and alone, even in the company of others. This is because the illness is not very well understood by those who do not have it. Most people who do understand the nuances of Lyme infection are those who are themselves infected; are family or friends of someone infected; or are a physician who actively treats Lyme patients. If you say to a Lyme patient "I too have Lyme" you need say nothing more, because to those among us who have it no explanation is required.

Unfortunately some family members or friends are far less than supportive than they could be. Lyme patients often struggle to communicate when words are flopped by dyslexia. The word "fine" becomes the default response when asked if you are "still" sick; or the code word when it is too tiring to give an updated health status. Some Lyme patients speak in rapid-fire motion. It is usually only another Lyme patient who understands that the run-on sentence is a symptom of infection and not a sign that the patient loves to hear their own chatter. Some of the most infected patients have no ability to check themself in conversation. Patients may even sound angry or argumentative, even when they are not, simply because they are passionate about a topic. This rough approach to conversation is caused by alterations in speech patterns and cognition. And it can make communication difficult, even between doctor and patient. Patients don't want sympathy, they want kindness and patience.

Lyme is so complex and individualized that any doctor unfamiliar with its symptoms may miss it even during thorough examinations. Diagnostic tests for many reasons are far less than ideal or accurate, as patients who are infected can test falsely negative (seronegative). The good news however is that some very clever researchers are working hard to bring forth more meaningful diagnostic tests. I have been fortunate enough to play a small part in the development of a new diagnostic test, and hopefully soon these more accurate tests will be readily available and affordable to the ill public and their doctors.[2]

It is the hope of many that these tests will become the new gold standard for Lyme disease testing. They certainly should, because for a patient (me) who tests negative on Lyme disease tests that were "standardized" by public health agencies in 1994, the ability to culture and photograph *Borrelia burgdorferi* spirochetes in under a week is an astonishing feat. Not surprisingly, the scientists and labs working on these new tests are not funded by government grants – neither do their methods necessarily support the current public health consensus that there is no chronic Lyme disease.

The politics of Lyme disease are contentious. By 2004 when I began to seriously research Lyme disease, I had learned there are two "camps" of medical professionals with differing methods of treating the infection. One of the camps, identified as the International Lyme and Associated Diseases Society (ILADS), is comprised of physicians and other medical professionals who are typically of the belief that Lyme disease is a complex illness that requires a flexible treatment approach. Many of these physicians believe that a chronic form of Lyme disease exists. They also feel that for some Lyme patients, longer treatments using multiple antibiotics and other therapies are necessary to successfully eradicate Lyme disease and its many "co-infections." The organization publishes diagnostic and treatment guidelines that were written by New York physician Dr. Joseph Burrascano, Jr., an ILADS member. The ILADS guidelines for Lyme disease are available on the organization's web site at www.ilads.org and they include valuable information that is useful for physicians and patients alike.

Short-term antibiotic therapy (roughly a month or less) for Lyme disease is the recommended treatment protocol of another group of medical experts who are identified as the Infectious Diseases Society of America (IDSA). This professional medical organization includes infectious disease doctors and researchers. A handful of "IDSA" members believe that a chronic form of Lyme does not exist, although many IDSA members believe that it does. Patients often make the mistake of placing the "blame" for their frustration on the entire IDSA group, and this is simply unfair. There are IDSA members who are also ILADS physicians, and who are on the front lines helping patients battle the disease, as well as its politics. However there is a small group of IDSA members and their peers who have been at the center of political controversy for the past several decades for their stance against "chronic" Lyme disease.

The general lack of credence afforded Lyme disease rubs patients, families, and medical professionals entirely the wrong way. Some infectious disease and public health experts claim that patients are suffering with "something else," or from delusional disorders for believing they remain ill after antibiotic therapy. And yet symptoms in so many people who have detectable infections are not mental fabrications. It is obvious that politics and conflicts of interest play a role in such blatant denials; therefore the public is understandably angry and sometimes even occasionally hostile.

Patients are fighting for their lives and for the right to be heard and acknowledged, and they do not understand why they are being forced to fight. The average ill Lyme patient or "Lymie" too soon becomes overwhelmed and exhausted by the amount of effort required to find a physician knowledgeable in treating Lyme. There is such a shortage of doctors willing to treat beyond public health consensus standards. Physicians are expected not to treat outside the "standards of care" outlined by a select group of medical experts who are often patent holders or part-time industry employees. Those who follow other standards (including their own) often wrongly face the scrutiny of state medical boards and the possibility of losing their license to practice simply for upholding the Hippocratic Oath.

Patients from Europe, Canada, and other countries are forced to flock to the US for highly specialized treatments that are unavailable in their country for political or economic reasons. Sadly, some of the sickest patients require expensive long-term treatments that are cost prohibitive for many – costs rarely covered in their entirety by medical insurance if the patient even has insurance coverage. Due to costs or principals, some patients attempt herbal and other alternative protocols with differing results. While some of these treatments are curative or supportive, others that are illegitimate are downright dangerous.

Physicians who treat Lyme patients and those who do not war between short and long-term antibiotic therapies while federally funded scientists claim there is "no benefit" to long-term antibiotics. Those who might be able to prove otherwise must carefully edit their research results or face losing federal or private research dollars on future projects; or sudden cut backs in their professional careers. Despite these problems, ill patients are often having their lives returned to them through longer and alternative treatment therapies despite the current medico-political war of so-called "evidence-based" medicine. The truth is that evidence-based medicine is subjective to the opinions or whims of those who interpret the evidence under consideration. If medicine were based on clinical patient evidence instead of mathematical formulas and laboratory techniques, patients might fare better in both the diagnostic and treatment categories.

The end result is that many patients are caught between warring factions over who is "right" or "wrong" regarding disease definitions and treatment protocols. The patient's income is also affected by the high costs of medicines, alternative treatments, and medical specialists outside of insurance networks. Insurance companies that are dictating medical and prescriptive treatments are practicing unfair cost management techniques to protect profit margins and biotech-laden investment portfolios. Disability payments are denied to patients who have legitimate infections that are at best poorly defined, or at worst openly ignored or difficult to quantify; yet are absolutely debilitating.

The situation is getting worse for patients the longer the Lyme disease epidemic remains unacknowledged, not only in the US, but in other countries as well. To make matters worse, foreign countries are now adopting "standardized" testing and treatment guidelines drafted by US "experts" – individuals who often do not treat patients. Many of these individuals are patent-holders or gatekeepers for "all things" borrelia-related. For outside observers it would seem that there are a few in public health service who are deliberately keeping the secret of Lyme disease's origins and pathology entirely to themselves. We have to wonder therefore if the reason for such efforts if they exist, is to protect reputations, liabilities, and/or millions of dollars in research funding, patent royalties, and other agendas.

It is clear from the research and clinical experience that Lyme disease should be diagnosed based upon clinical symptoms, and not upon the result of one or two or even ten diagnostic tests. Lyme disease or *Lyme borreliosis* is an illness complex because when patients are infected by an insect vector, multiple infections (co-infections) are transmitted by the insect into the patient's body in addition to Lyme disease. Persistence of tickborne infections is understood by patients and their Lyme-treating physicians, who are sometimes called "Lyme-literate" physicians. Some of the most common co-infections to appear in Lyme patients include those of bacterial, fungal, microsporidian, protozoan, mold, and viral origins. Even microscopic worms called nematodes (filaria) can be found in the bodies of many Lyme patients courtesy of an insect vector.

At least one patent invention by spirochetologist Dr. Russell C. Johnson (University of Minnesota) reveals that *Borrelia burgdorferi* spirochetes have been isolated from mosquitoes, deerflies, and horseflies. This reveals that other important insects besides ticks may transmit Lyme disease. This information is something that public health experts have repeatedly failed to make known to the general public.[3-6]

We can see evidence of what scientists know about Lyme disease and when they knew it if we explore the text of patent inventions. It is unfortunate however that some scientists will not publicly admit what they have admitted to in "private." A Dr. Johnson patent from 1988 states:

> "The etiological agent of this disease is the spirochete *Borrelia burgdorferi*, which is primarily transmitted by *Ixodes* ticks...*Ixodes dammini* is the major vector of Lyme disease in Minnesota, Wisconsin, the northeastern United States and adjacent Canada...*I. pacificus* is the primary vector of this disease in the western United States, and in Europe the major vector of Lyme borreliosis is *I. ricinus*. The spirochete has also been found in deerflies, horseflies and mosquitoes."[6]

Although some scientists argue that other insects "cannot" transmit Lyme disease by bites, they can transmit Bb and other bacteriae via a contaminated stylet, as can aphids, leafhoppers, and other insects with these structures. The Johnson patent continues:

> "As many as two-thirds of the people that become infected by this spirochete are unaware of the tick bite because of

the painless bite and the small size (several mm) of the nymphal stage."

"The early phase of the illness often consists of the ECM, headache, fatigue, muscle and joint aches, stiff neck and chills and fever."

"This phase of the disease may be followed by neurologic, joint or cardiac abnormalities. The chronic forms of the disease such as arthritis (joint involvement), Acrodermatitis chronica atrophicans (skin involvement), and Bannwarth's syndrome (neurological involvement) may last for months to years and are associated with the persistence of the spirochete."[6]

"A case of maternal-fetal transmission of *B. burgdorferi* resulting in neonatal death has been reported ... For every symptomatic infection, there is at least one asymptomatic infection."

"Lyme disease is presently the most commonly reported tickborne disease in the United States. The infection may be treated at any time with antibiotics such as penicillin, erythromycin, tetracycline, and ceftriaxone..."

"Once infection has occurred, however, the drugs may not purge the host of the spirochete but may only act to control the chronic forms of the disease. Complications such as arthritis and fatigue may continue for several years after diagnosis and treatment."[6]

These are vitally important clues to the chronic form of Lyme disease. These statements also reflect what patients have been saying for decades, despite denials by some public health experts. I might mention that the Johnson patent admits that Lyme notable Dr. Allen C. Steere provided a human spinal fluid isolate of the Bb agent for Dr. Johnson's patent research. Dr. Steere is among infectious disease doctors whose previously published efforts typically contradict the statements made within the Johnson patent. Dr. Steere was among those who helped identify the Lyme disease agent back in 1981 before it was announced to the world the following year.

Now that we know that some scientists know and acknowledge that Lyme disease can become a chronic and serious infection, let's explore the history of this mysterious malady and find out what else we haven't been told. ❑

Hear No Evil.

Here is the modern version of a popular 1841 nursery rhyme.
There may be more truth to these lyrics than we think:

All around the mulberry bush, the monkey chased the weasel.
The monkey thought 'twas all in fun, Pop! goes the weasel.
A penny for a spool of thread, a penny for a needle.
That's the way the money goes, Pop! goes the weasel.
Jimmy's got the whooping cough, and Timmy's got the measles.
That's the way the story goes, Pop! goes the weasel.

One: Don't Ask, Don't Tell Policies of Biowarfare

What We "Know" About Lyme

Lyme disease is the fastest growing vector-borne disease in the world. Vector-borne for our purpose refers to the transmission of infectious diseases by a biting, stinging, or blood-sucking insect such as a wasp, bee, flea, mite, louse, fly, mosquito, or tick. Lyme disease is caused by a spiral-shaped bacterium (spirochete) that is said to be a distant cousin of the Syphilis spirochete, *Treponema pallidum*. The eastern US is considered to be the epicenter of the Lyme disease epidemic. The epidemic was first announced as "juvenile arthritis" in 1975 since it was discovered in people (mostly children) from three Connecticut communities. The victims all suffered from a mysterious illness that produced flu-like symptoms, a rash, and arthritis-like joint pains. The children lived in communities in close proximity, including Old Lyme, East Haddam, and Haddam. Each town is located along the Connecticut River just east of the Cockaponset State Forest. Years later the disease's causative agent would be identified as *Borrelia burgdorferi* and was announced to the world in 1982. The organism was named after one of the National Institutes of Health (NIH) scientists who first identified it, Dr. Willy Burgdorfer.[1]

The complex organism called *Borrelia burgdorferi* belongs to a phylum of spirochetal bacteriae that also contains the human pathogenic *Treponemes* and *Leptospires*. Lyme disease is considered to be a tickborne spirochetal infection that is caused by a group of cork-screw shaped, gram-negative, spirochetes named *Borrelia burgdorferi* "sensu lato" (or "s.l." meaning broad sense). It is often abbreviated as "Bb." The Bb genospecies actually contains four groups, although only three are said to cause Lyme disease. Group I consists of *B. burgdorferi* sensu stricto ("s.s." or "strict sense") strains which include the type strain called "B-31" from New York, and at least twenty-eight strains from Europe and the United States.[2,3]

Group II was named *Borrelia garinii* "species novel," and includes at least thirteen isolates from Europe and Asia. Group III is called *Borrelia afzelii*, and includes at least nine isolates from Europe and Asia. The fourth group, *Borrelia japonica*, contains spirochetes that were isolated from *Ixodes ovatus* ticks in Japan, but this group is not felt to transmit Lyme disease. I believe that there will be other *Borrelia burgdorferi* species to be identified in the future, and it is clear that scientists are also aware of this possibility. Scientists key to Lyme disease history are currently investigating a "new" strain of relapsing fever, *Borrelia miyamotoi*. It is however not new, having first been isolated in 1995 in Japan. *B. miyamotoi* is a non-Lyme disease strain from the *Borrelia japonica* group. I discuss this agent at the very end of this book because I believe it serves as a useful model of study for an entirely different purpose than what others may currently believe it to be, and because scientists are intensely studying it as I write this book.[2-4]

Borrelia burgdorferi s.s. is the predominant group of Lyme disease strains detected in patients from the US and Canada. *Borrelia garinii* and *Borrelia afzelii*, in addition to *B. burgdorferi* sensu stricto strains are detectable in patients from other countries. The Bb sensu stricto strains typically cause arthritic symptoms. Strains in the *B. garinii* and *B. afzelii* groups are more frequently associated with neurologic and skin manifestations. However the Bb sensu stricto group can also produce neurologic, cardiac, and psychiatric symptoms during disseminated disease. *B. afzelii* is the apparent exclusive group that causes late skin lesions called *Acrodermatitis Chronica Atrophicans* (ACA, or Pick-Herxheimer disease); and other skin manifestations called *Morphea* and *Lichen sclerosus et atrophicus*.[2,3,5]

The skin presentations from *B. afzelii* seem to occur mainly in Europe, although there are a few scattered cases that have been anecdotally reported in North America on both coasts, and in Canada. There are roughly four dozen species of borreliae that are known to cause human Lyme disease. This highly diverse selection of strains speaks to differences between insects in various regions, and to multiple environmental factors which we will examine in this book. It also tells us that the classic Lyme disease probably did not have its origins in the US which is something that the public and public health experts have wrongly believed for decades.[2,3]

The different species of borreliae are mainly classified by the insects or arthropods (i.e. tick) which carry them according to a book edited by University of Minnesota Spirochetologist Dr. Russell C. Johnson. Other borreliae strains such as *Borrelia hermsii, Borrelia duttoni,* and *Borrelia recurrentis* are considered to be strains that curiously enough are not known to cause Lyme disease according to Dr. Johnson. However these strains are known to cause human relapsing fever infections, and are transmitted by infected ticks, lice, and mites. According to a 1991 research paper written in part by Yale University's Dr. Paul Duray, none of the Bb spirochetes that were tested in a study reacted to anti-*Borrelia hermsii* relapsing fever antibodies. This means that they were not genetically similar enough in relation to this relapsing fever strain to react to the test.[2,6]

According to the Johnson and Duray sources, borrelia strains that cause Lyme disease are a unique genospecies that does not include the relapsing fever borreliae. Therefore we might have to assume that all Bb strains were placed into this genospecies simply because one of their main components is a tick-transmitted spirochete. These current spirochetes may be entirely different than what we have been told they are. Dr. Johnson revealed that different borreliae are classified by the vectors that carry them. This means that *Borrelia burgdorferi* are in the borrelia category simply because they are some sort of tick-transmitted spirochete. The name "burgdorferi" merely represents some kind of spirochete that was first identified by Dr. Burgdorfer. What that spirochete is and how it got here is the focus of this book. We will learn also that the Bb spirochete genetically has very little in common with other spirochetes, including the one it is supposedly related to: the spirochete of Syphilis, *Treponema pallidum*.[2,6]

The most commonly reported symptoms of early acute infection in modern Lyme disease include fever, headache, muscle pains, gastrointestinal issues, fatigue, and a centrifugally expanding rash, called a "bull's-eye." The scientific name for this type of rash is an *Erythema chronicum migrans* (ECM), also known as *Erythema migrans* (EM). Once the localized skin infection spreads, cardiac, joint, ocular, nervous system, gastric, arthritis, and psychiatric symptoms can appear. If the infection is left untreated or under treated, it can significantly impact the patient's life to the point of disability (and occasionally, death). Although public health officials do not report deaths from Lyme disease, anecdotal reports and death certificates of some deceased patients indicate that what we think of as Lyme disease was a causative or a contributing factor to death.[7]

Most Lyme patients who are diagnosed early on in their infections (if aware of a bite), and before the spirochetes disseminate throughout the body stand a good chance of receiving what may be curative medical attention. However because of a tick's tiny size, most people are unaware they have been bitten, and it is several days to weeks before symptoms of infection begin to appear. By the time the patient begins to feel ill, the spirochetes are already migrating to other parts of the body where they sequester in a number of areas to evade antibiotic treatment. Lyme disease then becomes a systemic infection which can affect any and every organ system in the body.

The disappearance of the rashes of untreated Lyme disease does not mean that the overall infection is necessarily cured. Instead, it may be evidence that the infection has simply disseminated. The patient may still have to deal with the rest of the Lyme complex, including co-infections and any remaining spirochetes not killed by antibiotics or other treatments. This is why patients may continue to have symptoms even after treatment with a drug such as doxycycline or penicillin.

Since the Bb spirochete sequesters itself inside the blood cells of the immune system (macrophages), it may be important to treat patients with antibiotics that can penetrate the intracellular spaces of the immune fighting cells, as well as treating with an extracellular antibiotic. This speaks to the benefit of combining antibiotic treatments during early infection. When the Bb organism is challenged with antibiotics, it will change into a cyst form to protect itself against chemotherapies. This makes the infection far more difficult to treat, which then requires longer durations of therapy.[8]

As any infection, a diagnosis of Lyme disease is a clinical one that should be based upon factors including tick bite risk and symptom presentation. Laboratory tests should be used as adjunctive and confirmatory and not as diagnostic tools to rule out infection. For many reasons patients may not make sufficient antibodies that can be detected in tests; and some patients will remain seronegative. This is when a patient is infected and either they do not produce antibodies, or all their antibodies are complexed (bound) with the infectious agents so none are free to be detected by the test probes. Treatments for Lyme disease should be extended for a period of time dictated by ongoing symptoms to the judgment of the physician, and not be restricted by published medical guidelines which are only suggestive and not doctrine.[8]

The best way to prevent Lyme disease is not to become infected. Apply natural repellants or pesticides; and wear long pants, long sleeves, light-colored clothing, and tuck pants into socks to avoid exposures and simplify tick removal. Remove any ticks as soon as they appear to prevent them from latching on and transmitting diseases. Ticks love moist, woody environments (i.e. leaves, brush, wood piles), as they cannot survive in open, sunny areas. This is why it is a good idea to provide a gravel barrier that is two to three feet wide along any wooded areas in your yard or where ticks might find a suitable habitat.

If bitten, proper removal of ticks is extremely important. Always use a pair of tweezers or special tick removal tool to grasp the head of the tick as close to the surface of the skin where it is attached. Squeeze gently and lift the tick firmly and directly out of the skin, taking care not to damage the tick, and to ensure proper removal of mouth parts. If the tick is damaged or startled during the removal process, it may dump its infective saliva and gut contents into the wound and cause infection. Be sure to clean the bite area and seek medical attention. Do not use any other method to remove an attached tick.

Ticks have three life stages, the larval stage, the nymph, and the adult. These arthropods (meaning "jointed legs") take a single blood meal in each life stage. The larval stage is about the size of the period at the end of this sentence. The nymphs are not much larger, at about the size of a poppy seed. The adults are visually larger, but their painless bite and delicate weight may make them undetectable, especially if they are not crawling upon bare skin. Always be sure to check yourself and your pets thoroughly when returning from outdoor activities. Removing clothing and running in a hot dryer cycle for at least forty-five minutes or longer should kill any that might remain on clothes (ticks can survive the washing machine and short dryer times).

Infectious agents of many kinds may be transmitted through biting; by contact with a tick's infection-contaminated stylus (the injected probe used to break the skin); when a tick excretes coxial fluid (tick urine/poop); in a tick's ovipositor (egg laying apparatus), or if the tick is squashed on the surface of the host's skin (animal or human). Never squash a tick, mosquito, mite, or other insect on human skin or you risk disease transmission through the porous openings of your body's largest organ, your skin.

In 1966 an astute German physician named Dr. Carl Lenhoff reported on skin biopsies that were taken from patients who had ECM rashes in 1948. The cultures revealed the presence of spirochetes. These were probably the very first reports of modern Lyme disease in the United States – a disease name that has been called a "misnomer" by Dr. Willy Burgdorfer, because of its presentation in other areas of the world. In Wisconsin a case of an ECM rash illness was reported in 1970 by Milwaukee Dermatologist Rudolph Scrimenti. His patient was a male physician who had been hunting grouse in the northern part of the state the year before. The patient was treated with penicillin and cured. Dr. Scrimenti has stated that in retrospect, there were many more cases of ECM rash illnesses in patients in the state, years before his 1969 case.[9-11]

By 1972, a cluster of patients from Connecticut who complained of an ECM rash and arthritis-like illness began to receive the world's attention. The outbreak, named after one of the Connecticut towns where patients lived, was dubbed juvenile arthritis. In 1982 the causative agent would be publicly revealed, although certain aspects from that period have never been publicly discussed. By 1985, the roughly fifty-nine cases of "juvenile arthritis" that had originally been reported in Connecticut in 1975 had increased to eight hundred and sixty-three cases.[7,12]

By 1987, several states had reported Lyme disease cases: Minnesota, Texas, and Wisconsin in the Midwest; north Atlantic coastal states from Massachusetts to North Carolina; and the Pacific coastal states of Oregon and California. What were referred to as "scattered" cases were reported in Arkansas, Florida, Georgia, Indiana, Kentucky, Maine, Michigan, Montana, Nevada, New Hampshire, Ohio, Tennessee, Utah, and Vermont.

State and territorial health departments report Lyme disease case numbers to the Centers for Disease Control (CDC) as part of the National Electronic Telecommunications System for Surveillance. Final data are published annually (www.cdc.gov). CDC estimates of Lyme disease cases in 1996 were placed at just over 15,000. By 2002 the case numbers had climbed to approximately 24,000. Despite a significant increase in anecdotally reported cases, the CDC numbers did not reflect much of an increase even in 2008 where "probable" cases were reported at 8,000 and confirmed cases at roughly 28,000. In 2009 the CDC reported 30,000 confirmed cases and another 8,000 possible cases.[7,12]

The newest records for Lyme disease case numbers indicate a reduction with only about 26,000 confirmed cases, and about 4,000 "possible" cases. This reduction simply reflects the reporting of clinical case numbers. It does not reflect any evidence that Lyme disease infections are on the decline. All case numbers are reflective only of how many cases were actually reported to, and recorded by the CDC. These are included only if they conform to very strict surveillance case definitions. These definitions have been considered so restrictive over the years that most Lyme patients don't qualify as being infected based on the definitions. The patient and physician population feel that the reported case numbers for Lyme disease may be ten to twelve times higher, or 300,000 annually in the US alone.[7,12]

Unfortunately the CDC web site provides only basic information on what historically was known only as an ECM rash illness. There is much more to the story of modern Lyme disease. For example, the agency only reports that Lyme disease is transmitted by the black-legged deer tick, *Ixodes scapularis*. While this is true, any number of indigenous tick species, both of the hard or soft-bodied varieties are capable of harboring and transmitting Lyme disease and other infections, which are often called "co-infections." Other insects have also been discovered to carry the "Bb" spirochete within their bodies. This may allow them to transmit the infection along with other pathogens. The CDC does not make any accommodations for Lyme disease transmission by other important routes, (i.e. saliva, blood, sperm, insects); or provide information that Lyme infections may be acquired by a child in utero or via lactation. I know plenty of families where every single child born into the family is infected with Lyme disease simply because their mother is infected. Spouses also test positive, lending credence to sexual transmission.[7]

The CDC promotes that Lyme disease is easily treated with a short course of antibiotics. This may be partly true if a classic case is caught early. However a large percentage of patients are unaware that they have the infection. Untreated, these patients go on to manifest chronic, debilitating infections which prove difficult or impossible to eradicate under recommended treatment therapies of short-course antibiotics. Ticks are "dirty" arthropods. They carry a wide range of infections, and can and do transmit any number of them upon taking a blood meal.[7,13]

Patients can go for years without meaningful symptoms, but when their blood or body tissues are seen under the microscope, low numbers of active (motile) spirochetes can often be seen and cultured. By the way, I am considered by the CDC "not" to have Lyme disease. This is because I do not meet the surveillance criteria as a reportable case, and I have routinely tested seronegative (negative) according to CDC standardized tests for Lyme disease. Nevertheless I have had debilitating symptoms for years. I am still medically disabled by Lyme disease, or perhaps I should say "by something else," even though Bb spirochetes are still culturable from my blood and can be seen under the microscope.[7,13]

Borrelia spirochetes have been found on every continent, and in humans on all continents where man is indigenous. Borrelia has been around for centuries, typically presenting as relapsing fever infections. The "new" *Borreliae burgdorferi* s.l. however; are very different than the relapsing fever borreliae. They are also not as closely related to Syphilis spirochetes as we have been told, except for a few housekeeping genes common among most spirochetes. Instead what we learn when we truly study the literature is that *Borrelia burgdorferi* or "Bb" more closely resembles another spirochete that hasn't been discussed, the *Leptospires*.[14,15]

Leptospires are ubiquitous to the environment, and leptospirosis infections affect animals and humans. In fact animal and human leptospirosis is quite common around the world and has been a problem for centuries. These infections can be acquired through contact with polluted soil or water, or by contact with the urine, blood, or body fluids of infected animals. Leptospirosis remains a definitive problem in livestock animals that are used for food and other products. From 1940 to the late 1950s, transmission of leptospires was studied at Rocky Mountain Laboratories to see if ticks could spread leptospirosis. The laboratory collected soft ticks (*Ornithodoros*) from New Mexico in 1940 and kept them in a tick colony for at least two decades.[14-19]

Modern Lyme disease has a slightly different history than what the public currently believes. To find out more about how a classic ECM rash illness from past centuries has brought forth the present politics of modern Lyme disease, we must study the history of American industries. In the process we will learn about a very different kind of biological warfare; the kind that has always been aimed at controlling pest insect populations. We will also examine a pivotal event that has helped fuel the firestorm of controversy over this thing we call Lyme.[14,15]

The Hallmark Infection

It occurred to me that the hallmark of Lyme disease, the "bull's-eye" rash, isn't entirely what we have been told it is. What was the odd, red ring-like rash that appeared on my shoulder, and which expanded with a normal skin-colored center until it covered my back? What were the multiple red blotches that appeared two weeks later? In the process of seeking answers, I studied some very old medical textbooks. In a book published in 1857 by London physician Dr. William Jenner, I found a virus called *Roseola annulata*. Today this disease is called "sixth disease," "rose rash," or "pseudorubella." According to Dr. Jenner's descriptions, here was a virus that had the ability to create the familiar bull's-eye rash found in one-third to one-half, though not all Lyme patients.

I thought about this and wondered whether a past childhood infection *could be reactivated decades later by an insect bite.* I had been vaccinated as a child with the usual fare, including measles-mumps-rubella (MMR) vaccines, smallpox, and polio. Was the bull's-eye rash of Lyme disease caused by a reactivated rubella, polio, pox, or other vaccine virus? The publication says:

> "On the lower extremities, and sometimes on other parts, we observe several rose-coloured rings, varying in diameter from a quarter of an inch to an inch. The colour of the skin within the rings is quite natural...several diseases of the skin have the same tendency to affect a ring-shape, the part within the ring being, in all respects, healthy."[1]

This description seemed to adequately describe a Lyme bull's-eye rash. I did not find this kind of infection described in any of my *Merck* medical manuals, and I have quite a few dating back to 1899. The source says that this form of roseola infection may last from days to several weeks. This period is consistent with the eruption, expansion, and disappearance of a Lyme bull's-eye rash. In 1857 Dr. Jenner recognized the constitutional symptoms that often presented with this form of roseola. The symptoms also happen to be similar to the "flu-like" symptoms experienced during the initial stages of acute Lyme disease.[1]

According to the text, another skin infection that can also form a ring-like rash is an infection called *Erythema circinnatum*, although its ring-like rash apparently has a yellow center instead of a natural skin tone. In *Roseola annulata*, the central portion of the rash is clear, although both illnesses can produce what was referred to as "acute rheumatism." The good Dr. Jenner also recognized a "chronic" form of the infection, which he called *Erythema marginatum*. Dr. Jenner went on to say something that I felt was important to include:

> "...there is little or no real difference between roseola and erythema...that variety of roseola which so closely resembles measles, the other varieties of roseola and erythema might well be grouped together into one genus..."[1]

Perhaps the *Erythema migrans* (EM) rash that is associated with Lyme disease is what Dr. Jenner defined as *Roseola annulata* more than one hundred and fifty years ago. Roseola is a virus that most people have been exposed to during their early childhood. The infection is felt to be caused by the HHV-6 or the HHV-7 human herpes viruses. Most Lyme patients test positive for antibodies to the HHV-6 virus. Most children have been vaccinated – vaccines that may be contaminated with monkey herpes viruses that at least in humans could manifest as a reactivated human herpes virus (roseola) infection. Perhaps an insect vectored infection really could reactivate latent viruses whether natural or from previous vaccines.[2-5]

Other viruses to think about are the *Herpes simplex* virus types 1 and 2. These infections can also be found within the blood of many patients who have Lyme disease. The question in my mind then is whether these herpes strains appear in patients from past natural exposures or because one or more were used to create insecticides, or animal or human vaccines. From the available research I discovered that a few of the symptoms of Lyme disease (especially those with neurologic effects), mimic symptoms of active herpes virus infections. Herpes viruses can cause something called limbic encephalitis (brain stem) upon invasion of the central nervous system. Herpes viruses are used agriculturally. There are patent inventions which use herpes simplex virus enzyme genes (thimidine kinase) to make transgenic cotton plants.[2-6]

The herpes viruses can cause seizures, fevers, neurological symptoms; and may create characteristic plaques seen on magnetic resonance imaging (MRI) scans. Such plaques appear in nearly 90% of patients with herpes simplex type 1 according to some sources. These plaques may be similar to those found on brain MRIs of patients with Lyme disease or Multiple Sclerosis – plaques that may disappear after antibiotic treatment. However if vaccine cell lines are made with or are contaminated by herpes viruses, this is another way that patients may become exposed to herpes rather than through natural infections.[2-5]

While the prospect of a reactivated virus is worth considering as the cause of a bull's-eye rash, not everyone has been exposed to the herpes, rubella, or other viruses around the world. Maybe this is why some patients never exhibit a bull's-eye rash, while others will. The variable presence of a bull's-eye rash, a modified ECM rash (no central clearing), or no rash at all during acute *Borrelia burgdorferi* infections may instead depend upon whether a fungus is transmitted by an insect vector. Perhaps no rash will develop in a bite from an insect uninfected by fungi. Likewise no rash may form in persons whose latent natural or vaccine viruses remain subclinical do not become reactivated.

If a bull's-eye or other rash of Lyme disease has fungal origins, then it is easy to see why it may quickly disappear upon treatment with the tetracycline antibiotic doxycycline. This is an antibiotic that is heavily recommended by the IDSA guidelines and its authors to treat the acute stage of Lyme disease. Tetracyclines like doxy are also effective against certain fungal strains including those that are found naturally, and those that have long been used as agricultural and industrial insecticides. While we will learn the nuances of the history of Lyme, let's begin by examining a public health event that has changed the way Lyme patients are diagnosed and treated, and that would cause decades of confusion about what would become a global epidemic.

The Dearborn Conference

Lyme disease is probably the most politically contentious infectious disease epidemic on the planet. To understand the scope of the negative politics behind the history of Lyme, it is helpful to know of a precedent-setting event that took place in 1994. For more than a decade and a half, the culmination of decisions from this event would change the way patients with Lyme disease were to be diagnosed to the present day. The criteria established at this event would also restrict the manner in which Lyme disease cases are reported to, and recorded by the CDC. While the event did not establish all political issues encircling the topic of Lyme disease, it certainly has played an integral role in the denial and complication of an epidemic that affects thousands across the globe.

The "Dearborn Conference" for Lyme disease was held in Dearborn, Michigan on October 27-29, 1994. It was officially called the Second National Conference on [the] Serologic Diagnosis of Lyme Disease. The conference was sponsored by the Centers for Disease Control (CDC), the Association of State and Territorial Public Health Laboratory Directors (ATPHLD), and the Michigan Department of Health. It was co-sponsored by the US Food and Drug Administration (FDA), the National Institutes of Health (NIH), the Council of State and Territorial Epidemiologists (CSTE), and the National Committee for Clinical Laboratory Standards. Planning committee members included CDC employees. Other participants included a few scientists who will become important to Lyme disease history. In addition academic scientists with ties to the CDC; vaccine manufacturer representatives, public health officers, and representatives from private and public laboratories also attended the event.

The conference was held to establish the surveillance case definitions (criteria) for reporting emerging Lyme disease cases to the CDC; and to standardize laboratory diagnostic tests used to detect Lyme infections. Until then, laboratories across the country were using different diagnostic tests. Accuracy depended heavily upon the sensitivity and specificity of the individual test, which varied by manufacturer. The CDC also wanted to begin tracking what appeared to be an emerging human disease epidemic, and needed to establish criteria for surveillance purposes since Lyme was now a reportable infectious disease for public health purposes. Certain parties who attended the Dearborn conference would directly benefit from the manner in which the newly standardized criteria would become established, although this aspect of the event was not understood until years later.

Among those participating at "Dearborn" was a recent Epidemic Intelligence Service (EIS) "agent." Graduates of the CDC's EIS program are permanent employees of, and the eyes and ears of the Public Health Service. These sentinel individuals act as liaisons to the CDC, and are installed in key positions as lookouts for evidence of emerging infectious diseases and biological warfare threats. In 1975 when Lyme disease first surfaced in Connecticut, Rheumatologist Dr. Allen Steere was a recent EIS graduate. Therefore he was a natural selection to survey the Connecticut cluster of patients who were complaining of arthritis-like symptoms. He and his colleagues published a description of "Lyme arthritis" in 1977. They recognized that the classic "bull's-eye" (ECM) rash was a clinical marker for the new infection; and they also knew they were dealing with a multi-system disease.[1]

A federal research grant was awarded to Dr. Steere in 1986 to study *Lyme Borreliosis* in Russia. (This is the official name of the Lyme disease infection.) Dr. Steere was the principal investigator for the Russian project under a cooperative exchange program with physicians at the Rheumatology Institute of Moscow. Their work was performed under the auspices of the US/USSR Biological Health Agreement. This was four years after the Lyme disease agent was first named after Dr. Willy Burgdorfer as *Borrelia burgdorferi,* or more simply, Bb. Dr. Burgdorfer was the first scientist to identify the agent of Lyme disease. This was also five years after Dr. Steere and his colleagues cultured a peculiar mutant spirochete from a Lyme patient's ECM rash – a spirochete whose name was not made "publicly" known at the time Bb was first announced.[2]

Because the "bulk" of *Lyme Borreliosis* cases by 1986 were found in Europe and the former Soviet Union and not Connecticut, the three known borrelia families were being intensely studied with Dr. Steere's participation. These groups again are *Borrelia burgdorferi* sensu stricto, *Borrelia garinii,* and *Borrelia afzelii.* Dr. Steere would return to the states to make recommendations to the Dearborn conference work group committee with respect to which Bb strains should be used in the newly standardized Lyme diagnostic tests. Unfortunately as a Rheumatologist, Dr. Steere focused only on the Connecticut "arthritis"-causing strains with which he was most familiar, because that was the most common symptom in his patients. For some reason his recommendations at Dearborn would exclude other American Bb strains; and the two European Bb groups: *Borrelia garinii,* and *Borrelia afzelii.*[2]

There is a little known but important event which took place five years before Dr. Steere's Russian studies. In 1981 Dr. Steere was part of a small group of scientists who were trying to identify the causative agent of Lyme disease. The events of the day have been reported in their entirety to the public, or so people are led to believe. However there is one extremely important discovery that seems to have been left entirely out of the publicly communicated Lyme disease story line until now.

This event would not be publicly reported for over a decade, and only several years after the Dearborn conference took place. The timing of its publication is key since the study took place in 1981, thirteen years before Dearborn; and immediately prior to the announcement in 1982 of the causative agent of Lyme disease. If the event had been reported earlier, it would undoubtedly have changed not only the events which transpired at Dearborn, but probably also the entire Lyme disease history for decades to come. We will examine this "forgotten" event, and the role it may have played in some highly political events of the day.

It is important to point out that others who were responsible for identifying the agent of Lyme disease may or may not have been told about what Dr. Steere and his team had found. However it seems entirely likely that those involved could have known about the group's discovery as soon as it occurred. As often appears to be the case, those involved in certain aspects of Lyme history might have been willing to reveal all that was known to the public, but they may not have been able to do so for whatever reason, such as a directive from powerful players in the public health arena.

At Dearborn, Dr. Allen Steere presented what were called controversial recommendations for the CDC's "standardized" laboratory tests for Lyme disease. Colleague Dr. Frank Dressler and Dr. Steere had co-authored a paper which suggested that Lyme disease was "over diagnosed" and "over treated," even though human case numbers were rising. The paper was referred to as the "Dressler-Steere" paper, and Dr. Steere presented it at the Dearborn event. (Dr. Frank Dressler was also listed as a Dearborn attendee in the event's official program book.) Some conference participants disagreed with the recommendations made by Dr. Steere, but the objections were overruled and his recommendations influenced the standards established at Dearborn.[2,3]

A booklet from the Dearborn conference reveals that the strain recommendations used during quality assurance tests by the conference work group members included three Bb strains. One was a strain that had been laboratory-adapted from ticks collected on Shelter Island, New York in 1981. These were the same ticks that had yielded the Bb agent, and also the peculiar spirochete from the Lyme patient's ECM rash. According to the Dearborn conference booklet, the CDC felt that the selection of a single Bb strain would be most desirable for the newly standardized tests, yet declined to designate a specific strain. Because of the recommendations made at Dearborn, the newly standardized tests used probes that only detected east coast "arthritis" strains. Again these strains were only those found in patients that Rheumatologist Dr. Steere was clinically most familiar.[3]

Strains from other areas of the US and the world including those which cause neurologic, skin, cardiac, or other manifestations of Lyme disease were excluded from the Dearborn standards. This exclusion has been a terrible disservice to patients who are infected with any excluded strain. Patients who are tested using the CDC recommended two-tier system, ELISA* followed by a Western blot are often unlikely to have their infection detected, especially if their strain is excluded from the test probes. They may also test negative if they have the infection but do not yet, or won't make antibodies (seronegative).[3]

**ELISA stands for Enzyme-Linked Immunosorbent Assay, also called EIA, or Enzyme Immuno Assay.*

The new tests also excluded two of the most important Bb spirochetal proteins that should be included (detectable) by the tests, but are not. These two proteins represent the outer surface proteins "A" and "B" of the Bb spirochete. These are referred to as "OspA" and "OspB." Sometimes these are the only Bb proteins that are capable of stimulating antibody production in infected patients. If these antibodies are present in patients but unrepresented by test probes, then antibodies to these proteins cannot be detected by the tests, and therefore a patient will test falsely negative. If this occurs, a doctor may interpret a negative result to mean that the patient "does not have" Lyme disease. This is a "false negative" result, and may indicate that the patient is infected but there are no antibodies detected for any number of valid reasons; including that the test is not designed to detect the kinds of antibodies that are present.[3]

It is clear from the research including the official Dearborn conference booklet that patients do not always make antibodies to the Bb organism. When they do, sometimes the only ones produced are for OspA or OspB. Some patients won't make antibodies until a month or more after acute infection. If tested too soon, they will be negative. Tested later, patients may be found to be positive (seroconversion) or can remain negative. Others will never make antibodies, or will do so only after antibiotics lower their initial bacterial load. When diagnostic tests return "negative," patients are often told they don't have Lyme disease, and they are offered another diagnosis, which delays treatment. Patients are nearly equally told their result is a "false positive" if their test returns positive for Lyme. This is very strange indeed and I know of no other diagnostic tests that do not seem to allow patients to be genuinely positive for an infection. If this is the case, then what is the purpose of using "standardized" tests but to deny most patient infections?

Due to the newly standardized Lyme diagnostic tests, what are perhaps some of the most important Lyme antibodies in patients who have them cannot be detected even when present. You might think that Bb strains which produce the OspA/OspB proteins would have been mandatorily included in the Dearborn standards. It is felt by some people, including those who attended the conference, that had it not been for an upcoming Lyme disease vaccine that was in development and that was facing FDA approval at the time, the OspA and OspB protein "bands" may have been included in the tests.* At the time of the Dearborn conference, the new vaccine was about to go into clinical trials, for which Dr. Steere would also be lead investigator.[3]

**Diagnostic bands refer to the banding patterns that antibody proteins make when detected in serologic tests by the test probes. The bands are separated and recorded by molecular weight. This is expressed as kilodaltons, or kDa. Banding patterns in serologic tests place greater or lesser significance on particular proteins (i.e. 31kDa band represents the organism's outer surface protein A, or OspA; 34kDa is OspB).*

The way the Dearborn two-tiered test standards were established and are interpreted appears to lean toward the deliberate slow-playing and/or denial of an epidemic. Denial of illness in hundreds of thousands of people in North America and abroad by those who adhere to inaccurate testing methods appears stunningly illogical or even inhumane.

We can see how the "standardization" of diagnostic tests could be critical for an upcoming Lyme vaccine. In order for vaccine clinical trials to demonstrate a potential vaccine's effectiveness, researchers must differentiate between persons who are free of infection before vaccination; and those in whom new infections might be caused by the administration of a vaccine. By excluding key antibody bands from the diagnostic testing standards, natural infections would now be missed, but so would those caused by the failure of a vaccine that is based on the OspA/OspB proteins. This could make a vaccine appear highly successful even if it was not because important antibodies would be undetectable, even those of a failed vaccine.

Furthermore, a novel ELISA patent invention belonging to a CDC employee could be recommended for use under the new standardized two-tier process. CDC employee Barbara Johnson, a key Dearborn event organizer, is listed on a Dearborn-era ELISA patent. The ELISA is the first step of the standardized two-tier testing process recommended at Dearborn. This process is promoted by the CDC and is also recommended by the Infectious Diseases Society of America (IDSA). The Western blot is the second step. Despite the two-tiered recommendations, the CDC repeatedly states that Lyme disease remains a clinical diagnosis, and should not be based upon laboratory test results.

Despite the obvious shortcomings, the two-tiered process established at Dearborn remains in effect to the present day, and continues to negatively impact the Lyme community. The use of these tests, which are limited in scope; and the misuse of their results has led to misdiagnoses, treatment denials, insurance and disability benefit denials, and litigation. Unfortunately patients on more than one continent are called "crazy" for believing they are ill when laboratory tests fail to quantify infections that are often legitimately present, but are undetectable using the tests recommended at Dearborn and promoted by public health experts.[4]

Increasing numbers of Lyme treating physicians are using diagnostic tests that do not rely upon CDC standards to confirm cases of tickborne illness. As may be expected, substantially more patients are found to be positive for Lyme disease when such tests are used. Patients and physicians suffer backlash and ridicule by some public health officials and in the media on both sides of the pond for using diagnostic tests outside the CDC "standards." With few options to detect and quantify infections, physicians are hardly to blame for seeking better tools than those which simply cannot help. Unfortunately the tests are also relied upon too heavily by clinicians to diagnose an infection that should be diagnosed based on clinical symptoms. Laboratory tests may be appropriate as a confirmatory step, but should not be used to rule out infections. This is a statement that even the CDC now supports.

The Dearborn conference is considered by many to have been a distinctively negative turning point in Lyme disease history, especially for its patients. It is also the point in time where people claim the truth about Lyme disease became invisible. I have to disagree because the point of "no return" probably occurred very early on in the epidemic. After reading this book, we may understand perhaps why and when this occurred. If we look farther back into the history of Lyme disease, we may find evidence about its origins that until now has not been publicly discussed, especially by public health officials or those intimately involved in the discovery of the Lyme disease agent.

Had certain important information been disclosed by those in the know at the start of the epidemic (and at Dearborn), it would undoubtedly have changed the diagnostic test definitions and the way the disease has been, and continues to be acknowledged and treated. No doubt thousands more individuals would have had a more timely diagnosis and early treatment for an infection that once was a rare ECM rash-producing illness; but which over time has somehow managed to become a world-wide epidemic.[5-7]

Guidelines for a Silent Epidemic

There are currently two published sets of medical recommendations for the diagnosis and treatment of Lyme disease. The first set was prepared by members of the Infectious Diseases Society of America, and are referred to as the IDSA guidelines. In general these guidelines suggest that Lyme disease is a difficult to catch, easy to treat infection that is cured using short-term antibiotics; except for a small subset of patients who require short-term intravenous antibiotics. After the initial "curative" therapies, any patients who continue to have symptoms go on to have what the guidelines call a "post-Lyme syndrome" that is not an active infection, but an extended immune response to a previous infection.

Another set of published guidelines for Lyme disease were written by the International Lyme and Associated Diseases Society (ILADS). This is a medical professional organization whose members largely advocate on behalf of their patients – patients who claim not only to have the acute form, but a chronic form of Lyme disease. The ILADS guidelines in general promotes pulsed or mixed antibiotic therapies which represent longer treatment courses than what the IDSA guidelines recommend. There has been much controversy over the manner that the IDSA guidelines have been written, especially from patients who remain ill after their doctors attempt to use the IDSA guidelines recommendations as a tool to diagnose and treat them.

State medical boards, taking their cue from the CDC-promoted IDSA guidelines, have taken ILADS-friendly Lyme treating physicians to task for treating patients outside the so-called "standards of care." The IDSA guidelines are only one standard of care in a paradigm with multiple standards, whether published or perceived. Having multiple standards of care is not unusual in any medical field. For some reason it seems to be a serious problem for physicians who treat Lyme disease, and who are discouraged from following any other guidelines other than those written by the IDSA committee.

The stark contrast between the two sets of guidelines has created two opposing sides to the "war" that Lyme disease has managed to become. Public health and insurance agencies appear to take sides with the IDSA version, which was written largely by individuals who for the most part do not treat Lyme patients. ILADS doctors, those who support them, and their patients have been left to fend for themselves when the IDSA guidelines recommendations fail patients. The ILADS guidelines offer an intelligent approach to treating a multi-system infection, using therapies that have proven beneficial in the clinical environment. They don't necessarily use "evidence-based" laboratory tests to diagnose patients, and this has fueled political controversy, even in the media. Patients and physicians shout loudly that Lyme disease is often a complex, chronic, and persisting infection. However a core group of scientists with ties to public health and industry (some wrote the IDSA guidelines), may claim that patients and their physicians are "delusional," or that patients spend too much time on the Internet researching their ills.

However many registered patent inventions which were written under oath, contain comments which stand clearly in opposition to those who claim that there are "...self-proclaimed 'Lyme literati' that have used misinterpretations, misrepresentations, and bold fabrications to promote their ill-conceived and self-serving agenda regarding [Lyme] diagnosis and treatment." This horrible comment came from a web site that was promoting a new medical textbook co-authored by Drs. Jorge Benach, Ira Schwartz, Tom G. Schwan, Erol Fikrig, Alan G. Barbour, Stephen W. Barthold, Linda K. Bockenstedt, Gary P. Wormser, and Raymond J. Dattwyler. These individuals are among academic researchers who are sympathetic to the "IDSA" guidelines authors' consensus viewpoint. Three of these individuals were co-authors of the controversial IDSA guidelines for Lyme disease; several are listed on anywhere from one to one hundred patents for Bb-related products; several were present at the Dearborn conference, and at least three were part of the early search for the Bb causative agent.[1]

Some of these same individuals will publicly criticize Lyme patients and their physicians when they want to, yet will speak truths when necessary in texts that are far less likely to be read by the public. From the text of one patent application for a Lyme vaccine which lists Drs. Raymond Dattwyler and Benjamin Luft as inventors, we read important statements that were not included in the IDSA guidelines they sometimes helped to write. These statements speak in opposition to the unflattering comments that were made about "self-proclaimed Lyme literati:"

> "Currently, Lyme Disease is treated with antibiotics. However, such treatment is not always successful in clearing the infection. Treatment is often delayed due to improper diagnosis with the deleterious effect that the infection proceeds to a chronic condition, where treatment with antibiotics is often not useful. One of the factors contributing to delayed treatment is the lack of effective diagnostic tools."[2]

We can see that on the one hand certain individuals will establish guidelines which seem to minimize Lyme disease infections. On the other hand they may publish statements to the opposite effect when applying for a patent or license for an invention which is far more forthcoming than what they are willing to publicly reveal (i.e. as published in the guidelines or in the media). Those who sit on the sidelines observing the matter may feel that this approach may be protective of federally funded research, patent royalties, or perhaps something more.

Drs. Dattwyler and Luft were also part of the Dearborn conference planning committee where CDC standardized diagnostic tests were established – tests that Dattwyler and Luft's new patent application refers to as "ineffective." The truth about the serious nature of Lyme disease is also revealed in the text of another Lyme disease vaccine patent which was filed in 1992, two years before the Dearborn conference. According to the patent:

> "In the majority of cases Lyme Disease can be successfully treated with antibiotics, however, even with such treatment a number of cases will nevertheless proceed to chronic infection. At least 25% of the chronic disease does not the characteristic ECM response which means that a substantial proportion of chronic disease cases are presented to the clinician as advanced stages of the disease. In addition, approximately 1% of chronic disease patients either escape early stage detection or fail to respond to antibiotic therapy and consequently contract chronic Lyme Disease. Therefore, in a sizable number of instances, infection results in the development of debilitating late stage or *chronic* Lyme Disease."[1,3]

We can see how the truth about Lyme disease may be found within sworn patent applications. These texts are largely unread by the public; and some of the patents were written by some of the IDSA guidelines co-authors. There is a large body of published research (including patents) where chronic, persistent Lyme disease is openly acknowledged. Sometimes these same academic scientists will publish statements quite the opposite of those that may be found within the sworn testimony of their highly imaginative, and usually profitable patent inventions.[1,3]

It has been the experience of many Lyme patients that physicians who follow the recommendations of the ILADS camp of clinical physicians endow patients with the ability to fare significantly better in treatment than those whose physicians follow the more restrictive IDSA guidelines for Lyme disease. Nevertheless it is the IDSA guidelines co-authors and some of their colleagues whose ties and influence to industry and public health have a death grip hold on the diagnostic and treatment options for Lyme disease. Because the CDC in the US, and public health agencies abroad typically promote only the IDSA guidelines, patients around the world are being shortchanged on the unilateral promotion of one medical perspective – one that is based perhaps more on the conjecture of a core group of research scientists than they are based on clinical experience where actual patients can be found.

The divisional bias between treatment philosophies for Lyme disease has left a large number of lives broken and disillusioned due to the IDSA guidelines brand of "evidence-based" and "managed care" medicine. The other contributing factor has been the CDC's 1994 standardization of Lyme disease diagnostic tests that were established with the help of key IDSA guidelines authors and their colleagues. As a result, the public also suffers from the manner in which medical insurers deny their illness. These denials are based on the "evidence-based" brand of medicine that is often defined by those with industry ties and private agendas, and promoted by insurance companies. The idea that insurance companies are heavily invested in biotech companies that might be contributing to the diseases for which subscribers are requesting benefits, does not escape the most savvy of observers.

The Kaiser Foundation Health Plan Inc. of California is a non-profit corporation that shares a common board of directors with Kaiser Foundation Hospitals, and five health maintenance organizations in the system commonly known as "Kaiser Permanente." This is the largest private pre-paid healthcare program in the United States. According to tax returns, the Kaiser foundation provided financial benefits to institutions for "evidence-based research," to medical libraries, tumor boards, and cancer registries; and handed out "public policy" grants and expenses. It may be precisely these types of funding sources for academic researchers that are helping to fuel the denial of patient illnesses across the board.[4,5]

In what other disease category do we find patients literally forced to end treatments after only a month or so of antibiotics simply because a few public health experts suggest that an illness should be cured in that period of time? Patients with less physically devastating problems including chronic acne are allowed more potent antibiotics for indefinite periods. Meanwhile patients with debilitating and sometimes deadly tickborne infections are entirely dismissed, denied, and even ridiculed by

members of the scientific community and the medi- ating any disease are simply recommendations, not medical edict. Physicians
Any published guidelines for diagnosing and treating their patients, and then use their clinical expertise. They should not be
should consider all available guidelines wh- al boards simply for doing what they are trained to do. Lyme disease is a clinical
brought up on "charges" before state m- including exposure risk and symptom presentation. This is a statement that even the
diagnosis that is based on many fac- while it promotes the IDSA guidelines (which incidentally also support this statement)!
CDC is comfortable supporting- n for the third book in my Lyme series, *The Baker's Dozen & the Lunatic Fringe, Has Junk*
When researching the info- *se Paradigm?* I was hired by a well-known North Carolina AIDS/Lyme-physician. My task at
Science Shifted the Lyme assist in the presentation of evidence for Connecticut Attorney General Richard Blumenthal's 2006
the time was to researc- the Infectious Diseases Society of America's (IDSA) clinical practice guidelines for Lyme disease.
anti-trust investig- aborative venture and provided about three hundred pages of research from my then unpublished book.
I participated i- estigation the presentation was sent to the Attorney General's office for review. Some of this research was
Very late i- producers in production with the award-winning Lyme disease documentary film *Under Our Skin.**
also sha- *e Pictures*
*2006 A month after the materials were sent to the AG's office, on May 1, 2008, Attorney Blumenthal announced his findings
espect to the IDSA guidelines. These included a statement that there were:

> "...serious flaws in the Infectious Disease Society of America's (IDSA) process for writing its 2006 Lyme disease guidelines and the IDSA has agreed to reassess them with the assistance of an outside arbiter." A press release from the AG's office said "Insurance companies have denied coverage for long-term antibiotic treatment relying on these guidelines as justification. The guidelines are also widely cited for conclusions that chronic Lyme disease is nonexistent."[6]

Attorney Blumenthal's office also indicated that it had discovered:

> "...undisclosed financial interests held by several of the most powerful IDSA panelists. The IDSA's guideline panel improperly ignored or minimized consideration of alternative medical opinion and evidence regarding chronic Lyme disease, potentially raising serious questions about whether the recommendations reflected all relevant science."

In addition, Blumenthal said the guidelines process lacked procedural safeguards. A new panel was requested to review the guidelines as part of the settlement for the suit.[6]

A new review panel would be more independent said Blumenthal, and would consist of members selected by the IDSA and by Blumenthal's office. The panel would reassess the IDSA guidelines and determine whether they should be rewritten or let stand as written. This would be the first time in history that medical guidelines would be so heavily scrutinized. The panel reconvened in July 30, 2009 in Washington DC, at a public hearing that was publicized on the Internet. The public and academic researchers who had been excluded from providing input during the IDSA guidelines process were allowed to speak and to present their side of the story. My book *The Baker's Dozen* was sent to each panel member (twice), and was also presented at the hearing by a Lyme advocate since I could not attend myself. The panelists eventually determined that the IDSA guidelines should stand as written, despite evidence showing that chronic Lyme exists. Richard Blumenthal commented that his office would review the evidence to ensure that the IDSA had complied with the terms of their settlement.

While some media sources hailed the "successful" defense of the IDSA guidelines, many people came away from the second hearing dissatisfied that members of the hearing panel seemed determined not to change the guidelines at any cost. The weight of the evidence however is very clear, despite the outcome of any investigation; no matter how loudly any media source may crow (and there are EIS employees among media sources, and other important ties). The scientific and clinical evidence is real, palpable, and it agrees with the privately published patent texts of some of the IDSA Lyme disease guidelines authors – evidence that is not found within the IDSA guidelines for the disease. Those truths mirror the experience of the patients, and tell the real story about modern day Lyme disease and other tickborne infections.[6]

Biowarfare in History

Most people have heard of the terms "weapons of biological warfare" or "biowarfare." A significant number of people are aware that biological warfare has been practiced in one form or another for centuries around the world. In the modern day, biowarfare was recognized as an inhumane form of warfare, and over time restrictions to the kinds of warfare weaponry that could be used upon populations were severely restricted. While this is all well and good, very few people are aware that there has been an entirely different form of biological warfare that has been undertaken for the last century and a half. This kind of warfare is aimed at controlling insects of medical, veterinary, agriculture, and military importance.

I am talking about biological warfare against pest insects, or insect biowarfare, which uses the techiniques of chemical and microbial "weapons" to combat populations of pest insects which threaten crops, livestock animals, ornamental plants, forestry materials, food stores, and human populations with disease. This very different form of biowarfare is one that is actively practiced all around us; and of which the majority of people are completely unaware. Before we begin to study the history of insect biowarfare and its significance to the world of Lyme disease, let's examine a bit of history about the kinds of warfare of which most people are at least generally aware.

In 1940, the US Army decided to establish a comprehensive virus diagnostic laboratory which would focus on infectious diseases including those afflicting military personnel. The duties of the new laboratory staff were to extend beyond current research and diagnostic techniques typically practiced in traditional infectious disease laboratories. In 1941, the first military specialty laboratory was established at the US Army Medical Department's Research and Graduate School in Washington, District of Columbia. In the lab, diagnostic procedures for viruses and rickettsial diseases were brought together under one roof. A report refers to several such military virus laboratories that were initially established in the US in the form of the National Communicable Disease Center of the Public Health Service (PHS).[1,2]

In time the Army/PHS research grew to include other military laboratories around the world. Several of these laboratories were established in the State of California; in Philadelphia, Pennsylvania; in the City and State of New York; and in Atlanta, Georgia under the PHS name. The agency's name changed to the Centers for Disease Control and Prevention (CDC) in 1970.

As an offshoot of the US military, the CDC laboratories develop and implement infectious disease prevention and control techniques. The agency also handles issues of environmental and occupational health and safety; and provides educational activities to promote health within the US population. In fact the CDC's Laboratory Response Network website states that it is an: "...integrated network of state & local public health, federal, military, & international labs that can respond to both bioterrorism & chemical terrorism."[1,2]

From 1945 to 1950, the Army Medical Department Research and Graduate School assigned the responsibility of serologic (blood) diagnostics for certain infectious diseases to the military's new CDC virus laboratories. Many diseases were studied and samples tested at the new facilities on behalf of the Army. Influenza, epidemic and murine (mouse) typhus, Q fever, and psittacosis-lymphogranuloma venereum, a bird disease caused by *Chlamydia psittaci*, were studied. The medical school reportedly provided the Army laboratories with "standardized" antigens* and antisera, and also advised laboratory personnel on their use. A similar process to standardize laboratory tests would be undertaken four decades later with the CDC's "standardization" of laboratory diagnostic tests for Lyme disease.[1]

**Antigens are proteins that stimulate the immune system. Antisera is serum that contains antibodies.*

It is most curious that the emergence of a novel infection in Australian meat plant workers in 1935 that was eventually named "Q Fever" appeared to resemble typhus and psittacosis combined. Why would military scientists be studying these agents? Quite possibly because they are common livestock infections – illnesses that could be transmissible to the public through the ingestion of contaminated milk and meats. In my previous book *God Science,* I covered a basic history of the US military's biological warfare, and the establishment of the University of Chicago and the US government's military-scientific partnership called the War Research Service (WRS), which commenced in 1942. That was the year Harvard graduate and President of Merck & Co. Pharmaceuticals George W. Merck joined the WRS as head of its germ warfare advisory group. Biowarfare testing was headquartered at the military's Fort Detrick facility in Frederick, Maryland. As WWII loomed, Ft. Detrick scientists kept insectaries* and designed and tested chemical and biological weapons of warfare for offensive and defensive military and agricultural purposes. Concurrently in the background was the US government and military's research and development of nuclear weapons. The objectives of the War Research Service was to study and develop techniques and tools for use during the upcoming conflict. (Chemical and biological warfare for military use has a far earlier history not covered here.)[1,3,4]

**Insectaries were just as they sound; large enclosures where various arthropods (ticks) and insects were raised and maintained for laboratory and other testing purposes.*

Some of the same tools that were used as chemical and biological weapons of warfare during periods of conflict were also highly useful for controlling pest insects of agricultural, medical, and veterinary importance. These activities are highly significant to our story because biowarfare tools in the form of microbes and infectious insects can be dropped upon populations, agricultural fields, and livestock to cause epidemic diseases during conflicts. Likewise these tools may be deployed to protect the military, civilians, livestock, and agricultural crops from insects and diseases during non-conflict periods. This "non-conflict" period is of course the majority of the historical timeline, and the main focus of our story.

The protection of each of these vital commodities was and remains an important aspect of defending any nation against who might use similar weapons or tools in a "terroristic" manner. The development of any disease epidemics as a byproduct of nuclear, medical, agricultural, or other industries; or weapons or wastes either past or present, also fall under the same protections. For this reason nuclear, chemical, or agricultural weapons and biowarfare-related research of any kind (and the microbes of same), have now become matters of national and international security.

It is also important to understand that at the beginning of World War II, the main scientific institutions and their academic partners were one way or another studying nuclear, chemical, or biological warfare weapons (including nerve agents); as well as infectious diseases. These studies took place not only within the US, but in other significant powers around the world.

In the US, participating scientists at one time or another included individuals from Yale, Harvard, Stanford, Cornell, Columbia, Tulane, the University of Chicago, Massachusetts General Hospital, Northwestern University, Ohio State, Notre Dame, and the Universities of Wisconsin, California, Minnesota, Connecticut, Pennsylvania, Missouri, Illinois, Indiana, Iowa, New York, Nebraska, and Texas (and others). Governmental agencies at the highest levels were also involved with biowarfare research, and often helped finance same. Some of the federal agencies that have been directly involved in biowarfare research include the Centers for Disease Control; the laboratories of the National Institutes of Health (NIH); the National Institutes of Allergies and Infectious Diseases (NIAID), and even the Central Intelligence Agency (CIA).[5]

The appointment of George W. Merck to the WRS committee must have been a convenient relationship for the budding pharmaceutical company. This is because the use of chemical and biological weapons of warfare of any kind whether agricultural or military, would necessitate the manufacture of pharmaceutical solutions (i.e. vaccines, antibiotics) in response to any chemical or biological warfare agent deployments which could adversely affect humankind. In addition because of the nature of radioactivity, the use of nuclear energy for peaceful purposes was understood to be capable of causing cancerous diseases. It is impossible to think that the experts would not have fully understood that the global population would be among those affected by any deployed "weapons" no matter how benign the agent, or for what purpose it was deployed.

During and after WWII, in order to facilitate military studies of biowarfare agents, a huge metallic test sphere dubbed the "Eight Ball" was built by Chicago Bridge & Iron Company. The sphere was installed at Ft. Detrick for use during animal and human biological warfare experiments which were undertaken until such activities were banned. Sometimes biowarfare experiments were performed upon animal and human volunteers in the open air; and the military had special test sites for this purpose (i.e. Dugway Proving Ground southwest of Salt Lake City, Utah). In Canada and the UK, biological warfare programs were also underway since these countries were in collaboration with US scientists. One program included the design and production of 500-pound bombs that could deliver insects infected with diseases such as Tularemia or Rocky Mountain spotted fever. The fact that these programs existed does not provide comfort to civilians who have already been exposed to "simulant" agents for decades (by accident or otherwise) with or without their knowledge. The silence surrounding same also negatively enforces the public's mistrust in those whom we look to for protection in the public health arena.[6,7]

Infectious agents deployed or stumbled upon in the environment that are capable of causing disease epidemics in insect and animal populations could quickly become a danger to human health. Likewise anything deployed as an agricultural agent whether through an act of war or simply as an insecticide could accidentally cause problems within the human population. Chemical and biological insecticides were and are deployed as aerial releases over civilian populations; and as farm-based deployments for agricultural purposes. These deployments include "nerve agents" in the form of insecticides and other biocides which target insects, and which are strategically designed to force insect infections, also called *epizootics*.

There may be an increased risk to populations with the deployment of genetically engineered insecticides. If these tools would cause disease outbreaks, then pharmaceutical products and vaccines could be designed and delivered with the intent of fixing an emerging disease – even one caused by genetic engineering "accidents" that might arise. Such "accidents" caused by what appear to be inherently flawed recombinant constructs,* are "secretly" well-known, and clearly identified by scientists who patent the processes before they are produced and deployed. Despite any risks, the public is not usually informed about such matters because if they were, they would more than likely raise more than a few objections.

**Recombinant constructs are genetically engineered cells, also called chimera.*

Following World War II, a number of post-Nazi regime scientists were granted immunity from war crimes by the US government, and imported to expand and develop biowarfare tools for the US military's chemical and biological warfare programs. Some of these scientists were hired by prominent US chemical companies to design agricultural insecticides based ne nerve agents previously used to exterminate civilians during the Holocaust (i.e. massive killing of large military program associated with importing scientists into the country was called *Operation Paperclip*. he Paperclip program was granted in September 1946 by President Harry S. Truman. gress more than tripled its current military chemical and biological warfare budget. Newspapers of the day promoted a more "humane" type of warfare in articles claiming "war without death" – newspapers that may have been paid to publish such propaganda. By July of 1969, the military's secret chemical and biological warfare program and experiments on animals and human volunteers under a program called *Operation Whitecoat* was revealed on national television. The exposé included an interview with one of the program's participants, a Seventh-day Adventist volunteer.[8-10]

In 1969, President Richard M. Nixon declared the historic end to the use of biological warfare weapons through the establishment of the Biological Warfare Convention (BWC). Fort Detrick's US military scientists and their academic cohorts were forced to change gears midstream with this announcement, although not really by very much since most operations were already applicable to peaceful agricultural use. Scientists began to refocus research efforts toward matters involving cancers; and those pertaining to the military, agricultural, medical, and veterinary protection of animals, food crops, and people from pest insects. According to the text of the Convention treaty, scientists were still allowed to use "toxins" and "agents" for "peaceful" and "medical" purposes, including disease prevention. The use of nuclear energy was also converted to peaceful purposes, and nuclear efforts were now aimed toward agricultural, veterinary, medical, and industrial applications. The mitigation of potential diseases which might emerge as a result of agricultural deployments of engineered microbes, toxins, or even nuclear-related "pollution" is a poorly defined area of the BWC definitions, and one that has arguably been tested to its limits.

The study of cancers is also a natural offshoot of nuclear, industrial, and agricultural tools that were, and continue to be deployed. Whether these studies include the release of genetically modified insects (i.e. population replacement, irradiated "sterile" insect techniques), genetically engineered plants, or applied pesticides; the end result is that deployed microbes (especially viruses) can contain oncogenes. These are genes which can, and are known to cause cancers. The need for cancer studies may necessarily encompass the reactivation of latent (sleeping) viruses within an immune compromised human host; or the unintentional recombination (reassortment) of genes that accidentally or naturally occurs in an insect, animal, or human host. Reassorted, mixed infections are transmissible through the bite or sting of an insect. They may also be transmitted by ingesting genetically modified foods if genetic engineering techniques fail; or if nuclear wastes or agricultural chemicals bring about unexpected mutations in microbes or their insect or animal hosts.

Research has shown that sometimes viruses in genetic constructs get "kicked out" of the formula (also called viral vectors or expression cassettes). This describes a group of engineered genes that are spliced together to cause the expression or suppression of certain genes within a targeted insect host. The accidental escape of genes running rampant throughout the environment of microbes, insects, animals, or humans cannot at this time in scientific endeavors be either predicted or controlled.

The question to ask is what causes "accidents" of recombinant engineering to occur in the first place? The answers are complex but may include the introduction of applied microbes and toxins; industrial or agricultural chemicals, and/or the influence of radioactivity upon cells and the mutations that can occur. Even the organisms lying dormant in our own bodies can contribute to disease. Such organisms may be present as a result of past natural infections; as symbionts;* or from the receipt of recombinantly engineered vaccines, antibiotics, and other human products.[11]

**Symbionts in this book refers to host parasites that may be helpful or harmful to the host.*

What have been the findings concerning the deployment of agricultural chemicals such as those used over decades (i.e. Endrin, Chlordane, DDT, Heptachlor, Malathion, etc.)? These and other chemicals and nuclear wastes have been found to be highly mutagenic, teratogenic (malformations), clastogenic (break chromosomes), and/or are genotoxic (harms genes). This means they can break, reassemble, translocate, destroy, or otherwise alter or swap the genes of microbes, insects, animals, and/or humans because they are powerful chemical catalysts able to do so.

Scientists create chimera (blends of genes from more than one organism); and introduce toxins, bacteriae, viruses, and other microbial goodies in efforts to create natural insecticides. The unaware general public is going to be exposed to whatever is formulated and released into the environment, whether or not such constructs are tested or can be tested for safety. We will have absolutely no control over what happens to these agents once they are released into the unpredictable external world. Microbes are critters that are able to reproduce based on nutrients present. The reassortment of their genetic information (by mutation, transposons, plasmids) is highly adaptable after millions of years of environmental challenges. As the microbes change, so does the ability of the insects to resist the poisonous toxins to which they are exposed. Over time microbes through natural mutation, interfering viruses, and newly designed insecticides with potent neurotoxins become far more dangerous to insects, and to the animals and humans that are similarly exposed.

There is a cycle of infection and resistance that microbiologists and other scientists initiated during the 1880s when they began serious attempts to control pest insects that were destroying food crops, citrus trees, stored grains, textiles, and other products. With the importation of exotic insects meant to parasitize domestic insects, so too arrived natural infections caused by viruses, fungi, microsporidia, bacteria, and nematodes; all of which were covertly hidden in the imported insect guts. Little did scientists understand that by importing foreign insects as early "biological controls," they were introducing infectious microbes into areas which formerly did not have them. The result was the introduction and reassortment of Old World microbes into the New World. The effects of well-meaning scientists whose efforts were geared toward controlling pest insects seem to have caused or contributed to diseases that have become more difficult to control over time.

It might be argued that human disease is a constant and any biological control-related diseases could eventually be treated, if they ever surfaced. As we can see from current diseases of today (i.e. Lyme), if and when novel diseases have emerged, the tendency of some scientists or public health officials may have been to suppress and deny illnesses if they were discovered to have been inconveniently tied to insect or other biowarfare activities.

Others might argue that the entire idea of manipulating the environment was and is a dangerous game that should never have been played. It is not a stretch of the imagination to believe that those exploring biological warfare against insects probably knew ahead of time that human health would eventually be jeopardized to some degree. If so, this could very easily explain why the "new deal" agency of the War Research Service was to be shrouded in secrecy. We can see this sentiment described in then Secretary of War Henry Stimson's 1942 letter to President Roosevelt where he said, "…we must be prepared…and the matter must be handled with great secrecy and as well as great vigor." This was a period following the Japanese attack on Pearl Harbor, and the American mainland.[5,12,13]

The former quote is often cited by those who argue that it supports the laboratory fabrication of the Lyme disease organism as a biological warfare weapon. However this is unsupported by any evidence that such an endeavor was undertaken. The statement could have been made on behalf of the military's interests in creating "peaceable" weapons of nuclear and biological warfare for agricultural use, especially since at the time such weapons were about to be banned. These weapons included the use of nuclear energy-based techniques that were highly applicable for agricultural and industrial use.

Simply because some biological agents were fabricated for offensive or defensive purposes does not mean that the agent of Lyme disease was ever a biological weapon of warfare; or was fabricated within any laboratory, even in those that clearly used ticks for experimental studies. One example report cites tick experiments and possible aerial drops of insects at Plum Island, a military/US Department of Agriculture research laboratory located on a small island off the coast of Long Island, New York. Agricultural tools for biowarfare during periods of conflict were largely the very same tools that could be applied during non-conflict periods, and were only occasionally or sometimes never deployed during wartime. Even before "poison tick" experiments at Plum Island in the mid-to late 1950s, most agricultural agents had not been applied globally although they enjoyed limited regional agricultural use in multiple countries.[5,12]

Other popularly misquoted statements that are commonly cited to support a belief that the Lyme disease agent was a weapon of biowarfare are the July 1, 1969 declarations of Dr. Donald MacArthur, then Biological Research Administrator and Deputy Director for the Department of Defense (DOD) Research and Engineering agency. MacArthur testified at a hearing before the US House Committee on Appropriations concerning the state of molecular biology and the pursuit of possible bioagents which might: "incapacitate rather than kill large populations of people." The quote was,

> "…within a period of 5 to 10 years it would be possible to produce a synthetic biological agent, an agent that does not naturally exist and for which no natural immunity could have been acquired."[13]

Dr. MacArthur could have been speaking about biowarfare agents for use in the Vietnam War which was already underway. Of course that war would end in 1975, three years after former President Nixon banned such weapons for periods of conflict. The problem with citing this quote in an effort to link it to a current epidemic disease is in the timing and context of the program being discussed. The hearing took place just four months before President Nixon's termination of the US offensive biological weapons program, which took place in November of the year. The MacArthur quote typically continues:[13,14]

> "…it would probably be possible to make a new infective organism…Most important of these is that it might be refractory to the immunological and therapeutic processes upon which we depend to maintain our relative freedom from infectious diseases."
>
> "It is a highly controversial issue and there are many who believe such research should not be undertaken lest it lead to yet another method of massive killing of large populations."

Here the argument is valid that the topic of discussion could have been the synthetic creation of an agent that could have agricultural, medical, or military applications. But this statement could equally be attributed to the discussion of the use of nuclear energy for agricultural use. After all, the world was familiar with the power of atomic bombs; and the retooling of nuclear energy for medical, veterinary, and agricultural use would carry with it the same risks and processes that were used to create nuclear weapons.[13,14]

It is extremely important to say that just because a statement was made by a military officer just before the banning of biological weapons of warfare does not prove in any way nor suggest that any biological weapon was inferred, or was ever subsequently developed or released for the purpose of making any population ill. There simply is no concrete evidence proving that the Bb agent was entirely designed in a laboratory. When we look closely at the evidence that is readily available however, we find a very different kind of biological warfare that was undertaken over a century and a half against pest insects using weapons that are clearly described in the available literature. This very different class of weaponry when properly examined seems to have been fully capable of bringing about many kinds of human epidemics including modern day Lyme disease. However the emergence of Lyme disease as we shall see, appears to have been at least partly if not entirely by accident.

We will learn that ECM rash illnesses were already present in the US during the 1940s, before Plum Island was converted in 1953 from the military camp Fort Terry into a facility housing an agricultural research laboratory. It is interesting to postulate on the ability of past biowarfare weapons to spread diseases simply because they were tested in the open air. However even in areas close to a disease epicenter, we might consider that such deployments would thereafter have only a regional presentation and not a global one, unless similar agents were tested simultaneously on all continents. Since the history of Lyme disease seems to have begun during the 1800s, we can see how the Plum Island biowarfare argument does not hold up to scrutiny as the cause of Lyme disease around the world.

I am sure there are those who are vested in their beliefs enough to argue against these points ad nauseum. The fact remains however that there is no evidence to prove that any escaped "Plum Island" ticks were successfully carried to the mainland on the backs of swimming deer. Yes migratory birds may carry infected ticks a great distance. But the idea that one, two, or even ten ticks caused Lyme disease clusters that were clearly evident in Europe a century before Plum Island was ever built is illogical.

Accepting this critical point leaves us free to study the history of agriculturally deployed parasitoid insects and microbial cocktails which surpass a century of our collective world history. When we compare the use of these tools to the emergence of an ECM rash illness in all areas of the world, we can clearly see that the modern Lyme disease of today probably did not begin during the 20th century, but rather far earlier. There are differences however between the "classic" ECM rash illnesses and modern day Lyme, and I will attempt to describe them throughout this book from a hypothetical perspective.

While Dr. MacArthur was spouting off about a desire for the federal funding of biological weapons, the public got wind of the military dumping of its obsolete chemical and biological weapons off US coasts in multiple areas. In 1968 the public was still reeling from the discovery that the military had accidentally dropped toxic "VX" (mustard-based nerve agents) outside of Dugway Proving Ground, killing roughly 6,000 sheep in Skull Valley, Utah. At the time, a Harvard professor circulated a petition signed by roughly 5,000 scientists. The petition requested a moratorium on the use of chemical weapons in Vietnam, and for the oversight and examination of policies concerning the use of chemical and biological weapons of warfare during combat.

As a result of public outcry, the US, Canada, and Great Britain organized an international convention to ban such weapons. Newly elected President Richard M. Nixon hired National Security Advisor Henry Kissinger to advise him on the matter. The resulting declaration by Nixon for the US to renounce the use of chemical and biological weapons heralded the Biological Weapons Convention (BWC) treaty. It was ratified by the US Senate in 1974, and was effective March 1975. The Senate also ratified the 1925 Geneva Protocol which banned the wartime use of bacteriological weapons.

By 1977, US Senate hearings determined that roughly 239 populated areas of the US had been contaminated with biological agents over two decades from 1949 to 1969. This probably did not bode well for people who were coming down with an arthritis-like illness that had never been seen in the country before that time. Some of the areas that had been contaminated by such practices included Key West and Panama City, Florida; St. Louis, Missouri; Minneapolis, Minnesota; San Francisco, California; and Washington, D.C. It is clear that the environment and the microbes and insects within same were bombarded with weapons of military biological warfare, and also by agricultural weapons that often contained similar or more powerful microbial cocktails. The weapons appropriations requested by MacArthur were approved by Congress in July of 1969, but the declaration four months later by the President supports instead the pursuit of biowarfare weapons of an agricultural and medicinal nature. These practices are arguably allowable "peaceful purposes" under the new BWC definitions.[13,14]

Although the Soviet government signed the new BWC treaty, they allegedly carried out experiments irrespective of the agreement. It has not been proven yet whether the US military did as well; and we must take care not to assume that "everybody was doing it" was the order of the day. Still, an Institute of Medicine investigation into the WWII and Lewisite experiments undertaken in 1993 declared that an atmosphere of secrecy remains concerning the US WWII biological warfare testing program. We may never learn the truth about all that was undertaken unless in time such evidence is declassified.[15]

The literature describes a few rogue scientists who covertly performed less than humane experiments up [illegible] lized patients using radiation (uranium/plutonium) or surgery. It has also been revealed that there were those wh [illegible] agents into prison inmates and/or mental health patients. In 1972 the public was shocked by the expo [illegible] "experiment" where men infected with "Syphilis" were left to suffer from disseminated disease without tr [illegible] part, the US military's development and testing of chemical and biological weapons was centralized at pl [illegible]

Mountain Arsenal (RMA) in Denver, Colorado; at Dugway Proving Ground (Utah); Aberdeen Proving Ground (Maryland); Pine Bluff Arsenal (Arkansas); Edgewood Arsenal (Maryland); Huntsville Arsenal (Alabama); Fort Detrick (Maryland); or Plum Island (New York).[16-18]

After the BWC ban, the chemical and biological warfare weapons from conflict periods were realigned with cancer research and the agricultural and industrial use of such weapons. Indeed biological warfare against pest insects is described quite openly in many patent applications. Those who control the information flow about infectious diseases caused by anything agriculturally deployed (i.e. parasitizing insect, biocides) would require a small posse of infectious disease personnel to contain any epidemics that might arise from their use. Representatives of the CDC's public health elite EIS force might for example be used to contain and control information about an epidemic. Public health employees might be hired to protect genetic engineering profits, processes, research grants, patent royalties, academic funding, world-wide agricultural tools; and to promote public perceptions of the importance of such tools. But what if a militarily deployed agent accidentally combined with genetically modified agricultural tools? What if an accident of recombinant genetics caused a human epidemic now seen around the world? If this had occurred, then we can understand why there may be some in the public health sector who might work at the highest levels to conceal such events.

We might expect to see a small core group of individuals from the birth of any human epidemics to jump on board and to remain intricately involved throughout the lifespan of the epidemic no matter how long that timeframe might be. This would be most important if such epidemics were caused by or contributed to by any past nuclear, chemical, or biological warfare experiments or deployments for military, agricultural, or other purposes.

Unfortunately scientists of the day were rather shortsighted in their justifications to promote the global use of microbial and chemical agents that had not been "properly" tested before their release. According to a conference report,

> "Most insect pathogens (in fact, as far as we know; all true insect pathogens) are nonpathogenic for vertebrate animals. At least, this is true for all entomogenous microorganisms that have been tested. There have been no cases of spontaneous disease resulting in higher animals following application of microbial insecticides."[5,12]

I wonder whether regulators of the day were informed of any possible adverse effects of the agents about to be released. Would sporadic disease outbreaks be discovered to be linked to local or regional deployments of biological controls? Or were disease outbreaks which appeared post-deployment merely assumed to be random natural events? It is interesting to note that many scientists in earlier decades were well aware of specific microbes and of their effects upon many insect species. Did the scientific community suffer from a serious lack of communication with public health officials? Or was there a concerted effort by a few individuals with industry sponsors to keep adverse effects securely out of sight from public or regulatory bodies? The scientists who studied these controls were certainly not confined to US laboratories. Therefore we could hardly expect there to have been an "accidental" lack of communication, or even complete ignorance. US scientists collaborated with those abroad on the use of biological controls, so it may simply be that "everybody was doing it" was the mindset of the era, consequences be damned. It is anyone's guess as to the true origins of human epidemics. However upon careful study of the available literature and the past history of nuclear, chemical, and microbial tools; the light of truth may finally shine on what may have otherwise remained a closely guarded secret.

Ethics Violations Become Public Knowledge

The Tuskegee Syphilis experiment is probably the most well-known of the unethical infectious disease "studies" ever executed within the US. There are many others. In Illinois for example, prisoners of the Stateville Penitentiary in Joliet were injected with malaria and studied for the disease's effects during the 1940s. Often medical experiments of this nature were performed by unethical scientists upon "volunteers" under the defense that such experiments were for the expansion of scientific knowledge. Other examples were the use of prostitutes to infect prison inmates with sexually transmissible diseases; or the deliberate exposure of orphaned children, mental patients, and soldiers in 1946-1948 Guatemala to study "Syphilis" and other sexually transmitted diseases.

A fairly significant number of questionably ethical experiments have occurred; implemented by the Central Intelligence Agency (CIA), scientists from prestigious universities, the US military, and others. Some of these experiments were executed within the environment. Others were perpetrated against individuals from the 1940s to the 1970s to study biological warfare weapons and infectious diseases. Such studies could arguably have dual purposes, including as offensive and defensive weapons which might affect domestic or enemy troops. These tests could also arguably have had agricultural applications since recombinant microbes deployed in any manner could lead to animal or human disease epidemics.

any people are aware that bacteria called *Mycoplasmas* have been genetically engineered within the laboratory. At least ·e has been registered as a patent invention. There is a very different side of the story that hasn't been told with respect to the mycoplasmas. A US patent that has caused much controversy and conjecture regarding the practice of biowarfare human populations was issued in 1993, the year before the Dearborn conference. We now know that some covert experin using mycoplasma strains were undertaken under the guise of "military" defenses during past decades. But what we think of as biowarfare experiments may not always have motivations that are crystal clear.[4]

If scientists had discovered that cell lines used for insecticides and animal or human vaccines contained important contaminants, such revelations could force public health officials to isolate the agent(s) and study the pathology of same in human volunteers. Remember that CDC laboratories were first and foremost military laboratories. It has been revealed that there was experimentation upon human volunteers using recombinant formulas which contained mycoplasma agents. The purpose of such experiments could have been to test a novel human vaccine as a protective therapy against what had already been identified as a contaminant in animal and/or human cell lines or other biological products (i.e. interferon). Perhaps such contaminations had already spread to humans through infected medical products; or from animal meats and other products. It is also interesting that "covert" mycoplasma experiments were taking place in Texas during the First Gulf War.[3]

Recombinant (genetically engineered) mycoplasma agents could have been tested as a first generation military vaccine to protect against a food, water, or environmental threat that was expected to be present in the Middle East where troops were deployed. It may have also been "inconvenient" to obtain traditional permissions to test vaccine formulas upon human volunteers; but it may have been deemed necessary if there was an impending, unavoidable threat to military personnel. Public scrutiny will do much to detain science in an era already tainted by past covert biowarfare testing. There are government declarations which may supersede public laws and interests if a threat is militarily or strategically important to address. Historically speaking, certain "investigational" activities have been granted a green light by those at the highest levels of government for military purposes without the public's awareness beforehand. The public typically discovers such activities only many years later when files describing the activities are finally declassified.

Whatever the intent, scientists may have decided to forgo the usual ethics-permissions process. Or perhaps they received governmental dispensation to perform mycoplasma experiments upon human volunteers for militarily-important reasons. At least one book describes how Texas prison inmates and hospital and nursing home patients were used in this manner around the first Gulf War to test recombinant mycoplasma strains for military vaccines. However morally distasteful the experiments may be to the public, the fact remains that the government can and will grant permission for such undertakings if it deems them necessary.[3]

This covert approach probably saves scientists and/or military officials significant expense in time and energy, as well as public scrutiny and negative implications (liability) should such experiments fail. This of course in no manner speaks to the ethics of such activities. The fact that such formulas were tested upon humans speaks volumes about the kinds of covert activities allowed to continue post BWC ban. However the mere fact that an agent is tested upon civilians does not prove that the tests were connected in any way to other biowarfare "weapons" which might exist. It certainly does not prove that recombinant mycoplasmas were ever used or designed to make populations ill with disease-causing pathogens, although such claims have repeatedly been made.

Likewise it does not prove in any manner that the agents being tested had any other intended purpose other than as a protective military vaccine. All that past activities can prove is that at times, scientists and those who control the strings of biowarfare research have performed covert experiments in a manner that had questionable ethical standards. The common morality is that such experiments should never have occurred in the first place, and that is precisely why they would have been performed covertly. It is because public opinion carries tremendous weight that it is often avoided at all cost. As long as "we" are unaware of such activities, the easier it is for them to be undertaken without opposition from the public.

Two patent inventions describe methods of detecting some very "Lyme-like" illnesses, Chronic Fatigue Syndrome (a/k/a Myalgic Encephalomyelitis or ME); Fibromyalgia, and Rheumatoid Arthritis. The patents are for diagnostic tests to determine if mycoplasma genes or antibodies are present, including those belonging to *Mycoplasma fermentans, Mycoplasma penetrans,* or *Mycoplasma hominis* species. This implies that each of these illnesses have a common organism responsible for the physical symptoms of these illnesses – a *Mycoplasma* species. This also suggests that the illnesses are *valid infections* which are treatable because there is an infectious agent involved. According to one of the patents:

> "The mycoplasma species *M. fermentans, M. hominis* and *M. penetrans* have been isolated from individuals suffering from primary atypical pneumonia, urogenital infections, Rheumatoid Arthritis (RA) and AIDS-related infections."[1,2]

There are many people who insist that a US patent for a pathogenic mycoplasma is evidence that scientists engineered a mycoplasma strain as a biowarfare tool to cause people to become ill. I have investigated this patent which describes how scientists isolated a novel, pathogenic mycoplasma from patients who were suffering with Acquired Immune Deficiency atent describes a device to detect antibodies from the serum of AIDS patients; and also from those who emble AIDS. The device also describes specific DNA sequences that can be used within a laboratory nans or animals.[4]

believe from the patent text that there is any connection to military "biowarfare" experiments that were undertaken, ... conflict-related brucella or visna virus experiments (as some people claim); nor for offensive military use against "enemy" livestock or people. The fact that animals are mentioned in the patent is interesting however because *Mollicutes* including the mycoplasmas are well known pathogens of livestock animals (i.e. cattle, pigs, poultry, sheep, fowl). We must first ask why scientists are interested in these pathogens, and the answer may fundamentally have to do with contaminated cell lines for insecticides and vaccines, or the emergence of human pathogens from animal products or wastes.

Mycoplasmas can be transmitted to humans through the ingestion of contaminated animal meats, organs, milk, eggs, and biological products (i.e. vaccines, collagen, etc.). Many human biological products are derived from mycoplasma-infected animals because these pathogens are so tiny. If we test the population, we will find that many people are infected by many different types of mycoplasma strains. If scientists had genetically engineered any strains of mycoplasmas, the truth is that they may have done so to design a vaccine that would be useful in livestock animals, and/or to prevent the transmission of disease to the human population. Agriculturally speaking, the application of genetically engineered mycoplasmas for any purpose (i.e. insecticides, animal vaccines, military use, biowarfare simulants); if released or if they failed by design, could contribute to human epidemics. Mycoplasmas are also able to be inhaled as an airborne pathogen, so their presence in the applied pesticides might be able to infect animals and humans alike.

When we study the history of vaccines, we learn that vaccine cell lines have been repeatedly found to have been contaminated with "adventitious agents" since the earliest vaccine days. Sometimes when contaminants were found, public health experts made the choice to continue using them. Sometimes the contaminant was intrinsically present in the vaccine formula and could not be removed because it was part of the genetic material from a vaccinated source animal. The contamination of animal and insect cell lines useful for feed supplements (amino acids), antibiotics, animal and human vaccines, and applied biocides* is a problem that is clearly outlined in the text of numerous patents. From the look of things, cell line contaminants appear to be a problem that has already adversely affected generations of people on a global basis. It may also be an ongoing public health threat that should not be dismissed or ignored by anyone.

**Biocides are any microbial controls (biological controls) that may include animal vaccines, or applied pesticides including herbicides, insecticides, rodenticides, fungicides, algicides, acaricides, or similar formulas.*

Testing vaccine formulas in some manner would be critical to do if the military was intent on vaccinating troops against infectious diseases they knew the troops would be exposed to in a war theatre (i.e. foods, water, or environmental). Some might argue that testing agents in a covert manner might be necessary if the military did not want the public to know about biological weapons that had previously been sold to people about to be faced during combat.

A US Senate Banking Committee report was released in May of 1994 which discussed the sale of *Bacillus anthracis* (Anthrax) from the US to Iraqi government agencies from 1985 to 1989. The report was released just five months before the Dearborn conference event. The biological weapons that were sold were not weakened (attenuated) in any way before sale. It was later determined that weapons found by United Nations inspectors, and which were recovered from the Iraqi biological warfare program, were identical to those sold by the US. Former Michigan Senator Donald Riegle was quoted in an article blaming the US in part for the kinds of viruses found in the recovered weapons. Senator Riegle also conducted hearings on Iraq's biological weapons programs and on Gulf War Syndrome (GWS), a mysterious malady that affected military personnel who were deployed in the Gulf. Like Lyme disease, GWS is another illness that some military public health officials or government agencies have failed to properly acknowledge.[5]

In the 1990s, the US Department of Defense proposed an amendment to the US Food and Drug Administration's (FDA) regulations concerning informed consent for military personnel. The DOD was concerned for service personnel who might be exposed to chemical or biological warfare weapons. The agency sought to allow the administration of "new investigational drugs" to troops, whether they consented to them or not. The FDA reportedly granted the amendment and it was upheld by the courts. Investigational drugs are those that have not entirely made it through the FDA approval process; and is no indication of their safety status.[6-8]

The DOD then obtained waivers of informed consent for two new drugs, a botulinum toxin vaccine and pyriodostigmine bromide, which is a cholinesterase inhibitor (neurotransmitter enzyme) thought to be protective against chemical nerve agents including anthrax. If vaccines were experimented with using prison inmates at this time, such experiments could have been for the purpose of testing vaccines for military personnel about to be deployed in the Gulf. It is interesting that GWS patients are found to have mycoplasma strains in their body, and they could have been exposed to anthrax spores. Patients with Lyme disease also turn up with mycoplasma strains in their bodies, and they have also been exposed to the anthrax-related agricultural insecticidal toxins from the fermented soil bacteria *Bacillus thuringiensis*, or "B.t."[6-8]

According to a multitude of registered patent inventions, animal vaccine cell lines are routinely found to be contaminated with viruses or bacteria including mycoplasmas that are common to animals. They are also frequently contaminated with other agents including Newcastle disease, paramyxovirus, salmonella, retroviruses, arboviruses, spiroplasmas, and bacteriae. We incorrectly assume that vaccines and cell lines are 100% "pure." According to one patent:

> "In addition, many cultured cell lines carry endogenous infectious agents including mycoplasmas, low level bacterial contaminants, endogenous viruses, and the like."[9]

Despite the public's dislike of covert experiments, we must take great care not to assume that just because certain agents were designed, patented, or sometimes tested upon human volunteers; that they automatically were responsible for any infectious disease outbreaks anywhere in the world – or were intentionally used for such. It is likely that recombinant mycoplasma strains that were covertly tested represented a means to protect troops from biological agents the US military knew were present in the Gulf. As we can see, the line between what is considered to be a military weapon of warfare and what is deployed peaceably for agricultural purposes may be very thin indeed.

There were a few other weapons of "warfare" that were tested in the US during earlier periods of conflict, about which the public has not been made aware. These tests might have played at least a passive a role in the emergence of human diseases that would erupt decades later. The public discovered the "VX" nerve agent accident of Skull Valley, Utah in 1968 that killed six thousand sheep living near the military's Dugway Proving Ground where chemical and biological warfare tests were undertaken. Several fungal pathogens of plants were also pursued as anti-crop biowarfare weapons by various countries including the US during periods of conflict. The agents included rice blast, rice brown spot disease, soybean rust, late blight of potato, and wheat stem rust – all airborne fungi which destroy agricultural crops. A Fort Detrick scientist was credited with developing a rice blast fungus for use as an early anti-crop biowarfare agent. Rice blast fungus affects agriculturally important cereal crops including but not limited to rice, barley, wheat, and rye.

Using effective agricultural weapons against enemy crops or livestock would quickly decimate food stores and weaken a population. Publications reveal hundreds if not thousands of biowarfare experiments that were conducted on open air ranges at Dugway and other areas of the world. In the US, experiments were performed from 1951 to 1969 using infectious agents that cause anthrax, brucellosis, coccidioidomycosis, encephalomyelitis, echinococcosis (tapeworms), plague, psittacosis, Q fever, Rocky Mountain spotted fever, tularemia, Venezuelan equine encephalitis, and yellow fever. Fort Detrick scientists met in Chicago to discuss the military's progress with aerosolized microbes in 1968. Some of the agents deployed at Dugway during outdoor testing may have made their way into animal populations at the time. However scientists were also deploying nuclear techniques for agricultural purposes at the same time. It is clear that contaminants from nuclear or chemical applications could have substantially contributed to disease epidemics in animal or human populations. Although some biological weapons were developed, the evidence seems to point to another purpose for many biological weapons studies – there was already evidence of an emerging animal infection that would soon become a global public health threat.[10-15]

By the 1950s, the Second World War was over. During the period preceding the Korean and Vietnam Wars and while biological warfare weapons were still permitted, anti-crop weapons were produced. These included the sporulating agents "TX" the agent of wheat stem rust; and "LX" the agent of rice blast. Such agents were produced, dried, and placed into storage at Edgewood Arsenal in Middle River, Maryland; at Rocky Mountain Arsenal in Denver, Colorado; and Beale Air Force Base in California. A military report from Ft. Detrick as translated from a 1959 Bulgarian journal, described American aerial "deployments" during the Korean War. These included the alleged release of paper or metal cylinders; networks/lattices with built-in toxins; bombs of light metal or plastic that could be filled with infected insects (i.e. flies, spiders, beetles, fleas); animals (i.e. mice, rats, oceanic mollusks); and bacterial dusts that were allegedly disseminated from aircraft.[10-14,16-18]

The USSR biowarfare program during the 1970s also reportedly worked on anti-crop weapons including diseases of wheat crops. By 1972 when the US dismantled its anti-crop biowarfare program, nearly a ton of rice blast fungus had been amassed from 1951 to 1969 for potential use on overseas targets. The US military was left to dispose of weapons such as the M115 anti-crop bomb. This was a converted leaflet bomb that could be packed with bird feathers (feather bomb). These were to be tainted with fungal spores of wheat stem rust. About 30,000 kg of wheat stem rust was estimated to have been amassed for US anti-crop stockpiles. We cannot know for certain when biowarfare weapons were ordered destroyed, if anti-crop agents were destroyed. What if some were simply reassigned for "peaceful purposes" including as agents useful against agricultural pests? During the 1950s to 1960s, scientists were experimenting with many agents for agricultural purposes; some of which are strikingly similar to weapons of warfare.[10-14,16-18]

Wheat stem rust, from a family of "cereal" rusts is caused by *Puccinia graminis.* Fields infected with this agent are quickly and entirely decimated. Spores are scattered by winds, and most of the world's wheat crops are threatened by stem rust agents. The emergence of cereal rust stories in the media in recent months may be a preemptive effort to promote public acceptance of genetically modified wheat varieties that are engineered to be rust resistant. This is the current direction of Monsanto Company interests according to the company's web site. Epidemics of stem rust in the US have occurred from 1920 to 1960, including in Minnesota and the Dakotas.[19-25]

Stem rust resistance genes were engineered into commercial cultivars (plants used for breeding) around the world. A similar fungus called "yellow rust" emerged during the 1980s in eastern Africa. This fungus also caused a billion dollars in wheat losses in Asia and the Middle East. A new strain of stem rust emerged in 1999, and was named "Ug99." It first surfaced in Uganda, and then later in Kenya, Ethiopia, and Yemen. The strain is now found across the Middle East. Ug99 is predicted to be far more devastating than the yellow rust strain of the 1980s. We can question whether genetically engineered insecticidal formulas have included rust spores; or whether herbicides or other chemicals have caused mutations in resistance genes to create novel strains that cause new plant or even human infections.[19-25]

A 1964 US military report for a Canadian laboratory describes how wheat stem rust spores were incubated in a phosphate buffer of pelargonic acid-1-C14. Studies centered on the spore's ability to degrade pelargonic acid into acetyl CoA. *Pelargonic acid* is a fatty acid used in plasticizers (plastics), lacquers, and herbicides. Acetyl CoA is produced during cellular respiration, which takes place in the mitochondria (cellular engines). This is an important component to the neurotransmitter acetylcholine in the human body. Another patent uses a combination of insecticides and transgenic* plants to improve insect resistance.[26,27]
**Trasgenic plants are those that have been genetically modified; also called GM plants.*

The invention also uses acetylcholinesterase (AChE) inhibiting enzymes within its formula as an insecticide. If human neurotransmitters are altered by chemical or microbial insecticides, such applications could inadvertently contribute to neurotransmitter-affecting illnesses (i.e. Lyme disease, Multiple Sclerosis, Parkinson's, ALS, or depression) after exposures to same. The source of such exposures would not have to be a vectoring insect, but any exposure significant enough to cause a problem (i.e. foods grown in herbicide treated soils).[26,27]

A military report described stem rust infection and development studies undertaken in the US over a six-year period from 1960 to 1965 using artificially inoculated wheat fields. These inoculations occurred during a period when large-scale efforts to control aphid infestations across North America were underway. Aphids and leafhoppers carry a number of important infections; and one of the most important are the *spiroplasma* spirochetes. The use of chemical herbicides upon bacterially and fungally-infected crops could have contributed to the formation of novel spirochetes which would be detected just a few years later. Insects are fully capable of transmitting stem rust spores between plants; as well as other important viruses and bacteria, including spiroplasmas.[24]

According to a report, the epidemiology of stem rust was studied at Hays, Kansas in fields planted with Cheyenne wheat that was inoculated with wheat stem rust spores. Infections developed during each of the six years of testing. Additional outdoor field tests involving wheat rust spores occurred just three years before the discovery of a novel tick spirochete that would be isolated from rabbit ticks by NIH scientist Dr. Willy Burgdorfer.[24]

Other biowarfare experiments were undertaken in California skies. One of the most well-known involved the aerial release of a "harmless" bacteria. The official explanation was to study how wind currents could transport microbes of biological warfare weapons. The public often assumes this means weapons of warfare against humans or enemy crops. It may also have included weapons of agricultural warfare useful against pest insect populations. Above San Francisco, California in 1950, US naval aircraft performed biological warfare "simulant" experiments by releasing large quantities of the bacteria *Serratia marcescens* under a program named *Operation Sea Spray*. The releases caused many people to succumb to pneumonia or urinary tract infections. At least one person died from the experiments. The victim's family sued for gross negligence, but the outcome of the lawsuit favored the military.[28-30]

The serratia experiments continued for nearly two decades despite problems surrounding the releases. These bacteria are also employed agriculturally to control pest insects. For example, they are most useful against the corn earworm, a common crop pest. Patents describe the microbe's usefulness as an agricultural pesticide, and within virus and bacteria-containing gene expression systems. They also discuss tests designed to evaluate the pesticidal activity of microbes and toxins against select insects. This is certainly an agricultural application for a tool that was tested for "military" use. Let's not forget that biological warfare against pest insects is repeatedly described within patent applications. There is no reason to doubt the patents, which are sworn, truthful testimonials to the invention's objectives and design.[28-35]

Serratia marcescens (a/k/a *Bacillus prodigiosus*) bacteria are saprophytes, or organisms which gather nutrients from the host.

S. marcescens is common in soil. Certain strains are infectious to animals and humans. Several strains are common to insects such as moths, butterflies, bees, wasps, flies, mosquitoes, and ticks. *Serratia marcescens* is also found in silkworms, gypsy moths, and Rocky Mountain wood ticks (*Dermacentor andersoni*).[36,37]

S. marcescens produces two protein cutting enzymes (proteases); and chitinase, an enzyme that degrades fungal cells and insect exoskeletons. These enzymes are known to be toxic to wax moths. Although not typically infectious in the insect gut, if the bacteria migrate to the circulation (hemocoel), they multiply and kill the host in a few days through bacteremia. Co-infections in the insect gut (i.e. *Staphylococcus* species), enhances the infectivity of *S. marcescens*. Therefore agricultural chemicals and microbes in the exposed insect facilitates the reactivation of latent or sleeping infections.[38]

For over a century scientists have been deploying fungi agriculturally. For nearly as long, infectious soil bacteriae from the bacillus family have been used as insecticides. Scientists have employed *Bacillus popilliae, B. lentimorbus, B. sphaericus, B. megaterium, B. uniflagellatus*, and most importantly numerous strains of *Bacillus thuringiensis* (B.t.). This bacterium is closely related to the biowarfare agent *Bacillus anthracis* or Anthrax. What was shocking to me was the discovery of older research evidence which revealed that *Bacillus anthracis* can be fermented for a period of time under certain conditions in a process that will weaken it to create an attenuated form. This appears to describe an agent that is strikingly similar to the global agricultural tool *Bacillus thuringiensis*. Is B.t. an "almost anthrax"? Are the recent public health concerns over "bioterrorism," "anthrax," and the potential for infectious disease outbreaks related to the global use of *Bacillus thuringiensis* (B.t.) upon and within food crops? Or is there a problem with the applied insecticides which contain B.t., about which we have not (yet) been told?[28,39,40]

Bacillus thuringiensis can be distinguished from the related soil bacteria *Bacillus cereus* and from *Bacillus anthracis* by its toxic activity upon insects, and by the production of an intracellular parasporal crystal that is associated with spore formation. The bacterial spores and the protein crystals are what are used in the B.t. insecticides. However it appears that spores which remain in B.t. formulas may be responsible for causing infections in non-targeted species. More recent events have caused the creation of better insecticides which have significantly reduced the number of infective spores present in the formulas; while retaining the important B.t. crystal toxin proteins. However these formulas are not completely free of infective spores, so problems may still remain even in the newer formulas.[41,42]

The public is well aware that some past chemical and biological warfare experimentation has taken place using animal and human subjects. There have been hundreds if not thousands of biowarfare-related experiments deployed in the US and in other countries during periods which preceded the emergence of novel human epidemic diseases. We cannot discount these activities, but neither should we automatically suspect they are entirely responsible for human diseases. One day soon however, they may be proven to have played a larger role in some of the most important infectious diseases than we currently know.

Scientific errors and experiments are usually revealed over time by declassified documents or whistleblowers. Experiments continue to take place for various reasons, with or without the public's knowledge. Past experiments, no matter how questionably ethical, are sometimes inappropriately linked to emerging human epidemics without hard evidence that anything other than simple experimentation was ever achieved. The public must be careful not to assume conclusions based upon what is often only circumstantial evidence (i.e. patents, papers discussing experiments, human outbreaks, or reports of same). There may be experiments which continue in the present day, without the public's knowledge. However in this information age, it is probably a lot tougher to keep covert activities secret when undertaken.[43]

The "Secret" History of Lyme Disease

Fertilizers

The history of fertilizers began centuries ago with the use of potash (pot ash). To make potash, the ancients leached wood or plant ashes in iron or clay pots using water. When the water evaporated, it left a white residue of potassium carbonate. Potash contains organic materials such as plant remains because of its organic content. Potash in its crudest form was impure but useful for ceramics, glass, soap, textiles, and fertilizers. Potash would also be mixed with urine, blood, manure, and tinder to create saltpeter, a source of gunpowder. One of the most ancient potash sources is the Dead Sea. Today the term potash refers in general to mined and manufactured mineral salts which contain a highly soluble form of potassium.[1-10]

The very first US patent invention was signed by newly elected President George Washington in 1790, for a method to improve potash* and pearl ash for fertilizer. The patent was owned by Philadelphia resident Samuel Hopkins. The fertilizer industry is the largest global user of potassium; which is typically derived from caustic potash by electrolysis.[11]

**Potash is essentially Lye. It can be made from vegetable or mineral sources. Over time potash improved to mined formulas, which can be mixtures of potassium carbonate or potassium hydroxide. Today it is comprised of potassium chloride or other mined potassium salts. In 1861 the potassium fertilizer industry began using improved potash from mined sources in its commercial fertilizers.*

In 1769, Swedish Scientist J.G. Gahn discovered that human and animal bones were chiefly comprised of calcium phosphate, and that bone and bone meal was a useful fertilizer. Before about 1840, the principal commercial fertilizer around the world was bone dust, for its high phosphate of lime content. It was typically collected from human bones found at battlefields, or from discarded animal bones. However large quantities were necessary for widespread applications, making the use of bones impractical. In 1821, French Chemist P. Berthier discovered a store of aggregate rock near Les Baux, France that was named *Bauxite* (French for "beams"). This is a highly important sedimentary rock that is composed of minerals such as aluminum ores and iron oxides. Bauxite is commonly found in soils that also contain clays, silt, and silica. Bauxite is an aggregate from which alum is extracted to produce aluminum.* We should note that where bauxite is found, phosphates are retained at higher levels in the soil and water. Bauxite is also found in the presence of the radioactive rare earth elements uranium, thorium, and the metal zirconium (zirconium orthosilicate). Cryolite, which is sodium aluminum fluoride, can be found in bauxite groundwater.[1-16]

**Bauxite is highly valuable to the aluminum industry which began after 1854 when French scientist Henri Étienne Sainte-Claire developed a process to commercially produce aluminum from bauxite. Bauxite is used in many industries, including agriculture, wastewater treatment, brick making, and cement. The world's largest bauxite producer is Australia, an important location for many reasons we'll study soon.*

ALCOA, the Aluminum Company of America funded a University of Illinois-Urbana study in 1939 that showed that the fluorine content in cryolite was not appreciably different in toxicity than that found in calcium fluoride; both of which are found on foods and in drinking water as pesticide residues or water additives.[145]

It would not be until about 1831 that H.W. Köhler would suggest processing bones with sulfuric acid to create phosphate fertilizer for agricultural use. However helpful these findings were, they were still impractical for anything other than regional use due to the perpetual lack of source materials. Scientists of the day believed that phosphorus had to come from bone to be an effective plant fertilizer.[12,14]

In 1840 German Chemist Justus Von Liebig, the "Father of the fertilizer industry" discovered that when the lime in bone meal was treated with sulfuric acid, plants could more readily take up phosphorus from the lime. The continual shortage of available bone material for fertilizers led to the importation of bat guano (excrement) from Peru beginning in 1840. Bat guano is roughly 10% nitrogen, 3% phosphorus, and 1% potassium (10-3-1); which like other animal manures, is a good general fertilizer. In 1841, low-grade mineral phosphate rock in the form of fluorapatite was discovered in England and in France. The same mines that produce bauxite also produce raw rock phosphates including alumina, fluoride-containing rocks, limestone, and mudstone, other common phosphate-bearing rocks. Fluorapatite is also called phosphate rock or rock phosphate.[7,8,15-17]

In 1842, English agricultural scientist Sir John Bennett Lawes discovered that phosphate rock reacted to sulfuric acid in the same manner as bone meal. In 1842 Lawes developed a process whereby phosphorus could be extracted from coprolites. This extraction process created the early superphosphate fertilizers. Coprolites are fossilized animal or dinosaur feces, and are comprised chiefly of calcium phosphate and organic matter. Coprolites were not only used for fertilizer, they were also used to make ammunition and explosives beginning with the First World War. Lawes' superphosphates were manufactured in Harpenden in Hertfordshire, England at the Rothamsted Experimental Station which he established on his estate. This marked the origin of the chemical fertilizer industry. The first industrial plant for commercial superphosphate fertilizers was built in Liverpool, England in 1846. In 1854, an experiment station in Mockern near Leipzig, Germany was also established to explore the world of fertilizers. Following that successful venture, many such stations opened in the German countryside over the next several decades.[1-5,13]

In the US, bauxite was also discovered in 1842 at Fourche Cove, near Little Rock, Arkansas, but the Arkansas find was not considered valuable until a similar cache was discovered in Rome, Georgia years later. Large stores of rock phosphate rich in carbonate of lime were discovered in 1843 in South Carolina. By 1865, both North and South Carolina's phosphate rock deposits gave birth to the American phosphate mining industry. South Carolina mining began in 1860, and the first official phosphate mine owned by the Charleston Mining and Manufacturing Company was organized in 1867. Just three years later thirteen companies were mining phosphates and manufacturing fertilizers in the state. Phosphate rock became the first American "gold rush." South Carolina's phosphate rock stores are among the largest and are considered potentially inexhaustible.[1-5,13,16-20]

In Florida in 1881, huge stores of phosphate rock were also discovered, however Florida's cache would not become a contender in the phosphate industry until the 20th century. By 1887, the full potential of Arkansas's bauxite* stores would finally be recognized. A commission was established to protect South Carolina's phosphate stores, according to the January 29, 1891 edition of *The New York Times.* The State Treasury was already earning royalties from phosphate miners on a per-ton basis, and undoubtedly desired to protect this income. By 1889 South Carolina supplied roughly 90% of the world's phosphate fertilizers.[1-5,13-20]

**Radioactive rare earth elements uranium and thorium are found near bauxite/phosphate deposits.*

In 1889, American Chemist Charles Martin Hall patented a method of producing aluminum for commercial use, which allowed it to be processed from mined bauxite. In 1888 with Alfred E. Hunt, a wealthy financier named Charles Martin Hall founded the Pittsburgh Reduction Company; now known as the Aluminum Company of America (ALCOA).[15]

While the earliest fertilizer products were useful on a small scale, the sedimentary phosphate rocks did not have a high phosphate value (about 0.2%). Scientists found they could produce "artificial" superphosphate fertilizers, and not just from dinosaur poop. The superphosphates, a mixture of gypsum and mono-calcium, were being produced in England by 1843. When processed, they contain roughly 20% phosphorus. This period began the use of mined and processed phosphates for fertilizer instead of bone. The superphosphates were also far more soluble than first generation phosphate fertilizers, and their higher phosphorus content allowed plants easier access to nutrients. The countries with the greatest phosphate fertilizer use at this time in alphabetical order were England, France, Germany, and the US.[1-5,12,16,17]

In 1865, two decades after the introduction of the synthetic (mineral) superphosphates, and only five years after South Carolina phosphate mines were tapped; silkworms in the heart of Lyon, France became infected with a mysterious illness that threatened the French silk industry. The mysterious silkworm malady was named caterpillar wilt disease, although a causative agent was not isolated until five years later. Was the new silkworm disease triggered by viruses or bacteria in the bat-guano* fertilizers or the application of superphosphates of lime and the action of same upon the microbes found within the silkworm larvae? The combination of phosphates and insect symbionts† certainly could have led to the outbreak of caterpillar wilt disease. After all, DNA and RNA are composed of the same materials (phosphate, sugar) that were used to fertilize mulberry trees, the silkworm's food. The new phosphates of lime were also being used during the process of raising silkworm larvae.[1-5,12,16,17]

**Infectious diseases found in the bellies of bats (i.e. rabies) are significant to the story, since rabies and related viruses infect insects, the primary diet of bats. Centuries later Swedish American Scientist Dr. Willy Burgdorfer who studied rickettsias and Q fever in Sweden; and other scientists at Rocky Mountain Laboratories in Hamilton, Montana would study rabies virus in western Montana bats (1954), and in ticks (1957).*
†Insect symbionts are infections of any kind which live in the body of an insect; either in harmony or as parasites.

By 1855, superphosphate fertilizers were being produced in Germany, which also had a silk industry. Five years later Sweden's first fertilizer production plant was built in Klippa. (Scandinavian countries were some of the most ancient peoples to use potash and copper to form weapons.) In Germany in 1860, potassium salt deposits were opened. Due to the surge in phosphate fertilizer use, European cereal crops significantly increased in production from 1840 to 1880. By 1865, the year French silkworms became ill, the superphosphate fertilizer industry was a booming industry. The triple superphosphates came to the German market in 1870; and were commercialized in 1890. These were made by treating phosphate rock or limestone with phosphoric acid. The result was a purer, more soluble product with a phosphorus content above 40%.* In the 20th century until the mid-1940s, the superphosphates and triple superphosphates were used as fertilizers. The triple superphosphate nutrient content was approximately 0-46-0. In the US, the use of triple superphosphates was promoted by the Tennessee Valley Authority (TVA) and by land grant universities; which changed the face of modern agriculture in the states.[21]

**The N-P-K (nitrogen, phosphorus, potassium) content of superphosphates is expressed as 0-20-0, and triple superphosphates as 0-46-0.*

Because of its richer content, less could be used and therefore newer fertilizers were more costly. The downside of all fertilizers is that they leach micronutrients from soils; they wash into watersheds, and contribute to eutrophication (pollution) and algae growth. Another problem with the superphosphates is that phosphates bind with soil minerals including lead and calcium. They also bind important plant nutrients such as zinc, iron, and manganese, so these must be supplemented in soils during fertilization. A lack of soil nutrients contributes to the "yellows" diseases of plants.

More importantly, a nutrient imbalance encourages the growth and proliferation of plant bacteriae, including the *Spiroplasmas*. These plant spirochetes will become a critical part of the history of Lyme disease in upcoming chapters. For now we can see the role that fertilizers play in altering the mineral balance of soils, and in fostering environments favorable to plant viruses and bacteria. Today most rock phosphate is made into phosphoric acid and is used in processed phosphate fertilizers. Phosphoric acid, or phosphate rock are used as animal feed supplements after the rock's fluoride content is reduced (defluorinated). Phosphoric acid is also used in soft drinks for human consumption (i.e. colas) and as a dental etch solution.[22-24]

Agostino Bassi was an Italian bacteriologist after whom a fungal pathogen of silkworms was named (*Beauveria bassiana*) when he discovered it in 1835. Bassi would be called the "Father of insect pathology" and would join Louis Pasteur at the Pasteur Institute in Paris, France. Throughout the early 1840s, fertilizers were already highly popular throughout Europe, and of course so was the manufacturing of chemical dyes for various industries including silk textiles. The sudden 1865 emergence of caterpillar wilt disease was a serious problem, and silk industries suffered severe losses. Louis Pasteur was called on the scene to investigate the origins of the silkworm infections, and to finally solve the problem for French silk producers, which he did by 1870.[25-33]

During his investigations he discovered a contagious disease which was named *Pebrine*. The causative agents of this are the microsporidian parasites *Nosema bombycis, Variomorpha, Pleistophora*, and *Thelohania.** We will become familiar with these parasites in the modern day for they would be deliberately added to applied insecticides during the 20th and 21st centuries.

We might want to think about how intracellular infections that were normally latent (dormant) in silkworms were suddenly a problem. Was it something in the silkworm diet or in the water or soil in the form of a chemical or microbial "pollutant"?

**In 1996, two cases of central nervous system infection were noted in HIV-positive individuals. The organisms cultured from the patients were from the Thelohania family of microsporidiae. Microsporidiae are spore-formers that produce granules and which cause systemic infections. How did a silkworm microsporidia find its way into the human population – one suffering from an immune system-destroying "virus," and in a patient population that commonly has fungal infections?*

Another illness that occurs in silkworms is called *Flacherie*. This infection causes silkworms to die during heat spells. The flacherie virus is a member of the *Reovirus* family, a family that will be extremely important in future centuries. It is also called a CPV, *Cytoplasmic polyhedrosis virus*, or *Cypovirus*. Louis Pasteur would discover that there were several viruses responsible for the fatal flacherie, another is caused by a *Densonucleosis* virus. These infections are contracted when silkworm larvae eat virus-contaminated leaves of the mulberry tree; causing a lethal diarrhea. The flacherie viruses belong to three families:[25-33]

The *Bombyx mori infectious flacherie virus* (BmIFV) is from the *Dicistrovirus* family.
The *Bombyx mori densovirus* (BmDNV) is from the *Parvovirus* family.
The *Bombyx mori cypovirus 1* (BmCPV-1) is a member of the *Reovirus* family.

"Reovirus" stands for respiratory enteric (gut) orphan viruses. Reoviruses, which are CPVs, are associated with mined materials including bauxite, radioactive elements, and phosphate rock that is mined for fertilizers. However they are also found within insect populations including those that are important to Lyme history. Bacteriae can also contribute to the infectious flacherie process, including *Streptococcus, Staphylococcus,* and *Serratia marcescens*, another so-called "harmless" bacterium that we recently discussed. It will be the application of the CPV reoviruses and baculoviruses as insecticidal helpers that will be the underlying force which drives particularly virulent bacterial and fungal infections in the modern era.[25-33]

Silk in America

The story of the silk industry and the silkworm in America begins during the 1620s in the colony of Virginia. Settlers arrived with the intent of growing silkworms to supply English factories with raw silk. However they found tobacco easier to grow and far less labor intensive. Attempts to grow silk were again encouraged during the 1730s in Savannah, Georgia and in South Carolina, but silk growers struggled in both locations. By 1732 we find the white mulberry tree, a main food source of silkworms making its introduction into Georgia and Connecticut. In Georgia, settlers were granted land if they agreed to plant a large number of white mulberry trees on each land plot granted. A significant number of mulberry trees were grown on Long Island (NY), and nearby Brooklyn and New York cities, since the silk industry had a presence in these areas.[34,35,36]

In 1734 the Connecticut Assembly passed an Act to encourage interest in a budding silk raising industry. A Dr. N. Aspinwall imported silkworm eggs and mulberry trees into New Haven and Mansfield, Connecticut in 1762. Aspinwall met fellow silk enthusiast Dr. Ezra Stiles (later President of Yale University), who kept a diary from 1759 to 1790 of his work in silk culturing. In 1763 the two were able to obtain an Act from the legislature of the colony, offering a ten shilling bounty for every hundred trees planted and kept healthy for three years; as well as a stipend of three pence per ounce for all raw silk raised and produced in Connecticut. Dr. Stiles raised many silkworms and produced a good quality silk which he would weave into silk cloth for his official robes.[34-37]

By 1766 Georgia's silk was exported to England, and its quality was nearly as good as Italian silk. Largely due to Stiles and Aspinwall's work, this same year half an ounce of mulberry seeds were sent to every Connecticut parish to encourage the planting of mulberry trees. The state offered a bounty to plant trees, and to silk growers. As a result, silk processing grew throughout the state of Connecticut. Years later Stiles' diary could be seen in the Yale college library, with a cord made from his own silk tied around it. In 1749 an Act of Parliament declared that Georgia and South Carolina were silk colonies. A public "trustees' garden" was established with vines, mulberry trees, and a filature (for reeling silk).[34-37]

Dr. Aspinwall also introduced silk into Pennsylvania around 1768. Silk production flourished in the east for a time. In 1770 while in London, Benjamin Franklin wrote to the American Philosophical Society of Philadelphia to start a "public filature" which opened in June of the year. Unfortunately with the arrival of the Revolutionary War, the silk industry nearly collapsed due to lack of demand and because the colonists had to suspend silk production to literally feed an army. Some silk manufacturing continued, but silk quality was not as good as in earlier decades. By 1800 it was difficult to sell American silks abroad. Eventually silk growing revived as a cottage industry in Connecticut.[34-37]

Along with the importation of silkworms and the development of the silk (and cotton) textile industries in America, we find a parallel outbreak of infectious diseases. In Charleston, South Carolina and Philadelphia, Pennsylvania in 1699 there was an outbreak of yellow fever that killed many citizens. In 1721 there was an outbreak of smallpox in Boston. We can see how ports of entry into the US would be the most vulnerable to diseases that make their way into the country on foreign ships. By 1730, smallpox had taken yet more lives in Boston, New York, and Philadelphia.[38,39]

In 1732 there was another yellow fever outbreak in New York and in Charleston. Outbreaks of smallpox, plague, and German measles struck over the next few decades. We may imagine this was contributed to by improper manufacturing waste disposal techniques and poor personal hygiene. In 1747 a yellow fever outbreak was avoided by the off shore quarantine of a ship from Barbados (West Indies) when it was reported that sailors on board fell ill with the disease. However it would be another fifty years before the connection between yellow fever outbreaks on the mainland and seafaring vessels transporting diseases would be made.[38,39]

In the late 1760s, silk was arriving in Philadelphia, Pennsylvania. By 1771, the silk industry was well established in nearby Paterson, New Jersey ("silk city"). But again in 1793, roughly eleven thousand Philadelphia residents were killed by an outbreak of yellow fever. Even George Washington fled the city to escape the disease. The presence of water pollution (which was culturally accepted) was blamed on the outbreak. The connection to the silk industry and its diseased insects, and the effects of same upon mosquitoes and the viruses found within their bodies was not historically made. Paterson, New Jersey, besides being "silk city," was also home to Lyons Piece Dye Works, a manufacturer and dye operation which ran from 1898 until 1973. The firm's President was Dr. Ernest Cadgene, a chemist and inventor from Lyons, France who studied dyes and the silk industry in Zurich, Switzerland before coming to the US. We might note the Swiss reference here because it was a leading country for silk and dye manufacturing in Europe at the time.[25,34,38,134]

By 1810 the first silk manufacturing mill was built in Mansfield, Connecticut. Another was also opened in Philadelphia in 1815. Before this time, all silk processing and weaving had been done by hand. With the importation of new varieties of mulberry trees, came expansion for the silk industry in the northeast. Trees were introduced from China into the Philippines, then France, and finally to the US at Baltimore in 1826 where the first of a new mulberry variety was planted.[34-36,38]

The new species was the Chinese white mulberry (*Moris multicaulis*), and when compared to the black or Italian white mulberry, had a more vigorous growth and larger leaves. A large shipment of 70,000 trees was imported from Marseilles, France in 1836, although only about 15,000 survived the journey to be planted. When the new mulberry leaves were fed to the silkworms, their silk production increased. This caused a huge demand for Chinese mulberry trees in the states. Many were sold from the first nursery in South Manchester, Connecticut. The nursery was owned by the Cheney brothers, who also opened one of the first successful silk mills in South Manchester, Connecticut (Mt. Nebo Silk Mills).[34-36]

The Cheney brothers would soon expand into nearby Monmouth, New Jersey. State governments in Maine, Massachusetts, New Jersey, and Pennsylvania offered bounties similar to Connecticut's in an effort to expand silk manufacturing throughout the American northeast. In 1830 Congress proposed the establishment of a filature school in Philadelphia under a "Silk Bill." In 1831 the Massachusetts legislature provided a manual for silk culture, and most states offered bounties on trees, cocoons, and reeled silk.[34-38]

Unfortunately the new Chinese mulberry trees were not very hardy during northern winters. By 1839 most of the mulberry trees were struggling, and in 1844 a fatal blight affected nearly all mulberry trees in many parts of the east coast. By 1865 many silk manufacturers were failing although silk in Paterson, New Jersey survived. The US federal government attempted to help with the floundering silk trades by providing mulberry trees and silk worm eggs, but their assistance was insufficient to help boost manufacturing to any great extent. The early silk industry was present but hardly profitable in Scranton, Pennsylvania when the Scranton Silk Company was established in 1872. The company failed in a few years and was sold to the Sauquoit Silk Company in 1879 which eventually became the third largest silk producer.[34,35,36,38,40,41]

The owner of the Scranton Silk Company was John E. Atwood (Willimantic, CT); who associated with Charles Du Pont Breck of the Du Pont family. The Du Ponts attended the University of Delaware and helped financially support the institution over generations.* By 1869 when a French scientist named Trouvelot who lived in Massachusetts imported Asian gypsy moth eggs from a region not far from Lyon, France, it should not surprise us that his imports would be infected by the new caterpillar wilt diseases – diseases caused by bacteria and viruses that more than likely came from deep in the ground where the new phosphate fertilizers and potash made from lime had been recently mined.[41-44]

**By the 1950s the Du Pont family funded the University of Delaware's College of Agriculture's research into cattle and swine diseases.*

Although the silk industry had improved over time in the US, during the mid-1800s the silk manufacturing process was still somewhat crude. Raw silk which arrived at the factory had to be hand washed with saponified soap and olive oil; then wrung out and dried to remove impurities. Those impurities included virus and bacteria-infected silkworm larval bodies. Silks were then dyed using what today are known to be highly mutagenic chemicals, and which likewise became factory wastes. Those wastes entered the sewage systems or were discharged directly into local waterways, along with any spores and infectious agents that remained in the silkworm carcasses and silk remnants.

The saponified soaps were made using lye and animal fats or vegetable oils; creating alkali detergents called surfactants. Surfactants can be natural biosurfactants (animal or vegetable derived) or synthetic (petroleum based "petrochemicals" [i.e. coal tar]). Surfactants look like little round balls with tails. The ball is hydrophilic, meaning it is attracted to water molecules. Its tail is hydrophobic, meaning it will repel water molecules. On contact with water, the surfactants stick to the dirt and grime in the silk, remove it, and keep it from resettling on the fabric's surface.

Surfactants also lower the surface tension between substances including water. In still waters where mosquitoes normally lay their eggs, the surface tension of the water by surfactants will force the mosquito eggs to fall below the surface, where when they hatch, the larvae drown either from being unable to return to the surface, or from the surfactants or other chemicals that enter their respiratory system. There may also be an ability of enzymes, essential oils, and chemicals to permeate mosquitoes and other insects through their salivary glands, in the presence of surfactants. We will learn more about surfactants in an upcoming chapter.[30,31,42-65]

By the 1870s, French silk cloth made in Lyon had been imported into the US for many years; so much so that French silk goods ranked first in US silk cloth purchases. In 1898, the Duplan Silk Company was founded in Hazelton, Pennsylvania by Leopold Duplan of Lyon. In 1898, the Lyon firm J.B. Martin established a French subsidiary in Norwich, Connecticut, and in 1909 the firm formed the J.B. Martin Company in Portland, Maine, which purchased the Connecticut company. Another Lyon company, this time a silk dye firm, established a US subsidiary in Lodi, New Jersey, called the United Piece Dye Works.[66-68]

Incidentally, Russian and German silk manufacturers also had subsidiaries across Europe. The annual report from the Silk Association of American described Swiss investor Robert Schwarzenbach (Zurich) as the largest silk manufacturer in the world. His company had plants in Italy, France, Germany, Switzerland, and the US. Schwarzenbach was registered in New York but the silk factories were located in Hoboken, New Jersey. Later aniline dye companies would make New Jersey their home including the Calco Bound Brook site established in 1915 which was acquired by the American Cyanamid company. The chemicals used by dye companies which become environmental wastes may have played an integral role in human disease outbreaks.[66-68]

Because the infections from silkworms include soil-borne bacteria from a family of *Extremophiles,* (bacteriae that live deep underground in extreme conditions), the spores and viruses from the diseased silkworms easily remained infectious even in polluted water and soil sediments for more than a century. Some of the extremophile bacteria are the blue-green algae called *cyanobacteria* (blue-green algae). Others include those that are sulfur reducers, the *sulfobacteriae*. All that may be needed to "reawaken" sleeping bacterial spores is some kind of a catalyst, be it chemical, nuclear, fungal, or viral. The polluted waters of the mid-20th century would contain each of these important catalysts. In my book *God Science*, I discuss early disease epidemics and my belief that mutagenic chemicals used in dying textiles of military clothing (i.e. silk, wool, and asbestos fibers) were contributing factors to epidemics of *Encephalitis lethargica*, a polio-like illness beginning in 1915 in French, Romanian, US, English, and Russian soldiers. Similar factors may have contributed to the epidemics of Spanish Influenza beginning in the Spring of 1918 in the US at Ft. Riley, Manhattan, Kansas; and later in Spain (which also had a silk industry).[30,31,42-63]

French Silk, Dyes, and Human Disease

The silk industry in Lyon, France is but one critical element in the story of the early European ECM rash illnesses which emerged in the mid-to-late 19th century. We must also look at how silkworms were raised to find some of the hidden factors that could have helped this process along. Remember that in 1865 silkworms suddenly began to get sick. Silkworms come from Asia, and their main food, mulberry trees are also of Asian origin. The best trees for silkworm growth came from China since the Chinese mulberry trees provided larger, leafier canopies. China was also the leading silk producer in the world at this time, followed by Italy, India, and France.[69]

Silk-raising is an ancient industry, and by the 1860s Chinese silk and mulberry trees were grown in the Chinese Far East. This area is also home to geothermal veins. This is likely where French silkworms and mulberry tree imports, as well as those shipped to the US east coast originated. In the early centuries, mulberry trees were fertilized with animal manure. In the mid-1800s farmers began using sprayable liquid manures and insecticides made from dead, ground insect larvae.

More importantly however is the use of potash and lime (phosphates of lime) in the cultivation of silkworm larvae, moths, and their eggs. It is these basic ingredients potash (lye/alkylating agent), lime (phosphates), fungi (insecticides), and silkworm infections that would become the model for the early human ECM rash illnesses of the late 19th century. These came forward by way of sheep ticks which were exposed to agriculturally important soil bacteriae from the *bacillus* family; and to the earliest agricultural fertilizers and insecticides.[69]

In 1844, Englishman John Mercer discovered that caustic soda (lye) improved cotton and other textiles, including silk and silk threads. This process was called "mercerization" but it did not catch on until 1890. Potash however is essentially lye, and it is used extensively during the silkworm raising process. It was also used in the saponified soaps that were part of the silk cleaning and manufacturing processes. By 1860, highly toxic chemical dyes were already being used in the European and American silk industries. These included Prussian blue (a mixture of potash and copper iron salts), Quercitron (inner bark of oak trees); Picric acid* (an explosive, nitrated compound like TNT); Aniline† (from bleached coal tar); Indigo†† ("woad," a mustard plant); and noir de Lyon, a black dye derived from chestnut‡ wood. The industry also used chlorinated water for textile bleaching, as well as hydrogen peroxide, sodium peroxide, and sodium perborate.** Chlorinated compounds have since been shown to be mutagenic.[70,71]

**Picric acid was made by nitrating silk, indigo, and resins until 1841, when it was synthesized using phenol (coal tar). It was used in explosives since 1830, and by the 1890s for artillery shells. Picric acid was the primary high explosive for military use, and is a common contaminant near weapons manufacturers and test ranges.*

†Aniline was discovered in 1834 by German Chemist Runge during a search for the mosquito-borne infection, Malaria. Another source places its discovery in 1826 during the dry distillation of indigo. Aniline dyes can contain nitrobenzene, chromate, and other highly mutagenic chemicals.

††Woad is a plant used for indigo dyes until the late 1800s. It belongs to the Brassicaceae or mustard family where we find spiroplasma spirochetes. These plants were also used to create chemical mustard nerve agents (i.e. mustard gas).

‡Chestnut trees are parasitized by sawflies (and their CPV viruses) and are found in North America, Asia, Japan, and other countries.

***Sodium hydroxide, hydrogen peroxide, and disodium tetraborate pentahydrate combined make sodium perborate. When this comes into contact with water it undergoes hydrolysis, creating hydrogen peroxide and borate (boric acid). Boric acid is used in insecticides, in the lab, in nuclear pressurized water reactors, in electroplating, and pyrotechnics. Alkalis used in the chemical industry such as lime, potassium hydroxide (hydrated potash), potash fertilizers, and sodium hydroxide are in short, lye. When strong alkalis are mixed with animal fats or vegetable oils, saponification occurs. This process is used in soapmaking, and in the early silkmaking process, which used saponified soap to clean silk. Saponification, or fat necrosis, occurs during pancreatic disease (i.e. diabetes, pancreatitis, pancreatic cancers). Things known to damage the pancreas include viruses, microscopic worms, vasculitis, and scorpion toxins; all tools used in the modern insecticides.*

If there was a chemical culprit that could cause the sudden emergence of wilt disease in the French silkworm population, then it may have been the 1841-1845 development of the first synthetic chemical dyes made from coal-tar derivatives (phenol), especially *picric acid.* The manufacturer responsible for its development was the Lyon France firm, Guinon Marnas et Bonnet, which introduced picric acid commercially in 1845. By the 1850s, picric acid was the main yellow dye that was used in the French silk industry. It was followed by aniline purple, and "mauve"; created in 1857 by British chemist William Perkin. There appears to be a link between "yellows" diseases of plants, animals devoid of certain minerals, and the mined ores including coal, (used for coal tar) to make picric acid. A resource suggests that pure coal is devoid of the carbonate of lime, and calcium and magnesium salts. We know that plants with yellows diseases are unable to take up magnesium and certain other nutrients from the soil.[72-75]

Picric acid is an important aspect of our story, because of its wide use in many industries, and because it is highly unstable and explosive in its many forms. It is also called Melinite, Lyddite, or Schimose; and its chemical name is 2,4,6-trinitrophenol. Explosives containing picric acid were used in the Boer War and the First World War, then were largely replaced by TNT and other explosives. (This is interesting since Spanish Influenza began right after the First World War.)

When picric acid bonds with metals, it creates metal picrates, which can be more unstable than the first form. It can also degrade into dinitrophenol. Picric acid was first discovered around 1742, and was made by nitrating natural substances including resins, animal horns, or silk. French chemist Eugène Turpin patented a process using picric acid in artillery shells and blasting charges. Lyddite was composed of molten and cast picric acid, and was manufactured in southern England (Lydd, Kent) where it was also first tested in 1888. In 1889 the Japanese improved the formula and named their version schimose.[75,76]

Picric acid is also used in the laboratory for staining and other reagents. Oddly enough a picric acid-alum spray was used intranasally on monkeys and humans during a 1936 Alabama poliomyelitis outbreak as a preventative treatment, probably to bind the virus. However it was eventually discovered that picric acid is highly toxic to the human body. This makes me wonder whether picric acid was ever used within polio vaccine formulas. Even if it was not, the exposure to this chemical at a future date in people that have been vaccinated with live or attenuated vaccines might lead to instability of genetically engineered vaccine components which remain sequestered in our gut bacteria, or are incorporated into the human genome (DNA).[76,77]

In Europe in 1875, five years after the triple superphosphate fertilizers arrived on the scene in 1870, an odd human illness emerged and was described in *German Medical Weekly* (Deutsche Medizinische Wochenschrift). In 1883 a case of a "Lyme"-like infection would be reported by German physician Alfred Buchwald, who described it as a degenerative skin infection. It is now known as *Acrodermatitis chronicum atrophicans* (ACA). The earliest human cases of a rash-causing illness in Europe were associated with a bite from the sheep tick (*Ixodes ricinus*). The environment where the ticks were contacting the new fertilizers and applied insecticides might have had something to do with the emergence of a new tick-transmissible human pathogen.[78,79]

Next we examine a case report from a 1922 medical journal in Lyon, France. Although other countries were also silk producers, Lyon is our model location of study as it was the hub of the silk processing industry in the mid-1800s. It was also where textile manufacturers used caustic chemicals including mutagenic phenol and aniline dyes. It was also a country where decades later a male resident was bitten by a tick. Shortly thereafter the patient became ill with tick paralysis. The man had removed a tick from his left buttock, which he recognized as a kind commonly found on his dogs and sheep. Today the infection is known as tickborne meningopolyneuritis. It typically causes intense radicular (nerve root) pain. There is also peripheral nervous system involvement, and chronic lymphocytic meningitis; symptoms the man experienced. He entered the hospital Hôtel dieu Saint-Bruno in Lyon, France, complaining of leg pains. This infection has been repeatedly misidentified and assigned various names for the same illness including these:[82]

Tick paralysis (Paralysie par les Tiques)
Atypical polyradiculoneuritis with hyperalbuminemia and pleocytosis
Tick-bite meningo-myelo-radiculitis
Polyneuritis multiplex
Neuroradiculo-meningo-encephalomyelitis

Tickborne meningopolyneuritis as it is known today, is a manifestation of *Erythema Chronicum Migrans* disease, which is a tickborne spirochetal infection that can be considered to be the "classic" ECM rash illness of Lyme disease. If we take a look at what French scientists were studying in Paris at the time (another silk producing city), we may find clues to the infectious diseases of today including Lyme. From about 1861 to 1885, scientists Louis Pasteur, De Bary, Kline, Koch, and others were working at the Pasteur Laboratory of the École Normale Supérieure, in Paris. These gentlemen experimented with pathogenic microbes for agricultural use, and the creation of preventative vaccines for animals and humans. In 1877 Robert Koch* was the first to grow *Bacillus anthracis* the anthrax agent, in culture. Anthrax was also the first bacteria to have been identified as a disease-causing agent. Koch demonstrated that anthrax produces spores (endospores). He also performed anthrax experiments by injecting it directly into animals. Louis Pasteur would claim to invent a method of creating anthrax by exposing it to air and potassium dichromate, a hexavalent chromium compound that is highly mutagenic.† The method proved unsuccessful, but was eventually solved albeit a bit differently than what Pasteur had attempted.[80-99]

**Koch is also important because he established "Koch's postulates" which were specific techniques that scientists could follow to validate disease agents using "evidence-based" scientific processes. This becomes important in today's "evidence-based" research techniques and diagnostic guidelines including those which defined the parameters of Lyme disease treatment.*

†Hexavalent chromium is used in nuclear reactors and some chemical plants as (chromium VI or chrome-6). Chromium compounds are found in cement, treated wood, tanned leathers, magnetic tape emulsions (i.e. audio cassettes and video tape), and photography; and in mobile phones and surgical implants. Chromium compounds are carcinogenic and highly mutagenic, and appear at high levels in many municipal water supplies such as Madison, Wisconsin which is home to the University of Wisconsin-Madison and several important industries that have used chromium in their products and/or processes.

In 1877 Koch published a memoir that described anthrax as *splenic fever bacillus*. Pasteur and Kline wrote papers describing their 1881 experimental animal inoculations using a cultured, weakened (attenuated) anthrax strain. They were attempting to create a preventative anthrax vaccine for livestock animals (i.e. sheep, cattle, swine, poultry). As we shall learn, "anthrax-related" bacillus strains would become an important part of livestock and agricultural insecticides in the decades to come. These pesticides would be fermented from soil bacteria. Anthrax would also become a tool of biological warfare for prospective use beginning with WWII by scientists from the US and her allies.[89-91]

The Pasteur Institute opened November 14, 1888. There Louis Pasteur and Italian bacteriologist Agostino Bassi performed experimental insect studies upon honey bees and silkworms. They also experimented with rabies, chicken cholera, and vibrio cholera for animal vaccines. When we think about the manner in which laboratory wastes were discarded into existing sewage systems centuries ago, we will realize that whatever left the experimental laboratory would have made its way downstream into the surrounding countryside. Infectious wastes could have travelled into the Fontainbleu Forest region (southeast of Paris), an area from where the early parasitoid insects would be imported into the US in future centuries.[90,99-108]

Cells, cell lines, animal tissues, and who knows what were contaminated with *Fowl Cholera* (*Pasteurella moltocida*), Newcastle* disease (a *paramyxovirus* or avian flu). In addition, anthrax, the microsporidiae of honey bees (i.e. *Nosema, Theileria, Babesia*), silkworms and their bacteria and viruses, and rabies (related to reovirus and encephalitis viruses), were discarded via laboratory wastewaters. There like many laboratories, infectious agents freely floated through Parisian sewers into nearby rivers to disseminate throughout the region. The Pasteur Institute was located blocks from a tributary of the Seine River. Since anthrax, rabies, and other vaccines were created at scientific laboratories, we may imagine the worst with regard to what was probably merrily floating along French waterways after departing the laboratory.[90,99-109]

**Newcastle disease was first seen in Newcastle upon Tyne, in northeast England in 1926. The region was a major coal mining area; an important center for wool trades; and a large shipbuilding (aluminum, steel) centre. Newcastle disease is a paramyxovirus, also known as Avian parainfluenza virus 1, or "avian flu." We can see connections between mined ores, metals, phenols, viruses from deep underground, and animal diseases.*

The Pasteur Institute was not only a research laboratory, but also a rabies treatment center. During the late 1800s, Russian microbiologist Ilya Ilyich Metchnikov was appointed by Louis Pasteur to a position at an Odessa (Ukraine) laboratory where he also studied rabies. He had worked previously in a private laboratory in Messina where he studied comparative embryology and phagocytosis. (These are phages which infect bacteriae and viruses.) In 1888 Metchnikov came to the Pasteur Institute upon appointment by Louis Pasteur. While there, Metchnikov created an ointment called calomel (mercurous chloride) that was used to prevent Syphilis.[99-108]

It was in 1878 that Metchnikov proposed using the fungus *Metarhizium anisopliae** as an insecticide to control the wheat cockchafer. This beetle pest had caused tremendous economic losses to Russian cereal crops. In the US, scientists were attempting to disburse Agostino Bassi's fungus, *Beauveria bassiana* in regional efforts to control pest insects. In the early days (post 1835), *Beauveria bassiana* was called *Botrytis bassiana.* This very effective fungus would go into mass production in 1888 for use as an agricultural insecticide, although it was tried before that period in regional applications. The fungus is found naturally in infected silkworms, where it is called "the reds," and where it manifests in red blotches and stains the larval skin and silk. It is just one of a number of silkworm diseases capable of manifesting colored pigments in infected insects.[99-108,110,111]

**In modern times, the Metarhizium anisopliae (green muscardine) fungus would be deployed agriculturally on a grand scale in Africa, in a program called Green Muscle®.*

A bacterial "wilt disease" of silkworms would not be scientifically identified until 1902 by Japanese scientist Shigetane Ishiwata, who named it *Bacillus sotto*. The infection would be rediscovered soon however, and would be renamed. The first cases of European patients who were suffering from a new illness were described by Swedish Dermatologist Dr. Arvid Afzelius on October 28, 1909 at a meeting of the Dermatological Society in Stockholm, Sweden. There he described a severe skin rash and an illness following a bite of a sheep tick (*Ixodes ricinus*). These findings came just seven years after the initial discovery of the novel bacterium *Bacillus sotto*, and about a decade after the arrival of the triple superphosphate fertilizers in Europe.[25-31]

Over a decade later *Bacillus sotto* would again be isolated in 1915 in Thuringia, Germany by a German scientist named Ernst Berliner. This time it was found in the bodies of flour moths. Although *Bacillus sotto* and Berliner's agent were the same microbe, it would be renamed after the scientist as *Bacillus thuringiensis* or "B.t.," and the "sotto" name was all but forgotten. *Bacillus thuringiensis* is a sporulating bacteriae that creates crystal endotoxins (Cry toxins). Its spores are similar in toxic action to those of *Bacillus popilliae* the agent of another "wilt"-like agent that causes the "blue" disease of Japanese beetles.[112-116]

To be effective as a pesticide, B.t. crystal toxins must be ingested, where they are released in the insect gut by digestive enzymes. B.t. would become one of the first microbial pesticides to be deployed as a "natural" insecticide to control the European corn borer and the gypsy moth in different parts of Europe; and later in North America. The B.t. strain *Bacillus thuringiensis* variety Berliner, and the fungi *Beauveria bassiana* combined were the most successful combination to be deployed in the early days of agricultural insecticides. The fungus *Metarhizium anisopliae* was also combined with B.t. as an early insecticide. Other bacteria used in the early insecticides were *Bacillus popilliae* and *Bacillus lentimorbus*, the agents of "milky spore" diseases. The milky spore agents are similar to silkworm wilt diseases but they target different insects including gypsy moths and Japanese beetles.[25-31,118-121]

By the 1920s, several papers had reported cases of ECM rash illnesses in European patients. Could the application of superphosphate fertilizers and the new fungal/bacterial insecticides be the cause? The US Department of Agriculture and collaborators around the world have played a central role in the initiation of the microbial insecticides for agricultural use. These biological control programs were firmly established in the US and European countries by 1900.[25-31,117-121]

Additional cases of ECM rash illnesses were reported by Hellerström in 1930, and Gelbjerg-Hansen in 1945 who both described a rash illness in patients with tickborne meningopolyneuritis. "Inflammatory arthritis" (what the 1975 Connecticut outbreak was originally felt to be), was also reported in Europe in 1934 by Stadelmann. Tickborne meningopolyneuritis is considered to be very similar to Lyme neuroborreliosis. However the latter is more severe, it more frequently involves the nervous system, and has a longer course with frequent relapses. During the 1940s on the heels of the initial applications of milky disease spore insecticides in the US, came the first human cases of an arthritis-like illness in New York. According to serological surveys of New York during this period, cases of a spirochetal infection called leptospirosis were also on the rise.[25-31,80-88,117-123]

Those practicing the earliest insecticidal techniques were not based solely in the states. American scientists were learning agricultural techniques from European collaborators. The use of fungi as an insecticide was firmly established in France, Germany, and the US by the late 1800s. Scientists were also performing sporadic field tests with the bacteria *Bacillus thuringiensis* (B.t.) during the first decade of the 20th century. The first widespread applications of B.t. as a microbial insecticide began in Hungary* during the 1920s, and in the former Yugoslavia by the 1930s. European B.t. field tests were extensively undertaken during the 1930s.[25-32,118]

**Hungary borders Romania. Its watersheds will be critical in upcoming decades when a mutated spirochete is pulled from Romanian waters.*

The application of microbial and chemical pesticides and the implementation of superphosphate fertilizers contributed to the over nitrification of the soil and watersheds. This upset the pH of soil and water, and also the populations of microbes in the environment (eutrophication). With the arrival of industrial pollutants (i.e. surfactants, radioactive elements), came a parallel course of ECM rash-like illnesses in areas where agricultural tools were deployed. It may be concluded that the development of novel agricultural tools and concurrent human disease outbreaks was far more than a coincidence in timing.

The early ECM disease cases of 19th century Europe appear to have been different than classic tick paralysis cases reported in Australia by 1915. The difference between tick paralysis and the classic ECM-neurologic/skin disease could possibly be found in Lyon, France, and other areas well known for silk and wool textiles, chemical fertilizers, and (coal tar) aniline dyes. (By the way, Australia and Europe are huge phosphate producers.) When European and American companies sprang up to make fertilizers, chemical based dyes, and explosives, all of which used picric acid,† we can see how the emergence of human diseases could begin in a relatively short period of time in multiple countries under similar influential factors.[124-128]

†Picric acid is also called 2,4,6-trinitrophenol, picronitric acid, carbazotic acid, 2,4,6-trinitro-1-phenol, and 2-hydroxy-1,3,5-trinitrobenzene.

We might reexamine the early investigations into animal viruses that were undertaken by Louis Pasteur and his colleagues at the Pasteur Institute during the late 1800s. In southern and eastern France, rabbits were a common agricultural pest. They were also an important food animal. (In the 1800s in Spain, rabbit carcasses were placed into the wooden casks that were filled with sherry to enrich the alcohol. This practice was discontinued around the turn of the 20th century.) Rabbits are agricultural pests in many countries, including Europe, Australia, and the US. On the American east and west coasts, rabbits were a particular pest of viticulturists, just as they were abroad in French vineyards. The viticultural area in the northeast included Providence Rhode Island, Massachusetts, Connecticut, and New York, including the shorelines of Martha's Vineyard and Chappaquiddick Islands.[135-144]

Louis Pasteur was the first to suggest using the microbes of *Chicken cholera* to control rabbit populations. A French viticulturist was the first to experiment with Pasteur's chicken cholera theory; and allowed him to place these microbes on top of wine cellars as a contact poison to control rabbit populations in 1887. This technique was adopted by the Australian government in Sydney, New South Wales after seeing Pasteur's article about the method in the November 1887 Parisian Journal *Le Temps*. It was felt that a two gallon broth infected with chicken cholera microbes was enough to kill 20,000 rabbits. Liquids were preferred because solid pellets became inactive after about three hours exposure to the sun's ultraviolet rays. Experiments began in Australia in 1888 and continued for at least five years.[135-144]

In rabbits the chicken cholera virus produced a scarlet fever or smallpox-like infection that was rapidly fatal. Australia is of course well known for its *sheep,* and its coal, phosphate mines, and in the day, tobacco, wine, and silk production. By 1895, muscovy ducks and other fowl were suddenly dying in Brisbane. The microbes isolated from the dead fowl proved to be identical to Pasteur's microbes of chicken cholera (also called *septicaemia haemorrhagica*). The presence of this disease in Australia was blamed on the importation of fowl from European countries, not from the early open field experiments where chicken cholera was used to kill rabbits.[135-144]

Extremophile bacteria such as chicken cholera, which is caused by *Pasteurella multocida, an important gammaproteobacteria,* are found deep in the earth, and along with related family members, are exhumed during mining processes. This is vitally important to grasp because chicken cholera and its bacterium not only would infect local insects, but also those that would be imported into other countries including the US. *The chicken cholera microbe was also the basis for the earliest poultry vaccines, and may have contributed to the development of chicken retroviruses that would contaminate poultry stock and vaccine cell lines in future decades.* Birds pluck soil bacteria and insects from the ground, and these microbes are also taken up by grazing animals including ruminants such as cattle and sheep. We can therefore better understand how important microbes make their way into the human food chain through a variety of means, none the least of which is from applied microbial insecticides, animal products, and vectoring insects.[135-144]

Various mulberry tree varieties grow well in Australia, and mulberry fruits contain *anthocyanins* that are used not only as edible fruits, but also to tan leather hides (tannery). We know that anthrax or "wool sorter's disease" is a problem for those who handle sheep hides and process textiles from wool to silk, which of course is produced by silkworms that eat mulberry leaves. Mulberry trees take up bacteria and have beneficial cyanobacteria and nitrogen-fixers in their root systems. It was perhaps Pasteur's familiarity with the leather tanning process (his father was a tanner) that led him to explore chicken cholera and anthrax in the first place, as early as 1870.[43-53]

Natural anthrax outbreaks emerge all over the world. When we study the location of such outbreaks, we typically find them near the explosive residues of mines or weapons, textiles, and ruminant animals. In the fermentation tank that is a sheep's gut, we can see how bacteriae and viruses combine under influence of nitrites to create the "explosive" nitrosamines and an anthrax infection. When a blood meal is taken from an infected animal, bacteriae and viruses will reassort as mixed infections in an insect's gut before being transmitted to an unlucky human.[124-128]

Cutaneous (skin) anthrax has been called "wool sorter's disease." It is unclear whether the infective bacteriae are found on the wool fibers or in the hide (leather), but they are probably influenced by the nitrites, benzenes, surfactants, and other chemicals used during processing. The skin manifestation of anthrax creates ulcerating lesions, and can sometimes be fatal. This seems also to describe the kinds of skin lesions that are found in Morgellon's disease, a Lyme-like illness that produces ulcerative sores. Unlike anthrax however, Morgellon's lesions have additional, colored "fibers" or "hairs" which are found in, or which protrude out of the lesions or hair follicles.[124-128]

We can understand how bacterial spores acquired by animals during grazing might be carried into processing plants where workers could be exposed to them. There infected animal fur or hides are exposed to various mutagenic chemicals during wool/hide processing. Sheep are ruminants whose digestive processes continually ferment. As they graze they are exposed to soil bacteriae including spirochetes, viruses, and plant parasites. They also consume mulberry and other tree leaves that may be infested with virus-harboring silkworm, gypsy, and other moth eggs and larvae as well as specific *cyanobacteria* that are highly tolerant of their environment. In addition, airborne fungal spores and/or insecticides can be consumed during grazing, especially those that are taken up first by plants.[124-128]

Military experimentation with anthrax upon sheep led to the quarantine of tiny Gruinard Island in the Scottish Highlands after 1942 airborne anthrax experiments were undertaken there by British scientists. Anthrax spores can survive for hundreds of years in soils under optimal conditions. It is said that the experiments came about under suspicions that the German army would unleash anthrax upon European populations during WWII. This could have been a legitimate threat, given the extensive German fertilizer industries of the day. This was not the only biowarfare experiment to be undertaken on Scottish or English soils. One reason why the Gruinard Island tests were undertaken may have had to do with the current conflict, to develop a human protective anthrax vaccine.[124-129]

During the late 1800s, important insect and animal diseases were being studied at the Pasteur Institute to create the earliest animal and human vaccines. Laboratory wastes could have played an enormous role in disbursing important pathogens which would have been able to contribute to disease outbreaks under the right conditions, including aniline dyes or other industrial chemicals. The Pasteur Institute lends clues to how an aggregate spirochete could be created. This seems especially true when we observe the pathogens that were studied at the Pasteur Institute were also being studied by Ft. Detrick scientists nearly a century later, but this time as aerosolized infectious agents.

Did tickborne infections from early agricultural and industrial tools create a virulent infection in Europe called ECM disease; and one that would become far more pathogenic in decades to come? Was the early European ECM disease model used by Ft. Detrick scientists during aerobiology experiments of the 1960s? If so, did their studies become necessary after the discovery of novel animal epidemics? Did military scientists already know about an aggregate spirochete that was already detected in Romania and the US, and they were studying it long before the Connecticut outbreak was reported in 1975?

Due to the development and success of the modern chemical insecticides in the 20th century, the early practices of using bacteria and fungi as insecticides were largely discontinued until after WWII. By the 1940s, although occasional microbial insecticides were applied, chemical pesticides in the form of powerful nerve agents* became globally popular; and soared past the early microbial formulas.

**Nerve agents are a class of phosphorus-containing organic chemicals, also known as organophosphates. They interfere with nerve signal transmissions through the blockage of the enzyme acetylcholinesterase, which controls the activity of the neurotransmitter acetylcholine. Nitrogen and sulfur mustard gases are not only toxic; they are carcinogenic and also highly mutagenic. They are classified as "weapons of mass destruction" according to the United Nations Resolution 687. Nerve agents were banned by the Chemical Weapons Convention of 1993, which took effect April 29, 1997. Nitrogen, ammonia, and phosphate fertilizers and agrochemicals may exert similar mutagenic and neurotoxic effects upon soil and water-borne microbes as their weapons-grade chemical relatives, because they are similar to the banned chemical nerve agents developed for war-time use.*

In 1949, Swedish Dermatologist Dr. Sven Hellerstrom presented a paper at the 43rd annual meeting of the Southern Medical Association in Cincinnati, Ohio. The paper was titled *Erythema chronicum migrans Afzelius with meningitis*. He described how as early as 1930 he had successfully treated patients with ECM rashes using penicillin. He reportedly copied a technique that Dr. Carl Lenhoff and assistant Einar Hollstrom had attempted as a treatment for ECM. These individuals were probably the least known, but perhaps most influential people to the history of the ECM rash illness called "Lyme" – an illness that would emerge in multiple countries decades later.[79,123,130-134]

By 1962, a Lyme-like illness was quietly emerging on Great Island, a private estate on the south shore of Cape Cod, Massachusetts. A 1986 article by Rheumatologist Dr. Allen C. Steere and colleagues including Dr. Andrew Spielman (Yale) showed that in retrospect, the first official case of Lyme disease in the US came to a physician's attention in 1962. The case involved an adult woman who had experienced intermittent arthritis in her knee for three years; and hand stiffness and marked fatigue over a period of fifteen years. This puts the onset of her illness anywhere from 1947 to 1962; when agriculturally applied chemical and microbial agents surged forward in the US, especially in the northeast.

In 1969 in Wisconsin, another case of ECM rash disease emerged and was treated by Wisconsin Dermatologist Rudolph Scrimenti. As we can see, Lyme disease appears to have had very different origins than what has been announced to and believed by the world for many decades. While on the one hand these events may seem startling to some people, each aspect of the story fits the historical accounts of ECM and Lyme disease. We will see that it also fits with the story of how a simple, classic ECM disease came to become the complex, multi-system, infectious disease epidemic found around the world today. To fully appreciate the history of the "classic" versus the modern day Lyme disease, we must continue the story. ❑

> *"On the other hand, where human life or essential supplies of food and fibre can be protected only by the use of a particular [biological] control agent, it may be necessary to risk a certain amount of ecological disturbance."*
>
> Ray F. Smith. Considerations on the safety of certain biological agents for arthropod control. Bulletin of the World Health Organization. 1973;48:685-698. Prepared by participants in the Conference on the Safety of Biological Agents for Arthropod Control held at the Centers for Disease Control, Atlanta, Georgia (USA) on April 16-19, 1973.

Two: Weapons of Mass (Pest) Destruction

The global human population has grown exponentially over the past two hundred years. In previous centuries humans had to surmount many obstacles. Physical labor, famine, wars, and pestilences contributed to a vastly shortened human life span. As time advanced, the germ theory of disease arrived, and with this knowledge and the application of modern science and technology physicians became more adept at treating and curing human illness. As a direct consequence of these advances, the mean expiration date on the human species increased, and people began to live decades longer than their ancestors. However this increased the demand for living space, materials, agricultural foods and animals. A significant amount of plants, animals, and their products are required to provide enough food and raw materials for people around the world each day. Producers of crops and livestock for consumption, and wood and other materials for construction, textiles, and other goods continue to face the same problems that societies dealt with for centuries – insects, microorganisms, and disease.

Insect pests such as Japanese and potato beetles, corn borers, cotton bollworms, fall armyworms, tomato hornworms, brown-tail moths, gypsy moths, and many others cause severe destruction of crops, textiles, and stored foods and other products. Accidentally introduced pests also contribute to the defoliation of industry and habitat-supplying forested areas. Plant diseases affect turf, human and animal food crops; and fruits, vegetables, herbs, trees, and ornamentals. Resources such as timber and parks are destroyed by boring and leaf munching insects as they are pushed out of their natural environments into unfamiliar territories when housing and industrial developments arrive. As a result of pest insects, billions of tons (and dollars) of plants are spoiled; and agricultural animals and stored crops are lost each year to insect-borne diseases.

Outside of the known weapons of chemical and biological warfare that have been useful for military purposes, there is extensive evidence that a very different form of chemical and biological warfare has taken place throughout the world, and the intended targets have not been the human population. This kind of biological warfare may be arguably legal under the guidelines of the Geneva Convention since it falls under the category of "peaceful" or "medical purposes."

When the public thinks of the words chemical and biological warfare, the knee-jerk reaction is typically to attach the phrase "against people" to the idea. However until we look at these topics from a more objective perspective, we may never consider that these words and activities carry a very different yet highly significant meaning. This oversight has probably contributed to much of the conjecture about how epidemic diseases have arisen in the world.

There is however, a very real possibility that during the process of pursuing the perfect "bioweapons" useful against insect pests, that human disease epidemics may have accidentally come about. We will be studying a very different kind of biological warfare. That is the *biological warfare against pest insects of medical, veterinary, agricultural, industrial, and military importance.* This "war" has not only been waged in the past, it has been actively pursued for the last century and a half. The microbial pathogens that have been used as weapons of insect warfare are referred to in this book as biological controls, bioagents, insecticides, pesticides, or biocides. Many of these are just as potent, or perhaps more so than weapons that were developed for military use or potential use during periods of conflict.

For a pathogen to be considered a useful biological agent, it must be virulent, specific, culturable, and easily and inexpensively disbursed. Each of these objectives was achieved with the early releases of naturally parasitic insects to control insect pests. Insects that parasitize other insects are called *parasitoids.* Since the early days of biological controls, many insects were considered for their potential as parasitoids. Scientists studied black flies, deer and horse flies, house and stable flies, tsetse and sand flies; cockroaches, lice, spiders, midges, mites, wasps, mosquitoes, ticks, poisonous moths, and fire ants. Many of these insects have been released over decades as biological controls. Later tools included the use of microbes such as fungi, bacteria, viruses, protozoans, microsporidians, and nematodes (microscopic worms) to enhance the applied chemical and biological controls. For many years fungi were deployed as insect controls around the world. Sometimes fungi were provided for no cost or at low cost to area farmers to encourage application onto farm fields.[1,2]

In the US, parasitic wasp releases began in 1882 when exotic species were imported from Ontario, Canada into the US under direction of W. Saunders to control the gooseberry sawfly. The following year exotic wasps were imported by the USDA to control imported cabbageworms. In 1883, parasites of the cabbage butterfly became the first species to be shipped intercontinentally into the US by British-born Entomologist Charles Valentine Riley, the USDA's Chief Entomologist; and G.C. Bignell of England. In 1888 vedalia, coccinellid beetles, and other natural enemies from Australia were imported to control cottony-cushion and black scale insects on southern California citrus (and wine) crops, again with Dr. Riley's help.[3-5]

After the initial parasitoid releases, other insects were sought and used to control agricultural pests. Since then flies, mites, wasps, mosquitoes, and even ticks have been released over decades as biological controls, beginning at the turn of the 20th century. Later, disease-producing organisms such as fungi, bacteria, viruses, microsporidia, and nematodes were also applied in addition to chemical controls. According to a patent invention's text, biological control of harmful insects is described as:

> "the introduction, encouragement, and artificial increase of predacious and parasitic insects, other animals, and disease… the concept of biological warfare against insects has been tested at various times, and many natural enemies and parasites have been introduced in the natural habitats of pest insects." [5,6]

The first international conference for insect pathology and biological control was held in Prague in 1958. There, American scientists met with Russian insect pathologists to learn about insect control techniques that were already being deployed in Russia. These early lessons were shared with western scientists who then implemented similar practices. Whatever problems were encountered with the use of biological controls in the Russian model then, would likely have also been mirrored in the west, at least to some extent.[7]

We may learn about the scientific thinking of the day from a report of a two-day conference on the biological control of insects of medical importance held February 3-4, 1960. The conference was sponsored by the Office of Naval Research, the American Institute of Biological Sciences, the Armed Forces Pest Control Board, and the Army Chemical Corps. The report was date stamped June 28, 1961 Naval Medical Field Research Laboratory, Camp LeJeune, North Carolina. Conference attendees convened at the Armed Forces Institute of Pathology at the Walter Reed Army Medical Center in Washington, DC. Speakers at the event included representatives from the following organizations, in alphabetical order:

American Institute of Biological Sciences*
Armed Forces Pest Control Board
Bioferm Corporation (Wasco, California)**
Canadian Department of Agriculture/Entomology Research Institute for Biological Control (Belleville, Ontario)
Commonwealth Institute of Biological Control (UK)
Department of Zoology at Southern Illinois University (Carbondale, Illinois)
University of California-Berkeley Laboratory of Insect Pathology, Department of Biological Control
University of North Carolina
USDA's Laboratory of Insect Pathology and the Entomology Research Division

**AIBS was part of the National Academy of Sciences but became independent in 1950*
*** Considered the first industrial-based comprehensive biotech firm in the US.*[7,8]

The conference had been scheduled for Spring 1959, but was delayed to follow a joint meeting of the Entomological Society of America and the Entomological Societies of Canada and of Ontario that was held that winter in Detroit. Dr. Steinhaus moderated the conference and had this to say about biological methods of control:

> "…biological control is the action of parasites, predators, or pathogens on a host or prey population which produces a lower general equilibrium position that would prevail in the absence of these agents...the potentialities of biological control, are truly great. That is, 'biological power,' if I may use such a term, is truly as great, in its way, as atomic power is in its way."[7]

The World Health Organization (WHO) began its long-term biological control investigations in 1961 as part of a comprehensive vector biology and control program. For a decade from the mid-1950s forward, there was a substantial jump in the research concerning entomophagous (insect-eating) arthropods; microorganisms as pathogens of arthropods; and the development of autocidal controls (i.e. sterile insect techniques). According to documents, this interest was fueled in part by the development of chemical pesticide resistance within the insect populations.[9,10]

Fungal Feasts for Insect Pests

In 1878, Russian microbiologist Ilya Ilyich Metchnikov proposed the use of a green muscardine fungus called *Metarhizium anisopliae* to control the wheat cockchafer. This is a beetle that had caused tremendous economic loss to Russian cereal crops. The fungus naturally infects about two hundred different insect species including locusts, weevils, gnats, thrips, grasshoppers, leafhoppers, and beetles. It is also listed as a fungus that is useful as a biological control agent against ticks. Presently this fungus has been widely used against grasshoppers and locusts, especially in Africa. We might consider the massive famine and diseases in Africa, and which biological controls, natural viruses, fungi, bacteria, and other parasites are prevalent. We might also think about how each factor interacts in nutritionally compromised populations. If we do we may find interesting connections to some of the most important human disease epidemics of our day.[1,2]

Early attempts at biological controls in the US using chinch bugs infected with the fungus *Beauveria bassiana* were attempted in 1867. This fungus was demonstrated as a parasite to silkworm larvae by Agnostino Bassi of Lodi, Italy in 1835. In 1888, scientist Lugger applied the process to a wider area by distributing infected chinch bugs to Minnesota farmers in an effort to promote regional controls. The same year, University of Kansas scientist Frances H. Snow also introduced *Beauveria bassiana* fungus in a manner similar to Lugger's. After acknowledging Snow's experiments, the Kansas state legislature established an experiment station at the university so *B. bassiana* variety conidia could be mass-produced and provided to regional farmers at no cost. Once produced, about fifty-thousand fungal packets were distributed. Through the program in seven surrounding states, farmers could exchange live, uninfected insects for those that were fungally infected. Then the infected bugs could be released into the field as natural biological controls. In later years, chinch bugs in the Mississippi Valley were manually infected with the fungus *Sporotrichum globuliferum* to be used in a similar manner.[3-7]

Biological controls released in Florida have included the fungus *Beauveria bassiana* to combat citrus crop pests. In the 1890s, the Florida State Experiment Station sold *B. bassiana* fungus packets for seventy-five cents to treat whiteflies, one of several newly emerging pests. Similar attempts to market fungi to California citrus growers were unsuccessful. Sources reveal that entomopathogenic fungi were the main biological agent used throughout the latter part of the nineteenth century and into the twentieth century, until the bacteria *Bacillus thuringiensis* (B.t.) became the commercial leader.[8,9]

Entomopathogenic fungi create what are called aflatoxins. These are extremely potent toxins that are pathogenic to insects, animals, and humans. In 1930 a scientist named Burnside explored the susceptibility of honey bees to the fungus *Aspergillus flavus.* According to a WHO bulletin, in-vivo (in the body) mass production of strains of fungi by 1973 finally became possible. Whatever latent infections that the insects harbored likely contaminated the fungi grown on or in their bodies. In 1958, the WHO sponsored investigations to study a new fungus called *Coelomomyces stegomylae* in the South Pacific. This is an interesting area of the world since it is part of the US military's nuclear and biological testing area called the Pacific Proving Grounds.[8,9]

From 1968 forward in the southeast, small and large-scale field trials were undertaken using a fungus called *Coelomomyces punctatus* which infects mosquito larvae. Coelomomyces species are best used for mosquito control, and are not necessarily effective against other insects. Eleven of the twenty-one known species of coelomomyces were collected during World War II. Coelomomyces are a genus of aquatic fungi from the order *Blastocladiales*. These parasites infect mosquitoes in the larval stage. The fungi also lack a cell wall (cell wall deficient) and are unlike any other known fungi, even structurally. In some species thin and thick-walled sporangia (produces spores) are observed, although the thick-walled variety are more common.[8,9]

Beauveria bassiana has infected scientists who work with the fungus. Symptoms of short-term exposures cause mild to severe allergic reactions to the spores; neck, head, or other pain; and weakness, fatigue, or giddiness. *B. bassiana* is known to infect and kill *Ixodes* ticks. For this purpose it was studied as a tick control agent. Fungi that are pathogenic to mosquitoes are also highly pathogenic to most tick species. Of the pathogenic fungal strains we find *Beauveria, Aspergillus, Paecilomyces, Verticillium, Entomophthora,* and *Metarhizium* species. *Beauveria* and *Metarhizium* are the fungi most commonly applied as a biological control. Ticks were treated with these two fungi with relatively good success. Entomopathogenic fungi are commonly present in insects and ticks. This suggests that people who have been bitten by ticks are probably exposed to one of these fungal infections as well.[10-12]

The entomopathogenic fungi act as parasites by engulfing the insect body, and disabling or killing them. Species of *Beauveria* and *Verticillium* are fungi commonly found inside the tick gut. Fungal toxins from *Beauveria bassiana*, or Roseotoxin B from *Trichothecium roseum* are also found upon moldy corn and may be transmitted by vectoring insect. Toxins called destruxins from the fungi *Metarhizium anisopliae* are pathogenic to ticks and other insects. A 1967 patent describes the use of pathogenic fungi to control insect populations:[13-15]

> "The present invention involves the purposeful introduction of entomophagous fungi and certain bacteria into areas which have become contaminated by or which are susceptible to insect colonies, such as termites, cockroaches, silverfish, booklice, clothes moths, carpet beetles, ants, water bugs, etc."
>
> "The method of the present invention provides for insect control by deliberately fostering disease epidemics by combinations of fungi and bacteria which are shown to be lethal and more effective than with either organism alone. The combinations of the present invention produce disease more readily within groups of insects, disease which is communicated from infected individuals to a healthy group. Moreover, the presence of the combined organisms where the insects have died render the area uninhabitable to other susceptible insects."[13]

Early textbooks described the extensive use of fungi as insecticidal controls, including these strains that are commonly used:

Beauveria bassiana (f/k/a *Tritirachium shiotae*)	*Beauveria tenella*
Metarhizium anisopliae	*Paecilomyces farinosus*
Entomophthora spp.	*Coelomomyces Indiana*
Coelomomyces stegomyiae	*Spicaria rileyi* [15]

In 1922 a new genus and species of fungi was reported by Bogayavlensky and named *Zografia notonectae.* It was the only coelomomyces species not found in mosquitoes. Additional varieties were identified beginning in 1930. Early experimental infections with these fungi began in the 1940s in the field, and in the 1950s in the laboratory.[16]

The WHO and the New Zealand government jointly sponsored the first intercountry biological control pilot program in 1958. Their first introduction was a coelomomyces fungi from Singapore onto a Polynesian tiger mosquito (*Aedes polynesiensis*) in an experimental release program on the small Pacific Island of Tokelau (New Zealand). In 1966 another pilot project was undertaken on the island of Nauru, where *Aedes aegypti* and *Culex pipens fatigans* mosquitoes were released. (Nauru is the most famous phosphate mine in the South Pacific, since the island is composed entirely of rock phosphate.) These islands are also close to Australia (ring of fire) and the Pacific Proving Grounds. These and similar sites were important to the emergence of human diseases, encephalitis viruses, and nuclear testing that occurred during this period. We will examine the history of nuclear testing later in this book. While public health experts experimented with mosquito releases in the Pacific, various biological control applications were underway around the world in agricultural and forestry settings; and reached greenhouses by 1967.[15]

The fungus *Coelomomyces punctatus* was also deployed against mosquitoes (*Anopheles quadrimaculatus*) at University Lake in Chapel Hill, North Carolina in 1968. The fungus reduced mosquito populations by half. When we observe the history of biological controls, we find participation by academic institutions, militaries, the CDC, state and federal governments (including abroad); various industries, public health and agricultural organizations, and national and international nuclear agencies. These institutions have worked as a united front to reduce the number of vectoring insects and their associated infections around the world. Unfortunately the results of such efforts are somewhat difficult to appreciate since we now live in a world encumbered by novel infections, increased insect populations, contaminating chemical and nuclear wastes, and engineered microbes. Today biological organisms continue to be deployed in increasingly toxic combinations that are nevertheless declared "safe" and "effective" to use, when neither claim is probably entirely true. Early scientists even cautioned against the use of fungi as biological controls. According to an important book of the day: **"There might be risks for man and other vertebrates in the practical use of insect-pathogenic fungi..."**[15]

In the 1980s, scientists began to use the fungus *Entomophaga maimaiga* against gypsy moth populations although it was only effective under favorable weather conditions. Another fungus that was used as a biological control against ticks is *Lecanicillium psalliotae.* A manufacturing plant was built in Russia to manufacture mass quantities of the soil fungus *Beauveria bassiana.* This fungus was used to treat about five million acres. *B. bassiana* is used to control whiteflies, termites, grasshoppers, aphids, fire ants, flies, mites, beetles; and caterpillars of the European corn borer, codling, silkworm, and fir tussock moths. This fungus infects the insect cuticle (shell), and resembles white mold. Fungal spores can cause human respiratory problems, and human infections have been reported. *B. bassiana* is an acid-favoring endophyte, meaning it lives inside a plant for part of its life cycle without causing disease in the host plant. This fungus can also carry its own parasitic fungus called *Syspastospora parasitica.* This is an example of a natural, nested fungal pathogen inside of another fungus as a mixed infection.[17-19]

Fungi are particularly attractive to scientists as insecticides because they attack all life stages and penetrate the cuticle, even in ticks. The drawback of fungal agents is in their delivery which requires the use of a carrier agent. Oil-based applications proved more effective than water-based formulas. Another consideration is that horizontal transmission of fungal infections occurs in insects (i.e. insect to insect), plants, animals, and people. *Fungi can also share their genes with other microbes.* As fungally infected insects proliferated and transferred their infections to crops, chemical fungicides became necessary before and after harvest. The deployment of entomopathogenic fungi to reduce insect populations creates a larger problem of fungally infected foods, chemically treated foods post-harvest, and the development of antibiotic-resistant fungi.[20-22]

Studies were undertaken to find natural toxins and fungal proteins that can degrade insect cuticles (hard outer shell). Such proteins are produced by the muscardine fungus *Metarhizium anisopliae*. The saprophytic *M. anisopliae* fungus lives in the soil and affects insects such as ticks, termites, whiteflies, malaria mosquitoes, tsetse flies, thrips, grasshoppers, locusts, and beetles. This fungus has been widely used for tick control in livestock animals (i.e. cattle). In fact, *Metarhizium anisopliae* is a particularly virulent intracellular fungal infection in tick species including *Ixodes, Amblyomma, Rhipicephalus*, and *Argasidae*. This group includes species that commonly transmit Lyme disease to humans and livestock. Lyme patients should be examined and treated for any of these fungal infections if present.[23-34]

Scientists developed applications which use entomopathogenic fungi against livestock ticks, and *Ixodes scapularis*, another carrier of Lyme disease. Some tick species including dog tick (*Dermacentor variabilis*) and Lone Star tick (*Amblyomma americanum*) are said to "display a level of resistance to fungal infection." This resistance is easily overcome with modification of the insect cuticle. To do this, scientists engineered insecticides to contain a cuticle degrading protein called chitin ("kite-in"). This allows fungi to invade the more resistant tick body. Remember that pathogenic fungi have been deployed as insecticides since the earliest days of insect biowarfare – prior to the earliest reported case of a strange ECM-rash illness that was first described in Europe.[23-34]

Invasion of the Gypsys

One of the most important insect pests to agricultural world history has been the Gypsy moth. It is from the genus *Lymantria* and has the scientific name *Porthetria dispar* or *Lymantria dispar*. The moth has Eurasian origins although its name in Greek means "to ravage." The Asian gypsy moth is native to Russia, Germany, China, Korea, and Japan, where it has several natural enemies. Gypsy moth predators include wasps, flies, spiders, birds, beetles; and mammals such as raccoons, chipmunks, squirrels, shrews, and white-footed mice. Favored food sources for these moths are deciduous and citrus trees. In the US these insects thrive on oak, poplar (tulip tree or cottonwood), aspen, cedar, pine, and other trees at all elevations.

By 1909 in Russia, gypsy moths were a problem in the orchards of Bessarabia and Mishighari (now Moldavia and Romania). Scientists were considering parasitoid controls as the most effective way to deal with the problem. US scientists including Trevor Kinkaid travelled to Japan and Russia to hunt for useful predators. Kinkaid was key to the importation of parasitoids into the US in 1908 and 1909; and again from 1922 to 1933. All told, about forty species of natural gypsy moth predators were imported. These were colonized in the US from 1905 to 1933, and included about 1.8 million wasps, tachinid fly parasites; and predatory beetles from 1905 to 1911. With all of these parasitoid imports, it should be no surprise if natural infections covertly carried in their bodies initiated human disease outbreaks, at least in pocketed areas where they were first released. We have no way of knowing whether this occurred, but we can see the timely emergence of "poliomyelitis" or "encephalitis" outbreaks and the later emergence of "Lyme" disease, an infection with symptoms strikingly similar to those of either disease.[1]

The highest concentrations of trees favorable to the gypsy moth diet in the US are found in the Appalachian and Ozark mountains; in the pacific northwest Rockies; in the southwest and eastern states: Alabama, Mississippi, Oklahoma, Texas; and Apalachicolas in Florida; and in the upper Midwestern Great Lakes states: the Dakotas, Michigan, Minnesota, and northern Wisconsin. Each of these areas has subsequently become endemic for Lyme disease. Lyme was detected as early as 1948 in the US, before the first case in Wisconsin and the subsequent cases in the '60s and '70s on the eastern seaboard.[2]

In 1969 in Wisconsin, Dermatologist Rudolph Scrimenti treated another physician for an ECM rash illness who had been grouse hunting in northern Wisconsin. This appears to have been the first recorded case of a Lyme-like infection in the US. However some people on the east coast, especially in the Connecticut area, were already experiencing similar rash, arthritis, and other Lyme-like symptoms as early as the 1940s. Of note to the story is that the upper Midwest, northwest, south, southwest, and along the east coast, especially Connecticut, are home to large natural copper deposits that have been mined for centuries using nitrite-based explosives. These areas are also heavily forested, providing a perfect habitat for flies, mosquitoes, ticks, mice, and deer; all hosts of Lyme spirochetes.[2,3]

Other areas of the world have similar geographic features (forests, mineral, metal, and phosphate mines); and have become endemic for Lyme disease. Metals such as copper have been used within fungicides, fertilizers, dyes, and insecticides to kill algae, insects, and to enhance crops. Chromated copper arsenate (chromium, copper, arsenic or CCA) is used to preserve wood (i.e. piles, railroad ties, utility poles, timber). Metals of all kinds are used in many industries (i.e. aluminum, steel), and to create everything from weapons to semiconductors. We must note the association of microbes to mined and agriculturally applied minerals and metals (and their wastes). Each may play a significant role as catalysts for new animal and human epidemics under ideal conditions. This is because copper for example, helps metal-resistant bacteriae thrive. Certain bacteriae will be more prolific in the presence of certain metals and minerals and therefore will also be more readily available to be taken up by the resident microbes and the plants and insects which thrive in these environments. Copper is also used in the textile industry for dyes (i.e. copper sulphate), and has been used for coins and crop treatments; and is equally important for wire and computer circuit boards. Copper and aluminum alloys are some of the most valuable to industry.[2]

The initial introduction of silk producing gypsy moths into the US began during the American Colonial days of 1619. Nearly two hundred years later there was a sizeable textile cottage industry in the northeast. During and after the Civil War, cotton as a textile was largely unavailable. As an alternative, wool and silk were in high demand. In order to improve US silk quality, in 1869 French-American naturalist Étienne Léopold Trouvelot shipped Asian gypsy moth eggs from southern France into the US in an effort to enhance his ongoing silk moth breeding experiments.[2,4,5]

Trouvelot had planned to cross resident silkworms with his imported gypsys to produce a better quality commercial silk. (Lyon, France was the hub of the silk industry at the time, and it was also a location with a huge copper mining industry.) Trouvelot was already raising roughly one million *Polyphemus* moths of the giant silkworm family in the states, but was unhappy with their silk production and quality. Silkworms were already considered to be the best silk-producers in the world, but they were not hardy in the northern climate, and were difficult and expensive to obtain from abroad.[2,4,5]

Trouvelot felt that hybrids of silkworms and gypsies would be hardier than their Chinese relative, the silkworm *Bombyx mori.* Unfortunately Trouvelot's imported gypsys suffered from a natural viral infection that causes "wilt" disease in moths and other insects. Wilt is a nuclearpolyhedrosis (RNA) virus that has been identified as "LdNPV." The "Ld" stands for *Lymantria dispar,* the Asian gypsy moth's scientific name. The terms nucleopolyhedrosis and nuclearpolyhedrosis are interchangeable, and refer to the shape of the virus capsule. These viruses are abbreviated as "NPV" and they are also members of the *Baculovirus* family. The family of baculoviruses will become extremely valuable tools to be deployed in later centuries as agricultural insecticides.[2,4,5]

Trouvelot conducted his experiments outdoors in a carefully constructed enclosure. However within a few years some of his larvae escaped from their Medford, Massachusetts home. Without natural predators, by 1868 the gypsys were firmly established in the state as an important defoliating pest. By 1880 about four hundred square miles around Trouvelot's home were infested with descendants of the initial escapees. The defoliation of fruit and shade trees by these moths was so pervasive that the state of Massachusetts issued funds to the US Department of Agriculture in an effort to eradicate them.[6-10]

In 1892 a program was undertaken to kill the moths using lead arsenate, manufactured by the Federal Bureau of Entomology. Two years later the very first reported US human polio outbreak occurred in Vermont in 1894. This was just twenty-five years after Trouvelot's gypsy moths escaped from their compound in Massachusetts to spread in all directions; especially northward along the Atlantic coast. It was also a period which corresponds well with the application of the first US-mined phosphate fertilizers. Despite eradication attempts, by the early 1900s gypsy moth populations had increased to numbers which caused the defoliation of twenty-two hundred square miles of woodlands in Massachusetts and neighboring New England states. In Canada, while a few Asian gypsy moth egg masses were detected upon cedar trees that were imported from Japan in 1911, gypsy moth infestations that far north would not become a significant problem until the late 1970s.[6-10]

By 1905, US programs began under legislative direction to locate natural gypsy moth predators. The following year the US Secretary of Agriculture was authorized by Congress to rapidly initiate eradication methods. At the turn of the century, an estimated ninety-three million predatory insects were released into the US to specifically target gypsy and brown-tail moths; another serious defoliator.[8,9,11]

On August 12, 1912, Congress passed legislation which required that all imported plants should undergo quarantine upon import arrival to prevent accidental insect introductions into the US. Despite the quarantines, moth eggs accidentally entered the country prior to the law's full implementation, and were discovered upon young trees. By 1914, gypsy moth infestations stretched from Bangor, Maine to New Hampshire; and into Vermont, Massachusetts, and eastern Connecticut.[8,9,11]

Beginning in 1906 scientists began to deploy natural parasitizing insect predators (parasitoids) as a means to control the moths. Their first attempts included a tachinid fly (*Comsilura concinnata*) which was meant to target gypsys and brown-tailed moths. This fly's habits and host range (and natural parasites) were poorly understood before being imported from Europe. Nevertheless it was released continuously for eighty years. Scientists were unconcerned that the flies would target multiple insect species (polyphagic).[12-16]

Within a short period of time, the flies were observed attacking native giant silkworm moths of the *Saturniidae* family (i.e. luna moth, polyphemus moth); and other non-targeted species in addition to the targeted gypsys and brown-tails. Ground beetles were also shipped to New England from abroad as parasitoids of gypsy moths at the turn of the century. The forest caterpillar hunter (*Calosoma sycophanta*) and the convergent lady beetle (*Hippodarnia convergens*) were likewise released in huge numbers at different sites on both coasts, including the California foothills. Each of these insect species naturally harbored important viruses and other agents; and were free to distribute these infections to any insects they parasitized.[12-16]

By the mid-1800s, scientists abroad were using microorganisms to control insect pests in Europe. At the turn of the 20th century, gypsy moths were quite at home with other forest and crop defoliators. In 1827, young German scientist Theodor Hartig was the first to suggest the mass rearing of caterpillars so that their parasites could be harvested and used as insecticides. The first field tests using predatory ground beetles to control gypsy moth larvae on willow trees were undertaken in 1840 in Europe. In 1843 an Italian Society for the Promotion of Arts and Crafts offered a gold medal for any scientist who managed to conduct scientifically useful breeding tests of predatory insects that could be used as biological controls.[17,18]

In 1863 Agostino Bassi suggested the use of sprayable infectious liquids made from deceased larvae as useful insecticides, but the idea did not catch on until 1873. At that time scientist J.L. LeConte proposed the use of the muscardine fungus of the silkworm as a biological control. The following year Louis Pasteur, who had been studying the diseases of silkworms called pebrine and flacherie, suggested that microbes might be useful against the grape *phylloxera.* These are aphid-like insects that were eating their way through French vineyards. At the same time in Odessa, Russia, Metchnikoff was experimenting with diseases of the wheat cockchafer. His publications led Isaak Krassilstschick to develop spores from a metarhizium fungal species, which was subsequently field tested against sugar-beet curculio larvae near Smela, Ukraine.[17,18]

By 1920 Russia was just one area where gypsy moth infestations were extensive enough to warrant the use of parasitic wasps as biological controls. In later decades the Russian Plant Quarantine Service, the Russian Forest Service, the US Forest Service, and the US Animal and Plant Health Inspection Service (APHIS) entered into a comprehensive monitoring program after it was determined that ships arriving in North America from the Russian Far East were infested with gypsy moth egg clusters.[17,18]

In 1923, an Entomologist named R.T. Webber scoured European countries in search of natural parasites that would be useful to control rapidly expanding gypsy moth populations. Webber visited parts of Austria, France, Germany, Hungary, Italy, Poland, Romania, and Spain for this purpose. When he found significant infestations of gypsy moths in two countries, he established temporary laboratories there, and set about solving the problem of insect defoliation. Webber soon realized that the bacterial strains *Bacillus popilliae* and *Bacillus lentimorbus* appeared able to solve the gypsy moth problem.[6]

These infective soil bacteriae enter the insect larval gut when caterpillars eat plants that are exposed to the bacterial spores. The spores are activated in the insect gut through digestive enzymes. These sporulating bacteria create bacterial endotoxins in a crystal form which are harmful to the insects. Upon release, the spores bind to the gut brush border membranes (gut tissues), and create new channels or holes in the membranes. This allows the bacterial endotoxins to gain entry into the insect's circulation, and the insect subsequently dies as a result of bacterial septicemia (bacteremia).

While scientists were attempting to use soil bacillus strains as insecticides, they were also cultivating nematodes (filaria, or microscopic worms) from many species of moths and butterflies (lepidoptera), beetles and weevils (coleoptera), and other insects. Nematodes are highly effective microscopic insect parasites that have been widely deployed as biological controls.[6]

By 1920, heavy gypsy moth infestations could be found in Connecticut, Maine, Massachusetts, New Hampshire, New Jersey, New York, Ohio, Pennsylvania, Rhode Island, and Vermont. Two years later the first conference on gypsy moth control was held in Albany, New York. It was attended by agricultural scientists from the US and Canada. The following year a minimal gypsy moth control barrier zone was established to prevent the further northward advancement of these destructive pests. The zone was established just east of the Hudson River, and averaged twenty to thirty miles in width. Then it continued across Long Island Sound, and northward to the Canadian border; a distance of about two hundred and fifty miles. Individual states were expected to treat regions with pesticides and predatory insects; the latter provided by the Federal Bureau of Entomology. Despite these precautions, gypsy moths continued to spread west and northward into Quebec, Canada. Thereafter the barrier zone was increased in an attempt to slow their northward advancement.[8,9]

As the 1930s loomed, despite the releases of parasitoids, moth populations grew. As a result, US Congress appropriated additional funds to deal with the problem. Eradication efforts had already exceeded twenty-five million dollars. New Jersey spent roughly $1.2 million dollars on eradication programs over two decades. By 1930, gypsy moth control programs were centered at the Northeastern Forest Experiment Service in New Haven, Connecticut. Multiple bodies participated in collaborative efforts to rid states of moth infestations. Some of those working on this problem were from the Federal Bureau of Entomology and Plant Quarantine Service, state forestry services, the USDA, the US Department of the Interior, and other agencies.[21-25]

Throughout the 1930s, serious attempts were made to control gypsy moths using regional applications of the soil bacteriae *Bacillus popilliae* and *Bacillus lentimorbus*. These soil bacteriae caused diseases in gypsy moths and other insects, and are known as "milky spore" diseases. These bacteriae are classified within a bacillus-like group called *Paenibacillus* (Latin for "almost"). This group of agents includes the bacteria *Paenibacillus larvae* which causes American foulbrood disease in honey bees. (It is probable that the recent disappearance of honey bees is due to their incidental exposures to one or more applied agricultural controls which employ similar microbes to target other insect species, and which force latent infections to reactivate into virulent infections.)[21-25]

There are roughly seventy species of paenibacillus, which are considered to be members of the same species (morphotypes) of *Bacillus subtilis*, a common soil bacteria. As spore-forming bacteria they are also related to *Bacillus cereus, Bacillus sphaericus, Bacillus anthracis* (the agent of anthrax), and *Bacillus thuringiensis* (B.t.). This group of bacteria also includes the *Thermobacillus*. These are also called *thermophiles*, bacteria that live in extreme temperatures, and are members of the overall *Extremophile* group. They may be found in hot springs, deep underground, near mined minerals and ores, and in surface and subsurface acid mine wastes. This class of bacteriae is salt tolerant and highly antibiotic-resistant, including against ampicillin, spectinomycin, streptomycin, vancomycin, teicoplanin, and tetracycline. This resistance to tetracycline is key if human Lyme disease or other infections are caused in part by these agents, since treatment with the tetracycline drug doxycycline may be ineffective. Thermophilic bacteria and the agent of Lyme disease both have enzymes which contribute to antibiotic resistance (these are called ß [beta]-galactosidase).[22-24]

By WWII, gypsy moths had defoliated nearly one million acres of woodlands in the northeastern US. From around 1945 until 1972 when it was banned by the EPA, the chemical pesticide DDT (DichloroDiphenylTrichloroethane) was used to control gypsy moths and other insects. The chemical was perhaps the most successful insecticide against crop and forestry defoliators. Unfortunately the chemical was also found to be highly toxic and mutagenic, and was subsequently banned abroad in 1969 and in the US by 1972. With the disappearance of effective chemical pesticides such as DDT, gypsy moths and other insects made a strong come back. Once again their populations rapidly expanded west and southward across New England. Other countries that had banned DDT during the late 1960s also saw a resurgence of gypsy moths and other defoliating insect populations post-ban.[26]

We may learn much about the manufacture of sporulating bioagents from registered patent inventions. A 1971 patent describes the manufacture of *Bacillus popilliae* spores in mass quantities for use as a biopesticide (biological pesticide). Another patent describes the use of milky disease spores to control Japanese beetles and other insects. We may read how spores may be grown upon cane sugar refinery wastewater or "char." (The name is derived from animal charcoal-filled tanks which filter sugared syrups.) Now a food industry waste could be recycled to produce agricultural insecticides – undoubtedly good business for both industries.[27,28]

A 1968 patent assigned to the USDA describes the destruction of vegetative, but not sporulated cells of spore-forming bacteria which could be used as insecticides. The patent is assigned to the Amstar Corporation of New York. In 1970, the American Sugar Company (Domino Sugar) became the Amstar Corporation. The company is based in New Haven, Connecticut. The patent refers to other processes which use *Bacillus popilliae.* There are many US government patents for important biological controls. Other governments reserve similar patent royalties or licensing rights which are earned from agricultural inventions with global applications, including patents for *Bacillus thuringiensis* (B.t.) strains.[29]

By the 21st century, the Argonne National Laboratory* in Illinois was working in cooperation with the Illinois Department of Agriculture, the USDA Agricultural Forest Service, and the USDA Forest Service Northeastern Area, State & Private Forestry Unit in St. Paul, Minnesota. The group was scheduled to treat gypsy moth populations with pesticides in seventeen areas of Illinois. One proposal included treating a dozen sites with *Bacillus thuringiensis* variety kurstaki (B.t.k) through two applications in mid-May to June. The name of the initial operation was the Gypsy Moth Slow-the-Spread (STS) pilot project. It initially ran from 1993 until 1999, and became fully operational in 2000. This is just one example of the kinds of programs undertaken to treat these pests.[30,31]

**Argonne National Laboratory in Willowbrook (Argonne), Illinois was the first US national laboratory. It is a descendant of the University of Chicago's Metallurgical Laboratory and was part of the WWII Manhattan Project – the program that developed the first atomic weapons.*

Could there be an international "conspiracy of silence" about the negative consequences of using chemical and microbial insecticides that may have caused human epidemics? If so, revelations of these relationships would undoubtedly feel threatening to patent holders, academic scientists, industries, and government bodies. After all, if industries were forced to cease the production of their highly profitable tools, there would be no useful alternatives to protect the public from insects of medical, military, agricultural, industrial, and veterinary importance.[32]

Wasps as Insect Controls

Parasitoid insects have been used in efforts to control insect pests around the world. There are seven species of chalcid wasps (*Hunterellus hookeri*) that were identified from 1907 to 1977 as natural tick parasites. Chalcid wasps belong to the order of hymenoptera. They parasitize the eggs, larvae, or pupae of other insects; including lepidoptera (butterflies/moths), diptera (flies/mosquitoes); coleoptera (beetles/weevils), some arachnida (spiders, mites); and at least one family of parasitic nematodes. Scientific studies of chalcid wasps as parasitoids can be found as early as 1910. The most common species to have been released were the chalcids; including *Hunterellus theileri, Ixodiphagus hirtus, Ixodiphagus mysorensis,* and *Ixodiphagus texanus*.[1-7]

Initial field studies and mass-releases of chalcids to parasitize US ticks took place beginning in the 1920s, and continued for a decade. In 1926, nymph marsh ticks (*Dermacentor reticulates*), the American dog tick (*D. variabilis*), and the brown dog tick (*Rhipicephalus sanguineus*), already pre-parasitized by a wasp (*Ixodiphagus hookeri*), were obtained from the Fontainebleu Forest in France (about 60 km southeast of Paris) and released in the states. This same wasp species had previously been used to successfully control tick infestations in France during the early 1920s. This means that French ticks that were parasitized by wasps (which harbor latent polydnaviruses, reoviruses, and other parasites) were released into the US. At the turn of the 20th century, the first significant case numbers of an ECM rash illness began surfacing in Europe in areas where parasitoids, fungal insecticides, soil bacteria, and the superphosphate fertilizers were also deployed.[1-5]

In 1926 in the US, imported French nymph ticks that were already parasitized were released on Naushon Island, Massachusetts; and on adjacent islands in efforts to control the American dog tick. Unfortunately initial control methods with the wasps were considered only mildly successful, as dog ticks and deer ticks (*Ixodes scapularis*) continued to occupy the islands in large numbers. Upon field collections, various tick species demonstrated that they were parasitized by the previously released wasps. Although the majority of the wasps failed to establish, a few survived the cold winter climate and colonized.[2-5]

In 1927, a program to release more than four million parasitic wasps was undertaken. It began with the release of significant wasp populations in Montana, home of the National Institutes of Health's (NIH) Rocky Mountain Laboratories. The wasps were meant to control the Rocky Mountain spotted fever (wood) tick (*Dermacentor andersoni*), which was common to the area. In 1932, the balance of four million parasitic wasps was released in Colorado, Idaho, and Oregon. As in previous mass insect releases, the overall establishment of the wasps was once again considered to have been largely unsuccessful.[8]

In 1933, only a few wasp larvae were found in parasitized ticks removed from a Montana ground squirrel. Despite the early failures, from 1937 to 1939 nearly one hundred-thousand female *Ixodes hookeri* wasps were released on the east coast, and on *Martha's Vineyard* Island to control dog ticks. By 1942, studies again showed that parasitoid attempts had failed to reduce tick populations in a significant manner. However now parasitized ticks (and animals) were probably harboring important new viruses and other microbes to which they were not previously exposed.[8]

Similar attempts to control ticks using parasitic wasps were also attempted in the Soviet Union during the 1940s. Leningrad scientists released nearly forty thousand wasp-parasitized nymph sheep ticks (*Ixodes ricinus*) and roughly three thousand adult wasps. Once again control efforts were unsuccessful, probably due to the cold climate. Parasitized nymphal bont ticks (*Amblyomma variegatum*) were also released in Africa during field experiments by members of the International Center for Insect Physiology and Ecology, with somewhat encouraging results. Some of the pathogenic protozoan infections that are found as parasities in these ticks include *Haemogregarina, Nosema, Babesia,* and *Theileria.* At least one of these intracellular infections (babesia), has been detected in many patients who are co-infected with the Lyme disease agent.[9,10]

In general, significant numbers of parasitized ticks survived to spread various infections including microsporidiae, protozoae, bacteriae, fungi, nematodes, and viruses. The parasitic wasps that were released, and those managing to colonize were naturally infected with a number of pathogens that were not necessarily deadly for the ticks, but which remained transmissible to other species. After being inoculated with wasp viruses, ticks were free to feed upon hosts and to spread their new infections which percolated inside their midguts. Now ticks would become vectors of new disease agents with not only a wider host range, but which carried terrific host gene and metabolism-altering talents. The only issue keeping them at bay from animal and human populations was the necessity of accessing these infections by way of the gut or salivary glands; and this problem would be overcome by industrial, agricultural, and nuclear wastes found in soils and watersheds.[8,11-13]

Parasitoid wasps lay their eggs inside the bodies of nymph ticks. Scientists have discovered that the presence of wasp eggs inside the parasitized tick body seems to render the nymph tick hosts "unsuitable" for *Borrelia burgdorferi* (Bb) spirochetes and *Babesia microti** infections. It is most curious that scientists would study this possibility, unless they suspected that the early parasitoid insects were partly responsible for spreading Bb infections. What the results seems to say is that parasitized nymph ticks cannot harbor either babesia or Bb infections. If this is true, then this may only be incidental to the idea that the wasps only lay their eggs in ticks that are still in a nymphal stage. A lack of pathogens at this tick life stage means very little actually, since they only take one blood meal per life stage. Perhaps the nymphs studied simply haven't eaten yet. In addition, what happens in the laboratory is very different than what happens in the environment. There may be other factors that play a role in sustaining infectious diseases in any of a tick's life stages.

**Babesia is a protozoan that causes animal and human babesiosis, a malaria-like infection.*

Parasitic wasps lay their eggs in other insects including moth and butterfly larvae, and occasionally in plants. Moth larvae harbor their own infections which include but are not limited to the granulosis viruses* (GV), nuclearpolyhedrosis viruses (NPV), and cytoplasmic polyhedrosis viruses (CPV); as well as polydna, polydna-like, and other viruses. It would appear that insects and animal hosts are the point of origin for many mixed infections. Wherever vectoring insects obtain their pathogens, it is obvious they carry an assortment of mixed infections from multiple hosts and the environment; a world heavily influenced by pollutants and applied chemical, biological, and nuclear weapons of insect biowarfare.[8]

**The GV and NPV viruses are members of the baculovirus family. This is a group of viruses that not only appear naturally, but were and are used extensively as insecticides, alone or within genetically engineered formulas. CPVs are not baculoviruses, but RNA viruses that are commonly associated with baculoviruses. When stimulated by a baculovirus, the CPVs will reactivate and become highly infectious, and this synergy has been exploited within insecticides.*

Japanese Beetles

USDA scientists began to explore ways to control another important pest insect, the Japanese beetle (*Popillia japonica*) beginning around 1920. These beetles are from the *Scarabidae* or scarab family. They are native to Japan and Korea, and the family consists of about three thousand species. Japanese beetle larvae were accidentally introduced into the US, probably as stowaways in a shipment of flower bulbs which arrived at Riverton, New Jersey before the US Plant Quarantine Act was established in 1912.[1-5]

In less than a decade, Japanese beetles became firmly established as a defoliating pest due to a lack of natural predators. They quickly became important pests, particularly with respect to agricultural crops and ornamentals. Following the same parasitoid techniques employed to control gypsy moths, scientists discovered a natural beetle predator and parasitoid wasp called *Tiphia popilliavora* Rohwer which was imported from China, Japan, and Korea. These parasitic wasps were released with the intent of targeting Japanese beetles beginning in 1921 starting with New Jersey and nine other states. Another wasp species, *Tiphia vernalis* Rohwer was also released four years later in New Jersey. This wasp became distributed as far south as North Carolina, and eventually invaded fifteen states.[2-5]

In 1922, scientists also tried to control Japanese beetle infestations with a new natural beetle predator, a diptera "winsome fly" called *Istocheta aldrichi*, imported from northern Japan. The flies were released in thirteen states beginning with New Jersey where the original Japanese beetle outbreak began, and subsequent locations northward. Again in 1926, another parasitoid tachinid fly called *Dexilla ventralis* was imported from Korea. It was released in New Jersey and subsequently in Connecticut, Illinois, Maryland, New York, and Pennsylvania. Another attempt at controlling the beetles was made from 1923 to 1929 in New Jersey using a third Japanese fly import called *Prosena siberita*. From 1920 to 1933, over a dozen species of parasitic insects from China, India, Japan, and Korea were released in fifteen US states through the departments of agriculture in a massive effort to control Japanese beetle populations.[5-11]

In 1930, there was a sudden eruption of what was called "infectious polio virus" in Middletown and New Haven, Connecticut. In 1931, a Yale poliomyelitis study group was organized to investigate the outbreak. Unbeknownst to the public, the outbreak occurred just a few years after the initial releases of parasitic wasps, flies, and ticks to control various insect pests. These activities of course had been undertaken near the outbreak areas, and on nearby Long Island. The Yale group tested patient samples using research monkeys, and determined that the polio virus was present in sewage samples and flies found feeding upon sewage. As of 1930, in addition to parasitoid insects, new microbial insecticides were also being deployed in the area. Any chemical or microbial controls, fertilizers, and/or released insects could have contributed to any poliomyelitis outbreaks.[12]

In 1933, a new fatal disease of Japanese beetles called "milky spore" was discovered in New Jersey, although scientists did not know whether the infection had come from the imported insects, or from indigenous origins. Milky spore disease is caused by the paenibacillus class of bacteria that includes but is not limited to *Bacillus popilliae* and other thermophile bacteria. These bacteria infect not only Japanese beetles, gypsys and other moths, but also the parasitoid wasps. The thermophiles were being studied by USDA scientists from 1935 to 1937. Scientist Dutky reasoned that the failure of some of the released parasitoid wasps to thrive in certain areas where they had been released might have had to do with the presence of milky disease within the wasp populations. It is unclear however whether tiphia wasps were transmitting the infection to other species, or if something else had created the new disease that was now infecting many insect species.[5,11]

A 1943 scientific study revealed that tiphia wasps which were used as early parasitoids, can become infected with the milky spore agent. At the time of the study it was felt that the wasps were not largely affected by the bacteria, but they were able to spread it to their parasitized hosts. Such transmissions may have greatly contributed to insect, animal, or human disease outbreaks.[1-5]

The two kinds of milky spore disease that have been identified are "type A" *Bacillus popilliae*, and "type B" *Bacillus lentimorbus*. These infections are related to the soil bacteriae *Bacillus subtilis* and *Bacillus cereus.* The name "milky disease" comes from the milky white appearance of the larval insect's abdomen when infected. The abdomen of uninfected larvae has a normal grayish hue. In modern times this infection has been renamed *Paenibacillus popilliae*. When infected larvae die, their bodies become desiccated, and this releases fungal spores into the soil and air where they become airborne spores. In soil, spores remain infectious for many years. Spores can be found in the environment either as a result of natural infections or from applied insecticides which use these bacteria.[13-15]

Airborne spores may be inhaled by any living creature, and may remain infective. The exact mechanism of toxic action is unknown, but the crystal toxins of *Bacillus popilliae* are felt to be similar in function to those of another globally important agricultural bacterium called *Bacillus thuringiensis* or "B.t." The B.t. agent is created for insecticidal use by fermenting related soil bacteria. The activity of B.t. is similar to that of *B. popilliae* spores, as B.t. also sporulates and permits the infiltration of potent neurotoxins through the insect gut wall. Once it enters the circulation, bacteremia occurs (bacteria in the blood), and the insect dies. Depending on the presence of other infections in the insect body or in the insecticidal formulas, B.t. infections slowly progress or rapidly kill their hosts.[13-15]

From the 1930s forward, agricultural insecticides that contained viruses and bacteria were being tested as applied insecticides. Dead, and live diseased insect larvae were collected, dried, ground, and dispensed upon fields and turf, beginning on a New Jersey golf course. *Bacillus popilliae*, the agent of milky spore, was the first microbial agent to be registered in the US as an insecticide. However it was used only sporadically from the 1930s to 1949 against beetles and moths. The formula could be applied to plants or turf where Japanese beetle larvae (grubs) live.[8,13,16-18]

It has been estimated that the US government allowed more than 100 tons of *Bacillus popilliae* spore powder to be applied to over 160,000 sites within the US from 1939 to 1953; including in thirteen eastern states and the District of Columbia. In 1940 Maryland, *Bacillus popilliae* was applied to a golf course fairway, and the spores could be detected over the next nine years. In Connecticut, *B. popilliae* spores were first applied over various regional areas beginning in 1942. The earliest ECM rash illnesses in humans in the US were detected from patient ECM rash skin samples that had been collected in 1948. These were the first detectable ECM-rash producing infections in the US – far earlier than the 1969 Wisconsin patient, or the 1975 Connecticut outbreak for which Lyme disease was made famous.[9,18-24]

Releases of imported Japanese parasitoid wasps took place in New England during the 1930s by the USDA (and years later in the 1980s in North Carolina by the state's department of agriculture). Early parasitoid insect releases also correlate with President Roosevelt's attack of "polio" in 1921; and subsequent polio outbreaks in the US beginning in Connecticut in 1930 and Los Angeles in 1934. By the 1930s, California had for several decades also imported many parasitoid insects to control important citrus pests including scale, gypsy moths, and Japanese beetles. The question is whether any of these imports and/or the microbial insecticides truly correlated with outbreaks of human diseases. When parasitoids are included in the broad term of applied biological controls, the answer is in the affirmative. This concept is of course markedly different than historic accounts of the emergence and subsequent "control" of polio and other animal and human disease epidemics.[1-5]

In October 1940 in Nottingham, Pennsylvania, a scientist named P.S. Clarke was the first to note another fatal infection in Japanese beetle larvae. The agent was subsequently named "blue disease." In 1951, blue disease of Japanese beetles was again studied by scientists Dutky and Gooden of the Agricultural Research Administration in Moorestown, New York; and Beltsville, Maryland. The authors submitted their findings to Dr. Edward A. Steinhaus, formerly at Rocky Mountain Laboratories, but subsequently was at the University of California. Dr. Steinhaus's opinion was that the organism resembled a rickettsial agent than any known insect virus. He suggested placement of the blue disease organism into the order *Rickettsiales*. The organism is now known as *Rickettsia popilliae* or *Coxiella popilliae*. This means that the "blue" disease of Japanese beetles is a rickettsial infection.[25-30]

The organism's shape was described as being similar to *Vibrio* bacteriae, which are commonly found in sewage and polluted water sources. However the organism's small size and intracellular growth pattern seemed to exclude it as a vibrio bacterial strain. However it had characteristics similar to the polyhedrosis viruses that are found within the bodies of moths and butterflies, or those being applied as microbial insecticides. Dr. Steinhaus considered the organism to be a novel rickettsial infection; and observers may guess as to its origins.[25-30]

What was leading to the emergence of a new fatal illness within the Japanese beetle population? Was it a mutation of the milky spore disease agents or a virus from the gypsy moths or Japanese beetles that were targeted by early chemical and microbial controls? Could the diseased insects or the chemical and microbial agents that were applied in the environment have mutated a soil bacterium that was taken up by Japanese beetle grubs resting therein? If we explore this thought, we may understand how a soil bacterium, a fungus, and a *reactivated latent insect virus* could create the new "blue disease." Once again this occurred during a period where triple superphosphate fertilizers and other agricultural chemicals (i.e. herbicides) had entered the picture. Outbreaks erupted where soils were not only over-nitrified, but also contaminated with agricultural and industrial microbes, and radioactive and other mutagenic wastes.

We know that the blue disease organism was shaped like vibrio bacteria which are found in wastewaters. Among the vibrio species are *Desulphovibrio* species, which are sulfate (sulfur) reducing, extremophile bacteria. We also know that it was similar to the polyhedrosis viruses found in moths. It is not hard to imagine that a mutant bacteria and a moth virus could be created by agents collected from an agricultural or wastewater environment.

When baculoviruses (NPV or GV), and RNA viruses (CPV) are put into the same environment, the baculovirus will activate CPV reoviruses. Furthermore polyhedrosis viruses are enhanced in the presence of nitrates, including fertilizer nitrates. We can guess that the viruses, bacteria, and fungi from applied insecticides or from the soil which contained spores from deceased insects donated the necessary genes to create a mutant infectious new beetle pathogen. What is noteworthy is that vibrio bacteriae are also nitrate reducers. Nitrates bind to hemoglobin, the oxygen-carrying proteins in the blood, which causes cyanosis, or the "blue" tint seen in infected beetles. The beetles probably died of an infection that starved them of oxygen. A similar process may occur in the cattle pathogen "blue tongue" disease, because its agent is also a CPV or reovirus.[31-36]

By 1955, scientists from the New York Agricultural Experiment Station and the USDA Agricultural Research Service were studying the Japanese beetle and the European chafer. They were seeking a method of mass-producing the popular milky spore agents so they could be used as agricultural insecticides. In 1966 USDA scientists from Riverside, California; and the New York State Agricultural Experiment Station compared all globally collected milky disease species and strains from beetle larvae isolations. Their studies included US strains of *Bacillus popilliae* and *Bacillus lentimorbus* variety Maryland – strains that were already being applied in the states. They determined that the organisms could not be mass produced upon artificial media for global use. While small-scale efforts to control insects using *B. popilliae* viruses and similar tools continued regionally, scientists would need a different agent capable of being mass-produced in order to have an effective biological control insecticide for agricultural use on a global scale – and they set about developing one.[13,18,37,38]

Mosquito Manipulations

One example of agricultural tests that were undertaken in the environment for "peaceful" medical applications involved millions of mosquitoes that were infected with dengue and yellow fevers. The insects were released over Avon Park, Florida, and Savannah, Georgia. The latter is a site that will become important to us for the CDC's interests in its resident fauna. In my book *God Science*, I also discuss the many sterile insect techniques that were used upon insects such as mosquitoes and ticks, to study infectious disease transmission, and to control global pest insect populations.

In summary sterile insect techniques (SIT) included the use of chemicals, genetic engineering, and/or nuclear irradiation before release of sexually sterilized males (i.e. mosquitoes). Many harbored "deleterious genes" that were first manipulated within the laboratory. These altered mosquitoes were released with the intent that they would replace indigenous mosquito populations within a given area through selective breeding. These techniques are considered "population replacements." Some of the releases occurred outside of the US, but a great number were performed on domestic soil. Such "new and improved" genetically altered insect species carried genes that some scientists warned, worried, and communicated might be wrongly transmitted to other insect species. They had legitimate concerns that the altered insects could negatively impact other insects, animals, or humans. Unfortunately nobody seemed to heed these warnings because a multitude of experiments and releases have, and continue to occur.

In 1950s Florida, a sterile male mosquito release program took place over a five square mile peninsula on the south side of Lake Okeechobee at a field test site for sterilized "malaria" mosquitoes. Scientists also studied the effectiveness of gamma irradiation toward mosquito mating habits. Sterilized male insects were released at a rate of roughly fifteen hundred to two thousand individuals per square mile every week. Other research was conducted on irradiated boll weevils, codling moths, European corn borers, and tsetse flies.[1]

One document describes how Harvard researchers may have been part of a group of collaborators who released and/or planned to release mosquito and tick vectors that were carrying deleterious (harmful or destructive) genes into the environment as agricultural biological controls. These experiments were scheduled to take place at least one year before the Lyme disease organism was officially "identified." The program reportedly ended in May of 1985.[2]

Mosquitoes were released by the University of Maryland and collaborative researchers from Lahore (Pakistan medical research center), and in other countries. There were also planned releases of ticks which harbored deleterious genes during the 1980s. I located an NIAID grant abstract titled "Arthropod-borne diseases and their control." The grant was awarded fiscal year 1980 for a five-year project. The abstract described how scientists had genetically altered mosquitoes to a stage where "…field release trials of lab-reared populations, carrying deleterious genes, are currently in progress."[3]

This means that by the time of the grant award, researchers were already releasing genetically manipulated mosquitoes into the environment and these events were far from novel. The abstract also declared that future research into tick vectors (and their release) with manipulated genes would be a "possibility." According to the text:

> "Additionally, field studies of mosquito predators and pathogens as control agents are continuing. A clinical component is being established that will relate these control projects directly to malarial and viral diseases. In a like manner, a tick project is proposed, in order to define the role of ticks in the transmission of viral, rickettsial, and protozoal agents."[3]

A substantial number of research grants were awarded to academic scientists to study mosquito and tickborne diseases, and many of those studies included field release experiments. For example a five-year program was undertaken from 1970 to 1975 by the University of Maryland's ICMR unit in Brazil. Researchers were studying the genetic manipulation of mosquito vectors.[4]

In 1974, another grant was awarded to the university for genetic studies on the control of insect arbovirus vectors, especially mosquitoes. The grant abstract discusses the "bioregulation of human disease" based on genetic studies of culex mosquitoes as vectors of Japanese B encephalitis, West Nile, and Chikungunya fever arboviruses. Scientists were searching for a genetic means to control or eradicate mosquito infections and to reduce mosquito populations. They raised mosquitoes at the university's Pakistan Medical Research Center in Lahore. An additional objective was to monitor a genetic control release program, and to develop a compound chromosome strain that could replace those found in natural mosquito populations.[5]

Another grant issued to the University of California at Irvine indicated that certain genetically altered mosquito strains could be used to test disease control protocols. The abstract discussed the "…low frequency, *illegitimate recombination* that has been demonstrated to take place in mosquitoes." This appears to address natural recombinant events that might lead to the creation of infectious agents which accidentally infect mammals. Such recombinant events are considered "illegitimate," or in other words, they are unplanned and undesired genetic changes. Scientists were developing transgenic mosquitoes with specific genes that might prevent such "unacceptable" gene reassortments. This was an attempt to create mutant mosquitoes that cannot create certain diseases in their bodies, through the manual manipulation of their genes.[6]

Genetic reassortment of microbes in the insect gut is important to understand as a natural process that takes place in mosquitoes, ticks, and other insects – but perhaps more so from the effects of gamma irradiation, which was often used on released insects. Scientists felt it was important to "fix" this gene problem by creating mosquito populations that could not transmit certain infections. We might note that "unacceptable" recombinant events may also occur in vertebrate animals including livestock and humans who are similarly exposed to mutagens (i.e. infections, chemicals, radiation).[6]

Other grant awards reveal that parasitic diseases transmitted by mosquitoes are a major threat to life and health across the globe. The objectives of some studies were to develop mosquito strains that were highly resistant to parasites. Strains were developed with genetic alterations, and then the altered mosquitoes were released. From 1998 to 2003, scientists at the University of California-Irvine were working on transgenic mosquitoes while studying the yellow fever mosquito. From a grant abstract we read how: "The development of mosquito transgenesis has made possible the production of mosquitoes that have been altered by the stable insertion of exogenous genes."[7]

Many research papers have been published about the mass-production of insect parasitoids, including using mites for field trials against houseflies; and mosquito cultivation and maintenance, the latter in an insectary in Mexico City. The WHO also published many bulletins on biological controls and infectious diseases.[8-15]

Some publications discuss the mass propagation of bacteriae that are pathogenic to insects; parasites of black flies and mosquitoes; and the application of genetic technologies toward mosquito rearing. WHO reports mention that *genetic manipulations up until 1964 also took place during the breeding of silkworms and honey bees*. While honey bees have mysteriously vanished (and this has been blamed on *Nosema* protozoan infections), gypsy moth populations have remained highly problematic. A 1960 report states that "only very recently" was there much interest in autocidal control, which is the use of insect parasitoids. However this is categorically untrue when we know that insect parasitoids were released since the turn of the last century to control pest insects. Furthermore insects have been extensively studied during WWII and beyond as potential weapons of biological warfare, including billions that were irradiated before their release.[8-15]

For nearly a century wasps and other insects have been mass-released to parasitize other insects in efforts to control agricultural and industrial pests. The transmission of the pathogens they carried into their parasitized hosts is a given, as this was an objective of the release programs. The introduced parasitoids co-evolved with a myriad of infectious microbes in their bodies. Following the first attempts at autocidal controls came the manual manipulation and application of microbes to augment the earliest microbial insecticides. Every step of the way scientists promoted or tampered with insect diseases to reduce insect populations. However no methods were effective in the long-run. Therefore scientists studied other methods of eliminating disease transmission in insects, including genetic engineering.[8-15]

Scientists have manipulated insect genes using transgenic viruses. These are literally transplanted, laboratory-manipulated viruses. A Canadian-assigned patent by California inventors describes a "new kind" of transgenic virus that uses insect transcription factors to control molting and metamorphosis. The invention is useful as a biopesticide. The patent discusses how a transgenic insect virus from a group of *Entomopoxvirus A, B*, or a baculovirus family is made with insect developmental or hormone-regulated genes. An example of a baculovirus gene that blocks an insect's molt process is the alfalfa looper virus *Autographa californica* nuclearpolyhedrosis virus (AcNPV). This virus has already been used extensively within microbial insecticides for many decades.[16,17]

Nuclearpolyhedrosis viruses (NPVs) are members of the baculovirus family. These are enveloped viruses that are large and rod-shaped. The group also includes the insect granulosis viruses (GVs). Baculoviruses are large DNA viruses. There are cytoplasmicpolyhedrosis viruses (CPV) which are not baculoviruses but are instead reoviruses, a large group of RNA insect viruses. Even though they are different, RNA viruses including the reoviruses are commonly found in association with baculoviruses. The baculoviruses and the reoviruses infect the insect gut tissues, and cause a slowly progressing fatal infection. If humans are infected with any of these, such infections may contribute to a chronic wasting syndrome (i.e. AIDS or Lyme).

Baculoviruses and reoviruses have been used extensively over many decades as microbial controls to augment the applied insecticides. Today baculoviruses and reoviruses are genetically engineered directly into food crops as insecticides. Putting these viruses together causes the RNA viruses to become active and highly virulent which is why they are exploited in insecticides; and more recently in genetically engineered crops. Together they provide a faster kill time, either on or in the plants. A Canadian patent describes a "safer" alternative to the bio-insecticide B.t.:

"...some recent concerns over the specificity of B.t. have resulted in the recommendation that it not be used in areas where there are endangered Lepidoptera. Ecological interests have resulted in a shift in emphasis to examine and develop other microbial products, including the insect viruses. Insect viruses are naturally occurring insect pathogens that are considered to be host specific and environmentally safe. They can persist from year to year to impact on several generations of insects. There are over 1200 insect viruses (nucleopolyhedroviruses, granulovirus, entomopoxviruses, cypovirus and others) that have potential for insect control."[16,18-20]

The patent also describes the use of scorpion or mite toxins, enzymes, neuropeptides, and hormones that can be engineered into the alfalfa looper virus. These neurotoxins will enter the insect's gut and act upon its nervous system to rapidly kill it. Another process describes the modification of silkworm moth genes as part of the genetic engineering of insecticides.[16,18-20]

According to a grant abstract we learn: "Replacement of wild mosquito populations with genetically modified counterparts that cannot transmit disease provides an alternative approach to disease prevention." Scientists are attempting to create "disease-free" mosquitoes "to bring population replacement technology to the stage where it can be applied successfully, and the communities involved will have enough confidence the technology can be controlled to allow its use." Scientists are worried that the public will not like them tampering with the genes of insect populations, and they are undoubtedly correct. The idea that genes that are manipulated by the laboratory can be controlled once they are released into the environment is something the public should indeed question.[16,18-20]

If you think that mosquito population replacement attempts are all in the past, think again. In an October 2011 article from the *New York Times* we learn that scientists are again attempting to introduce the public to the idea of mosquito population replacement. The truth is however that these techniques are not even remotely new, despite the positive spin placed on the program by the media. What is alarming in the article is that scientists reported "initial success" with the release of mosquitoes that contain a gene that is designed to kill only male mosquitoes before they grow to adulthood. The article admits that other insect populations are targeted for population replacement and deleterious gene programs as were performed decades ago.[21]

It seems a bit naïve to believe that only the male mosquitoes which the genes are supposed to target will be affected. This is because mosquitoes harbor many different infectious agents in their bodies. Even if they are microbially sterile upon release, they will contract infections upon a blood meal. There is simply no scientific way to predict the consequences of the release of genetically modified insects. A comment at the end of the article is also troubling. A scientist was quoted saying that the research was for a "good cause" and that people do not eat insects. But eating insects is not what matters. More likely the public should worry about what happens when genetically altered insects collide with infectious agents and pollutants found outside the laboratory. That environment includes other insects, animals, humans, and a myriad of chemical and microbial pollutants with proven potential to reassort genes – and to produce infections that are transmissible to animals and humans by vectoring insects.[21]

The process of irradiating insects for agricultural release is just one aspect of *radiobiology*. This is the process of using nuclear energy for peaceful agricultural, medical, veterinary, and industrial purposes. Over the past several decades many insect species have been studied for their use as population replacers that will breed with indigenous species to create non-fertile offspring. As of the 1960's before the Lyme outbreak emerged in Connecticut, the following insects had been studied under an 84-nation membership in the Joint FAO/IAEA* cooperative program to eradicate insect pests from the face of the earth. The insects that were studied, irradiated, and/or released during field trials include at the very least these species:

New Guinea screwworm
Mediterranean fruit fly
Olive fly
European corn borer
Australian sheep blowfly
Mediterranean flour moth
Carribean fruit fly
Onion fly
Yellow fever mosquito (*Aedes aegypti*)
Filariasis† mosquito (*Aedes scutellaris*)
Filariasis mosquito (*Culex pipiens fatigans*)
Malaria mosquito (*Anopheles gambiae*)
Cotton bollworm
Japanese beetle
Coco capsid
Locust
Grape phylloxera
Tropical ox warble
Mexican fruit fly
Codling moth
Pink bollworm
Fall armyworm
Melon fly
South American fruit fly
Gypsy moth
Human bot fly
House fly
Bean weevil
Coffee leaf miner
Rice-stem borer
Hornworm
Honey bee
Cave-dwelling ticks
Colorado potato beetle
Tsetse fly
Queensland fruit fly
Sugar cane borer
Boll weevil
Drosophila
Oriental fruit fly
Vinegar flies
Aphids
Hornfly
Rhinoceros beetle
Cockchafer
Tobacco budworm
Cotton red stainer
Cabbage looper
Stable fly
Braconid wasps
Leopard moth

**FAO/IAEA stands for the Food and Agriculture Organization of the United Nations and the International Atomic Energy Agency. Its headquarters are in Vienna, Austria. †Filariasis is a nematode infection.*

As we can see, population replacement was practiced with many insect populations over many decades as of today. These techniques are hardly new, they are just not publicly known. These processes were also not limited to irradiating insects using sterile insect techniques. They included the use of hormones (pheromones); and the insertion of recombinant genes followed by extensive release programs in many parts of the world including the US. While we can appreciate the efforts of scientists who desire to undertake such exploits, it is difficult to appreciate how well such designs could have been tested before the insects were released to ensure that "no harm" could ever come to non-targeted insects, animals, and humans who contact altered insect populations. Unfortunately there is no possible way to ensure safety. Similarly there is no way to ensure that deleterious genes cannot or will not become reassorted with natural genes, or transmitted to human populations to cause novel, important infectious disease epidemics similar to those desired in the targeted insect populations.

Fire Ants and Lone Star Ticks

A paper described the arrival of fire ants in Alabama during the 1920s as an "accident." Another source revealed that the importation of South American red fire ants began in Mobile, Alabama; and Pensacola, Florida between 1933 and 1945. The USDA claims that fire ants arrived during the 1930s when they accidentally climbed aboard as ship ballast. Still another source says the ants were accidentally introduced into the Gulf region during the 1920s when they arrived as stowaways on imported plant materials.[1-3]

However they arrived, fire ants have expanded their territory in their new environment, reaching Texas by 1950. Today they are present in roughly a dozen states including Arkansas, Florida, Georgia, Louisiana, Mississippi, North and South Carolina, Texas, and Tennessee. They may also be found in Arizona, New Mexico, and southern California. Fire ants are native to Argentina, Brazil, and Paraguay; and were introduced into Central America, the US, and the British Islands of Bermuda, the Virgin Islands, Puerto Rico, Trinidad, and Tobago. The imported red fire ant (*Solenopsis invicta*) has continued to spread throughout the southeastern US where they have contributed to the loss of biodiversity. They are also renowned for harming the livestock of commercial feedlots; and of native ground nesting birds, snakes, and lizards.[4,5]

Fire ant colonies may contain a single, or multiple queens. According to sources this may be a result of organophosphates or other pesticide applications and their mutagenic effects upon insect genes. Fire ants use hormones called pheromones for navigation and communication and to facilitate breeding. Scientists have engineered pheromones into insecticides to attract insects to a specific area where insecticides are applied. There have been extensive efforts over decades to control what was once considered to be a beneficial insect. Such efforts began with the Federal Fire Ant Quarantine Act, enacted in 1958. Hay, turf grass, and ornamental plants are now subjected to inspection and insecticidal treatments before they may be transported or imported. Tiny parasitic worms called nematodes have been used as biological controls to reduce fire ant populations.[2,6-11]

According to two WHO reports from December 1962, a cooperative study was undertaken in 1959 with the Game and Fresh Water Fish Commission of Florida and the Division of Plant Industry of the Florida Department of Agriculture. The study concerned the use of the chemical heptachlor to eradicate imported fire ants. It also analyzed the effects of the chemical upon non-target species. A test plot of 1,250 acres in northwestern Florida was selected for the studies. One of the reports detailed the application of DDT dust for tick control that was applied to a 206-acre test plot of Texas prairie in 1949. It also described a study the same year of the effects of airplane applications of DDT upon forest invertebrates in Pennsylvania.[12,13]

In Florida, Louisiana, and Texas, fire ants *Solenopsis invicta* Buren and others have been released in efforts to control tick populations. In Louisiana, introduction of these ants was proven to reduce cattle *Anaplasmosis* infections. Anaplasmosis is an infection that is also found in many Lyme disease patients as a co-infection. In Baton Rouge and Pine Grove, Louisiana, various stages of Lone Star ticks (*Amblyomma americanum*) were released in areas that were heavily infested with fire ants. They were also released in test areas that contained anti-ant bait traps. The Lone Star ticks were released in August and September of 1970. By March of 1971, nearly three quarters of the released ticks were recovered from control areas; while none of the ticks were recovered from fire ant-infested areas. Therefore the whereabouts of about one quarter of the released ticks was unknown. Survivors probably went on to populate naturally and their offspring continue to propagate along with any infectious pathogens they harbored. Perhaps this is one way that Lone Star ticks became so well established in the southeastern US.[12-23]

Or perhaps populations of Lone Star ticks that were already present for several decades before these tests were simply augmented by the increased numbers of relatives that were released in the area to control fire ants. One can only speculate about the infections carried by ticks or fire ants, including which infections might be transmissible to humans. It is known that a Lyme-like illness called *Southern Tick Associated Rash Illness* or "STARI" is an infection that is carried by Lone Star ticks.

Several infectious disease experts claim that Lone Star ticks cannot transmit Lyme disease. A number of other reliable sources including military and USDA reports indicate however that Lone Star ticks are certainly able to transmit Lyme disease. It is obvious from at least the 1970s that the Lone Star ticks and whatever infections they carry have continued to spread north, east, and westward as they expand their host range. We will soon learn about the Lone Star virus – a virus carried by Lone Star ticks, and which may be partly responsible for the very Lyme-like STARI infections.[14-23]

A CDC/NIAID report from May 2004 indicates that the DNA for STARI was "first" characterized by Dr. Alan Barbour, et al. in 1996. A patent dated August 3, 1999 is for a diagnostic test for the "new" spirochete *Borrelia lonestari*. This is the spirochete that causes STARI. The Barbour patent discusses the organism's flagellin (tail) gene proteins, and a test that can detect the lonestari spirochete which the patent calls "unculturable." That this spirochete cannot be cultured is strange, especially since Dr. Barbour was able to specially modify a culture medium to isolate related *Borrelia burgdorferi* spirochetes in 1981.[19-23]

Why hasn't the patent been developed into a meaningful test if it can detect the STARI illness better than current diagnostic tests? Information about Lyme disease-transmitting Lone Star ticks was available from the military and the USDA during the 1980s, yet for some reason public health experts seem to continually overlook some of the most important information that is available about tickborne diseases. The government retained certain rights to the NIH-funded Barbour invention.[19-23]

The reference may suggest that *Borrelia lonestari* is not a true aggregate Bb spirochete, but another kind of spirochete that is very fragile; and one that is perhaps just a part of a complex infection. In other words, it is just one part that causes a Lyme-like illness, but it may be missing key ingredients that are found in Bb spirochetes. Perhaps STARI is a lot like Bb except that its fungi, viruses, and bacteriae are members of similar but different microbial families than those belonging to an aggregate Bb spirochete. We will learn more about another fragile so-called "unculturable" spirochete in upcoming chapters.[19-23]

Insect symbionts are infectious parasites that are found in an insect's body and which may or may not affect their host. There are a lot of them out there, and there are thousands of insect species. For example the red fire ant typically has a symbiont virus that has been identified as *Solenopsis invicta* virus or SINV-1. This virus contains structural proteins that are similar to the *Dicistroviridae* group. These are *Picorna*-like viruses (think polio). Florida researchers surveyed fire ant populations and found that SINV-1 was fairly widespread. Additional viruses have also been isolated and identified as SINV-2 and SINV-3. Scientists have also found sporulating microsporidian infections from mosquitoes in these ants. At least two strains were isolated from fire ants, including *Thelohania solenopsae* and *Mattesia* microsporidians. If fire ants now harbor what are typically mosquito infections, what happens when virus genes from genetically modified mosquitoes transfer into other insects, animals, or humans?[3-10,24-27]

Future fire ant control efforts will involve the laboratory rearing of South American fire ant decapitating flies (*Pseudacteon*, a phorid fly). Once permits are obtained, field releases will be undertaken. One study reportedly began September 2009 and will end September 2014. This research includes releasing at least two species of microsporidia-infected decapitating phorid flies (*Vairimorpha invictae* and *K. solenopsae*). The SINV-1, -2, and -3 viruses are carried within the decapitating fly guts as symbiont infections. The presence of these agents renders the flies useful trojan horse vectors of fire ant-infecting viruses. The question is whether humans or animals will also play host to vectoring insects with newly applied viruses. If so, in what way and how soon will unusual animal or human epidemics begin to emerge? If they do emerge, will anyone bother to tell the public or will they simply join the ranks of other "unknown" human infections?[28-30]

Filariasis – Nematode as Biological Control

Helminths, filaria, or *nematodes* all describe tiny parasitic roundworms. The worms vary in size from several inches in length to microscopic in size. They naturally reside in the upper layers of soil where they come into contact with ticks and other insects that crawl through their habitat. Nematodes naturally infect plants, mosquitoes, ticks, flies, beetles, other arthropods; and animals, birds, marine animals, and humans. Nematodes are also natural parasites of moths, butterflies, and their larvae. Nematodes are among the first natural parasites to be widely applied as biological controls against pest insects; and they have proven to be highly useful employees. Their application was initially attempted only in a few areas since they were difficult to culture (reproduce) in large numbers within a laboratory. It was not until the 1930s before efforts to mass produce nematodes as biological controls were considered successful. Despite the difficulties, studies were well underway in Russia and in the United States on the potential use of nematodes for insect control prior to World War II.[1]

Nematodes of agricultural importance are of the species *Merminthidae, Steinernematidae*, and *Tylenchida.* Any of these pathogens may be spread to the human population by any of thousands of species of vectoring insects. Nematodes were reportedly first observed in 1912 in southern California orange groves by scientist J.R. Hodges. A year later they were found in citrus groves in Alabama and Florida. They could have easily arrived in the bellies of the early parasitoids. Nematodes were first investigated in 1929 by Glaser and Fox when they studied the mortality of the Japanese beetle grub on a New Jersey golf course. A USDA Nematology specialist named Steiner later identified a species of nematode and named it *Neoaplectana glaseri.* According to the literature, only *Neoaplectana* were used as biological controls until 1960. The Rockefeller Institute for Medical Research scientists began studying nematodes as biological controls a short time later. Some nematode species that have been collected and identified, along with their place of origin are these:

Culicimermis sp. – Manitoba
Culicimermis schakhovii – USSR
Empidomermis cozii – West Africa
Hydromermis churchilliensis – Manitoba
Octomyomermis muspratti – Zambia
Octomyomermis troglodytis – CA, FL, LA
Paramermis Canadensis – British Columbia
Perutilimermis culicis – Louisiana, New Jersey[2-4]
Romanomermis communensis – Manitoba
Romanomermis culicivorax – California, Florida, Louisiana
Romanomermis hermaphrodita – Manitoba
Romanomermis iyengari – India
Romanomermis kiktoreak – Northwest Territories
Romanomermis nielseni – Wyoming
Strelkovimermis peterseni – Louisiana

The first scientist to suggest the use of nematodes for biological control work was Oldham in 1933. Field tests using nematodes commenced in the US in 1935 at ten locations, starting in New Jersey. The following year about four dozen applications were made in the field. In 1939, a statewide colonization program for nematodes was established in New Jersey. Releases took place at five hundred and sixty-three locations in the state; and were repeated in other New England states until scientists were able to verify that the parasites were well established.[2,5-8]

During the 1940s, field experiments using nematode species *Steinernema carpocapsae* were undertaken at Belleville, New Jersey during attempts to use them to parasitize Colorado potato beetles. The *Neoaplectana* species of nematodes are more easily infected with microbes, and can be efficiently mass-produced. It was discovered that *Neoaplectana* and *Heterorhabditis* species of nematodes are prolific parasites of fall armyworms. Therefore these nematodes were exploited as natural control agents of the armyworms, which are highly pervasive and destructive agricultural crop pests.[2,5-8]

During the 1950s, nematode species *N. glaseri* was applied to field plots in Alabama, Florida, Louisiana, Mississippi, and North Carolina to control white fringed beetle larvae. By the mid-1950s, about 90% of California citrus crops were considered infested with the *Tylenchulus semipenetrans* nematodes. By 1962, about half of Florida's trees were also infested.[2,5-8]

What must be considered with respect to nematodes is that they are not pathogenically sterile parasites. In fact they can be parasitized by medically important rickettsiae, protozoae, microsporidiae, bacteriae, viruses, and fungal infections that affect not only insects, but also mammalian hosts. In addition, nematodes may harbor spirochetes such as borreliae, leptospires, and spiroplasmas. According to a 1970s textbook, merminth nematodes found in tsetse flies may cause human infections. This is very concerning since the presence of multiple infectious agents living inside of the parasites and parasitoid insects that are used as natural biological controls can distribute multi-tiered, mixed infections and cause human diseases. According to a WHO International Conference report dated 1973, some nematode species that were employed as biological controls include these species:[5]

Mermithidae (parasites of terrestrial and fresh-water insects)
Reesimermis nielseni (used extensively in field trials against mosquitoes. This species was mass-produced by the USDA. Southeast Asian field trials occurred under WHO auspices by 1973 using this species.
Steinernematidae (including *Neoaplectana* and the DD-136 strain of *N. carpocapsae*)
Allantonematidae (including *Heterotylenchus,* used to control flies, sterilizes host)
Neotylenchidae (natural parasites of wasps and weevils)[9]

Some of the ways humans can contract nematodes are by mechanical inoculation through an insect bite or sting; contact with an infected animal, or infected human body fluids or feces. Various species of parasitic nematodes are also found naturally in the soil and water, so some contact with these parasites may be unavoidable. Ingestion of foods which contain these organisms or their eggs may subject us to infections or allergies, and nematode eggs are commonly found on produce. Fish and shellfish including herring, cod, frogs, prawns, snails, clams, other crustaceans; and freshwater, brackish, and ocean fish all contain various species of worms, nematodes, and flukes. Many people are unaware that they have a nematode infection.[10-17]

During scientific efforts to identify the agent of Lyme disease, on November 13, 1981, *Ixodes dammini* ticks were collected from Shelter Island, New York vegetation and provided to Dr. Willy Burgdorfer at Rocky Mountain Laboratories in Hamilton, Montana. Inside the body of one of the ticks, Dr. Burgdorfer reportedly discovered thirty or more microfilaria (nematodes) that were approximately 0.70 to 1.32mm in length. Dr. Burgdorfer assumed they were ingested during a blood meal when the ticks were larvae or nymphs, and that the worms persisted without development. Their presence in ticks has essentially been dismissed by many scientists. However patients with Lyme disease typically have nematodes as co-infections. Furthermore they respond favorably to treatments of anti-helminths including Ivermectin, Stromectal, diatomaceous earth, or iodine treatments. (Iodine also kills bacteria such as leptospires according to sources with as little as 1 ppm after 10 minutes in vitro [the lab].)[16,17]

An antibiotic called Alinia (Nitazoxanide) has been used to try to kill nematodes and other intestinal parasites. The tetracycline antibiotic doxycycline sterilizes the worms, which prevents their reproduction, by killing an important nematode reproductive symbiont parasite called *Wolbachia.* The nematodes thereafter live out their life cycle and eventually die. Since they make their home in the tissues of the eye, destroying them too rapidly can cause a loss of vision. When I could no longer suddenly tolerate foods that contained large amounts of iodine, and my body reacted adversely whenever I held a tube of Ivermectin to deworm our horses, this became a major clue as a Lyme patient that I may have a nematode or an iodine-sensitive spirochetal infection; or both.[16,17]

Rodents and other insects besides ticks carry nematode parasites including *Acanthocheilonema viteae*; a microscopic round worm common to soil. Ivermectin has shown effectiveness against a wide range of parasitic worms including *A. viteae*, but it is not lethal to adult forms except at higher doses (200 mg/kg for 5 days) where it killed 74% of adults. Other gut parasites of importance worth mentioning are *Capillaria* and *Angiostrongylus.* These worms are found in certain species of birds and rats respectively. These parasites also have fish, prawns, crabs, and snails as intermediate hosts. The latter parasite has been known to cause cases of meningitis in human infections. Nematodes may be one of the more important infections in Lyme patients.[14,16,17]

Because nematodes are parasites of insects such as flies, mosquitoes, ticks, and higher animals, scientists have been studying their usefulness as biological control trojan horse delivery systems. This means that nematodes or other gut residing pathogens can be used against targeted insect populations as biological controls by harboring their own (nested) infections.[18]

At present the biological properties of nematodes are being studied for their antibody-provoking ability for use within future animal and human vaccines. From several current patents assigned to the Heska Corporation (Ft. Collins, Colorado), we learn about the role of nematode transglutaminase. These enzymes initiate bonding between proteins and peptides (two or more amino acids). In two patent inventions are references to multivalent protective compounds useful for vaccines and diagnostic tests. Multivalent means having multiple (>3) antibody and/or antigen-binding sites.[19-23]

Patents describe nematode transglutaminase proteins which can be attached to one or more compounds. They are designed to protect against infections caused by viruses or bacteria. Some of the pathogens targeted by the inventions include borreliae, leptospirae, *E. coli,* helicobacter, mycoplasmae, neorickettsiae, rickettsiae, bartonellae, bacilli; fungi such as aspergillus, blastomyces, candida, chlamydia, coccidioides, cryptococcus, histoplasma; and parasites leishmania, cryptosporidium, babesia, giardia, plasmodium, or trypanosoma. We could see a future vaccine against Lyme for example that incorporates nematode proteins. The reason Bb would be included in this list is because the pathogens listed here are transmissible by vectoring insects, including ticks. This means that each of these infections is found inside vectoring insects and arthropods (i.e. ticks). Because of this fact, any of these pathogens may be found among patients bitten or stung by same.[19,20,23-25]

There are roughly eight "useful" nematode enzymes identified since 1959, including blood coagulation protein factor XIII, which was discovered in 1948. Factor thirteen is a plasma enzyme that helps hemophiliacs with blood coagulation. We might think about how *the early blood products were made using nematode proteins*; and consider that nematodes carry infections including mycoplasmas, spiroplasmas,* and viruses; each of which have been implicated within patent inventions as causing diseases including AIDS. It is not difficult to imagine how blood products might have become contaminated with any number of viruses, since nematodes are present or were used within insecticides upon food crops such as cassava, a tuber similar to a potato; and a main staple of the African diet.† Likewise we can see how the subsequent outbreak of hepatitis and HIV/AIDS in human populations may also have occurred through the use, or contamination of blood products with co-infected nematodal enzymes.[22-24]

**The tickborne spiroplasmas are in the same Mollicute class as the animal mycoplasmas.The mycoplasmas are found in the blood of patients affected by many of the infectious diseases of our day including Lyme disease, Chronic Fatigue Syndrome, Fibromyalgia, Gulf War Illness, Alzheimer's, Lupus, Multiple Sclerosis, Parkinson's, Rheumatoid Arthritis, AIDS, and other illnesses.*

†*Cassava plants are frequently infected with Gemini viruses, which are renowned for reassorting with other viruses. I discuss cassava's importance to global industries and to human diseases including AIDS in my book "God Science."*

Transglutaminases are natural protein polymers that act as stabilizers and structural solidifiers. These are found in human hair, nails, skin, and the prostate. Catalytic reactions caused by these proteins are considered to be irreversible and according to scientific documents, they must be monitored carefully when used within genetic processes. (This may mean that if genetic constructs that use these enzymes fail, whatever harm they cause might have the potential to become permanent.)[23]

When we think about people who have immune or other gut problems, and we remember that nematodes are ubiquitous to the environment (either naturally or from applied biological controls); we might understand that food grains that have been contaminated with nematode proteins might irreversibly bind with genes or tissues in the human gut, to create permanent food allergies. Antibodies to tissue transglutaminase are sometimes found in people who suffer from digestive disorders such as celiac disease, a serious disorder of the small bowel. Perhaps such tissue-specific antibodies are formed in response to nematode infections, for example in Lyme patients with a celiac-like colitis. Elimination of gliadin-containing foods from the diet is typically helpful for these people. (Gliadin is gluten.) Therefore, perhaps it is not the wheat gluten that is the problem, but the nematodal proteins that may be attached to same, that the immune system recognizes as a foreign invader (antigen).[23-25]

Whether a person is genetically susceptible to a true "celiac disease" appears to be dependent upon the presence of at least one of two genes. However any organism or disease process that damages the gut lining can cause a celiac-like "leaky gut syndrome" whether one carries celiac genes or not. Of interest is that many Lyme patients (even those who do not carry celiac genes), suffer from leaky gut syndrome or a pseudo-membranous colitis. Removing gluten from the diet (or the foods that contain gluten and possibly nematodal proteins) usually helps a damaged gut to heal over time. But a greater contributor to gut damage may be the pore-forming, gut-degrading B.t. insecticides and other toxins sprayed or engineered into our foods.

Patients with certain neurological diseases may have high levels of tissue transglutaminase in their bodies (i.e. Parkinson's or Huntington's). Tissue transglutaminase has also been hypothetically described as a protein aggregator or joiner. An example of this kind of protein building occurs within the brains of Alzheimer's patients, where plaques are formed and deposited in brain tissues. Again I question whether tissue transglutaminase was first and foremost of nematodal or bacterial origin, and which becomes permanently attached to human tissues. Some Alzheimer's patients upon autopsy and examination of brain tissues had *Borrelia burgdorferi* spirochetes within the tissues; and many Lyme patients harbor covert nematode infections.[21-25]

What we may discover is that certain pathogens allow plaque building because they act as protein aggregators. Such plaque-building is also accomplished by spirochetes such as Bb; by parasitic nematodes; and with plant and insect spirochetes called *Spiroplasmas*. NPV viruses from insects (which are baculoviruses), also serve as efficient aggregators and plaque builders. Remember that baculoviruses have been engineered into, and applied as agricultural insecticides to which we have all been exposed. Viruses which infect spiroplasma strains, including a tick spiroplasma 277F agent, also produce plaques. The spiroplasma viruses are assigned different numbers, but are in general identified as SpV1-type viruses. These viruses are naked, rod-shaped, or filamentous viruses which resemble coliphage f1-type viruses. Coliphages are phagic viruses that infect bacteria such as *E. coli*, a gut bacteria found in wastewaters and in the human bowel.[21-25]

A paper describes the susceptibility of the western cherry fruit fly to at least five species of nematodes. Yet another describes how temperature differences affect the ability of various nematode species to infect moths. Nematodes and other organisms including *Borrelia burgdorferi, Borrelia japonica*, babesia, and rickettsiae species have been found within the bodies of soft and hard-shelled Egyptian ticks according to a 2008 study. Collaborative research experiments have taken place using Egyptian camel ticks and mosquitoes as shuttle vectors for biological controls. Shuttle vectors are the proverbial trojan horse where the shuttle agent is a bacteria, virus, or nematode that harbors either single or multiply-layered infections.[24-32]

A grant was awarded to University of Kentucky scientists to study the eradication of filariasis (nematodal infections) in endemic field sites. The studies were to transition from field trials into a full vector eradication program in Polynesia. The grant's scheduled end date was listed as mid-2011.[33]

A 1987 patent for membrane-coated hydrogel encapsulated nematodes was granted to a California company. The device includes the use of a virus and a fungus that are inserted into nematodes. The co-infected nematodes are subsequently released as shuttle vectors. Just like the chemical pesticides, shuttle vectors can be sprayed or delivered by other means to targeted areas. The tiny nematode-containing capsules can also be aerially rained upon our heads, released from above cloud cover.[34]

Nematodes are highly antigenic (immune stimulating) organisms. Patients with zinc deficiencies may have impaired immune responses to nematode parasites in their intestinal and peripheral sites. The paper discussed the Th1 to Th2 shift in immune response in patients with nematode infections. This is a similar immune event often found with Lyme patients. This makes sense if patients are exposed to insects that are co-infected with nematodes. A deficiency in zinc supports the growth of parasites in the gut including nematodes, and many Lyme patients suffer from zinc deficiencies, as well as food or medicine intolerances. Such intolerances may be caused by weakened epithelial cells of the gut membrane, as zinc deficiency contributes to membrane atrophy. In short, Lyme patients and people who are low in zinc may have difficulty absorbing essential nutrients from their diet since the gut is too damaged from parasites – organisms that were probably originally applied as biological controls.[34,35]

Sawflies and Suspensions

Serious pests of heavily forested regions of the world are the numerous species of sawflies. Sawflies are thought to have accidentally arrived in North America, and their populations have been monitored since 1939. About seventy years ago sawflies threatened the spruce forests of southeastern Canada, and those of the northeastern US. Some of the first records regarding sawfly introductions into North America revealed their presence in 1925 in New Jersey; and in 1939 in Windsor, Ontario. One species, the European pine sawfly or fox-colored sawfly (Neodiprion sertifer), was already causing serious damage to pine trees in Michigan, New Jersey, and Ohio by 1943.[1-3]

There are several insect nuclearpolyhedrosis viruses (NPV) which typically infect sawflies. One is *Borrelina diprionis,* and is abbreviated as "NeseNPV" after the insect's name (*Neodiprion sertifer*). This virus typically kills young larvae; and infects, but does not kill older instar* larvae. Borrelina viruses can remain latent (inactive) in adults until populations increase. There stressors from overcrowding and food competition cause them to activate. Many sawfly species are infected or are susceptible to viruses which destroy the midgut epithelial tissues. Because of this, DNA baculoviruses and RNA viruses are considered to be the most effective biological controls. Remember the RNA viruses and the baculoviruses typically associate with one another. Alone they are infective, but together they are superinfective.[4-7]

**Each phase of a caterpillar molt cycle is called an instar.*

The virus classification *Borrelina Paillot* includes two genera: *Borrelina,* and *Morator mora.* (The rice beetle, a scarab, is *Dyscinetus morator*). Czech parasitologist Stanislaus Josef Matias von Prowazek originally described the yellow (jaundice) disease of the silkworm as *Chlamydozoon bombycis*, although it was later renamed *Borrelina bombycis.* In a manner of speaking, perhaps silkworms get a version of yellow fever, which has a mosquito-borne version that is infectious to humans. *Borrelina Paillot* members include the NPV virus *Borrelina bombycis* (BmNPV) or jaundice milky disease which attacks silkworms. Viruses in this family also attack gypsy moths as *Borrelina reprimens*; the nun moth as *Borrelina efficiens*; and there are those which infect sawflies. This group of borrelina viruses and the baculoviruses are among the most important microbes to have been used in microbial insecticides. They are also the most important to the world of genetic engineering, and possibly to the evolution of many infectious diseases of this era.[8-13]

Dr. von Prowazek discovered the agent of epidemic typhus. He would also study rabies, vaccinia, and scarlet fever among other important infectious diseases. *Vaccinia* is a satellite virus which helps other infectious viruses such as polio or smallpox become complete, infective agents capable of causing disease. Without this satellite virus, polio or smallpox viruses may infect but not cause disease. A virus that lacks a satellite virus helper is called an incomplete virus, or a focus-forming agent. When a satellite helper is present, the incomplete virus becomes a complete, infective virus. Focus forming agents can cause cancers because they try to replicate without key proteins they would get from their satellite. This causes protein folding errors, and the cells that are infected by them begin to grow erratically. If the body does not keep these cells in check, cancer occurs.[8-16]

The *vaccinia* virus has been used within smallpox and some polio vaccines as an interfering virus* (satellite). This satellite helps the body become resistant to one aspect of a duo of infectious viruses that together cause disease. Scientists cannot use an infectious agent such as smallpox in a vaccine for obvious reasons. Instead they use a virus that is a satellite helper, which allows the body to develop immunity to one virus of what would be a duo of viruses that form a complete infectious virus pair. This is a similar pattern that occurs with other infectious diseases. Perhaps von Prowazek was the first to discover the cooperative action of viral satellitism. This is the association of tiny viruses to larger infectious agents (i.e. viruses, bacteria, or fungi) to cause diseases.[8-16]

**In simple terms, an interfering virus is an infectious virus which blocks viral replication by being the dominant virus during mixed infections. Interfering viruses also dominate mixed infections inside the insect body. For example mosquitoes which harbor La Crosse, EEE, and WEE viruses will have one virus as a dominant infection, while others may contribute symptoms (or not). Symptoms of the passive viruses will be less noticeable than those of the dominant virus. This common natural process is exploited in genetic engineering and insecticidal formulas.*

Incomplete or focus-forming agents are viruses that lack a satellite partner. These partly infective viruses are capable of causing cancer since they lack genes they normally receive from a donor satellite virus. Therefore when they try to duplicate, the process is faulty (improper protein folding). Folding seems to work correctly only in the presence of a satellite helper, which donates the necessary genes or other components. Infectious viruses do not only have a single satellite partner, they may pair with any compatible RNA virus to create what is called a pseudovirus. This pairing with an infrequent partner allows the dominant virus to create an infection similar to, but different than polio for example. Although the result will be infectious, it will produce a slightly different disease than a "normal" polio virus paired with its typical satellite virus.

The *borrelina* viruses are examples of important satellite helper viruses that were exploited by placing them into the environment to augment natural insect infections and the early applied insecticides. These applications were bold but unpredictable because their release allowed them to freely associate with any infectious agents naturally found in the environment and in insects. But then again, they were released specifically to create insect epizootics (disease outbreaks).[8-16]

What was probably a polyhedrosis virus was recorded as early as the sixteenth century. The silkworm virus *Borrelina bombycis* is a filterable RNA virus which produces ultramicroscopic granules. It may be visualized under darkfield microscopy, and was characterized as: "Viruses [which induce] polyhedral, wilt, and other diseases; hosts, Lepidoptera, so far as known." Jaundice or yellows disease of silkworms was the very first insect virus ever to be scientifically described. Scientists are said to know more about this one insect virus alone than perhaps any other.[8,17,18]

It is interesting to fully investigate the relationships between the insect yellows diseases and the yellows diseases of flowers (i.e. aster yellows) as compared to yellow fever, the human infection transmitted by mosquitoes. Aster yellows is caused by a mycoplasma-like phytoplasma (a plant spirochete), and possibly also *Spiroplasma citri* (another spirochete). Yellow fever is caused by *Flavivirus fibricus*, an insect virus, and a leptospira spirochete. Perhaps the "yellows" viruses are simply satellite viruses that bind with spirochetal bacteriae to cause yellows diseases of plants, insects, animals, and humans.[8,17,18]

The borrelina virus (NeseNPV) was first introduced into the US in 1950 from Sweden, to be tried as a biological control agent. This was the same year that extensive field trials of the fermented soil bacteria *Bacillus thuringiensis* (B.t.) were also taking place throughout the world. The presence of B.t. and other microbial insecticides as global facilitators of insect infections may be key to understanding the emergence over a century and a half of novel diseases of insect, animal, and human origin. After all, their method of infection is to degrade gut tissues and to introduce and reactivate latent infections.[4-7]

Countries abroad such as Finland also treated pine sawfly infestations using borrelina viruses. Early products which contained these viruses were developed and sold under the trade names *Neocheck-S* and *Lecontvirus*. The microbial control "B.t." is now typically used to control sawfly infestations in many areas. Remember that NPV and GV viruses of insects are baculoviruses (DNA viruses). As such, they are members of the same group of viruses that have been extensively used as microbial enhancers to agricultural and industrial insecticides, especially in the genetically engineered formulas.[4-7]

The sawfly as a globally important pest insect cannot be understated. In Europe the largest population explosions were observed in southeastern forests from 1936-1938; 1947-1951; and from 1957-1960. In the Ukraine, the common pine sawfly was more harmful than the European pine sawfly, and caused significant outbreaks from 1945 through 1966 in forests in the Asian, Siberian, Tomsk Oblast, (Russia), Belorussia, Austria, Czechoslovakia, Finland, and Hungarian regions. The first outbreak was recorded in eastern Siberia in 1938, although the European pine sawfly virus was first described in 1913 by Escherich. From 1950 to 1955 scientists P.A. Polozhentsev and N.I. Korovina studied diseased pine sawfly larvae from the Voronezh region. They suggested that in both outbreaks larval death was caused by bacteremia from *Bacillus septicimiae lophyri.* Scientists V.Y. Shiperovich and P.P. Maslakovetz in 1925, and other scientists from 1939 to 1964 also noticed a similar bacteremia taking place in sawfly species.[19]

In studies performed in the Tomsk region by L.I. Burtseva, the strain *Bacillus thuringiensis* was found in larvae, although it was felt not to have been very virulent. In that instance, B.t. was probably a bacterial infection that facilitated bacteremia caused by an additional pathogen such as a virus. Note that this is the exact reason why B.t. is used as a global insecticide. By introducing B.t. bacteria into the insect's environment through insecticides or genetically engineered plants, these phagic bacteriae facilitate the erosion of the insect's gut membranes; introduce the accompanying insecticidal cocktails, or reactivate naturally latent insect viruses to cause disease. The questions to ask then are how are the microbial insecticides that are used on a global scale impacting the non-targeted animal and human species whose gut tissues might also be degraded? What if the phagic bacteria from B.t. are able to bind with other bacteria in the environment, to cause a new method of entering the human body and systemic infections that differ from the way B.t. infects insects?[19]

The sawfly viruses *Borrelina reprimens* and *Borrelina diprionis* were both introduced as biological controls in the US beginning with limited field tests undertaken by scientists from the USDA Forest Insect Laboratory in New Haven, Connecticut in 1951, a year after they arrived from Sweden. At first the sawfly virus *Borrelina reprimens* was deployed in test areas near the lab. This baculovirus is the agent of "wilt" disease in gypsy moths. These first applications were followed by the release of *Borrelina diprionis*. Take note that these field trials took place in an area of the US where the first clustered cases of Lyme disease emerged. We must remember also that these viruses occur naturally, and can be transmitted by infected insects. Other polyhedral sawfly viruses could also have been attempted at this time since they were mentioned in another scientific paper from this period. Some of the viruses that were released may have included *Neodiprion lecontei* (NeleNPV) from the red-headed pine sawfly; and an NPV from *Neodiprion pratti*, another sawfly species.[4-7,20-23]

In 1949, diseased sawfly larvae were sent to Ontario, Canada from Sweden for testing. By 1950, limited field trials were undertaken to determine if the *Neodiprion sertifer* NPV would be an effective biological control. After the Connecticut field trials, larger trials began in 1953 using pressure sprayers, mist blowers, and aircraft as insecticide delivery vehicles. Effective sawfly controls were fully developed by 1953. Note that this period preceded all reported cases of a Lyme-like infection that would emerge over the next three decades in this same area. (There were a few New York patients who experienced an ECM rash during the late 1940s; and from whose skin lesions, spirochetes would be isolated.) Remember that milky disease viruses (NPVs) were also being deployed at this time. The cytoplasmic polyhedrosis viruses, also called cypoviruses or CPVs, include the reoviruses. Borrelina viruses are members of the reovirus family. CPV family members were added to microbial insecticides beginning in the 1950s in New Haven, Connecticut according to the literature.[1-3,5,22,24-26]

Diseased sawfly larvae from Maryland were used to mass-produce their viruses by 1956. About twenty-five to fifty acres of the Beltsville Experimental Forest in Laurel, Maryland were sprayed by helicopter with the new biological controls according to a 1961 paper. With indications that field trials were successful, the new insect viruses were put into use over wider areas by 1962. In fact, their arrival had been quite timely because by the 1950s, sawflies had already damaged pine forests in the eastern US including in Virginia and North Carolina. The sawfly decimated areas covered approximately fourteen million acres. Such applications help spread these viruses across wider areas, allowing them to become potential satellite virus partners to the baculoviruses used in the applied insecticides.[1-3,5,22,24-26]

In a 1965 published report from the USDA Northeastern Forest Insect Laboratory in New Haven, Connecticut; Entomologist Dr. Franklin B. Lewis indicated that by 1960, the insect pathology section of the station's lab had a quantity of sawfly insect virus (polyhedral virus from *Neodiprion sertifer*) that it was willing to provide as a sample to interested scientists. The station was also willing to provide a starter culture for scientists who were undertaking a laboratory rearing method to build a supply of insect baculoviruses for use in the field as microbial insecticides. Additional information was also available upon request from the New Haven laboratory on how to collect and process small and large polyhedral virus suspensions. We have no idea what other agents might have been lurking within the insects or the formulas used for these early insecticides.[22]

The USDA New Haven laboratory was one of the central points for biological control agent testing in the US. Scientists at the facility appear to have been the first to widely deploy the sawfly borrelina viruses during regional field trials undertaken as early as 1951. It appears that American scientists obtained their initial samples from Sweden. Other countries (i.e. Romania) which held cooperative agreements with the US may have obtained their own virus stocks from the USDA lab as early as 1951, or they also may have obtained samples from Sweden. We must take notice of these activities as they may have played a role in the global dissemination of important insect viruses. These viruses may have been capable of causing the emergence of not only insect, but also animal and human epidemics.[4,5,22]

From a 1970 registered patent text we may see that insect polyhedrosis and granulosis viruses are sometimes freed from their inclusion bodies (capsules) in the laboratory. This process creates infectious protein particles that might help explain the origin of "prions." These naked virus particles are mixed together in a lab to fabricate viral concentrates for insecticidal use. Once the viral particles are removed from their capsules, they are capable of binding to other viruses or bacteria to establish new, complete, and highly virulent agents. This binding activity significantly ramps up the killing effectiveness of insecticidal formulas where they are applied. If these virus particles are transmitted to insects, animals, or humans, they may lie dormant as proviruses. There they will remain quiescent until reactivated at a later point by a triggering agent (i.e. another virus or bacterium).[27]

The patent also refers to a patent that is assigned to the National Cash Register Company of Dayton, Ohio. This patent describes a formula to protect virus particles from ultraviolet degradation. UV light kills viruses in insecticidal formulas unless they are first encapsulated within a protective coating. These shells prevent deactivation of the viruses, which prolongs their use in the field. The viruses intended for the invention include NPVs (polyhedron in shape, and which contain rod-shaped virus particles); CPVs (polyhedrons with spherical virus particles); GVs (granular shaped with one rod-shaped virus particle in each granule); and non-inclusion viruses (unenclosed, and spherical or polyhedron shaped).[27-34]

The 1970 patent also mentions the sawfly virus *Neodiprion sertifer*; and references older patents including a 1958 USDA-assigned patent. The invention describes a process of dehydrating biological materials (i.e. microbial cultures) which can be stored for lengthy periods without a loss of infectivity. It also references an early B.t. spore pesticide patent from 1963; a 1967 patent for "termite control by induced epizootics of entomophagous microorganisms" and a patent for anhydrous liquid suspensions of "biologics" which is assigned to the American Cyanamid Company (Stamford, CT). The latter patent may be significant because it describes how insect viruses can be mixed with chemical propellants or refrigerants (some of which may be mutagenic), to be used as organic pesticides or soil inoculants. The compounds may use dichloro-tetra*fluoro*ethane (cryofluorane), dichloro*fluoro*methane, trichloro*fluoro*methane (freon-11), trichloro-tri*fluoro*ethane, or dibromotetra*fluoro*ethane (halon); or a pesticide tetrachlorodi*fluoro*ethane (anti-nematode and anti-fluke). Notice the fluorine (fluoride) compounds. Fluoride is a significant organic chemical that not only produces strong chemical bonds, it may also be shown to negatively impact the enzymatic activities of the microbes of the internal and external environments in which they are found.[27-34]

A 1973 patent assigned to the McLaughlin Gormley King Co., a Minnesota pesticide and agrochemical chemical manufacturer founded in 1902, is an early polyhedrosis (NPV) and granulosis virus (GV) formula for use in biological controls. These are certainly not the only patents to describe methods to protect insecticides from ultraviolet radiation and other elements, such as natural or chemical pollutants. The patent describes how the viruses are liberated from their inclusion bodies (removed from shell). The virus is then joined with a protein to produce a virus concentrate that is useful as an insecticidal oil. (Some oils contain petroleum-based hydrocarbons.) Some of the NPVs or GVs that can be utilized by the patent include these from the following insects, (insect's common name in parentheses):

Lymontria monacha (nun moth)
Choristoneura fumiferana (spruce budworm)
Spodoptera frugiperda (fall armyworm)
Prodenia eridania (southern armyworm)
Heliothis virescens (tobacco budworm)
Pseudaletia unipuncta (armyworm)
Porthetria dispar (gypsy moth)
Heliothis zea (corn earworm)
Trichoplusia ni (cabbage looper)
Colias eurytheme (alfalfa caterpillar)
Autographa californica (alfalfa looper)
Spodoptera exigua (beet armyworm)

Pieris rapae (imported cabbage worm)
Diprion hercyniae (european spruce sawfly)
Neodiprion pratti banksianae (jackpine sawfly)
Peridroma margaritosa (variegated cutworm)
Prodenia praefica (western yellow-striped armyworm)[37]
Pectinophora gossypiella (pink bollworm)
Neodiprion sertifer (european pine sawfly)
Tipula paludosa (crane fly)
Prodenia ornithogalli (yellow-striped armyworm)

An American Cyanamid patent for anhydrous liquid suspensions is useful for biological controls or vaccines. Once deployed into the environment, insecticides which contain engineered microbes meant to target insects could initiate animal or human epidemics for which vaccines and antibiotics thereafter become necessary.[33]

Another patent for an oil-based insecticide describes large DNA viruses including GVs and NPVs that are freed from their inclusion bodies. This freedom of naked viral particles in an oil suspension makes the viruses more stable and capable of withstanding storage for longer periods. When altered in this way, the virus particles are capable of infecting greater numbers of insects than their naturally encapsulated counterparts. According to the patent:

> "The total number of individual virus particles in that body would be potentially capable of infecting a large number of target insects if the virus particles were liberated from the polyhedral inclusion body before application to the insects. Thus, by freeing the particles from the polyhedral inclusion bodies, the infectivity titer is greatly increased by a factor which is theoretically proportional to the average number of virus particles within each body."[27]

The list that follows describes viruses that were applicable to the oil-based pesticide patent. The list provides readers with a glimpse of some of the many insects being targeted by biological controls by 1970 when the patent was filed.[27]

Lymontria monacha (nun moth)
Trichoplusia ni (cabbage looper)
Heliothis zea (corn earworm)
Prodenia eridania (southern armyworm)
P. praefica (western yellow-striped armyworm)
Heliothis virescens (tobacco budworm)
Colias eurytheme (alfalfa caterpillar)
Pieris rapae (imported cabbage worm)
Neodiprion sertifer (european pine sawfly)
Diprion hercyniae (european spruce sawfly)
Peridroma margaritosa (variegated cutworm)[27]
Porthetria dispar (gypsy moth)
Choristoneura fumiferana (spruce budworm)
Spodoptera frugiperda (fall armyworm)
Pseudaletia unipuncta (armyworm)
Spodoptera exigua (beet armyworm)
Prodenia ornithogalli (yellow-striped armyworm)
Autographa californica (alfalfa looper)
Pectinophora gossypiella (pink bollworm)
Neodiprion pratti banksianae (jackpine sawfly)
Tipula paludosa (crane fly)

A recent patent discusses methods of detecting the DNA of "bioagents." Bioagents according to the device includes these pathogens; most of which have been used within applied insecticides; and some of which have been studied during periods of conflict for use as biowarfare weapons.

Bacillus anthracis (Anthrax)
Franciscella tularensis (Tularemia)
Burkholderia mallei (Glanders)
Rickettsia typhii (Epidemic typhus)
Coxiella burnetii (Q fever)
Escherichia coli
Clostridium botulinum
Borrelia burgdorferi (Lyme disease)
Yersinia pestis (Pneumonic plague)
Brucella suis, B. abortus, B. melitensis (Brucellosis)
Salmonella (Typhoid fever)
Rickettsia prowasekii (Endemic typhus)
Chlamydia pneumonia
Bacillus cereus
Pseudomonas aeruginosa
Vibrio cholera[35]

With the exception of *Borrelia burgdorferi,* many of these agents are commonly engineered into biological insecticides, although it is entirely possible that Bb is actually an aggregate organism that has been formed through the aggregation of several applied bioagents. The patent also identifies *Coccidioides immitis,* which causes coccidioidomycosis (San Joaquin valley fever), an important fungal infection that is endemic in the American west and southwest, and present throughout the US. The patent describes "biological warfare toxin genes" that may be detected by the invention including:[35]

> "...botulism, T-2 mycotoxins, ricin, staph enterotoxin B, shigatoxin, abrin, aflatoxin, *Clostridium perfringens* epsilon toxin, conotoxins, diacetoxyscirpenol, tetrodotoxin, and saxitoxin."

The biowarfare genes it mentions however sound much more like those found within the agricultural insecticides. We might also consider that the term "biowarfare" usually refers to the "natural" infections which come about as a result of the deployments of insecticides on or in agricultural crops and livestock animals.[35]

According to the patent, the invention may also be used to test livestock animals for diseases such as foot and mouth or mad cow disease. The latter is a prion disease. The human form of prion diseases is CJD or *Creutzfeldt-Jakob disease*. The variety found in wild deer is called *chronic wasting disease* (CWD). In sheep it is called *scrapie*, and in cattle, *mad cow disease* or bovine spongiform encephalopathy (BSE). The prion diseases are collectively called transmissible spongiform encephalopathies or (TSE). *The patent also describes how RNA viruses are all related, and how they are able to mutate.*

> "Biological warfare viral bioagents are mostly RNA viruses (positive-strand and negative- strand), with the exception of smallpox. Every RNA virus is a family of related viruses (quasispecies). These viruses mutate rapidly and the potential for engineered strains (natural or deliberate) is very high."[35]

Such mutations may occur not only under direction of *other viruses*, fungi, or bacteria, but also under the action of agricultural chemicals, industrial, or nuclear wastes, which act as catalysts. These pollutants affect not only the microbes in the environment, but those within applied insecticides, insects, animals, and humans. The extremely complex techniques of genetic engineering design mixed infections that are far more virulent and effective insecticides. Because insects, animals, and humans have similarities to our bodies and nervous systems, we are each in our own way vulnerable to the chemical and microbial cocktails that are and have been deployed – even those considered to be "safe" to use.[35]

For nearly a century and a half scientists have applied a wide variety of infective agents across the globe for the purpose of biological warfare against insect pests. They began these efforts long ago using fungi and parasitoids. Imported insects introduced natural epizootics into targeted insect populations. Once the use of microbial insecticides went global, the incidence of animal and human epidemics also rose. Historically speaking, several novel animal and human epidemics "coincidentally" appeared shortly after the introduction of each biological control method attempted.[36]

Since bioagents have been deployed around the world, the tools used could certainly explain the so-called "Lyme" disease, as well as other arthritic, neurologic, skin, "autoimmune," and immunodeficiency diseases in the global patterns that have emerged over a similar period. Although some reports claim that Lyme disease originated in Connecticut, this may be only partly true since similar microbial enhancements were applied in Europe and elsewhere up to a century earlier.

In those countries, Lyme-like illnesses also emerged during periods that preceded the Connecticut outbreak by roughly a century. The various deployments of microbial controls also easily explains why epidemics with seemingly similar origins differ in composition and pathogenicity, depending of course upon the regions where the pathogens and the vectoring insects are found. Such variability may be driven more by the different biological control formulas that were deployed. This variability includes whatever microbes were added to insecticides, and those that are found naturally in insects and the environment. This also reasonably explains the regional differences between *Borrelia burgdorferi* sensu lato (broad sense) strains, as well as why symptom presentations vary so much between continents, or even within a similar geographic region.[36]

When observing the various techniques of biological controls that were deployed over a century and a half, it is only natural to wonder whether these applications are responsible for many animal and human infections around the world. This question is more important to explore when we realize that despite assurances that biological controls are "safe," there have been repeated demonstrations of novel diseases emerging with each new technique deployed. Each process carries with it a certain amount of risk. There is often also a shocking lack of long-term safety data or independent scientific analyses which can prove safety and reliability of any insecticidal formulas. Of course there is no possible way to predict the long-term effects of releasing any genetically engineered insects. We must remember that the techniques and tools of genetic engineering are relatively new, and at best, poorly understood. Without proper legislation and oversight in place, the non-targeted human population will be among those impacted by global biological controls – with "untold" consequences.

The Tail of the Scorpion

Fungal spores have proven useful since the earliest days of biological warfare against pest insects. In recent years however, genetically modified fungi have been engineered to harbor potent natural toxins. These nerve agents are derived from the venom of scorpions, spiders, wasps, mites, and sea urchins to increase the killing effectiveness of fungal insecticides. Killing times of toxin-augmented fungi are markedly increased over those of wild-type fungi. The new engineered fungi also require fewer spores to be effective against the same number of insects; as tested on pine caterpillars and wax moths. Now more clever toxins appear inside the applied and engineered insecticides, and must be considered as important co-factors in patients who display neurologically toxic states, even after all evidence of bacterial infections have cleared.[1]

Coffee berry borers, one of the world's most devastating pests of coffee crops, are controlled by both fungi *Metarhizium anisopliae* and *Beauveria bassiana.* Both of these fungi have been genetically modified to express the scorpion toxin "AaIT." This combination greatly increases virulence. (Think about how many people drink coffee!) The "AaIT" toxin is the *Androctonus australis* Hector toxin from the Algerian scorpion. It is a protein peptide (think chain) that neurologically targets and binds to an insect's voltage-dependent, excitable sodium channels of cells. This connection affects nerve conduction by modifying the gating mechanisms. This in turn interferes with electrical signaling. Similar combinations were used to control the malaria-carrying *Aedes aegypti* mosquitoes, and the larvae of *Manduca sexta*, the tobacco hornworm moth. These same kinds of pathways are present in the human body and are responsible for nerve conduction, brain function, and muscle contraction and relaxation.[2-6]

Various fungi have also been genetically manipulated in the lab using insect baculoviruses, B.t. endotoxins, and scorpion toxins to produce some of the most effective insecticides ever imagined. The question is whether these toxic blends are also leading to more severe human neurological diseases upon exposure to the human population. An infective baculovirus construct (genetically engineered insecticide) can translocate, or insert the genes of a scorpion toxin directly into the cells of an insect's central nervous system. What if this also occurs in humans by vectoring insects that are infected with these recombinant constructs? AaIT scorpion toxin is especially toxic to yellow-fever mosquito larvae, and because of this is useful in controlling them. Can these scorpion toxin genes likewise be incorporated into the genes of human cells to cause permanent neurotoxic states? Furthermore what happens when these scorpion toxins meet the genetically modified mosquitoes or other insects that are being released in today's world as "population replacers"?[2-6]

The AaIT scorpion toxins and other toxicants like pyrethroids, sea anemone, local anesthetics, and anticonvulsants all cause various physiological effects when bound to receptors in the human body. Depending on the toxin and the receptor binding site, toxins can stimulate sodium ion influx. The chemical trypsin from the human pancreas works in the intestines to degrade some toxins. Plant, insect (i.e. spider, scorpion), animal (snake), and bacteria (i.e. borrelia) which express neurotoxins act as trypsin inhibitors. This allows their toxins to contribute to neurologic symptoms as seen in Lyme and other infectious diseases.[5-11]

Another baculovirus that has been used as a biological pesticide is the *Helicoverpa zea* Boddie nuclearpolyhedrosis virus (HzNPV). This one is useful against the tobacco budworm, cotton bollworms, and corn earworms. "HzNPV" is considered a more effective agent than the widely used alfalfa looper baculovirus *Autographa californica* (AcNPV). Patent inventions describe the use of the HzNPV virus in conjunction with scorpion toxins so we know that insecticides contain these formulas.[12-15]

One patent describes how some *A. australis* scorpion venom toxins which negatively affect humans have no such value against insects. This may be directly true however an unexpected indirect mechanism might produce a different result. Scorpion toxins "AaIT" and "AaHI" are those which are felt to be useful against insects. Here is a statement that can be found within four scorpion toxin-related patent inventions: "Understanding the molecular basis of this selectivity may lead to the development of chemical insecticides with reduced effects on mammals and other non-target organisms." The words "reduced effects" implies that non-targeted species have already been adversely affected by these toxins, and not that these toxins have proven to be safe.[12-15]

Several patents describe the earliest engineered baculovirus expression system (recombinant construct) that is identified as "pAc373." This system was apparently widely used before scientists realized that a key gene sequence was missing. Once they realized their mistake, scientists designed baculovirus expression systems based on the *Autographa californica* nuclearpolyhedrosis virus (AcNPV). *The Texas A&M University System (College Station, TX), and the University of Georgia Research Foundation are patent assignees on baculovirus expression systems.* The University of Georgia established a research laboratory to study the effects of radiation upon microbes. Perhaps the studies included the recombinant insecticides that are used agriculturally and industrially to treat water before it enters or exits nuclear plants; where water used in the cooling process is irradiated.[16-20]

Several patents describe spider or wasp toxins which may be engineered into biological controls or transgenic plants. In addition to scorpion excitotoxins that are stimulatory to the nervous system, depressant scorpion toxins may also be used. Toxins have also been cultivated from the venom of the Israeli yellow scorpion *Leiuirus quinquestriatus hebraeus.* There are two well-known toxins from this species, which are identified as "LqhIT1" and "LqhIT2." The venomous mechanisms from these toxins affects insects in a depressant manner similar to the AaIT toxins; although "AaIT" is considered to be an excitatory toxin. Both LqhIT toxins share similar receptor binding sites, but each has a different toxic activity.[21-24]

One fairly recent patent assigned to Australian scientists describes the use of funnel web spider venom to treat insects, larvae, and plants. Two spider species mentioned are from the genera *Atrax* and *Hadronyche.* These are highly aggressive funnel web spiders whose venom is toxic to mammals and humans. It is not enough that scorpion or snake venom has been exploited as an insect control. Now scientists use toxins from deadly spiders and retrovirus-like proteins (pro-retroviral DNA, pro-retroviral-like DNA and recombinant chimera derived therefrom) that are designed to provide transgenic soybeans and other crops with resistance to diseases, herbicides, and insects.[6,25,39]

What happens when such toxins enter the human body? How do we repair genes which wrongly express or are adversely affected by toxins that incorporate into the human body to permanently express neurotoxins? What happens if insecticidal formulas contribute to the formation of new human retroviruses?

Many patents describe the use of multiple toxins as insecticides. For example biopesticides are designed with the *Autographa californica* virus (AcNPV) and with scorpion endotoxins. The combination of these two agents is abbreviated as "AcNPV-AaIT." Evidence of scorpion toxin and baculovirus constructs for use in GM crops is widely available and described within numerous patents.[6,25]

The AaIT scorpion toxin has been shown to cross the midgut tissues of the flesh fly *Sarcophago falculata* through a distinct segment in its midgut. This hints that these toxins may be able to permeate other insect gut tissues as well. This will allow the transfer of insecticidal toxins to insects that may pass on these constructs to animals and humans. Various studies were undertaken to determine the paralytic potency of the AaIT toxin against all kinds of insects including house flies, fruit flies, and blow flies.[5,25-27]

When this toxin is used with a baculovirus, proteins are expressed directly within the insect. When this design was tested on silkworm larvae, it caused tremors consistent with sodium channel blocking. It also caused the insects to stop feeding and increased the period between initial infection and death. Could such designs affect human hosts in a similar manner, and cause tremors or other neurologic symptoms from similar sodium channel disruptions? Human diseases which produce neurotoxin-related symptoms (including tremors) are Lyme disease, Multiple Sclerosis, Parkinson's, Alzheimer's and Amyotrophic Lateral Sclerosis (ALS). Perhaps even in patients whose infections have been cleared, the lingering effects of pesticidal scorpion and other toxins may continue to cause symptoms because of damaged receptors, nerve pathways, or continual gene expression.[5,25-27]

An insect baculovirus called *Trichoplusia ni* (TnNPV) is another example of a virus that has been combined with AaIT scorpion toxins to improve killing speed. Chinese studies revealed that genetic constructs using *Helicoverpa armigera* (HearNPV) virus were used as pesticides against cotton bollworms. This virus could be recombinantly modified to become more toxic by deleting one gene and replacing it with an AaIT scorpion toxin gene. Remember that the insecticidal cocktails that use viruses and "natural" neurotoxins are used in insecticides which also contain the bacteria "B.t." B.t. acts as an introductory mechanism into the insect's gut where it degrades the gut membranes, allowing entry of the highly potent insecticidal toxins into the insect's body.[28]

While scientists do not appear to understand the mechanisms of how B.t. or scorpion toxins work, they do understand the importance of manipulating sodium and calcium channels in insects. Those who design insecticides know that by incorporating calcium salts or other calcium modulators into B.t. preparations, that the effects of B.t. endotoxins can be regulated in insects.[29]

In the human body, the cardiac, skeletal, muscle, brain, aorta, and lung systems have what are called dihydropyridine receptors. These are voltage-dependent, calcium channel receptors that are controlled by a human gene (CACNA1S). Persons with an error in this gene suffer muscle weakness or paralysis, and decreased potassium levels in the blood. Infections such as Lyme disease and other neurotoxic states which affect these channels produce similar symptoms. Perhaps this is caused by the negative effects of recombinant neurotoxins, and/or suppression of the CACNA1S gene during infection.

There are a number of scientific papers which describe how scorpion toxins negatively impact the human body. They activate macrophages of the immune system; alter intracellular functions; and damage the cells of the kidneys and pancreas. Most notably, scorpion toxins exert negative actions upon the pancreatic islet cells. It is entirely possible that scorpion toxins like those used in the agricultural insecticides may damage organs. This may be the reason there has been an increase in pancreatic-related diseases. These illnesses include pancreatitis, pancreatic cancers, hepatitis, and diabetes. It is important to state that CPV (viruses) have been found in scorpions, and it is possible that latent scorpion viruses and toxins are contributors to human diseases.[29-38]

Can the genetically engineered insecticides which include scorpion and other neurotoxins affect human genes enough to cause neurotoxic states even after an infection is cured? If so, could this be why some Lyme patients who have undergone experimental gene therapies (i.e. stem cell transplants) have occasionally improved? Is "gene therapy" to be the medical cure of the future? Do new stem cells help to replace defective genes that now wrongly contain insect viruses and toxins in our DNA? If so, we should be asking if the intense scientific interests toward the expansion of stem cell technologies has been brought about due to genetic damage that may be caused by the potent, recombinant insecticides that are supposed to be aimed only at insects – formulas that unfortunately appear to be harming the non-targeted human species as well. ❑

Three: The Elements of Surprise Epidemics

Arboviruses and Multiple Infections

In 1940 Yale scientists found an "adventitious agent" (contaminant) in cell cultures that was labeled in a paper as a "mystery virus." The new virus was uniquely different than St. Louis and Japanese B encephalitis viruses. Until 1940, human tickborne encephalitis viruses were thought to be restricted to the thick forests of the Taiga region of the Russian Far East. Now scientists were wondering if tickborne encephalitis viruses had come to America. What was once thought of as "polio" or "atypical poliomyelitis" infections was proving to involve tickborne encephalitis and other arboviruses which produce polio-like symptoms. Arboviruses are arthropod-borne viruses where "arthro" means jointed legs.[1-4]

In 2010, scientists from Columbia University published a paper that discussed polymicrobial infections of New York ticks. Their focus was to determine through PCR* testing, the percentage of ticks that carried mixed infections. Approximately 70% of ticks tested had at least one organism from a group which included *Borrelia burgdorferi, Anaplasma phagocytophilum, Babesia microti, Borrelia miyamotoi,*† and *Powassan* virus. Anaplasma is an intracellular infection. *Borrelia miyamotoi* is a human relapsing fever, and babesia is a malaria-like intracellular infection. Powassan virus is a tickborne encephalitis virus that is related to West Nile virus, and is similar to a deer tick virus found in wild deer.[7-14]

**PCR is polymerase chain reaction testing. †We will examine this agent in a later chapter.*

The *Powassan* virus was first isolated in 1952 in Colorado. In 1958 it was found to cause a human infection. It was renamed after its second place of origin, Powassan,* Ontario. The isolate was found to be antigenically related to the *Russian Spring-Summer Encephalitis* group. This means the immune system sees the two infections as the same. Powassan virus was also found in cottontail rabbit ticks and rodent ticks. Mixed infections were also found in marine bird ticks from the eastern US. Their mixed infections included Bb, human monocytic ehrlichiosis (HME), Rocky Mountain spotted fever, and several arboviruses (including mosquito-borne flaviviruses).[5-15]

**Powassan, Ontario is home to a long-established copper mining industry.*

The powassan virus is closely related to another infectious encephalitis virus of animals, the deer tick virus. Ticks from northeastern Massachusetts and northwestern Connecticut are found to carry the deer tick virus; which is about 84% similar to powassan. Powassan provides an important clue that ticks that are exposed to gut-degrading insecticides are transmitting important infections. This is because tick digestion, called *heterophagy* takes place inside the tissues of the tick midgut (epithelial cells). This type of digestion is used because tick saliva lacks the enzymes required to digest blood meals.[5-19]

Inside the gut, blood and cellular components are absorbed and digested directly into the gut lumen. This sort of direct intracellular digestion is known to occur in ticks and possibly other acari (i.e. mites), but is unknown in other arthropods. This process also favors the introduction of recombinant bacteria and viruses from insecticides directly into the tick's circulation. This therefore allows the infectious agents to become amplified or increased in strength (host amplification) the longer they circulate inside the infected tick. Thereafter the infections may be transmitted upon the next blood meal.[5-19]

In 1966 and 1968, California group arboviruses were isolated from Florida rabbits and from mosquitoes collected in Simsbury, Connecticut. This was the first time that California group arboviruses were found in a New England state. A survey was taken in Simsbury in March of 1966 by a Dr. Whitman who was collecting mosquito larvae and pupae. Another study by Whitman et al., while with the Yale Arbovirus Research Unit (YARU) in New Haven, detailed the Simsbury collections where one of the scientists lived. Serologic (blood) surveys elsewhere suggested that California group encephalitis viruses were also present in the Rocky Mountains of the northwestern US, in southern Canada; and in Wisconsin, Ohio, and Florida. Another scientist named Whitney isolated a California group arbovirus from New York State, from an aedes mosquito.[20-23]

Perhaps one of the reasons the surveys were completed in Simsbury was because of its connections to mining, atomic energy, the silk industry, and/or the early agricultural insecticides; each of which have greatly impacted the region. By the late 1960s, scientists were probably already aware of mutated spirochetes that had surfaced in Romania and in the US Midwest beginning a decade earlier. Perhaps there were concerns that mutated spirochetes were being created with the help of an insect arbovirus such as a mosquito-borne powassan virus. Or perhaps they were worried that the borrelina (sawfly) viruses that were used as insecticidal helpers from 1951 onward were causing problems. Since the nuclear age was well underway during this period, another consideration could have been whether nuclear wastes were contributing to the mutation of water or soil-borne spirochetes to create novel strains, whether those wastes were located in agricultural soils, nuclear wastewaters, or were airborne.[20-23]

Since 1963, YARU scientists had been in Connecticut conducting field surveillance for eastern equine encephalitis (EEE).

Animal EEE infections were concentrated in the upper Hammonasset River region about twenty miles west of the Lyme, Old Lyme, and East Haddam areas where the first human "juvenile arthritis" cluster had not yet appeared but was soon to arrive. Was there a connection between the early applied agricultural controls, the outbreak of animal diseases, and the emergence of novel human spirochetes? Perhaps that is precisely what scientists were studying.[20-23]

In a 1985 French paper scientists discussed blood tests from one Canadian and three French patients who presented with symptoms of Lyme disease. Patient serum was tested for the presence of rickettsiae, *Borrelia burgdorferi*, and insect (alpha)viruses. When testing patients for antibodies, a few returned positive to the Eyach virus and a Nairovirus. Eyach and Nairoviruses are members of the *Reovirus* group, and can be tick or mosquito-borne. The Eyach virus is commonly found in France and in other parts of Europe, especially Tschechien in the Czech Republic.[24-27]

Finding evidence of reoviruses in Connecticut where a Lyme disease epidemic was already smoldering is highly significant because these viruses may be a potent contributing factor to the emergence of this disease. If we are wondering why this may be so, it is because reoviruses are associated with mined materials, minerals, and metals, and Connecticut has a huge copper vein and mine, and nuclear plants in the state. The bacteria and viruses found in acid mine wastes are significant to our story. The serologic tests previously mentioned were reportedly performed with the assistance of Dr. "N." Magnarelli, Department of Entomology, Connecticut Agricultural Experiment Station, New Haven, Connecticut. This is a misspelling however, as the only record of a "Dr. Magnarelli" at the Connecticut station is Dr. Louis A. Magnarelli, who is a colleague of several of the IDSA Lyme disease guidelines co-authors, and an assignee on more than one *Borrelia burgdorferi*-related patent.[24-27]

After translation, the French paper also described insect arboviruses, in particular those transmitted by mosquitoes which are members of the African Sindbis virus group. Infection with these viruses causes symptoms which resemble Lyme disease. These include fever, fatigue, encephalitis, conjunctivitis, adenopathies, and arthralgias. The paper mentioned the sindbis virus-caused Ockelbo disease of Sweden, and a polyarthritic rash illness of Australia called Australian-X disease. The report also described how at least five mosquito-transmitted arboviruses are known to cause similar arthritis-like diseases in humans. During arbovirus infections patients frequently manifest multiple odd-shaped rashes that are more or less disseminated; and do not necessarily appear in a bull's-eye pattern. *The paper suggested that differences in clinical presentations between Lyme disease and arbovirus infections are not always evident.* This is interesting because many Lyme patients experience similar odd rashes during acute infections.[25,28-32]

This supports the idea that Lyme infections may involve an arbovirus infection such as a tickborne flavivirus or reovirus. The viruses may initiate the reassortment of genes during mixed infections inside the insect body. The newly created infection is then transmitted to a human by blood-feeding insects or arthropods (i.e. tick, mite, mosquito). If we are wondering from where Eyach virus came, we might recall the nymph ticks that were imported from the Fontainebleu Forest in France during the 1920s. These ticks were released on Naushon Island, Masschusetts and adjacent islands to control dog/wood ticks in 1926. They certainly could have spread the Eyach virus to northeastern tick populations within a few short decades. Then again so too could any of the millions of other imported wasps, flies, beetles, and other insects that were deployed in the US as parasitoids.[25,28-32]

In a similar manner, in the early days of textiles in the northeastern US, diseased silkworms were being imported into silk factories, and textile and tannery wastes were dumped into sewers and nearby rivers. Japanese beetles and other imported beetles brought their own menu of infectious viruses. I might also point out that France was not only home to a large silk industry during the 1800s, and from where Monsieur Trouvelot found his gypsy moth imports; it is also a region that has a geothermal vein below it, like Connecticut and other New England states. Geothermal and hydrothermal veins are home to thermophilic bacteria and reoviruses. Hydrothermal veins are found in the ocean, and geothermal veins upon land. What comes up from deep within the ground whether by natural or man-made (mining) methods is essential to understanding what kinds of microbes are able to help create infectious diseases and a particularly odd little spirochete named *Borrelia burgdorferi*.[25,28-32]

In New York State, California group arboviruses were isolated from aedes mosquitoes collected in St. Lawrence County, July of 1965. Antibodies to these viruses were also detected in humans, wild animals (woodchucks, deer); and in dairy cattle from several counties. In addition, eastern equine encephalitis and *Flanders* viruses were also found on Long Island, New York. EEE is an alphavirus, while flanders is a *Rhabdovirus*. This family includes important livestock viruses (vesicular stomatatis virus, rabies); and plant viruses (orchid fleck virus, lettuce necrotic yellow virus, potato yellow dwarf virus).[22,33-35]

The Rhabdoviruses, like the paramyxoviruses are members of the Order of Mononegavirales. This is a group of viruses which includes the related *measles, mumps,* rabies, Ebola, marburg, J virus, rinderpest, sendai virus, parainfluenza, *yellows and mosaic plant viruses, simian* virus 41 (SV41), vesicular stomatitis virus (VSV), and *avian bornaviruses.* We discuss many of these viruses in this book, including those that may reactivate from human vaccines. Bornavirus was first detected in horses in 1970, and these are similar to rabies and sindbis (think recombinant constructs). What is interesting is that bornaviruses may not only be found in horses, poultry, and other birds; but also in rodents, primates, and in their mosquito and tick vectors.

Bornaviruses have been found in the genomes of insects and arthropods (i.e. ticks) as remnants of ancient infections (i.e. viruses or retroviruses). These old latent viral genes are sometimes called "fossilized" gene fragments, or gene fossils. The introduction of bornaviruses into human patients has been seen in Lyme patients. This virus family can cause serious mood disorders, depression, bipolar disorder, schizophrenia, and other psychiatric presentations. Bornavirus has been shown to invade brain tissues in voles; and has been detected in birds suffering from *psittacosis* infections and in rabbits and sheep. Bornavirus antibodies have been found in human patients who suffer from alcohol and drug addiction. We might think about how ancient animal and insect viruses are being reactivated from dormancy. The answer may simply be through the exposures of insects, animals, and humans to the very powerful recombinant genes of insecticides and other formulas. What is supposed to be "safe" for non-targeted populations may be anything but.[44-53]

In Wisconsin and Minnesota, California group arbovirus antibodies appeared in the blood (sera) of forty-six Wisconsin residents, and twenty-five Minnesota residents surveyed in 1978. This was just three years after the outbreak of "juvenile arthritis" was first announced in Connecticut. The states that reported the highest case numbers of California group arboviruses were Wisconsin, Minnesota, Ohio, Indiana, Iowa, and Illinois. California group arboviruses became reportable infections to the CDC in 1963. About thirty to one hundred and sixty cases were reported annually by 1975.[22,33-35]

Scientists might have felt it appropriate to track suspected human arbovirus infections to see if there were any new epidemics emerging where any of these viruses might play a role. By 1978, the Minnesota department of health requested that physicians from surrounding states report all suspected cases of California group viruses. This may have been ordered if public health agencies felt that viruses from this group were contributing to the emerging "juvenile arthritis" cases in Connecticut.[33-35]

They also requested that serum specimens from infected patients be sent to and analyzed by the Minnesota state laboratory. In Illinois, a major outbreak of West Nile and St. Louis encephalitis virus occurred in 1975. A larger outbreak took place in Illinois in 2002 according to a cooperative paper written by the CDC's Epidemic Intelligence Service (Atlanta); the IL Department of Public Health; the Cook County Department of Public Health (Oak Park, IL); and the Chicago Department of Public Health. The paper considered mosquitoes the vectors of the West Nile virus with crows as the infection's amplifying host.[33-35]

The crow is also a common host of the African sindbis virus in Egypt. Sindbis is an important virus that has been used to create genetically engineered microbes for vaccines and applied insecticides. The reoviruses and other arboviruses found within biting and blood-feeding insects (i.e. rabies, West Nile, St. Louis encephalitis), are all related to their Old World parent virus, sindbis. Do insect infections trigger accidental recombinant events inside the bodies of infected humans? If so, are genetic engineering "accidents" the result of defective vaccine constructs or agriculturally applied insecticides that contained a defective sindbis virus? Were the genetic constructs reawakening sleeping ancient viruses in the insects and arthropods exposed to recombinant insecticides? Were they being transmitted to humans and emerging in Connecticut patients?[33-35]

A similar surveillance program was established by the State Department of Health for southeastern Minnesota in an exercise that involved nine hospitals. Wisconsin also established a hospital-based surveillance program through the WI Department of Health with the CDC's assistance. The program was undertaken at ten major hospitals in the southwestern part of the state, which included Gunderson Lutheran in La Crosse, Wisconsin. This is a hospital where we find a group of scientists who have publicly dismissed chronic Lyme disease patients. Both the MN and WI State laboratories provided diagnostic screening for all serum specimens, and screening for all virus specimens received from surrounding states for each patient with acute central nervous system disease (i.e. meningitis, encephalitis). Similar symptoms are sometimes found in "chronic" Lyme patients who are suffering from serious neurologic complications.[23,33,34,36,37]

This survey process is an important clue as to why at least one Lyme patient's serum samples were re-routed from the physician's office in Illinois to the Minnesota-based Mayo clinic laboratory when the patient tested CDC positive for Lyme disease based on standardized ELISA and Western blot tests. Was the patient's blood being examined for the presence of a California group arbovirus strain? If so, this could provide a clue that current standardized Lyme tests include at least one probe that is used to detect an arbovirus such as a reovirus (i.e. Eyach) – one that can reassort in the bodies of mosquitoes or ticks to cause new vector-borne infections. The surveillance programs may also explain why the patient received a personalized phone call from a CDC employee who wanted to ask the patient questions when their test results turned positive. It might also explain why around the time of the Connecticut "juvenile arthritis" outbreak, Yale scientists were examining patient sera for the presence of specific arboviruses.[37]

Arboviruses were studied by scientists during the 1950s following outbreaks of St. Louis encephalitis in Miami in 1958; and in Tampa Bay in 1959, 1961, and 1962. A new virus called *Tensaw,* a member of the *Bunyavirus* group was isolated from one hundred and fifty-six mosquitoes examined between 1960 and 1963. The mosquitoes were collected in southern Florida, southwestern Alabama, and southeastern Georgia. Were these mosquito viruses a result of the mosquitoes from early mass release programs that used sterile insect techniques including irradiation and/or genetically engineered genes?[38-42]

Note the Georgia location which may have been near the Savannah River nuclear site, and where mosquito release programs had been undertaken in previous years. Irradiation would have not only sterilized the mosquitoes about to be released, but could have led to the mutation of the viruses and other bacteria alive in the mosquito gut cell genomes. Field and laboratory studies of St. Louis encephalitis virus took place in McLeansboro, Illinois after a 1964 epidemic. The studies were expanded to include the metropolitan area of St. Louis, Missouri after a similar outbreak occurred there. McLeansboro is located in the southeastern part of Illinois, just north of the Shawnee National Forest. This is an area I discuss later for its importance to mining, nuclear research, and deer repopulation efforts.[38-42]

A 1969 paper co-authored by Dr. Daniel E. Sonenshine* describes testing ticks that were collected from wild birds in the eastern US. The ticks were tested for the presence of bacteria and viruses. In 1965, migrating birds were captured in Maryland at Kent Island (Chesapeake Bay), and at Ocean City on the Atlantic coast. Over a three-year period, scientists in Massachusetts, New York, Delaware, North Carolina, Arkansas, and Missouri, tested more than ten thousand birds from one hundred and fifty different species. There was evidence of Rocky Mountain spotted fever virus in the birds. But curiously the paper also claimed that no viruses were isolated. The idea that no viruses were found could be a reflection of a poor culture medium or faulty test methods. It is hard to believe this many birds harbored zero viruses. A total of four thousand two-hundred and sixty-six ticks were grouped into one hundred and eighty nine pools and tested. To be unable to isolate a single virus from this large of a tick pool seems incredibly odd if not virtually impossible.[43]

**Dr. Sonenshine is a colleague of the IDSA Lyme disease guidelines co-authors; Professor of Biology at Old Dominion University (Norfolk, VA); and National Scientific Advisor for the American Lyme Disease Foundation (ALDF). He also has a history in biological warfare research at Ft. Detrick.*

Leptospires, Reoviruses, and Reassortments, Oh My

I revealed earlier that yellows diseases of plants and insects may involve a combination of a virus and a spirochete. Some of the most important clues there may be a viral component to the Lyme disease organism might be found in an annual report published by the Yale Arbovirus Research Unit. This is the University's agency that is responsible for cataloging and supplying the majority of the world's most infectious organisms. The report discloses what may be important Lyme-related research that took place during the mid-1970s.

It covers a period from July 1, 1976 to June 30, 1977, immediately after the announcement of the juvenile arthritis outbreak in Connecticut. The paper also discusses medical research conducted on behalf of Yale's New Haven School of Medicine for the US Army Medical Research and Development Command at Ft. Detrick. The paper was written by Dr. Robert E. Shope, a former colleague of Lyme notable Rheumatologist Dr. Allen C. Steere. At the time the paper was written, Dr. Steere was already aiding in the collection and analysis of serum samples from Connecticut patients who were presenting with the new arthritis-like illness.[1]

From the Yale report we learn that eighty-four new arbovirus strains were received from twenty-one countries. The viruses were identified, catalogued, and studied by Yale scientists from 1975 to 1976. The question to ask is why would Yale scientists take a sudden interest in such an extensive number of new arboviruses? The obvious reason is there may have been a suspicion that an arbovirus was playing a major role in the new outbreak that would eventually be named Lyme disease.[1]

Two new viruses were isolated in Mayenne, France in the spring of 1981, the year the Lyme disease agent was identified by Dr. Willy Burgdorfer and colleagues, and a year before it was publicly announced. The viruses were found in two species of ticks, the sheep tick (*Ixodes ricinus*) and the rabbit tick (*Ixodes ventalloi*). This was the region of the French countryside from where the first parasitoid insects and parasitized nymph ticks were exported for release into the US northeast during the 1920s. The chalcid wasp-parasitized nymph ticks were collected from the Fontainebleu Forest near Mayenne. Were scientists certain of an imported arbovirus component to the new outbreak in Connecticut? If so, maybe this is why a massive sweep was undertaken to search for the origin of a suspected arbovirus.[1]

Serologic testing by Yale scientists uncovered the two new viruses from the French ticks; and these isolates were added to the Colorado tick fever virus family. The new viruses were considered to be indistinguishable from the Eyach virus, a tickborne virus first described in 1976 in West Germany. Eyach is an RNA virus which belongs to the reovirus family of the coltivirus subgroup. These viruses are carried by *Ixodes, Dermacentor, Haemaphysalis,* and *Otobius* tick species. Colorado tick fever virus is considered to be endemic in northwestern North America, and it is closely related to Eyach virus.[1]

The reoviridae group includes the genera reovirus, orbivirus, rotavirus, *plant reoviruses*, and *cytoplasmic polyhedrosis viruses* (CPVs). Remember that reoviruses associate with baculoviruses. They are also found among mined metals, mineral ores, and rock phosphates. The CPV reoviruses have been found in over one hundred and fifty insect species, including the silkworm (as flacherie). There are also plant reoviruses (phytoreoviruses) such as the maize rough dwarf reovirus, all of which cause significant agricultural losses.[1-7]

CPV reoviruses are also associated with respiratory infections in animals including monkeys. This means that monkeys culled for vaccine purposes may be naturally infected with these viruses. Reovirus agents that are part of the rotavirus group cause diarrhea in calves, foals, and mice. Reoviruses of this group also cause fatal gastroenteritis infections in children, especially in third world countries. Another group of reoviruses are the *Orbiviruses,* which cause disease in animals and humans. Some of the most important animal reoviruses in this group cause *Bluetongue* disease in ruminant animals, and African horse sickness, which is found in Africa, the Mediterranean, and the Middle East. The CPV reoviruses should be an item of interest to us with respect to modern day "influenza" vaccines as well.[8,9]

CPV reoviruses have been engineered along with baculoviruses in the globally applied agricultural insecticides. In the company of baculoviruses, reoviruses are made far more virulent. Most, if not all of these viruses have segmented genomes. Segmented genes facilitate the reassortment (recombination) of genes between compatible viruses within the guts of insects that carry mixed infections. These mixed infections include the genetically engineered pathogens of agricultural insecticides.[1-7]

Compatible plant reoviruses which belong to this same group are found in seed plants and in their insect vectors (i.e. leafhoppers, aphids, moth larvae, mites). The insect reoviruses of major importance here are found in the silkworm moth, the gypsy moth, the parasitoid wasps, and the sawflies. In short, the Lyme disease story includes one or more insect viruses as part of a mixed infection that is transmissible by ticks, mites, and other blood-feeding (hematophagous) insects.[1-7]

The brome mosaic virus is an example of a plant reovirus that has a segmented genome. Brome mosaic virus (BMV) was first isolated in 1942 from bromegrass. BMV also infects agriculturally significant cereal crops including corn, wheat, and barley. It is a member of the alphavirus-like super family of *Bromoviruses* which includes more than two-hundred and fifty animal and plant viruses. This family also includes the tobacco mosaic virus (TMV). Many reoviruses have been genetically engineered into insecticides to cause infections.[10-24]

Researchers at the University of Wisconsin-Madison's Department of Plant Pathology published a paper in 1982 that detailed how bentonite clay, a material useful in fertilizers, is known to strip proteins from the tobacco mosaic (reo)virus. Bentonite is also used to backfill underground storage facilities for nuclear wastes. Studies show that radiation changes structural and physical properties of the clay depending on composition and radiation dosage. This also means that viruses can be broken open by the clays used in agricultural fertilizers, wastewater, construction, nuclear waste storage, pond liners, and other bentonite-related products. This may cause the release of naked virus proteins. Once free of their virus capsule, they may infect local bacteriae. When nuclear wastes leach into soils and watersheds; viruses, bacteria, and other microbes that have been attracted by the clay become part of the "waste" equation. Microbes take up nuclear and other wastes and metals into their cells. The stripping of protein coats to remove viruses from their capsule is a technique that is exploited by genetic engineers.[10-27]

Studies have analyzed the ability of bentonite clay to degrade the brome mosaic (BMV) and tobacco mosaic (TMV) viruses. It was found that bentonite clay adsorbed the BMV virus coat. Bentonite was shown to degrade the virus into individual proteins, each of which contained one piece of infectious RNA. This "naked" RNA remained infective while the proteins were free to horizontally transfer with any compatible virus, fungi, or bacteria in the area. Another paper described how the tobacco mosaic virus was degraded to RNA virus and proteins in a bentonite-buffered solution. The RNA and DNA viruses are important to our story because viruses can reassort. This is more easily achieved under the influence of gene-damaging radiation and/or chemical wastes, especially in the presence of baculovirus partners.[10-15,28-32]

Bentonite clays, which also contain aluminum compounds, are used in pesticides, fertilizers, and in pond and wastewater pond liners. In pesticides, bentonite clays act as virus stabilizers and binders. (This is also why aluminum is used in underarm deodorants.) Examples of important segmented viruses include those from mosaic (RNA), and gemini (DNA) virus families:

Cassava mosaic	Alfalfa mosaic	Beet mosaic	Tobacco mosaic
Plum pox virus	Tulip breaking virus	Carrot mosaic	Clover mosaic
Marigold mottle	Peanut mottle	Plum pox	Potato Y or V viruses
Soybean mosaic	Chickpea bushy dwarf	Panicum mosaic	Wheat mosaic
Cotton leaf curl	Cabbage leaf curl	Tomato golden	Potato yellow
Maize streak virus	Cassava latent	Tomato pseudo-curley top virus	

Vine mosaic viruses (pumpkin, squash, zucchini, watermelon, etc.)[10-15,28,32]

When we consider that plant, insect, and animal viruses in wastewaters can reassort with the microbes that were, and are globally deployed in agriculture, then the number of new pathogens we may see emerge in insect, animal, or human hosts may be staggering. This ability to reassort genetic information means viruses will infiltrate bacteria (i.e. leptospires) that are degraded by the chemicals that pollute them, facilitating mutations and the "pollution" of leptospires or other bacteria. Reassortment happens more easily with bacteria that have segmented genomes (like beads on a chain) such as leptospires. The reassorted bacteria becomes a mutant leptospira for example, that contains genes from bacteria, fungi, or viruses found in the polluted water or microbially fertilized soil where they live. When we consider that insect larvae are found in water and soil, their viruses, fungi, bacteria, and other pathogens can become part of a mixed infection. Inside an insect's gut, new mutant bacteria may continue reassortment during fermentation. Thereafter they may be transmitted to animal or human hosts during a blood meal. This creates novel pathogens that are excreted as animal wastes into the soil and groundwater. When these infections enter an animal or human body, they may reactivate sleeping infections, including quite possibly those that were part of recombinant vaccines. Like the latent viruses of insects that are targeted for reactivation by insecticides, the latent viruses of vaccinated humans may have the potential to spring back to life upon exposure to recombinant genes introduced by vectoring insects, from ingesting GM foods or animal products, or even pharmaceuticals. With the advent of chemical and recombinant microbial insecticides, the reassortment of microbes became an unwelcome reality for all species exposed to same.[10-15,28-32]

The pathogenic *Leptospira interrogans* serovar "Lai" is an example of a bacterium that can remove DNA from its segmented genome and donate it to other microbes. This talent was found in all leptospira species studied. One laboratory created an *E. coli*-leptospira "shuttle vector" using this principle. If this can be done in a lab, it can certainly occur in wastewaters or soils with a little help from agricultural chemicals, transgenic microbes, or nuclear or other industrial wastes.[10-15,28-32]

According to a paper, segmented gene "islands" or plasmids play an important role in spreading genes, including virulence factors among bacterial populations. The segmented genomes of more than two hundred and fifty plant and insect viruses including all of the reoviruses; and the segmented baculoviruses of insecticides are highly important. Each may swap genes in the microbial soup of industrial or agricultural chemicals and radioactive elements found in contaminated soils and waters. The *Borrelia burgdorferi* genome contains a mixture of more than twenty linear and circular plasmids. This is a large number, and we can understand how this may occur if we accept that Bb is an aggregate formed by reassorted microbes.[10-15,28-33]

RNA viruses can quickly adapt to changing environments through genetic variation by mutation, reassortment, or recombination. It appears that the genes of bluetongue diseases (an orbivirus from the reovirus family) are remarkably similar across strains. This virus was first described in the late 1870s and may have been exhumed from early bauxite/metal ore or phosphate mines anywhere in the world. A reovirus such as bluetongue could have infected a vibrio-like soil bacterium as described in early papers on "blue disease" to create the fatal "blue" disease of Japanese beetles. Although it was labeled as a rickettsial infection (*Coxiella popilliae*), in its simplest form it may represent a bacterium that is infected with a bluetongue reovirus and a soil bacterium. (bacterium + reovirus = rickettsial infection).

Blue disease of Japanese beetles emerged in the US just after the dust bowl, at the beginning of the widespread use of mined phosphate fertilizers and microbial insecticides. Blue disease was first described in scientific literature in 1951, but it was identified as early as 1940; and appeared in areas where fertilizers and early insecticides were being applied. Could this have been Yale's 1940 "mystery virus" that was found in cell cultures? Perhaps the viral aspect of a beetle blue disease is a bluetongue or related virus. While this idea may seem far-fetched to some, it is interesting to read early publications by the Viral and Rickettsial Research Section of the American Cyanamid Company (Pearl River, New York).[34-42]

American Cyanamid was a chemical manufacturer founded in 1907, and which produced the Sabin type polio vaccine. (Lederle Laboratories is its pharmaceutical division.) American Cyanamid provides products for aerospace, water treatment, agriculture, plastics, coatings, and mining industries. These include phosphine and phosphorus specialty chemicals useful for fertilizers and insecticides. The company also produces chemicals for rubber, polystyrene, fibers, polymers, additives, and adhesives. American Cyanamid has been involved in phosphate mining for many decades and has sold chemicals to the dye industry. It has also produced malathion and parathion herbicides; provided explosives and mineral flotation products for mines and quarries; and antibiotics including aureomycin (a tetracycline). The company also created resins, including a urea-formol (Beetle) resin as early as 1923.[34-42]

A March 1972 report described ten species of *Ixodes* ticks that were collected one year earlier. One hundred and seven collections were made in Indian River County, Florida by members of the Entomological Research Center of the Florida Department of Health. The tick species gathered included *Amblyomma dissimile, A. maculatum, A. tuberculatum, Dermacentor variabilis, Haemaphysalis chordeilis, H. leporispalustris, Ixodes brunneus, I. cookei, I. minor,* and *Ixodes scapularis*. The American dog tick was the species most frequently found. Rabbit ticks were also frequent although they were nymphal in form, and noticeably abundant on Florida migratory birds. The role of birds in tick transmissions is key since reoviruses were first recognized as bird pathogens in 1957. This was a few years after a mutated leptospira spirochete would emerge from a highly polluted Romanian river. Indian River County is rather "coincidentally" also where we find the St. Lucie nuclear power plant.[43-46]

The avian (bird) reoviruses cause malabsorption syndromes, inflammation of the heart, gastroenteritis, immune suppression, brittle bone syndrome, hepatitis, thigh bone destruction, and acute and chronic respiratory syndromes. Neurologic signs include tremors, twitches, and incoordination. Arthritis is common. The malabsorption syndrome is related to intestinal, liver, and pancreatic abnormalities. There is also a reovirus-associated viral arthritis of birds. In 1966, seventy-seven bird reoviruses were isolated in Japan; a country that has suffered huge agricultural losses due to avian reoviruses.[43]

In 1975, US scientists classified nine avian reoviruses and placed them into four distinct serotypes (distinct variations in the species). There are also four distinct serotype groups for *Borrelia burgdorferi* sensu lato. Each group contains multiple strains. Three of the Bb serogroups cause Lyme disease, and a fourth found in Japan is not known to cause Lyme disease in humans, but typically infects mice. The "juvenile arthritis" that is now known as Lyme disease was also announced in 1975 as a human infection. In 1995 a fifth serogroup, *Borrelia andersonii* was added to the Bb sensu lato groups, isolated from rabbit ticks *Ixodes dentatus.* Since this tick rarely bites humans, it has not been identified as a Lyme disease vector. Lyme disease may be spread by ticks that feed on migratory birds. Avian reoviruses are very similar to human reoviruses, which makes them compatible gene-swapping partners during mixed infections. It may also make them compatible when introduced into an animal or human that has been inoculated with a vaccine that contains a reovirus contaminant (which can be reactivated).[43-50]

Another five avian reoviruses were found in the US, Germany, and the UK by 1980, and more have been identified since then. Remember that avian reoviruses include those which affect poultry, including chicken embryos that are used to create animal and human vaccines. By 1980 there were at least eleven reovirus subtypes identified. Today there are several hundred avian reoviruses that have been isolated and identified, although they are very difficult to classify. Since scientists say that additional Bb strains are likely to appear in the future, we can imagine this may be because there is such a huge variety of reoviruses available.[43-50]

Clearly the application of reovirus CPVs within agricultural insecticides and the wild-type CPV infections found in insects being targeted by these controls plays an important role in the reassortment and transmission of infections to animals and humans. The viruses found in chicken embryo-grown vaccines for animals and humans may also play a role in the reactivation of human diseases, because they are compatible partners to the viruses in the insecticides. In 1981, Yale Arbovirus Research Unit's Dr. D.L. Knudson was studying reoviruses from the orbivirus group (i.e. bluetongue) at the same time that his colleague, Dr. Willy Burgdorfer was studying the relationship between rabbit ticks and reoviruses.[5,51]

A paper authored by Dr. Knudson was accepted into publication just before Dr. Allen Steere et al. isolated a novel spirochete from the ECM rash culture of a Connecticut Lyme patient. According to a Yale article on Colorado tick fever virus (a reovirus), scientists were studying other reoviruses including reovirus type 3 Dearing strain; orbivirus changuinola strain BT 766 (found in *turtles,* armadillos, and sloths); a human rotavirus (from a reovirus family, rotaviruses are "flu"); CPV reovirus from *silkworm* caterpillar larvae; and a *plant* reovirus called wound tumor virus (WTV). According to the document, WTV was not a "wild-type" isolate but possibly a variant. A "variant" may represent a recombinant version such as has been used within transgenic plants or insecticides. Changuinola is a location in Panama, Central America where Caribbean sea turtles travel to lay their eggs. The turtle connection to reoviruses will become important in an upcoming chapter.[5,52]

Dr. Knudson's (Yale) reovirus studies are interesting since they occurred right before the agent of "juvenile arthritis" was formally identified by Burgdorfer et al. in 1982. Yale's Dr. Robert Ellis Shope was acknowledged in the article for "suggestions and advice." The wound tumor virus samples were supplied by B. Kobilka (Yale University School of Medicine); from Y. Furuichi (Roche Institute of Molecular Biology); and L. Stanker and R. MacLeod of the University of Urbana, Illinois. The latter is the very same university campus where Illinois turtles and bulls would produce mutated spirochetes during the 1950s and 1960s. No doubt those spirochetes also had reovirus connections. From the published studies it appears that just about "everyone" was aware of novel animal pathogens or aspects of their composition before the agent of Lyme disease was formally named in 1982. Since I hypothesize that *Borrelia burgdorferi* is an aggregate organism which contains microbes including a reovirus and at least one mutated spirochete, it is probably no coincidence to see similar studies by Yale's Arbovirus Unit or important individuals such as Dr. Burgdorfer just before the announcement of the causative agent of Lyme disease.[5]

In 1998, the Indian River County, Florida area was again studied for its arbovirus-hosting mosquitoes. Why were scientists looking at the California group of arboviruses and their host-vector relationships from 1963 to 1972? There was a 1962 outbreak of St. Louis encephalitis in Tampa Bay, and they were probably attempting to see if a reovirus had contributed to the outbreak. Even Central America is not a long distance over time for mosquito-borne infections to arrive in Florida. We know there were mosquitoes experimentally released over several years of past biological control programs undertaken in El Salvador. There were many mosquito release programs and field studies undertaken in the US during the 1950s to 1970s; and in other regions including El Salvador. For example field tests were performed at Lake Apastepeque, Florida and the surrounding valley in 1972 where sterilized male mosquitoes were released. Similar programs were implemented in 1974. Since mosquitoes are carriers of many arboviruses, we can understand transmission cycles between vector insect and animal or bird host; and how reassortment during mixed infections varies depending on host factors.[53-62]

Dr. Willy Burgdorfer should be well acquainted with the Colorado tick fever group and other reoviruses, as we know it was an area of his studies. Drs. Burgdorfer and colleague Eklund were investigating the Colorado tick fever group in 1959 in ticks collected from Lost Horse Canyon near the Montana NIH laboratory. For the next several decades, Dr. Burgdorfer would be one of the key investigators into tickborne infections. He would of course also be bestowed with the honor of having the Lyme disease agent named after him in 1982.[10-15,29-33,43,65-67]

It is interesting to read the literature published in May of 1981 on the reassortment of bunyaviruses. This family consists of three groups: togaviruses, flaviviruses, and bunyaviruses. The following month (June 1981) colleague Dr. Allen C. Steere and team members would isolate a novel spirochete from a Connecticut Lyme patient. However the name of this particular spirochete would not become part of the fanfare in 1982 which announced the spirochetal agent of Lyme disease. Many mixed mosquito and tickborne bunyaviruses were examined prior to the announcement of the Lyme disease agent. Obviously scientists were trying to determine which family of insect-borne viruses was involved in the human disease outbreak. Since any of these viruses may represent a degraded version of a reassorted reovirus, any of these viruses may play a role in Lyme disease.[10-15,28-33,64-73]

Only later on would there be clues that a transmissible flavivirus was isolated from *Ixodes scapularis* ticks in New England and in the upper Midwest. The new agent was said to be related to the powassan encephalitis virus, and was named "deer tick virus." Several viruses are found in ticks that are able to transmit Lyme disease. It is obvious from research papers that Yale, Harvard, and other scientists were studying arboviruses and their relation to Lyme disease. Why scientists have not spoken up about "deer tick virus" or the possibility of an arbovirus or reovirus connection to Lyme at any time since the announcement of the Bb agent seems very odd. If we recall that for decades scientists have manipulated mosquito populations using radiation (mutation), chemical pheromones, and "deleterious genes;" and we remember that for a century microbial insecticides were applied agriculturally, we can understand why such connections are not, or perhaps cannot be made. Decades ago scientists worried about the ramifications of irradiated or genetically engineered insects being released into the wild. Were their worst fears now being realized? Were the reoviruses of applied insecticides, those found naturally, or those that may contaminate vaccine cell lines converging to cause animal or human diseases?[10-15,28-33,64-73]

Scientists on both sides of the globe were studying members of the encephalitis group of viruses. These viruses have a close kinship with the African sindbis virus, and the important plant and insect reoviruses. The sindbis virus was determined by Russian scientists Shubladze and her colleague Margulis to be antigenically identical to the rabies virus during the 1950s. This means the immune system cannot tell them apart. Drs. Margulis and Shubladze were developing a vaccine for Multiple Sclerosis/tickborne encephalitis at the time using an "S.V." strain of acute encephalomyelitis. This was probably a street virus strain of rabies, or its ancestor, sindbis.*[74-76]

**The sindbis virus was first isolated from mosquitoes in Sindbis, Egypt in 1952, the same year that polio vaccines were first developed. Sindbis has been widely used in recombinant vaccines and insecticides since then. The virus and its clones are heavily patented by academic institutions. We will learn that when it is used recombinantly, sindbis constructs may be highly flawed.*

In 1965 Russian scientists investigated a fatal case of Russian spring summer encephalitis (RSSE) in the village of Aleksee-Nikol'sk that had occurred two years earlier. Cases of leptospirosis (leptospira infections) had also been found in the region. What was this curious correlation between insect reoviruses and the bacteriae known as leptospires? This was just a few years before the announcement of a juvenile arthritis outbreak in Connecticut; and just four years before a Wisconsin man would be treated for an ECM rash illness by Dermatologist Rudolph Scrimenti.[74-76]

By 1972, three years before the Connecticut outbreak was reported in the US, Russian scientists were studying the antigenic features of West Nile, sindbis, and related viruses. In 1968 and 1970, a new tickborne group B viral agent related to RSSE was isolated from ticks collected from pigeon pet shops in Kabul City, Afghanistan; and from pigeon houses on the Royal Farm near Kabul (here is the avian reovirus reference again). The new virus was named Royal Farm virus, and was found to be closely related to powassan and langat viruses, two North American insect-borne viruses. Each of these viruses are closely related to one another and to rabies; with sindbis being the putative parent virus. Any of these viruses may reassort inside an insect during mixed infections because their similar and segmented genes are easily traded with the highly compatible segmented reoviruses.[74-79]

We might wonder what were the objectives of the Burgdorfer et al. studies of rabies, WEE, and tickborne leptospirosis when they were undertaken. Was there a novel organism that was already appearing in eastern Europe (i.e. Russia, Romania) as well as the US (i.e. Georgia, Illinois, Montana ticks)? Were scientists of the day already aware of and attempting to identify novel agents and how they spread among animal populations long before Lyme disease emerged in the human population?[80]

Wolbachia as Symbiont

Microsporidiae are not the only parasite symbionts found within the bodies of fire ants and other insects. *Wolbachia* is a small gram-negative bacterium of the rickettsial family. The agent was first isolated in 1924 from culex mosquitoes by scientists Hertig and Wolbach. These bacteria infect most arthropod species and nematodes, as well as animals and humans. Indeed they are the predominant reproductive parasite in the world. This is a very important infection to consider as we observe the rising rates of human infertility and consider what may be a causative infection in a percentage of cases. The presence of wolbachia in fire ants is an example of a symbiotic relationship between parasite and insect. According to a source:

> "...every species in the *Solenopsis saevissima* species complex to which the *Solenopsis invicta* belongs is infected with Wolbachia." (In other words, nearly all fire ants have wolbachia infections.)[1]

The rate of infection in other insect species is also significant. Wolbachia-infected mitochondria (cell engines) contain genes which provide resistance to pesticides or parasites. These genes can be donated to other species. Wolbachia infections also frequently *alter sex ratios* in infected offspring. Scientists have already begun manipulating wolbachia genes in the laboratory as part of long-standing mosquito "population replacement" programs. Up to seventy-percent of all insect species are thought to be potential hosts of wolbachia.[2-6]

Wolbachia persica was isolated from the malpighian (waste) tubules and gonads of the Egyptian fowl tick in 1961. In earlier decades, *W. persica* was studied frequently since it is a member of the *Francisellaceae* lineage where we find the tickborne *Francisella tularensis*, or tularemia (rabbit fever). Tularemia was a weaponized agent of US biowarfare during the War Research Service years. Ft. Detrick scientists were studying the aerosolization of this agent as late as 1968.[5,7]

Wolbachia strains have been isolated from Rocky Mountain wood ticks and studied at NIH Rocky Mountain Laboratories in Hamilton, Montana. Organisms frequently found to be infected with wolbachia are mosquitoes, spiders, mites, ticks, flies, and nematodes. Wolbachia can also infect humans and animals, and may contribute to other important diseases including elephantitis or river blindness; as well as heartworm infection in dogs.[5,8-11]

Wolbachia causes infected male insects to die. It can also cause feminization of infected males so they develop into females, or into infertile males. Some insects and nematodes are so dependent upon wolbachia as a symbiont that they cannot successfully reproduce without its participation. Wolbachia are very susceptible to the tetracycline antibiotic doxycycline. This drug is also used to control nematode infections in humans. Doxycycline will usually not kill the nematodes, but it will render them sexually sterile, because it kills their wolbachia symbiont. Once the nematode life cycle is complete the worms die, and this ends the nematodal infestation if all the worms are sterilized. It is perhaps a bit curious that the IDSA medical guidelines for Lyme disease heavily recommend the administration of doxycycline to treat Lyme disease, even though patients and doctors feel the drug does not cure Lyme infections. Perhaps this recommendation is partly aimed at treating the nematodes and their wolbachia infections that are commonly found in Lyme transmitting ticks; and as co-infections in Lyme patients.[2,5,6,10,12-22]

Modified wolbachia strains have been used to control malaria and dengue fever in transgenic mosquitoes. This means there may be genetically engineered versions of wolbachia out there that may be introduced by vectoring insects. In addition, a virus-like super infection dubbed "bacteriophage WO" has been found within all wolbachia-infected insect hosts that have been examined. This is evidence of nested infections, and an important clue that patients bitten or stung by insects may harbor important, undetected, and possibly recombinant infections that must be addressed, including wolbachia and its phage "WO."[19-25]

In 1975 and 1977 respectively, the National Institute of Allergy and Infectious Diseases (NIAID) awarded research grants to Dr. L.P. Brinton to study Colorado tick fever (reo)virus development in Rocky Mountain wood ticks. He also studied gut structures of normal ticks, and those infected with Rocky Mountain spotted fever (RMSF). Dr. Brinton has published nearly a dozen articles from 1970-1975 along with colleagues including Dr. Willy Burgdorfer. Two of Brinton's grants covered comparative work on the fine structure of wolbachia-like organisms in various tick species; and the structure of Rocky Mt. spotted fever and rickettsia species in vero* cells from Mississippi brown dog ticks. Brinton's 1970s studies also investigated an important *spiroplasma*† called the "277F" agent. This was first isolated from cottontail rabbit ticks by colleague Dr. Burgdorfer in 1967.[26-28]

**Vero cells are from a 1962 established cell line, isolated from African green monkey kidney epithelial cells.*

†Spiroplasmas are spirochetal bacteria that are cell-wall deficient, and have flagellum — characteristics in common with the agent of Lyme disease, Borrelia burgdorferi. Spiroplasmas are found in plants and are transmitted by insects where they live as symbionts. Some spiroplasma strains are known to be virulent vertebrate pathogens.

Dr. Willy Burgdorfer published many papers about mites, ticks, and infectious agents while employed at NIAID/NIH Rocky Mountain Labs. Dr. Burgdorfer also studied the tick symbiont wolbachia and a spiroplasma "277F" agent that he, E.G. Pickens, and R.K. Gerloff first isolated from Montana cottontail rabbit ticks in 1967. Studies by RML scientists undertaken in 1973 revealed that wolbachia infected nearly all Rocky Mountain wood ticks that were collected from the Bitterroot Valley, which spans Idaho and Montana. Several wolbachia-like organisms have been isolated from tick species *Dermacentor, Ixodes, Amblyomma, Rhipicephalus, Haemaphysalis, Hyalomma, Argas, Ornithodoros,* and *Boophilus*.[29-37]

The Bitterroot Mountains are of great interest to our story because copper was discovered in Butte in 1880, in one of the largest US deposits. A smelter was built to handle the ore, and the Anaconda Copper Mining Company (ACM) was built by owner Marcus Daly (a "Copper King"). The purchase was financed with the help of George Hearst; father of newspaper magnate, and former House of Representatives member William Randolph Hearst. During the 1950s open pit mining began, and during the mid-1970s the Atlantic Richfield Company (ARCO) bought the ACM Company, which closed in 1982, the year the Lyme disease agent was formally named. Open pit copper and other mines remain today in Montana. When we take a look at what Dr. Burgdorfer et al. were studying during the 1950s and 1960s, we can see how it serves as a model for the 1970s emergence of a Connecticut outbreak that emerged in an area of the US that has similar deep copper (and other mineral and elemental) deposits.[38]

There is also a Bitterroot strain of California encephalitis virus according to a publication from 1968. Connecticut is also a state where California group arboviruses were isolated for the first time in 1966 and 1968; discovered in mosquitoes from Simsbury. The fact that Dr. Burgdorfer would receive ticks to study for the causative agent of the Connecticut outbreak tells us that some individuals probably knew a lot more about the connections between Lyme, insect arboviruses, and agricultural and industrial "tools" than we have ever been told.[39-42]

I discovered ninety-six scientific research grants in an NIH database for wolbachia; awarded from 1972 to 2009. Immediately before the Lyme outbreak in Connecticut, scientific eyes were focused on wolbachia as a biological control agent. From 1973 to 1976, scientists from the University of California-Los Angeles studied the exploitation of cytoplasmic incompatibility to eradicate mosquito populations using a sterile incompatible male method. This is one of the sterile insect techniques that has been used as a biological control. *Cytoplasmic incompatibility* is the inability of sperm and egg to form a viable offspring. This reproductive problem can be caused by an active wolbachia infection. Scientists would infect mosquitoes with the agent to hinder reproduction. A recent anecdotal report from a couple who were both diagnosed with Lyme disease, and who had failed to conceive a child despite years of efforts; were able to do so after taking the tetracycline doxycycline for several weeks. Was this a "coincidence" or evidence that one or both partners were infected with wolbachia?[43]

During the 1990s, Yale scientists received research grants to study mosquito transinfection with wolbachia. The goal of their research was to develop cytoplasmic incompatibility as a tool to genetically manipulate "insect disease vectors." The design would also attempt to reduce the ability of the genetically engineered mosquitoes to transmit infections to humans. This was not a new discovery as scientists knew about wolbachia as a human pathogen, and were taking steps to eliminate it from mosquito populations before Lyme was reported in 1975. A 2009 grant awarded to Michigan State University scientists described mosquito control and dengue fever studies using wolbachia as a transgene driver. This describes the use of bacteria to plant wolbachia genes inside an insect host. The process was designed to reduce mosquito populations once the genetically engineered bugs were released and allowed to breed with native populations.[26,44-51]

In 1993, the year before the Lyme-related Dearborn Conference in Michigan, Yale scientists received a research grant to study the sindbis virus and insect symbiont viruses including wolbachia, in a plan to engineer mosquito viruses to make their infections less likely to be transmitted to vertebrates. The grant was titled *Trans-infection of mosquitoes with Wolbachia pipientis*.[51,52]

A Yale University predoctoral student received a 1997 grant to test a strain of genetically engineered mosquitoes with a reduced ability to transmit La Crosse virus. La Crosse is a leading cause of mosquito-borne encephalitis, especially for children. The genetically altered "chimera" (genetically combined microbes) used the sindbis virus to produce antibodies which block or inhibit virus transmission. Another goal was to design a way to introduce wolbachia infections to maintain cytoplasmic incompatibility genes within mosquito populations. In other words, wolbachia would be used as a tool to manipulate and reduce the reproductive and disease-transmitting capabilities of mosquitoes.[51,52]

From 1992 to 1996, Rocky Mt. laboratory scientists were again studying wolbachia-like organisms in Rocky Mountain wood ticks harvested from the Bitterroot Mountains. They found another symbiont of the francisella line. The agent was described as "wolbachia-like." Scientists also determined that around 96% of Rocky Mountain wood ticks carried the infection.[53]

Perhaps it is no coincidence that along with the importation of, and the manipulation of insects infected with wolbachia and other agents; and the application of recombinant insecticides, that we have seen a significant rise in human diseases and infertility. Perhaps one factor behind these increases is an epidemic of subclinical reproductive infections caused by wolbachia or other insect symbionts – pathogens transmitted by mosquitoes and other vectoring insects. It is perhaps of interest that a few esteemed physician/scientists who studied infectious organisms including wolbachia, left academic careers in the southeast to establish fertility clinics.[54-61]

Certain infectious disease experts including a few involved with the Lyme epidemic are obviously aware that wolbachia, spiroplasmas, reoviruses, and other infections are present in mosquitoes and ticks which transmit Lyme disease. USDA, NIH, SUNY (State University of New York-Stony Brook) and French scientists were actively studying and publishing information in a Yale journal about the tick spiroplasmas by 1983; the year after the Bb agent was named after Dr. Willy Burgdorfer. It is perplexing then why a public discussion of these and other important insect symbionts that are important human pathogens in their own right, remains noticeably absent in today's highly contentious Lyme disease medical and political arenas.[54-61]

The sheep tick *Ixodes ricinus* is common to Europe and the UK. According to at least one study sheep ticks are a common vector of *Borrelia garinii.* They not only carry wolbachia infections, but also *Candidates neoehrlichia mikurensis, Candidates midichloria mitochondrii,* and *Rickettsia australis* infections. Laboratory testing has revealed that each of these agents and the borreliae species *B. afzelii, B. garinii, B. valaisiana, B. lusitaniae,* and *B. ruski* are found among forest ticks from The Netherlands. The most common Bb strain found in these ticks is *B. afzelii,* which produces unusual skin manifestations during disseminated infections. Individuals from The Netherlands who are ill or having reproductive issues might ask their physician to consider the previously mentioned albeit less commonly known tickborne infections.[62,63]

From a 1984 study scientists learned that ticks harbor other rickettsia-like organisms that are rod-shaped symbionts of wolbachia. This means that even the tiny wolbachia can be infected with nested infections. These superinfections include chlamydia, ehrlichia, cowdria, and neorickettsia. And yet to date very few of these aforementioned infections have been openly acknowledged as possible co-infections in people with Lyme or other tickborne illnesses.[62,63]

NIH studies reveal that wolbachia infections were found in Pacific coast ticks (*Dermacentor occidentalis*), and in the blood of chipmunks. Wolbachia has also been isolated from African green monkey kidney cell cultures. This means the organism is able to grow in animal and insect cell lines as a contaminant – and also in animals useful for animal and human vaccines. Wolbachia has also been found within some moth species that have been sampled. This lends new credence to a highly important insect pathogen that can be transmitted through a variety of routes. These include vectoring insects, agricultural insecticides, and products made using wolbachia-contaminated insect cell lines.[64,65]

March of the Spiroplasmas

The *Mollicutes* are the smallest self-replicating organisms known to exist. They were placed into a phylum of bacteria called *Tenericutes* as a new division in 1984, two years after the announcement of the causative agent of Lyme disease. The mollicutes were formerly classified with swine erysipelas, which is a swine gut infection (swine flu). This family also includes gram-positive organisms that have cell walls. The mollicutes are a newer group of plant and animal bacteriae which lack a cell wall (wall-less). A cholesterol-like membrane surrounds the cell in these organisms. They are phylogenically related to the gram-positive bacteria, and may have evolved from *Clostridia* species through a process called degenerative evolution (loss of genes). This is a process that probably also occurred with the saprotrophic leptospires (saprophytes or saprotrophs are considered non-infectious). Mollicutes tend to be plastic-like (pleomorphic), they are often penicillin-resistant, and they have phages or viruses that commonly associate with, or infect them.[1]

The mollicute class contains the genus *Acholeplasma, Ureaplasma, Mycoplasma,* and *Spiroplasma.* We will focus on the spiroplasmas here although Lyme patients are often co-infected with mycoplasma strains. Most of the mollicutes move about by gliding, although the spiroplasmas are typically helical (helix). Since they move by twisting, they are considered to be true spirochetes. The mollicutes can spread actively through plant and animal tissues. Even nearby cells not associated with invasion are known to be adversely affected. Mollicutes are similar in structure and form to the rickettsiales and mycoplasmatales. The mycoplasma, spiroplasma, and rickettsia-like organisms are felt to contribute to the various "yellows" diseases of plants, insects, and humans. Research into the plant yellows diseases may prove a relationship to the mosquito-transmitted human yellow fever. Perhaps a leptospira spirochete when infected with a yellows disease virus causes human yellow fever.[1-6]

The spiroplasmas and acholeplasmas are considered to be the earliest species of mollicutes. Their genomes are larger than those of the mycoplasma or ureaplasmas, which appear to be more recent evolutions. Spiroplasma sizes vary between species. The largest spiroplasma genome belongs to the *Spiroplasma ixodetis Y32*, which is a tick spiroplasma. The reason for this genetic diversity is because of regressive evolution, or the reduction of genome size through a loss of genetic information over time. This can occur during normal evolutionary processes, or by mutation caused by chemicals, UV light, or other radiation. Sources describe a method of killing spiroplasmas by keeping them from escaping from a growth phase called the lag phase, which has several stages.[6-8]

Spiroplasma infections have been associated with more than two hundred diseases of plants, insects, and animals around the world. Not only do they live within the plant xylem and phloem, but they also replicate inside of insect vectors. They are said not to be culturable outside insect or plant hosts, but that is probably because they are sensitive and require a special nutrient medium. This is a similar problem with the Lyme disease spirochete. When plants are infected with mollicutes in general, they are less able to take up nutrients from the soil. When infected with spiroplasmas in particular, the uptake of magnesium from the soil is particularly affected. This is curious since most Lyme patients are also virtually depleted of magnesium and manganese;

requiring oral supplementation of these nutrients.* The Bb spirochete thrives in the magnesium rich human body where most magnesium is stored in the bones. Spiroplasma-infected plants show symptoms that are similar to those of plants grown in magnesium-poor soils. This provides a clue that just like the Bb spirochete, spiroplasmas consume a host's magnesium stores. Perhaps this is because Bb is (theoretically) part spiroplasma.[8-10]

**Many Lyme patients add magnesium-based epsom salts to bathwater to increase absorption of magnesium through the skin. This relieves muscle pains and twitching from cellular magnesium deficiency. Lyme patient blood levels of magnesium can remain normal even though cellular magnesium levels are depleted.*

Citrus trees and other plants are naturally infected with a spiroplasma spirochete that research says under darkfield microscopy looks exactly like the spirochete that causes Lyme disease. However the spirochete that causes citrus stubborn disease is identified as *Spiroplasma citri*, or the citrus spiroplasma. It was one of the first strains of spiroplasmas ever to be identified, along with the corn stunt spiroplasma (*Spiroplasma kunkellii*), and a few others. There are about three dozen species of spiroplasmas that have been identified to date. These include plant, insect, and vertebrate pathogens. Like the spirochetes of Lyme disease, the spiroplasmas are also helical, motile, wall-less, filamentous, and culturable only with specialized media.[11-12]

The spiroplasmas are cell-wall deficient mycoplasma-like organisms that were reportedly first discovered in 1972. I say reportedly because although this discovery date is often quoted; reliable sources show that these agents were actually discovered as early as 1944 in citrus trees. In 1964 scientists were studying the SMCA spiroplasma collected from pooled rabbit tick sera. By 1967 even Dr. Burgdorfer, after whom the Lyme disease agent was later named, had isolated a novel rabbit tick spiroplasma. There is an interesting image of *Spiroplasma citri* cells published within a citrus industry pest control textbook. The photograph demonstrates that these spirochetes also create sac-like "blebs" similar to the blebs created by Bb spirochetes.[13-19]

Spiroplasmas are considered to be highly motile (mobile) and to have a helical membrane tube. Attached to the inside of the tube is a flat ribbon of parallel fibrils. Spiroplasma fibrillar proteins are similar to the fibrillar proteins of the agent that is thought to cause a human prion disease called Creutzfeldt-Jakob disease (CJD). This may be an important link to understand, as transmissible spongiform encephalopathies (TSEs) including CJD, bovine spongiform encephalopathy (mad cow disease); sheep scrapie; and chronic wasting disease of deer are all important, fatal diseases that may have a spiroplasma component involved with their disease pathology.[13-23]

Organophosphate chemicals have also been implicated as a cause of TSE diseases. We know that certain chemicals mutate bacteria. If they force spiroplasmas to break apart and if spiroplasma proteins are part of Bb spirochetes, it may explain how these factors are implicated in brain infections including the TSE "prion" diseases. Just like the spiroplasmas, Bb spirochetes have been implicated in brain affecting diseases including Alzheimer's and ALS. Spiroplasmas have an unusual adaptation for mammalian host brain tissues and so may spread rapidly into brain and nervous system tissues. Bb spirochetes have also been found in the brain tissue cultures of deceased patients with these diseases. It is reasonable then to suspect there may be a spiroplasma at the heart of an aggregate Lyme disease agent. This does not automatically mean that Lyme disease is a prion disease, but there may hypothetically be factors involving a Bb aggretate which could lead to prion diseases in susceptible patients under the right conditions.[13-35]

When spiroplasmas are treated with non-ionic denaturing detergents or surfactants such as those used in industrial cleaners, biocides, or agricultural chemicals and fertilizers, *spiroplasmas will cast off their cytoplasmic (cellular) contents including their fibrils.* This means they will disassemble their cells under environmental or chemical pressures. Those agents may include phosphates, detergents of agrochemicals or industrial wastewaters, or other factors. Some example chemicals are sodium deoxycholate, Triton X-100, Tweens, Nonidet P-40, and amines. The spirochetes of Lyme disease will do the very same thing in the insect body during a temperature change. Within the human body under environmental stress (i.e. temperature, antibiotics, radiation) and as a survival mechanism, the Bb spirochete will change its outer surface protein structure by casting off one kind of protein to assume another form that is more compatible with the changing environment.[36,37]

The Bb spirochete can assume motile, helical, wall-less L-forms, S-forms, cysts, or blebs. It can aggregate into plaques or utilize the kinds of slimy biofilms that are established by other organisms within the gut. There it will sequester itself and hide among other microbes like a boat seeking shelter in a storm. Similar forms and activities are assumed by spiroplasmas. We should not assume that the casting off of spiroplasma parts occurs only in the external environment. It likely also occurs in an animal or human body; as well as a laboratory upon exposure to chemicals or detergents, including those used to create vaccines.[36]

A number of spiroplasmas infect plants and animals that eat spiroplasma-infected plants. Spiroplasmas may be found in the circulation of nearly all insects including mosquitoes, flies, bees, beetles, mites, and ticks. Spiroplasma strain *S. citri* harbors its own satellite virus, identified as "SpV1-R8A2B." This is a single-stranded, rod-shaped DNA virus, (baculovirus), and another example of a spirochetal bacteria that is co-infected with a baculovirus.[13-15,38]

Spiroplasmas are lethal to honey bees, and are found on the surface of many trees and flowers. According to an article from

1979, tick spiroplasmas can kill chicken embryos. They can also cause cataracts, neurologic problems, and death in neonatal rats. Some spiroplasma strains are known to cause mastitis infections in cattle. Spiroplasmas have been isolated from infected stunted corn plants; from rice plants infected with yellow dwarf virus; from cacti, lettuce, citrus, and other crops; and from ornamental plants and flowers. Corn (maize) plants have been shown to be infected with spiroplasmas and avian mycoplasmas (a bird mollicute or perhaps a cause of "bird flu"). Some of the spiroplasmas are serologically related. Spiroplasmas and phytoplasmas cause significant agricultural diseases in plants. Efforts to prevent and treat these infections are hampered by a lack of knowledge about the agents. There were twenty-eight strains of spiroplasmas listed in a 1995 published source. Included among known strains are tick, bee, leafhopper, syrphid, deerfly, beetle, tabanid, and firefly spiroplasmas.[2,39-47]

Spiroplasmas are regularly seen with blebs and spherical attachments. Much like the Bb spirochete, during cultivation spiroplasmas change their structural form (morphology). Spirals elongate and collapse until all that remains are non-helical filaments and a few round structures. The spirochetes of Lyme are also very fragile, and break apart during cultivation. The filaments and other structures when broken remain infective for Bb and spiroplasma alike. The non-helical spiroplasmas are related to the *Spiroplasma citri* strains. In younger cultures, spherical forms may dominate, followed by helical forms which increase and divide through a process of constriction. The new shorter segments resemble other mycoplasmas. Filaments can produce chains of spherical forms that produce segments. The spiroplasmas also produce phytotoxins. These are bacterial toxins similar to those found in Pierce's disease of grapevines. *Xylella fastidiosa*, a *gammaproteobacteria*, which is the agent of Pierce's disease of grapevines.[2,13,48,49]

There is a relatively new patent that is assigned to the Los Alamos National Security Company.* The patent describes compositions and methods to treat Pierce's disease. The patent reveals how human neutrophil elastase may possibly kill *Borrelia burgdorferi*. Neutrophil elastase is thought to target outer membrane proteins of organisms such as Bb. Pierce's disease typically attacks vineyards and citrus trees. The patent uses recombinant human antimicrobial proteins to treat Pierce's disease. *Xylella fastidiosa* belongs to the same class of bacteria where we find the enterobacteria *Escherichia coli* (*E. coli*). Xylella species are transmitted by plant juice-sucking insects including leafhoppers, mites, and aphids. These are the same insects that transmit spiroplasmas. Since xylella also infects citrus trees, it is interesting that the citrus spiroplasmas were noted to be similar to the 277F tick spiroplasma detected by Dr. Burgdorfer in 1967. If Bb contains a spiroplasma, perhaps this is why the two agents can both be treated using the same method.[50-53]

**Los Alamos Laboratory received the first refined batch of plutonium in 1945 for the Manhattan project. The Los Alamos National Security Company is a private company formed by Bechtel, Babcock & Wilcox Technical Services, the University of California, the US Department of Energy, and the National Nuclear Security Administration. The group took over operations and management of the Los Alamos National Laboratory from the University of California.*

The Los Alamos patent describes a way to genetically engineer plants to secrete antimicrobial agents in their xylem where insects feed and spiroplasmas live. Plant juice-sucking insects take up microbes during feeding, whereafter plant pathogens replicate in the insect gut. In a plant that has been treated with chemical and microbial insecticides, the microbes in the formula will also be taken up by the insect. The presence of chemical surfactants, nuclear residues, and bacterial spores of insecticides creates an environment in the insect gut which promotes reassortment of genes between plant and insect host. In chemically treated plants, the infections that lie within the plant's cells become part of the mixed infection as chemicals degrade cells and release the contents from the cell cytoplasm.[52-54]

The Los Alamos patent also describes a method to kill *Borrelia burgdorferi* spirochetes. Since the patent targets plant pathogens, this is an important clue that Bb spirochetes have one or more plant pathogens at its core (i.e. spiroplasma). The patent states, "Recent research has shown that human neutrophil elastase can kill the causative agent of Lyme disease, *Borrelia burgdorferi*... Neutrophil elastase is also known to target outer membrane proteins..." This patent could be an indirect admission that Bb contains a spiroplasma similar to *Spiroplasma citri*; just like the 277F tick spiroplasma that was discovered by Dr. Burgdorfer.[53,55-57]

Decades ago scientists found helical spiroplasmas within the bodies of *Ixodes* ticks from Germany, the USSR, and the US. Their emergence may have had something to do with the microbes that were being applied all over the world as insecticides; and the chemicals and/or residual radioactive elements in the formulas and/or the enviornment. The spiroplasmas copy themselves (replicate) inside the cell (cytoplasmic vacuoles) in a similar manner to that of *Coxiella burnetii*, the agent of Q fever. Spiroplasmas were sometimes isolated during Q fever studies. The spiroplasmas were shown to be distinctly different from coxiellae, ehrlichiae, and chlamydiae species of bacteria.[58-61]

The *Ixodes* tick spiroplasmas tend to be non-helical, wall-less filaments, although they can also be helical in shape. Spiroplasmas can be detected using broad-range PCR-TTGE testing (temporal temperature gradient gel electrophoresis). A new spiroplasma was isolated in 1981 from Oregon western black-legged ticks (*Ixodes pacificus*). The strain was found to be distinctly different than other known spiroplasmas. The new organism could also be isolated from tick cell cultures. Of course 1981 was the same year that NIH scientists isolated the spirochetal agent of Lyme disease. Dr. Burgdorfer was the first to identify a novel, mutated spirochete in rabbit ticks back in 1967, which he would identify as a spiroplasma similar to the citrus spiroplasma.[58-61] According to a paper's abstract:

> "...discovery of a new fastidious mycoplasma in ticks offers opportunities to explore the possible role of these agents in human and animal diseases."

Another agriculturally significant spiroplasma is the corn stunt spiroplasma *Spiroplasma kunkelii.* It was the first spiroplasma to be identified in 1946 by Kunkel, although it was found in Texas and California two years earlier. Corn stunt spiroplasmas are a significant agricultural pest of corn and other crops in the US and abroad. There is a reovirus called the Maize Rough Dwarf Fiji virus or cereal tillering disease. This is a reovirus that contributes to stunting of corn, wheat, and rice. It also represents a (satellite) virus that is known to associate with corn stunt and other spiroplasma strains. This means that spiroplasmas can be infected by reoviruses. This is significant to the Lyme story because reoviruses are not only found among mined ores, insects, and plants; they were also deployed separately and within insecticides as the CPVs, or cytoplasmic polyhedrosis viruses. Both spiroplasmas and reoviruses are found in ticks, so we may assume they are part of a Bb aggregate spirochete.[62-68]

There was a serious outbreak of corn stunt in Florida during 1979 and 1980. At least five viruses and two mollicute plant pathogens were isolated. Depending on the type of crop pest present in a given region, any number of spiroplasma strains may be found in the bodies of insects including ticks. In my book *God Science* I list a significant number of spiroplasma species including a pathogenic strain that causes cataracts and neurologic damage in suckling mice, *Spiroplasma mirum* (SMCA) or the suckling mouse cataract agent. Since spiroplasmas are found in many tick species, it is apparent they are an important aspect of neurologic diseases, including that seen in "chronic" disseminated Lyme.[62-65,69]

The very first Bb strain to be identified was named "B31." It was isolated from ticks collected on Shelter Island, New York. There also happens to be a bee-flower strain of spiroplasma that is also identified as strain "B31." Are the names a mere coincidence? As we will learn, there is much more to the story of the identification of the causative agent of Lyme than has ever been publicly revealed to an audible degree before now. The "B31" strain of *Borrelia burgdorferi* was also considered to be from a strain that causes an arthritic form of Lyme. A lab-adapted strain of B31 was used during the work group sessions for the Dearborn conference where Lyme disease diagnostic tests were standardized.[69]

Spiroplasmas have also been shown to contain a very specific Outer Surface Protein (Osp) that has been identified as *Spiralin.* This protein has the ability to adversely affect human immune function. In humans and animals, bacteriae in the mollicute group cause respiratory, urogenital, and arthritic diseases; and are considered contributing factors to other viral and bacterial diseases through the activation or suppression of immune function. Spiralin proteins are the most abundant outer surface protein of spiroplasmas. They are not required for infection (pathogenicity), but they are required in order for the spiroplasma to be transmitted by insect vectors.[62-65,70-73]

Spiroplasmas display antigenic variation. This process describes the ability to swap outer surface proteins to avoid immune detection within a host. This technique is also used by the Bb spirochete to do the very same thing. The Lyme disease agent requires its outer surface protein A (OspA), to be transmissible to insects from plants. It also requires its outer surface protein B (OspB) in order to adhere to, and to survive within the tick body. In order to be infective to mammals, Bb requires its outer surface protein C (OspC). The difference in necessary proteins demonstrates that the organism has adapted to multiple hosts. Such adaptability is found in both Bb and spiroplasma spirochetes.[62-65,70-73]

A study described how mouse spleen cells could be made to react and proliferate in the presence of spiroplasma spiralin protein. This is the same stimulating ability demonstrated by the OspA and OspB proteins of the Bb spirochete. In mouse spleen cells, spiralin proteins caused "T-cell-independent blastogenesis of the B-cells." This is reproduction by budding in response to the presence of spiralin antigens; which are highly immune-stimulating substances.[64]

Bacterial lipoproteins (LPS), which are endotoxins; and a synthetic OspA lipopeptide designed for the first Lyme vaccine (called Pam3Cys)* was unable to activate mouse B-cells without a co-stimulating molecule. This means that the synthetic vaccine protein "Pam3Cys" alone was insufficient to cause an immune response to bacterial endotoxins. An additional co-factor was probably involved in the activation of the B-cell immune response in patients who received a Lyme vaccine. LPS, lipopolysaccharides, or lipoproteins, are bacterial endotoxins that are found in the outer surface proteins of bacteria. These proteins stimulate antibody production during infection. Studies demonstrated that spiroplasma spiralin proteins activated a larger number of resting B-cells than either bacteria or synthetic LPS alone.[64]

**The scientific name for the synthetic Lyme vaccine peptide is Pam3CysSer(Lys)4-OH. There is also a synthetic Pam2Cys formula.*

If the Bb spirochete contains spiralin proteins, then this may explain the kind of B-cell hyperactivity often seen in the dysfunctional immune systems of Lyme patients. A spiroplasma outer surface protein gene would be considered useful in vaccines and diagnostic tests to detect spiroplasma infections. We might note also that a gene for spiralin was recombinantly cloned and expressed within *E. coli*, (a gut bacterium) according to a study published in 1985.[62-65,70]

The questions to ask are whether this recombinant clone was used within laboratory test probes that were standardized to detect Lyme disease; or whether spiralin proteins or other spiroplasma antigens were part of the first generation of OspA-based Lyme disease vaccines. Perhaps the Bb diagnostic tests that carry a horseradish-based probe do so partly because these plants are commonly infected with *Spiroplasma citri*.[62-65,70]

As of 2010, spiroplasmas were found in about 80% of all flies (*Drosophila neotestacea*) collected from upstate New York. This lends a clue that spiroplasmas from this area (or any other) may contribute to Bb mixed infections. Bb spirochetes have been found within the guts of mosquitoes and various fly species, although these additional vectors are almost never discussed as able to transmit Bb infections. One paper revealed that "museum specimens"of this mosquito were collected in the 1980s (after the announcement of the Lyme disease agent), and that they do not have spiroplasma spirochetes. This doesn't really make a difference in the tick model however. It simply means that the flies probably weren't picking up spiroplasma infections from animal wastes or wastewaters before 1980. However these mushroom-eating flies are known to be infested with nematodes and wolbachia.[74-76]

Documents provide rough estimates of what scientists felt was the prevelance of spiroplasmas in NY flies at the time – about 14%. This means that spiroplasma infections have grown substantially in number over the past several decades. There was a corresponding increase in commercial insecticide use during the same period. It is important to reveal that fruit flies were the first flies identified as having genes called transposons. These special genes are capable of causing the reassortment of fruit fly genes – genes that may be transmissible to other fly species. According to sources, fruit flies across America are evolving more rapidly than they would have if left to the devices of Mother Nature. What may be driving their evolution is the natural or genetically engineered genes, and/or infections such as wolbachia or spiroplasmas.[73-77]

A Yale Evolutionary Biologist commented in an article about the spread of beneficial microbes. Symbionts allow flies a kind of horizontal gene transfer which provides them with special adaptations they might not otherwise acquire. In one case the adaptation is bacterial resistance. Bacteria are noted to be "ultra-adaptable" organisms capable of picking up new genetic material over their life span. This helps drive mutations in insects and other bacteria when they share reassorted genes.[74,76]

The Gates Foundation recently provided a grant for scientists to study whether spiroplasmas can be used to control human parasitic infections. This is a good question, and the answer may not only be disappointing, but closer than we realize. They may already be part of a pathogenic aggregate spirochete that causes persistent human infections called Lyme disease (and Morgellon's). But then again, perhaps the studies may also address a known human epidemic already affecting people around the world.[74,76]

Spiroplasmas have been observed attached to the midgut tissues of Colorado potato beetles collected from Alberta and Quebec, Canada. They have also been found in beetles from the US (Arizona, Maine, Maryland, Massachusetts, Michigan, Minnesota, New Jersey, New Mexico, New York, North Carolina, Utah, and Washington). They were likewise observed in chrysomelid beetles from Texas. In 1973, scientists were studying the mycoplasma-like citrus spiroplasma, and noted under darkfield microscopy that it produced helical and non-helical forms; that it presented with surface projections; and that it produced a tailed, type-B bacteriophage that attaches to its outer layer. By 1984, three years after the Bb spirochete was isolated, spiroplasmas were being discussed in relation to biological controls but not necessarily for their usefulness as insecticides.[78-80]

While the spiroplasmas are not known to be pathogenic to Colorado potato beetles, the fact that they are easily transmitted was explored as a tool into which *Bacillus thuringiensis* subspecies tenebrionis and its delta-endotoxin genes might be incorporated as an insecticide by 1982, the year the Lyme agent was announced. Perhaps an existing B.t.-spiroplasma model that occurred naturally in ticks was being studied as a model for a new B.t.-spiroplasma insecticide. The general idea was to use spiroplasmas as a host for the B.t. insecticide toxins; and then to infect insects with the formula. After the initial study, seven spiroplasma isolates were made available for further studies. A 1991 French study suggested that *Spiroplasma taiwanense* would make a good biological control agent against mosquitoes. The B.t.-spiroplasma studies took place two years before the Dearborn conference.[80-84]

By 1984, two years after the announcement of the Lyme disease agent, spiroplasmas were already being studied for their potential as insecticides. Does this timing lend a clue that those who were studying the agent of Lyme disease understood the presence of spiroplasmas in Lyme disease-transmitting ticks, and thereafter decided to keep this secret; quietly exploiting this accidentally-formed agent as a novel insecticidal tool? We have only to examine the various agricultural patents filed on or around the period that the Lyme disease agent was identified; and the events which transpired at Dearborn to elucidate what could have been "secret" motivations behind keeping certain aspects of Lyme disease history entirely absent from the public's awareness.[81,82]

A Fungal Spiroplasma is Born

In 1882 parasitic wasps were first introduced into the US from Canada to control the gooseberry sawfly. The following year parasites of the cabbage butterfly became the first parasitoid species shipped intercontinentally into the US. Beginning in 1888 in order to protect citrus groves, US agricultural scientists imported coccinelid and vedalia beetles (ladybirds or ladybugs) from Australia to California. These were the first major attempts by the USDA to control agriculturally important pests through the use of parasitoids. We might inquire about the types of fungal, viral, spirochetal, and other agents that were covertly hiding in the bodies of these early imports. One answer may have been a fungal infection called *Coccidioides immitis,* the agent of coccidioidomycosis infections.[1-3]

Coccidioides immitis is a sporulating fungus that begins with "flu"-like symptoms and a simple skin infection. Untreated it spreads systemically to other tissues. This fungus is common to the American southwest including California (as San Joaquin valley fever). It is also found in Mexico and Central and South Americas. Fungi are notoriously unstable organisms capable of gene swapping with other organisms including bacteria; especially under direction of chemicals or viruses that promote such events. We know that experimental coccidioidomycosis was an area of interest as a biological weapon of warfare by Ft. Detrick scientists during the 1950s and 1960s. The "cash" strain of this fungus received the military name "OC." It was however known to be a lethal fungus, so it was never formally weaponized, although limited field trials were undertaken. Most of the military studies for this fungus concerned vaccines and the study of fungal spores as airborne pathogens. This fungus remains on the CDC's list of select agents (potential biowarfare weapons).[4-15]

In 1968, coccidioidomycosis was one of the least known diseases in Poland. However it was already endemic at this time in the US, northern Mexico, and South America (Bolivia, Argentina, Venezuela, Paraguay). It was also present but to a lesser degree in Hawaii and Alaska. Abroad it was found in Italy, Great Britain, the USSR, and Africa. This fungal infection affects the lungs, skin, oral cavity, and the digestive tract. It is most commonly found in humans, domestic animals, rodents, and lizards. Some infections are asymptomatic. The *Erythema nodosum* lesions seen on patients with the skin version of coccidioidomycosis look exactly like the "atypical" (non-bull's-eye) rashes seen during acute Lyme infections. It is entirely possible that by 1968, this fungus was already part of a mutated spirochete that was emerging within animal and human populations. Was it also part of a mutated tick spiroplasma that was first identified by Dr. Burgdorfer in 1967?[4-18]

When I considered how a novel tick spiroplasma strain might be created, I realized that this fungus, which likely arrived during the 1880s in the imported parasitoid insects, was already endemic on the west coast by the 1940s. It would have been highly prevalent upon citrus crops where the early parasitoid beetles were released. One of the most common plant pathogens of citrus trees today are the spiroplasmas. We can see how an important spiroplasma/fungal pair could be present as a mixed infection in plants and insects. The fungi and the spiroplasmas probably mutated to create a novel mutant spirochete that infected ticks and other insects. In order to understand how this might occur, we must remember that scientists and farmers were dumping fungi and insect baculoviruses into the environment. They were also placing mutagenic agricultural chemicals upon citrus and other crops, and there were radioactive trace elements involved in the process, as well.[16-18]

The presence of a spiroplasma-fungal mutant such as may be found in the tick 277F spiroplasma may explain some of the varied symptoms during Lyme infections. In other words symptoms could depend upon which fungi mutated with a bacterium to make a pathogenic spiroplasma strain. What is the spiroplasma? It could be a plant spirillum-gammaproteobacteria-fungal mutant. The *Spirillum* are gram-negative soil and water-borne spirochetes. One strain, *Spirillum minus* is associated with rat-bite fever. In that case, the spiroplasma may be a spirillum-fungi-rickettsial bacterial mutant.[19]

The kind of pathogenic spiroplasma created could vary depending on the type of fungi and bacteria applied to, or found in the environment. A spiroplasma-fungal hybrid could emerge since fungi are notably genetically unstable. Spiroplasmas have segmented genomes, and so do other bacteria and viruses. This means they may easily swap genes with other microbes including fungi. We may take this a step further to find a spiroplasma-leptospira mutant in soil or water if a leptospira bacterium becomes polluted or infected with other microbes. This may occur due to bacteriophages or the mutagenic action of chemicals and toxic wastes.

Spiroplasmas are pathogenic to ticks. Patent inventions for vaccines now routinely screen formulas for spiroplasmas although earlier vaccine formulas did not. We must wonder then if spiroplasmas were found to contaminate insect or animal cell lines for animal or human vaccines, animal feeds, or insecticides. If so we may see the subsequent creation of new insect cell lines at some critical point in time (and we will).[20-32]

Let's look at the fungal connection for a moment. In Kern County, California, viruses were collected from desert arthropods and wild vertebrates between 1961 and 1968. They were also collected from adjacent irrigated agricultural fields in the San Joaquin valley and the Sierra foothills within fifty miles of Bakersfield, California. Additional collections were obtained near the Kern River in the Mohave Desert. Coccidioidomycosis (San Joaquin valley fever or Valley fever) was already a problem on southwestern military bases by 1941, since it was endemic in the southwest by the 1930s. At the time, new arrivals and resident military personnel were screened for this fungus at training bases including Bakersfield; and at Kern County airport by scientists from Stanford and the California Department of Public Health.[33-36]

Perhaps collections made in this same area two decades later were designed to check the spread of an important fungus. Were scientists concerned that the fungi had mutated in the bodies of insects? Or were they worried that military field trials of aerosolized *Coccidioides immitus* had helped spread the fungi? Remember that in 1968, Ft. Detrick scientists would meet in Chicago to report progress on the aerosolization of mosquito-borne pathogens including yellow fever, Rocky Mt. spotted fever, Venezuelan equine encephalitis, and coccidioidomycosis. I find it incredibly interesting that each of these pathogens includes a family member that according to my theories also makes up an aggregate spirochete called *Borrelia burgdorferi.*[33-37]

Aerosolization experiments could have been studying whether the components of an aggregate spirochete were spreading as airborne contaminants because of agricultural or industrial pollutants – not necessarily that they would make an attractive biowarfare weapon. During the late 1960s there was ongoing research into the role of aerosolized pathogens and human viral respiratory diseases. These studies were undertaken by scientists at the US Army Biological Center (Ft. Detrick), and the National Institute of Allergy and Infectious Diseases, National Institutes of Health. Investigations were probably studying the cause and effect of agents, and the development of useful vaccines. I say this because by this time it was known that *Coccidioides immitus* fungi "targets" certain ethnicities more than others. This factor was actually considered to be an undesirable trait for a "covert" biowarfare tool (perhaps because the race aspect is too obvious). Therefore any interests in this fungi were probably geared toward developing vaccines and studying its ability to combine with other airborne and insect-borne pathogens.[33-37]

The introduction of *Coccidioides immitus* into the US may have occurred in 1882 when USDA scientists imported the first wasps from Canada or the coccinellid and vedalia beetles from Australia a few years later. Then again spores could have been introduced quite simply following a major earthquake, such as one that shook California in 1865. The prevalence of this fungus was shown to be measurably increased after at least one earthquake. In the US, coccidioidomycosis infections are endemic along the Pacific coastal states; and in Arizona, New Mexico, and Texas. The first human case of coccidioidomycosis was documented in Buenos Aires in 1892 in an Argentine soldier who had been sick since 1889. (Remember the 1840 imports of bat guano from Peru?) This fungus is prevalent in insect populations, including the imported Australian parasitoid beetles. Australia, Japan, the Russian Far East, and the Pacific coastlines of North and South America are located along the "Pacific Ring of Fire." This area has a long chain of active volcanoes. It is also home to hydrothermal and geothermal veins which harbor thermophile and sulfur-reducing bacteriae and reoviruses. The microbes from deep underground are brought to the surface through volcanic activity, earthquakes, natural springs, and industrial mining.[38-41]

This fungus was thought to have arrived in the San Joaquin valley of California (where it is highly endemic) by migrant workers. However we can see that early biological control attempts using bat guano fertilizers or beetles upon citrus crops is a more likley culprit, since the fungi are not commonly transmitted by person-to-person contact.* Some reports indicated that Valley fever may have been introduced from the midwest following the Dust Bowl of the 1930s (the "Dirty Thirties"). However we know the infection was already endemic in California by then. The more likely scenario is that the infection rode on or in the imported Australian beetles that were agriculturally deployed.[38-44]

**Human sexual and in utero transmission has been documented for this fungus.*

Soil microbes from seismic activity that become airborne may include the paenibacillus, thermophiles, coccidioides fungi, and reoviruses. The presence of these agents in insects also makes sense where there are radioactive elements, metals, phosphates, and aggregate rocks. Fungal infections are a side effect of radiation and could be a common problem for insects found near radioactive ores. (Australia is a huge exporter of mined minerals by the way, including bauxite, phosphates, and uranium.) We can understand how a bacterium and a regional fungus could mutate and be transmitted by insects, especially since bacteria are essentially fungi. Nuclear wastes cannot be ruled out as a mutagenic factor as they appear in agricultural products, wastewaters, and soils. They are also found as airborne contaminants from cooling towers, steam vents, and atmospheric fallout. Exposures to radioactive wastes could certainly foster fungal infections in insects exposed to them as well as reassortments between fungi and bacteria.[38-41]

During the summer of 1948 in California's San Joaquin valley, testing and field trials of NPV baculoviruses from imported cabbageworms were undertaken on four plots which ranged in size from .2 to 6.2 acres. Tests were repeated the following year. The applications effectively reduced larval populations in the trial areas. In the fall of 1949, aerial and ground sprays were again deployed. In 1968 and 1969, scientists conducted additional experiments with orange and tangelo seedlings to study natural *Spiroplasma citri* infections. Test plots were located at University of California field stations including Mareno Ranch east of Riverside; two in the San Joaquin valley; one at the Citrus Research Center, Riverside; and one at South Coast field station, Irvine.[42,43]

Extensive field applications of baculoviruses were undertaken across the US and Canada from the 1940s through the mid-1970s. Baculoviruses caused insect epizootics (infectious disease outbreaks) in the areas where they were applied, and spread up to twenty miles from their point of origin. Did the early applications of baculoviruses and fungal agents used on agricultural fields contribute to the formation of the novel fungus/spiroplasma mutants?[42-44]

Mutagenic herbicides and insecticides are applied to crops including citrus, field corn, and ornamental flowers. Either may have caused the mutation of a plant spirochetal bacterium such as a spirillum and a fungus. The fungus could be either naturally derived (*C. immitis*), or one from an applied insecticide (*Beauveria bassiana*). For example the citrus spiroplasma, corn stunt spiroplasma, and the bee spiroplasmas could have each been created by a different fungus which mutated with a single plant spirochete. These could form the various spiroplasma strains such as *S. citri* (citrus spiroplasma); *Spiroplasma kunkelii* (corn stunt spiroplasma); and *Spiroplasma apis* (bee spiroplasma). Bees and other insects carry multiple plant pathogens as they pollinate; and that which reassorts inside a bee gut could create a bee-flower "B31" spiroplasma, and likewise for the corn stunt and citrus strains. A similar tick-transmissible agent was identified by Dr. Willy Burgdorfer as a 277F spiroplasma. Since the Bb agent was named after him, it would not be surprising to find a spiroplasma/fungal component in an aggregate Bb spirochete. (Does the "F" in 277F represent a fungus?)

A 1964 US military report for a Canadian laboratory described how fungal wheat stem rust spores were incubated in a phosphate buffer that contained pelargonic acid-1-C14. Scientists were probably studying the fungi's ability to degrade pelargonic acid into acetyl CoA. Pelargonic acid is a fatty acid used in plasticizers (plastics), lacquers, and herbicides. Acetyl CoA is produced during cellular respiration, which takes place in the mitochondria (cell engines). This is an important component to the neurotransmitter acetylcholine in the human body. Another patent describes the use of insecticides and transgenic plants to circumvent insect resistance. The invention uses acetylcholinesterase (AChE) inhibitors within its insecticidal formulas.[45,46]

What if human neurotransmitters are altered by exposures to chemical or biological formulas, including herbicides, plasticizers, plastic wastes, plastics in bottled water, or insecticides? Can the plasticizers of fertilizer microbead formulas adversely affect the microbes contained within them or the natural fungi found in the environment? It is possible that insecticides contribute to human neurotransmitter-affecting illnesses (i.e. Lyme disease, Multiple Sclerosis, Parkinson's, ALS, or even depression). Remember "TX" (wheat stem rust) spores were part of the US military's anti-crop biowarfare arsenal post WWII. Any stem rust or other spores could be used agriculturally as "nerve agents" to target insect populations, and still arguably be considered to have a peaceful use. We know that for years insecticides have been deployed above civilian areas, and spraying continues today to control gypsy moths for example. Could outdated anti-crop weapons have been reassigned for agricultural use?[45,46]

A military report described stem rust infection and "development" studies undertaken from 1960 to 1965 using artificially inoculated wheat fields. The studies occurred while large-scale efforts to control aphid infestations across North America were well underway. Aphids carry a number of important infections including spiroplasmas. Such experiments could have contributed to the formation of novel insect infections that would be detected just a few years later in animals in Illinois. According to the report, the epidemiology of stem rust was studied just two states west in Hays, Kansas in fields which contained Cheyenne wheat that had been inoculated with wheat stem rust spores.[47]

Plant infections developed during all six years of testing. Outdoor field testing of wheat rust spores also took place just three years before the discovery of a novel tick spiroplasma that would be isolated by Dr. Willy Burgdorfer. Is it possible that a novel agent from plants and insects, agrochemicals; and experimental wheat fungus spores produced a genetically mutated microbe only to be detected three years later? If so, it is entirely possible that such pathogens may have contributed to an infection that would emerge in animals during the mid-1960s, and in human patients at the end of the same decade.[47]

In 1983, just a year after the Bb agent was formally announced, a paper was published in a Yale Journal by NIAID, USDA, and French scientists. The paper described the spiroplasmas of Group I, or the *Spiroplasma citri* cluster. The authors proposed that Group I, which includes the citrus, honeybee, and corn stunt spiroplasmas, be further divided into seven subgroups as determined by DNA. The Yale article describes the first International Congress on Mycoplasmas that was held in Bordeaux, France in 1974. This was just one year before the declaration of an arthritis-like outbreak in Connecticut. It seems that scientists were already studying the spiroplasma for several years before the Connecticut outbreak was officially announced – an epidemic that may yet prove to include a spiroplasma. We might wonder why the French conference was held; probably because there was a new mutant bacterial/fungal spirochete that was attacking grape vines in the region. It is curious that the mycoplasma conference was held the year before the Connecticut outbreak was announced, and Yale scientists published a paper about the French May disease the year after the Bb spirochete was "identified." However "nobody" said anything about Bb possibly containing a spiroplasma, either then or at any time since.[48,49]

At the time of the 1974 mycoplasma conference, only three helical spiroplasmas had been identified. These were the agents of citrus stubborn disease, the corn stunt spiroplasma, and the drosophila (fruit fly) sex ratio agent. According to a Yale paper, during the 1960s the agents of citrus stubborn or corn stunt had not yet been identified; but they actually had been, and so had another spiroplasma, the 277F tick agent isolated by Dr. Burgdorfer in 1967. This agent resembled the citrus spiroplasma, *S. citri*. Two additional spiroplasmas were isolated from rabbit ticks (SMCA and GT-48). These were grown in chicken embryos, and described as viruses or mycoplasmas by the early 1970s. In 1980 after all currently known spiroplasma strains were analyzed, the agents were reclassified. This was just one year before the "discovery" of the causative agent of Lyme disease, and the year before the isolation of a novel spirochete from a Lyme patient's ECM rash – another spirochete no one has "talked" about back then, or any time since in relation to Lyme disease.[48-52]

According to a 1983 Yale paper, among the newly discovered spiroplasma strains were some unclassified strains, including the green leaf bug spiroplasma (LB-12), the Coco spiroplasma (N525), and the Maryland flower spiroplasma (M55). By the time the report was published, none of the unclassified strains or the 277F spiroplasmas were identified in the report as the cause of any disease. This is curious even though it was known that spiroplasmas had been isolated from Lyme disease-transmitting ticks. Instead, a chart in the paper indicated that the status of spiroplasmas as pathogens was "unknown." In France, the well-known honeybee "May" disease had already been identified and associated with spiroplasmas from Group IV. By the conclusion of the Yale study, it was clear that the spiroplasmas *S. citri*, the honeybee, and the corn stunt subgroups were considered to be pathogenic organisms. It is however strange that they were not considered to be connected to any current human disease outbreaks. Other members of the spiroplasma subgroups showed remarkable similarity, so we must consider whether these were pathogenic, including the 277F agent originally isolated from Montana rabbit ticks by Dr. Burgdorfer, decades earlier.[48-53]

Another 1981 paper suggested that spiroplasmas may be more widespread in insects than previously believed. At the time the paper was written, forty percent of the fruit fly *Drosophila hydei** population in Ito, Japan, was thought to be infected with spiroplasmas. A large percentage of leafhoppers surveyed in Florida also showed evidence of spiroplasma infections. In order for spiroplasmas to fulfill a life cycle, they must pass through and multiply within at least two cell types. These include the gut epithelial cells, and the salivary glands. Spiroplasmas are found mainly in the insect hemolymph (circulation). Rabbit ticks have yielded both the 277F and SMCA spiroplasmas.[54]

**These fruit flies are attracted to gardens, orchards, decaying vegetation, and livestock areas.*

In 1981, although the SMCA spiroplasma had not yet been isolated from vertebrates, they were nevertheless assumed to be pathogenic. In contrast, the 277F agent cultured from Dr. Burgdorfer's rabbit ticks in 1967 was not associated with any vertebrate infections. Another 1981 report described spiroplasmas that were isolated from *Ixodes* ticks. These spiroplasmas were referred to as "helical mycoplasmas." The Bb organism is also helical in shape. According to the paper:

> "...the vertebrate pathogenicity of spiroplasmas raises questions about their potential pathogenicity for man. Spiroplasmas recovered from rabbit ticks may have limited potential for transmission to humans, since these arthropods infrequently bite man."[54]

This statement is a bit short-sighted since rabbit ticks are not the only species to harbor spiroplasmas or that bite humans. It was proposed that spiroplasmas were infectious to humans prior to the announcement that the Bb agent had been isolated; and yet spiroplasmas were not, and have never been *audibly* mentioned in association with the agent of Lyme disease; nor that Lyme-transmitting ticks harbor them at any time at an *audible* level up to the present day.[54]

The article goes on to say that other North American tick species including *Amblyomma, Dermacentor*, and *Ixodes* represent a "more serious pathogenic potential" due to the presence of spiroplasmas in these human-biting ticks. This is acknowledgement that there are spiroplasmas in these ticks and also that they may be pathogenic. The paper refers to a "human disease of unknown etiology, the so-called 'Lyme disease,'" which according to the paper's authors, "directed our attention to the possibility that spiroplasmas may occur in this tick genus. *We now report the discovery of a new spiroplasma from Ixodes*."[54]

It is obvious that scientists have known about spiroplasmas for the past half century. It is curious though why scientists might remain so intransigent against the possibility that spiroplasmas found in Lyme disease transmitting ticks are transmissible and infectious to humans. We must wonder why those who have known about the spiroplasmas have failed to publicly and openly discuss many infectious agents that have been isolated from Lyme disease transmitting ticks. It is strange that spiroplasmas have never been publicly associated with the Lyme disease agent even though four decades have passed since the tick spiroplasma was identified by the same scientist after whom the Bb agent was named.

In 1975 and 1977 soon after the announcement of a "Lyme arthritis" outbreak, the NIAID awarded two grants to Dr. Burgdorfer's colleague, Dr. L.P. Brinton. Dr. Brinton published nearly a dozen articles from 1970-1975, sometimes with Dr. Burgdorfer as co-author. Brinton's grant studies included Colorado tick fever (reo)virus development in *Dermacentor andersoni* ticks,* and the structure of the gut from normal, and Rocky Mt. spotted fever infected ticks of this species. The two grants also funded comparative work on the fine structure of wolbachia-like organisms in various tick species; the structure of *R. rickettsii* and rickettsia species in brown dog ticks from Mississippi; and the investigation of the spiroplasma 277F agent from cottontail rabbit ticks. Here was Dr. Burgdorfer's colleague studying spiroplasmas before the Lyme agent was formally announced![55-58]

**The "Colorado tick fever" studies could have included other reoviruses, which may have led to the Lyme disease outbreak that was just announced. Did scientists already suspect a reovirus-spiroplasma component to the as yet unidentified Lyme disease agent?*

Remember that in 1968, Ft. Detrick scientists met in Chicago to study the progress of aerosolized "biowarfare" agents which included Rocky Mt. spotted fever, yellow fever, Venezuelan equine encephalitis (a possibly degraded reovirus), and the "experimental" fungi coccidioidomycosis. Were the Ft. Detrick aerosolized biowarfare agents studied for agricultural use? Were military scientists already aware of an emerging animal pathogen that was beginning to affect humans? Did that pathogen emerge as a result of industrial and agricultural pollutants?[55-57]

If tick-carried spiroplasmas, fungi, arboviruses, or reoviruses have absolutely nothing to do with Lyme disease, then it is curious that "everybody" was so fascinated with them at the time of the Connecticut outbreak, including colleagues of Dr. Burgdorfer. Remember that Dr. Burgdorfer had also studied a former biowarfare agent Q fever; an agent that resembled the livestock diseases typhus and psittacosis, and one sometimes found in the presence of spiroplasmas.

Top US military personnel were well aware of San Joaquin valley fever during the 1940s. The staff of military laboratories were alerted to the infection as scientists visited military hospital and bases across the country to study the disease's epidemiology. Reports reveal that military installations in California, Colorado, Georgia, Louisiana, Michigan, New York, New Mexico, North Carolina, Tennessee, and Washington were visited for this purpose. Infections were noted in Florida, Iowa, North Carolina, and at Walter Reed Hospital in Washington, DC during the mid-1940s. Service personnel were routinely tested for this fungal infection upon return from overseas duty, especially soldiers returning from Australia where the fungus is found in humans and insects.[58-60]

Animal experiments with coccidioidomycosis were undertaken upon monkeys, mice, and dogs from 1949 until the 1960s, and vaccines were attempted. This could explain the aerosolization progress reports discussed by Ft. Detrick scientists in Chicago in 1968. One military report revealed that five fungal strains were possible vaccine candidates. Some of the Ft. Detrick cutaneous (skin) fungal studies included pulmonary vaccination (aerosolization and inhalation in an aerosol chamber); or forearm inoculation. Cutaneous studies used five strains with varied virulence upon humans and experimental animals. These experiments may have used Operation Whitecoat volunteers to test military vaccines.[61-71]

By 1968, not only had a novel tick spiroplasma strain been identified by Dr. Burgdorfer, but the military's interest in Rocky Mt. spotted fever may have included other members of the *alphaproteobacteria* family where *R. rickettsii* is found. This may include bacterial families such as the *Caulobacterales* (caulobacter) water bacteriae, and the *Rhizobiales* (nitrogen-fixing plant root bacteriae). Among the genera in this group are *Agrobacterium tumefaciens,* which is highly important to genetic engineering and to crop science. A familiar Lyme co-infection called *Bartonella henselae* is also found in the rhizobiales (plant) pathogen category. Yes plant bacteria are turning out to be pathogenic to animals and humans. Also in this group are the *Brucellaceae*, a family that includes an important insect and animal infection, brucellosis. This is another agent that was studied by the military as a potential "biowarfare weapon," for its livestock significance.[72,73]

As for the agents of yellow fever that Ft. Detrick scientists were discussing in Chicago in 1968, the yellow fever studies may have disguised another mutated pathogen in the form of a *leptonema.* It seems plain that military scientists may have been trying to determine the origins of an emerging animal pathogen that might soon become a human public health concern. Their aerobiology experiments could have had an agricultural focus to determine how an aggregate animal pathogen had been created, not how to create an aggregate Bb spirochete. They may have already known about and were actively tracking important animal spirochetes that had formed from agricultural and environmental pollutants. Indeed contrary to popular belief, most military experiments appear to have revolved around agricultural tools and the creation of vaccines for pathogens that already existed, and not solely for the design and fabrication of human "biowarfare" agents for military deployment.[72]

Did a mutation or a horizontal gene transfer occur between indigenous bacteria and an airborne fungus? Were airborne contaminants the result of agricultural deployments, or industrial pollutants from discharged nuclear wastes or mixed fuel coal-burning? Was an environmental pollutant responsible for the mutation of soil or water spirochetes? We can understand why scientists studied aerobiology and disease transmission; to determine the origins of infectious agents and to create meaningful vaccines for emerging pathogens. With the extensive field experiments in California and other areas that deployed viruses and fungi, we can see how pathogens under the influence of catalysts may swap genes in co-infected plants. We might also expect to see public health agencies and military scientists tracking the progress of emerging pathogens over time; especially if they were emerging as a result of agricultural chemicals, industrial pollutants, or recombinant insecticides that had been deployed.[74]

Spirochetes and Yellows Diseases

Fertilizers support crop and microbial growth. Modern fertilizers are purer in form, highly concentrated, and are more soluble to plants. They also contain trace elements which can exert radioactive stressors upon microbes. The superphosphates, nitrogen, potassium, and chlorine-containing fertilizers have greatly contributed to the over fertilization of soils. The addition of chemical herbicides, fungicides, and insecticides also contributes to imbalanced soil micronutrients. These products purposely skew the microbial content of the soil and waters where applied. In soils, the binding of valuable minerals (i.e. zinc, iron, manganese) by applied chemicals fosters the proliferation of bacteriae and viruses, depending on soil nutrient quality. The correct balance allows plants to stay free of disease, while an imbalance encourages disease. When using agricultural chemicals, soil supplement becomes necessary to replace whatever lacks from the nutrient binding ability of fertilizer formulas.

Various soil bacillus strains are capable of taking up heavy metals from the environment (i.e. copper, mercury, silver). This uptake can adversely affect the division of chromosomes in cells because the metals cause the chromosomes to become "sticky" and this prevents proper cellular division, leading to mutations. The bacilli produce a capsule that takes up metallic ions such as zinc, magnesium, manganese, iron, and calcium; whether these ions are in the external; or the internal environment of the body. Soils depleted of certain nutrients will produce plants suffering from yellows diseases. Mosquitoes, aphids, white flies, and leaf and planthoppers can transmit yellows diseases of crops and ornamental plants (i.e. aster yellows) – diseases that may infect animals and humans (i.e. yellow fever). The yellows diseases of plants typically involve a mollicute bacteria such as a phytoplasma, a mycoplasma, or a spiroplasma. Aster yellows of plants is caused by a mycoplasma-like spirochete, *Spiroplasma citri* (which has its own satellite virus). Other yellows diseases are caused by related spiroplasmas and phytoplasmas in association with yellow's viruses (i.e. potato yellow mosaic virus). Yellows diseases can also be caused by related mosaic or compatible viruses in combination with other spirochetes. Yellow fever of humans for example is caused by *Flavivirus fibricus*, a mosquito-borne arbovirus and a leptospira spirochete.[1-18]

When silicon is added to soils as an amendment, certain plant diseases are reduced, including rice brown spot, rice sheath blight, and rice blast fungus. Iron-rich soils reduce wilt in peanuts and mangos. Iron applied to fruit trees reduces silver leaf infections. Increased iron contributes to fusarium wilt in tomatoes. Copper added to the soil significantly reduces fungal diseases such as stem melanosis in wheat and barley crops (by *Pseudomonas chicorii*). Copper also reduces ergot diseases.[19-23]

Excess copper supports the growth of *E. coli*, vibrio, pseudomonas, and *Bacillus cereus*. These bacteriae demonstrate extracellular proteins which detoxify copper. The addition of manganese reduces late blight of potatoes and stem rot, but increases corn leaf blight, tobacco mosaic, and fusarium wilt in tomatoes. Plants that are diseased with spiroplasmas (i.e. corn stunt), do not consume as many nutrients from the soil as their healthy counterparts. This may be because the soil lacks these nutrients or because the spiroplasma agents are robbing the nutrients from the plants they parasitize. Magnesium uptake from soil is noticeably altered in spiroplasma-infected plants. This may be a clue that people whose infections involve a spiroplasma may demonstrate lowered levels of magnesium and manganese in their bodies – a condition often seen in Lyme patients.[19-23]

Gemini viruses are important plant viruses which cause serious crop damage, and which commonly reassort in coinfected plants and insects, giving rise to new virus combinations. Members of this family include the *African cassava mosaic virus* (cassava latent virus), the brown streak virus, potato yellow mosaic virus, maize streak virus, bean golden mosaic virus, beet curly-top virus, and the tomato pseudo-curly top virus. These viruses are transmitted by plant and leafhoppers, mites, and whiteflies.

Monsanto and Smithsonian scientists were collaborating in Panama; bioprospecting for novel biological control agents useful against whiteflies. Another of their objectives was to establish diagnostic tools to detect HIV and cancer. This is a clue that whiteflies, the plants they infest (i.e. cassava, corn, beets) and the geminiviruses (i.e. cassava latent virus, mosaic viruses) may indeed play a significant role in human diseases including the HTLV/HIV family of viruses.[24-33]

What was probably a polyhedrosis virus was recorded as early as the sixteenth century. Jaundice or yellows disease of silkworms was the very first insect virus to be scientifically described. Researchers are said to know more about this insect virus than perhaps any other. This silkworm virus, *Borrelina bombycis* became the center point of nomenclature for all other insect viruses. The silkworm virus *Borrelina bombycis* is a filterable* RNA virus that produces ultramicroscopic granules. It can be seen under darkfield microscopy and was characterized according to a publication as: "Viruses [which induce] polyhedral, wilt, and other diseases; hosts, Lepidoptera, so far as known." The literature leans toward the inclusion of the polyhedrosis viruses of wasps, flies, mosquitoes, and honey bees as members of the *Borrelina paillot* group. The release of borrelina viruses by New Haven, Connecticut scientists beginning in 1951 proved they were useful for agumenting baculovirus-containing insecticides. However their subsequent promotion for global use may prove to have been a highly problematic, animal and human disease-causing endeavor.[33-37]

**Filterable refers to the ability of tiny viruses to pass through laboratory filters.*

Grasserie disease in silkworms (jaundice), another form of "wilt" that causes a spotty yellowing of the skin and inner putrification, is caused by a baculovirus. The baculoviruses have been used extensively as biological insecticides. This particular nuclearpolyhedrosis virus multiplies in the circulation, trachea, silk glands, and adipose tissues of the silkworms. Infection is believed to begin when the insect ingests the virus from infected leaves (i.e. mulberries). Digestive enzymes release the virus particles into the gut where they enter the tissues. If this process can occur naturally in insects, it may also take place in animals or humans under the right conditions.[36,38]

In 1983 a Yale report attempted to dismiss the spiroplasma connection to plant yellows diseases on the grounds that helical spirochetes could not be found in aster yellows affected plants. Was this study a coincidence or an attempt to distance the plant spiroplasmas of aster yellows diseases (*Spiroplasma citri*) from a human agent of Lyme disease which might also contain a spiroplasma agent? Remember this disease agent was just formally announced only a year earlier, without mention of spiroplasmas.[39]

At the time of the 1975 Connecticut outbreak, scientists analyzed patient sera for arboviruses (i.e. reoviruses). This was somewhat problematic since some viruses are easy to detect while others do not bind easily to test antigens (i.e. bunyavirus). As a result, those which bind poorly produce very low titers (results). This could also be a reason why some Lyme patients don't register "positive" on Lyme diagnostic tests if their infections involve a virus with poor binding ability.[40,41]

A Yale annual report written by Drs. Robert Shope, Allen Steere, Steven Malawista, and colleagues described patients from the region where the Connecticut outbreak occurred. From June 1972 until March 1976, forty-eight residents from three towns presented with similar rash/arthritis illnesses. Cultures from synovium (joints) and synovial fluid, and patient sera were screened for pathogens known to cause arthritis. However none suggested bacterial or mycoplasma infection. (The results may have been influenced by the type of test or by viral binding ability.) Sera was tested for powassan and arena (rodent) viruses, but was negative. These are encephalitis-causing flaviviruses that are related to the alphavirus-like reoviruses. Indeed, they may be degraded forms of reoviruses which lost genes after reassortment.[41,42]

Another Yale report from the same period revealed that the sindbis alphavirus was not tested against the patient sera, although it was detected in the serum of Senegalese (African) birds. Scientists also discovered a new species of phlebotomine sand fly in the East Haddam, Connecticut area at the time of the Lyme outbreak that was previously unknown to the US. During the Connecticut outbreak, scientists collected thirty times the number of *Ixodes scapularis* ticks, and an increased number of deer from the east side of the Connecticut River, than the substantially fewer numbers of deer and ticks collected on the west side of the same river during the same period.[41]

Cryoglobulinemia (CG) was a "predominant" finding in Connecticut arthritis patients according to a Yale report. This is a medical condition that is classified into three types, and which causes blood proteins to become insoluble at colder temperatures. CG is usually associated with multiple myelomas, and hepatitis C virus infection. CG proteins may also be found in *Mycoplasma pneumonia*, leukemias, "autoimmune" diseases (i.e. lupus, rheumatoid arthritis); and quite possibly in Lyme disease, especially since Lyme patients often carry mycoplasma co-infections. A condition called hyperviscosity is associated with CG, and is caused by blood and immunoglobulin (antibody) malignancies. This "thick blood" is a condition commonly seen among Lyme patients. Two of the three CG classifications are associated with a hepatitis virus.[41]

There are other important soil and water bacteriae in a family called *Leptothrix* which we should discuss. This is because they are ubiquitous to the soil and water, and because they may play a role in or serve as a model of study for a component of a Bb aggregate spirochete. The leptothrix are separated into two groups (genera): the *Leptotrichia* and the *Bacterionema.* These organisms are very similar to the *Mycobacteria.* Examples of mycobacteria are the agents of tuberculosis (*Mycobacterium tuberculosis*); cattle tuberculosis (*Mycobacterium bovis*), and bird and swine tuberculosis (*Mycobacterium avium*). *Mycobacterium tuberculosis* and *Mycobacterium butyricum* have been used in Freund's complete adjuvants, which are adjuvants used within animal vaccines (Freund's incomplete adjuvants are used in human vaccines).[43-49]

Mycobacteria and organisms related to them contain special proteins (lipids) that are unique to all organisms which lack a cell nucleus (prokaryotes). These lipids are not found in other natural objects or organisms. Leptothrix bacteria are found in aquatic environments that contain sufficient organic matter (i.e. polluted water, underside of water lilies). Some species live in wastewater treatment plants. For example there is a group of "iron bacteria" called *Sphaerotilus-Leptothrix* that are often found in polluted wastewaters.[43-50]

We might find *Mycobacterium tuberculosis* in wastewater contaminated by urine or feces from the manure of vaccinated livestock. In a 1989 study, antiserum against *Mycobacterium tuberculosis* (heat shock proteins) reacted with two *Borrelia burgdorferi* proteins. This suggests there may be Bb proteins that are derived from *Mycobacterium tuberculosis* or *E. coli* which is used in vaccine formulas and is found in wastewaters. We also find leptothrix from the *lactobacillaceae* family in wastewaters. This family also includes certain human and oral (dental) spirochetes.[43-50]

The leptothrix can oxidize iron, magnesium, and manganese sets (i.e. stainless steel). In the process, they can add minerals to their bacterial sheaths. This means they take up metals as a kind of interior suit of armor. The leptotrichia/leptothrix for the most part is unable to branch like fungi, although a strain called *Bacterionema matruchotii* is able to do so. Because of this, it is felt to belong to the family of *Actinobacteria.* This family also includes the subclasses *Bifidobacteriales* and *Actinomycetales.* Remember that bacteria are essentially fungi.[43,44]

The *Actinobacteria* are gram-positive organisms that have a high G+C content and which can sometimes stain weakly gram-negative. (G+C refers to guanine and cytosine, constituents of DNA and RNA.) The Bb spirochete also stains weakly gram positive even though it has been labeled as a "gram negative" bacteria. The leptotrichia and the bacterionema are natural aggregators and plaque builders. This is a talent that is also found in the *Borrelia burgdorferi* spirochete.[43,44]

According to a paper co-authored by Yale's Dr. Paul Duray et al., there was insufficient evidence that the Bb spirochete is truly gram negative, although scientific papers label it thusly, probably because it stains weakly gram-negative. Changing the culture conditions can affect spirochetal form/structure, as will the age of the culture. Bb gram-staining is said to be "generally unsuccessful." It is entirely possible that the Bb spirochete has a bacterionema or leptotrichia component to its genetic makeup. Whether that component comes from wastewater, or a mycobacterium from vaccinated animal wastes remains to be seen.[51-53]

I found the tick spiroplasma 277F agent listed in the index of a 1976 publication. Again this is an important spiroplasma first isolated from rabbit ticks by Dr. Burgdorfer in 1967. It is listed under the category of *Actinomycetes* (actinomycetales), which are the fungal-like bacteriae that includes the bacterionema. Dr. Burgdorfer wrote an article about the 277F agent under this category, which unmistakably labeled the rabbit tick 277F spiroplasma as an actinomycetes. The bacteriae in this category are best known for their ability to produce antibiotics. They are typically isolated from marine sediments. Patients who have Lyme disease often develop "allergies" to antibiotics, fish, shellfish, or marine products. Perhaps the patient's body has become sensitized to the bacteria found on or in these products because similar bacteria are part of an aggregate Bb spirochete.[43,54-61]

The 277F agent could be a form of mollicute that naturally aggregates with pathogens in ticks like those studied by Dr. Burgdorfer. While at Rocky Mountain Laboratories, Drs. Burgdorfer and Brinton analyzed the 277F agent and felt that it had serological properties similar to the spiroplasmas of the *Spiroplasma citri* group. These are tiny plant spirochetes that infect plants and insects and which cause significant damage to crops including citrus. More recently and not incidentally, multiple strains of spiroplasmas were recovered from *Ixodes pacificus* ticks from Oregon. Does the Bb agent contain a spiroplasma that is part fungi, part bacterionema? Is this one half of a mutant spirochete that will be detected in the 1950s?[43,54-61]

Q Fever-Spiroplasma Connection

A human Q fever agent (*Coxiella burnetii*) first surfaced in employees of a meat-packing plant in Australia in 1935. Q fever is the only species in its genus (group). It is an intracellular protozoan *gammaproteobacteria* that is closely related to other rickettsial agents, including the intracellular *Ehrlichia*, the agent of animal and human ehrlichiosis. This is curious since according to my research, ehrlichiosis may have emerged subsequent to the deployment of agricultural and military herbicides. Decades ago, Q fever was studied as a possible biowarfare agent; probably because it was first found in contaminated livestock meats and milk. Human exposures to Q fever were linked to contact with livestock and their products. Typical patients were individuals who worked in meat and dairy industries; those who wove or processed textiles; and those who sheared sheep or were involved with livestock breeding.[1]

During the 1930s, the Q fever organism was thought to be a virus, although a rickettsia-like agent was identified in the spleen of infected animals. The illness resembles typhus or psittacosis, a bird respiratory infection. Cattle, sheep, and goats are the primary reservoir for Q fever. Human infections occur after inhalation of aerosolized organisms, or ingestion of raw milk or cheese. Most Q fever infections occur during the birthing season because the organism is associated with parturient animals. Spiroplasmas were discovered during Q fever studies. Ticks that transmit Q fever also transmit Lyme disease, so we can see important connections here if the Lyme disease agent contains a spiroplasma and Q fever component. It is interesting that Wisconsin's health department has recently clamped down on family farms that sell raw, unpasteurized milk. Since Wisconsin is endemic for Lyme disease, if cattle transmit infections that contribute to the Lyme disease agent, this could explain the unwanted attention that dairy farmers receive over the sale of raw milk on organic, non-commercialized farms. Unfortunately however, pasteurization of milk and dairy products does not kill all bacteria, and destroys essential milk enzymes found in raw milk.

German studies of Q fever in north Rhine-Westphalia revealed an intracellular organism in an *Ixodes* tick pool. Researchers isolated the Z/16* spiroplasma as a potential vertebrate infection. Perhaps scientists at Ft. Detrick when studying Q fever as a potential biowarfare weapon during the 1940s first learned of spiroplasmas during their studies. If they did, we can imagine that they would have studied their sudden appearance around the time that agriculturally and industrally important chemicals were being deployed. Dr. Burgdorfer studied Q fever as early as 1951. A paper revealed that Q fever was identified as early as

1946, about the time the first spiroplasma was discovered; and several years after agricultural chemicals were deployed around the world. Some of these chemicals and the radioactive elements of fertilizers are capable of causing microbial mutations such as may have created the unique spiroplasmas of the 20th century.[8-12]

**There is a Bb strain called "ZS7" that was first isolated from Ixodes ricinus ticks. These ticks were collected from dragging the Freiburg, Germany area during the 1980s. Remember that sheep are also hosts to Q fever infections. Does a gammaproteobacteria such as Q fever and a soil bacteria help to create the infective anthrax? If Bb contains a gammaproteobacteria (or related extremphile), and people digest B.t. bacterial toxins, is it possible that "anthrax" may be created in the guts of humans? Is this the huge "anthrax" threat we face today?*

In 1963, Dr. Burgdorfer also isolated Q fever from rodents in western Montana, and continued to study Q fever for several decades. It is clear from papers that Q fever and Rocky Mountain spotted fever were important animal infections during the 1950s and 1960s; especially in goats, cattle, and rodents. By 1965, Rocky Mountain Lab scientists were studying Q fever among residents of infected dairies in Montana. This may have occurred because since 1951, Q fever vaccines that were prepared at RML to immunize livestock and humans were formulated from either the California AD strain of Q fever (Phase I); or from a Phase I strain that was isolated from Ohio dairy cow milk.[13-16]

A human vaccine was developed for those exposed to livestock or their products, or to laboratory Q fever agents because they had an increased risk of contracting the infection. Studies in Idaho, and from the Crimea (Ukraine), indicated that a high percentage of dairy cattle showed evidence of Q fever infections at this time. The question is where did the Q fever organism first originate? Could it have come from a microbial mutation caused by an agriculturally applied chemical/biological pesticide to which cattle and other livestock were exposed (i.e. *Bacilla popilliae, Bacillus thuringiensis,* or related agent)? Remember these agents were first deployed to kill other insects that were destroying agricultural crops, like the Colorado potato beetle – an insect also found among Idaho potato crops.[13-17]

The Q fever agent, *Coxiella burnettii* may have been isolated in 1925 by Hideo Noguchi, but those samples did not survive. During the late 1930s scientists from Australia and Rocky Mountain Labs published a description of the Q fever agent. It is possible that the infection came about due to the early applications of parasitoid insects, fertilizers, or agricultural fungal agents used as insecticides. Then again, it is possible that the infection first came about because of the pollution of ground or surface waters by radioactive elements (i.e. uranium mine or milling tailings/wastes). It is noticeable that phosphate, metal ore, and uranium mines or enrichment plants exist in Australia, the Ukraine, Ohio, and in Idaho where Q fever was isolated.[13-17]

Were scientific concerns over human Q fever infections geared toward epidemics caused by contaminated milk and meats? Or were Rocky Mt. scientists investigating the role of contaminated milk from Ohio and the emergence of animal and human infections because cell lines that had been created using the milk may have been contaminated with animal and human transmissible agents? Were the early vaccines also grown in chicken embryos? An early paper reported that scientists routinely fed blood-sucking arthropods upon chicken embryos to transmit diseases to them so they may be studied. Arthropod studies included mosquitoes, flies, and ticks. But there may have been a hidden infection in chicken embryos that was an item of interest to these scientists. Was it a chicken cholera retrovirus, bornavirus, or gammaproteobacteria; and part of all chicken DNA?[3-7]

In 1949 Dr. Burgdorfer's colleague E.G. Pickens attempted to infect Rocky Mt. wood ticks and Lone Star ticks with spotted fever rickettsia bacteriae. These are tick species that in the present day also transmit Lyme disease. A few years later, scientists would be successful at infecting soft-bodied ticks with *chicken embryos* that were infected with Q fever, tularemia, the infectious leptospira strain *Leptospira icterohaemorrhagiae,* and the insect reovirus-like western equine encephalitis virus. This is roughly the same combination of pathogens that may make up part of the aggregate Bb organisms found today.[3-6]

According to a paper, "The successful results of the described feeding experiments indicated that this method might be employed as a practical means of infecting argasid ticks with certain pathogenic microorganisms which grow well in cell cultures." There was a lot of research by 1961 which attempted to define what was referred to as the "Q fever problem." We may wonder whether each of these agents or members of their families and the spiroplasmas found in these ticks were already understood to be a problem caused by agricultural and/or industrial pollutants.[3-6]

Remember I just told you that Q fever studies during the 1950s in Germany, the USSR, and the US revealed intracellularly growing microorganisms in an *Ixodes* tick pool. In Germany the Z/16 spiroplasma strain was identified. A paper says that these organisms replicate within the cytoplasmic vacuoles of cells in a manner similar to Q-fever. This means simply that they are intracellular infections. Were cattle in the US and elsewhere showing evidence of spiroplasma/Q fever infections? Were these infections now found in animals due to the global application of insecticides which degrade the guts of insect vectors?[3,9,18-42]

French scientists found that when the "A56" *Spiroplasma melliferum* of honey bees was injected into suckling mice, it persisted in brain tissues for up to nine months. Other spiroplasma strains were isolated from other insects including beetles, fleas, fruit flies, wasps, deer flies, mosquitoes, and dragonflies. Several of these insects have been shown to harbor Bb spirochetes. The question is of course, how did these insects become infected with Q fever and/or spiroplasmas? The answer may prove to be simply because they came into contact with infected crops and animals that had been sprayed, inoculated, or otherwise fed chemical and microbial insecticides. Such contact may have facilitated infectious diseases through catalytic chemicals and digestive fermentation.[3,9,19-21,23-42]

From 1953 forward, CDC, NIH, Illinois, and Romanian scientists were already tracking the emergence of novel animal infections. Some very odd spirochetes had already been isolated from a Romanian river, and from US bulls and turtles. Components of these spirochetes may have been actively studied since the 1940s following the application of chemical fertilizers, particularly after the emergence of an *Ehrlichiosis*-like infection in Texas soldiers we will examine soon. But this was also a period when early nuclear energy studies were undertaken; and uranium, tritium, and plutonium processing was underway around the world. There were small particle accelerators already being used for nuclear medicine, industrial, agricultural, and other purposes. We may wonder what was happening to their wastes and to the wastes at radioactive fuel mines or processing plants. The evidence shows that these wastes were making their way into waterways and water tables around the world.

Mollicutes and Swine Diseases

The mollicutes were considered to be meaningful biological control agents for mosquito control. Some insect species have an "aggregation phase" to their life cycle, during which they are more susceptible to spiroplasma infection. This facilitates spiroplasma infections, and makes them part of transmissible mixed infections. Spiroplasmas are well adapted to specific insect hosts. One example is the plain tiger Monarch butterfly which naturally harbors a male offspring-killing spiroplasma. This particular spiroplasma is closely related to two ladybird beetle male-killing spiroplasmas; and also to the tick symbiont *Spiroplasma ixodetis*, which was isolated from Oregon *Ixodes pacificus* ticks. Just as the Bb spirochete was found in blood-sucking diptera (deerflies, horseflies, mosquitoes); it has also been found in ticks and lepidoptera (moths, butterflies).[1-3]

Remember that the German Q-fever studies recovered Z/16 spiroplasmas from tick pools; and it was shown to be a potential vertebrate pathogen. Dr. Burgdorfer studied Q-fever in the 1950s, and again in 1963 in western Montana rodents. In mice, French scientists found that when the *Spiroplasma melliferum* strain A56 of honey bees was inoculated into suckling mice, it persisted in brain tissues for up to nine months. (This may have been the SMCA spiroplasma or suckling mouse cataract agent). Other spiroplasma strains have been isolated from other insects including beetles, fleas, fruit flies, wasps, and dragonflies.[4-23]

Although the use of mollicutes for mosquito control was referred to in a 1960 conference paper, not many publications revealed evidence of the release of these agents except during experimental studies. However even field trials could have introduced spiroplasmas into the environment where they could spread. If genetically engineered mosquitoes were inoculated with spiroplasma-contaminated cells, they certainly could spread the pathogen far and wide over decades, especially since mosquito releases occurred around the world. By 1982 when *Borrelia burgdorferi* was formally announced, two new spiroplasmas had recently been isolated during a search for microbial agents useful against Colorado potato beetles. A later (1991) French study suggested that *Spiroplasma taiwanense* had "considerable potential" as a biological control against mosquitoes.[24,25]

Mycoplasmas, a member of the mollicute family and cousin of the spiroplasmas, were implicated in 1985 along with chlamydia as contributing agents to human female infertility according to a study. One paper revealed that women with a history of infertility for two or more years were examined for antibodies to *Chlamydia trachomatis, Mycoplasma hominis,* and *Mycoplasma genitalium.* Out of forty-five women, 33% had antibodies to *C. trachomatis* and 35.5% to *M. hominis.* Antibody to *M. genitalium* was found in 20% of patients. The results indicated that *C. trachomatis* was an important cause of infertility in women; and *M. hominis* was also implicated. The US Armed Forces Institute of Pathology in Washington, DC discovered *Mycoplasma incognitus* infections in AIDS patients. This mollicute is felt to be an opportunistic infection but we might inquire about its origins.[26,27]

What is interesting with respect to *Mycoplasma genitalium,* is that researchers from the University of Utah (Salt Lake City), the Institute for Genomic Research (Rockville, Maryland), and a Maryland company were studying this mycoplasma as compared to *Borrelia burgdorferi.* Such studies are important because Bb and *M. genitalium* are said to be "distantly related." What is generally unknown is that in 1917 scientists Inada and Ito identified a pathogenic leptospira called *Leptospira icterohaemorrhagiae* that was isolated from British soldiers in Flanders who were suffering from infectious jaundice (slime fever).[4,35-38]

In 1918 Dr. Hideyo Noguchi from Rockefeller Laboratories discussed this leptospira (*Leptospira Noguchi* 1917) in relation to the spironemas and treponemes that are found on the oral, alimentary, and genital mucous membranes. *L. Noguchi* 1917 was classified as a new leptonema strain (mutant, intermediate spirochete). Noguchi's leptonema was placed into the same class as modern leptonemas isolated from the environment, from animals, and from a human Lyme patient's ECM rash in 1981. The connection between Bb, mycoplasmas, and the scientists studying them now seems far more interesting.[4,35-38]

Back in 1966, military scientists at the Aerospace Medical Research Labs at Wright-Patterson Air Force Base (Ohio) published a report that discussed experiments from 1962-1964 with a Texas isolate of *Mycoplasma hycarthrinosa.* The strain was injected into Hampshire and Yorkshire pigs that weighed between forty and one hundred pounds. Some of the pigs developed pathogenic lesions. The pigs that had not been deprived of colostrum at birth had the greatest response to the injected organism. Colostrum* therefore may provide protective antibodies which helps animals resist mycoplasma infections. The *Mycoplasma hyoarthrinosa* organism was demonstrated in swine tissues using indirect fluorescent antibody (IFA) laboratory techniques.[28-30]

**Some Lyme patients have tried colostrum as a treatment. I wondered if children who were not breastfed fared worse during infections than those who were breastfed. Colostrum is produced in the first days after delivery. It provides beneficial antibodies and digestive enzymes which become part of the adaptive (long-term) immune system; and provides resistance or immunity to certain pathogens over a lifetime.*

Mycoplasma hyorhinis is also called swine arthritis. These organisms invade pig joint cavities and synovial tissues, even in pigs that lack skin lesions. Mycoplasmas were isolated from joint fluid of what were described as "normal" joints in young pigs weighing less than one hundred pounds. When the organisms invaded the joints of pigs weighing more than this, microscopic and gross lesions were found. Scientists claim that mycoplasmas have poor antigenicity.* They also indicated that the onset of immunologic maturity (the age of the pigs' immune systems) was a determining factor to the development of lesions.[28-30]

**Antigens are proteins that stimulate antibody formation. Antigenicity is the ability to provoke an antibody response.*

Research into swine arthritis is the model for human rheumatoid arthritis. There may be a link between pigs that produce antibodies to a severe swine respiratory syndrome virus called PRRSV ("swine flu"), and those with lung lesions where PRRSV and *Mycoplasma hyorhinis* antigens were detected.[29-31]

A 1971 paper described a link between *Mycoplasma hyorhinis* and *Hemophilus suis*, a swine influenza virus. According to the paper, cows and pigs infected with just the pig pneumonia (*M. hyorhinis*), had only moderate damage to tracheal (airway) cells. However when co-infected with the swine "flu" virus, animals experienced increased airway destruction. Another paper described how ten mycoplasma strains were isolated from synovial cultures and from cultures that were inoculated with synovial fragments from patients with rheumatoid arthritis or osteoarthritis. None of the patients showed positive for mycoplasma antibodies.[29-33]

We can wonder about the purpose of the 1962 military swine arthritis studies which seem curiously similar in scope to early Lyme arthritis studies. In the latter, synovial fluid and tissues were examined for evidence of Bb spirochetes. This would prove more intriguing if Bb proves to be an aggregate spirochete that contains a mollicute (spiroplasma). We might venture a guess that the early military studies were to develop vaccines and antibiotics to treat agriculturally important food animals for insect pests and the diseases they carry.[30-34]

More than a dozen mycoplasma species are known to cause arthritis; including chronic disease in animals. Some infectious disease researchers have acknowledged chronic forms of arthritis in Lyme disease patents, so this may be an additional clue that Bb contains a mollicute pathogen. The animal and human links between arthritis and mycoplasmas were known for certain by 1983, one year after the announcement of the Lyme "arthritis" causing-agent, *Borrelia burgdorferi.* The presence of spiroplasmas in ticks was also known for decades before a cluster of Lyme disease cases erupted in Connecticut. However these important ideas have never really been revealed to the public or to their treating physicians to date – both of which have been left to figure out the Lyme disease picture largely by themselves.[29,30,32,33] ❏

Speak No Evil.

> *"Biological warfare viral bioagents are mostly RNA viruses (positive-strand and negative-strand), with the exception of smallpox. Every RNA virus is a family of related viruses (quasispecies). These viruses mutate rapidly and the potential for engineered strains (natural or deliberate) is very high."*
>
> Source: World Health Organization Patent #WO/2008/147879 – Automated Method and Device for DNA Sequence Determination, and Identification. Filed 5/22/08, published 12/4/08(US).

Four: What We Are Told (or Not) Matters

Secrets of the Agricultural Biocides

In 1955, researchers from the New York Agricultural Experiment Station and the USDA Agricultural Research Service studied the larvae of the Japanese and European chafer beetles. Both insects are susceptible to milky spore diseases, and researchers were looking for a way to mass-produce the milky spore agents as biological controls. Soil inoculation with milky disease spores was impractical, so alternative methods were studied to enable the development of a more efficient and cost-effective insecticide.[1-3]

In 1965, USDA researchers tried to inject *Bacillus popilliae* directly into insect larvae as a method of mass-producing these sporulating bacteria. This process was inefficient however, and it became clear that a more effective method would have to be devised. One problem with these agents is their rapid degradation under ultraviolet light (within minutes), and in temperatures above 30°C (86°F). They may persist in soils for a decade or longer. Therefore these agents were not considered to be as "environmentally safe" as a related soil bacteria, *Bacillus thuringiensis* (B.t.). This bacterium has been in use since the late 1920s as an agricultural pesticide, although it was not widely used until after World War II. In 1966 USDA scientists from Riverside, California, and the New York State Agricultural Experiment Station compared available milky disease species and strains from beetle larvae collected from around the world. However these agents were not reproducible on the artificial media required for mass production. The agricultural industry would have to find a more efficient bacteria to control pest insects that could be commercially produced and easily applied to agricultural fields.

The most promising *Bacillus* strain as an insecticide was *Bacillus thuringiensis* or "B.t." B.t. is a gram-positive organism that lives on the dark surface of plants, and thrives within the guts of caterpillars of moths and butterflies. *Bacillus thuringiensis* sporulates, and its spores are similar in toxic activity to those of the milky spore diseases.

A wilt-like disease in silkworm larvae was first identified in 1902 by a Japanese scientist named Ishiwata, who identified it as *Bacillus sotto.* In 1915, German scientist Ernst Berliner identified the agent for the second time, and named it *Bacillus thuringiensis*. Berliner discovered the agent in Thuringia, Germany within the bodies of flour moth larvae. Without knowing it both scientists had identified the very same organism. The latter name has become the accepted term for a group of spore-forming bacteriae which create insect-specific toxic crystals during sporulation. B.t. affects other insect species in addition to the flour moth, including *Lepidoptera* such as the silkworm and gypsy moths. Incidentally, Thuringia, Germany is also an area that has long been home to various mining industries (i.e. malachite, alum shales, iron ores, potash, uranium).

Widespread applications of B.t. insecticides began in Europe, in Hungary at the end of the 1920s; and Yugoslavia the following decade. The product entered the commercial market in France under the trade name of *Sporine* in 1938. With the onset of World War II, B.t. use was still somewhat limited in Europe. However by the end of the war (in the US at least) B.t. field tests had moved toward mass-production of what was considered to be an environmentally friendly insecticide, and a good alternative to toxic chemical pesticides such as DDT.[4,5]

In 1948, bacteriologists at Cornell University and RCA Laboratories (New York) were studying spore germination in a related bacterium, *Bacillus megaterium.* This agent's spores can also survive for years under desert-like conditions. Beginning in 1950 and due to the development of insect resistance to chemical pesticides like DDT, B.t. found its place as an effective global bioagent through the work of Dr. Steinhaus. Even though B.t. became the agricultural product of choice to control widespread insect infestations around the world, *Bacillus popilliae, Bacillus lentimorbus, Bacillus sphaericus,* and related sporulators were still used in select areas. If human diseases were to be a consequence of bacterial insecticides, then infectious disease outbreaks would have emerged in the countries where these agents were being applied. We may catch a glimpse of such a correlation if we study the history of disease outbreaks and follow the trail of applied insecticides around the world.[6-9]

After WWII, widespread applications of the chemical pesticide DDT were used to control insects. Outbreaks of novel diseases appeared sporadic and unrelated, probably because chemical pesticides could be applied as soon as an outbreak occurred. Whenever chemical pesticides were used during an outbreak, an epidemic could be curbed by exterminating local insect populations responsible for the outbreak. Unfortunately with the removal of chemical pestcides from the equation, and with the use of microbial insecticides, new and unusual disease outbreaks began to erupt in animal and human populations.[7-9]

Today microbes and toxins are genetically engineered as topical insecticides; and also into food crops for animal and human consumption. These engineered formulas also contain chemicals that are bacterial aggregators (joiners) and catalysts for the introduction of, and mutation of microbes. Not only are insect guts deliberately being infected with B.t. and other microbes and toxins; but the ovipositors, stylets, and stingers of insects also become contaminated with bacterial spores. This facilitates the transmission of infections to other hosts including humans. The literature clearly shows that B.t. is used to activate latent infections in insects to cause disease. B.t. has also been shown to produce intestinal infections in animals and humans.[10-13]

Scientists know that organisms including B.t. in either synthetic or natural formulas will join microbes together, and that it may assist in the *alteration of the genes* of exposed insects. A patent states:

> "For instance, in the case of B.t., the vegetative cells, spores, and proteinaceous crystals are all effective in directly or indirectly killing host insects susceptible to B.t..."
>
> "It is also known that *naturally occurring and synthetic vectors such as plasmids, phages, and various DNA/RNA constructs have potential for functionally modifying higher organisms*, and therefore are also included herein as being within the scope of the term 'biocontrol agent.'"

This is a huge statement which seems to admit that microbial insecticides may be able to initiate novel animal and human diseases. These diseases may come about through genetic mutations and/or the reactivation of infections in the plants, insects, animals, or humans exposed to these insecticides. With the transfer of plasmids, infection by phages, or mutation with recombinant genes, we can expect compatible fungi, bacteria, and viruses to incorporate this DNA or RNA into new infectious strains to cause diseases in any organisms, regardless of their location on the tree of life.[14]

Some of the phagic viruses that were found during milky spore infections include the "Pj" iridescent virus of the Japanese beetle (*Popilliae japonica*). The "Pj" virus is a member of the *Iridopox* virus family of iridescent viruses. This group also includes viruses such as *Tipula,* which is found in mosquitoes and gypsy moths. Most agricultural pests are hosts to iridescent (reoviruses) and other insect *poxviruses.* There are roughly thirty iridopoxviruses alone. The iridescent or opalescent color that is produced in the body of an infected insect is caused by the large quantity of virus particles found in the cytoplasm of infected cells. There is another factor that we need to consider that may be the most important aspect of Lyme disease:[15-17]

Latent (dormant) or dead poxviruses can be resurrected during a mixed infection by another live poxvirus.

This can occur even if the two strains of poxvirus are different. This happens because the live virus contributes valuable genes to the dead virus, resurrecting it into an active infection. According to a patent:

> "The virus yield from cells infected with inactivated virus of one strain and active virus of another strain contains infectious particles of both strains, and also, if the viruses are sufficiently closely related, recombinants. Inactivation by heat, therefore, does not inactivate the [DNA] of the virus particles, since all known genetic markers are preserved."

Again this means that a new infection from a compatible poxvirus is able to reactivate or bring to life the remnants of an older, inactive infection in a host's body. It may make no difference whether the formerly inactive infection was from a previous natural infection, or if it came from a former recombinant vaccine or was an ancient, latent virus. Since poxviruses replicate in the cell's cytoplasm, any infections in the cytoplasm may contribute genes during reassortment in a mixed infection.[15]

A synergistic effect between pathogens and chemical insecticides has been observed with the microbial insecticide "B.t." Czechoslovakian studies demonstrated how the intracellular microsporidian parasite *Nosema* accelerated the effects of certain contact insecticides within weevil populations. Nosema was first collected from European corn borer larvae in Hungary in 1927. Microsporidiae have been widely deployed over decades to control mosquito populations. Nosema infections are common among insect populations. They have also been proven to infect honey bee populations; causing rapid declines in population numbers.[15,18]

Other microsporidian infections also accelerate the effects of applied insecticides. *Ovavesicula popilliae* is a microsporidia that has been isolated from Japanese beetles in Michigan and Connecticut. These intracellular infections typically affect the trachea, skin, fat, and pericardial cells, and cause an intense inflammatory response. As of 2007 there were nine microsporidian groups, any of which may be present as unidentified co-infections in patients with tickborne diseases. This particular infection is found in the malpighian (waste) tubules of insects. This is interesting because another infection found in the pine resin gall moth is *Larssoniella.* This agent also affects the malpighian tubules, and the silk glands, adipose, and connective tissues. Spores may be found in both eggs and sperm.[19-22]

Ovavesicula is a huge problem for bark beetles in the Czech Republic, and other heavily forested areas of the Euro-Siberian Taiga region. It is also found in areas of the US known to be endemic for Lyme disease, and yet the Lyme-infected public has never been told of this infection. Other microsporidian infections are caused by Ips species (i.e. *Ips typographa, Ips duplicatus, Ips amitinus*). A patent for an insecticide that is suitable as a growth regulator and ovicide for insects mentions these microsporidiae. It is possible that applied insecticides which contained chemical or microbial "growth regulators" (ovicides) may have contributed to the menu of intracellular infections that may reassort in the insect gut and be transmitted to humans. The microsporidian infections that are transmitted to humans are assisted by the application of gut-destroying B.t. insecticides. As the gut membrane degrades, intracellular infections are released where they are free to reassort and be transmitted as mixed infections to animals or humans.[19-22]

A 1963 Canadian B.t. insecticide describes how chlorinated chemicals such as DDT, endrin, and heptachlor were incorporated into animal, vegetable, or petroleum-based oils for aerosol use. As a result of these chemical/microbial suspensions, B.t. "unexpectedly" became far more effective against lepidoptera. B.t. has been paired in this manner for decades to shorten on-contact killing time. Irrespective of this efficiency, scientists continue inventing more potent, cost-effective formulas. In recent decades, natural toxins are engineered into B.t. insecticides to help circumvent the continual problem of insecticidal resistance. Scientists have also attempted to use different but related soil bacteria within the insecticidal formulas to see which will prove to be the most effective.[23]

Certain soil bacilli are closely related, such as *Bacillus cereus* and *Bacillus megaterium. Bacillus cereus* causes food-borne illness, and skin and eye infections. *Bacillus megaterium* is used to make the antibiotic penicillin,* but it has also been used as an insecticide. *Bacillus subtilis* is also a related soil bacterium of hay and grasses. *B. subtilis* is considered a model organism for laboratory study, and at least one strain has been used as a fungicide. A paper describes how the flagellar (tail) antigens of *B. cereus* and the agricultural agent *Bacillus thuringiensis* "overlap" (are identical). This indicates that certain "non-toxic" strains of B.t. which do not form crystal or Cry toxins, are strains that are derived from *Bacillus cereus.*[24]

**B. megaterium is also used to make a high-quality brewer's yeast. Sudden penicillin allergies are common for Lyme patients. If "Bb" is an aggregate that includes insecticidal genes, (i.e. B. megaterium, B.t.), than this makes sense in a body pre-sensitized to related bacillus strains, perhaps due to a cross-reactive sensitivity.*

The related *B. cereus* and *B. subtilis* are only slightly different from another close relative, *Bacillus anthracis. Bacillus anthracis* is the highly toxic and infectious agent of *Anthrax,* an infection that not only occurs in ruminant animals and in humans who process their hides; the agent was manufactured and stockpiled as a weapon of biological warfare for use during periods of conflict. According to scientific texts, *Bacillus anthracis* and *Bacillus subtilis* may both be descendants of *Bacillus cereus.* When anthrax endotoxins are manipulated in the laboratory, they become *virtually indistinguishable* from those of the less harmful *B. cereus* or *B. subtilis* soil strains. According to a Canadian-assigned patent, *Bacillus thuringiensis* subspecies *israelensis* is the exact same organism as *Bacillus cereus* subspecies *israelensis.* Therefore B.t. israelensis or "B.t.i," is simply a fermented mutant of the soil bacteria *Bacillus cereus,* and both are closely related to the anthrax agent.[25]

The relationship between fermented soil bacteriae, whether in a manufactured setting or through a natural occurrence is important to our story. With the global application of "B.t." insecticides, the odds increase for future "anthrax" outbreaks. This is because there are environmental factors which combine to create infectious anthrax, among which is fermentation. The other factors include agents and/or elements that are applied agriculturally, or that are naturally found in contaminated areas. This may explain the intense interest by public health officials toward protecting the world from "bioterrorism." However "bio" more frequently may represent the biologically deployed insecticides; and "terrorism" may refer to bacterial agents that of their own accord may transform into an infective anthrax agent. *This is more than likely the most important "bioterrorism" threat we face today, although the public is not informed about this aspect of "homeland security."*[25]

Bacillus cereus and *Bacillus anthracis* are known to be transformed by bacteriophages (phages) that are found in the soil. For example, phages can cause soil bacteriae to mutate. (A bacteriophage is an organism that infects bacteria. There are also virophages which infect other viruses.) Because phages are also engineered within microbial insecticides, they are capable of transforming insecticidal bacteria into *Bacillus anthracis* under optimal conditions. B.t. has phages, and two have been identified as "CP-51" and "CP-53." These phages are also recognized as a possible prophage (latent infection) in certain strains of *Bacillus cereus*. Since the Lyme disease spirochete has also been found to harbor a phage, it makes sense to consider whether the Bb phage is the same agent found in other soil bacteria. It also makes sense to consider if the Bb phage is the same phage that may be found in B.t. insecticides and genetically engineered B.t. crops. Many of the bacillus subspecies (but not necessarily their mutants), are aerobic spore-producers. This means their spores thrive in oxygen-rich environments.[26-30]

A number of patents exist which discuss methods of delivering B.t. insecticides into the environment. The most common is aerial high-pressure spray systems (aerosol). B.t.-containing herbicides and insecticides have been globally marketed for agricultural use upon crops and livestock. Animals have been dusted, dipped, sprayed, and had B.t. formulas applied in their feeds.[54-59]

Several B.t. patents are assigned to E.I. du Pont de Nemours and Company (Wilmington, DE). One of the earliest is assigned to one of the first biotech companies in the US, the Bioferm Corporation. That company was founded by Jerry M. Sudarsky under the name Pacific Yeast Products. Mr. Sudarsky, a 1939 University of Iowa graduate, pioneered the production of vitamin B-12, and created and marketed the first bio-insecticides. It is probably no coincidence that a number of Lyme patients are severely depleted of B vitamins, if they are exposed to microbial insecticides that are causing disease.[54-59]

An older B.t. patent by a Canadian scientist is assigned to the Esso Research and Engineering Company (an affiliate of Standard Oil Company). The patent describes in great detail the aerial spraying of B.t. upon agricultural crops. Another 1963 patent is assigned to the Rohm & Haas Company, Philadelphia, PA (a wholly owned subsidiary of Dow Chemical Company). A Canadian patent filed in the 1970s describes the use of B.t. and the enzyme *chitinase*, which helps degrade the chitin (hard shell) of insect bodies. A 1970 patent assigned to the Cornell Research Foundation, Inc. (Ithaca, NY) describes the addition of specialized fatty acids to *Bacillus popilliae* spores to promote sporulation and to extend its useful life in the field as an insecticide.[60-65]

According to a textbook published in 1971, B.t. endotoxins are capable of activating latent infections such as the granulosis virus (GV) of the fall webworm (*Hyphantria cunea*). The main reason why B.t. is used agriculturally is that it promotes latent insect infections and delivers additional recombinant infections and toxins to targeted insects. According to an early text that proved highly significant to the biotech industry, various pathogens will:

"...induce activation of latent virus infections, activated by application of B.t. to late larval instars."[66,67]

This is possible since B.t. acts as a phage and transcription promoter, which initiates natural gene recombinations (mutations). B.t. also facilitates the entry of systemic toxins by degrading the insect's gut tissues (epithelial cells) through the action of enzymes called *bacteriophage lysins.** The introduction of B.t. alone is enough to cause problems in the target insect, but the addition of other infectious agents ramps up and significantly increases B.t. toxin killing time and activities.[68,69]

**The release of B.t. bacteriophage lysins disintegrates the gut tissues. This creates new ion channels (holes) in the cellular membranes; changes cellular calcium levels, and causes cytotoxic effects. On a large scale this forms large holes in gut tissues. The holes lead to an influx of water, causing osmotic shock and death. The destruction of gut tissue is a gateway for opportunistic microbes to enter the circulation. If a similar process occurs in humans, such holes may lead to a celiac-like disease, nutrient malabsorption, allergies, septicemia, anaphylaxis, and wasting diseases. A side note is that ion channels are the voltage-regulating processes which mediate nerve signals. They are present in the nervous, cardiac, skeletal, smooth muscle, mammary, pancreatic, and (gut) epithelial cells; and are used for ion and nutrient transport. They also activate T-cells of the immune system, and manage insulin resistance. If insecticides adversely affect ion channels and enzyme systems, this may cause immune and disease states, including the noticeable rise in human diabetes, Lyme, and AIDS-like diseases.*

According to an early WHO bulletin, although bacterial septicemia is the end stage of every natural insect infection where B.t. is present; only in so-called "well-defined" cases is B.t. felt to be directly responsible for an insect's death. An "indirect" defense however might be considered woefully inadequate if the bacteriae otherwise lead to disease in animals and humans. According to the paper, secondary factors play an important role in the ability of pathogens to penetrate the gut wall; however the paper fails to state what those factors might actually entail.[68,69]

They may include tissue destruction from chemical and microbial toxins, metabolites, heavy metals, viruses, recombinant genes, parasites, and infections which open the door for insecticidal pathogens to enter the circulation. A paper written some three decades after scientists became aware of B.t.'s gut-damaging and virus-reactivating abilities reveals this:

> "*Bacillus thuringiensis* is being used worldwide as a biopesticide, although increasing evidence suggests that it is *emerging as an opportunistic human pathogen.* Despite a long record of being safe, there is increasing public concern about the potential pathogenicity of *B. thuringiensis* to humans. This is due to the sporadic but sometimes severe infections caused by this organism, which include diarrheal food poisoning…corneal ulcer…cellulitis…and burn…as well as war wound…infections. Moreover, the pathogenicity of *B. thuringiensis* has been demonstrated in an animal model of infection by administering spores to mice via nasal inoculation."[68,69]

The aforementioned WHO paper reveals that **B.t. is known to be potentially harmful to humans and animals.** According to the 1963 report, the mass-produced B.t. was felt to be of only "limited potential" to the public health field at the time of the report. Nevertheless B.t. has proven over more than a half century to be the most useful tool for the global control of insects; especially when used in conjunction with other microbes and toxins. However at the same time over the last half century, there has been a significant rise in human diseases of "unknown" cause. Other microbes described in the WHO report as "useful" bioagents include the bacteriae *Serratia marcescens* and *Pseudomonas aeruginosa.* The "important" fungi were *Coelomomyces, Beauveria, Isaria, Spincaria* and *Metarhizium;* with *Beauveria bassiana* the most commonly applied fungi to reduce *Ixodes ricinus* tick populations. In the protozoan category, *Lankesteria culicis, Caulleryella, Nosema,* and *Thelohania* were notably "useful" for insecticides.[69]

A scientific paper describes how a strain of *Bacillus thuringiensis* subspecies *konkukian* is responsible for a superinfection in a human, and in immune-suppressed mice. According to the paper, the human infection was considered "unusual" although it was noted that *gastrointestinal tract infections do occur from human exposures to B.t.* This is a significant statement since it once again recognizes that B.t. causes human disease. Furthermore, superinfections from an aggregate spirochete that happens to harbor a B.t. component (i.e. bacteriophage) may help introduce more infectious components of an aggregate spirochete into a host.[70-72]

A fermentation process similar to that used to produce *Bacillus anthracis* (anthrax) is undertaken to create *Bacillus thuringiensis* (B.t.) toxins for insecticides. A problem with fermentation however is that certain toxins may be produced that are considered to be "undesirable." These toxins must be removed from the finished products before use; and are described by the US Environmental Protection Agency (EPA) which regulates B.t.-containing pesticides. The agency expects manufacturers to carefully self-monitor B.t. batches, and to perform quality testing to ensure that unwanted toxins are absent from finished B.t. products.[70-72]

The brewer's yeast *Saccharomyces cerevisiae* is used during the B.t. fermentation process. This yeast can create its own toxins, depending upon strain. There are killer, neutral, and sensitive yeast strains which are classified by size as P1 to P3. The killer strains produce a toxin that is lethal to sensitive yeast strains. Neutral strains do not produce this toxin nor are they susceptible to it. The killer strains are said to be associated with the presence of viral particles that are 41 nm (nanometers) in diameter. These strains are dependent upon the presence of virus particles in order to synthesize their toxins. This means that under the right conditions in the presence of satellite viruses of a certain size, that killer strains of *S. cerevisiae* yeasts can use the viruses to replicate and to produce extremely virulent toxins. There are many compatibly sized viruses in the environment that may be used as satellites, including some of the genetically engineered viruses found within B.t. insecticides, or the large and small RNA viruses that have been released by scientists as insecticidal helpers.[77-78]

The combination of yeast + virus augments B.t. formulas, but it may also leave humans susceptible to toxic yeast strains and to their virus infections. The virus size that is helpful to killer *S. cerevisiae* strains is roughly 41 nm in diameter. Any compatible viruses of about this size may bind with the yeasts of a fermented B.t. product to create a toxic killer strain capable of initiating virulent infections when delivered in B.t. formulas. The yeasts do not have to reside in the insecticidal formulas; they may be taken from wild yeast or fungal strains from the environment (or host) wherever B.t. is present. Yeasts and fungi are able to be infected by other viruses, and we will find this may be how a *spiroplasma* component of a Bb spirochete originally formed. The bad news is that in humans with an overgrowth of yeasts in their gut, toxic yeast strains may be formed upon consumption of B.t.-containing foods. This scenario if accurate, may involve resident yeast, introduced B.t. toxins, and latent viruses or other infections that are already present in the virus-vaccinated host. Any of these agents may reactivate latent infections.[73-78]

The silkworm *Borrelina bombycis* virus is of an appropriate size, and it produces ultramicroscopic granules that may bind with toxic yeast strains. Other viruses that may bind include the borrelina viruses such as were released by scientists from New Haven, Connecticut to enhance insecticides; and the viruses released by others who adopted these techniques. Bacterial strains which are largely yeast anyway, if they produce granules may also bind in this manner. *Leptospires* and *Spirochaeta aurantia* are examples of spirochetes that form granules of approximately the right size, and which may bind in a similar fashion.[73-79]

It appears possible from the literature that viruses from genetically engineered chimera may bind with toxic yeast strains only to break apart and be "kicked out" of the construct after binding. If so, this could cause genetically engineered chimera to fail, and to contribute to active infections. This might occur in an insect, or a vaccinated animal or human host. It is also known that active infective spores remain in the B.t. formulas when creating Cry toxins. This allows the spores to bind with wild-type yeasts, fungi, or bacteria to cause active infections in non-targeted populations.

The *Nudaurelia* ß virus (a betatetravirus), and the *Astroviruses* (enteroviruses) of lepidoptera are small RNA viruses that also fit into this size category. Fungi are hosts to viruses, and this is important when we consider that fungi, baculoviruses, and the small and large RNA viruses have been deployed agriculturally to augment B.t. insecticides. The idea that fungi, yeasts, and molds may become infected by viruses from a variety of agents is helpful to understanding the highly varied and often nested infections that are introduced by vectoring insects into the human body. [75-78,85]

Fungal viruses may include or be closely related to the *Reoviruses,* and may vary in size from 33 to 41 nm. For example, the fungi *Candida albicans* harbors a *polyoma* virus; and the yeast *Saccharomyces cerevisiae can harbor polio virus, polyoma virus, tobacco mosaic virus, and encephalomyocarditis viruses.* Indeed wild or recombinant yeast strains from B.t. insecticides can become infected with any number of microbes, including the reoviruses or their genetically degraded relatives. When we find patients suffering from encephalitis or polio-like illnesses, we should consider the influence of B.t. insecticides upon latent viruses in the human body. This is even more critical to evaluate in animals or humans who are exposed to microbe-containing insecticides when they have been vaccinated with virus formulas (i.e. leptospirosis, polio), especially when vaccine formulas contain live or attenuated viral proteins. This is because inactivated viruses can be brought back to life by the donation of live genes during a mixed infection with a compatible virus. Such a virus might be supplied by a recombinant B.t. insecticide.[75-78,85]

Many scientists were and are concerned about the global applications of recombinant insecticides to the environment, and the consequences of these applications upon the human population. According to a patent, the commercialization of biopesticides using baculoviruses "...has given rise to a perception that there may be a second potential impediment to their widespread acceptance." The patent specifically named the release of recombinant viruses into the environment with unforeseen consequences to the ecosystem; which undoubtedly includes the human body. We learn from many sources that B.t. residues persist upon foods that have been treated with these insecticides. The other constituents of their formulas may also remain in residual form.[79,82-84]

Exactly fifteen strains of *Bacillus cereus* variety *thuringiensis* (B.t.) were originally isolated from diseased insect larvae. These were then manufactured into the earliest B.t. insecticidal formula models. This means that B.t. strains that are in use today may fundamentally contain nested insect viruses, phages, and other pathogens which may include GVs, NPVs, CPVs (reoviruses), iridescent viruses, yeasts, fungi, protozoans, microsporidiae, or even nematode eggs. Since B.t. formulas are engineered to contain viruses and other pathogens, their influence is not only exerted upon targeted insects, but also upon the microbes in the environment. Here is a list of what appear to be the fifteen fundamental B.t. (parent) strains, as collected from multiple databases. This is by no means a complete list of all B.t. formulas ever applied agriculturally.[28-30]

Subspecies - ATCC	**Source of isolate**
Berliner	Mediterranean flour moth – *Ephestia kihniella*
thuringiensis	Indian-meal moth – *Plodia interpunctella*
thuringiensis	Larva of moth (unspecified species)
alesti	Silkworm moth – *Bombyx mori*
dendrolimus	Siberian coniferous silk moth – *Dendrolimus sibericus*
entomocidus	Stored nut moth – *Aphemia gularis*
subtoxicus	Indian meal moth – *Plodia interpunctella*
finitimus	Forest tent caterpillar – *Malacosoma distria*
sotto	Silkworm moth – *Bombyx* species
- NRRL (USDA Agricultural Research Service Culture Collection)	
Penicillium simplicissimum	Soil fungi
*Penicillium chrysogenum**	Soil fungi from Zimbabwe
Penicillium citrinum	Soil fungi

- NRS
1441 Information on this B.t. strain is not available
1442 not available
1455 not available

**Selected from Wis. 49-133 strain after N-mustard exposure. (1950) High-yielding, sporulating, penicillin strain. P. chrysogenum has been used to produce enzymes; penicillin, xanthocillin X; and to treat (paper) pulp mill wastes. Wis. 49-133 is a non-pigmented mutant strain of Penicillium chrysogenum that is fermented to make antibiotics. It was isolated from soil samples by Dr. Martha Christensen in Umtali Africa (now Mutare, Zimbabwe) in the fall of 1961. Samples were stored at the University of Wisconsin's Botany department.*[31-33]

The establishment of exactly fifteen original B.t. insecticidal "parent" lines is interesting. In a 2007 patent for a Lyme vaccine and diagnostic test that was filed by Drs. Raymond J. Dattwyler, Benjamin J. Luft, John J. Dunn, and Maria Gomes-Solecki; exactly fifteen strains of *Borrelia burgdorferi* are addressed. The patent is assigned to the Research Foundation of the State University of New York (Stony Brook, NY); and Brookhaven Sciences Associates, LLC (Upton, NY).* The patent describes a Lyme vaccine that incorporates the outer surface proteins A and C (OspA, OspC) of Bb spirochetes. The vaccine formula attempts to avoid a situation that occurred with the first generation OspA-based Lyme vaccine; whereby a treatment-resistant arthritis developed in some vaccine recipients. The male inventors listed in the patent were each co-authors of diagnostic and treatment guidelines for Lyme disease.[34]

**According to their web site, Brookhaven Sciences Associates was established "for the sole purpose of managing and operating Brookhaven National Laboratory." BSA is a 50-50 partnership between Battelle and the Research Foundation of State University of New York [SUNY]. BSA's board of directors includes individuals from Columbia, Cornell, Harvard, Massachusetts Institute of Technology, Princeton, and Yale Universities.*

What is curious is that exactly fifteen strains of European and North American *Borrelia burgdorferi* were used in the study of antibody binding domains described by the Dattwyler et al. patent. Note that these Bb strains came from various regions of the world; just as the original fifteen (parent) lines of B.t. Cry toxin-containing insecticidal formulas have been globally applied. The new patent incorporates strains of *Borrelia burgdorferi* sensu stricto, *Borrelia afzelii,* and *Borrelia garinii* groups in the vaccine. These are the three recognized Bb serogroups known to be pathogenic to humans; and which are found around the world. Is the number "15" a coincidence or something far more revealing?[34]

As of 1995, scientists who analyzed the eighteen known Bb s.l. genotypes found that sixteen had significantly different types of OspC gene sequences. Of these, thirteen strains corresponded to one of the OspC types that were detectable using existing monoclonal antibodies. Of those remaining, one represented a similar type, while two represented completely new types. One of the new types was divided into two groups with different gene sequences but with the same antibody pattern. Therefore a total of *fifteen* different types were analyzed and are probably the same genotypes that are referred to by the Dattwyler et al. patent; and which we discuss in the following section.[150]

It is also interesting that co-authors of at least one set of Lyme disease guidelines authors (Luft, Dunn) and their colleagues would publish an article regarding exactly *thirteen different* isolates of Bb spirochetes in 2011. These probably represent the OspC variations discussed in the Dattwyler et al. patent that are identifiable using monoclonal antibodies. The reason the number isn't fifteen instead of thirteen may simply be because two monoclonal antibodies have yet to be developed for the two novel strains; or the two newest strain types are close enough genetically that they may be detected by cross-reaction of two existing monoclonal antibodies already in use (or some other method).[178]

The new Dattwyler et al. vaccine patent describes the following fifteen *Borrelia burgdorferi* strains (noted in bold). After each strain name is the strain's initial point of origin. I also describe interesting connections between the Bb strains, and the kinds of natural and industrial issues (resources, wastes) that may have influenced the development of the particular strain type.[34]

B31 - This strain was isolated from *Ixodes dammini* (a/k/a *Ixodes scapularis*) ticks on Shelter Island, New York in 1981. Shelter Island is not far from Brookhaven National Lab (Riverhead, NY), which has had several particle accelerators (since 1953's Cosmotron Synchrotron) at its Long Island facility. There is also a landfill at Brookhaven that is said to be a long-time leacher of nuclear wastes and other toxins into the soil and groundwater. The B31 strain of Bb was placed in a culture database by Dr. Alan G. Barbour, who obtained it from Dr. Willy Burgdorfer.[35-37,179]

ZS7 - This strain was isolated from *Ixodes ricinus* ticks in Freiburg, Germany during the 1980s. This area is home to a sizeable silver mining industry, the Black Forest, uranium mines, vineyards, and nuclear power plants. Freiburg is located on the east bank of the Rhine River, which is an area formed by a volcanic ridge.The area is also home to fruit orchards and several *Max-Planck Society* (science) institutes, formerly called the *Kaiser Wilhelm Society* or *Kaiser-Wilhelm Gesellschaft* (KWG).

N40 - This strain was isolated from an adult deer tick (*Ixodes dammini*) in Westchester County, New York, down river from Knolls Atomic Laboratory on the Mohawk River, which discharged nuclear wastes directly into the air, soil, and the Mohawk River – the largest tributary of the Hudson River. The Hudson empties into New York Bay; in the part of the Atlantic that forms the New York Harbor.[37,38]

PKa1 - This strain was isolated from a human cerebral spinal fluid (CSF) sample in Germany. We will examine the German-derived strains in more detail.

25015 - This strain was isolated from *Ixodes scapularis* and *Ixodes persulcatus* ticks in Millbrook, NY, one of the first areas to fluoridate water in the US. Millbrook is also near nuclear generating stations that are collectively called Indian Point.

K48 - This is a strain of *Borrelia garinii* that was isolated from *Ixodes ricinus* (sheep) ticks in former Czechoslovakia, where B.t. insecticides and fungicides were first applied. The Temelín, Dukovany, and Bohunice nuclear power stations are also located there.

DK29 - This strain was isolated from a human patient from Denmark who had an ECM rash. Denmark is home to the Niels Bohr Institute (f/k/a Institute for Theoretical Physics), which began nuclear fission experiments as early as 1939. The Risø National Laboratory for Sustainable Energy is home to nuclear research, and there is also a Cyclotron at Hevesy Lab.[86,87]

PHei - This strain was isolated from a human CSF sample from Germany.

Ip90 - This European strain was isolated from an *Ixodes persulcatus* tick from Khabarovsk, Russia by American Lyme-notable Dr. Alan G. Barbour. *Ixodes persulcatus* is the Taiga tick, named after the heavily forested Taiga region. The area is home to the Amur Shipyard where nuclear submarines were built. It is also off the coast of the same seaways shared by Japan's Fukushima and other nuclear plants (i.e. Sea Okhotsk, East China Sea). The area is also home to the Siberian silkworm and to nuclear weapons facilities, coal mining, agricultural and oil industries, and uranium mines.

PTrob - This strain was isolated from human skin in Germany.

ACAI - This *B. afzelii* strain was isolated from a patient with ACA* in Sweden.[144]

PGau - This *B. afzelii* strain was isolated from a patient with ACA in Germany.

Ip3 - This strain was isolated from an *Ixodes persulcatus* tick in Khabarovsk, Russia. (See Ip90 notes)

PBo - This strain was isolated from a human CSF sample from Germany. The Gudremmingen nuclear power plant is located on the Danube in Bavaria; and the Biblis nuclear power plant is found on the Rhine River in Hesse.[93]

PKo - This strain was isolated from a patient's ECM rash in Germany.[58,59]

**ACA = Acrodermatitis chronica atrophicans, a chronic skin manifestation of Bb infection by B. afzelii strains; ECM = Erythema Chronicum Migrans; CSF = Cerebrospinal fluid of a patient with Lyme disease*

Each of the "Bb" strain types could have come from insects that feed upon animals – animals that would also have been affected by applied insecticides; or from humans who were exposed to insects or insecticidal residues which persist on fruits and vegetables were applied or engineered. We can imagine that B.t. insecticides targeted not only the desired pests, but possibly also non-targeted microbes in the environment. Another important connection to these isolates is that each was found near an area where mineral, phosphate rock, or radioactive elements (including acid mine wastes) or pollutants are found. This is significant for two reasons.[40,41]

First, because sulfur-reducing, metal tolerant (thermophile) bacteria and blue-green algae live in these areas, and because scientists use genetically engineered sulfur-loving bacteria to bioremediate acid mine wastes and to help leach metals from ores during mining and related processes. Scientists also designed insecticides with metal tolerances that were useful industrially and agriculturally, including for nuclear plants which use synthetic polymer coatings, corrosion inhibitors, insecticides, and surfactants in their normal course of operations – and which for decades expelled nuclear wastes into the environment before better pollution control measures were enacted.[40,41]

To help "debug" what makes up a Bb spirochete, I searched through culture databases looking for *different* microbial strains which share the same *borrelia* strain names as those listed in the Dattwyler et al. patent. A few searches did not return a result, but we'll examine the strain and I ask questions after each strain. The possible origins of the strains should enable observers to detect patterns that may noticeably repeat for each and every *Borrelia burgdorferi* strain, not just the fifteen serotypes described by the Dattwyler et al. patent (or the thirteen serotypes that have monoclonal antibodies).

B31: One strain of *Spiroplasma apis* and strains of *Borrelia burgdorferi s.s.* emerged under this search term. *Spiroplasma apis* is the honey bee spiroplasma. A culture is on deposit from France which represents the French May disease of honey bees. "B31" is also the name of a bee-flower spiroplasma, a plant spirochete. The "B31" Bb strain came from Shelter Island, NY ticks, and was deposited by Dr. Alan Barbour (from Dr. Willy Burgdorfer). The 60kDa antigen from the B31 strain is listed in a database as *Borrelia coriaceae.* This is a Bb strain that is transmitted by the soft tick *Ornithodoros coriaceus* – an insect that harbors the relapsing fever agent *Borrelia parkerii.* Does this mean that B31 is a mutated spirochete that contains some genes from a relapsing fever strain? According to phylogenic trees, it certainly could; and Bb could also be a strain that was passed through rodents on its way to becoming a human pathogen.[152]

During my search, a bacteriophage also returned under "B31" that contained *Escherichia coli* and so did a strain of human DNA that had a "unique subtelomeric region." This could represent a recombinant B.t. insecticidal formula that made its way into wastewater. There it could have combined with human gut *E. coli* to form this unique species. There is also a yeast species *Saccharomyces cerevisiae* "telomorph" (sexual form of a fungus) that returns under this strain; as well as a cloned B31 strain that is used in PCR (polymerase chain reaction) and other diagnostic tests to detect the Bb-B31 strain. The yeast strain could have been used in fermentable products including the insecticide "B.t.,"or pharmaceutical or other industrial products. The patents for PCR probes are owned by Hoffman La Roche, Inc. We know that Lyme-notable and 2000 Lyme disease guidelines co-author Dr. Benjamin Luft reported that he was on the speaker's bureau of Roche Laboratories.[42,89]

An alternative explanation of the "unique subtelomeric region" may represent a bacterium that contains synthetic polymers such as "C8." C8 is also known as the endocrine-disrupting, and persisting pollutant "APFO" or ammonium perfluorooctanoate. This chemical polymer is used to manufacture fluorinated plastics, high temperature thermoplastics, and elastomers. It is also a surfactant and dispersing agent used in many fluoropolymers. Fluoropolymers such as PTFE have been used to capture beetles. DuPont and 3M have both manufactured polymers from C8, which is an organic pollutant that persists in the body (POP). Pesticide dispersants typically contain some kind of fluoropolymer agent.[90-92]

When we think about the Dattwyler et al. patent, we might also consider that the Brookhaven National Laboratory, the Shoreham Nuclear Power Plant, and Stony Brook University are all located on Long Island. Long Island is a major Atlantic coastal estuary that abutts New York and Connecticut. It is also home to pollutants from dump sites, wastewater treatment plants, industrial runoff, and nuclear pollutants. Some of these may have been derived from the Brookhaven Laboratory which according to many public documents has a history of nuclear-related clean air and water pollution violations. These may also include similar wastes from the radiation therapy facility operated by Stony Brook Hospital.[43-51]

Industrial and nuclear wastes from the Connecticut and Thames Rivers; and from the Hudson River including its main tributary the Mohawk, which is adjacent to the Knolls Atomic Power Laboratory in Niskayuna; and Indian Point's nuclear plants on the east bank of the Hudson in Buchanan, also likely contributed to the variety of nuclear and other toxic effluents discharged into the air, soils, and waters around Long Island. Water currents that circulate highly contaminated waters in the Sound flow past Shelter Island, Plum Island, and into the Atlantic Ocean. Obviously the toxic water quality is directly responsible for the kinds of sulfur-reducing extremophilic bacteria and other microbes that are found in this environment.[43-51]

The disposal of solid, gaseous, and liquid wastes from laboratories, hospitals, and other facilities that use nuclear technologies (i.e. nuclear medicine, particle physics); and the discharge of industrial and municipal wastewaters remains a hugely impactful public health issue. Sediments contain toxic contaminants, including some that originated during the early part of the 20th century (i.e. "Black Tom" explosion) or far earlier (i.e. textiles, metal working, dyes).

One of the most prolific of the sporulating bacteriums to be isolated from Long Island Sound is *Clostridium perfringens.* This bacterium is normally found in the intestinal tracts of animals and insects. It is also found among decaying matter and in marine sediments. A more familiar strain of *Clostridium* called *C. botulinum* produces toxins and is used to make the cosmetic *Botox.* We might think about the presence of these toxins in the human body, and whether they are able to bind with the microbes of ingested B.t. insecticidal formulas. Long Island is also largely marshland, and in the 20th century it was home to fish processing plants. *Clostridium botulinum* toxin is a hazard found in fish and fish products. In addition, silkworms and gypsy moths can also harbor clostridium species, and these moths have historically been a huge problem in the northeast.[94,95]

Some bacteria produce extracellular enzymes, including *Penicillium roqueforti* Thom. These enzymes destroy the vegetative, but not the sporulated cells of *Bacillus popilliae* (milky spore), and other spore-formers including B.t. These enzymes are used to help generate large quantities of spores in the laboratory for insecticidal use. The spores are then used in conjunction with *Clostridum, B. popilliae, Sarcina,* and other spore formers to ramp up the effectiveness of pesticides. [44,94-95]

Question: *Does the American B31 strain of Borrelia burgdorferi include a bee-flower "B31" spiroplasma from plants that have been exposed to recombinant B.t. insecticides? Does the B31 Shelter Island strain of Bb harbor a mutated Leptonema like the one isolated from a Lyme patient's EM rash in 1981 by Dr. Steere's team – something also found on Shelter Island? Does the B31 strain contain a sporulating clostridium bacterium with a "nuclear waste" element or persisting pollutant (i.e. polymer component) such as may be isolated from Long Island Sound or any similiarly contaminated water source?*[52]

ZS7: Although no strain returned under this name in one database, there are uranium and silver mines in the German Black Forest. There is also a nuclear power plant in the town of Wyhl, Freiburg. The city of Freiburg im [in] Breisgau lies in the heart of wine-growing country in the Black Forest. Germany has also been home to various vulcanised rubber, cellulose, film (cellulose nitrate), and plastics industries. Nitrocellulose (cellulose nitrate, flash paper) uses nitric acid to create a propellant or explosive. It was also used as a film base for photograph, motion picture, and X-ray films (nitrate film). It was used in gun-cotton, and later in smokeless powder (gunpowder); as a blasting (mining) explosive (i.e. cordite); and in underwater mines, torpedoes, warheads, and certain diagnostic tests (Western blots, and other antigen-binding tests).[97,98]

Nitrocellulose lacquers were used on band instruments, furniture, and automobiles. DuPont is just one company that manufactured this kind of lacquer. These lacquers were used until the 1950s when synthetic polymers were developed (i.e. acrylic resins, enamels, polyurethane, other solvent-based lacquers). Indeed lacquer was originally a resin that was made from insect pests of the *Acacia catecu* (mimosa), a Malaysian thorny tree; from the Ficus (fig); or the Butea (parrot tree) another Asian, Malaysian, and Indonesian tree. Common pests of these trees are thrips, cottony cushion scale, beetles, glassy-winged sharp-shooters, leafhoppers, spittlebugs, looper caterpillars, citrus long-horned beetles, cable borers, mites, and whiteflies.

Acacia wood is used as livestock fodder; while wood extracts are used for leather tanning, dyeing, preserving fish nets, and for oil drilling. The fig is used for latex and food; and the butea for dye, resins, timber, tannins, charcoal, and pharmaceuticals. Obviously the insects that are used for resins and lacquers are important to consider for their resident microbial infections. Lacquer was used as early as 5,000 BCE in China. In the 1600-1700s, Asian and Indian lacquered items of a process known as "japanning" were popular in Spain, England, France, and The Netherlands.[99-103]

A "Z/16" spiroplasma was also isolated from *Ixodes ricinus* ticks in Freiburg, Germany. A US patent refers to the Bb "ZS7" strain as "DSM 5527." I found *Saccharomyces cerevisiae* (brewer's yeast) and *Streptomyces ardus* (f/k/a *S. verticillium* and *S. caespitosus*) in databases under a similar number. *Streptomyces caespitosus* is an *Actinobacteria* that produces the antibiotic and chemotherapeutic agent Mitomycin C. I also found a Bb 31-kDa OspA antigen gene for the Lyme disease vaccine under this number.[49,104]

The US patent mentioned is for antigens associated with Lyme disease. The patent is assigned in part to the Max-Planck Society (Max-Planck-Gesellschaft). The Max Planck Institute for Nuclear Physics (Max-Planck-Institut für Kernphysik [MPIK]), is one of eighty institutes and research establishments of the Max Planck Society which focuses its research in astro-particle physics and quantum dynamics. Here again is the nuclear research link to Lyme disease. The Max Planck Society is listed as assignee on a number of *Borrelia burgdorferi*-related patent inventions. Their patents include vaccines and diagnostic antibodies, antigens, and recombinant DNAs and vectors related to Lyme disease. Why would scientists who study nuclear physics hold patent rights on Bb-related products or processes if nuclear energy or its fuels or wastes did not have some kind of participatory link to the creation of the Bb agent? According to one of their patents which discusses the isolated ZS7 and B31 strains of the Bb organism:[104]

> "It is assumed that the pathogen passes over very quickly from the blood circulation into the tissues and can there no longer be directly reached by the immune system."

The pathogen referred to in the patent is the Bb spirochete. This speaks to the inability to detect Bb spirochetes in blood samples except for a very brief period. Several Max Planck Society patents are co-assigned to the German Cancer Research Center at Heidelberg. There is a close association between the University of Heidelberg and the Heidelberg Ion Beam Therapy Center, which provides particle therapy for cancer using protons and heavy ions (radiation). We might wonder what happens when cancer radiation therapy wastes make their way into wastewaters; and what those radioactive ions might do to resident microbes and their cells, or the insects that take up radioactive elements into their bodies.[104-111]

It is also interesting that two "Z4" strains of Bb exist (Z41293, Z41493), as isolated from German *Ixodes ricinus* ticks. These strains are *mutant relapsing fever strains* that are described as mutants of a bird strain and a mouse strain. In other words, these strains probably developed after passage through birds and mice into an insect vector which delivered mixed infections to humans.[152]

Question: *Is Bb ZS7 a strain found near silver and other metallic ore mines or nuclear science facilities; and where "B.t." formulas with a spiroplasma and an Actinobacteria (which degrades insect chitin and cellulose) were deployed (i.e. Black Forest or nearby vineyards)? Did this strain pick up polymers or bacteria from agricultural dispersants or nuclear wastewaters? The Bb strain "ZS7" may also be found in people who received the Lyme vaccine, and in whom the vaccine failed to protect them. If this is true, it could explain why the OspA "31kDa" and OspB "34kDa" bands were excluded at the Dearborn Conference in standardized Lyme disease diagnostic tests. Do these Bb strains contain a B.t. fermented yeast?*

N40: A strain of *Listeria monocytogenes* returned under this search term. This is a virulent food-borne pathogen that causes *Listeriosis.* The organism causes meningitis in newborns; and meningoencephalitis in ruminant animals including deer. It is also highly pathogenic to rodents such as mice and rabbits. Listeria produces adhesive proteins which bind to the intestinal wall, and can cause septicemia (bacteremia). It also crosses the placenta and the blood-brain border to cause meningitis in newborns and adults. The N40 strain also appears to have been adapated to birds and mice as hosts.

What is also important to state is that deer were repopulated in the northeast and in the midwest. Animal vaccines sometimes use radioactive tracer elements (radiotracers). Did deer and livestock receive animal vaccines that contained radioactive tracers? Animals are also fed corn and other crops. The crops have sometimes been genetically engineered with radiotracers. Crops have also had chemical herbicides and insecticides applied to them; and the formulas can contain dispersants, radioactive trace elements and persisting chemicals.[96]

A soil bacterium called *Mycotypha indica* that was isolated from India also returned under this number. I also found a wild yeast strain called *Saccharomyces paradoxus* that was isolated from oak wood (*Quercus* species) from Yalta, Ukraine. These are interesting for several reasons. First, *Mycotypha indica* is a sporulating fungus that is found in the soil and in manure (i.e. turkey dung). Strains have been isolated from the US (CA, DC, IA, KS); and from Finland, Venezuela, Africa, India, and Japan. All species form yeast cells when grown in the lab.[167-174]

Second, wild yeast strains from the *Saccharomyces paradoxus* family are important when we realize that yeasts are part of the fermentation broth that creates B.t. insecticides. The ability of wild yeast strains to bind with the applied yeasts of insecticides may play a role in the creation of toxic yeast strains that cause human-affecting neurotoxic illnesses. This wild yeast + lab yeast connection cannot be stated loudly enough for its importance to agriculture and to the development of Bb strains. There were more than three dozen wild yeast strains of *Saccharomyces paradoxus* known by Russian (Moscow) and American (MI State Univ.) scientists by 1997. It was also known that these strains could produce infectious hybrids when crossed with other yeast strains, as tested using an isolate from Denmark upon strains from Japan and the Russian Far East.[167-174]

There is an important natural fungus of oak trees called *Endoconidiophora fagacearum,* which has been renamed *Ceratocystis fagacearum,* or the *oak wilt fungus.* It is a highly prevalent fungal infection of oak trees, having been detected in Wisconsin in 1944 in the US. It covers twenty-one states from the midwest (Minnesota, Wisconsin, Michigan, southward through Kansas into Texas; eastward from Missouri through Virginia down into South Carolina; and from Iowa to almost the eastern coastline. There is no cure for this fungal infection in trees, which is naturally transmitted by sap and bark-feeding beetles. The tick that bit me in 1992 came from our backyard which had a stately oak tree. I would not be surprised at all if I prove to have this fungal infection.[198-200]

Research proves also that oak wood such as that used to make wine barrels has become contaminated with organochlorine biocides including those which *form naturally from the application of various organochloride pesticides through a process which was felt to be "impossible" in nature.* One example is the formation of TCA and 2,4,6-trichloroanisole. TCA is used as a fungicide, and trichloroanisole is a fungal metabolite of TCA. When airborne fungi or bacteria come into contact with chlorinated phenolic compounds (chlorophenols), they convert the compounds into anisole derivatives. This process can also be seen with pesticides, wood preservatives, and chemicals used to bleach paper, or in wood pulp. The biochemical formation of toxins in woods (and other plants) through the uptake of chemical pesticides is a problem that has also been seen in cork woods. If we study the science, we will find that the biochemical formation of toxins by the uptake of multiple chemical toxins is not restricted to trees, but is the process after which the industrial bioremediation of harmful, persisting pollutants in the environment is actually modeled.[167-174]

Not only plants and trees have this ability to take up harmful chemicals and toxins, but also the microbes in the environment. Microbes which commonly produce TCA metabolites are the *Actinomycetes, Rhizobium, Streptomyces, Botrytis, or Aspergillus* species of bacteria and fungi; including wild and recombinant strains. Since we know that the early applied fungi *Beauveria bassiana* was formerly known as *Botrytis bassiana*, and we grasp the relationship between these microbes and their ability to biosynthesize toxic chemicals, we may begin to understand the kinds of microbes and toxins that may be at the heart of Bb strains. *Borrelia burgdorferi* strain N40 has the same number as the N40 strain of *Saccharomyces paradoxus,* which has family members that have been isolated from Denmark, Russia, Ukraine, Finland, Japan, the Netherlands, Spain, Estonia, Lithuania, and the US.[167-174,180]

<u>Question:</u> *N40 was one of the first American Bb strains isolated. While this strain is present throughout the world, it probably formed an organism that contains wild yeast, fungi, and chemical toxins which were probably first gathered from the environment by oak or other tree species. Does the American N40 strain of Bb also include strains that came from vaccinated livestock that ate contaminated wood pulp-augmented feeds? Can these strains also contain a ruminant (i.e. white-tailed deer, cattle) meningoencepahlitis bacterium (i.e. deer tick, powassan, or related arboviruses)? Does this group include diseases from failed livestock "vaccines," or from repopulated deer that were vaccinated before release? Could animal feeds contaminated with wild yeasts or fungi have led to the failure of an animal leptospirosis vaccine to create a mutated leptonema that could be excreted in livestock urine and solid wastes? Were animal vaccine cell lines or animal feeds contaminated with radioactive tracers, or did this particular bacterium become contaminated with nuclear wastes from the Hudson River or other similarly polluted waters?*

PKa1: Four samples of *Schizosaccharomyces pombe* come up under this search term. These are "fission yeasts" used in molecular and cellular biology. They are also useful when studying cellular responses to DNA replication and damage (i.e. gene damage from nuclear fallout or nuclear wastes). The strains on deposit at the culture database may be a recombinant clone of *Acetobacter S. pombe.* This organism suppresses temperature-sensitive mutants in yeasts (*S. cerevisiae*) during B.t. fermentation. This may be used because without it, after fermentation, B.t. spores that should not remain infectious are able to be so despite fermentation. This seems to have been a problem with earlier B.t. products – spores remained infectious in the environment, and not just to insects that ate them. Using a recombinant clone seems to avert this problem by producing spores that are only infective upon ingestion. But this does not necessarily mean that the spores will only infect insects when eaten. If Bb is an aggregate, the PKa1 strains may include a recombinant clone used to ferment B.t. insecticides.

When we look for fission yeasts, we also find those that are able to convert ethanol into acetic acid. This technology may represent the production of *corn amylase.* This Bb strain may come from a B.t. formula that is applied to corn, or engineered into (GM) corn. The B.t. genes could be engineered with special "output" genes that when harvested, faciliate the manufacture of corn-derived biofuels. Since this Bb strain was isolated from a human patient's cerebral spinal fluid, the patient could have become infected by ingesting contaminated food, or by an insect vector that transmitted the infection.[112-114]

<u>Question:</u> *Is the European PKa1 strain of Bb associated with the yeasts of B.t. insecticides applied to GM corn with a future intended as biofuel – and which harbor the corn stunt Spiroplasma kunkelii that may have been created with the help of nuclear isotopes? Such wastes could be derived from uranium mining, military ranges, nuclear fallout/blasts, nuclear accident or isotope contaminated wastewaters. Since radiotracers are sometimes engineered into B.t. formulas, these strains could represent infections caused by bacteria that carry radioactive markers from insecticides. Note: biofuels that contain viable spores will become aerosolized when burned; further increasing the likelihood that such spores will continue to spread via an airborne route.*

25015: It is interesting that the US Army Corps of Engineers-Marmet Resident Office is located on Dupont Ave., in Belle, West Virginia, with the postal code of 25015. Among its advertised products are glass and laminates which include bullet and bomb blast-resistant windows and window films. The DuPont Washington Works plant is among the largest DuPont manufacturing facilities in the world (located in Parkersburg, West Virginia). The DuPont Works manufacturers many products including polymer modifiers, fluoropolymer additives, carpet and flooring, safety glass interlayers, Teflon© (non-stick materials), sandblasting materials, and chemicals that include cleaners, disinfectants, lubricants, and fluorochemicals. We will learn more about the Washington Works site in the upcoming chapter on persisting pollutants. Remember that herbicides and other agrochemicals are sold in plastic containers. For now, we might consider whether PFOAs or other persisting organic pollutants (POPs) are part of this particular Bb strain that was found in a polluted stream in Millbrook, NY. DuPont's Epidemiology Review Board on PFOA "safety" has included scientists from the following Universities: Yale, Johns Hopkins, Georgetown, the University of Washington, and the University of Massachusetts-Lowell according to a DuPont press release. The POPs including PCBs are well-known pollutants of water sources in this area of the country.[115,115a]

There is also a strain of *Francisella philomiragia* in a culture database that is listed as *Yersinia philomiragia* under the number "25015." This organism was isolated in 1959 from a dying muskrat, found on the shore of the marsh at the Bear River migratory bird refuge in Brigham City, (northern) Utah. The animal was sent to the Bear River research station in July 1959. A small gram-negative *Y. pestis*-like bacillus was isolated. It was similar to, but smaller than other *Pasteurella* strains.[51,175-177]

There is also a fungus called *Sporotrichum globuliferum* that was identified in 1914 near Salt Lake City, Utah, and this may also play a role in Bb isolates under the 25015 strain group, as it is a common fungus of the alfalfa weevil. However, nuclear wastes for the Hanford, Washington site were stored in northern Utah and near the Idaho border according to reports. There they await interrment in Yucca Mountain, a permanent high-level nuclear waste storage facility that was being built and studied for such suitability inside the volcanic ridgeline just outside of Las Vegas, Nevada. Yucca Mountain was a "deep geological disposal" solution for spent nuclear wastes and fuel elements in response to the 1982 Congressionally-passed Nuclear Waste Policy Act (NWPA). The Act addressed the growing problem of the disposal of high-level radioactive wastes. 1982 of course was also the same year that the "Lyme disease agent" was officially announced to the world from a Montana lab, and this may be no coincidence.[116-118,120a]

A 1969 paper was published by researchers at the Bear River research station and Rocky Mountain Laboratories in Hamilton, Montana about the 25015 strain of bacteria mentioned previously. Research experiments undertaken at the time indicated that the 25015 "muskrat pathogen" was similar to a *Yersinia pestis** strain and a *pseudotuberculosis* strain. This is interesting because there is a new patent that was filed in part by Lyme notable Dr. Raymond Dattwyler which describes a novel vaccine for this very same plague agent. Dr. Dattwyler is one of the IDSA co-authors of medical guidelines for Lyme disease, and of course an inventor of the patent that described to us the fifteen different strains of Bb that we previously examined.[34,50,51]

**Yersinia pestis is an enterobacteria that causes plague, the infamous "Black death."*

Yersinia pestis is considered by the Centers for Disease Control to be a biological warfare agent. It should be, as the most recent pandemic began in China, travelling along the Silk Road in the mid-1300s, and was responsible for killing about half of Europe's population then, and in earlier centuries. This agent was allegedly deployed by Japanese forces over China prior to WWII. In 1960, NIH researchers at Rocky Mountain Labs were studying the presence and distribution of *Francisella novicida* (*Pasteurella novicida*). The organism had originally been isolated from water samples collected *a decade earlier* from the Ogden Bay refuge, a marshy area just a few miles from the Bear River research station where the "25015" agent was also found in a dying muskrat. A pathogen isolated from four water samples at the time, *Yersinia philomiragia* turned out to be the same pathogen that would be isolated from the dying muskrat in 1959.[50,51,54]

The presence of a plague-related bacterium is not particularly unusual as *Y. pestis* is prevalent within US rodent populations. However, a mutant of a plague bacterium could come about as a result of a natural horizontal gene transfer, or perhaps through the deployment of a recombinant biological warfare agent that was first created in a laboratory and then deployed in open-air biological agent field experiments. Such deployments would not be outside the scope of the biowarfare tests that were undertaken in 1951 by the US military at Dugway Proving Ground (Utah) or other locations. This testing range is not geographically far from where the mutant 25015 agent was originally isolated.[50,51]

Within roughly a hundred miles of the marsh at the Ogden Bay Refuge (and the Bear River Research Station), is the Dugway facility where many biological warfare open-air experiments were performed. The marsh at Ogden Bay refuge is also part of the Wasatch-Cache National Forest. It is located just south of the Great Salt Lake, along the path of prevailing winds for the area. The US military experimented with all kinds of biological agents at Dugway. To find this agent in a muskrat in the Dugway area may be either insignificant, or highly significant, depending on how the animal was exposed (natural vs. descendant of past military experiments). There are also nuclear wastes found in the area that are natural components found in salt deposits; from uranium or vanadium mining; or from nuclear fallout from weapons testing that was undertaken in the region during the 1940s and 1950s.[53,54]

If nature, nuclear, or biological warfare experimentation led to the formation of mutant bacteriae (*Yersinia pestis-tuber-*

culosis) in the environment; and it was subsequently contracted by a muskrat (and other wildlife); such microbes may be transmited by marsh mosquitoes. If a biological warfare agent was tested and it migrated into the environment to infect insects and animals, it could explain the emergence of a strain of pathogenic animal bacteria, even decades later. If one or more such pathogens are a component of a Bb strain (if gene bank numbers are the same as the "strain" number indicated by the Dattwyler et al. patent), then this may help prove that Bb is an aggregate organism.[50,51,53,54]

Other items also returned in databases under this number, including a human kidney hypernephroma cell line and a human fetal brain tissue sample. This may indicate that this strain may in part have involvement with human neurological disease or tumors perhaps caused by a problem with human cell line-grown vaccines or other pharmaceutical products.[176,177]

At least indirectly in the case of one strain group, Bb could be a possible byproduct of biological warfare and nuclear testing that meets the body of a vaccinated human. Different Bb strains may incorporate different bacterial agents to form a virulent mutant aggregate organism in a like manner. In this example however, the end product might possibly include a natural or recombinant plague-tuberculosis virus that is either a natural mutant; a descendant of weapons of biological warfare tested at Dugway; and wild yeasts such as *Sporotrichum globuliferum* that were donated by mining or nuclear wastes. We might also think about how closely related is anthrax (another formerly weaponized biowarfare agent that was experimentally tested in the area); and the agriculturally applied "insect biowarfare" agent called *Bacillus thuringiensis* or B.t.

Question: *Is the 25015 strain of Bb associated with a Yersinia (plague) strain that was transmissible by animals that eat insects that are exposed to B.t. pesticides; and/or biological and nuclear wastes of past warfare tests? Does this group include a wild yeast found near uranium/vanadium mines or stored nuclear wastes as found in Utah? Is this group also a manifestation of the many aluminum, or nuclear plants located near the Millbrook, New York area where the 25015 strain of "Bb" was first isolated? (After all, aluminum contains radioactive trace elements, and nuclear wastes contain radioactive elements and POPs.) Does this group contain a radioactive element found in nuclear wastes – elements and metals that contaminate the microbes carried by rodents (i.e. field mice, rats, or rabbits)? Can these strains also contain a nuclear isotope from fallout or wastes caused by previous nuclear testing, mining, or production in any part of the world?*[51,116-118]

K48: This search term returned as fungi, yeast, and yeast genetic stock in a database. It also revealed an organism numbered 44779. This is the same number as the B.t.-fermentation yeast *Saccharomyces cerevisiae,* but this strain has an "alternate state" that is called *Candida robusta.* This pathogen is thought to be an "imperfect" strain of *Saccharomyces cerevisiae* and is typically found in flower nectar. Since this strain was isolated from Czech sheep ticks, we might look at the pest insects of sheep and the viruses from same, or the forage they eat (i.e. flowering clover). One virus that is registered as a pesticide is *Cydia pomonella granulovirus,* a GV baculovirus of the codling moth. K48 also returned as a genetically engineered clone that was isolated from lung tissues of *Rattus norvegicus,* the brown rat, sewer rat, or Norway rat. This strain may represent a spiroplasma found in rodents, which also feed upon insects including moths and moth larvae. These rats are widespread in the US in Texas including marshy areas; and in other parts of the world, including Europe.[119,120,120a]

Question: *Is the European K48 strain of Bb associated with a fermented yeast strain of S. cerevisiae as found in B.t. deployed in the former Czechoslovakia (where there are uranium mines and nuclear fallout)? Or do these strains contain wild, imperfect yeast strains of the Candida family? Rats are found around sewers, mine waste stacks, and mines; as they live in lowlands, wetlands, and marshes. Strain K48 is a Borrelia garinii strain that is associated with rodents, wastewaters, and/or mines. These animals were likely exposed to B.t. formulas which included (moth) baculoviruses. Alternatively, could these strains be related to the release of irradiated codling, gypsy, or other moths which were meant to be used as "population replacers"?*

DK29: No strain returned for this name, but Denmark is a supplier of horticultural plants to the world. It is also a country where biological controls are used to control pest insects, in fields and greenhouses. Important pests found upon imported plants from The Netherlands include for example gypsy, pine shoot, and tussock moths. More simply, twenty-nine Bb strains were isolated from patients with Lyme borreliosis and compared in a 1994 study performed by scientists from the University of Munich (Germany); and the Borrelia Laboratory in Copenhagen, Denmark. The strains analyzed could represent each of the DK29 European and American strains with a common origin – one that is probably agriculturally related. The twenty-nine strains were members of each of the pathogenic Bb sensu lato groups: *Bb s.s., B. garinii,* and *B. afzelii.* Also noteworthy is that as of 2010, Denmark had a total of twenty-nine plants which burn tons of household garbage and industrial wastes, including that which contains toxic pollutants (i.e. dioxins).[52,120a,121,122]

Question: *Is this Bb strain group a manifestation of a Netherlands strain of spiroplasma or another flower, tree, or plant spiroplasma found for example in ornamental tulips or tulip trees that have had B.t. pesticides sprayed upon them, and which are grown in ground that has been contaminated with applied or aerosolized nuclear or persisting chemical wastes? Does this spiroplasma include a virus from gypsy moths? Are these strains the result of irradiated gypsy moths or other insects which were released agriculturally; and the effects of irradiation upon insect viruses? Dr. Burgdorfer would classify a spiroplasma from a rabbit tick in the Ascomycetes family – which is among the fungi/yeasts that are able to biosynthesize toxic pollutants into toxic metabolites. Is this strain the result of a waste-contaminated airborne fungus that met the yeasts of applied B.t. products upon ornamentals?*

PHei: No strains returned under this number, however once again we may find a fluoropolymer called PEI, or polyethyleneimine. In this strain name, perhaps the "H" represents human, since the strain was isolated from a human CSF sample. These polymers contain amines and are used in cell cultures to aid weak attachments, most commonly in cell lines PC-12 and HEK-293. The PC-12 cell lines are derived from rat adrenal tumors (pheochromocytoma) that are treated with nerve growth factor. The HEK-293 cells are derived from human embryonic kidney cells. These cells are used in gene therapy, to create adenoviral vectors, and can be used in genetic engineering to transfect plasmids using the SV40 (simian) virus. Proteins of interest with these cell lines include those which affect acetylcholine receptors. There have also been studies of these cells in relation to environmental toxicants – studies which included *Saccharomyces cerevisiae.* Another HEK-293-related patent describes the use of its peptides (proteins) within B.t. transgenic plants. This means exactly as it sounds, that human and rat tumor cells that have been treated with nerve growth factors, or which may adversely affect acetylcholine receptors have been engineered into B.t. insecticides or B.t.-toxin engineered plants.[125-129]

Of interest is that UT-Battelle (Oak Ridge, TN) is assignee on more than one patent that discloses recombinant *agouti* proteins derived from human and mouse cell lines. These cells are described as "inhibitors of agouti activity" and "for altering fatty acid synthetase activity and intracellular calcium levels in transformed cells." This sounds like a rodenticide that could be used within B.t. formulas. But more likely it refers to the use of these proteins in transgenic plants that are likely to be eaten by insects and mice, which are each important crop pests.[130-134]

One Battelle patent references a paper that describes the significance of "loops" in the receptor binding domain of B.t. Cry toxins. The patent also references a transgenic animal patent assigned to Harvard, and a virus-resistant transgenic mice patent assigned to Ohio University. The Battelle patent claims to be for the detection and treatment of diabetes, neoplasms (tumors), hyperinsulinemia, and obesity. In the invention, agouti hair genes are targeted. This is interesting as hair is one location where heavy metals and persisting organic pollutants are stored by the body. The invention also discusses a chromosomal protein called HMG-1. When these proteins activate antibodies during infection, they play an active role in inflammation, arthritis, colitis, sepsis, endotoxemia, influenza, and systemic lupus.[130-134]

The HMG-1 antibodies secreted during inflammation are the HMGB1 cytokines, and these bind to TLR4, the toll-like receptors of the human immune system. These same toll-like receptors are also activated during Lyme disease infections. HMGB1 cytokines have been studied as a vaccine adjuvant. The Battelle patent also describes the use of agouti-derived polypeptides *within insect cell lines that include Trichoplusia ni cells.* These insect viruses have been engineered into insecticides.[129-133]

Question: *Is this a loose admission by the patent that this insect Ascovirus, which is common to the Cabbage Looper, a targeted pest of B.t.-transgenic crops, is responsible for important human infections? Are the PHei strains of Bb due in part to transgenic crop formulas that have in a sense, failed? Do these strains include the cabbage looper virus Trichoplusia ni, an agricultural yeast; and exposure to a recombinant B.t. insecticide? Are these strains found among fluoropolymers?*

IP90: Several human Coxsackie virus A strains returned under this number and so did a mouse hepatitis, and a polyomavirus strain from *Mus musculus* (house mouse). The human strains were isolated from Texas flies in 1948; from stool from a two-year old Mexican child in 1952; stools from children in South Africa (1950-1952); and in 1952 from a five-year old Japanese boy with a paralytic illness. Dr. Alan Barbour first isolated the Bb-IP90 strain, and he also works in the Texas University System. This is curious since in 1948 Texas flies were found to carry the coxsackievirus A strain. We will also study a human rickettsialpox outbreak in New York in 1946 that involved the coxsackievirus; and we know that polio virus was also isolated from Connecticut flies during the 1930s. Do the IP90 strains involve wild or vaccine-derived coxsackie and polio virus strains that have been reactivated inside the human body?

A hepatitis strain was isolated from mice that were infected with a *Nidovirus,* a group 2 coronavirus from a family that includes SARS (severe acute respiratory syndrome). The *Nidovirales* group also includes viruses that infect crustaceans (i.e. shrimp). Livestock animals are also infected with nidoviruses of the *Torovirus* genus. These viruses affect horses, cattle, and pigs, and can be made to encode 30-kDa recombinant virus proteins. The coxsackie virus A is a *picornavirus* and enterovirus (think polio). The mouse polyomavirus was isolated from lymph nodes from mice with ascites tumors. The polyomavirus was isolated from a mouse tumor grown cell line that was injected with SVEC4-10EHR1, or SV40-virus transformed endothelial cells. What this means is that a genetically engineered cell line uses SV40 cells, mouse tumor cells, and a hepatitis-polio causing nidovirus/coxsackie virus. Perhaps this combination is part of a recombinant B.t. insecticide.[135-139,146,147]

The OspA genes from the plasmid of the IP90 strains from Russia (and the US) were found to be 86% identical to those of strain B31, according to Dr. Barbour and colleagues. Could these strains possibly also include an "Ips" species of microsporidia (i.e. *Ips typographa, Ips duplicatus, Ips amitinus*)? An IP90 strain of Bb was provided for studies by the Gamaleya Institute, Moscow, Russia. According to their web site, the Institute is comprised of four WHO collaborating centers and nine centers of excellence of the Russian ministry of health and social development. Scientists at these facilities study the following diseases, which also coincidentally appear in co-infected Lyme patients: *Leptospirosis, Brucellosis, Tularemia, Clostridiosis, Mycoplasmosis, Legionellosis, Chlamydiosis, Rickettsiosis.* The Gamaleya Institute scientists mainly study food production using *genetically modified organisms*; but they also produce vaccines, diagnostics, nutrient media, and immunomodulators. This is interesting because polio viruses are entero (gut) viruses, and we are discussing genetically modified foods and food crops. This makes me wonder about GM foods that have had B.t. insecticidal formulas applied or engineered onto or into them; and which might contribute to the reactivation of viruses in animals, or vaccinated humans.[19-22,135-145]

There is a paper that describes a number of Bb strains, including those from France that are listed under strain numbers "IPT." Roughly three dozen of these strains were derived from Limousin, Alsace, Auvergne, Meuse, and Normandy, France. IPT may stand for Instantaneous Power Theory or more simply, "IP" or Instantaneous Power. In physics, this is the rate at which electrical power is transformed, or used. I find the power reference interesting because the area where the "IP" Bb strains were isolated is an area of France that was home to uranium ore treatment plants, uranium oxide and tailing wastes (dump sites), uranium mines, and uranium testing laboratories. The "IP" referenced strains could also involve uranium-associated wastes that are derived from nuclear power plants or from spent nuclear fuel storage facilities or abandoned mines.[152,154]

Under the IP90 strain number 20047, *Borrelia garinii* returned, isolated from *Ixodes ricinus* ticks from France. Also a soil fungus *Aspergillus flavus* returned, as did a UV-induced mutant, recombinant mouse genes, and a fungus called *Kluyveromyces lactis.* This fungus has a teleomorph called *Kluyveromyces drosophilarum* that was isolated from the fruit fly *Drosophila azteca.* Several patents describe the use of these kinds of fungi to produce enzymes that can convert uric acid into *allantoin.* Allantoin is also found in cosmetics, oral hygiene products, and pharmaceuticals. This enzyme has been produced by yeasts including *Aspergillus* and *Kluyveromyces* species collected from fruit flies in places such as southern and central California. It has also been cloned to produce genes necessary for *killer toxin production* (i.e. B.t. insecticides). There is a transformation system derived from the circular plasmid pKD1 that was developed for *K. lactis*, and which was "essentially equivalent" to that used for the yeast *Saccharomyces cerevisiae.* Using *K. lactis,* the KEX1 gene was studied in relation to the creation of killer strains for insecticidal use.[181-191]

Question: *Do the IP90 strains involve a hepatitis-causing virus, killer toxins, and wild or recombinant fungi first derived from fruit flies? Are the IP90 strains those that may contain nidoviruses, coxsackie, polio, or related viruses? Is this group caused by the release of irradiated fruit flies that harbored deleterious genes – recombinant genes that can reactivate human latent infections including important viruses from past vaccines? Are these strains found among nuclear wastes or irradiated insects that were released as population replacers?*

PTrob: No strain returned under this number, however there is an international petroleum company called Petrobras that is headquartered in Houston, Texas as the business unit of Petrobras Brazil. The company is responsible for deep water (oceanic) well drilling (i.e. Gulf of Mexico); and for exploration, production, refining, and related activities. The company also participates in US gasoline, ethanol, and fuel oil markets. Their business is conducted on the Gulf, west, and east coasts (in the US) and the company has storage tanks in the New York harbor. They also supply the US, Mexico, Central American, and Carribean markets with crude oil and gasoline.[148,149]

The *Borrelia garinii* strain PTrob is also called *Borrelia bavariensis.* The PTrob sample was isolated from the skin of a Slovenian patient. This means the patient was probably bitten by a vectoring insect. The strains that belong to this group include those associated with mice; and that are mutated descendants of relapsing fever spirochetes *Borrelia duttoni, B. hermsii,* and *B. turicatae* according to phylogenetic trees.[150-153]

Question: *Are these strains derived from areas where petroleum products are drilled, stored, processed; or are the result of deep well or borehole drilling and their acid mine wastes that have leached into groundwater? Are the mutagenic agents the chemicals and microbial biocides that are injected into bore holes to leach and recover petroleum or other resources?*

ACAI: No strain returned under this number, however these Swedish-derived strains contain OspA genes on a plasmid that were found to be 85% identical to the OspA gene of strain B31; and 86% identical to Russian IP90 strains. The OspB sequences of ACAI and IP90 were found to be 79% identical to the OspB gene of B31; and 81% identical to one another. Scientists had by

1992 already identified that the OspA and OspB genes of each of these Bb strains were duplicated before the strains dispersed globally. This means simply that the OspA and OspB genes probably became part of mobile plasmids (gene islands) before they started to appear globally in various strains (so they have a shared origin). It should be no surprise to scientists if Bb proves to be an aggregate organism that contains the globally-applied B.t. insecticide and other fungal/spirochetal agents that converged to form different Bb strains. We already suspect that B31 strains are related to the uptake of toxins by oak wood.[155,156]

Question: *Do the IP and ACAI strains represent wastes (including nuclear wastes) that have been taken up by other wood species? Are these woods used to make paper, or other products including fodder for livestock animals?*

PGau: No organisms returned under this search term in the database. However what is interesting is that PGAU or "Play Golf America" University is a PGA college and university golf program. Among PGA-active higher institutions, we find most of the key American universities that have connections to the Lyme disease arena. Strain P/Gau is a *Borrelia afzelii* strain that is adapated to mice. Since golf courses have been irrigated with wastewaters; have been dyed with turf pigments; and have had B.t. and other insecticides applied to them, it would not be a surprise if these strains are associated with turf grasses including golf course turfs. However since the P/Gau strain was isolated from a human skin sample in a German patient, we might look more closely at the "Gau" portion of the word. In French, "gau" means "grape," and is another word for the French wine grape Gouais blanc. We already know there is a copper-grape connection to spiroplasmas. In Germany, Gau (Größter Anzunehmender Unfall) is a German term to describe nuclear accidents including the 1986 Super-GAU Chernobyl disaster in the Ukraine.[157,158]

Question: *Are the P/Gau strains of B. afzelii those that are in part, the result of microbes that are found upon turf, vineyards, or other locations that have been contaminated with nuclear fallout from Chernobyl or other nuclear waste sources and the regionally applied B.t. insecticides or biocides used in mining or bioremediation?*

IP3: While no strain returned under this search term, we discussed the "IP" connection to Bb in the IP90 section. What is curious is that "IP3" in biological terms also represents *Inositol trisphosphate,* which is used by cells as a cellular messenger and lipid signaling mechanism. It was discovered by scientists that radioactive chromic phosphate (^{32}P or phosphorus-32), is a radioactive phosphorus that can be incorporated into cellular membranes of pancreatic cells when stimulated with the neurotransmitter acetylcholine. This neurotransmitter is used in the autonomic, central, and peripheral nervous systems of the human body. Perhaps these strains of Bb are organisms that have taken up radioactive phosphorus from the environment into their cellular (lipid) membranes. In the human body, IP_3 may alter calcium channels and therefore lead to neurodegenerative diseases such as Huntington's or Alzheimer's. In sea urchin eggs, IP_3 opens calcium channels. We know from patents that sea urchin toxins have been engineered into some B.t. insecticidal formulas.

Question: *Are the "IP3" strains responsible for neurologic diseases and which include engineered "natural" marine neurotoxins in B.t. formulas? Do these strains also include a radioactive phosphorus? Are these strains the result of the use of barium sulfide or other phosphates that may be used in nuclear medicine (radio contrast), copper casting, pyrotechnics, paint pigments, or drilling fluids? Or are these strains associated with phosphate mining, and/or the sulfate minerals hematite (i.e. hot springs), baryte, such as may be used in "heavy" cement as in oil drilling?*[159-162]

PBo: No organisms returned under this search term. However, it is highly interesting that polymers and plastics have a rich history that appears to be connected to our Lyme story. There are several kinds of plastics of interest, including plastic-like rigid-rod polymers. These types include PBI, PBO, and PBZT polymers. If we study their chemical structure, we might find interesting correlations with the genetic structure of certain Bb strains. Rigid-rod polymers were among the first polymers synthesized; including polyaniline, polyacetylene, polypyrrole, and their co-polymers. Rigid-rod or conductive polymers are organic polymers that are capable of conducting electricity, and can be used as semiconductors. These not-quite-plastics contain aromatic hydrocarbons including the luminescent fluorene from coal tar (not elemental fluorine), nitrogen, or sulfur. Polyfluorene also reportedly contains the highly mutagenic chemical benzene.[163-165]

Polyfluorenes are found in many industrial solvents, and are useful to academic and industrial research. Superconductors are used in dye/pigment industries; in electronics, and in nuclear medicine for magnetic resonance imaging (MRI) and nuclear magnetic resonance (NMR) machines. They are also used in mass spectrometers, and in nuclear particle accelerators. It is interesting that when we study the abbreviated names of some of the polyfluorenes that they are curiously similar to the names of some *Borrelia burgdorferi* strains. For example there is a "PBo" strain of Bb, and a "PBO" polymer. There is a "PBi" strain of *Borrelia bavariensis*, and a "PBI" polymer. There is a "PKo" strain of Bb (see next section) and a "PKO" polymer.[163-165]

Question: *Are certain Bb strains formed in the presence of nuclear wastes that contain polyfluorinated chemicals (or other industrially-important plastics/resins)? If so, do they also include bacteria or yeasts that are able to degrade polymers?*

PKo: Several organisms returned under this search term in a database, and the Bb-PKo strain is from the *Borrelia afzelii* group. Isolates also returned in the database under *Mus musculus* (house mouse) and *Rattus norvegicus* (brown rat) liver tissue cultures. We just discovered there is a polymer with the name PKO. But PKO also stands for Palm Kernel Oil, a product that is used in the food industry (mainly supplied by Indonesia and Malaysia). Acacia oil, kernels, and plant wastes are used for food, cosmetics, soaps, disinfectants, livestock feeds, agricultural mulch, and other industrial purposes around the world, and the connection between Malaysian rubber plantations, chemical herbicides, and palm oil should not be overlooked; in particular because palm oil is a major food staple in Africa, Brazil, and Indonesia. Palm oil ranks second in the world's most internationally traded edible oils. Palm kernel shells are used in aggregates for asphalt concrete and cement; in activated carbon water treatment processes, and are burned as charcoal, as biomass fuel, and as mixed fuels in boilers and electrical power generators. Palm kernels and related products are known to habor *Aflatoxin B1,* which is a mycotoxin produced by *Aspergillus flavus* and *Aspergillus parasiticus* strains of wild fungi. This aflatoxin is highly toxigenic and can lead to cirrhosis or liver cancer. These and other mycotoxins contaminate stored grains, and crops including cassava, potatoes, peanuts, rice, sorghum, sunflower seeds, corn, cotton seed, millet, tree nuts, spices, and wheat. Aflatoxins can also be present in milk products or animals fed toxin-contaminated grains.[166]

Aflatoxins have also been the target of clay formulas that can adsorb these fungal toxins, for example for water treatment processes. In one patent we can learn that tests were run using water samples that contained heavy metals and diazinon (phosphate pesticide), aflatoxin B1 (mycotoxin) and diethylstilbesterol (DES-hormone). These are pollutants that are also commonly found in municipal and industrial wastewaters. Curiously, I found patents which describe the use of "*aspernomine,"* a terpenoid metabolite that was isolated from the fungus *Aspergillus nomius. This fungus produces aflatoxins and is related to other aflatoxin-producing Aspergillus strains.* The metabolite *nominine* is used in insecticides to control corn earworms and other lepidoptera (moths, butterflies) and coleoptera (beetles, weevils). Insecticidal patents that use these and other toxic metabolites are assigned to several entities including the USDA. Interestingly enough, patents describe the antibiotics *Neomycin sulfate* and *Amoxicillin trihydrate* as inhibitory for the aflatoxins produced by *Aspergillus* fungal strains.[192-197]

<u>Question:</u> *Is the PKo strain of Bb associated with rodents of laboratories, mining, sewers, and palm-processing industries in Germany and other parts of the world? Do these strains include organisms derived from white-footed mice, rats, or rabbits of forests and agricultural crops that come into contact with nuclear wastes? Do these strains have to do with palm oil or other agricultural crops that are used for water treatment or are burned for fuel and whose particulates contaminate surrounding areas? Do these strains contain important Aflatoxins such as those found on food crops that have been sprayed with B.t. insecticides?*

There seems to be a pattern among Bb strains that is clearly associated with insecticides, nuclear, polymer, chemical, and other wastes, and which repeats throughout our story. While these connections are only hypothetical at this point, we must admit their continued emergence is worth more than a casual glance.

B.t. is Widely Deployed

In 1953 President Eisenhower reorganized various federal agencies to create the Agriculture Research Service (ARS). The ARS is the research arm of the USDA. The USDA and the ARS are responsible for research pertaining to infectious diseases of animals and food crops, especially those that are transmissible to humans. The USDA operates a huge research campus in Ames, Iowa which houses the ARS and the Animal and Plant Health Inspection Services (APHIS). Together these agencies comprise the National Centers for Animal Health.[1-11,11a]

Shortly after the 9/11 attack on the World Trade Center, and right before Congressional leaders signed an "anti-terror" bill called the *US Patriot Act,* the "*Ames"* strain of anthrax was found applied to letters that were mailed anonymously to Congresspersons and news personnel; causing five deaths. The letters carried a Trenton, New Jersey postmark, which in and of itself seems strange, unless we consider that New Jersey was one of the first states where agricultural agents including *Bacillus popilliae* and *Bacillus thuringiensis,* and the early parasitoids were first applied in this country to control insect pests.[1-11,11a]

Several people were investigated for possible ties to the anthrax letter mailings, and one suspect died under "mysterious" circumstances. Despite lingering doubts as to suspects, the FBI declared a suspect and closed the case. Trenton is home to a company that makes electronics for aerospace, avionics, communications, and defense industries. Trenton is also home to the National Terrorism Advisory System or NTAS (www.dhs.gov/alerts), which seems a coincidental arrangement since the anthrax letters were postmarked in Trenton before the anti-terror bill was presented to Congress to promote "homeland security."[1-11,11a]

The US military reportedly developed a highly sophisticated weapons-grade anthrax formula of the USAMRIID-regulated

Florida or *Ames* strain of anthrax, and had it in its possession since at least 1992. Resources show that samples of the Ames strain of anthrax were shipped between the laboratories at Dugway and Ft. Detrick. While some people speculate that US biological warfare programs continue beyond the scope of the Geneva Convention, this research might nevertheless be considered arguably within the confines of "peaceful medical purposes" outlined in the Convention; especially when used for agricultural or medical purposes.[6-16]

Such studies could have been related to scientific attempts to understand how a bioagent that *may first and foremost be related to applied insecticidal toxins useful against insects* may affect human populations if deployed by those who might *convert and use such tools* in a terroristic manner. Similarly, they could have been investigating the ability of a global insecticide to arbitrarily and naturally cause human infections when combined with naturally present microbes from the areas where they are applied. Studying such agents in a covert or quiet manner would be advantageous so that the public or public health agencies would not feel it necessary to speculate about any relationship between anthrax and agriculturally deployed B.t. insecticides. This would similarly protect the "safety" status of B.t. and other recombinant formulas.[6-16]

A 1948 paper reported on studies of the sugar compounds of apple juice, egg whites, and sheep blood. This seems a peculiar unrelated mix. Perhaps scientists were looking at the effects of how B.t. bacteria sprayed upon apples affected the blood of sheep that were inoculated with an anthrax vaccine that had been grown in chicken embryo cells (egg white membrane).[17]

The areas of the US that reportedly apply the most B.t. upon fruits and vegetables are California, the Pacific Northwest (Washington, Oregon), and Florida to the south. The other regions most affected by agricultural and forest applications of B.t. are the New England states (Ohio, Pennsylvania, New York, and Maryland into the Carolinas); the midwest (Michigan, Wisconsin, Illinois, Minnesota, Missouri); and Texas to the south. From 1987 through 1996 alone, about two million US acres of agricultural, nursery, and greenhouse crops were treated with B.t. products. We may recognize that the areas of the world which deploy B.t. insecticides are also known to be highly endemic for illnesses including Lyme and Multiple Sclerosis.[17]

Mosquito, black fly, and gypsy moth control is practiced annually using B.t. to the tune of about 1.5 million base acres, with another 1.5 million for forests and parks. Base acres are those where B.t. is applied only once. Many areas receive multiple applications. The largest agricultural sites to have B.t. externally applied are typically crops of corn, cotton, leafy vines, (grape, raspberry, blackberry); and vegetables such as artichoke, spinach, cabbage, and celery. Despite these applications, in 1981 alone, a record thirteen million northeast acres were decimated by gypsy moths, just one important agricultural pest insect.[18,19]

A 2006 Danish study evaluated one hundred and twenty-eight *Bacillus-cereus* like strains isolated from fuits and vegetables on sale in Danish grocery stores. Out of these, fifty were found to have insecticidal residues of the same subtype as the commercially-applied B.t. pesticides. The study "strongly" indicated that *B.t. residues can be found upon fresh fruits and vegetables, and that the residues are potentially enterotoxigenic* (toxic when eaten.)[18,19]

A patent describes B.t. strain kurstaki that can contain a radio label (radioactive element) that enables the insecticide to be tracked (i.e. by satellite). It also declares that the formula "doesn't cause secondary contamination to silkworms." This means that B.t. pesticides in traditional formulas may be able to produce "interfering spores" when all that is desired are Crystal toxin proteins, not the spores. It is acknowledged in B.t. patents that during the production of B.t. Cry proteins, spores are released that may contaminate the finished formulas. In earlier formulas, these spores were allowed to remain because they were costly to remove. Spores that do remain in B.t. formulas are infectious and could cause disease in the guts of insects, animals, or humans that consume these spores. The newer formulas are considered to be "substantially free" of the problematic spores, but they are not entirely free of them. A B.t. insecticide patent states this:[20]

> "Bacillus thuringiensis produces crystals of .delta.-toxin and spores in the cells. The crystals and spores are usually released out of the cells when cell walls naturally rip at the final stage of cultivation and strengthen activity available as insecticide. The whole culture broth is usually dried and applied directly without separating the crystals from the spores when *Bacillus thuringiensis* is used as an insecticide because the separation procedure is very complicated."
>
> "Unfortunately, however, the application is extremely restricted since *there is the possibility that the spores in the preparation will be multiplied in the natural world after application* and cause hazard on the sericulture. The creation of an asporogenous strain of *Bacillus thuringiensis* was attempted to remove the defect and an insecticide containing Bacillus thuringiensis but not causing secondary contamination to silkworms was developed."[21-28]

In 1964, *Biospor* became the first licensed B.t. pesticide product for use in Germany. However older B.t. patents were filed in 1959 and the 1960s. One of the earliest insecticide patents describes the use of *Bacillus thuringiensis, B. sotto,* and *B. entomocidus* strains. Additional B.t. strains were discovered in 1965 (*B. sphaericus*), and in 1976 (*B. israelensis*), as well as others since then (*B. kurstaki, B. galleriae, B. aizawai, B. tenebrionis, B. san diego,* etc.). Each has been implemented as an insecticide. The WHO published a 1964 report discussing *the likely profitability of the early B.t. patents*. Although the organization declared a year earlier that B.t. was of "limited use," the 1964 report freely commented on the B.t. patents that had been issued in five countries over the previous four years, stating: "It is difficult in most cases to estimate the dividends that insect pathology, in particular, and biological control, in general, will receive as a result of the interest shown by industry in the mass propagation of a single pathogen."[29-34]

Other older B.t.-like patents describe the use of *Bacillus uniflagellatus,* a *B. subtilis* related soil bacteria and the fungus *Agaricus bisporus* in a 1-2 punch insecticide. This follows along the formula used for B.t. and fungi (i.e. B.t.-*Beauveria bassiana*) that is employed agriculturally. While the patents do not reveal where such formulas were applied, they do reveal the timeframe and the organisms involved. When I researched related patents I discovered that *Agaricus bisporus* is an airborne fungus from the common button mushroom (i.e. salad mushrooms). California has many mushroom farms, and their spores escape to become airborne pathogens. This combination of bacteria-fungi was also used in insecticides to control tobacco mosaic virus disease upon crops.[35-37]

It is apparent that the World Health Organization was keenly aware there would be a reasonable market for B.t.-containing insecticides, although the paper does not fully acknowledge the significance of B.t. patents. With the banning of harmful chemical pesticides, came an explosion of B.t.-related products over the past half century, as well as substantial profits from their global use. If B.t.-related products were suddenly proven to be contributing to human infections, this revelation could thoroughly drive the silencing of global epidemics and the denial of ill patients for many decades. Such silence could assure the preservation of substantial profits; the reputations of the companies that make these products; the patent rights and royalties earned by patent holders; and the ability to utilize potentially faulty products the longer they are believed to be safe. According to the WHO document, the earliest B.t. patent interests were held by the following institutions:

Institute	Patent Country and No.	Date
Pasteur Institute, France	French Patent #1,225,179	02/15/60
	Canadian Patent #630,687	11/07/61
	US Patent #3,071,519	01/01/63
Bioferm Corporation, US	Canadian Patent #639,333	04/03/62
	British Patent #907,030	09/26/62
	US Patent #3,073,749	01/15/63
Roussel-Usines Chimiques des Laboratories Français		
(French Chemical Lab)	French Patent #1,284,026	01/02/62
Institute of Biology, Prague	Czech Patent #105,416	1962 (estimate)[31]

As a result of research by the early patent holders, the scientific community felt confident there was enough experience working with applied insect pathology that B.t. was "generally regarded as safe." B.t. was first commercialized in 1958, but in 1961 the B.t. industry finally surged forward on a grand scale after it was registered as a pesticide – first in Germany and then in the US. This was shortly before the first outbreaks of human Lyme disease were reported (1969 in WI; and 1970s in CT). Despite the early confidence in B.t.'s safety, WHO scientists expressed a general concern over the manner that new B.t. isolates might be brought to a field-testing stage. It is curious that there is a distinct lack of discussion about the potential for B.t. to reactivate latent infections in the documents of the day.[30,31]

According to scientific texts, this reactivation ability was known at the very least by 1962, which was two years before the aforementioned WHO report was published, and only four years after B.t. was first commercialized. However there is no discussion of this aspect of B.t. within the WHO document, or in any other public health document I studied for that matter. It is entirely possible that those who were formulating B.t. products for industry may have withheld this important information from public health officials and regulators alike. If they did not, perhaps no one considered the possibility that latent infections might be reawakened in non-targeted populations – at least not by the routes that were studied.[30,31]

Although early field trials and applications of B.t. actually began during the 1930s and 1940s in sporadic areas of the United States, more widespread use of this biological agent commenced in 1951, including in Connecticut. Small US field trials with B.t. began during the 1950s, including limited "safety" studies which sometimes required testing the agent using animals and human volunteers. From 1956 to 1958, the FDA granted a temporary exemption and an experimental permit to test the use of B.t. upon vegetables and forage crops. In April of 1960, the US began the widespread use of B.t. as a commercial pesticide. Again this period was just before the human outbreak of an arthritis-like illness that would later be named Lyme disease.[38-44]

Once B.t. was recognized as a useful insecticide, the more cost-effective B.t. quickly increased in popularity over other microbial and chemical insecticides. Insect resistance to chemical pesticides was already a well-known phenomenon, and chemical pesticides were soon shown to contain harmful and mutagenic compounds. But just as happens with chemical pesticides, insects become resistant to B.t. formulas over time, although this takes longer to manifest for B.t. than for chemicals. Scientists work to circumvent this problem by designing increasingly toxic microbial cocktails.

The initial applications of B.t. in the forests of Europe and the USSR during the 1950s demonstrated not only reasonable success, but also affordability. B.t. products cost 4.5 to 10 times less than DDT to control the Siberian silk moth for example. The convenient and economic B.t. powders and liquids for agricultural and forestry use quickly gained global popularity over a short period of time.[41,43]

In 1961, the first microbial pesticides based on B.t. were registered in the US with the EPA. From 1957 through 1973, the EPA only classified one isolate of B.t. In 1974 one isolate became eleven based on *differences in antigen serotypes found on the flagellum* of the organism.* This discovery allowed the individual delta endotoxins (toxic proteins) to be identified and subclassified. (This same difference between flagellin proteins is also used to differentiate between *Borrelia burgdorferi* strains.) Delta endotoxins that are created using genetic engineering techniques are registered separately with the EPA. Highly specific B.t. toxins may be created from different bacillus strains, with each toxin effective against one or more insects depending on the toxin.[45]

**Flagellum (plural) or flagella (singular) means "tail."*

In recent decades B.t. and its crystal (Cry) toxins have been genetically engineered into numerous foods and industrially important crops to provide insect resistance to genetically modified plants. When insects consume or contact the GM plants, they become infected with B.t. toxins and recombinant microbes, and they quickly die. Now B.t.-laced foods that are extremely common among grocery store shelves, and which are unfortunately *never labeled as such*, contain genetically engineered toxins and microbes that are specifically designed to kill pest insects.

These same genetically engineered insecticides may also have the potential to infect animal and human guts to cause systemic infections. Do you think that if the world's most critical agricultural tools were discovered to be infecting the public, that scientists would redesign such tools – tools that are reaping billions in profits each year they are deployed? Do you think that royalty-receiving institutions would be keen on revising these highly profitable tools?

The presence of B.t. and other new, genetically engineered toxins (i.e. scorpion, mite, spider, sea urchin); and bacteria, viruses, fungi, protozoans, hormones, enzymes, and organisms (i.e. nematodes); have helped expose insects, animals, and humans to a myriad of infectious agents which may otherwise not have been harmful. Such powerful insecticides are designed specifically to gain entry into the insect's body through the alimentary tract and to create pores or holes in the insect's gut. Likewise consumers who choose to eat foods that are sprayed with, or are genetically modified using B.t. and other toxins and microbes run the risk of exposure to these toxins. The difficulty is in finding foods that are unaffected by these pesticides, as even organic foods can contain microbial insecticide residues.

If we study B.t. insecticide patents carefully, we will find clues to the ingredients that may be contributing to chronic illnesses including Lyme. For example, the yeasts *Beauveria bassiana*, and *Metarhizium anisopliae, Metarhizium flavoviride,* and *Streptomyces avermitilus* are fermented into some B.t. formulas to ramp up the insecticidal activity against insects. Yeasts under fermentation produce substances that effectively block insect neurotransmitters. For example *S. avermitilus,* an actinomycete, produces the antibiotic avermectin under fermentation. When made part of a B.t. pesticide, it blocks GABA neurotransmitters, and is toxic to rodents orally and dermally (on contact).[46-49]

Citrus nematode parasites and molds (*Pasteuria penetrans, Pasteuria thornei, Paecilomyces lilacinus*, and *Paecilomyces penetrans*) when used in combination are effective against nematodes and have been used in field trials beginning in the late 1980s. Scientists used any combination of molds, yeasts, soil bacteria, viruses, in recombinant constructs that contain "natural toxins" in B.t. insecticides to control insects and nematodes. To believe that any of these potent mixtures will remain entirely harmless to humans who consume treated crops and animal products; or who are subjected to insect bites, stings, and blood feeding pests seems naïve or even absurd.[46-47,49]

In 1998, the EPA declared that all uses of B.t. were not to cause "unreasonable" risks to either humans or the environment. However the EPA seemed only to address B.t. toxins produced naturally by the bacteriae. It does not appear to address toxins that are recombinantly made and inserted into genetic constructs or plants. It is unclear whether these categories have ever been properly regulated. It is clear there are no regulations requiring the labeling of foods or other products to alert consumers if a product or food contains an insecticide of any kind, including applied or genetically modified B.t. toxins.[46-49]

The EPA requires manufacturers to eliminate or minimize "undesirable" toxins. One example is a heat stable beta-exotoxin called *thuringiensin.* This was shown to be toxic to rat pulmonary tissues. Therefore this toxin is required to be eliminated from all production batches or the batches must be discarded. This toxin is a particular problem during manufacture of the B.t. strain *aizawai.* Heat labile toxin impurities also occur in other B.t. strains that are widely used including strains *israelensis* (B.t.i), and *kurstaki* (B.t.k).[50-53]

B.t. products with technical grade active ingredients are manufactured using a standard fermentation process. The growth medium used in the process appears to be at least partially involved in the creation of undesirable toxins. This may refer to the toxic "killer" strains that can be created by the yeast *Saccharomyces cerevisiae,* or another component; and must be closely monitored. Registrants are not required to adhere to a standardized fermentation process, but they must control and delete the undesirable elements. While these problems occur and can be controlled during manufacture; the binding of viruses to yeasts which can create toxic killer strains occurs in nature, far beyond laboratory control. The evaluation and regulation of undesirable toxins recommended by the EPA includes a standard production batch quality control test, and may include mouse toxicity studies.[51-53]

The manufacturing batch testing process appears to be standardized, but the performance of these tests seems virtually left to the individual manufacturers to monitor. Information reveals that the EPA simply requires batch test results to be readily available should the agency wish to examine same. Acute toxicity data sets are required for the registration process and there may be other controls required. In addition, the agency requires updated labeling on each product being reregistered, yet there is no requirement that foods or other products be labeled if they contain these insecticides.[51-53]

Over time the EPA found that the toxicity levels for mammals required adjustment. Established levels were demonstrating mortality for bacteriae otherwise considered non-toxic or nonpathogenic, especially *Bacillus subtilis.* The agency acknowledged that registered B.t. products might produce diarrheal enterotoxins similar to those typically associated with *Bacillus cereus,* a soil bacteria that produces foodborne illness. The EPA does not appear to publish evidence linking B.t. use and human cases of diarrhea after consumption of B.t.-containing foods on its web site, so it is unclear whether they are aware of a link.[51-53]

The agency does not at this time appear to require manufacturers to provide any information about the human endocrine effects of B.t., simply because no known metabolites have been shown to act as endocrine disrupters or immunotoxicants. This lack of evidence may simply be due to insufficient studies. Despite a lack of scientific evidence, the agency does not expect any ill effects toward immune or endocrine functions in humans from any B.t. products.[51-53]

If we consider that product safety studies may be performed by those with a keen interest in a positive outcome for such test results, we might find studies that are hardly independent. We might also find individuals who at times are not entirely forthcoming with unfavorable results when or if found. So-called long-term data studies may not truly be long-term; often covering weeks, months, or at best two years post-study, if ever undertaken. This timeframe is sometimes insufficient to assess cumulative damage, or to uncover unpredictable toxicology results. For example, from one document we learn that less than a dozen men were exposed to a half-year's exposure of fermentation broth, moist bacterial cakes, finished powders, and waste materials from B.t. production. The men were said to have "no complaints." Animal studies revealed some toxicology problems but these were hardly disclosed as serious; and animals are not human. We might wonder whether follow-up studies were performed upon the exposed men over decades to see if any ill health effects manifested over time, either to themselves or their offspring.[51-53]

The EPA acknowledges that B.t. spores may remain on harvested agricultural products and foods, although the agency appears to assume that the risks associated with consumption of residual insecticides is negligible. The EPA position on ground water exposure of B.t. toxins is also apparently negligible with the justification that B.t. has been used as a pesticide for a half century without any "known" ill effects. While the EPA recognizes that B.t. toxins affect insects through the mechanism of binding to receptors in their gut cellular membranes, the agency does not feel that a similar process may occur in the human body.[51]

This may simply be because there are no *known* identical receptor sites in the human digestive system. Or the EPA may simply be unaware of receptors which bind B.t. toxins directly or indirectly. In addition, the binding of B.t. toxins may be unnecessary in the human gut to cause disease, especially if microbes in the formulas can reactivate latent infections in humans in a manner that differs from that which is exploited by insecticides to kill insects. The EPA document I read concludes with the general assumption that B.t. is "harmless" to humans because "long-term" data has not revealed any harmful effects. Despite a good faith effort by the EPA including the establishment of strict requirements, we may wonder if manufacturers will comply as stringently as regulators hope. Some of the main manufacturers of B.t.-containing products listed within an older EPA source document are these:[51]

- Abbott Laboratories (North Chicago, IL)
- Ecogen, Inc. (Langhorne, PA)
- Thermo Trilogy (Columbia, MD)
- Becker Microbial Products, Inc. (Plantation, FL)
- Novartis Crop Protection (Greensboro, NC)
- Troy Corporation (Florham Park, NJ)

Other documents list Sandoz Crop Protection Corp. (Des Plaines, IL) as a B.t. manufacturer. Sandoz is a division of Novartis, a company that Lyme notable Dr. Allen C. Steere has revealed has provided him with at least one research grant. Dr. Steere, the Rheumatologist and CDC/EIS "agent" first on the scene at the outbreak of juvenile arthritis in Connecticut during the 1970s, was a co-author of two sets of IDSA Lyme disease clinical practice guidelines. He also helped establish the CDC surveillance case definitions after studies in Russia; and assisted with the standardization of diagnostic criteria for Lyme testing at Dearborn.

Dr. Steere recently appeared before a public web cast in July of 2009 in Washington, DC. The event was the IDSA guidelines review panel hearing that was held as part of a settlement in the historic Connecticut anti-trust case. Dr. Allen Steere indicated that Lyme patients are indeed ill, but that they are not ill with Lyme disease, but with "some other" disease. Dr. Steere did not identify then, and has yet to identify what that "other" disease might be. From the content of this book we may be able to guess what that answer might be. Dr. Steere's colleagues and Lyme disease guidelines co-authors Drs. Gary Wormser and Raymond Dattwyler have each disclosed that they have been paid speakers for Pfizer. Dr. John J. Halperin another co-author, was a paid expert witness for Glaxo SmithKline's Lyme disease vaccine. Dr. Steere was instrumental in the FDA approval of the Lyme vaccine, and he appeared before the committee as a vaccine manufacturer representative. He also ran clinical trials for the vaccine and has disclosed that he has received consulting fees from pharmaceutical company Baxter.[51,54-56]

Baxter is assignee on Lyme vaccine patents including a 1992 patent. Dr. Benjamin Luft, also a 2000 IDSA Lyme disease guidelines co-author and recent speaker at the Washington, DC hearing with Dr. Steere, has received grants from Abbott Laboratories. Dr. Luft was on the speaker's bureau of Roche and Abbott Labs; and has reported to be a stockholder in Brook Biotechnology. These firms directly or indirectly have ties with B.t.-containing products and/or with *Borrelia burgdorferi*-related tools or its history. With the main characters of the Lyme disease controversy potentially aligned with agrochemical, pharmaceutical, and/or biotech firms, it is easy to see how conflicts of interest, should they exist, might prevent scientists from revealing all that they know about an illness; especially where profits or research dollars may be involved or affected by the point of view adopted.[57,58]

Brook Biotechnology may in fact be Stony Brook Biotechnology LLC, which was founded in 2004 to develop and commercialize a diagnostic test based on proprietary biomarkers that were discovered by scientists at Stony Brook University. The company is heavily funded by the NIH and the NIAID branches of the US government. Dr. Benjamin Luft is Professor of Medicine at Stony Book University Medical Center, where a team of researchers report that they have determined the "genetic blueprint" of thirteen strains of the bacteria that causes Lyme disease. Are those strains related to thirteen strains of B.t. that are used in global insecticides? While there are hundreds of strains of B.t. available, up until 1977, only thirteen B.t. strains had been described. These thirteen strains were toxic only to certain species of lepidoptera. If we consider that the Bb agent may be an aggregate bacterium, we can see that it is possible that it may contain a B.t. insecticidal bacteria.[59,60]

One of the largest companies to produce insecticidal products is the Monsanto Company. Sources indicate that Monsanto and G.D. Searle merged in 2000 with Pharmacia & Upjohn to create the Pharmacia Corporation. In 2002, Pharmacia completed the spin-off of its agricultural subsidiary, which became the new Monsanto Company and focused on agricultural products. Pfizer reportedly acquired Pharmacia in 2003. Pfizer's Global R&D laboratory in St. Louis, Missouri reports that it concentrates on arthritis, osteoarthritis, and inflammatory pain research. These are conditions that are associated with "chronic" Lyme disease, a manifestation that Dr. Allen Steere and others seem to repeatedly claim "does not exist." In 2009, Monsanto announced that it was purchasing the Chesterfield Village Research Center from Pfizer in Chesterfield, Missouri, as the company increases its robust pipeline to reach its goal of doubling crop yields by 2030.[61,62]

It should not be surprising to find a few Lyme disease guidelines co-authors who have declared to be, or have otherwise been paid speakers for Pfizer, SmithKline, Novartis, Abbott, or other pharmaceutical firms with agricultural "interests." And it is no stretch of the imagination to consider perhaps why some infectious disease researchers might insist that Lyme disease is an "autoimmune disease." It may be easy to conclude why paid speakers might claim that Lyme patients are sick with "something else" that is not Lyme disease; especially if some of the companies that employ or have employed them are studying "autoimmune" diseases or hold interests in products that may contribute to Lyme or other important disease states.

Scientists are not content designing B.t. applications for the exterior of ornamentals and food crops; they now pursue the genetic engineering of plants that can grow with the B.t. pesticidal toxins already inside the plant. This saves the costs and effort associated with the physical application of pesticides; and reduces non-point source pollution. *Transgenic* (transplanted gene) crops have been genetically altered to contain foreign DNA and/or RNA, and to produce a desired insecticidal effect within the plant. These effects may include pesticide, antibiotic, and/or insect resistance. B.t. toxins are genetically engineered into various food crops, including plants such as tobacco, potatoes, tomatoes, corn, soy, rice, or cotton; with wheat as the "next" crop to be targeted.[63-69]

B.t. endotoxin genes may also be introduced externally into plants through a variety of methods including *electroporation.* This is the process of running an electric current through plant cell membranes to insert genes. Scientists might also apply microinjection techniques using a fine needle to inject DNA directly into cell lines that are used to cultivate GM plants. Another technique to introduce B.t. toxins into plants is by nanoparticle gun. A 0.22 caliber gun contains "bullets" with ultra-tiny metallic particles of silver or zinc oxide that are coated with DNA. The bullets are shot directly into plant tissues. About six hundred nanoparticle-containing products are currently on the market from food storage containers to computer peripherals. There appears to be absolutely no requirement for these products to be labeled as genetically modified, in case consumers wish to avoid them. Unfortunately there also does not appear to be any FDA or EPA regulations to ensure that adequate safety studies are performed before such products are made available for human use.[63-71]

The bad news is that laboratory studies have already shown that some nanoparticles are harmful to human lung tissue and to liver and brain cells of laboratory rats. Nanoparticles are also being targeted for delivery by vaccines and for cancer therapies. In 2006 the EPA began the process of regulating nanosilver under its Federal Insecticide, Fungicide, and Rodenticide Act. Currently companies that manufacture nanosilver particles must register them as a pesticide. Registration is a step in the right direction, but as long as safety studies or labeling requirements are missing, consumers have no way of knowing if the products they consume or use contain pesticides, nanoparticles, or anything else that may be proven later to be harmful.[63-71]

Another technique to engineer plants to confer viral resistance is by inserting recombinant viral coat proteins (capsid proteins or "CP") directly into the plants. In a process called *transfection,* a non-virulent viral protein coat or capsid is added to a plant's genome (DNA). Plants that have CP genes are more resistant to virus infections. Since CP-transfected crops have fewer protein binding sites in their host cells to which wild viruses may bind, viruses must be present in greater numbers in order for the disease-resistant plants to succumb to infections.[63-71]

The first experiments with CP genes were performed using the tobacco mosaic virus CP gene which was transfected into tobacco plants. Over time many crops have received transfected CP genes. Examples in alphabetical order of plants approved for CP gene field tests in the US from 1987 to mid-1995 include: alfalfa, barley, beets, cantaloupe, corn, cotton, cucumbers, lettuce, papaya, peanuts, plum trees, potatoes, rice, soybeans, sugarcane, squash, tobacco, and tomatoes. Researchers who performed experiments on these crops included those from the USDA, Monsanto, Frito-Lay, the New York Experiment Station, Cornell, and other universities in Florida, Hawaii, Idaho, Kentucky, Michigan, North Carolina, Oklahoma, and Oregon.[72-74]

Because of its global use, we must ask whether B.t. and other genetically engineered crops are safe for human consumption, and whether B.t. is truly safe for the environment. The answers may depend upon point of view. Manufacturers and the EPA say that genetically modified crops are safe, non-toxic, and non-allergenic. The contents of this book should help shed light on what goes onto and into our environment, and this information may make us reconsider such claims of safety when we realize that new human disease states are emerging along a similar timeline as the application of chemical and microbial agricultural products.

Pioneer Hi-Bred International, Inc. (Johnson, Iowa) is assignee to several patents for B.t. toxin receptors and methods of use. In general the patents are designed to allow the manipulation of B.t. Cry 1A (crystal or Cry) toxins in genetically modified corn crops, to provide resistance against lepidoptera. B.t. Cry proteins are said only to affect certain insects with specific receptors in their bodies. There have been some limited studies but these appear inadequate to definitively prove overall safety for B.t. as an insecticide upon crops for human consumption. Documents exist which indicate that B.t. is perhaps not as safe as some manufacturers, agencies, lobbyists, or even researchers might like us to believe.[75-78]

From the standpoint of the manufacturers, B.t. is supposed to augment crops so farmers can profit from higher yields. The use of B.t. cry genes reduces the amount of pesticides required, which would theoretically be beneficial to harmless insect populations. B.t. also reduces fungal toxins such as *fumonisin,* which is kidney and liver toxic to animals. Some species of insects are already showing resistance to B.t. in the laboratory including the Colorado potato beetle, the tobacco budworm, and certain moths. Some registered patents discuss how B.t. toxins are used in combination with pesticide genes. The Flavr Savr® tomato (Calgene-1994), Zeneca's tomato (1995), and Monsanto's (1996-2007) cotton, potatoes, and maize have reportedly all introduced B.t. toxins into plant genomes.[79-82]

Monsanto also created *Roundup Ready*® soybeans, canola (rapeseed) and cotton (1995-1996); all of which were genetically engineered to be resistant to the herbicide *glyphosate*. When fields are sprayed with herbicides that contain glyphosate, weeds die but the herbicide resistant crops do not. Glyphosate in commercial herbicides has been implicated in human diseases including hairy cell leukemia, Parkinson's, and Non-Hodgkins lymphoma. Case numbers for Non-Hodgkins lymphoma have reportedly increased nearly seventy-five percent in the US since 1974; the year glyphosate was first marketed. When I searched through US patents registered under various B.t. trade names, it became clear that the extent by which B.t. is used covers everything from terrestrial food and non-food crops (i.e. tobacco, cotton); aquatic and greenhouse foods and non-foods, forests, and even domestic indoor and outdoor stored products.[66,75-83]

As far as genetically engineering plants within the laboratory, B.t. toxins are isolated and inserted into a plasmid vector, which is a double-stranded DNA-carrying molecule capable of entering and replicating inside of a host plant's cells. The vector also contains a gene promoter which enables the construct to activate gene expression within the plant. The vector, now called a "recombinant DNA molecule" is inserted into host plant cells where it replicates. An antibiotic marker allows selection in the lab of only the cells that have successfully taken up the transferred genes (transgene plasmid). These markers sometimes use organisms that fluoresce (glow) under UV light. The cells that survive the genetic engineering process contain B.t. toxins and antibiotic resistance genes. The cells can then be used to culture plants. This is where the name "transgenic plants" is derived, since they now carry transferred, foreign genes.

The safety of GM crops and animals has been hotly debated for some time. As far as GM food crops go, problems can occur in plants that use modified viruses and other pathogens. When a plant is naturally invaded by a virus that is superinfected with another virus, the invading virus becomes enclosed in a protein coat that belongs to the initial virus, in a process called *transencapsidation.* This alters the host/vector relationship between plant viruses and plant. It may also affect the insects that feed upon the infected plants, and may continue to affect the insects, animals, or humans that feed upon, or are bitten or stung by the mixed infection and altered gene-carrying insects.[84]

There seems also to be a very real risk that a transgenic virus may infect other plants and create a new infection within unintended plants or their insect vectors. There is already a well known problem with transgenic seeds blowing into non-GM farmlands, and which contaminates the non-GM crops; causing problems for innocent farmers. Farmers have been held responsible for patent "infringements" even when innocent, simply because GM seeds accidentally blew into their fields. As a result, some have paid heavy fines and have lost their entire crops or farms as a result of such unwelcomed invasions by GM crops upon non-GM fields.

Plants that contain engineered viruses can also cause an insect to become a carrier for a new virus that does not normally affect that insect. Such viruses may be passed onto animals through ingestion or vectorization. Some scientists believe this process occurs no more frequently with a lab-created virus than it does for natural plants; but others categorically disagree. Research has shown that transgenic DNA is far more likely to transfer horizontally to other species than non-transgenic DNA. Horizontal gene transfers occur between two genetically unrelated cells, or two unrelated species, in a manner other than sexual reproduction. Evidence of the ability of transgenes to cross species barriers is surfacing more frequently in scientific literature over time.[67]

Under normal circumstances, natural transgenes from a different species which accidentally enter a cell are quickly degraded and destroyed. However, sometimes this material is not completely broken down and it simply becomes part of the host genome. This happens in nature quite often with viruses, but more typically in the laboratory with man-made genetic constructs. Situations such as heat shock (stress), heavy metals, and other pollutants can also interfere with natural foreign DNA degradation. Genetically engineered DNA however, is designed to specifically transfer its DNA into cells and genomes as a deliberate vector of horizontal gene transfer. These chimeras (genetic constructs) often contain more than one set of altered genes, and special signals to facilitate gene transfer between species. This allows the chimera to overcome species barriers that natural chimera are unable to overcome.[85]

Once inserted into the genome of cells, foreign genes become permanent fixtures. Sometimes it alters cellular function and turns off natural processes that would otherwise auto-kill mutated cells. This can lead to the creation of *immortal* cells, or cells that will not naturally die at the end of their replication processes. This is one way that cancerous cells may be formed. Other problems that arise with recombinant constructs are protein folding errors. When this occurs, the result may be a "prion" disease. The reactivation of dormant or latent viruses already present in the body or those which may appear at a later point in time may also occur. The more foreign agents in the body, the greater the chance of reactivating an infection, causing a mutation, activating virus oncogenes, or forming a new, *host-derived aggregate organism* that causes an active disease state.[85]

Genetically engineered crops have incorporated viral protein coats and antisense RNA (which blocks the translation of genes). These genes may confer resistance to fungi or include late-stage genes that allow plants to grow to seed, but which will produce sterile seeds (i.e. "terminator" technology). Examples of plants that have been genetically altered to carry antisense RNA genes are the proprietary GM tobacco, tomatoes, corn, and soybeans. This technology allows agricultural companies to patent seed technologies. If the public allows companies to monopolize our seeds and grains, in time the lack of diversification of food crops will dwindle to one or two or ten types. Limiting food choices to such a narrow field contributes to famines around the globe – especially if or when diseases arise in the remaining crops and there are no alternative crops left to eat. Common sense encourages us to push for continued diversity, although multinational companies promote standardization and profits.[87]

The literature reveals that *the presence of antibiotics within genetic constructs increases the frequency of horizontal gene transfers ten thousand-fold.* This raises the stakes in terms of "accidental" diseases, and makes them harder to treat because of antibiotic resistance. If we include GM plant, animal, and insect genes, the presence of foreign DNA in the body may potentially lead to novel genetic mutants, especially under influence of long-term antibiotic treatments. Microbial insecticides or mixed infections from vectoring insects may lead to chronic disease states that cannot be cured without the invention of new antibiotics. When infectious disease guidelines frown upon the use of long-term antibiotics to treat infections such as Lyme, we must consider the possible underlying reasons behind such recommendations. Perhaps one concern is of preventing accidental horizontal gene transfers of lab-created viral constructs from biological controls now present in the infected individual; and any gene transfers that might occur during the long-term use of antibiotics.[86,87]

Concerns over the safety of transgenic crops and other products have fueled anti-GM food and GMO (genetically modified organism) campaigns around the world. In California in 2004, three counties banned the production of GM crops (the first state in the US to do so). This was done partly in response to anti-GM food consumer groups, and because transgenic crops have been shown to contaminate non-transgenic crops that are grown for animal and human consumption. Genes from transgenic crops can be transferred by insects, wind, or by sporulating soil bacteriae.[88-95]

In North America there currently are no food labeling requirements for GM foods, although other countries require labeling. Countries around the world have also banned imports of, or the growth of GM foods or agricultural fiber crops including in Australia, Austria, Bulgaria, Croatia, France, Germany, Greece, Hungary, India, Japan, New Zealand, Pakistan, Poland, Romania, and Wales.[89-95]

Since about 1990 genetically engineered baculoviruses have been used in various cell lines for vaccines and other processes. Beginning in 1951, New Haven scientists released borrelina viruses in Connecticut and provided samples and instructions for other interested parties. These viruses associate with baculoviruses, and they were exploited for insecticidal use because together they are far more virulent. Baculoviruses have been applied even earlier, beginning around the turn of the 20th century through various attempts at field inoculations using dessicated, diseased insects. Two centuries ago the applications of fungi in the environment enabled natural insect viruses to cause infectious disease outbreaks, especially in areas where industrial chemicals assisted their mutation. Less than a decade ago, scientists learned that *baculoviruses in the presence of a suitable promoter including B.t. can transduce, or change mammalian cells.* Scientists have exploited not only the baculoviruses *Heliothis zea* and *Autographa californica* viruses for agricultural insecticides, but also other viruses in combination with B.t., toxins, and enzymes. These applications have been useful in many formulas, including agricultural, industrial, and pharmaceutical products.[96-100]

We have established that B.t. can alter cells. Novel combinations of viral, fungal, and bacterial genes are not only applied agriculturally, but are engineered into foods and medicines. What happens if B.t. interacts in an unexpected manner with human cell receptors, causing us to express unintended enzymes, proteins, or toxins that will manifest as new epidemics or so-called "autoimmune" states? What happens if B.t. becomes a catalyst for other organisms that gain entry or are already present within the human body? What happens if the microbes of biological controls, vaccines, antibiotics, or foods trigger latent infections in our bodies, or cause other unexpected recombinant events? The answers are that scientists have no idea to what extent genetic engineering techniques may fail, while the non-target species are left to fend for themselves. As members of the public affected by scientific processes and the diseases they may cause, we have a right to know the truth about the inhabitants of this planet that are far smaller than ourselves. We also have a right to know who is manipulating which organisms and why. We already have the right and responsibility to decide whether we wish to allow such manipulations to continue largely unregulated and/or unchallenged; the only problem is how soon, and to what extent will we be willing to do so?

The effects upon the human species of genetically engineered crops with herbicide and insect-resistance genes cannot be determined before these foodstuffs or insect controls are introduced into animal or human environments. The diseases of present and future generations that may surface once genetic constructs and agricultural tools are deployed remain unpredictable. We cannot simply assume that bioengineered foods are automatically "safe" just because those who eat them are not dropping immediately dead like so many targeted insects.

Brucellosis

A little while ago I mentioned that B.t. isolates have been registered with the EPA based upon the differences in antigen serotypes that are found on the flagellum of the various organisms. The discovery that flagellum are different allowed individual toxic proteins (endotoxins) to be identified and subclassified. Now highly specific B.t. toxins are formulated to exert a toxic action upon individual insect species. What is interesting is that Lyme notable Dr. Alan Barbour is listed as inventor on a *Borrelia burgdorferi* patent for a "flagella-less" *Borrelia burgdorferi* diagnostic test. Some of Dr. Barbour's other patents seem to hint at connections between Bb, *Pseudomonas aeruginosa* (another recombinant tool), and the soil bacteria *Leptospires.*[1-5]

A 1993 patent filed under an NIH grant by Barbour et al. is assigned to the University of Texas System in Austin. The patent describes recombinant vaccines and diagnostic tests for many Bb strains. Among the flagella-less strains of *Borrelia* considered useful for the invention are *Borrelia coriaceae,* the putative agent of epidemic bovine abortion; *Borrelia anserina,* an avian spirochete; and relapsing fever spirochetes. These borrelia strains are said not to be closely related to Bb according to the experts, however they serve as useful models since they may be more related than we are told.[1-5]

Brucellae abortus is an important livestock disease of cattle, particularly in California. If we peek at the past history of the agent of bovine abortion to which the Barbour et al. patent refers, we find that a tick-amplified *brucellosis* may be at the heart of a leptospira/brucellae aggregate spirochete that causes epidemic bovine abortions (EBA). This spirochete was named *Borrelia coriaceae,* which means "tick-transmitted" (borrelia) and "coriaceus" from the *Ornithodoros coriaceus* soft-bodied tick from which the agent was isolated in 1985. Brucellosis is also infectious to humans. We can see how a tick-transmitted brucellosis/leptospiral aggregate (a mutant, or intermediate leptospira form) might be named *Borellia coriacei.*[6-18]

There are also clues that the EBA agent may have genetic sequences that are very similar to the *Borrelia burgdorferi* strain "CA4." Perhaps a cattle-derived brucellosis plays a role in the overall picture of some Lyme disease infections. Perhaps this is why some Lyme patients test positive for *Brucellosis* – because an animal infection that is transmitted by ticks plays a role in an aggregate organism for some Bb strains. Remember that cows and other livestock eat B.t.-containing grains or are treated with B.t. insecticides. The brucellosis agent is an intracellular infection that hides inside of phagocytes* such as *macrophages* in cows and humans; and like the Bb spirochete, has circular plasmids. Dr. Barbour's "flagella-less" patents refer to scientific articles which discuss the flagellum of *leptospires,* another infection of ruminant livestock and other animals. This is another clue that Bb strains may include a leptospira spirochete as an aggregate organism.[1,5-11,16,19-54]

**Phagocytes are white blood cells that protect the body by eliminating foreign proteins and dead or decaying cells. Macrophages are large white blood cells that destroy foreign invaders and stimulate the production of lymphocytes, other cells important to immune function and disease resistance.*

Like the Bb agent, the *Brucellae abortus* agent causes symptoms similar to Lyme disease including weight loss, fever chills, headaches, backaches, and fatigue. Treatments include the antibiotics doxycycline and rifampin in combination. This is a combination that is increasingly used to treat Lyme disease. During early acute Lyme infection, the immune response is to infiltrate the ECM rash lesion with macrophages and neutrophils. Perhaps this is the point at which a brucella-containing Bb spirochete infects macrophages, which go on to infect the rest of the body. If so, then it may appear that a useful antibiotic therapy during early acute infections that contain a brucellosis component might include a doxycycline/rifampin combination to eradicate intra- and extracellular pathogens before they spread throughout the body.**[6-18,55]

***Statements about the use of doxycycline and rifampin are simply commentary on the use of these drugs based upon what is stated within the literature. It is not a medical recommendation for treating any disease.*

We may use a similar rationale to analyze the *Borrelia anserina* strain from the flagella-less patent described previously. In an older medical dictionary I learned that *Spiroschaudinnia audinnia* is the agent of avian spirochetosis or bird septicemia. *Spiroschaudinnia* means "relapsing" and "anserina" refers to geese or goose, which are the birds from which the *Borrelia anserina* spirochetes were first isolated by Sakharov in 1891. *Borrelia anserina* is a tickborne relapsing fever of geese. Likewise we find *Spiroschaudinnia recurrentis*, which has been renamed *Borrelia recurrentis,* the tickborne agent of human relapsing fever. These relapsing fevers however are not the same infections caused by the Lyme disease agent, *Borrelia burgdorferi.* But they appear to be distantly related, more so than the spirochetes of Syphilis called *Treponema pallidum.*[6,8-11,19]

Many references discuss the difference between relapsing fever spirochetes and the spirochetes of Lyme disease. Even the Barbour patent for flagella-less strains says this:

> "Many present immunoassays use whole spirochetes or a crude sonicate of the cells. However, those assays suffer from complications resulting from cross-reactions with *other spirochetes, especially Treponema pallidum and the relapsing fever Borrelia species.* (Magnarelli and Anderson, 1988)..."[4]

Later the patent again shows there are differences between Bb spirochetes and those of relapsing fevers:

> "Accordingly, with the aid of the present disclosure, *flagella-less mutants* of other Borrelia species, e.g., *B. coriacei,* which causes epidemic bovine abortion, *B. anserina,* which causes avian spirochetosis, and *B. recurrentis* and other Borrelia species causative of relapsing fever, such as *Borrelia hermsii, Borrelia turicatae, Borrelia duttoni, Borrelia persica,* and *Borrelia hispanica,* can be prepared and used in accordance with the present invention...."[4]

Perhaps the reason Dr. Barbour et al. created a flagella-less diagnostic test under this method (and a vaccine tool), is because not only is the test useful to detect "Lyme disease" in patients, it is useful precisely because the test can detect infections that are first and foremost, derived from animals. These animals typically harbor the non-mutated spirochetes of relapsing fever and other infections, which are cross-reactive. The patent nearly acknowledges that Bb spirochetes are mutations of these agents. The terms "epidemic bovine abortion" and "avian spirochetosis" are used within patents in place of mentioning the ticks which transmit these infections – namely the *Argasidae* (soft ticks) and the *Ixodidae* (hard ticks). These are ticks which also transmit Lyme disease and relapsing feveres. Lyme disease is different from the relapsing fevers, but perhaps only because it is a mutated, aggregate organism whose genes were partly derived from relapsing fever agents.[4]

Remember that bovine abortions can be caused by the common cattle disease, *brucellosis.* What if infections that contain this agent can lead to miscarriages in pregnant human patients? Women who have difficulty carrying to term might consider asking to be screened for *brucellosis* and Lyme infections. The brucellosis agent is transmissible from contaminated meats to humans.

Brucellosis was also a biological warfare weapon that was tested in open air experiments on military ranges (until 1969) since it could be aerosolized. A Harvard paper reveals that the antibiotic *Moenomycin A* is the only known natural antibiotic to inhibit this agent through a specific enzyme-binding process.[4,12-15]

What I also found interesting from several Barbour et al. patents are comments about the *time frame required to successfully culture Bb spirochetes within a laboratory*, as well as the expense and difficulty isolating Bb from patient cultures. The patents describe a far longer time frame for culturing the Bb spirochete than what is achieved by "standardized" CDC-recommended diagnostic tests. Perhaps this is one reason why so many patients test "negative" for Lyme disease – simply because cultures are not grown long enough for the organisms to be *properly* detected. According to the patents:

> "Recovery of *Borrelia burgdorferi* from patients is possible and should be considered diagnostic. However, the medium is expensive to keep stocked, *cultures require up to 4 weeks of incubation for routine detection of spirochetes*, and the frequency of isolating bacteria from the blood of acutely ill patients is less than 30%. Consequently, cultivation for *B. burgdorferi* is only done in a few institutions." Fortunately for patients, new tests are on the horizon to improve detection even in seronegative patients who display Lyme symptoms.[4,56,57]

It is clear from the research so far, that the links between the globally applied agricultural tool *Bacillus thuringiensis* (B.t.), and the agent of Lyme disease are tightening. In order to explore further the possibility that the "Bb" agent might have come about from the industrial and agricultural tools of the last century and a half, let's examine the kinds of catalysts that had the potential to bring about what is perhaps the most mysterious organism in infectious disease world history.

Pleuropneumonias and Animal Feeds

In 1898, scientists Nocard and Roux cultivated a livestock disease agent that was widespread among cattle. The agent was named *Contagious Bovine Pleuro Pneumonia* (CBPP). Pleuropneumonia was a huge problem by the end of the 19th century, and one outbreak caused the British to impose a trade embargo. No cattle or their products were allowed to be exported to Great Britain or Canada. As a result the USDA established the Bureau of Animal Industry in 1884. The agency combined the powers of the Treasury Cattle Commission and the veterinary division of the USDA. The duties of the new agency were to conduct scientific investigations; enforce regulations to eradicate livestock diseases and improve herd quality; and to protect the public from the receipt of infected (diseased) livestock products. The agency was abolished in 1953, when the Agricultural Research Service (ARS) was established.[1]

Pleuropneumonia is caused by the bacteria *Mycoplasma mycoides mycoides.* This is a member of the *Mollicute* class. Mycoplasmas affect warm-blooded animals and can become airborne or be transmitted many ways including by infected meat products or milk. It is interesting that in March of 1968, US military scientists from Fort Detrick in cooperation with the Illinois Institute of Technology (IIT) in Chicago, Illinois held Fort Detrick's Second International Conference on Aerobiology. Aerobiology is the study of inhaled pathogens and pollutants.[2-4]

Conference papers from the event discussed the military's progress with aerosolized biowarfare agents including tularemia (rabbit fever), Venezuelan equine encephalitis (flavivirus), Rocky Mountain spotted fever, yellow fever, and experimental coccidioidomycosis (San Joaquin valley fever). The latter is an infectious fungus that was already prevalent in the US and known to have contaminated military bases in the southwest. Each of these agents is tick-transmissible; and yellow fever is particularly interesting since it appears to involve not only a mosquito-borne flavivirus, but also a leptospira spirochete. If we use these studies as a model, we may imagine a Lyme disease organism that contains a degraded reovirus, a bacterium, a fungus, a rickettsia, and a leptospira spirochete. We may find later that these studies may have been related to an epidemic that was already smoldering in the Midwest and on the US east coast, although it was not yet known to the public.[1,3,4]

Mollicutes are slow-growing bacterial infections that are transmissible to humans by vectoring insects including flies, fleas, mites, mosquitoes, and ticks. Mycoplasmas were called pleuropneumonia-like organisms, or wall-less bacterial L-forms, until 1962 when a new human infecting strain *Mycoplasma pneumoniae* was first isolated. It is now known that mycoplasmas cause arthritis in animals, and acute and chronic disease in human joints, lungs, and the genitourinary tract. There are nearly 200 kinds of arthritis including mycoplasma arthritis, which are connective tissue infections. Rheumatoid arthritis was once called chronic infectious arthritis, although it is now called "autoimmune" disease or collagen vascular disease. Mycoplasmas are capable of causing a wide range of symptoms depending upon which part of the body they infect. For example in one person you may find juvenile arthritis, in another systemic lupus erythematosus (SLE); and in another, inflammation or cardiac issues.[5]

Mycoplasmas are both parasitic and saprophytic, and they are *pleomorphic* which means they assume many forms. Because these agents lack a cell wall, they are able to bind with host cells and exchange genetic information; setting the stage for an "autoimmune" disease. Mycoplasmas also suppress the host immune response, especially peripheral T-cells. In animals the attachment of mycoplasmas to nerves, lymph vessels, and blood cells is thought to be responsible for plaque formation and impaired circulation. This can lead to a restriction in milk flow in animals; and in plants, capillary fluids which causes "wilt" diseases. The latter may also be caused by the related *citroplasma.* The mycoplasmas can remain attached to host tissues and remain dormant for months, or be transmitted in utero without activity until a later date where the infection activates.[5]

Treatment with doxycycline produces a *herxheimer* effect. Scientific papers reveal that mycoplasmas are "frequently" transmitted among families. Although arthritis is not usually considered to be contagious, all family members should be considered for treatment if one or both parents are mycoplasma-infected. Females are usually more heavily and more frequently infected than males. Minocycline was considered an effective therapy for Rheumatoid Arthritis, another name for mycoplasma-caused arthritis according to some papers. What is interesting is that a paper suggests the use of oral and intravenous antibiotics. Lyme patients are commonly prescribed both doxycycline and minocycline, since many Lyme patients have mycoplasma "co-infections."[5]

A scientific paper described various mycoplasma species. I list them with the host from where the isolations were made.

Mycoplasma pneumonia	Human
Mycoplasma hominis	Human
Mycoplasma fermentans	Human
*Mycoplasma gallisepticum**	Bird
Mycoplasma iowae	Bird
Mycoplasma pulmonis	Rodent
Mycoplasma muris	Rodent
Mycoplasma arthritidis	Rodent
Mycoplasma neurolyticum	Rodent
Mycoplasma bovigenitalium	Cow
Mycoplasma californicum	Cow
Mycoplasma mycoides	Cow, Goat
Mycoplasma agalactiae	Goat
Mycoplasma capricolum	Goat
Mycoplasma putrefaciens	Goat
Mycoplasma sualvi	Swine
Mycoplasma hyopneumoniae	Swine
Mycoplasma hyorhinis	Swine
Mycoplasma ellychniae	Insect (firefly beetle)[6]

**Mycoplasma gallisepticum was used in sulfonate fungicides (herbicides).*[101]

A US Patent assigned to E.R. Squibb & Sons, Inc. (Princeton, NJ) describes the use of antibiotics to inhibit mycoplasma growth in livestock animals with mastitis infections. The patent is designed to be used in animals with the following infections:[7]

Mycoplasma hyorhinis (swine upper respiratory infections)
M. hyopneumoniae (chronic pneumonia in swine)
M gallisepticum (chronic respiratory disease in poultry)
M. synoviae (infectious synovitis and air sacculitis of chickens)
M. meleagridis (skeletal lesions in turkeys)
M. agalactiae (mastitis in sheep, cattle, goats)
M. bovigenitalium (contagious pleuropneumonia in goats)
M. mycoides v. mycoides (contagious bovine pleuropneumonia)
Mycoplasma species which cause *Endometriosis* in cattle, sheep, and goats

A 1989 paper classified mycoplasmas into six distinct groups. These groups include the hominis group (*M. hominis, M. lipophilum, M. pulmonis, M. sualvi,* and *M. neurolyticum*); a pneumoniae group (*M. pneumoniae, M. muris*); a *Spiroplasma* group (*Mycoplasma mycoides, Spiroplasma citri* (citrus pest), *Spiroplasma apis* (bee pest); and *Spiroplasma strain Y-32** (blood-feeding insects). There is the *Anaeroplasma* group which includes *Anaeroplasmas* and *Acholeplasmas*. There is also a group that has the single *Asteroleplasma anaerobium;* and a group that contains gram-positive walled relatives including *Clostridia, Lactobacilli, Streptococcus pleomorphus,* and *Erysipelothrix rhusiopathiae.* There are many mycoplasmas that affect livestock animals and humans. Some of the better known strains include *Mycoplasma hyopneumoniae, M. hyorhinis, M. californicum, M. fermentens,* and *M. arthritidis.* Some of these infections are being discovered in patients who suffer from Lyme disease, HIV/AIDS and illnesses of "unknown cause."[8,9]

**Spiroplasma Y-32 strain was isolated from western black-legged ticks Ixodes pacificus collected in Oregon in 1981 and again in 1995. A 1981 paper indicated that Y-32 could be isolated from tick cell cultures. This may be a clue that certain insect cell lines were found to be* *contaminated with tick spiroplasmas/mycoplasmas. Spiroplasmas are helical spirochetes, one of the forms that Bb, the spirochete of Lyme disease most commonly assumes.*

Mollicute infections are frequent among livestock animals including poultry, cattle, sheep, and pigs. Each of these animals has been subjected to feed supplements, fungicides, larvicides, miticides; as well as hormones and vaccines for many decades. They have also been treated with pesticides whether by organophosphate dips; or by powders, sprays, implantable devices, feed supplements, or fodder that contains B.t. or chemicals. Livestock have also been used to create human vaccines, products, and cell lines. We can see many routes by which animal pathogens migrate into the human population. Animal pathogens are also transmissible through vectoring insects infected with agricultural chemicals and microbes; by human vaccines or medical products made with contaminated cell lines; or contaminated foods and animal products (meat, dairy, eggs, gelatins, tallow/lard, etc.).[10]

One of the most important individuals to the history of Lyme disease and its recombinant patents, Dr. Alan Barbour, is assignee to many *Borrelia burgdorferi*-related patents, and works in the University of Texas and University of California systems. In 1994, Dr. Barbour also attended the Dearborn Conference, a key event to the history of Lyme disease public health. We must not overlook important details such as the establishment of the CDC surveillance case definitions; and the standardization of laboratory testing for human patients with Lyme disease. Besides establishing test criteria, this event would significantly impact the emergence of a novel human vaccine that was meant to prevent Lyme disease in the human population. What if an animal pathogen (i.e. a tick spiroplasma/leptonema) influenced how the guidelines were established at Dearborn? If it did, then we might find clues within patent inventions and other events of the day when examined closely.

If infectious diseases were emerging from the use of contaminated animal or insect cell lines, then the ramifications of this news could have been too great for "those in the know" to reveal to the public. We might expect to see covert experiments, media silencing, and public health efforts to control the information flow about a globally emerging human epidemic. We might also expect laboratory tests to be standardized so specific populations of infected patients might be "overlooked" during testing to keep reported case numbers low. We might even find certain public health experts working overtime to silence public discussions of a disease epidemic that has an untoward relationship to globally important agricultural tools.

Remember that insect cell lines were recombinantly engineered for use as applied biological controls to target insects. The cell lines that were created from infected insects established the most powerful and globally applied biological insecticides in existence. These insecticides were used within animal feeds, were applied to forests, industrial products, were sprayed agriculturally, applied to animals, and genetically engineered into foods and textile crops. Scientists may also have used contaminated cell lines to create "deleterious genes" which were placed into mosquitoes or other insects as population replacers. Insect cell lines are used to create animal vaccines, and for human products. If the cell lines that were being used for insecticides or other products were contaminated with agents that cause disease, then any products made with them could transmit infections into the finished products.

Despite the perspective of some people, this next patent does *not* describe the creation of a biowarfare tool that is useful against people. It does reveal however that *Mycoplasmas* and *Mycoplasma-like organisms* (including *spiroplasmas*) of many different strains may be partly responsible for diseases of our day including Lyme, HIV/AIDS, Fibromyalgia, CFS/ME, Wegener's disease, Sarcoidosis, Respiratory Distress Syndrome, or "autoimmune" diseases such as Lupus, Arthritis, and Alzheimer's. According to the patent invention, *Mycoplasma fermentens incognitus* may be either a causative agent or a key co-factor in the diseases mentioned. While a recombinant mycoplasma strain may have been created, experiments with this agent could have been geared toward the strain's usefulness to a human vaccine, not as a biowarfare weapon. Mycoplasmas with other strain names are often found in patients who have chronic infections, including Gulf War Syndrome, Endometriosis, Rheumatoid Arthritis, Lyme disease, and other illnesses. Not all Lyme patients test positive for *Mycoplasma fermentens,* but they may test positive for other mycoplasma species, such as *Mycoplasma pneumonia.* Again the mycoplasma and mycoplasma-like infections (MLOs) are incredibly common *livestock* pathogens, and they may also become airborne, to be inhaled by animals or humans.[11,12]

Animals and plants may be the origin of most human mycoplasma infections, but then again so might vaccines. For example a Merck assigned 1969 patent for a mycoplasma vaccine uses *Mycoplasma pneumonia,* or many other insect, animal, or plant mycoplasma strains (i.e. *M. hominis, M. arthritidis, M. bovigenitalium, M. fermentens*). The invention describes the reduction or removal from calf serum of an anaphylactic factor. The invention appears to describe mycoplasma strains useful within animal or human vaccines to make them more immune-friendly and less able to provoke allergic reactions. We have no way of knowing how many human vaccines use or may be contaminated by mycoplasmas. Either could explain why immunized people around the world test positive for various mycoplasma strains. It is already known that a number of important human diseases of our day have mycoplasma strains as part of their infective process (Lyme, Gulf War Symdrome, HIV/AIDS). We may want to consider whether animal and human vaccines have unwittingly exposed generations of people to "harmless" disease agents that in the end, may prove to be anything but.[11,12]

What is curious is that the agent of bovine pleuropneumonia used to be called *Asterococcus mycoides* before it underwent a name change. Asterococci are algae that are either planktonic or benthic in freshwater (found at lowest levels). They have flagella, they form vegetative cells, and they sporulate (create spores). If there is a bovine pneumonia that is caused by exposure to dirty water which contains algae, we can see how aerosolized spores may be passed to other animals or humans. If animal meats or milk are contaminated, or these agents are found in animal and/or human vaccines, we can see where some infections might originate. If food supplements fed to livestock animals are contaminated with plant-based mycoplasmas or their related phytoplasmas or even algae, we can see how easily animals can become infected with an agent to cause bovine pleuropneumonia. We can also understand how the presence of mycoplasmas and mycoplasma-like infections will complicate treatment in human diseases such as Lyme or HIV/AIDS.[13,14]

Something called *Ionophores* are used in the laboratory and in animal feeds as antibiotics and growth enhancers (i.e. poultry, swine, and cattle). Ionophores help penetrate plant membranes to form new ion channels or pores (holes). A similar process occurs at the hands of several bacterial species, to gain access to plant tissues or insect gut membranes. It is for this ability that B.t. toxins are utilized as insecticides. *Rumensin* (monensin sodium) is a well-known natural ionophore antibiotic that is used in the dairy industry to increase milk yield and feed efficiency, and to prevent acidosis. Rumensin is produced by the bacterial strain *Streptomyces cinnamonensis,* and it is fed to the cattle in the form of a sodium salt. (Acidosis occurs in animals fed a diet too high in mycotoxins, corn silage, or other highly fermented feedstuffs, and is common in feedlot animals.)[15,16]

The food company *Tyson* has reportedly used ionophores in their factory-farmed chickens. The USDA required the company to remove labeling that claimed its chickens were raised "without antibiotics" even after the labeling had been approved by the agency. The agency may have misunderstood the purpose of ionophores, which technically falls under the classification of antibiotics. Once the error was realized, labeling requirements were updated. In the European Union the use of ionophores was to be entirely banned by January 1, 2006. This occurred because a relationship was shown to exist between the use of *avoparcin*, an ionophore used as a growth enhancer in livestock feed, and the development of vancomycin antibiotic resistance in animals fed the substance.[17-20]

In the US, food animals are still fed ionophore-containing feeds. Ionophores were originally used to prevent *coccidiosis* infections in livestock. Coccidia are single-celled, spore-forming protozoan parasites that infect the intestinal tracts of mammals. One example is *Cryptosporidia,* a common infection in cattle which can also be a water-borne human infection due to its presence in sewage. In 1993 in Milwaukee, Wisconsin, raw sewage made its way into municipal water and infected approximately a half million people with cryptosporidiosis. Cryptosporidiosis is an important parasite in immune compromised patients. Other examples of coccidia are *sarcocystis* infections of horses, dogs, or cats; and *toxoplasmosis* infections in cats, fish, reptiles, or amphibians. (Either may infect humans.) During the late 1970s to 1980s, the CDC classified toxoplasmosis, cryptosporidiosis, and coccidioidomycosis infections among a group that today remains on the substantial list of immune-suppressing infections *that are considered to cause "AIDS."*[21,22]

The ionophores that are present in the environment as agricultural applications or feed supplements will come into contact with soil and water sources and the microbes that reside there, from animal wastes and agricultural run-off. Such applications may contribute to the ability of microbes to become more efficient human pathogens. The transmissible infections and infectious animal wastes from industrialized feedlots is important to think about since their wastes come into contact with insecticides, fungicides, the microbes of feed supplements, and the insects present in these environments.

Animal feed supplements and chemicals may expand the natural host range of infectious organisms; allowing an opportunity to enter the human system when we consume animal products. Feedlot cattle were routinely exposed to Dow ET-57 (trolene) or Co-Ral (Bayer 21/199) as a treatment for ticks, cattle grubs, lice, horn flies, and screwworms. The chemicals don't remain inert, but enter into food products that consumers eat, passively transferring chemical and microbial pesticides from animals into the human body. Poultry houses have used antibiotics, organophosphates, and other compounds (i.e. larvicides) to treat birds for insect infestations (i.e. house and soldier flies, mites, lice, ticks, screwworms). The chemicals diazinon, dipterex, Dow ET-57, trithion, malathion, kepone, calcium arsenate, baytex, phenothiazine, polybor, thiourea, naphthalene, and deodorized kerosene have all been used upon feedlot animals including poultry according to reports.[23-29]

Diseased feedlot animals that die are sometimes ground up and fed back to feedlot or other animals in an effort to dispose of carcasses. Animal wastes are routinely sold as fertilizers to be applied by spray upon agricultural fields. Industrial wastes since the late 1940s have also been used to irrigate and fertilize farm fields (i.e. tannery wastes). These disposals began during the 1860s when raw sewage wastes were disposed of in this manner. Fruit, vegetable, and fish cannery wastes have also been used as agricultural fertilizers over many decades.[30-33]

In 1978, the National Research Council's committee on animal nutrition convened a scientific task force to discover new sources of cost-effective feedstuffs for the livestock industry. Examples of industrial wastes that have been used or studied as animal feed supplements include: winery wastes, cacao (cocoa) processing wastes, fruit pit and nut shell wastes, animal by-products (i.e. diary whey, seafood, poultry), and red meat processing wastes. The group also considered the regulatory aspects and animal and human health issues including pesticide residues and heavy metals. In the non-food waste categories, reviewers examined the potential of organic chemicals, products from the fermentation industry, and municipal solid wastes. Forestry residues studied include whole and fractions of tree wastes, pulpmill and papermill residues, spent sulfite liquor, wood residues as roughage substitutes in ruminant diets, and even animal wastes. The group also studied pathogenic organisms and other harmful substances typically found in animal wastes. Crop residues from grain crops (i.e. corn, soybean, wheat, straw, sorghum, small grains) were also reviewed as potential food additives, as were aquatic plants including seaweed.[34,45-61]

Livestock experiments were undertaken whereby laying hens were fed B.t. spore powder to control house flies which emerge from their feces. The success of the agents in the experimentally fed hens was only studied for twenty months. The studies suggested that B.t. consumption had "no effect" on egg laying production. No testing appears to have been undertaken to determine the overall effects on the health of the hens beyond twenty months. And no studies appear to have been undertaken to determine the health effects upon persons who eat eggs or meats from B.t.-fed hens. Chicken embryos are infected with avian viruses or retroviruses that cannot be removed because they are part of a long line of vaccinated poultry stock. Therefore we should be concerned about feedlot animals that are treated with chemical and microbial insecticides, and what those applications may mean to the microbes living on and within the animals that will be passively transferred onto people who eat animal products.[35-37]

Scientists should have understood there could be a broad range of effects from microbial pesticide use in animals. Simply because the effects were inadequately studied does not mean that products were or are "safe." Studies from California indicated that by using a similar method of feeding B.t. to cattle, house flies could also be controlled in cattle manure. B.t. has also been used as an external powder to control lice on commercial chickens and other livestock. It was felt to be useful when applied externally to pets or humans to control fleas or ticks. From a patent, "...for example, the feeding or injection of livestock with biologically produced materials for controlling dipterous parasites. Similar treatment of pets for the control of fleas, or of human beings for fleas or ticks may be possible."[35-37]

A 1991-filed patent describes the use of spiroplasma enzymes in genetic engineering. According to the patent, which refers to a spiroplasma strain that was isolated from a Maryland potter wasp (*Monobia quadridens*) we learn that:

> "The Spiroplasma sp. strain MQ1 is a member of the Spiroplasmatacea family which belongs to the class Mollicutes of wall-less bacteria. This bacterium is a plant parasite which grows very slowly in culture and reaches a very low cell density (at confluency 10^8 cells/ml). Also the culture medium is relatively complex and expensive. There is, therefore, a commercial incentive to obtain strains of bacteria through recombinant DNA techniques that synthesize this methylase in abundance..."

The North American potter wasp is a vespid wasp found on the eastern seaboard of North America, in Canada, and in the midwest (Wisconsin, Illinois, Kansas) to New Mexico; and south into Mexico. The wasps live in old bees nests, and within plant stems. The wasps eat plant pollen and caterpillar larvae.[86]

Livestock feed additives have employed polymers and antibiotics in microbead-containing formulas. Patents from the 1950s forward describe how antibiotics from the *pleuromutilin* family were used within animal feed compositions to control *spiroplasma*, *mycoplasma,* and other infections in poultry, swine, sheep, or cattle. This means that these infections were known to appear in feed animals before the Lyme disease epidemic emerged in the human population. It also supports the idea that public health officials could have been tracking these infections within wild and livestock animals for many years. A number of other antibiotics have also been used to control these spirochetes, including nystatin, penicillins, streptomycin, and tetracycline. The widespread use of antibiotics in animal feed supplements has probably contributed to the rise of antibiotic resistant bacteria, fungi, and viruses; since the microbes which infect animals can mutate when exposed to antibiotics. We might want to note the antibiotics used to treat animal spiroplasma infections in case they might be useful in treating patients with tickborne infections that may contain a spiroplasma and/or mycoplasma component.[38-44,100]

Segmented polymers are used in nanotechnologies. It has been scientifically proven that *bacteria adhere to polymers.* For example this has been demonstrated with long-term urinary catheter polymers in the human body. Polymer blends directly impact the adhesion properties of bacteria including *E. coli, Proteus mirabilis*, and *Staphylococcus epidermidis*. We can assume this binding occurs with other bacterial species, including the leptospires found in wastewaters, or those of an aggregate Bb spirochete. If so, this could demonstrate that bacteria can introduce persisting pollutants into the human body, or similarly bind to pollutants that are stored in the skeletal structures, allowing them to persist.[93-96]

Proteins such as fibrinogen, fibronectin, serum albumin, and collagen are genetically engineered to coat synthetic materials to improve their biocompatibility, and to improve the ability to degrade in the human body. SELP and SLPF polymers are fibrous biodegradable polymers that are being used in medical devices such as sponges or dermal wound care wraps. SLPF is a silk-like protein polymer that can be synthesized by genetically engineered *E. coli* bacteria. The proteins are made using amino acids and are modeled after those used for silk fibroin. They include a cell attachment domain (gene) from human fibronectin. Altered fibronectin expression affects wound healing and connective tissue/collagen function. Spore-forming and other bacteria have also been used to scavenge oxygen from plastic materials; and to scavenge metals to protect plants from fungal diseases. Polymers and plant bacteria are found in animal feeds and supplements, and bovine serum albumin has been used within a number of human biological products including but not limited to interferon and vaccines. It has also been used in B.t. agricultural insecticidal toxins (Cry proteins) including those used upon feedlot livestock and their foods.[93-98]

According to a 1949 paper, cattle were fed *raw rock phosphate* as a feed supplement in place of feed-grade bone meal. The substitute proved disastrous and caused the animals to suffer toxic effects from the fluoride-containing phosphates. Tricalcium phosphate was substituted, providing a feed supplement with a reduced fluoride content. Sodium hexafluorosilicate is used to control lice, mosquitoes, roundworms and whipworms of feedlot animals. Before it was banned by the FDA, animal feeds contained gentian violet, a carcinogenic substance that was used as an antifungal agent. Gentian violet (an aniline dye) is used in laboratories as a gram-staining agent. We might think about the mutagenic potentials of the chemicals used on or in animal feed supplements as insecticides and antibiotics, and their effects upon the microbial infections present in these animals.[45,46]

Other chemicals have also been applied to feedlot cattle to control ticks, cattle grubs, lice, flies, and screwworms. These chemicals included Dow ET-57 (trolene) and Co-Ral (Bayer 21/199). Such chemicals do not remain inert, but can passively enter food products and transfer chemical or microbial agents from animal tissues into the human body. Poultry houses have used antibiotics, organophosphates, and larvicides to treat birds for insects.[23-29]

An older report on the topic of diseases of feedlot cattle showed that the industrialized processes of "growing" beef cattle and other food animals has actually produced higher incidences of animal diseases including nutritional diseases, respiratory and intestinal tract diseases, clostridium bloat, pink eye, foot rot, actinomycosis, actinobacillus, shipping fever, and swine erysipelas. The latter is a serious infection that occurs in a large percentage of pig populations intended for food.[62-66]

Patents describe livestock pesticides that use bacteria or fungi. The bacterium *Serratia marcescens* can be used as an insecticide in the same way *Bacillus thuringiensis* is used. This may bring new meaning to the biowarfare "simulant" experiments that took place over San Francisco, California in 1950 under *Operation Sea Spray.* Was *S. marcescens* being tested as a biowarfare agent for insects? A B.t. pesticide patent states that "*B. thuringiensis* insecticides are quite specific and are harmless to non-susceptible orders of insects, and relatively safe to animals and humans." Note it does not say "safe" but that B.t. insecticides are "relatively safe."[67-71]

A 1968 patent was filed by Corn Products Company International (CPC), a corn refining company now owned by Bestfoods (New Jersey); and one of the largest food companies in the world. Bestfoods' history includes acquisitions of food lines from SmithKline Beecham PLC and Kraft Foods. (SmithKline Beecham's pharmaceutical division sponsored the first Lyme disease vaccine.) In 1997 the company spun-off its corn refining business to create Corn Products International. As we know, corn appears in virtually every processed food, commercial animal feed, and many non-food products. According to the 1968 patent, scientists were trying to extract RNA from treated cells including brewer's yeast *Saccharomyces cerevisiae.* Yeasts are important in the fermentation of the agricultural insecticide B.t. This is also a microbe whose toxins are applied onto and genetically engineered into corn crops. According to the patent:[76]

> "Such mode of treatment would be particularly useful in extracting ribonucleic acid from yeast cells. ...For example, it has been found that the extract from yeast cells may be used as *additives to fermentation media, as cattle and poultry feeds*, and so forth."
>
> "The term 'microbial cells' as used herein is to be broadly applied and to include the cells or mycelia of diverse micro-organisms such as yeast, bacteria, fungi, algae, etc. Thus, any cell which is found in various micro-organisms may be treated through contact with ammonia, which cells may be then utilized in the food, feed, pharmaceutical, fermentation and other industries."

The ammonia discussed in the patent may include the applied agricultural anhydrous ammonia or ammoniated fertilizers or other agrochemicals such as *quaternary fluorinated ammonium salts* (amines).[76]

These chemicals are also used as disinfectants and surfactants, and can appear in formulas with chloride salts. Amines may adversely affect microbial genes and cellular membranes. It is curious that during the 1950s, the Battelle Memorial Institute performed large-scale tests on acidulation and ammoniation. Be assured that where amines are applied (i.e. soil or water), these chemical catalysts kill certain bacteria while leaving others untouched. Those that survive are usually the *Pseudomonas* species, *the non-enveloped viruses,* and *Bacillus thuringiensis,* or B.t. The non-enveloped viruses of course include the RNA viruses which associate with the *baculoviruses* of the applied microbial insecticides.[72-84]

It is most interesting that a company (3M) that holds a patent on a Lyme disease diagnostic test to detect *Borrelia burgdorferi* in urine (i.e. wastewater) also holds a patent for quaternary fluorinated ammonium salts (amines) that are useful in water, soil, and industrial applications (i.e. health, medicine), including as animal insecticides. We know that chickens are vaccinated, and that they carry important retroviruses. We might want to know that quaternary ammonium compounds are widely used as germicides (i.e. Roccal D Plus,® Gluquat) when treating poultry or swine feedlot drinking water lines; washing eggs; or cleaning housing and slaughter facilities, livestock trucks and trailers, and processing equipment (i.e. poultry eviscerators, hatcheries, smokehouses). It is perhaps also interesting that the University of Connecticut is assignee on a 1968 patent for a poultry conveyor system. In the end, what goes onto and into the animals and the plants we use to sustain ourselves, will significantly impact human health either in a beneficial or an adverse manner. Such effects are both unpredictable and virtually unavoidable.[72-84]

Minerals and Reoviruses

Malachite is an example of a mineral that is created by the weathering of ores; in this case, copper. Minerals and ores of many kinds are found deep in the earth and are mined for many industries, including fertilizer and nuclear industries. Malachite and other minerals are found in the same area where we find metals; and rocks such as limestone, granite, phosphates, and bauxite. Malachite is useful in the laboratory for staining; and in dyes and for copper smelting. It is a useful model to describe the association between mined minerals and ores, and the bacteria and viruses that live underground and which may be found in their presence.

Malachite is found worldwide, and has been mined in areas that have significance to the story of Lyme disease. This includes the Ural mountains of Russia; in Africa, Mexico, New South Wales, Australia (Broken Hill mine); Lyon France, and Israel in Timna Valley (King Solomon's Mines where it has been mined and smelted for over 3,000 years). Malachite is also mined in the US, especially in Loudville mine in Massachusetts (near Trouvelot's gypsy moth studies). It is also mined in Arizona, Colorado, Michigan, Nevada, New Mexico, Utah, and Montana; where Rocky Mountain Lab scientists first identified important tick agents such as spiroplasmas and *Borrelia burgdorferi.*[1,2]

Perhaps malachite and copper are why Dr. Burgdorfer and his colleagues found rabbit ticks from the Bitterroot mountains so interesting. The fact that Connecticut also has a large vein of copper flowing underneath the region is significant. Where there are metals and mining, there will also be malachite, and other industrially important materials; as well as reoviruses and extremophilic bacteria that thrive deep underground. Malachite green (MG) is a triphenylmethane that is used to dye silk, cotton, wool, jute, leather, paper and fiber industries. In the dye industry, *chromium fluoride* has been used to dye fabrics, including silk, wool, and aesbestos fibers (that also contained alumina). Malachite green (an aniline dye) has also been used in aquaculture since the 1930s as an antifungal/antiprotozoal agent. It is also used as a veterinary drug for ornamental fish, but not in fish for human consumption.[3,4]

Malachite green is considered an industrial contaminant, and it is converted by the fish body into a persistent, colorless agent called *leocomalachite green* (LMG). Residues of MG and LMG are retained in fatty fish and are known to enter the human diet. This chemical has been shown to be toxic and carcinogenic to animals; and it binds to DNA. This means that it will persist within cells and can be passed on generationally as a contaminant. Salmon from Chile and Scotland have been found to be contaminated with malachite green, and residues have been isolated from many species of freshwater fish including catfish, trout, and eels.[3,5-8]

Traditional wastewater techniques are unable to entirely remove synthetic dyes including malachite green and its structurally related compounds. Some fungi can partially metabolize dyes. Intestinal bacteria including *E. coli, Clostridium perfringens,* and *Peptostreptococcus anaerobius* convert the dye to a derivative. Scientists investigated sprayable granular formulas for B.t. insecticides that contained malachite green oxalate salts. Baker's yeast *Saccharomyces cerevisiae* also decolorizes malachite green, and we know this yeast is part of the fermentation process in the manufacturing of B.t. insecticides.[3-8]

Large quantities of malachite may be found in Lyon France, which was the hub of the silk industry during the 1800s, and from where gypsy moth imports were harvested for silk entrepreneur Trouvelot. It was also the region from where the first parasitic wasps and parasitized ticks were imported into the US during the 1920s. Areas such as this are home to large geothermal veins where thermophile bacteria live. These are bacteria that are capable of living in extreme temperatures. We must carefully study the different kinds of microbes that are commonly associated with malachite and other minerals, metals, and elements found underground – materials that are mined for their global usefulness in agriculture and other industries.[4,9,13-19]

Among mined minerals and their elements we also find fluorite (fluoride), and the radioactive element *uranium. Bauxite,* an aggregate material is useful for many products including fluoride-based agricultural chemicals and fertilizers. I might also point out that bauxite, which is useful within fertilizer compositions and in sewage treatment, has the *ability to enhance the infectivity of viruses including Reoviruses*. Scientists were studying this important association in 1985, just three years after the causative agent of Lyme disease was publicly announced. Indeed the research shows that the *persistence of reoviruses*, hepatitis A, and other enteric (gut) viruses in soil or water depends heavily upon the type of organic matter or clay materials that are in contact with these viruses. For example in soils that have a high organic carbon content, we will find elevated levels of coliphages (bacteriophages that infect *E. coli*).[9-13]

Reovirus type 3 is found naturally within rodent populations, and is especially prevalent within laboratory rodents. **Reovirus type 3 is also a common contaminant in transplantable tumor cell lines and other biological materials.** In rodents, reovirus type 3 infections cause a multi-system disease. Symptoms include necrotizing hepatitis, pancreatitis (inflammation of pancreas), myocarditis (inflammation of heart), and meningoencephalitis (inflammation of brain and spinal column). In addition, a condition called steatorrhoea (excess fat in the feces) develops after the onset of liver disease during this infection. This causes an "oily skin" appearance. A similar condition is seen in celiac disease, pancreatic cancer, bacterial overgrowth, and malabsorption syndromes including those seen in Lyme disease or HIV/AIDS.[14]

Such information seems entirely relevant when we observe the organisms studied by public health officials in fauna around wastewater treatment plants, and nuclear and agricultural facilities during the 1950s and 1960s. Laboratory-manipulated organisms and chemicals, applied agrochemicals, nuclear wastes, and natural rodent viruses make their way into water sources and the insects in these environments. Under optimal conditions viral infectivity is enhanced by the organic matter of nutrient-rich sediments, toxic chemicals, and clays of filtration ponds, river/pond sediments, and agricultural and industrial retention ponds.[14]

Uranium of course is one of the most valuable elements to nuclear physics and industries around the world. There are productive uranium mines in many countries including Africa, Europe, England, France, Hungary, Israel, Italy, Japan, Korea, Kazakhstan, Malaysia, Mexico, the Middle East, The Netherlands, Romania, Russia, Sweden, Spain, and the US. In nearly every major country we find nuclear reactors, nuclear power plants, research reactors, nuclear medicine, nuclear fuel production plants, and fuel storage facilities. We will study important connections between uranium mining/processing/usage, the agricultural agent B.t., and a new strain of tickborne relapsing fever *Borrelia miyamotoi* in one of the last chapters of this book.[9,13-19]

Plutonium is also produced in nuclear reactors through a fission process, which releases neutrons; converting Uranium-238 into plutonium. Plutonium is most useful for nuclear weapons. Metallic plutonium is created through a chemical reaction that includes plutonium tetrafluoride (fluoride). Plutonium-aluminum and plutonium-uranium are useful components in nuclear fuels. Plutonium was first synthesized in 1940 at the University of California-Berkeley laboratory. The production of plutonium for wartime use was a major aspect of the Manhattan Project. The first nuclear test took place in July 1945 (Trinity). The disposal of plutonium wastes from nuclear power plants, weapons plants, or research facilities is a huge issue of environmental concern, as is the disposal and recycling of post-war nuclear weapons.[20-22]

What is also important to understand about mined materials, is an important *thermophile* (*thermoacidophile*) that was isolated in 1995 from a uranium mine in *Thuringia, Germany,* that was named *Metallosphaera prunae* species novel. This bacterium is a natural bioleacher and metal mobilizer from the family of sulfur-reducing bacteriae. It was discovered on a smoldering slag heap in a uranium mine. The thermophiles are extremophiles that are capable of withstanding extremes in temperature and soil conditions, deep within the earth's crust. Thuringia, Germany is the exact same place where the original microbial insecticidal agent, *Bacillus thuringiensis* or B.t. was isolated for the second time in 1915 by German Scientist Ernst Berliner. Remember he discovered the agent inside the bodies of flour moth caterpillars. The thermophilic bacteriae are also found in association with reoviruses that are not only in the ground, but that also reside within the bodies of insects and animals as latent infections.[4]

We have already studied the reoviruses of mined materials, and of insects. Reoviruses are a subject with which Dr. Willy Burgdorfer and his colleagues appear intimately familiar, due to their studies of these viruses at Rocky Mountain Labs. Reoviruses of course are highly important to the *baculoviruses* that have been applied as agricultural insecticides, because they commonly associate with these bacteria as satellite viruses; and because reoviruses are *intracellular infections* which ramp up the killing action of insecticides that contain baculoviruses. Reoviruses are capable of infecting both the wild-type fungi and the fungi of applied insecticidal formulas. Now we may better envision a B.t.-reovirus-fungi-baculovirus-extremophile aggregate.

When reoviruses are put into an environment that encourages them to reassort (i.e. insect bodies), they can create new mutant (mixed) infections that are highly virulent. Some of the members of the reovirus family are the *Orbiviruses*. Orbiviruses are also found deep in the ground, in soil and water, and in the bodies of insects and animals. The orbiviruses are RNA viruses, and they include the animal infections equine encephalitis, bluetongue, and epizootic hemorrhagic disease of deer virus, among others. Orbiviruses have been found to cause persistent infections in American dog tick cell lines in the laboratory. Insect cell lines are of course useful for agricultural and industrial insecticides and for animal vaccines.[2,9,13,15-19]

One member of the orbivirus family is the Colorado tick fever virus. The reovirus family includes the *Cytoplasmic polyhedrosis viruses* (CPVs) which are found within the bodies of insects including gypsy moths and other silkworms. Other reoviruses include *bluetongue,* a disease of cattle; *rice dwarf virus, rice ragged stunt virus,* the *Eyach* virus (found in France); and the *corn stunt* virus of corn plants that is associated with the *corn stunt spiroplasma.* Because CPVs are ineffective to be used alone as microbial insecticides, they are often genetically engineered into *baculovirus* constructs to purposely increase their virulence in the insecticidal formulas. Some of the most important CPV reoviruses to our story come from the sawfly, silkworm, and gypsy moth species.[9,13-19]

We may now more easily appreciate the connections and the 1920s efforts by USDA scientists to import French nymph ticks that were parasitized by indigenous wasps collected south of Paris in the Fontainebleu Forest. And we can see how these parasitoids could have inadvertently spread one or more important bacteria and viruses into the US (i.e. Eyach), beginning on the east coast where these insects were first released. Subsequent releases of imported insects could have further compounded the problem, and accidentally contributed important viruses to future epidemics. This is because the Eyach virus is a close cousin of the rabies virus. Eyach was isolated years later from persons living in Mayennes, France, not far from the Fontainebleu forest where the imported wasps and ticks originated.[24-30]

An article described the "ultimate goal" of scientists who engineer B.t. Cry proteins for maximum toxicity to insects (while making them non-toxic to non-targeted species). Scientists feel they have attained this goal through the use of *shuttle host cells* or *shuttle vectors.* These are genetic constructs that are specially designed to carry toxic genes into microorganisms, and that are delivered by applied insecticides. Shuttle vectors are made to work (propagate) inside the bodies of two hosts – namely plants and insects. Some of the most frequently engineered toxin-expressing genes used within shuttle vectors come from the bacteriae *Pseudomonas aeruginosa, Serratia marcescens,* and *Bacillus thuringiensis* variety Berliner. Other B.t. varieties include *kurstaki, tenebrionis,* or *israeliensis.* Any species of *Bacillus* (i.e. *subtilis, cereus, sphaericus, popilliae* etc.) may be used as each may produce its own unique toxins that are useful in recombinant insecticides.[31-38]

A registered patent describes a way to identify genes that encode previously unknown toxins, or toxins for which genes were previously unavailable. Those genes are then engineered into plants. Among the microbes that can be used to create insecticides are B.t. strains; and *Serratica marcescens, Bacillus popilliae,* mycoplasma/spiroplasmas, fungi, nematodes, and viruses including insect arboviruses, baculoviruses, *Poxviruses, Picornaviruses* (think polio), *Iridoviruses* (insect iridescent viruses), *Polydnaviruses* (found in parasitoid wasps); and the reoviruses such as those found underground and in insects, animals, and birds including *poultry. The polydna viruses of parasitoid wasps are able to infect and alter the genes of the host cells of the organisms they invade.*[31-38]

Reoviruses are also very closely related to the African sindbis virus, a virus that has been critically important to scientists who genetically engineer viruses and bacteria, especially for vaccines. Sindbis is a highly patented insect virus that has been the model alphavirus for genetically engineered vaccines, biological controls, human biologicals, and cancer research. Sindbis apparently has a dark side, making it possible under certain conditions (including recombinant vaccines), for the virus to be "kicked out" of the genetic construct. What this means inside the body is that it may leave an animal or human susceptible to the reactivation of latent viruses if a defective, genetically engineered vaccine fails and creates a disease state.

The vulnerability of sindbis vectors is described in the literature and registered patents; and appears to be a huge problem. It also helps illustrate that some genetically engineered tools may be highly flawed. According to a patent:[39,40]

> "...insofar as applicant is aware, a problem with the Sindbis vector is that the heterologous insert is unstable therein and is 'kicked out' of the vector..."

The question is whether recombinant constructs break apart and contribute to the reassortment of genes in transgenic crops, applied insecticides; insects, or vaccinated animals or people to create infectious diseases. The sindbis virus has proteins in the 41 nm range, which makes it ideal for binding with the yeast proteins of the B.t. insecticides to produce toxic "killer" yeast strains. Perhaps such viral binding is what "kicks out" the sindbis virus from the recombinant construct in the first place.

Interferon is a pharmaceutical product that is used to treat viral infections and diseases such as Multiple Sclerosis. Most of the early interferon patents including one assigned to Imperial Chemical Industries Limited (ICI), describe the production of interferon in chicken embryos, and in calf and monkey kidney tissues. If cell lines used to create animal or human vaccines or applied biological controls harbor contaminants, then patent holders and their parent companies would certainly not be pleased when or if such information was discovered or revealed.[41-47]

Imperial Chemical Industries Limited (ICI) supplied herbicides to British military forces including chemicals that were sprayed in Malaysia during the 1950s. In 1955 ICI began to produce *Paraquat,* a quaternary ammonium herbicide that was widely used in agriculture. In the 1980s ICI became one of the largest international seed producer and agrochemical companies in the world. ICI is now owned by Syngenta, a division of Monsanto. ICI was founded under a merger of four companies: British Dyestuffs Corp., Brunner Mond, United Alkali Co., and Nobel Explosives. The latter was the Scottish nitrogen-based propellant and explosives company founded by Alfred Nobel in 1866. During the 1830s the Ensign-Bickford Company (EBCo) was built in Simsbury, Connecticut to manufacture safety fuses and detonating cord for the mining industry. Today Ensign Bickford and Dyno Nobel Inc. are both located in Simsbury. The area has a large underground copper deposit. It is also where in 1966 and 1968 California group encephalitis viruses were isolated for the first time in mosquitoes by Yale scientist Dr. Whitman. Connecticut was one of the first areas where RNA viruses were released to augment agricultural insecticides; and where a cluster of Lyme disease cases first emerged in the US.[48-54]

The Syngenta Company (Monsanto) is considered to be the largest agribusiness company in the world, and the leading manufacturer of agrochemicals. Syngenta is also the third largest owner of plant-based biotechnology patents, and a major seed supplier. Its parent companies, Novartis and AstraZeneca also promote GM crops, and produce agricultural chemicals. Syngenta was formed as a spin-off company following the merger between Novartis' seed and agrochemical divisions. British chemical and biotechnology company Zeneca was one part of ICI. Zeneca merged with Swedish pharmaceutical company Astra AB to form AstraZeneca in 1999. During the late 1990s, seed and biotech companies held by Novartis and AstraZeneca merged their pharmaceutical, chemical, and agricultural divisions.[55-61]

By 1999 there was a civil movement against GM crops, so the company Syngenta was formed, and is headquartered in Wilmington, Delaware. Its lawn and garden, crop protection, and biotechnology headquarters are in North Carolina; while its seed headquarters are in Minnesota. Some of the co-authors of the IDSA guidelines for Lyme disease have accepted research grant funding from companies such as Novartis; and academic institutions such as the University of Minnesota and Yale University have been awarded multi-million dollar research grant awards from major agricultural companies.[55-61]

It's Elementary Dear Watsons

One of the most striking aspects of the Lyme story is the presence of radioactive elements in the air, soil, and water; and their effects upon microbes and higher organisms including humans. We may also consider what happens when these wastes make their way into wastewaters, surface water supplies, and underground aquifers. In this section I address the naturally occurring radioactive uranium and thorium, just two of thirty rare earth elements (and byproducts of their decay). These and other elements are commonly found along geothermal veins deep in the earth's crust, in igneous rocks from the Jurassic period of world history (roughly 200-145 million years ago). Elemental and mineral deposits vary according to geographic region, and so do accompanying materials including metal ores, clays, sandstones, granites, pitchblende, bauxite, fluorapatite, and phosphates. Among these rocks are industrially important metals (tin, alumina, copper, silver, zinc, gold, etc.), viruses, and extremophile bacteria. These microbes are able to withstand extreme temperatures, and acidic soil and water conditions.

Uranium is a naturally abundant metal; and thorium to a far greater extent, both of which are mined. A significant amount of uranium can be found in coffinite, a uranium-bearing silicate rock; while thorium is found as thorium-232. The latter is a byproduct of rare earth extraction from monazite sand, which is a phosphate mineral that contains other elements. There was a monazite mine in Shelby, North Carolina, but most is mined in India, Australia, South Africa, or Brazil. There is a large cache of coffinite in the US, especially in the "Copper King" mines of Utah, and in the Colorado plateau. This area is a mineral belt that belongs to the Morrison Formation, which is a large deposit that covers the western portion of the United States. It is the most fertile source of dinosaur fossils in North America (and no doubt coprolites, or fossilized dinosaur poop).

The formation's center lies in Colorado and Wyoming; and there are outcroppings in Arizona, Idaho, Kansas, Montana, Nebraska, New Mexico, North Dakota, Oklahoma, South Dakota, Texas, and Utah. Yellowstone National Park in Wyoming is part of this formation and has one of the world's largest collections of geothermal hot springs and geysers (i.e. Old Faithful) in the world. Similiar formations are found in Canada. The Morrison Formation has been a major source of uranium and other mined ores over the past century. Uranium is of course accompanied by the extremophile sulfur-reducing, acid-loving bacteria.[1,2]

Similar formations created the Great Rift Valley of Africa, and the Alpine Valley of Europe, as examples. There are uranium deposits in many countries including Australia, Argentina, Brazil, France, India, Eastern Germany, Russia, Switzerland, and Romania. Australia has the world's largest uranium reserves. It is interesting that major uranium or thorium deposits, geothermal veins, hot springs, and sulfur-reducing bacteria and their viruses are found in areas of the world where Lyme disease is endemic.

Uranium is also found in carnotite, a radioactive potassium-uranium-vanadian mineral rock mined in the US, Australia, France, Kazakhstan, Morocco, Russia, and Zaire. Uranium and thorium are both useful for nuclear weapons and fuels; as are plutonium and tritium. Uranium is also present under the Great Salt Lake of Utah and surrounding marsh area, which is important since a mutated bacterium was isolated from a dying muskrat near a Utah salt marsh.[3]

Coffinite, which is also found in Kazakhstan, is a uranium-bearing rock that is highly important to the development of nuclear energy or weapons, as a source of uranium. Coffinite was discovered in the La Sal No. 2 mine in Mesa County, Colorado in 1951. Torbernite is a radioactive phosphate of uranium and copper, and can be used for uranium extraction. Torbernite was found in Connecticut in Haddam, Middlesex County, in Rock Landing Quarry. In the 1920s to 1930s this particular quarry produced granite, uranium, and columbite, and is the area of the state where the Connecticut cluster of Lyme disease cases emerged. Today other quarries operate in the area. The presence of uranium is important to our story, as is the mining of other industrially important rocks (i.e. limestone, sandstone, clay, granite, gypsum, fluorspar), minerals and metals (i.e. alumina [aluminum], silver, tin, copper, gold) which are used for everything from weapons to paints, plastics, fertilizers, pharmaceuticals, canned goods, and other goods important to nuclear, agricultural, and other industries.[3]

During the 1950s, scientists from the US Geological Survey (USGS), the US Atomic Energy Commission (USAEC), and Harvard University attempted to create synthetic coffinite for the US Atomic Energy Commission (AEC). They succeeded in 1956. Besides the natural decay of uranium and the byproducts thereof, the nuclear age brought forth nuclear weapons and synthetic elements which could be created in nuclear reactors. These elements are called actinides, and are found in the environment as nuclear fallout, nuclear wastes from metal ore processing and manufacturing; and in wastewater that has been contaminated by spent fuel wastes. Synthetic actinides have been created using nuclear reactors by Russian, Swedish, and American scientists including at the University of California-Berkeley. Laboratories that have used betatrons, synchrotrons, cyclotrons, and other particle accelerators for nuclear science and industry are among the facilities that have produced nuclear wastes. More significant is that these wastes have been carelessly discharged into the environment over decades.

The first cyclotrons were used for X-ray therapy to treat cancer patients beginning in the late 1950s. However the betatron was created in 1940 and a unit was housed at the University of Illinois Urbana-Champaign until it was replaced. The Case Institute (now CaseWestern) in Cleveland, Ohio also had a betatron during the 1950s. There is a cyclotron in Hevesy Laboratory in Denmark, and we have already discussed Brookhaven's accelerators. It is estimated that there were about two hundred of these machines in the world. They were used for nuclear medicine, particle physics, and weapons development beginning in the mid-1940s. By 1946 units were operational in Switzerland and Germany. The Paul Scherrer Institute in Zurich now operates several particle accelerators including a cyclotron. Switzerland is now home to the CERN laboratory near Geneva, and the world's largest particle accelerator, the Hadron collider. **Copper is an integral mineral for nuclear and renewable energy sources,** and is used in the Hadron Collider. The kinds of microbes that are present in areas where copper, aluminum, and other ores are mined are key to understanding how microbes may aggregate to cause infectious diseases such as Lyme.[27,42,43]

In the US, General Electric and Allis-Chalmers built betatrons. Other particle accelerators also came online from the 1950s forward, and were used during the Manhattan Project by subcontractors of Battelle. For example, quality control work included taking X-rays of uranium ingots to detect metallurgical flaws during the manufacture of reactor fuels. This task was undertaken by General Steel Industries in Granite City, Illinois (northeast of St. Louis, Missouri).[27]

Fermi Laboratory and Argonne National Laboratory are located in suburbs of Chicago, Illinois. These facilities house particle accelerators and are owned by the University of Chicago, the institution which began nuclear research in the US. These two laboratories also happen to flank the community where I grew up. Other famous nuclear reactors in the US are at Hanford Works (WA), Savannah River (SC), and Three Mile Island (PA). There are many laboratories with particle accelerators, and there are nuclear plants, and nuclear medicine-related machines around the world. We have come a long way since the world's first nuclear reactor, the Chicago Pile-1 graphite/uranium block reactor of 1942. And yet the presence of nuclear wastes in soils, air, and wastewaters is an integral part of the story. Where we find radioactive elements and their products of decay, whether natural or synthetically created; we will find bacteria and plants which take up these pollutants, and whose genes may mutate as a result of such exposures.[4-10]

Uranium and thorium are also naturally found near bauxite and zirconium, a radioactive metal that is mined as zirconium orthosilicate, and then manipulated in nuclear reactors. The crystal form is called cubic zirconium, as the diamond substitute worn as jewelry. Since zirconium is extremely resistant to seawater and acids, it is used in highly corrosive environments, especially by chemical companies. It is also used in steel making, explosive primers, flash bulbs, and bulb filaments, high temperature crucibles, metal furnaces, ceramics, as refractory material, and for nuclear fuels. Most of the zirconium in use today is for nuclear power generators.[72,73]

Zirconium, chromium, and other nuclear wastes (as some escapes into wastewaters or steam vapors) can be taken into the body through inhalation or ingestion, where it deposits into organs and skeletal structures. It has a radioactive half-life of up to twenty-five years, although other radioactive wastes decay far more slowly. Since zirconium is used in some dental implants or ceramics, the radioactivity of this and other materials may present health risks. A 1960 article written with the cooperation of scientists from ALCOA and the Rice Institute (Houston, Texas) reveals that after processing bauxite for its alumina content, roughly seventy percent of uranium or thorium is excreted as "red mud," which is then recycled for bricks and other construction materials.[11,12]

Small amounts of radioactive elements are found in alumina, which is processed to make aluminum. Steel also contains small amounts of radioactive isotopes, according to a report that sampled bauxite from two mines including the ALCOA mine in Bauxite, Arkansas. The concentration of thorium in red mud samples from an East St. Louis alumina plant demonstrated that up to forty thousand pounds of uranium might be recovered annually from one alumina plant alone. This points the finger at the aluminum and steel industries as providers of radioactive uranium or thorium. The latter is currently being eyed as the "new" (old) nuclear fuel in upcoming decades. Any diseases which might be caused or contributed to by the presence of nuclear "wastes" in the environment, could be considered a huge threat to several important industries whose eyes are undoubtedly on the future prospects of nuclear energy use and their associated profits.[11-13]

Radioactive elements in the form of identification tracers (identification chemicals) have been used in various industries since the late 1950s. At the beginning of the Cold War, as nuclear techniques for "peaceful purposes" were pursued instead of atomic weapons, new and exciting applications for nuclear energy emerged, as did the need to safely eliminate nuclear wastes. In the plastics industry, some polymers are formed using nuclear radiation techniques. Agricultural chemical insecticides such as chlorpyrifos and phosphates contain(ed) radiolabels or natural uranium that is radioactive.[10-13]

Even animal vaccines and the microbes within them (i.e. nematodes) were irradiated before use; and sometimes they contain radioactive tritium tracers (radiotracers). Insects of all kinds have been irradiated under *sterile insect techniques*. This rendered them sexually sterile before they were released in the billions around the world to mate with indigenous populations. The irradiated insects may carry genes that are damaged from these techniques. Furthermore, the microbes within their bodies could also mutate from the irradiation.[14]

Mutations can lead to new infectious diseases that are transmissible. As techniques evolved, radiolabelled genetically engineered crops were grown, and foods and pharmaceutical products became irradiated to inactivate viruses and bacteriae. The use of radiation techniques for industries and agriculture is not inert. Radioactive isotopes decay at various rates, are stored in our bones and teeth, and may contribute to gene damage, cancers, bone loss, or other health problems.[14]

Scientists have found that environmental contaminations of uranium, thorium, and byproducts of their decay are elevated in areas where nuclear production, processing, storage, mining, and nuclear power plants and reactor sites are located. Soil, air, and water contaminations occurred over decades simply beause environmental pollution regulations were sorely lacking, even with the implementation of the Federal Water Pollution Control Act of 1948. In 1972 in the US, the Environmental Protection Agency (EPA) implemented major changes to pollution control standards. In 1977 those changes became known as the Clean Water Act (i.e. clean and wastewater quality standards). However uranium, thorium and other decaying synthetic elements have long half-lives. This means they will persist and remain radioactive in the soil or water, for a very, very long time. (The half life of natural uranium-238 is roughly four-and-a half billion years.)

It is likewise difficult to assess the long-term effects of nuclear fallout from deployed weapons, testing, manufacturing, power plants, or natural nuclear accidents (i.e. Three-mile Island, Chernobyl, Fukushima). It is apparent however that radioactive fallout and other discharged wastes play a role in the exposure of organisms to radioactive, gene-damaging radicals. Uranium or tritium have also appeared in agricultural chemicals (i.e. organochlorides); and other ag-related tools (i.e. animal vaccines, insecticides, GM crops). As well, natural radioactive elements are present in the phosphate fertilizers that have been applied over centuries, but especially during the late-nineteenth century forward with the use of mined phosphate rocks.

In the US after the Dust Bowl, Congress formed the Tennessee Valley Authority (TVA) which helped promote modern agricultural techniques in the states. Over time the peaceful use of nuclear energy has expanded to a point where today radiation exposures are far greater than they have ever been. What has also increased in number are cancers and infectious diseases. Because of this, nuclear medicine has also gained importance. Food irradiation and the use of radioactive elements in industries (i.e. plastics, power, particle physics, wastewater irradiation, medicine, veterinary science) also creates nuclear wastes. The use of nuclear energy and fuels for "peaceful purposes" presents a unique challenge in the modern arena. It is increasingly important to prevent unnecessary radiation exposures, and to avoid spontaneous gene mutations in insects, plants, animals, and their microbes. Insecticides, animal vaccines, and genetically engineered chimera (blended genes) have also employed radiolabels, and the bacteria in those formulas can take up these elements. Fertilizers contain radioactive elements and their residues remain upon the foods we eat and drink.[15-21,25,26]

The literature clearly demonstrates that *up to eighty-percent of radioactive particles taken up by insects remains within the mid-gut*. There resident microbes are penetrated by radioactive ions. In a similar manner, tobacco plants were shown to take up significant levels of radioactive elements not only from the soil, but more frequently from the air. According to a patent:

> "Experiments with moderate doses of 0.4 .mu.g larva of C^{14} labelled inclusion protein indicate an uptake of protein measurable by 10 minutes and peaking by 20. Counting of dissected larvae show that 80% or more of the radioactivity is held in the mid-gut region." (C^{14} is Carbon 14.)[16]

Soil bacteriae including bacillus species and the sulfur-reducers are also able to take up radioactive elements along with metals from their environment. These organisms are ubiquitous and are found near mines, acid mine wastes, gypsum stacks, smelters, metal processing plants, nuclear test sites, reactors and processors, geothermal veins, agricultural soils, and polluted waters. Radioactive particles are able to mutate the microbes in the insect or animal gut to create complex mixed infections and aggregate organisms.[15-21,25,26]

Sulfur-reducing bacteriae are helpful in the formation and decomposition of rocks and minerals. These include the extremophile and thermophile bacteriae that are found underground in the presence of phosphates, sulfur, uranium, coal, shale, oil, and other deposits. These bacteria are typically anaerobic (without oxygen), and many are spore-formers. Among the most important bacteria to our story are those from the phyllum *Thermotoga*. Examples are *Petrotoga* (oil reservoirs), *Firmicutes* (clostridium, bacillus, mollicutes), *Synergistetes* (periodontal, soft tissue and gut infections), *Deinococcus-Thermus* (*Deinococcus radiodurans, Thermus aquaticus*), and *Fusobacteria** (similar to bacteroids that cause skin ulcers, periodontal disease, ulcerative colitis; and that are found in colon cancer cells).[22-24]

**Clindamycin is revealed in sources as an antibiotic that is useful against fusobacteria. This is not a medical recommendation.*

Thermophilic bacteria are not only present in mines, they have been genetically engineered to be copper and metal tolerant for the purpose of leaching metals from ores, and for bioremediation of acid mine and radioactive nuclear wastes. A few of these agents are described in mining-related patents that are assigned to companies such as Minnesota Mining and Manufacturing (3M) and Amoco. These patents are for diagnostic tests to detect *Borrelia burgdorferi* spirochetes from wastewaters and urine samples. The patents specifically mention thermophiles and rodents that might be found around mines and wastewaters. I will discuss these patents in detail in an upcoming chapter.[28-30]

Among the thermophiles that may be detected by these diagnostic tests are *Deinococcus radiodurans* and *Thermus thermophilus*. Since these patents also detect *Borrelia burgdorferi* and *leptospires*, we may rightly suspect there is a thermophilic and a leptospiral bacterial component involved with Bb spirochetes. *T. thermophilus* produces an enzyme in the presence of manganese that has reverse transcriptase ability. *T. thermophilus* enzymes may cause the mutation of viruses or other organisms under optimal conditions. This may occur in wastewaters, or within the bodies of insects or animals to reactivate latent infections including perhaps the viruses of past vaccines that are part of the host's DNA (genome). Bb is another organism that has enzymes which use manganese. It is obvious that patent holders are well aware that Bb spirochetes are detectable from wastewaters and urine samples. They more than likely also understand the relationship between wastewaters, mined materials, thermophiles, and the leptospira spirochetes that after aggregation and host amplification, will become the spirochetes of Lyme disease.[28-30]

The literature shows that genetically modified extremophile bacteria were specifically designed for, and placed into the environment to remediate acid mine wastes. Although this may have been a benevolent idea, these recombinant microbes and their wild relatives manage to leach into ground and wastewaters where they are free to reassort with leptospires and other bacteria in polluted environments. Genetically engineered thermophilic bacteria if sought, might be easily isolated from *Borrelia burgdorferi* spirochetes. If so, this could explain the "veil of secrecy" that has surrounded Lyme disease and leptonemas for decades.[28-30]

It could also explain the extremely low reported case numbers for Lyme disease, if and only if public health officials are only tracking one group of Lyme disease cases – those that are fully CDC-positive. Fully CDC-positive laboratory results are rather rare among Lyme patients, and when found, typically warrant a personal phone call from a CDC-representative. If the standardized Lyme disease tests were established to largely detect only Bb strains that are caused by *recombinant thermophiles* or those that have taken up *synthetic elements*, it may explain why most Bb strains were summarily excluded from the Lyme disease diagnostic test criteria established at the Dearborn conference. The remaining Bb strains that are found in the world may represent those that have been formed by wild-type thermophiles, and thus may be considered less of a "liability" if they were formed with the help of industrial chemicals or processes. If true, this may also mean that the B31 and N40 strains are those that involve a recombinantly created thermophile bacteria (i.e. Taq pol enzyme of blue-green algae), or elements first created in laboratories or nuclear reactors (i.e. physics, power, research, medical, fuel production, industrial use).[28-30]

Extremophiles are radiation and dessication resistant. As such, they live among radioactive elements in the worst temperatures and environmental conditions. **They also have a unique feature that includes multiple copies of their DNA in each cell.** This allows them the ability to repair cellular damage, and to persist where other bacteria would perish, such as under assault of nuclear radiation or antibiotics. When damaged, they simply repair their DNA with one of the extra copies. Other important bacteria that are also extremophiles are found in the environment and in insects that are targeted by insecticides, including paenibacillus, clostridium, and pseudomonas species.[31-33]

Patent inventions reveal that thermophiles and sulfur reducing bacteria have been used since before the beginning of the Lyme epidemic to extract metals from ores, and during milling procedures. One example is a 1955 patent that is assigned to the Salt Lake City, Utah Kennecott Copper Corporation. Another patent from 1935 is a process by which biological materials (i.e. animal or vegetable cells, drinking water, or organisms) may be purified by treatment with oxidizing or reducing agents (disinfectants). The patent also names pathogenic organisms including anthrax, which may be removed from skin, fascia, muscle, bone, hair, hemp, cotton, linen, hides, leather, wood products, ivory, wool fur, cloth, etc. This seems to loosely admit that the anthrax agent includes a sulfur-reducing extremophile bacterium.[38,39]

Another Kennecott Copper Corporation (NY) patent filed in 1972 describes the recovery of metals including copper from wellbores (deep well bore holes) which access copper ores from sulfur deposits hundreds of feet below the earth's surface. From the patent we read important statements about sulfur-tolerant extremophiles:

> "Detailed investigations have demonstrated that two strains of bacteria, namely the *Thiobacillus ferrooxidans* and the *Thiobacillius thiooxidans, are present in mine water*...The *Thiobaccilus ferrooxidans* are capable of oxidizing dissolved ferrous iron to the ferric state, while the *Thiobaccillus thiooxidans* are capable of oxidizing elemental sulfur to sulfuric acid. Both strains will oxidize thiosulfate to sulfuric acid." The patent continues: "In addition, for as yet unknown reasons, *some organic compounds help increase their activity; one such compound is Tween-20.*"[40-41]

We will discuss Tweens and their ability to aggregate and enhance the growth activity of bacteria – in this case the sulfur-reducing extremophiles found in acid mine wastes (sulfidophiles), and water, mineral, oil, or gas wellbores. This technique of recovering minerals or metals from bore holes drilled into underground deposits is called *in situ* mining. Chemicals or other leaching solutions are pumped into the bore holes, after which the dissolved minerals are pumped to the surface. Other techniques used to leach materials use bacteria, air/oxygen, sulfur dioxide, electrolytic oxidation, ultrasound, and photochemicals. Xray diffraction (scattered Xrays) are used to detect subsurface deposits, and may include Xray cameras (fluoroscopes*) or other devices. [40,41,59-64]

**Thomas Edison is credited with developing the first fluoroscope which used Xrays to produce radiographs. Edison's associates were Henry Ford and Nikola Tesla. His rival George Westinghouse established General Electric. GE eventually absorbed Edison General Electric in 1892, a company that Thomas Edison founded in 1878 in New York with J.P. Morgan and the Vanderbilt family. GE of course would go on to become part of the Manhattan Project and a major player in the development of nuclear energy and atomic weapons.*

In the laboratory, synchrotrons are used for Xray diffraction to analyze core samples and mineral crystals. This is important because Xrays produced in the lab are thousands or millions of times more powerful than those of typical medical Xrays. Uranium can be mined using the in situ method, and this is one of the most common methods used for subsurface mining in many countries including the US, Canada, Kazakhstan (Russia), Czech Republic, UK, and Australia. The problem however is that this mining/leaching/removal process acidifies the groundwater, and pollutes underground aquifers, the microbes that live there, and the rivers and streams fed by these water tables.[40,41,59-64]

When we discuss the extremophiles, we must consider there are at least three genetically engineered strains of *Deinococcus radiodurans* which were isolated and cloned from wild strains of the sulfur-reducer *Thiobacillus ferrooxidans.* Perhaps the three genomic groups of *Borrelia burgdorferi* are those that are delineated by their wild or recombinantly created thermophiles. Since a number of thermophiles and extremophiles exist, more than likely the various Bb strain types include some kind of a thermophile or extremophile bacterium (i.e. paenibacillus, thiobacillus, deinococcus, clostridium, etc.), either natural or recombinant in origin. We will discuss how the recombinant *Deinococcus radiodurans* may also incorporate genes from a thermophile blue-green algae that is highly valuable and important to genetic engineering, and that is called *Taq polymerase*.[34-37]

The *Cyanobacteria* are also extremely important to our story. These are the blue-green algae-like bacteria that are found in water and soils. Some cyanobacteria live in animal fur or in plants. Cyanobacterial colonies may form filaments, balls, or sheets. They have a gelatinous cell wall, and they are nitrogen fixers which convert nitrogens into a form that can be readily taken up by plants. One example of a nitrogen fixer useful for fertilizers is *Anabaena*, a symbiont of an aquatic fern that is used to fertilize rice paddies in northern Italy. Some cyanobacteria produce *cyanotoxins* which are neurotoxic to animals and humans. Other cyanobacteria have been known to cause Amyotrophic Lateral Sclerosis (ALS or Lou Gehrig's disease), and this is important because *Borrelia burgdorferi* spirochetes are found in some Lyme patients who suffer from ALS. But then again this may simply prove that Bb spirochetes have incorporated the genes of cyanobacteria. The question is whether these bacteria are wild, or lab-created clones that contain cyanobacteria from genetically modified thermophiles.[44-48]

Anabaena and other nitrogen-fixing bacteria (i.e. *Klebsiella, Rhodospirillum, Clostridium*) have been cloned into *E. coli* to increase nitrogen fixation for agricultural crops such as soybeans; and have been used within insecticides. Nitrogen fixers are used not only to improve crop yields, but when combined with yeasts and fungi, help degrade chemicals in the pesticidal formulas including persisting organochlorine compounds. The cyanobacteria are also a target of disinfectant formulas which contain amines, and that are used to clean industrial water systems, paints, oils, rubber, fabrics, bandages, coatings, potable water, swimming pools, hot tubs, and nuclear cooling towers. From one disinfectant patent:[49]

> "The biocidal efficacy of poly-1,3-dichloro-5-methyl-5-(4'-vinylphenyl)hydantoin (1a) against microorganisms which are potential pathogens in potable water on spacecraft during long-term missions was evaluated..."[50]
>
> The patent continues: "The species tested were *Pseudomonas cepacia* (a gram negative rod), *Klebsiella pneumoniae* (a gram negative rod that forms capsules), *Staphylococcus epidermidis* (a gram positive coccus), *Methylobacterium radiotolerans* (a large gram negative rod that forms vacuoles), and *Bacillus thuringiensis* (a gram positive rod that forms endospores)."[50]

Methylobacterium is an important soil bacteria found in potatoes and other tubers like cassava that are treated with B.t. and fungi-containing insecticides. Methylobacterium infections have been reported in HIV/AIDS patients, and readers may want to study the section on HIV/AIDS in my book *God Science* for its connections to cassava, geminiviruses, and agricultural pesticides.[50-54]

The thermophile *Thermus aquaticus* is widely used for its DNA polymerase enzyme, for example in polymerase chain reaction (PCR) diagnostic tests. The organism lives in geothermal vents and springs; it can synthesize filaments, and withstand elevated temperatures. Its enzyme is known as *Taq polymerase* or *Taq pol* and is *one of the most profitable agents of genetic engineering science*. Patents for this enzyme are currently held by Hoffmann-La Roche. Taq polymerase is widely used in forensics, PCR testing, and HIV virus testing. It is also used to manufacture DNA at higher temperatures, for all kinds of industries. This is intensely important to our story if *Borrelia burgdorferi* spirochetes are ever proven to contain Taq polymerase genes from genetically engineered thermophile bacteria; especially if those bacterium came from nuclear, mining, bioremediation, or agricultural products or processes.

Is the presence of recombinant Taq pol enzymes from insecticides or other formulas one reason why PCR tests are frowned upon by public health experts for the detection of *Borrelia burgdorferi* spirochetes? Do Bb spirochetes contain Taq polymerase genes from genetically engineered thermophiles; and/or Cry toxin proteins from recombinantly engineered B.t. insecticides?[55]

A while ago I mentioned the synthetic actinide elements, which are created in nuclear reactors. There are fifteen of these, and they may or may not be important when we explore the number of *Borrelia burgdorferi* sensu lato strain groups that were known by the time a patent to detect Lyme disease was filed. Remember that the number fifteen may also be important to us because it may represent the number of original B.t. "parent" insecticidal formulas that have been globally applied. We do not know whether Bb strains include radioactive elements from wastewaters or soils. If they do, perhaps they include one each of the actinide elements that have been created in nuclear reactors or particle accelerators (or more rarely as nuclear fallout). Note there are also natural uranium, plutonium and thorium elements. These are the synthetically created actinides, along with their atomic name; all of which are radioactive:

Actinium (Ac)	Thorium (Th)	Protactinium (Pa)
Uranium (U)	Neptunium (Np)	Plutonium (Pu)
Americium (Am)	Curium (Cm)	Berkelium (Bk)
Californium (Cf)	Einsteinium (Es)	Fermium (Fm)
Mendelevium (Md)	Nobelium (No)	Lawrencium (Lr)

Synthetic actinides and other radioisotopes are only present in the environment because of detonated nuclear weapons, or as discharged nuclear laboratory or reactor wastes. Synthetic transuranium elements can also be synthesized in nuclear reactors. The following transuranium elements were artificially created in nuclear reactors, followed by year of creation.

Neptunium, 1940	Plutonium, 1941	Curium, 1944	Berkelium, 1949
Californium, 1950	Einsteinium, 1952	Ferrinium, 1952	Mendelevium, 1955
Nobelium, 1965	Lawrencium, 1961, 1971		

A Russian article described a study that was undertaken to determine the concentration of radionuclides (radioisotopes) and heavy metals and their effect upon the chromosomes of submerged plants found in the highly polluted Yenisei River, in Central Siberia. The river has been subjected to the effects of radioactive mining and production wastes from one of the largest nuclear weapons production facilities in Russia, the fully underground Mining and Chemical Combine (MCC), which was founded in 1950. Artificially created radionuclides present real dangers to public health, and the MCC produced weapons-grade plutonium from irradiated uranium for many years, which leached wastes into the soil and groundwater. The MCC is located in Zheleznogorsk, although it was previously secretly known as Krasnoyarsk-26, PO-9, or SocCity. The reactors there were used continually in the post-war period to provide electricity and heat to the Tomsk-7 and Krasnoyarsk-26 regions. The decommission process began in 2003 when the Russian and American governments signed an agreement to shut down the facility's reactors over the course of the next decade.[65-70]

The results of the Russian study may serve as a model to understand the negative impact of nuclear wastes and heavy metals when combined upon the chromosomes of microbes in soils and water tables. What is produced as radioactive wastes, fallout from nuclear weapons deployments, or nuclear accidents (i.e. Chernobyl), includes cesium, strontium, plutonium, and other radioactive isotopes that exert powerful activity upon the microbes and higher organisms that are exposed to same. In the presence of heavy metals and POPs, these isotopes have increased mutagenic effects upon chromosomes of all living organisms, from the smallest microbes to those of the human race.

Another important contributing factor to nuclear "wastes" is the presence of uranium and thorium in agriculturally applied fertilizers, chemicals; and the plants that have been "engineered" to contain radioactive tracers. Wastewaters have been irradiated to kill bacteria. Seeds, microbes, insects, spices, and foods are irradiated to kill microbes. Any of these nuclear elements have the potential to alter the genes of microbes and the insects that come into contact with them.

According to an International Atomic Energy Agency (AIEA) report, the induction of mutations using culture techniques in the laboratory is a process commonly used to improve (crop) plant resistance to diseases and insects. The report calls mutation induction a successful way of widening genetic diversity in crops; although mutation is referred to as a "random phenomenon." The report reveals that gamma irradiation is applied to pollen, beans, and vegetative buds; and to cocoa plants. It also cites gamma irradiation as a means to breed cocoa plants to be resistant to the cocoa swollen shoot virus (CSSV). This disease was noted as early as the 1930s in Guana (British Virgin Islands).

It is most curious that along with the irradiation of plants and insects, products, and foods; has come the emergence of new spiroplasmas including the Cocos spiroplasma. This is a spiroplasma strain that was said in a 1983 Yale Journal publication to be derived from *Cocos nucifera* or the coconut palm. It also has a plasmid (mini chromosome) that is similar to other spiroplasmas including corn stunt, and the tick spiroplasma 277F agent. We know now that spiroplasmas are found in the bodies of ticks that transmit Lyme disease and other infections. What we don't know for certain is whether Bb spirochetes and their possible spiroplasma component are a product of agricultural, industrial, and nuclear wastes – but they certainly appear to be.[56-58]

The Fluoride Whitewash

When we examine the industries responsible for the production of bauxite, phosphates, aluminum, uranium, and other important commodities; we see a lengthy history that involves fluorides. We find organofluorides, chlorides, and phosphates in agricultural products; in fluoridated water to "prevent cavities"; and in industrial wastes. Many industries over the past century and a half have generated substantial quantities of fluoride as industrial waste, as byproducts of manufacturing nuclear fuels (i.e. ingot production, enrichment, reactors); from mining, smelting; and as industrial and agricultural chemicals. In earlier days, fluoride toxicity lawsuits were successful because of the known toxic effects of fluoride wastes upon crops, animals, and people. Expensive lawsuits would have continued unchecked and likely ruined industries unless something could be done to stop them.

The only way to end the ongoing threats to numerous industries which belched out toxic fluoride wastes was to change the public's perceptions. To do so, industries set about changing public opinion through a positive public relations campaign and the initiation of public health education campaigns about fluoride. Without these efforts, the truth about the hazards of fluoride could have threatened industries ad nauseum. Such a situation would have been the downfall of many industries, none the least of which were the Manhattan Project and the fertilizer industry – the latter which the US government entered into with the Tennessee Valley Authority Act of May 18, 1933. The TVA was part of President Franklin D. Roosevelt's "new deal" in Congress.[1-5]

The TVA agency was created to be "a corporation clothed with the power of the government but possessed of the flexibility and initiative of a private enterprise." The tasks assigned to the TVA included malaria prevention, flood control, improved crop yields and wildlife habitats; power production, navigation, reforestation, and erosion control. The latter was necessary following the 1930s Dust Bowl which affected the Great Plains and Midwestern states. The new TVA agency was established at Muscle Shoals, Alabama: "in the interests of the national defense and for agricultural development, and to improve navigation in the Tennessee River and to control the destructive flood water in the Tennessee River and Mississippi River Basins."[1-5]

In the US, potassium fertilizer production began during World War I, increased in 1931, and surged again in 1958. A US bureau of mines survey during the mid-1990s showed that potash producers were located in New Mexico, Mississippi, Utah, Texas, California, and Michigan; and in Canada (Toronto, Saskatchewan). Overseas mines were located in Russia and Belarus; and Chile, China, Great Britain, Japan, Jordan, and Thailand. The largest region of potash consumers in the US has been the midwest (Illinois, Indiana, Iowa, Missouri, Ohio); followed by the Great Lakes region (Michigan, Minnesota, Wisconsin). In third place are the southeastern states (Alabama, Florida, Georgia, South Carolina).[6-14]

German nitrogen and ammoniated fertilizer production began in 1898. The first synthetic fertilizer was made using calcium nitrate in 1903. The first manufacturing plant using the *Cyanamide* process was constructed at Westeregeln, Germany in 1905. An Italian plant was built in 1906, and the fertilizer industry came to North America with the construction of a plant at Niagara Falls, Ontario by North American Cyanamid Limited. By 1913 the first synthetic ammonia plant began operations in Oppau, Germany. By 1920, Germany I.G. Farben entered the urea fertilizer industry. In the US, an ammonia nitrate fertilizer plant was constructed at Muscle Shoals, Alabama in 1918. Two years later, the Atmospheric Nitrogen Corporation built an ammonia fertilizer plant in Syracuse, New York.[15-18]

By the 1930s, Du Pont in Belle, West Virginia was also producing urea fertilizers. The Shell Chemical Company began researching ammonia-amended soil and irrigation water in 1932, one year before the establishment of the Tennessee Valley Authority Act that would significantly impact the fertilizer industry and allow the government to join this booming industry.[15-18]

The TVA was given the power to develop better agricultural fertilizers and to convey or lease two of its nitrate plants and its Waco, Texas quarry with the approval of the War Department and the President. It also allowed the TVA board to manufacture and sell fixed nitrogen, fertilizer, and fertilizer ingredients at its Muscle Shoals plant. Under TVA authority the board could donate or sell fertilizer products to: "the agency of county demonstration agents, agricultural colleges, or other as the board may direct, for experimentation, education, and introduction of the use of such products."[15-18]

Besides phosphate rock, another agriculturally important rock is the aggregate bauxite, which is found near phosphates. Bauxite is the main source of *alumina,* which is commercially processed to make *aluminum* products. The clays where it is found typically contain high levels of phosphate, uranium, other radioactive minerals; fluorites (fluoride); thermophile bacteriae, and reoviruses. Even before bauxite is processed, this essential material is as precious and valuable a natural resource as gold, which is often found nearby. Bauxite is also found near granite and phosphate rock. During bauxite processing, the alumina is mixed with a flux made of *sodium fluoride* and cryolite, which releases the aluminum. Toxic waste gases such as hydrogen fluoride are expelled during metal processing.[19-25]

Bauxite is used in resin coated sand (proppants), to reduce viscosity of liquids for the gasoline and oil industries. It is used in wastewater treatment plants, brick manufacturing, as a catalyst; and in abrasives, cements, absorbants, and fertilizers. Bauxite is used to treat acid mine wastes, and in refractories (i.e. kilns, crucibles, incinerators, reactors). It is an excellent soil amendment, because it sequesters metals. Bauxite has anti-caking and anti-sticking properties and is used in fertilizer as a filler and stabilizer. It has high alkalinity and contains iron oxides, aluminum, and titanium.[19-25]

In fertilizers, bauxite helps maintain and control the growth rate of bacteria, and the growth rate of *crystalline* substances. This may include the crystal (Cry) toxins which belong to the globally applied insecticide *Bacillus thuringiensis* (B.t.). Bauxite is also used to process manufactured food sugars including beet sugars and sugar cane (sucrose) because it aids in crystal formation during the refining process. The Defense National Stockpile Center sells tons of refractory-grade bauxite from its stockpiles. We can see now how bauxite is one of the world's most important natural resources.[19-25]

In 1938 President Franklin Delano Roosevelt began the restoration of the country's phosphate-deficient agricultural soils following the great American Dust Bowl by encouraging farmers to use phosphate fertilizers. In a manner of speaking the US government would enter the fertilizer industry. Phosphate rock is made into fertilizer, and is processed and sold in an ammoniated form as well. Between the mined phosphates and the synthetic chemicals, agricultural fertilizers became a booming global business by the 1930s.[26-33]

The TVA board also developed a process to defluorinate rock phosphate (remove fluorides) which could be fed to cattle as a feed supplement because there was a shortage of food-grade bone meal. Early attempts at feeding cattle raw rock phosphate were "usually met with disaster" due to the toxic effects of high fluoride level phosphates. Cattle developed poor health, stiffness, and joint problems, badly worn and cold-sensitive teeth, reduced milk production, and a decreased appetite. As a result tricalcium phosphate was used as a phosphorus supplement for cattle because of its reduced (but not absent) fluoride content. Tricalcium phosphate also appears in human food products today including table salt, baking powders, and oral healthcare products.[34]

During World War II, fertilizer plants were converted, and additional ammonia plants were built to provide the ammonium nitrate necessary for ammunition production. As the war ended, fertilizers returned to their agricultural purpose as manufacturers concentrated on increasing crop yields to feed the expanding global population. Industries that manufactured and processed these materials, and those that produced fluoride wastes rapidly became implicated as contributors to *fluoride poisoning* in workers, crops, animals, and people living near these industries.[15-18,35]

The phosphate fertilizer industry has been a long-term producer of uranium. From 1952 to 1962, a Joliet, Illinois phosphate plant produced roughly two million pounds of uranium for the US government's nuclear program.* With the US atomic energy program underway before and during WWII, the successful elimination of its toxic wastes including fluorides and other byproducts of plutonium, uranium, or tritium use was critical. Nuclear wastes for decades were disposed of through direct discharge into local water sources, land burial, and through steam emissions. The elimination of fluoride wastes was, and remains an enormously important issue for industries around the world. In order to properly pursue the manufacture of atomic weapons, industries had to establish a "safe" waste disposal system; although standards from decades ago underwent revisions over time, and nuclear wastes that have been improperly stored or disposed of have become a global, not a regional problem.[36-42]

**The Joliet, Illinois reference is interesting, as prisoners incarcerated at Joliet's Stateville Penitentiary were injected with a mosquito-borne malaria during the 1940s, and studied for disease effects. Such early "biowarfare" experiments on humans with an intracellular parasite may have been geared toward vaccines, or studying the effects of fluorides upon insects and the microbes reassorting within them.*

With the help of the aluminum manufacturers, scientists went about attempting to find a disposal method for industry-generated fluoride wastes. Some of the industries who were the worst fluoride producers and those that would be immediately impacted by a positive spin on fluoride wastes were those that mined phosphates for fertilizers; and those that mined or employed ores, aluminum, coal, uranium, bauxite; and other industries. This included coal-burning industries as coal is notoriously responsible for the release of toxic airborne fluorides and harmful particulates.[38]

The Mellon Institute in Pittsburgh, Pennsylvania, was founded by Andrew W. and Richard B. Mellon, former owners of the Aluminum Company of America (ALCOA); a company with large bauxite mines in Arkansas. In the late 1920s in Bauxite, Arkansas, ALCOA chemist Harry Van Osdall Churchill was asked to test water samples from abandoned mining wells because area residents were suffering from yellow stained and mottled teeth. Churchill determined that high levels of fluoride in the groundwater caused the dental problems. He also detected the presence of cryolite, a fluoride-halide aluminum oxide used to produce aluminum, grinding wheels, flux, and other products. (Cryolite is also used in agricultural biocides.) Mottling and staining are symptoms of *fluorisis* or fluoride poisoning. This was not the first time that fluorides were connected to mottled teeth. German dentist Kuehms discovered the link in 1888. In 1901 the mottling of teeth by fluoride would be revisited by Assistant Surgeon J.M. Eager, and reported by Dentist Frederick McKay.[43-48]

ALCOA Chemist Churchill was said to have connected the tooth mottling to fluorides after reading two articles about how calcium fluoride was used to sterilize beer vats because it killed "undesirable" yeast strains. Those who drank beer from the sterilized vats were afflicted with odd bone problems, so brewers stopped using the compound. Beer is made from brewer's yeast, *Saccharomyces cerevisiae,* the same yeast used to ferment agricultural insecticides. Is it possible that calcium fluoride is also used in the fermentation process of B.t. to kill undesirable *S. cerevisiae* strains including "toxic killer strains?"[38-40,43,47-49]

Another problem at this time was a decrease in the public's consumption of sugar in the US. Representatives from the Sugar Institute of New York on behalf of sugar refineries supervised a program by Gerald Judy Cox to invent new uses for sugar. At the end of the program, Cox and colleague Mary L. Dodds invented and patented new industrial sugar applications. These new sugar cane derivatives were marketed by the Niacet Chemicals Corp., aided by the ALCOA-founded Mellon Institute. Some of the new uses included as perfume additives and lacquer dissolvers. We must not dismiss the sugar refining industry or its source plant, sugar beets. Neither should we forget the insects that are their pests (i.e. leafhoppers, planthoppers) and the pathogens found within them (i.e. mosaic viruses, yellows diseases, spiroplasmas, phytoplasmas, etc.).[50-59]

The Mellon Institute was an industry-friendly laboratory where a flurry of research was undertaken in efforts to demonstrate a beneficial use for industrial fluorides. Academic laboratories such as the Universities of Cincinnati, Tennessee, and Wisconsin were provided with grant funding from 1940 through 1960 by chemical giants to "create a favorable climate of opinion" for fluoride use. Some of these companies included ALCOA, the American Petroleum Institute, E.I. du Pont de Nemours Co., Harshaw Chemical Co., Kaiser Aluminum and Chemical Corp., Pennsylvania Salt Manufacturing Co., Reynolds Metals Co., Tennessee Valley Authority, and Universal Oil Products Co. Some of these companies were already among the worst industry offenders responsible for dumping fluoride compounds, fluorine gases, and other toxic chemicals into the environment.[48]

At this time Cox was looking at animal consumption of fluorides. He studied the effects of feeding fluorides to pregnant and lactating rats, and the effects of fluorides on the teeth of their offspring. It is said that when Cox interpreted his data, he may have mistaken his findings, which when interpreted differently, may have changed the outcome of recommendations he and other scientists made about the "safety" of fluoride. Cox and colleagues also undertook experiments with rats fed a diet of waste liquors from the milk industry that was donated by the Borden Company. Borden held a new patent for chemically separated dry skim milk which used fluoridated water. At this point in history, the use of fluorides in food products including the inexpensive powdered milk was still negatively stigmatized by fluoride's widely-known tooth mottling effects.[50-55,60-65]

Although Cox was not the principal individual responsible for implementing water fluoridation, he was one of its most influential advocates. In the early 1940s, Cox became a member of the Food and Nutrition Board of the National Research Council and subsequently other state health departments, and continued advocating for water fluoridation. A small group of scientists from Harvard, the American Dental Association, the National Academy of Sciences, and the Kettering Laboratory of the University of Cincinnati, were also heavily promoting water fluoridation. (The US government had by now passed the TVA Act and had its own interests in fluoride waste-producing fertilizers.)[50-55,60-65]

Dr. Robert Kehoe was by then Director of the Kettering Laboratory and medical director for the Ethyl Corporation. He was also a consultant for the TVA (which owned or operated three nuclear plants to generate electricity); and for the Atomic Energy Commission, the US Air Force, and the Division of Occupational Medicine of the Public Health Service. The aforementioned scientific group provided what may appear to some to be biased statements that were highly favorable for fluoride use in a booklet the team jointly created. The booklet was published by the Public Health Service (PHS) and the American Dental Association (ADA). The group called itself the *Committee to Protect Our Children's Teeth* and was largely funded by the US government's public health service.[41,48,60-74]

The Kettering laboratory's specialty was the investigation of the hazards of industrial chemicals. Its research was funded in part by some of the top fluoride waste-producing companies including ALCOA. In the booklet, a list of signators in support of water fluoridation included individuals from chemical or mining companies. Companies listed in the booklet included Merck, DuPont, American Cyanamid, International Minerals and Metals, Minnesota Mining and Manufacturing (3M), Allied, Harshaw Chemical, Armour and Carbide and Carbon Chemicals; and the Atomic Energy Commission at Oak Ridge. Kettering scientist E.J. Largent also published a book titled *Fluorosis: The Health Aspects of Fluorine Compounds* which was designed specifically to "aid industry in law suits arising from fluoride damage" according to the verbiage on the cover of the book. The booklet strongly minimized or discounted the toxic effects of fluoride on the human body. This booklet was used to thwart all further industrial fluoride-related lawsuits for decades. Dr. Largent subsequently became a consultant for the Reynolds Metals Company.[41,48,60-74]

In 1931, the head of the laboratory of the Dental Hygiene Unit at the National Institutes of Health, Dr. H. Trendley Dean looked into tooth mottling from fluorisis and began epidemiological surveys. Once the idea of adding fluoride wastes to drinking water was adopted at a "safe" level of <1 ppm (parts per million), field studies began in 1945 in Grand Rapids and Muskegon, Michigan; in Newburgh and Kingston, New York; in Evanston and Oak Park, Illinois; and Brandford and Sarnia, Ontario, Canada. The road to public water fluoridation proved to be rocky, mostly because of those who opposed the chemical treatment of drinking water for its possible adverse health effects.[49,75-78]

Strangely enough, Dr. Dean who at first opposed water fluoridation due to its potential toxicity, changed his mind about its negative health effects, and became a fluoridation advocate. He subsequently became the first Director of the National Institutes of Dental Research (NIDR) and in 1953 he was a key official at the American Dental Association (ADA). Both of these organizations, probably under the influence of Dr. Dean, became strong advocates of water fluoridation. Observers speculate on the relationship of Dr. Dean and his employer's interests and the change in his stance on the matter.[48,79]

From 1950 to 1951, the ALCOA Company advertised their fluoride products in a water works industry magazine, although the company claimed later that it was not promoting fluoride for water fluoridation, nor was it selling the product directly to municipalities for that purpose. And yet an ad in the publication had this to say: "Fluoridate your water with CONFIDENCE. Use high purity ALCOA SODIUM FLUORIDE."[51]

It may appear that the company was vying for municipal sales however it could also have been advertising the use of its fluorides to the dye industry, which used chromium fluoride. According to testimony before the US Congressional hearings on water fluoridation, Committee on Interstate and Foreign Commerce, ALCOA was behind the tremendous push for water fluoridation. Perhaps this is because it would profit upon the disposal of industry wastes in a kind of waste "recycling" process. In 1944, attorney Oscar Ewing was placed on the ALCOA payroll at an annual salary of $750,000, a tremendous sum in those days. This placement was curious since ALCOA had no meaningful litigation pending at the time of his appointment. Was the move precautionary, or for future interests? A few months later Ewing became Federal Security Administrator for the Public Health Service. Prior to Ewing joining the PHS, Andrew Mellon, one of ALCOA's co-founders, had been US Treasurer.[41-44,46,51,52,78-81,86,103]

Observers may speculate as to how the roles of Trendley Dean and other colleagues of the Dental Division of the PHS under direction of Ewing may have played a role in promoting water fluoridation as a public health "benefit." Once limits for water fluoridation were established at <1 ppm, then deemed a "safe" level to prevent fluoride intoxication (poisoning), Ewing gave the green light to begin prospective field studies with fluoride-treated drinking water despite a lack of long-term safety studies.

It is easy to see how the byproducts of aluminum smelting, nuclear, fertilizer, textiles, foods, and other manufacturing processes could produce "favorable" and "safe" research study outcomes, especially where conflicts of interest might enter the process. The Kettering laboratory, like many academic and government laboratories, depended in part on government grants from sources such as the National Institutes of Health and the Public Health Service. It seems that even to the present day, the influence of government and industry persists as we witness industry-sympathetic executives installed at the highest levels of government regulatory agencies. There key individuals make important decisions that will not only affect a nation of citizens and industries, but which could be biased toward industrial desires or long-term objectives above the needs of public health.[44,51,74,75]

For something so often cited as "safe," the evidence appears overwhelmingly in opposition of the "fluoride is non-toxic" party line. Most of the initial scientific evidence proving fluoride's "safety" for human use was generated by scientists of the atomic energy program. This included scientists at the University of Rochester where covert human radiation experiments were undertaken. Dr. Harold Carpenter Hodge helped orchestrate human uranium and plutonium experiments; and was a leading defender of water fluoridation. He was also Chief toxicologist for the *Manhattan Project.* There his responsibilities included the investigation of the "safety" of the toxic chemicals used to make nuclear weapons, including the fluorides and other byproducts that would be discharged in nuclear wastewaters and in evaporative cooling towers or steam vents. Extensive fluoride-related investigations were undertaken as they applied to nuclear research and to the Manhattan Project, but the results of those studies have remained strictly confidential for decades under claims of "national security."[87-101]

Central Florida is a huge producer for the US phosphate industry, and its gypsum stacks (phosphate/fluoride slurry and wastes) are estimated to be nearly one billion metric tons in size. These wastes, which contain radioactive elements (i.e. radium/radon, uranium) sit around in huge piles because there is no place to dispose of them without further processing. As these products degrade, caustic compounds leach into the soil and groundwater. Some of these wastes are buried underground, some are recycled, and others sit degrading in the Florida sun. For every pound of commercial fertilizer, approximately five pounds of contaminated phosphogypsum slurry remains. The waste compounds considered useful after processing are sold to US communities as water fluoridation agents. These agents are the *silicofluorides* which typically include *hydrofluosilicic acid, sodium silicofluoride,* or *sodium fluoride.* There these otherwise toxic waste compounds are suddenly not considered to be either toxic wastes or pollutants. In a manner of speaking, what is considered to be toxic industrial waste is recycled to treat human drinking water and table salt that people the world over have been consuming for generations in the name of "public health."[20,49,54-58]

Fluoride Pollution and Toxic Effects

An important subject to discuss is the effect of fluorides upon the microbes that are important to public health; and the effects of fluorides in the body. The flood of fluoride-supportive research articles over decades is startling when we consider the conflicts of interest that were likely present with academic scientists who were supported by industry grant funding. We can only speculate on whether these individuals might manufacture or massage research papers to a predetermined, industry-favorable "consensus" endpoint. Such an endpoint is hardly unexpected if we consider that fluorides and the products which contain them have a direct impact upon the microbes that reside in the soil, water, foods, and industries upon which we depend to live.

After many decades of water fluoridation, in 1975 the US Food and Drug Administration determined that fluoride was suddenly *"not generally recognized as safe."* However fluoride in several forms today remains an additive to municipal and industrial water supplies in nearly 70% of American cities and in a few foreign countries. It is also routinely added to foods, oral health products, and table salt. The CDC has called the fluoridation of drinking water "one of the greatest public health achievements in the 20th Century." It may instead prove over time, to have been one of the most unfortunate practices ever undertaken.[41,44,46,51,52,78-82,86]

It is most curious that in 1975 the FDA would suddenly declare fluoride to be "unsafe." This was the very same year that the "juvenile arthritis" outbreak in Connecticut was announced – an outbreak that would later be called Lyme disease. Lyme disease is also an illness that produces most of the symptoms seen in cases of fluoride toxicity, or *fluorosis*. With respect to microbes, we need to know that research papers clearly demonstrate how *in the presence of fluorides, bacteriae such as Streptococcus species are able to mutate.*[51,53-58,102-111]

From the very beginning of the Connecticut outbreak, did public health experts discover a link between the pollution of soil or water-borne spirochetes, water fluoridation, and the interactions of fluoride agrochemicals, industrial fluoride wastes, and microbes that cause human disease? It is strange to think there may be a connection, or perhaps it is merely coincidental, that those who became ill with "juvenile arthritis" (Lyme) also happened to live in communities on the shores of the Connecticut River. There they would be among the first in the country to be exposed to the newly implemented public health policy of water fluoridation.* This was also the first population to be exposed to the new viruses that were released in the area during the 1950s as insecticide boosters. By the way, the outbreak of Lyme disease in Connecticut occurred not far from the Millstone nuclear plant on the Thames River in Waterford.[102-109]

**US water fluoridation began in 1945 in New York and Michigan. Wisconsin began adding fluoride to water in 1946. Connecticut became the first state to implement state-wide water fluoridation in 1965, all periods of time which preceded cases of Lyme disease in Wisconsin (1968), and the juvenile arthritis outbreak in Connecticut.*

A slide presentation that discussed the WHO guidelines for recreational water environments indicated that the public health safety hazards of water environments are gastroenteritis, acute febrile respiratory illness, and ear infections. These infections are said to arise from the *pollution of water leptospires (spirochetes),* and from human contact with toxic bacteria in fresh and marine waters. This "pollution" of water leptospires and the presence of toxic microbes are important facts to which public health officials have long been aware. Just three years after juvenile arthritis was announced, from September 1, 1978 to September 30, 1979, scientists from the Connecticut University Health Center in Farmington studied the effect of low levels of fluorides upon bacterial metabolism, bacterial attachment, and dental caries.[112-114]

The "dental" reference would certainly have also applied to skeletal structures, including the study of microbes that can bind to the fluorides that bind to our bones and teeth. The report abstract had this to say about stannous fluoride, a compound used in toothpaste, "Hence, at the therapeutic release goal of 1-2ppm, the effect of fluorides would not be due to killing of the organisms." The idea that animal leptospires can be opened by the action of agricultural and industrial chemicals (and other microbes) will become important to the story when we learn about a novel mutated leptospira that was found in the body of a Lyme patient from Connecticut immediately before the Lyme disease agent was formally announced. This spirochete was identified and named, however it was *never announced as being part of the Lyme disease spirochete.* A study by Dr. Allen Steere and his colleagues which would reveal this mutated spirochete would not be published until several years later. The agent was not discussed at the Dearborn conference in 1994 where Dr. Steere's recommendations would help standardize surveillance case descriptions and diagnostic testing for Lyme disease for decades to come.[112-114]

Any so-called "beneficial" effects of fluoride against the sugars which cause tooth decay appear to come from an inhibition of bacterial enzymes, or mutagenic action toward bacterial cells. From a 1979 grant abstract we read:

> "The next phase of the study was to establish the lowest level of various fluoride solutions which had an effect on the bacterial acid production of *Streptococcus mutans,* a known cariogenic organism which produces caries by its release of acid...Electron dense bodies, identified as tin by electron microprobe, found in bacterial cells exposed to 5ppm fluoride as SnF2, gives strong indirect evidence that *fluorides, even in trace amounts, become concentrated in the bacterial cells.* Furthermore, the bacterial cells exposed to 5ppm SnF2 showed *other ultrastructural changes within the cell compatible with altered growth of these cells.*"[113]

The quote admits that *microbes take up fluorides into their cells*, and that *fluorides cause mutations*. We might think about the concentration of fluorides, nuclear isotopes, heavy metals, and persisting pollutants in microbial cells, and what their presence means in terms of altering cellular chromosomes to create mutant microbes. The public health service raised the standards for "safe" levels of fluoride in drinking water from <1ppm to <2 ppm during the 1960s, but then suddenly increased these "safe" levels to <4 ppm in 1985. We can see from studies that at 5 ppm, bacterial cells which also contain tin were structurally affected by fluoride. Other bacterial cells that contain other metals may also be adversely affected. Perhaps the PHS <4 ppm limit was changed as a best-guess estimate of the most effective limit for bacterial inhibition, while hopefully avoiding the mutation of living bacteria. This significantly higher level could also facilitate the disposal of increased levels of industrial fluoride wastes, and unfortunately correspondingly raise the levels of fluoride exposures in animals and humans.[113,114]

Double and triple superphosphate fertilizers were developed and began global use during the 20th century. We will learn more about their activity upon soil minerals and plants later. Their technical names include calcium dihydrogen phosphate, and monocalcium phosphate. Non-agricultural uses of triple superphosphates include animal feed supplements (monocalcium phosphate) and as an ingredient in baking powders for baked goods (tricalcium phosphate). Our bodies are made up of phosphates in our bones and teeth, and we need phosphorus to synthesize B vitamins. Synthetic tricalcium phosphate is added to sugars, salts, dry mixes, granular foods, and packeted and bottled sauces. Organofluoride products also include dyes, poisons, agrochemicals, pharmaceuticals, refrigerants, persisting organic pollutants, and surfactants. I find it most interesting that some Lyme patients are highly reactive ("allergic") to tricalcium phosphate, phosphoric acid dental etch, foods which contain synthetic phosphates; and medical phosphate salts. Either there is a contact allergy or perhaps the microbes react adversely to these chemicals.[85]

In 2005 the FDA withdrew its approval of fluoroquinolone (fluoridated) antibiotics used in poultry to treat respiratory diseases. *The indiscriminate use of fluoride-containing antibiotics in chickens and turkeys led to the mutation of bacteriae which have also become antibiotic resistant.* This includes a fluoroquinolone-resistant strain of *Campylobacter,* which produces gastrointestinal infections. We may wonder what other poultry microbes might have been adversely affected by fluoridated antibiotics, or fluoridated drinking water fed to poultry. The literature clearly shows that *bacteriae and viruses can mutate in the presence of fluorides.* This may be related to the chemical itself or because fluorides are found in geothermal veins where we also find radioactive elements and their byproducts of decay. [115-124]

This mutation process can also occur in the soil as a result of the applied chemical and microbial fertilizers, herbicides, and pesticides that contain fluorides, trace amounts of uranium or tritium; from radioactive elements used in agricultural chemicals as radiolabels (i.e. chlorpyrifos/tritium); and from the discharge of industrial fluoride wastes. This interest in fluorides makes me wonder if the real problem that scientists are worried about has something to do with chicken cholera gammaproteobacterial genes or retroviruses from recombinant vaccines and the ability of fluorides to mutate in the avian, or human body from a lifetime of exposures to fluoridated water, foods, and oral products.[115-124]

Fluorides can also calcify in the soft tissues of the human body. Because of the uptake of fluorides, people become fluoride toxic over time, which is called *skeletal fluorosis*. The first clue to this was the mottled and yellow-stained teeth of people who drank water with high fluoride levels. Fluoride toxicity produces many of the symptoms that make up chronic illnesses including Lyme disease, Fibromyalgia, Chronic Fatigue Syndrome, etc. When we understand that the *carbon-fluorine bond is the strongest bond in organic chemistry,* we can also understand that what becomes bound to our body tissues and structures, may include chemicals that readily bond with fluorides; as well as the microbes that are mutated by, and which also take up fluorides into their cellular structures.

This means that fluoridated pesticides, herbicides, fungicides, water-repellent oils, pharmaceuticals, anesthetics, laboratory reagents, cancer drugs (5-fluorouracil), catalysts, solvents, surfactants, synthetic and aniline dyes, synthetic polymers, PTFE, PFOA, CFCs, etc. will be taken up by the body along with heavy metals, radioactive particles, and other pollutants. There they will persist as toxins within the soft tissues, teeth, and bones of our body unless and until they are released. Even plastic water bottles may leach perflourinated chemicals into the water we drink, allowing persisting chemicals the opportunity to bind to our skeletal structures.

Of the pharmaceutical products which contain fluorides are *Ciprofloxacin* (Cipro), *Fluconazole* (Diflucan), *Mefloquine* (Lariam); each of which are used to treat Lyme disease. Other fluoride-containing drugs are *Flunitrazepam* (Rohypnol) to treat insomnia, a symptom of Lyme; and *Paroxetine* (Paxil), *Fluoxetine* (Prozac), and *Bupriprion* (Wellbutrin) which are SSRI antidepressants. These drugs are used to treat Lyme disease and a range of mood disorders, including OCD, anxiety, ADD, ADHD, and pre-menstrual disorders – any of which may be exacerbated by fluorosis and the presence of persisting pollutants. The fluorinated molecules from these drugs are commonly found in municipal wastewaters, even after wastewater treatment. From an FDA document that described buproprion use:[83,84,122]

> "Two main ingredients are fluoride and hydrochloric acid, the most caustic, corrosive substances known. These neurotoxins poison the brain, triggering adrenaline, masking symptoms."

While some highly problematic fluoride molecules have been found in mined rocks (i.e. CFCs, a potent greenhouse gas), what may be more important to us is their ability to *bind with fluorides and to be deposited within skeletal structures and soft tissues in the human body.* There they will only be released over time as the demineralization (removal) process occurs in the absence of fluoride intake. Since our bones take up fluorides through dietary and other exposures, they continue to mineralize (add) fluorides at a rate that is much faster than the rate by which our bones demineralize fluorides.

Whatever is bound to the fluorides we take up (chemicals or otherwise), becomes a permanent part of our body unless and until those chemicals are remediated. This may occur naturally over time through the loss of bone; through chemical chelation; or at the hands of spirochetal or other microbial activity (i.e. binding, enzymatic action, or physical drilling). Once released, the levels of circulating fluorides, toxins, and microbes formerly bound to skeletal structures or tissues may contribute to many symptoms. These symptoms may vary each day and are similar to those experienced by people with many chronic illnesses, including those of "unknown origin." Such symptoms may occur in the absence of laboratory detectable infections simply because the body demineralizes skeletal structures over time, which may release stored fluorides and any bound chemical toxins into the body.

5-FU is a fluoride-based anti-metabolite medicine that is used to treat cancers. 5-FU is highly toxic and produces kidney damage, bone marrow suppression, and *central nervous system damage to the myelin sheath and to the spinal cord and peripheral nerves in patients with skeletal fluorosis*. This process is called toxic neuronal injury. In a similar manner, dietary fluoride exposures may also degrade the myelin sheath of the spinal cord, and contribute to diseases such as Multiple Sclerosis in some individuals – especially if the body produces antibodies to circulating myelin proteins.[51,82,123-131]

A friend of mine who lives in Ireland and who has tested positive for several Bb strains, demonstrated antibodies to several myelin proteins which baffled doctors. I wondered whether fluoride-based antibiotics were causing damage to myelin, or whether damage from the physical activity of Bb spirochetes upon skeletal structures was releasing fluorides into the body. There they could have produced a corresponding immune response to the freed fluoride ions in the patient's body. The patient of course would have a lifetime exposure to fluorides from fluoride containing foods, pesticide residues, oral health products, and fluoridated drinking water and table salt.[132,133]

It is interesting to note that the symptoms caused by fluorosis in the following list, are identical to symptoms experienced by people with Lyme disease and other chronic illnesses. Many of these symptoms may be reduced or alleviated over time after removal of all fluoride sources from the diet and personal care products. Symptoms of fluoride toxicity (poisoning), are derived from many scientific sources and include the following:

Mouth ulcers	Stomach and intestinal complaints
Abdominal pain	Flatulence
Nausea	Bloating (possible "IBS")
Muscle weakness	Migraine-like headaches
Visual disturbances	Tinnitus
Mental depression	Hyperplasia of Parathyroid glands
Convulsions Chronic	Fatigue not relieved by sleep
Excessive thirst	Dryness of mouth or throat not relieved by water consumption
Frequent urination	Arthritis-like aches, pains in back, neck, jaw, arms, shoulders, legs, knees
Urinary infections	Muscle twitches, spasms
Nervousness	Tingling sensations (paraesthesias) in hands and feet
Loss of balance	Dizziness
Brittle hair, nails, hair loss	Blind spots in visual field
Diarrhea	Skin rashes or itching, especially after showering
Flu-like symptoms	Inability to focus
Loss of cognitive function	Inability to concentrate
Behavioral disorders	Lumbar disc disease of the spine
Osteoarthritis	Chronic emphysema
Gastroduodenitis	Polynephritis
Diabetes	Legs that frequently collapse
Hematuria (blood in urine)	Memory Lapses
Progressive malaise	Dropped articles from numbness, hand pain, or inability to grasp objects
Burning pains in skin	Acute gallbladder attacks not caused by stones or other dysfunctions
Cardiac muscle breakages	Cardiac irregularities, low blood pressure
Calcifications in arteries	Vertigo
Bony protrusions	Muscle atrophy
Underactive thyroid	Enzyme inhibitions
Excess parathyroid hormone	Enlarged pituitary glands in animals
Retinitis	Cataracts
Skeletal fluorosis	Mottled teeth, dental problems
Chromosome damage	Birth defects
Menstrual irregularities	Increased leutinizing hormone levels
Genital irritations	Early onset of menses in children, early breast development
Dermatitis	Urticaria (hives)

Food and medicine "allergies" in people who were formerly not allergic
Hypersensitivities to fluoride dental preparations
Increased inflammation (pro-inflammatory cytokines)
Cancers of thyroid, kidney, stomach, esophagus, colon, rectum, bladder, bone, breast, and leukemias
Chizzola maculae skin bruises that are round/oval, and disappear in 7-10 days. Bruises appear without injury.[51,134-153]

We might consider the Bb spirochete's affinity for bones and other skeletal structures which upon penetration or enzymatic action, may release stored fluorides (and any bound toxins) from our skeletal structures and soft tissues into the blood stream. There the increased levels of circulating fluorides may contribute to the symptoms that Lyme and other chronically ill patients experience. Because the organism itself may have mutated in the presence of fluorides, Bb is probably highly fluoride tolerant. If so, this tolerance may promote resistance to fluoride-derived antibiotics.

Symptoms of Lyme disease (and fluorosis) are highly varied from day to day, and from patient to patient. For obvious reasons, symptoms alone will be only generally helpful in the search for a diagnosis. Still, many of the symptoms for Lyme disease may be derived from an underlying fluorosis problem. This problem may be suddenly activated by the actions of bacterial enzymes. Patients who present with many of these symptoms may be prescribed anti-depressants to help alleviate them. Other patients are offered anti-depressants simply because some physicians wrongly believe that the chronic "illness" being described by the patient, and which happens to be difficult to quantify under standardized laboratory tests, is "all in their head." The real culprit as we can see may be related to the activities of fluorides, bound persisting pollutants, and the activity of fluoride-tolerant, mutated microbes and their enzymes upon the fluoride-soaked skeletal structures and tissues of the body. ❑

> *"The potentialities of biological control, are truly great. That is, 'biological power,' if I may use such a term, is truly as great, in its way, as atomic power is in its way."*
>
> Dr. Edward R. Steinhaus is quoted in a technical report from the November 1, 1960 Conference on Biological Control of Insects of Medical Importance at the American Institute of Biological Sciences (Washington, DC).

Five: Paving Roads with Unknown Intentions

International Interests and the OPs

The first international meetings on microbial controls for agricultural and industrial use (biological controls or biocides) occurred in Prague in 1958. At the time, scientists shared information about microbes and insect pathology and international networking opportunities. The first Commission Internationale de Lutte Biologique* (CILB) meeting was held the same year in Paris. After 1960, national teams were established in the US to study microbial controls and insect pathology on a larger scale than what was previously undertaken. The focus of the studies was agricultural insecticides. Similar large-scale efforts were also undertaken across Europe in France, (former) Czechoslovakia, Germany, and the former USSR.[1-7]

**The first International Commission for Biological Controls.*

In order to share their discoveries, new scientific journals were established including *Entomophaga* (Organisation Internationale de Lutte Biologique) and the *Journal of Invertebrate Pathology*, founded by Dr. Edward A. Steinhaus. Dr. Steinhaus was a former NIH scientist. In 1942 while at Rocky Mountain laboratories in Hamilton, Montana he studied the microbial flora of the Rocky Mountain wood tick. In 1945 Dr. Steinhaus joined the laboratory of insect pathology at the University of California where he and his colleagues studied insect diseases and their usefulness as insecticides. In fact, it would be Dr. Steinhaus who would say the following at a 1960 conference:

> "...the potentialities of biological control, are truly great. That is, 'biological power,' if I may use such a term, is truly as great, in its way, as atomic power is in its way."[1-8]

In 1944 Dr. Steinhaus worked with a virus of the orange sulfur or alfalfa butterfly (*Colias eurytheme*). Successful field trials took place just four years later in an effort to control these pests. Rickettsial organisms identified during the Steinhaus studies included several strains of Rocky Mountain spotted fever, American Q fever (*Rickettsia diaporica* Cox, or *Coxiella burnetii*), and a so-called non-pathogenic rickettsia-like organism. As a result of Steinhaus' studies, it was determined that the alimentary tract of ticks is "invariably sterile." This means they contract infectious microbes from host animals during feeding stages but are otherwise considered to be fairly clean before such infections occur. It was felt that whatever the ticks come into contact with may be transmitted to them, and passed to subsequent hosts during blood meals. Alternative routes of infection are through contact with tick fecal matter, mating, or by passage of infections to offspring through infected eggs.[9-12]

In 1962, a scientific committee was formed to select a work group for a future conference. Two years later with British and French support, the CILB held a meeting in London to coordinate international research efforts and to establish basic techniques for applying a new microbial tool, *Bacillus thuringiensis* (B.t.) as a global insecticide. Also discussed was the importance of safety toward non-targeted species including the general population; and the establishment of manufacturing standards for B.t. toxicity and purity. The CILB entrusted the identification of currently known B.t. strains and the standardization of tests to scientists at the Pasteur Institute in Paris, France.[3]

Four international work group meetings were held between 1958 and 1970. The first group met in Prague in 1958, with participants from seventeen countries. The second meeting was held in Paris in 1962 with more than two dozen countries represented. The third meeting was held in Wageningen, The Netherlands in 1966, and included scientists from fourteen countries. The fourth and final meeting was held in Beltsville, Maryland in 1970, and included one hundred and seventy-seven participants from thirteen countries. Among those who organized the final meeting were individuals from the companies Nutrilite Products Inc.,† the International Minerals and Chemical Corp.,* the International Commission for Biological Controls, the International Union of Biological Sciences, and the USDA Society for Invertebrate Pathology.[3,13,14]

†Nutrilite Products Inc. was a vitamin company founded in a California laboratory that sold America's first multivitamin and mineral supplements. In 1972, controlling interest in Nutrilite Products Inc. was purchased by the Amway Corporation which was already using Nutrilite's marketing plan to sell household products. It is interesting that a vitamin company would have interests in B.t. Consider the effects of B.t. upon the enzyme and hormone systems of the body and the necessity of supplementing nutrient imbalances caused by the effects of the applied insecticides which contained microbes and toxins.

**The International Minerals and Chemical Corp. was founded by a Tennessee phosphate mining entrepreneur named Thomas C. Meadows, then the leading phosphate and fertilizer producer; just behind agricultural giant Cargill. In 1941 the company changed its name and moved from Atlanta to Chicago. In the 1990s the name changed again to IMC Global with >$2 billion in annual revenue. IMC Global and Cargill eventually merged their fertilizer businesses. Now the leading producer of phosphates and fertilizer, the company has plants in Florida.*

Cargill, the largest privately owned agricultural corporation in the world, is based in Minnetonka, Minnesota. It is just southwest of Minneapolis/St. Paul and not far from La Crosse, Wisconsin, its former home. La Crosse is also the home of the former

Cargill-MacMillan homesteads and Gunderson Lutheran Hospital, which is an assignee to a *Borrelia burgdorferi* diagnostic test patent. A Gunderson researcher co-authored a recent article refuting the existence of chronic Lyme disease.[13-16]

A 1970 patent is assigned to the International Minerals & Chemical Corporation (IMC) for a virus insecticide. The invention describes a powdered insecticide formula that contains baculoviruses and iridescent viruses including nuclearpolyhedrosis (NPV), cytoplasmic polyhedrosis (CPV), granulosis (GV), and insect poxviruses. Like many fertilizer and agricultural companies, IMC's history is intrinsically connected to the organophosphate industry.[13-16]

Organophosphates have been declared by the EPA to be highly neurotoxic to animals and humans. "O-Ps" as they are called, have been implicated as the cause of birth defects, leukemia, lymphoma, and childhood brain tumors. Mild or chronic exposures may lead to learning and memory disorders, depression, irritability, headaches, nightmares, sleepwalking, numbness or weakness, tremors, slow reflexes, liver and stomach inflammation, and other symptoms. Acute exposures cause diarrhea, vomiting, cramps, dizziness, blurred vision, confusion, twitching, paralysis, or death. OPs negatively affect the brain and central nervous systems of insects, animals, and humans; and are considered to be endocrine disrupters. Research has even linked OP insecticides used on corn (chlorpyrifos) with attention deficit hyperactivity disorder (ADHD). This pesticide is still used on a wide variety of fruits and vegetables, although chlorpyrifos was banned for residential use in 2001.[16-21]

Rats exposed to the OP insecticide methidathion were shown in a study to suffer ill effects to kidney tissues. These effects were partly reversed after high doses of vitamins C and E. After exposure to this pesticide, decreased cholinesterase activity and increased malondialdehyde levels were observed. Cholinesterase is an enzyme that causes the neurotransmitter acetylcholine to change into choline and acetic acid. This is required for proper nervous system functioning in humans, animals, and insects. We can understand that they are toxic when OP chemicals were originally developed as potent nerve agents for chemical warfare use (i.e. sarin, VX). Inside the human body these agents are converted to metabolites, and they may bind with circulating fluorides. Since our teeth and skeletal structures take up fluorides, it is entirely possible that persisting organic pollutants will bind indefinitely to the structures in our bodies, or that they may be released through the enzymes of microbial infections.[17,22,23]

Two organophosphate insecticides were recently phased out by the EPA due to safety concerns after the implementation of the pesticide reform law of 1996. Diazinon, chlorpyrifos (dursban), and methyl parathion have been banned from foods, although some bug sprays and pest strips may still contain the latter. Beginning in the 1970s, dursban was used to control insects including ticks by spraying directly onto the backs of animals including feedlot cattle. It was also widely used in farm sprays to control crop pests. Its residues appeared on many food crops and remained on pesticide-treated foods. It was also widely used in homes to control fleas, roaches, and termites; and appeared in some animal flea collars. OPs have even been detected in children's toys, as described in a 1998 Rutgers University report. Under pressure from the public, the EPA is continuing to review OPs to determine whether safety concerns necessitate a full ban of these chemicals. Currently however, OPs are still used agriculturally. Like it or not OPs remain a source of exposure in our foods and environment.

Union Carbide (NY) owns one of the oldest organophosphate patents I could find. There are more than twelve hundred patents under the search term "organophosphate" in one database alone. I am certain there are many other patents registered worldwide. I also found an early patent filed in 1971 for purified antibodies. The inventors were from Maryland and the assignee is the US Secretary of the Army. The invention describes a process to recover heterogeneous (non-native) antibodies against a specific antigen or ligand. These are antibodies that belong to different species or substances. Ligands are molecules like antibodies, hormones, or drugs which bind to cellular receptors in the body. According to the patent, the claim is:

> "A method for isolating the total heterogeneous antibody population against antigens…thereby recovering a heterogeneous antibody population against moieties of organophosphates, aromatic acids, sugars, small peptides or neutral antigenic determinants."[24-26]

The patent appears to describe antibodies that can recognize organophosphates. Examples from the patent were these:

> "…the moiety of organophosphate is diethyl-p-nitrophenyl phosphate." (Parathion)
> "…the moiety of organophosphate is 0-pinacolyl methylfluorophosphate." (Soman, a nerve agent)
> "…the moiety of organophosphate is 0,0'-diethyl-0'-p-nitrophenylthiophosphate." (Ethyl Parathion)

The patent also claims: "A total heterogeneous antibody population against a specific poisoner." The invention identifies nerve agents that have since been banned, and seems to describe how to produce nerve agent antibodies for use in preparations such as vaccines. These may be useful for military service personnel, civilians, or livestock animals to help the immune system seek out and destroy OP residues when ingested or otherwise encountered. If this explanation is valid, such a process could have potentially made it "okay" to use hazardous and toxic chemicals upon our food and food animals or within the environment as agricultural chemicals; because in theory at least, any mammal could be vaccinated against these poisons. In other words, vaccines might conceivably be designed to help the body render OP or other poisons "non-toxic" through the activation of antibodies to such toxins.

Whether such an attempt was ever intended or deployed in past (or present) vaccines remains to be revealed.[24-26]

The top ten agrochemical manufacturers in the world are Bayer (Germany), Syngenta (Switzerland), BASF (Germany), Dow AgroSciences (USA), Monsanto* (USA), DuPont (USA), Makhteshim Agan (Israel), Nufarm (Australia), Sumitomo Chemical (Japan) and Arysta Lifescience (Japan). Organofluoride and/or organochloride chemicals are globally applied in agriculture and industries of all kinds, from plastics and textiles to mining and nuclear fuel processing.[27]

**During WWII the Monsanto Company researched uranium for the Manhattan Project, and its company chairman was reportedly present at the first atomic bomb test. Dupont became the contractor for the construction of the Hanford and Savannah River nuclear facilities which were both part of the Manhattan Project.*

Once the pesticide DDT was banned abroad during the late 1960s and in the US by 1972, the emergence of novel animal and human infections became more visible. Now there were fewer chemical pesticides capable of substantially controlling insects and their infective agents. In earlier decades outbreaks of "rickettsialpox" or "polio" occurred. In later years, new epidemics with strikingly similar symptoms received new names including Lyme, CFS/ME, Fibromyalgia, Rheumatoid Arthritis, or "autoimmune" disease. In the absence of the chemical pesticide DDT, insects readily reproduced and epidemics in plant, animal, and human populations surged forward. While new disease names were being invented, the truth is that the old and the new outbreaks were probably related. The new diseases were probably formerly labeled as "polio," but their new identities cleverly disguised and protected vaccine programs which secretly may not have been as safe or effective as they were intended to be.

International biological control meetings continued during the 1960s. Scientists discussed diagnostic assays (tests) for pathogenic insect viruses and fungi; and studied insect pathogens in vertebrates. They also addressed how best to apply microbes for agricultural use. In 1965, the University of California's Division of Invertebrate Pathology held a meeting whereby researchers from American university laboratories, private industries, and the USDA discussed the use of the nuclearpolyhedrosis virus (NPV) as a biological control agent of a major agricultural pest, the corn earworm moth (*Heliothis zea*).

In 1967 a collaborative meeting was held in Kyushu, Japan between US and Japanese researchers regarding microbial insecticides. Until then most Japanese research was focused on silkworm diseases. Silkworms were an important agricultural pest in the US and other countries for centuries. After this period the exchange of information concerning biological controls began to take place freely around the world. Hundreds of microbes were studied among partnering academic institutions and research laboratories. Scientific investigations included bacilli and fungi, protozoans, nematodes, viruses, rickettsiae, baculoviruses, RNA viruses, cytoplasmic spindle inclusion viruses, and iridescent viruses. Other viruses that were studied included acute and chronic bee paralysis, "AV" virus, *Galleria mellonella*, flacherie virus of silkworms; a non-occluded virus of *Pseudaletia* (lepidoptera), and the sacbrood virus of the honey bee.[28,29]

Viruses and insects including ticks were made available for distribution to laboratories around the world for research and biological control use. The labs were located in Australia, Belgium, Bulgaria, Canada, Czechoslovakia, France, Hungary, India, Israel, Japan, the Netherlands, New Zealand, Pakistan, the Philippines, Switzerland, the US, and Western Samoa. Some of the American labs that participated in the early international exchanges of biological controls included these institutions:

American Type Culture Collection, Rockville, MD
Boyce Thompson Institute for Plant Research, Yonkers, NY
Cornell University, New York State College of Agriculture, Ithaca, NY
International Minerals and Chemical Corporation, Libertyville, IL
Mississippi State University, MS
New York State Agricultural Experiment Station, Geneva, NY
Nutrilite Products Inc., Lakeview, CA
Ohio State University, Columbus, OH
Purdue University, Lafayette, IN
Smithsonian Institute Museum of Natural History, Washington, DC
Texas A&M University, College of Agriculture, College Station, TX
University of California Berkeley, CA; and Irvine Center for Pathobiology
University of Wisconsin, Madison, WI
USDA Agricultural, Forest Experiment, and Research Service Stations
And other laboratories located in: Ankeny, IA; Beltsville, MD; Brookings, SD; Brownsville, TX; Charleston, SC; Corvallis, OR; Fresno, CA; Hamden, CT; Gainesville, FL; Lake Charles, LA; Peoria, IL; Research Triangle Park, NC; Riverside, CA; and State College, MS.[3,8]

A *Select Agent Program* workshop was sponsored by the CDC, USDA, and the USDA Animal and Plant Health Inspection

Service (APHIS). The program was held at the CDC Roybal Campus Auditorium in Atlanta, Georgia on August 12, 2009. From the event we may learn much about the direction and intent of the government and academic scientists regarding the creation of biological chimera that do not naturally exist. According to the European Commission, the term for creating artificial chimera is *synthetic biology*. This describes the process of engineering biologically based or inspired systems which display functions that do not naturally exist. Chimera are created for new vaccines and therapeutics, environmental remediation, improved agricultural crops and animals; industrial products, insecticides, and as new sources of energy (biofuels). The goal of synthetic biology is to extend or modify the behavior of existing organisms and to engineer them to perform new tasks.[30,31]

The federal government's National Select Agents Registry Program oversees all "activities of possession of biological agents and toxins that have the potential to pose a severe threat to public, and or plant health, or to animal or plant products." The agency has a federal advisory committee called the National Science Advisory Board for Biosecurity (NSABB). The board is comprised of twenty-five professionals from multiple disciplines, including biology, microbiology, genetics, and infectious diseases. These parties provide recommendations to the Health and Human Services Secretary on issues of "dual use" in research. In December 2006 for example, the committee prepared a report called *Addressing Biosecurity Concerns Related to the Synthesis of Select Agents.* The report described information and technologies used to generate biological agents which could threaten public health, agriculture, plants, animals, the environment, or other valuable materials.[31,32]

The committee has the unenviable task of identifying potential biosecurity concerns and advising the US government on whether current policies are sufficient to regulate and cover *de novo* (new) synthesis of select agents. It is also responsible for determining whether additional biosecurity measures and oversight are required. In the area of oversight, components of the oversight system most relevant to synthetic genomes may be found within the Select Agent Regulations (SAR).[31,32]

In the October 31, 2007 government newsletter *Federal Register* was an announcement that the NIH/DHHS/PHS* had approved proposals to conduct research involving *the deliberate transfer of a drug resistance trait into a microorganism that causes human disease.* This research was reviewed by the recombinant DNA advisory committee and was approved by the NIH Director on September 24, 2007. The problem of antibiotic resistance that is discussed among research scientists and infectious disease personnel today can now be seen for what it really is. This problem may have more to do with recombinant manipulations of laboratory microbes rather than as a creation of the usual scapegoats: the antibiotic consuming public, or some "random" microbial mutation.[33]

**National Insitutes of Medicine, Dept. of Health and Human Services, Public Health Service of the US Federal Government.*

Another *Federal Register* notice from September 22, 2009 revealed there were revisions to the NIH guidelines concerning influenza (flu) viruses that *"have either caused pandemics or are believed to have the potential to cause a pandemic."* The viruses included human H2N2 virus (1957-1968); the fully reconstructed (1918-1919) "Spanish flu" virus; and the "highly pathogenic" Avian influenza (HPAI) H5N1 within the Goose-Guangdong-96-like (H5) lineage. These agents were suddenly *upgraded* to risk group 3 agents that *"have the potential to cause serious or lethal disease in humans for which preventative and therapeutic measures may be available."*[34]

Up until this point all influenza viruses of the *Orthomyxovirus* family were classified as risk group 2 agents. This group describes agents that are associated with human disease but that *are rarely serious,* and for which preventative and therapeutic agents are often available. We may ask what prompted this sudden change in classification from "rarely serious" to "potentially serious." The answer may lie within the new guidance measures for containment of research using influenza viruses which are:

> "...generated by recombinant methods (i.e. reverse genetics of chimeric viruses with reassorted segments, introduction of specific mutations) containing one or more genes or segments derived from human influenza viruses."[34]

In short, because there are now genetically engineered products (including insecticides) which contain *influenza and other segmented viruses*; and/or that use reverse transcription processes to *reassort segmented microbial genomes,* now all of a sudden the diseases that can come about from their use may be far more virulent than ever before, and should be considered to be far more serious or deadly; or perhaps even more difficult to treat.[30,34]

This lends validation to the idea that recombinant insecticides cause the reactivation of viruses which can form more virulent mutants when they reassort with other live or latent viruses. It also explains the public health push for newer vaccines which may be inadequately (meaning long-term) safety tested before "outbreaks" or potential outbreaks occur. Recombinant viruses may be introduced into foods as insecticides or oral vaccines; by vectoring insects, animal vaccines, contaminated vaccine cell lines, or other routes.

Since scientists are fabricating vaccines and other products using recombinant genes from viruses that include influenza, the exposure of people to live viruses (even if natural), is raising alarm bells for officials. This is because they are recognized as able to *cause the reactivation of recombinant viruses and other pathogens in the human body upon exposure to genetically engineered insecticides.* This sounds as if we are now walking time bombs of disease reactivation based upon whatever recombinant products or insecticides we are exposed to from the past to the future. Public health scientists are finally beginning to *publicly* acknowledge what many have long been privately known – that genetic engineering techniques are inherently unpredictable and therefore may be considered, or one day proven to be highly flawed and potentially unsafe and causing human diseases.[30,34]

It is perhaps odd to find no evidence of the impending "swine flu" pandemic in the aforementioned September 22, 2009 *Federal Register* notice. This seems highly unusual if such an epidemic was already suspected to be under way. And yet a swine flu pandemic was declared just *one month later* by President Obama on October 25, 2009, when he announced a "national emergency" in the form of a swine flu outbreak in the United States. Suddenly there were "therapeutic agents" available in the form of "swine flu" vaccines that had conveniently been approved by the FDA on September 15, 2009, just one week before the September 22, 2009 *Federal Register* notice, and just one month before the President's declaration of a pandemic – a declaration made no doubt upon the advice of public health officials.[31,33,35,36]

Was the swine flu pandemic declared at the urging of public health officials simply because a new vaccine had recently been licensed and made available by a pharmaceutical company? Or was this declaration made in an effort to covertly close a recombinant loophole that was discovered or suspected to exist from the potential "failure" of recombinant vaccines or applied microbial insecticides? If so, what additional "pandemics" will suddenly be declared (even if only potentially so) as each novel vaccine is created to "fix" a recombinant accident or potential accident caused by newly designed microbial insecticides?

The agenda of public health agencies (as reflected in an Institute of Medicine book), appears to have the goal of ensuring the production and availability of vaccines into the twenty-first century. The reason for this need in fact may be due to the application of recombinant tools (i.e. recombinant insecticides, GM crops, animal/human vaccines, recombinant antibiotics). Each of the new recombinant tools may inadvertently import diseases to both targeted and non-targeted populations. However, the use of the new era of recombinant tools and the preservation of same despite risks or inherent flaws might be something we may be forced to live with whether we like it or not.

This is because there are no immediate solutions to the problems of controlling insects of medical, military, agricultural, industrial, and veterinary importance. The value of these new genetic tools at least at the present point in time seems to outweigh the value of abandoning their use despite serious inherent or potential flaws. At least this may be the point of view adopted by those who advocate for their use. The question is whether there is a middle ground that can be found so the benefits to public health may be enjoyed while the risks to same are significantly minimized.[31,33,35,36]

I need not remind readers that the science of biotechnology for agriculture and vaccines generates untold trillions of dollars in an industry that has grown exponentially over the last century. Despite this, even in the earliest days of genetic engineering, scientists had moral reservations about this new field. For example Polish Virologist and Immunologist Dr. Hilary Koprowski who worked at Lederle Laboratories* in Pearl River, New York, was said to have been "plagued by concerns" over the safety of his live polio vaccine, developed during the late 1940s. (He invented the world's first live and effective polio vaccine). That scientists must navigate and potentiate their excitement over new discoveries with the responsibilities and liabilities which may be created by their use is not a position to be taken lightly; nor one that anyone should particularly envy.[37-40]

**Lederle Laboratories is the pharmaceutical division of American Cyanamid. Parts of the company were spun off to form the Shell Oil Company, Shell International Chemical Company, BASF, Wyeth, and Criterion Catalysts & Technologies, a supplier of catalysts for refineries.*

In a paper on the topic of the "misuse of science" from 1970, we may read about one scientist's take on the developing biotech situation with regard to genetic engineering and recombinant viruses. Dr. Beckwith the article's author, discussed the special responsibility he and other scientists shouldered concerning genetic manipulation. He expressed concerns over how new processes would be used in society. He shared his concern for the misuse of science and felt it was imperative for scientists to take clear sides. He also pointed out the potential for government and industry to misuse science.[39]

Clearly one of his greatest concerns revolved around the pharmaceutical industry and what he felt was its propensity to exploit science for profit. He also remarked that those who make decisions about monetary awards must take care not to differentiate between serving the public and serving the interests of government and industries. A group of scientists attempted to make a political statement about the potential misuse of science including the isolation of pure *lac operan* DNA; which is necessary for successful gene manipulation. Many scientists including Dr. Beckwith recognized "capitalist exploitation as a means for oppression" and felt that science was being used to exploit and oppress people around the world even decades ago.[39]

Most people understand that regulators for the most part attempt to make responsible decisions that will affect industrial products and the insects, animals, and humans that will be affected by same. However the rapid design of recombinant tools that may be militarily, agriculturally, industrially, or medically important seem to outpace the ability of those who regulate these devices to control and analyze the impact of products before use. There are those at the highest levels of government who also seem to have conflicts of interest that could favor industrial and agricultural giants at a regulatory level.

At the present time there appears to be inadequate long-term safety studies and insufficient regulations for many recombinant products already long applied and consumed. There also seems to be inadequate regulations which mandate the listing of genetically modified organisms and pesticides upon foods and other products consumed by the public. There also seems to be a gross misrepresentation and shortage of information concerning emerging epidemics, and vaccines to "prevent" same. Each of these processes needs meaningful reform. With the proliferation of the new tools of modern recombinant science, how is the public expected to keep their freedoms of choice? How may we be assured that the products we select or that are applied to us or around us are healthy and safe? The answers may be that unless industries and the scientists who design their products are forced to answer to the ill public, we may never be advised as to the nature of what we are being exposed.

Chemicals and Mutated Microbes

Scientific papers reveal that bacteriae aggregate by attaching to other microorganisms and biofilms in the environment for survival. Spirochetes are not alone in their ability to aggregate. Many pathogens use this strategy to overcome host barriers. During the aggregation process, an organism may undergo subtle or drastic structural changes to its outer protein surfaces, depending upon the environment and the microbes to which it bonds. In addition industrially used mutagenic chemicals, surfactants, and other microbes can "lyse" (open) and degrade microbes. This allows natural reshuffling of genes (recombinant events), including the infection of bacteria by other organisms found in soils or wastewaters. These environments create aggregate organisms that may be difficult to identify when viewed under a microscope. The combining of multiple pathogens also creates far more virulent pathogens. Thus the identification of a novel spirochete may become a case of "mistaken identity" to those who are unaware of what they are observing under the microscope.[1]

Any organisms present in the body may become temporarily or permanently joined with the Bb spirochete to create a far more complex, virulent organism capable of a wider host range than what the individual microbes enjoy when unattached. While the Bb spirochete is not found in its entirety in the environment, its whole form has been documented in insect, animal, and human bodies. This means that *the Bb agent cannot sustain itself in the external environment;* or more simply that *it is a pathogen that is formed partly in the environment, and partly from microbes found in insects, animals, or the human body.*

There are a number of new human illnesses which do not seem to have a specific cause. Insects are multiply infected with a variety of pathogens, and these mixed infections are determined by the individual insect and by the microbes and toxins to which they have been exposed. Microbes, parasites, chemicals, pollutants, and metals in the insect and human body will further complicate the infections that are initially delivered by vectoring insect.

The process of Bb aggregation was shown to occur under high temperatures, low pH, and high cell density. These are the same environmental conditions that are favorable for the expression of the Bb Outer Surface Protein C (OspC). This protein is required to initiate human infections. When the Bb spirochete is present in a multiply-infected insect, it aggregates with any microbes that are present. These agents can adhere to Bb spirochetes like barnacles on a ship, to infect a human host when the insect transmits infections through the next blood meal. Since borrelia species have been around for centuries, we might ask why the "new" borrelia and their aggregates have become more problematic in modern times. The answers may lie not within the Bb organism itself as we know it to be described. Instead we must understand there are important environmental factors that play a role in the aggregation of Bb spirochetes, including the spirochetes themselves and other agents which infect and pollute them.

When studying a 1971 patent that described the mass culture of leptospires for a vaccine, I noticed that the patent recommended the use of several substances. One was a medium that used Dowex 1 or Dowex 2 resins. These are ion-exchange resins produced by the Dow Chemical Company. (Dowex is also used in dye manufacturing). Ion-exchange resins can be used in microbead formulas to separate, purify, or to decontaminate. Polysorbates or emulsifiers called "Tweens" are suggested by another patent from the Atlas Powder Company. *Tweens*™ are specialized mixtures which act as aggregators of chemicals and heavy metals. Tweens also work as nonionic detergents (surfactants) and as *bacterial aggregators and growth promoters*. They are also used for remediative purposes to clean up toxins such as toluene or *hexavalent chromium* (chromium-6 or chromium VI) from nuclear reactor wastewaters, for example.[2-7]

Hexavalent chromium, chromic acid, or chromium compounds have various forms and are used in paints, primers, inks, plastics, surface coatings, stainless steel welds, and electroplating. *Chromium fluoride* is used to dye textiles. Chromium can be found in phosphate and other fertilizers. Chromic acid is formed by reacting sulfuric acid to a dichromate compound. (Remember how sulfuric acid reacts with bone, and was added to fertilizers to make superphosphates?) Chromic acid can also be used to clean laboratory glassware, and chromium is useful during glass making, leather tanning, chrome and electroplating, as an anti-corrosive agent to metals including *aluminum* and *stainless steel*; and to manufacture alloys and bricks (refractory industry). It is also used in the textile industry as a mordant (set dyes). Chromium is used to preserve wood as chromated copper arsenate. Remember that when wood or pulp wastes are burned as fuel, their particulates become airborne. Leather tanning or tannery wastes are recycled as fertilizers and as livestock fodder.[8-11]

Fertilizers that contain toxic substances including chromium, dioxins, cadmium, arsenic, mercury, lead, and hexavalent chromium, are the target of investigative reports and lawsuits. Fertilizers have been tested for levels of heavy metals and toxicants and have been found to contain high levels of harmful contaminants. Heavy metals are naturally found in phosphate rock and may remain after processing as fertilizers. Fertilizers are one source for heavy metal exposures because they enter crops and livestock through the food chain. Equally important is that fertilizer manufacturers are not required to label the entire contents of their formulas. This leaves out some of the most important ingredients including heavy metals, radioactive elements, persisting chemical pollutants, and other toxicants.[8-11]

Chromium oxide acts as a catalyst to create polymer plastics (i.e. polyethylene-HDPE, LLDPE). During the 1950s German Scientist Carl Ziegler devised a way to create high-density polyethylene by using a catalyst (Ziegler process). In the 1960s, Phillips Petroleum Company developed a similar process to polymerize ethylene using the Ziegler catalyst. The process, which uses chromium oxide as the catalyst on a high-surface silica, was commercialized to produce high-density polyethylene (Phillips method). I think we can all appreciate the connections between metals and elements important to many industries; plastics, radioactive wastes, and what ends up as airborne particulates, at waste dump sites, and in surface and subsurface watersheds.

The most abundant sources of chromite ore are located in areas of the world where we find diamonds; South Africa and Kazakhstan (Russia). Chromite ore is leached or roasted to produce chromium and ferrochromium. Chromium is also the radiogenic (radioactive decaying isotope) product of *manganese*. Soil and aquatic-borne bacteria express manganese dependent sphingomyelinase/hemolysin enzymes, including *Bacillus cereus, Pseudomonas, Staphylococcus, Listeria,* and the pathogenic *Leptospira interrogans.* Another bacterium, *Chromobacterium violaceum* also has these manganese-dependent enzymes. *Chromobacterium violaceum* is a proteobacterium of the highly antibiotic-resistant family *Neisseriaceae* (i.e. meningitis, gonorrhea). A unique characteristic of *C. violaceum* is that it is able to decompose petroleum tarballs. These are aquatic pollutants that are remnants of petroleum (oil) spills in marine environments. When we look at where *Borrelia burgdorferi* is highly prevalent in the US, we find it along coastlines of marine environments, whether oceanic or freshwater. In these environments we find the highest number of persisting pollutants, heavy metals, oil and nuclear bioremediation; and petroleum-based, or petroleum-influenced "wastes" (i.e. plastics, insecticidal oils).[112-114]

When we analyze the Bb organism, we can see that it was probably formed in part from spirochetes that are able to survive in volcanic regions (geothermal veins) and acid mine wastes, because it too has replaced all of its iron-related enzymes with those which use manganese. These aggregate organisms may contain genes from bacteriae including leptospires, chromobacterium, and soil bacteria. Some of these genes may include those that are applied agriculturally in fermented B.t. products, or that are used to leach ores during in situ or other mining processes. Some of the enzymes produced by these microbes are highly significant.[112-114]

Sphingomyelinase enzymes (SMase) determine the degree of infectivity (virulence factors) of pathogens, and are known beta-toxins (ß-toxins) which cause anemia and hemolysis, or the destruction of red blood cells. An example of a microbe with these enzymes is *Mycobacterium tuberculosis,* an agent that causes tuberculosis, and that has been used within animal vaccines. In the case of intracellular blood-borne pathogens, the destruction of co-infected cells allows pathogens to be released, to reassort with other agents, and to be transmitted during blood meals by vectoring insects. Some of the same microbes used in insecticides are used in animal vaccines, presumably to protect them from the recombinant insecticidal formulas. We may imagine the microbes which may reassort in an animal if a vaccine "fails," thus providing microbes that can reassort inside the body and which may be deposited in the environment as animal wastes. Insects that harbor microbes with these enzyme toxins will have cells destroyed and intracellular infections dumped into the insect's circulation; which may then be transmitted to human hosts.[112-114]

Near the end of this book is a discussion of scientists who studied a frozen human approximately 5,300 years old, and from whom they claim to have isolated the DNA "footprint" of *Borrelia burgdorferi.* The mummy is felt to be from the *Chalcolithic Age*, a phase of the *Bronze Age.* During this era people manipulated copper, tin, and bronze using smelting processes. Chromium oxide was used over 2,000 years ago to *plate steel and to bronze weapons.* Lyme-notable scientists are currently concentrating their *Borrelia burgdorferi*-related studies of a related relapsing fever agent *Borrelia miyamotoi,* in Kazakhstan, Russia. These two subjects would seem to be unrelated if we did not fully appreciate their probable connections to Lyme history.[13-16,20]

Chromium VI is used in circulating water for nuclear cooling; and chromate compounds can be found naturally in rocks mined for their phosphates and uranium. In Greece, studies were undertaken in 2007 by scientists at the University of Athens to determine the groundwater status of chromium, especially in areas of heavy industrial activity. Results revealed that levels were higher than those deemed to be "safe." The increase in these pollutants was blamed on industrial processes that use chromium. Chromium VI or hexavelent chromium is known to be highly mutagenic and carcinogenic and was the subject of a popular Hollywood movie.[2-7]

A recent lawsuit filed in 2009 alleges that toxic wastes in the form of recycled wastewater sludge were spread over farm fields across four counties near Kansas City, Missouri. Chromium VI is known to cause brain and other tumors, and may be linked to a rash of brain tumors in residents in these areas. The chemical was alleged to have come from a local leather tannery. Hundreds of tons of chromium VI contaminated sludge were said to have been spread as fertilizers – a process which also allows the chemical to become an airborne contaminant. Chromium has been found in other tannery meal fertilizers according to 1994 studies. Wastes that are generated during the process of tanning leather are commonly added to some commercial organic fertilizers. Sewage sludge or animal wastes used as fertilizers also contain enteroviruses including poliovirus, reoviruses, adenoviruses, myxoviruses, and paramyxoviruses. The chemicals used to process hides are thus free to influence the microbes of soils and wastewaters.[17-19]

Conversion coatings are important industrial wastes. These are coatings that are produced by a chemical or electrochemical process to treat metallic surfaces (i.e. steel, aluminum, nickel, or other metals). For example, such coatings are used on films; and on aluminum, cadmium, copper, magnesium, silver, tin, and zinc alloys. Chromate can also be used for decorative finishes, or as a primer. These coatings are commonly found on tools, and aluminum alloys for ship building, automotive, aviation, or military industries. Chromate conversion coatings are also used over phosphate conversion coatings to enhance the phosphate coating. Phosphate coatings are applied to metals including steel, aluminum, zinc, cadmium, silver, and tin. Phosphate coatings are made from mined phosphates. The fertilizer industry produces large quantities of what is called a "wet process" phosphoric acid solution, which is a potential source of uranium since uranium may be extracted from phosphoric acid solutions.[20-22]

According to a 2004 environmental work group report, chromium VI was found in the drinking water of thirty-one US cities. The cities reporting the highest chromium levels nationwide included Honolulu, Hawaii; Madison, Wisconsin; Norman, Oklahoma; and Riverside, California. Many sources report that the tap water industry may have found clear evidence of chromium contaminations in drinking water as early as 2004. Despite a Senate environmental committee hearing on chromium VI pollution, industry representatives reportedly did not inform Congressional members about the contaminated waters. Chromium VI has been shown to be "common" in American groundwater, and again, is a known human carcinogen.[23,24]

We should be interested in chromium concentrations in natural and chemical fertilizers, in lime, and in animal wastes because chromium is found in each of these. As far as natural and commercial fertilizers go, chromium levels are detectable in nitrogen, phosphorus, and potassium fertilizers; in limestone, and in animal wastes including cattle, pig, poultry manures; and farmyard and feedlot manures. Chromium levels are significantly higher in phosphate fertilizers. What is also important is that chromium is found in leachates from mining wastes, from industrial lagoons, and from industrial metal processing.[25-29]

We can also find chromium in wheat germ, cheese, and brewer's yeast (*Saccharomyces cervisiae*). In California, chromic acid is registered as an insecticide and a fungicide. It is also used to treat wood and termites. Remember that chromium VI is mutagenic and carcinogenic not only to humans, but it is also taken up by microbes which lie in the soil and water. The reason it is mutagenic is because as it breaks down into chromium III, it generates free radicals. These radicals are able to mutate DNA, cause inflammation, malignant transformations, cell proliferation, and other toxic effects.[25-29]

Besides cleaning up after chromium VI and other harmful chemicals, Tweens were used in the Gulf of Mexico to try to bind free-floating oil above and below the ocean surface after the Deepwater Horizon petroleum accident of April 20, 2010. The accident was caused when an offshore oil drilling rig exploded and sank, resulting in a disastrous oil spill that took a long time to cap. Although biosurfactants such as *Pseudomonas aeruginosa* are sometimes used to bioremediate (clean up) petroleum contaminated sites, they were not used in this disaster. Instead, two surfactants called Corexit EC9500A and EC9527A were used, which contained Tween-80. Other dispersants were also used. Remember that Tweens aggrgate bacteria and promote their growth.[30,31]

Tweens including Triton X-100 and Tween 80, Polysorbate-80*, and Nonoxynol-9 are known to be immunosuppressive, and have been used in vaccines. The latter is also used in spermicides; and in an H1N1 vaccine. Tweens as surfactants have been used in DtaP, Tdap, and DTaP-combination vaccines (tetanus-diphtheria-pertussis); and in Influenza and *Gardasil*® (human papillomavirus) vaccines. In laboratory diagnostic tests, Tweens are used to break apart cell membrane components so they may be detected in tests. The Tweens family of detergents are well known for their ability to *break apart cellular components* (organelles) including mitochondria, chloroplasts, plasma membranes, endoplasmic reticulum, and nuclear membranes. This means *Tweens can disassemble the intracellular components of bacteria and viruses*. Such disassembly allows the dumping of genetic materials and intracellular infections into the environment whether that occurs in water or soil; or inside an insect, animal, or human body. Since Tweens are used in vaccine formulas, this may also create a problem with the microbes therein.[30,31]

**Polysorbate-80 is a surfactant that is also widely used in cosmetics, foods, and pharmaceuticals.*

Triton X-100 is a nonionic *surfactant* that was an original trademark of Rohn & Haas Co. (now Dow Chemical Company). This compound is also used in the laboratory and in cleaning fluids and compounds from detergents to industrial cleaners. When these and similar chemicals make their way into wastewaters, they will cause indigenous bacteria including spirochetes to break apart and to release their cellular contents. This facilitates the genetic reassortment of microbes. The literature clearly shows that this "lysing" or opening of spirochetes also occurs in the presence of bacteriophages such as those found in insecticides. This process is further augmented by agricultural chemicals and industrial biocides (i.e. fungicides, herbicides, algaecides). Animal feed supplements, GM plants, and animal and human vaccines often involve these same or similar chemical agents.[32]

Our bodies make biosurfactants in the air sacs (alveoli) of our lungs. The rise in asthma in recent decades may have a connection with the chemicals and insecticides being applied agriculturally or by aerial release. These formulas when aerosolized can be inhaled, although public health officials continue to deny any connection between insecticides, chemicals, and increased asthma rates. Tweens which coat nanoparticle drugs or other substances can penetrate the blood-brain barrier. This occurs through a reaction between the Tweens and brain endothelial cells. Brain cells are very vulnerable to inhaled substances. There, potent neurotoxic chemicals will take up residence in the central nervous system. Tweens are considered to be carcinogenic or are co-carcinogens; and have been shown to speed up the reproductive organ function and development of female rats.[33-38]

Tween-containing microbeads have been used in fertilizers, insecticides, and for bioremediation (i.e. remove sulfur from diesel oil). According to a 1961 article published by the American Society of Linnology and Oceanography, Tween 80 from the Atlas Powder Company was added to sea water samples collected off the east coast of Connecticut, and east of Fisher's Island, New York. Scientists were studying the role of bacterial aggregation in seawater under the influence of Tweens. Is the timing of the study a clue to the scientific awareness of the origins of an upcoming human epidemic in Connecticut?[39-41]

Dow Chemical Company is assignee to a 1972 filed patent for biuret-polyethylenimine resins. The invention is designed to slowly degrade in water and to encapsulate chemical insecticides and fertilizers. A 1979 patent assigned to the Battelle Development Corporation describes a microbial insecticide that contains insect pathogens of viral, bacterial, and fungal origins. The microbes are embedded in a microbead structure to protect them from sunlight-induced inactivation, since they can be killed upon exposure to UV light. Organisms described in the Battelle patent include B.t. cells, spores, and toxin crystals; the *Autographa californica* nuclearpolyhedrosis virus (AcNPV); and vegetative bacterial cells including *Pseudomonas fluorescens* (which fluoresces under UV light); *Serratia marcescens,* and *Escherichia coli.*[39-42]

The Battelle patent declares there is "little doubt" that any insect pathogens embedded in its special microbeads would fail to be protected from UV light. This microbead delivery system was designed for droplets or solid formats (aerosol or granules). The Battelle patent also refers to a scientific textbook that has arguably become one of the most important to understanding today's microbial insecticides. Within this book is sufficient evidence that *Bacillus thuringiensis* (B.t.) *can reactivate latent viruses*. Insecticidal formulas that use Tweens will allow bacterial aggregation and growth. The fluorides and other chemicals and mutagenic elements present may promote mutation. B.t. allows latent viruses to become viable, while baculoviruses and reoviruses partner together with B.t. toxins to become highly effective killing formulas.[42-46]

The Battelle Development Corporation is a subsidiary of the Battelle Memorial Institute, Inc. (the latter has headquarters in Columbus, Ohio). The institute manages laboratories and develops and commercializes technologies including diagnostics and agricultural products. Battelle conducts about $3.7 billion in annual research and development projects. Researchers there team with more than eight hundred federal, state, and local government agencies to provide science and technology for energy and the environment; for health and life sciences; transportation and space; national security; and homeland defense. "Homeland defense" therefore appears to include protection against agricultural pests, and problems which may arise from applied insecticides or industrial pollutants. Therefore matters of "national security" likely also encompass all matters of public health including infectious diseases.[43,44,46]

Battelle is in a 50:50 partnership with the Research Foundation of the State University of New York (SUNY). At this institution we find several Lyme disease guidelines co-authors and borrelia patent holders. This partnership, which is called Brookhaven Sciences Associates, was established solely to manage and operate Brookhaven National Laboratory, according to its web site. Brookhaven Sciences Associates Board of Directors includes individuals from Columbia, Cornell, Harvard, Massachusetts Institute of Technology, Princeton, and Yale Universities. When we look at the academic ties of some of the IDSA Lyme disease guidelines co-authors, we see interesting connections especially with respect to the events which transpired at the Dearborn conference. Many of these individuals are key patent holders of *Borrelia burgdorferi*-related products. For example Bb-related patents are assigned to the Research Foundation of the State University of New York at Stony Brook, and Brookhaven Sciences Associates, LLC – patents which involve Lyme disease vaccines.[47]

The Battelle Memorial Institute is reportedly also a contractor for the Pentagon and the CIA. In 1998, Battelle's Program Manager was biological warfare expert Dr. Kanatjan Alibekov (Ken Alibek), the author of the book *Biohazard.* Alibek, a Soviet defector and former First Deputy Director of the Russian biological warfare program *Biopreparat* from 1988 to 1992, became a consultant to the US government and *Anthrax* expert. He was President of Hadron Advanced Biosystems, a Virginia company that with links to American intelligence and to a firm that received an $800,000 grant from the NIH to study "anthrax defense." Hadron Advanced Biosystems was reportedly a subsidiary of Analex, a defense contractor which was incorporated into Bio-Rad Laboratories, Inc., a specialty chemical and life sciences company founded in 1952 by two University of California-Berkeley graduates; one of whom was working with the tobacco mosaic virus. The company provides tools for genetic engineering and diagnostic kits for infectious diseases including HIV and prion diseases (i.e. chronic wasting disease of deer, mad cow disease). Over decades the company expanded product lines to include pharmaceuticals. Bio-Rad systems are used for *Borrelia burgdorferi* detection by academic researchers important to the Lyme story. It is interesting that Dr. Alibek developed an immune system support formula (supplement) which offered similar ingredients to those now "prescribed" for Lyme disease patients. The organisms in the Alibek formula according to an ingredient label include vitamins A,C,E; B-6 and B-12; zinc, selenium, copper; and multiple strains of lactobacillus and bifidobacterium (as gut probiotics); the same bacteriae used in a Dattwyler et al. patent for an oral Bb vaccine. When we study the connections between scientists who are well-versed in anthrax-related bacteria such as B.t. and its effects upon the gut, we can see that an issue of great concern for the human population may not be "anthrax preparedness" as much as it may be *the need to protect our gut bacteria and membranes from the microbes of anthrax-related recombinant B.t. insecticides.*[48,116-120]

According to sources, Battelle conducted a "secret" biological warfare test in the Nevada desert using a genetically modified anthrax strain in early September, 2001. This was prior to the 9/11 attacks on the World Trade Center and the Pentagon. This test also preceded the US Postal Service anthrax letters incidents. The first letter was discovered a week after 9/11, and was stamped with a Trenton, New Jersey postmark – an event for which Dr. Alibek was allegedly considered as a suspect. New Jersey is interesting to us for many reasons nonetheleast of which is for its connections to the early applied insecticides. It is also home to Du Pont's Deepwater Point plant that has produced explosives, dyes, anti-knock gasoline agents (tetraethyl lead), and chemical intermediates. The pollutants which contaminate our environment may collide adversely with recombinant insecticidal formulas and the results may be important human infectious diseases for which we have no current cures.[48,49]

Battelle manages or co-manages laboratories for the US Department of Energy including those with the longest ties to the nuclear era. These include Brookhaven National Laboratory (Long Island, Upton, NY); Oak Ridge National Laboratory (UT-Battelle LLC-Oak Ridge, TN); the National Renewable Energy Laboratory (Golden, CO); Pacific Northwest National Laboratory (Battelle Northwest, Richland, WA); and Idaho National Laboratory (Battelle Energy Alliance-Idaho Falls, ID). Sources reveal that Battelle holds a use permit agreement with the Department of Energy. This relationship allows Battelle scientists to use government facilities and equipment. Battelle also holds a permit to operate the Pacific Northwest National Laboratory. UT-Battelle's Technology Transfer and Economic Development organization handles interactions with commercial businesses, researchers and facilities; collaborations, contracted research, and user facilities. Battelle also manages intellectual property, licensing, and patenting.[43,44]

In 1943, Battelle scientists began studying how to process uranium in connection with the Manhattan Project; and the institute became one of the country's leading nuclear research centers, including for weapons and for the 1948 research for the nuclear submarine *Nautilus.* (Remember that chromium and fluorides are part of nuclear wastes.) In 1950 Battelle also constructed the world's first privately owned nuclear research center. Tweens and other surfactants are used in nuclear power plants, as foaming agents, and to clean up nuclear radioactive wastes including chromium. They are also used in industries that produce *non-stick polymer coatings*; for wastewater treatment, oral health products, airlift and bioreactors for the chemical industry; in metal etching (fluorosurfactants), and as corrosion inhibitors for the aluminum and other metal industries. They are also used in the food industry, and are found in mine and quarry wastes, all of which may include chromium, picric acid, nitrates, and other important mutagenic or toxic chemicals.[43,44,50-57]

In 1990, the National Toxicology Program (NTP) published the results of a two-year Battelle laboratory study of rodents that were fed fluoride-treated water. The study revealed a dose-related increase in osteosarcoma in male, but not female rats. Observers might wonder if the studies were related to the use of fluorides within municipal water systems, animal feeds, or applied agricultural pesticides. We may see interesting links between Battelle and the State University of New York (SUNY) and other institutions if we look carefully at the literature and patents held by institutions and the co-authors of the IDSA guidelines for Lyme disease.[43,44,50,51]

Among the inventors listed on a patent for *Recombinant Constructs of Borrelia burgdorferi* are Drs. Raymond J. Dattwyler, John J. Dunn, Benjamin J. Luft, (co-authors of one or more clinical practice guidelines for Lyme disease), and their associate Maria J.C. Gomes-Solecki. The assignees on the patent are the Research Foundation of the State of New York (Stony Brook) and *Brookhaven Science Associates*, LLC (Upton, NY). The patent uses the outer surface proteins A and C (OspA, OspC) of the Bb organism to make diagnostic tests and a second generation Lyme vaccine. According to the transcripts of a 1998 FDA advisory meeting held in Bethesda, MD which discussed a then upcoming Lyme vaccine, Drs. Dattwyler and Luft were present at the meeting along with colleague Allen C. Steere, then lead investigator for a Lyme vaccine's sponsor, Glaxo SmithKline.[58-63]

Remember that Brookhaven Science Associates is in partnership with Battelle and the Research Foundation on behalf of

SUNY-Stony Brook. When we look at the Dattwyler et al. patent, we might consider it linked at least indirectly to Battelle. It is curious then that some IDSA Lyme disease guidelines authors and/or their scientific partners with connections to institutions or industries that have nuclear, biowarfare, and/or agricultural links, would carefully define medical guidelines that have been deemed "flawed" by some parties – guidelines which recommend treatment for a disease whose severity might be "ignored" due to its possible industrial, agricultural, nuclear, or biowarfare origins.[58-64]

A 1951 patent assigned to Dow Corning Corporation reveals a side of the story that is infrequently discussed. This is the possibility that pesticides that are applied to human skin can mutate bacteria that are present in or on our bodies, to contribute to disease states. From the patent we learn how *organopolysiloxanes** are used in an emulsion to create a long-acting pesticide that can be applied to human skin. In the invention, the use of "Spans" and "Tweens" are described. What happens when these chemicals are absorbed into the human body? What happens to the microbes in our bodies that are exposed to pesticides? This patent refers to older patents, including a 1936 patent assigned to E.I. du Pont de Nemours & Company which describes the use of normal and acid salts of *fluosilicic acid* (fluoride) with nitrogen-containing chemicals to make insecticides for textile use.[65-68]

**Organopolysiloxanes have silicon bonded hydrocarbon radicals (methyl, ethyl, propyl, butyl, phenyl, benzyl, vinyl, allyl, or chlorophenyls)*

E.I. du Pont entered the coal tar dye industry after June 25, 1917. An early announcement describes it best, "Our development during the recent years in the explosives and in several other branches of the chemical industry brings us now to the logical result of undertaking in a broad and comprehensive way the manufacture of synthetic dye-stuffs and kindred products." We can see how intricately connected are the explosives, mining, metal, chemical, dye, textile, and agricultural insecticide industries.[69]

What we might also consider is whether patents that describe how antibiotics with antibacterial properties useful against animal (livestock) diseases such as *Treponema dysentery* (swine dysentery) also contain chemicals that can cause *chemical reactions* within the animals' bodies (in this case a conversion of one chemical to another). Certain chemical changes are purposely sought after and desired. For example *dehydrogenation reactions* are desired for a patent that describes the use of antibiotics as feed supplements and insecticides for use in swine. The mixture is added to the pigs' drinking water. To dehydrogenate something means to detach hydrogen atoms from molecules. The dehydrogenating reaction produces heat (heat-shock). Heat shock proteins are released, which affects the protein folding/unfolding process of cells, including viruses. Protein folding errors have been identified as a possible cause of prion diseases. Prion diseases began to be identified in 1987 in Europe; and in 1993 in Alberta, Canada. If this reaction can occur in livestock, it most certainly can occur in humans who may be exposed to similar processes by recombinantly engineered foods, insecticides, or medicines.[65-68]

When studying Tweens, I read a letter from molecular biologist and Nobel Laureate Joshua Lederberg that was sent to the Director of Research Development of the Atlas Powder Company* in Wilmington, Delaware, the company mentioned in the earlier patent. The letter was dated November 18, 1946. It stated briefly that Dr. Lederberg was interested in obtaining a 20g sample of Tween 80 (polyoxyethylene sorbitan mono-oleate) after reading a report from Dubos and Davis which discussed factors that affected the growth of the tubercle bacilli in liquid media. Lederberg's letter described his keen interest in Tweens, and conveyed that Tweens were "exceedingly efficacious" in promoting diffuse growth in tubercle bacilli. Dr. Lederberg desired to study whether it would have the same effect on the growth of other bacteriae and yeasts, which he said would "greatly facilitate" ongoing research. Dr. Lederberg was no doubt interested in Tweens for their usefulness to agricultural insecticidal formulas.[70-72]

**Atlas Powder Co. is the sister to Hercules Powder Co., both were formed when DuPont was ordered to be broken up in 1912 according to the Sherman Anti-trust Act.*

In 1946, Joshua Lederberg and Edward L. Tatum (Yale) published the first paper on bacterial conjugation (bacterial sexual reproduction). Lederberg had studied at Columbia, received a PhD from Yale in 1947, and finished his medical studies at the University of Wisconsin-Madison. He then went to Stanford where he helped establish the Department of Genetics. Eventually he became President of Rockefeller University. Lederberg was also an advisor to several US Presidents; was involved in space exploration and "exobiology" (study of space microbes); and headed the US Department of Defense Task Force on Persian Gulf War Health Effects. The group investigated Gulf War Syndrome in 1994 and claimed there was "insufficient evidence" that the syndrome even existed. We might wonder if such beliefs were purely evidence-based, or whether the use of Tweens and any human epidemics emerging after the global application of same had anything to do with these conclusions.[72-74]

When Tweens are used within fertilizer and insecticidal formulas, they act as natural bacterial aggregators (joiners). Tweens also help bacteria degrade pyrethroid* insecticides (i.e. permethrin). Chemicals in the insecticides and fertilizers that are applied to the soil (and which wind up in water sources) are capable of aggregating, opening, and transforming microbes from the environment. Tweens are considered to be emulsifiers, and were extensively used, especially during the 1940s to 1950s when the pesticide DDT was globally applied. They are still used today in many industrial applications.[75-81]

**Pyrethroids, (pyrethrin/piperonyl butoxide), rotenone, carbamate insecticides, chemosterilants, or other chemicals were used extensively* *against ticks and other insects. Pour-on pesticides were used on livestock to treat flies and ticks. Piperonyl butoxide is a potent inhibitor of cytochrome P450 enzymes, which are important detoxifying (liver) enzymes found in insects and animals.*

Since the timeframe of Dr. Lederberg's letter and interest was 1946, it is not difficult to imagine that the mention of "other bacteria and yeast" in the letter may have referred to the fermentation of the biowarfare tool anthrax; the agricultural agent B.t., or other similar "weapons" being explored at the time. In September of 1946, just two months before Lederberg's letter was sent, President Truman signed into authorization *Operation Paperclip*. While some people assume that this research led to the creation of a biological warfare weapon that escaped from Plum Island to harm the human population, American scientists who worked on bioweapons for military purposes were keenly aware of the hazards of manipulating dangerous microbes. A few laboratory accidents were reported, and there have been releases of ticks and other insects and arthropods. However *there is no evidence to suggest that the Bb agent was ever specifically created within any laboratory* to be released upon an unsuspecting population. Indeed all of the evidence in this book seems to point to the fact that Bb has had very different origins and indeed a far earlier timeline that may yet prove its creation to have been an "industrial accident" on a global scale.[78-80]

Dr. Lederberg was a vocal advocate of the genetics movement, and the person thought to have been responsible for the word "Euphenics." However, a handwritten note proved otherwise. It should also be noted that Dr. Lederberg was highly instrumental in the process of *banning* weapons of chemical and biological warfare during the Nixon administration. Dr. Lederberg expressed "very grave fears" of what he called "virological warfare." He understood the importance of protecting the population from bioterrorism, and also from *infectious diseases of a natural origin.* It would be entirely ironic then if Bb turned out to be a "biological weapon" that nature herself created using the very tools that scientists manipulated by genetic engineering whether for warfare, agriculture, industry, or by the chemicals intended to "improve" public health or habitat.[82]

Dr. Lederberg wrote numerous articles about genetics and biological weapons, often covering both sides of the debate. He was a strong advocate for the exploration of genetic engineering for its potential benefits to medicine; and called Eugenics "the conscious betterment of man's genetic quality." He also called it a noble aim that "has been perverted to justify unthinkable inhumanity." In one paper Lederberg said that Eugenics is the design of a DNA sequence that will develop to a somewhat defined end goal. Euphenics according to Dr. Lederberg was man's control of his own development. He believed this development would pave the way for a more comprehensive eugenics, even if only begun through the expanded knowledge of genetics.[83-85]

Instead, we may find that these explorations into a little known science, even with good intentions, may have brought about some of the worst and most prevalent infectious diseases of modern times. When speaking of genetic engineering in a 1975 paper, Dr. Lederberg had this to say, and yet he was one of the first scientists interested in the use of Tweens to promote the growth of bacteria useful for industry:[83-85]

> "In the face of such a revolution, the primary concern of researchers in the field has been the public hazards that such a technology may create. While we may indeed inherit a Promethean dilemma, public policy decision can lead to social good only if we are equally well-informed about the potential risks and benefits of further work on DNA splicing."

According to a GlaxoSmithKline International patent for *Pandemrix,* the newest "swine flu" and other vaccines utilize Tweens as a detergent in a process called "Tween-ether" splitting. According to a swine flu vaccine patent, the preferred split flu vaccine antigen preparations "...comprise a residual amount of Tween 80 and/or Triton X-100 remaining from the production process, although these may be added or their concentrations adjusted after preparation of the split antigen. Preferably both Tween 80 and Triton X-100 are present."[86]

Agriculturally speaking, Tweens are and have been among the most powerful chemicals to have been applied to the soil and which migrate into water as non-point source pollutants. Among the microbes that may be found in wastewaters are B.t. toxins and spores, and *Agrobacterium tumefaciens.* Both of these bacteria have natural aggregation and infection talents and may initiate mutations, which helps to create new bacterial species. Chemical fumigants and bacterial growth promoters are applied to soils to raise soil nitrogen and ammonia levels, and to facilitate microbial growth. The combination of these components could absolutely play a role in the development of pathogens that would not naturally congregate and breed except under these exceptional circumstances.

Could Tweens have contributed to the development of an animal pathogen? According to a document published in 1967 by Spirochetologist Russell C. Johnson and colleague Virginia G. Harris (University of Minnesota), *some saprophytic leptospira strains* produce something called *mouse-erythrocyte hemolytic factor*. In mice, this toxic substance destroys blood cells. Perhaps soil or water-borne *leptospira* spirochetes combined or shuffled genetic information under the influence of agricultural chemicals such as Tweens to create this animal pathogen, especially since pathogenic leptospires and other bacteria (i.e. chromobacterium) have hemolysin enzymes. Could it have developed in an animal body from a failed leptospirosis vaccine? Tweens, as non-ionic surfactants, are ethylene oxide products. *Ethylene oxide is highly mutagenic, carcinogenic, and toxic to humans. It is also a precursor to both ethylene glycol (antifreeze) and to the chemical weapons called nitrogen mustards (i.e. mustard gas).* Tweens contain antifreeze-like proteins that may be acquired by insects including ticks, and which may confer a genetic ability to survive freezing temperatures. Did chemicals help create an important spirochete called the *Suckling Mouse Cataract Agent* (SMCA *Spiroplasma*)? Could a spiroplasma spirochete obtain a mouse hemolytic factor from a saprophytic leptospire under a process that involved an agricultural or industrial chemical like Tweens?[87-90]

The SMCA spiroplasma was discovered in 1954, only three years after New Haven scientists began experimenting with large and small RNA viruses (i.e. *borrelina* viruses). At the time, wide-scale deployments of fertilizers and insecticides that contained Tweens and other catalytic chemicals were being released around the world as herbicides, fertilizers, fungicides, and insecticides. Could a novel mouse pathogen or plant spiroplasma contain genetic information from a virus that was first applied as a biological control enhancer? Is the emergence of novel spiroplasma strains a result of man's manipulation of microbes and the deployment of chemicals? A study suggested that spiroplasmas originated from bacteriae. From the research I have examined, spiroplasmas have only recently emerged; noticeably arriving in the years since the application of biocides and chemical and microbial agents of industry and agriculture.[91,92]

Studies by Johnson-Harris during the 1960s observed the growth response and differences between saprophytic (*Leptospira biflexa*) and pathogenic (*L. pomona*) leptospires at low temperatures. Growth rates were measured in rabbit serum medium versus a modified Tween 80-albumin medium to temperatures as low as 10°C (50°F). The saprophytic *L. biflexa* spirochetes were found to multiply at lower temperatures while the pathogenic *L. interrogans* spirochetes grew little at lower temperatures. Strains that were tested included *L. australis, L. ballum, L. canicola, L. icterohaemorrhagiae, L. biflexa* (including a CDC strain), *L. grippotyphosa, L. autumnalis* and others. A great genetic diversity was noted among the aquatic leptospires studied.[91]

Johnson and Harris demonstrated that saprophytic leptospires that were maintained in a lab for some time were easily killed by low numbers of rabbit serum antibodies. However the pathogenic and saprophytic strains isolated from surface waters were completely resistant to rabbit antibody concentrations of more than 50%. This means that rabbit antibodies did not kill these strains, allowing them to remain available during a rabbit tick blood meal. The use of Tweens in these studies could have been a routine laboratory practice to enhance bacterial growth; or there could have been an unpublished goal to study whether Tweens enabled leptospires to flourish and remain infective in lower soil or water temperatures. Another objective could have been to see if Tweens provided leptospires protection from the rabbit immune system; allowing persistent infections. To some degree, the studies appear to show that this is possible. It would be interesting to know for certain whether Tween-enhancement contributes to persistence of pathogenic spirochetes that can be isolated from animals or humans.[91]

It is noteworthy that the Johnson-Harris studies took place in 1967, the same year Dr. Burgdorfer isolated the novel 277F spiroplasma from Montana rabbit ticks. Other scientists including Dr. Johnson in 1976 (the year after the announcement of Connecticut arthritis cases), were studying these very same processes. From a paper we learn that scientists placed leptospires in various polysorbate-based growth mediums including Tweens 20, 40, 60, and 80, to study their survivability. From a paper we read, "We need to understand what constitutes the endogenous nutrient stores of leptospires and how such stores are related to survival and possibly virulence."[93]

Were researchers studying the leptospires and the Tweens because these chemicals were felt to be contributing to an emerging animal infection that was first discovered during the 1950s? We saw how scientists in the 1960s were studying marine-based Tweens off the US northeast coastline. Would the Connecticut outbreak that was already being detected at this time be the first evidence that an animal infection had crossed over into the human population? A paper on Tween-based virulence of leptospires was written in part by Dr. Ellinghausen, a scientist at the USDA Animal Disease Center in Ames, Iowa. (We have already learned about the Florida Ames strain of anthrax.) Dr. Ellinghausen was among those who nine years earlier had supplied a 1966 CDC "A-177" turtle-cultured strain of *Leptospira biflexa* to Dr. Russell C. Johnson for his 1967 leptospira studies.[93-96]

Can chemicals cause the mutation of leptospires? The loss of genes by mutation (whether by chemicals or viruses) is a common process in bacteria. In fact, meiosis is the process of reductional division, where the numbers of chromosomes per cell are cut in half. The first stage of this process is actually called *leptonema.* In animals, this division gives rise to cells that fuse during reproduction. In other organisms, this process can give rise to spores. Meiosis is necessary for sexual reproduction, even for bacteria. Therefore a leptonema may be a description of a mutated or intermediate stage leptospira that has undergone the process of reductional division – to create a "sporulating" spirochete that has lost some of its genetic material.[97-101]

Borrelia burgdorferi may be such an example of an unusual mutant spirochete that has a correspondingly smaller genetic structure due to a similar loss of genes. Scientists will tell you that Bb does not appear to sporulate. However it seems to have retained the processes which support sporulation activities. Even if it does not produce actual spores, Bb divides into blebs and granules, which are similar forms made by sporulating fungi. Since bacteria are in fact fungal in origin, and agricultural fungi are routinely used in the field, it makes sense that Bb spirochetes have a fungal component as well as genes from a sporulating bacteria, such as is found in B.t. pesticides. We will also learn that a mutated spirochete would be found in a Lyme patient's ECM rash in 1981, the year that the Bb causative agent was first identified. This spirochete would be classified as a *leptonema*.[97-101]

A 1993 textbook discusses the genes of leptospires including strains found in animals and the mutant *Leptospira illini*. Ribosomal genes are special genes that can transcribe cellular RNA, for example from RNA viruses. In leptospiras these genes belong to *sphingomyelinase** enzymes. We discussed these enzymes in the last section, and their dependence upon manganese. In the presence of compatible viruses or bacteria, these enzymes may begin transcription, the first step toward gene expression. This means that leptospira genes can influence the genes of RNA viruses, such as those released into the environment to augment insecticides. This process may be further supported by the chemical Tweens, radioactive elements, or the phagic bacteriae found in global insecticides which lyse or open spirochetes including leptospires.[97-101]

**We already addressed sphingomyelinase enzymes. Sphingomyelin however is particularly abundant in the human nervous system. Sphingolipids are regulated by enzymes that respond to cellular stress (i.e. infection). When these enzymes are deficient, hosts are susceptible to fatal encephalitis viruses. When patients are infected with leptospirosis (or Lyme disease), the microbes utilize the host's sphingolipids. Lipids are important to all cellular processes including proliferation, apoptosis, and inflammation, and are required for viruses and bacteria to thrive. Disruptions in these lipids and enzymes cause diseases such as Crohn's, Tay-Sachs, Gaucher, inflammatory bowel disease, and lysosomal diseases that are common to people of Nova Scotian, Eastern European, and Ashkenazi Jewish descent. This may identify a genetic aspect of disease susceptibility, and explains why a large percentage of people with certain genetic backgrounds suffer more severe cases of Lyme disease than other populations.*

A textbook says there is *"longstanding direct and indirect evidence for genetic transfers between leptospires."* Such transfers include the exchange of virulence (infective) enzyme genes. It is possible for leptospires to transfer genes between other bacteria by packaging segments of its genome into mobile plasmids (smaller chromosomes). These little plasmid islands can separate to incorporate into other bacteria, because leptospires are segmented bacteria. This structure facilitates the transfer of genes between organisms. Such transfers are performed in the laboratory using chemicals including Tweens during genetic engineering. This can also occur in nature from the agriculturally and industrially applied chemicals and microbes found in agricultural soils or polluted wastewaters.[97-101,115]

In short, leptospira strains can donate their (plasmid) genes to other organisms, or incorporate other compatible genes during aggregation and mutation under favorable conditions. The question to ask is what might cause a leptospira spirochete to be opened (lysed) so that it can mutate under the action of agrochemicals and the microbes of insecticides? The answer is that phagic bacteria such as those found in insecticides, and in nature can open many kinds of spirochetes, especially under the influence of chemical pollutants including Tweens (surfactants). In addition, leptospiras have been found to harbor a *leptophage bacteriophage.* This means a phage may be found parasitizing leptospires, including mutant *Leptospira illini* strains. We don't know whether this phage was naturally acquired or was the result of the applied insecticides, but we may guess.[97-101]

Once opened by phagic bacteria, spirochetes are vulnerable to infection by other microbes including viruses, fungi, molds, and other bacteria. Under optimal conditions more than one spirochete can donate genetic information to another to create an aggregate organism that retains the virulence factors of one or more of its parents. These "superbacteria" (i.e. leptonema) are transmissible to insects or animals, where their final assembly will be completed under fermentation of the insect or animal gut. Since Bb spirochetes are unculturable from the environment in their entirety, host factors are likely involved in the creation of the final aggregate spirochete. Inside the insect gut, microbes and toxins from insecticides contribute to mixed infections by damaging the insect's gut membranes, and releasing resident intracellular parasites and latent infections.[97-101]

These parasites may include bacteria, fungi, viruses, protozoans, etc. Some examples that may be found as Lyme co-infections are arboviruses, babesia, ehrlichia, spiroplasmas, bartonella, theileria, coxiella, rickettsia, Q fever, brucella, and more. The variety of transmissible mixed infections varies depending on insect vector and the regional infections they acquire. This well explains why patients with Lyme borreliosis have individualized disease complexes; and common but non-identical co-infections that vary in every patient.[97-110]

Perhaps one reason scientists were studying what leptospires used as nutrient sources in 1976 had something to do with the recent discovery that *Leptospira biflexa spirochetes had contaminated sterilized, deionized water, and stock cultures that were used to make animal vaccines.* The contamination of commercialized water by leptospires is a particular problem in the lab since leptospires pass through conventional water filters (filterable) and often contaminate finished laboratory products. Perhaps scientists were concerned with the contaminant strains' stability and whether "non-pathogenic" strains might mutate in the presence of Tweens in vaccines to affect vaccinated animals. Or maybe they were worried that applied insecticides that contain Tweens and other important components would mutate in animals fed recombinant crops. There mutated bacteria would surely be excreted as animal wastes to contaminate soil and water. It is interesting to find a statement in a scientific paper that says this:[91,94-96]

"...if *Leptospira biflexa* are found in tissue culture media, or if they are found in live vaccines as a contaminant, that scientists believe they should pose 'no hazard' to either laboratory workers or to vaccine recipients."

Leptospira strains however are not exactly reliably classified as to whether they are pathogenic or non-pathogenic. For example a so-called "non-pathogenic" leptospira strain called *Leptospira Andaman correa* was isolated from the spinal fluid of a man; and was said to be serologically related to a "non-pathogenic" saprophytic *Leptospira biflexa* strain. If a spirochete had contaminated animal vaccine cell lines, it could survive in animals, mutate, and be excreted as animal wastes to infect other animals and insects. Such animal wastes would end up in soil, water, and could be recycled as fertilizers for use upon agricultural crops. If leptospira-contaminated animal cell lines were to become a problem, then we might expect scientists to eventually catch this error and to create new animal vaccine cell lines.[92,94-96]

Studies could have been used as a model to study contributing factors to a newly announced human "arthritis"-causing spirochete. What happens when a mutational event occurs between a non-pathogenic leptospire and other bacteriae to make it pathogenic? Scientists were possibly interested in this topic due to the emergence during the 1950s of novel, mutated, intermediate leptospires that we will examine shortly. These were detected in the livestock and fauna around wastewater treatment plants and other aquatic areas. The questions remain, were these mutant spirochetes being created inside the animal bodies from failed *leptospirosis* or other animal vaccines? If so, is that where other animals were picking up similar infections? Or was there another problem that was contributing to the creation of novel mutant spirochetes?[91,92,94-96]

A paper described how leptospires are "omnipresent" in fresh water. Another leptospira strain was isolated from deionized, filtered water in 1974. The strain was named WRAIR after the laboratory at Walter Reed Army Institute of Research where the organism was isolated. (Walter Reed has the largest biomedical research facility administered by the US DOD). The WRAIR strain was identified and confirmed as a *Leptospira biflexa* strain that was closely related to *Leptospira biflexa* strain "Wa Reiden." The source of the contaminant was not definitively traced to the laboratory tap water supply. Instead scientists thought the contaminant may have come from the tap water at the facility where the *resins* for the water filtration system were prepared. The report also referenced the contamination of a tissue culture medium with *L. biflexa* leptospires.[95]

The addition of Tweens to fertilizers and insecticides may not "seriously" affect the presence of some bacteriophages (i.e. in soil or insecticides) according to one research paper. However Tweens may inhibit the interaction of phages and some bacteria, yet not adversely affect the phage/bacteria relationships of others. These effects appear directly dependent upon the concentration of Tweens present. If Tweens enhance the relationships between phages and bacteria and act as aggregators and growth promoters, we can see how Tweens could encourage the aggregation phase of microbes from insecticidal formulas to create a human pathogen under the right environmental and host environments.[111]

In May 1978, a patient who was suspected of having a leptospirosis infection provided specimens for culture including cerebral spinal fluid, blood, and urine. Again in March 1979 another patient provided similar cultures. During the study of these culture sets, it was discovered that deionized water that was commercially prepared and labeled "sterile for tissue culture" was contaminated with a saprophytic strain of leptospira. At first the *Leptospira biflexa* strain that was isolated was thought to have come from the human cultures. However it was later proven to be a contaminant from the commercial water that was used to culture the specimens. An unopened water bottle was sent to the National Animal Disease Center in Ames, Iowa where it tested positive for the contaminating leptospires. The source of the contaminant was confirmed to be the sterile, deionized water for laboratory use. It was noted that *contamination by leptospires is considered to be particularly problematic when filtered deionized water is used in media preparations* since leptospires can pass through tiny (0.22-µm) membrane filters which ordinarily trap most bacteria (are filterable). We have to wonder what this means in terms of cell line creation and the possibility of leptospires or other contaminants which may remain in end products including animal or human vaccines.[97]

Herbicides and Amines to an End

Amines or *quaternary ammonium salts* are used as disinfectants, surfactants, shampoos, detergents, spermicides, and as soil amendments for agricultural fertilizers. Surfactants are used as phase transfer catalysts to force chemical synthesis. They are able to disrupt cell membranes and proteins of most organisms through a chemical reaction. They will kill most microbes except for the most part those found in the agricultural biocides that contain *Bacillus thuringiensis* (B.t.). They also do not kill *Pseudomonas, non-enveloped viruses,* or *Mycobacterium* strains including *Mycobacterium tuberculosis.* This will be key to understanding that bacteria which remain in the soil and water, including those that are discharged in the wastes of vaccinated animals, can remain untouched by the agricultural or industrial products that contain catalytic amines.[1,2]

Certain bacteriae and viruses will be found in abundance in soils and water where surfactants are applied or found since they are left unaffected by these chemicals. The non-enveloped viruses of course are those which include the CPVs, or *cytoplasmic polyhedrosis viruses.* For example this includes Colorado tick fever, bluetongue, rice ragged stunt virus, corn stunt virus, and the viruses of *silkworm* and *gypsy moths*. The CPVs are a genus of *Reoviruses,* a family which includes the *Orbiviruses*. The CPVs multiply inside the insect's midgut epithelial cells. CPVs naturally infect a number of insects in their gut tissues. There they are dissolved by gut enzymes under stress which releases the viruses. CPV infections progress very slowly but are eventually fatal. Because CPVs are ineffective alone as a bioagent, they are genetically engineered into baculovirus constructs that are used as insecticides. Adding them exponentially increases the killing action of the baculoviruses when the two combine. The borrelina viruses that were released in New Haven, Connecticut beginning in 1951 are also left untouched by surfactants, so they may remain available to mutate with other bacteriae in soil and water.[1,2]

There is a quaternary ammonium herbicide with the trade name of *Paraquat* (*N,N'-dimethyl-4,4'-bipyridinium dichloride*). The organic compound pyridine (which is related to toxic benzene), is a solvent and reagent that is mixed with sodium, chloromethane, and anhydrous ammonia to create Paraquat. This is a potent contact herbicide (weed killer). Paraquat was first used commercially in 1955, and was produced by a company called Imperial Chemical Industries (ICI). ICI is reportedly owned by Syngenta, a division of Monsanto. Paraquat not only acts as an herbicide, it also holds antimicrobial properties for example, toward some but not all soil bacteriae and viruses. Paraquat has been one of the most widely used quaternary ammonium herbicides across the globe. Paraquat is considered to be one of the "dirty dozen" of the world's most harmful pesticides. It has already been banned, severely restricted, and/or deregistered by at least ten countries. Paraquat is used as a cause of poisoning by suicide in some cultures, and Paraquat-induced toxicity in rats has been linked to a Parkinson's-like disease.[3-5]

Anhydrous ammonia is what farmers spray on their fields to increase the nitrogen content of soils and to help break down phosphate fertilizers. According to a patent, anhydrous ammonia also "upgrades" microbial cells in the soil to increase their protein content; and improves the taste and smell of plants grown in treated soils. Microbial cells in soil may consist of yeast, fungi, bacteria, viruses, and algae. This compound acts as a fertilizer and makes the crops grown in treated soils taste better. For example a corn field sprayed with *Bacillus thuringiensis* (B.t.) may have a bitter taste, but when these same fields are treated with anhydrous ammonia and B.t. together, the resulting crops will be more palatable in taste, odor, and color.[6,7]

Surfactants have been used in fertilizers at Battelle Memorial Institute in large-scale tests on acidulation and ammoniation during the 1950s. Ammoniation allows a product or drug to be delivered more efficiently into the body across the blood-brain barrier, (i.e. ammonia chemistry used to deliver nicotine by cigarettes.) The addition of surfactants to fertilizers was felt to benefit the curing of superphosphates and ammoniated products. It may have also facilitated the penetration of insect bodies, as well as the mutation of microbes by the chemicals being deployed.[11]

The Minnesota Mining and Manufacturing (3M) Company is assignee to a patent for *Quaternary Fluorinated Ammonium Salts*. These salts are also called quaternary ammonium compounds, or amines. These chemicals are used as disinfectants and surfactants. Off the field they are commonly found in shampoos and fabric softeners; in fabric sheets as antistatic agents (chloride salts); and as an ingredient to spermicidal jellies. These compounds are antimicrobials which break the surface tension of solutions. Soil and water bacteriae can be targeted by the invention, which can be used as an antimicrobial for water treatment, as a soil amendment, or for fertilizers. A problem with quats however is that their antibacterial properties may be altered depending upon which chemicals bind to them. Quats can be fluorinated according to a 1970 patent. This patent describes the surface tension lowering and antimicrobial abilities of these chemicals; particularly against microbes *Bacillus subtilis, Staphylococcus aureus, Escherichia coli, Streptococcus* species and *Aspergillus niger*. This particular invention is useful in many applications including soil amendments, pesticides, and fertilizers.[8-11]

In organic chemistry, quaternary ammonium salts are used as *phase transfer catalysts* to cause chemical synthesis. *Quats disrupt the cell membrane and proteins of microbes* through a chemical reaction. They kill most microbes except for *endospores* such as those found in B.t. insecticides. They also do not kill *Pseudomonas, non-enveloped viruses,* or *Mycobacterium tuberculosis*. The latter is the tuberculosis bacteria. If this microbe mutates under influence of agrochemicals or quats, it may become a virulent tuberculosis-like "flu." There are specific quat disinfectants that will kill *M. tuberculosis,* including a 3M brand, but these appear to be industrial disinfectants, and may not be used agriculturally.[13,35]

Quaternary ammonium compounds are also used in various vaccine formulas. This seems a bit strange since research shows that direct exposure to quats by skin or respiratory inhalation causes irritation. They are also known to degrade gut tissues, they may cause anaphylaxis during anesthesia, and yet such compounds may be injected into our bodies. One patent describes the rather unpredictable nature of these chemical compounds (quaternary halides) when coupled with fluorocarbon chains (molecules with multiple carbon-*fluorine* bonds). The result of this bonding is a modified activity toward bacterial flora. According to a patent:

> "Apparently, *when fluorocarbon chains are substituted* on the nitrogen [molecule] of a quaternary amine salt, *the pattern of antimicrobial activity becomes unpredictable*. It is a feature of this invention that a specific class of fluorocarbon-containing quaternary amines, i.e. that defined by Formula I, has been discovered that possesses the desired surface tension lowering ability and yet retains the antimicrobial activity sometimes attributed to quaternary amine salts."[10,13,35]

This simply means that in the presence of fluorides, the antimicrobial properties of quats are altered, and this patent formula attempts to overcome this problem. Quats are ineffective in the presence of organic compounds and may fail in temperatures above 100°F. They are deactivated by anionic detergents, soaps, and cotton fibers, which may also be found in wastewaters. It is perhaps noteworthy that a company that is assignee for at least one patent for *quaternary fluorinated ammonium salts* useful in water and soil applications would also be listed as an assignee for a diagnostic test for Lyme disease which can be used to test wastewater samples for the presence of leptospires and Bb spirochetes.

This seems less curious if we consider that the causative agent of Lyme disease may have its origins in high nitrogen, phosphorus, ammonia, organic matter, microbe, mineral, and metal-drenched environments. There, industrial and agriculturally applied chemicals may adversely influence microbes due to the action of fluorides, surfactants, nuclear wastes, and other pollutants upon microbes. Such toxic "soups" may be found in industrial and municipal wastewaters, in groundwater, or in the soil and subsurface water tables around commercial feedlots, mining and metal industries, nuclear plants, laboratories, and agricultural areas where chemicals mix with soil and water-borne pathogens to create mutant, aggregate spirochetes.

Beginning in 1975 under indirect financial support from the US government (about $30 million annually), the government of Mexico sprayed Paraquat upon poppy and marijuana fields to destroy these crops. The herbicide took several days to be effective, so Mexican workers reportedly harvested crops before they turned yellow. The drugs were then smuggled illegally into the US. As a result drug users were exposed to an estimated 3,000 tons of herbicide-contaminated pot and heroin. A few University of Illinois-Urbana students who had smoked the herbicide-tainted marijuana reportedly told a drug counselor that they had become sick after use.[3]

At the time, Illinois Senator Charles Percy pressed for an investigation to determine how much contaminated pot was circulating. The University of Illinois-Urbana has plant and animal genetics laboratories which are used (among other studies) for crop sciences and herbicides. This university also had connections to an llinois laboratory which isolated mutant leptospira spirochetes from bulls and turtles in the area a decade earlier.[3]

A Skokie, Illinois laboratory belonging to the G.D. Searle Company (a division of Monsanto), tested the marijuana samples for evidence of Paraquat. The tests revealed that thirty-nine out of forty samples tested positive for the herbicide. Twenty-one percent of pot samples in the southwestern US were tested and returned positive for the herbicide. Paraquat is capable of permanently damaging human airways. As a result there was widespread panic among people who had smoked the tainted pot. These circumstances resulted in CDC surveys and combustion tests which were designed to assess toxicity and exposure risks. Eventually the CDC declared there was "no risk" of lung damage from Paraquat-contaminated marijuana. In 1978, Senator Percy introduced an amendment to the Foreign Assistance Act of 1961 which prohibited the US from funding any future programs (even indirectly), which spray herbicides upon marijuana plants if the herbicides are harmful to humans.[12]

When Paraquat is present in the human body, it undergoes a process that converts it to a superoxide, also called a free radical, and which damages cells. Scientists have performed a number of studies concerning Paraquat and its effects upon plant, insect, and human systems. For example, a 1976 collaborative study at the pulmonary-toxicology laboratory and research services of the Veterans Administration hospital and the department of pharmacology at the University of Minnesota looked at the production of free radicals and the anorexic effects of Paraquat upon rats.[14-17]

A 1985 study from the University of Minnesota in partnership with the University of California-Davis studied the fruit fly gene variations which provide Paraquat and DDT pesticide resistance. Scientists determined that survival and resistance to pesticides is provided by specific genes. The study also discussed scientific efforts to extend the fruit fly life span by providing them with genes which create antioxidant enzymes that are important to maintaining pesticide resistance. Their findings correlated with an existing "genetic rescue" hypothesis. Genetic rescue is a technique that uses like species with beneficial genes to improve populations of similar species which lack the beneficial genes. We have already learned that scientists released millions of mosquitoes with the objective of "population replacement." Could some of those mosquitoes have been carrying important viruses that were capable of mutating in the presence of pesticides, herbicides, or other agriculturally applied weapons of insect biowarfare? Or were they possibly carrying lab-manipulated genes that conferred pesticide resistance – genes that could be transferred across species to cause interspecies pesticide resistance?[15-17]

Mycobacterium tuberculosis and *Pseudomonas aeruginosa* are two organisms that have rapidly developed antibiotic resistance. Pseudomonas bacteria attach to other bacteria to form *biofilm aggregates*. As an opportunistic pathogen, this bacterium is one cause of hospital-acquired infections. It might be suggested that the biofilms created by these organisms may contribute to chronic infections in certain individuals; especially when biofilms are formed in the mouth and which when swallowed, help colonize the gut. It is acknowleged within some scientific circles that Bb spirochetes may be found within biofilms, and one paper specifically notes how Bb spirochetes aggregate within laboratory cultures. Regardless of which microbes produce them, biofilms provide protection against unfavorable environments and antibiotics in the body in the same way they provide protection to multiple microbes which sequester inside of them in the external environment.[18-21,23]

What is interesting is that Dr. Allen C. Steere was lead author of a research paper that discussed a 1977 study of bacteremia caused by *Pseudomonas* species. The paper discussed the contamination of an *albumin* product which caused bacteremia after patients underwent surgery. The albumin when cultured from previously unopened vials yielded *Pseudomonas cepacia.* This described the contamination of albumin, a product that is useful in surgery (human albumin); and to create vaccines (bovine albumin). The paper cautioned that so-called sterile laboratory products can become contaminated by pathogenic agents (i.e. leptospires), which can of course contribute to infectious disease outbreaks.

> "Since sterility testing by manufacturers may not detect low-frequency contamination, surveillance of nosocomial infections, investigation of unusual disease clusters, and prompt reporting of suspect reactions are essential in the control of such outbreaks."[22]

Pseudomonas aeruginosa are slimy bacterial aggregates that form resistant biofilms, and which contaminate clinical and industrial environments. Copper and quaternary ammonium compounds (amines) are used to kill biofilms in vitro (lab) and in vivo (body). These compounds have been used for several decades in the forestry industry, in part to control biofilms left by bacterial biodegraders including *Pseudomonas aeruginosa*.[18,19,22,23]

Copper and quaternary compounds have been used as fungicides and insecticidal wood preservatives since the early 1990s. About 454,000 kg of ammoniacal copper quaternary (ACQ) was released in British Columbia, Canada in 1996. Gentian violet and ferric ammonium citrate may also be used to disrupt *Pseudomonas* biofilms. Gentian violet is a bactericide/antifungal agent used in the laboratory as a gram-staining agent. It is also applied topically as a weak solution.[24-32]

Gentian violet was used as an animal feed additive, but has since been banned by the FDA. Mice and rat studies demonstrated toxicity and carcinogenic potentials for gentian violet. In the textile industry, gentian violet is a general term which represents a group of *methyl violet* dyes which include any violet pararosanilin dyes which produce rich blue-purple hues (aniline dyes). Gentian violet is also used *as a marker dye in herbicidal formulas.* Marker dyes are simply used so farmers (or crop dusters) can see how much, and where herbicides have been applied to fields. Similar dyes have been used since the 1800s in the textile and printing industries (i.e. inks, marking pencils).[24-32]

Once again we see a connection between copper, quaternary herbicides, and aniline dyes that are active in the presence of fluorides, chlorides, and agrochemicals including Tweens. Commercial dyes are used as vegetation markers, for industrial purposes, and upon *golf courses,* which is where the earliest microbial insecticides were first applied (i.e. milky spore agents). These marker dyes are also used to track wastewaters in industrial flows; and many colors including *malachite green* are used. Remember that malachite is formed by degrading copper. There was malachite mining in Thuringia, Germany where B.t. was originally isolated in 1915. Incidentally, golf courses are often fertilized using recycled wastewaters or sludges.[24-32]

One report describes how scientists analyzed the microbial communities that thrived in different developmental stages of *Ixodes scapularis* ticks collected from Westchester and Dutchess counties, New York. They found many pathogens living inside of tick bodies including *pseudomonas, rickettsial* species (including *Ralstonia,* which causes *bacterial wilt* in plants)*, borreliae, anaplasmas, enterobacteriae* (i.e. *E. coli*, *salmonella*), *Moraxella* (a respiratory coccobacilli), *Rhodococcus* (mycobacteria), and other proteobacteriae. When we examine the history of what has been applied to the environment by many important industries, it is no surprise that Bb spirochetes can form, or that insects are now able to transmit a wide variety of mixed infections; including some which might "secretly" harbor recombinant genes.[33,34]

Chasing Rainbows

If we look a little closer at the history of the rainbow herbicide *Agent Orange*, we find links that are important to agriculture. In the 1940s American Botanist Arthur Galston, a graduate of the University of Illinois, studied the properties of the chemical plant growth regulator 2,3,5-T (TIBA or 2,3,5-Triiodobenzoic acid). His early research and a 1943 PhD dissertation centered on a search for a chemical which could accelerate soybean growth. During his work he realized that 2,3,5-T had dual properties as a growth-enhancer; and at stronger concentrations as a defoliating agent (causing leaf loss). Arthur Galston was drafted into the US Navy and served in Japan until his 1946 discharge. Thereafter he taught at the California Institute of Technology; and from 1955 forward at Yale as a Professor of Bioethics.[1-3]

In 1943, University of Chicago scientists were contracted by the US Army to study the effects of the herbicide 2,4-D and "Galston's" growth regulator 2,3,5-T upon rice and broadleaf crops. From February to April of 1945, aerial experiments were undertaken at the Bushnell Army Air Field in Florida using various mixtures of 2,4-D and 2,4,5-T over three hundred and eighty-two acres. When mixed in equal parts, these chemicals make *Agent Orange* (perhaps even if deployed separately). These herbicide deployments do not mean that the military did not experiment with tactical herbicides in 1942 or 1943 at Camp Bullis, Texas; or decades later at Fort Chaffee (both sites where novel human ehrlichiosis infections first emerged).[1-3]

Although rainbow herbicides were said not to have been deployed during WWII, they were studied by scientists in 1951 at Camp Detrick's laboratory for potential deployment during the Korean conflict. To that end, from May 1951 to March 1959, the US Air Force and the Army Chemical Corps conducted a series of herbicide tests that were aerially released by towers, balloons, and aircraft; and sprayed at Dugway Proving Ground in Utah. From May to October 1959 at Fort Drum, New York, thirteen drums of surplus Agent Purple, another herbicide, were aerially dropped over roughly 2,500 acres of Ft. Drum's forested areas. Agent Purple, like Agent Orange, contained dioxins from a chemical contaminant that was a byproduct of its manufacture. Agent Purple is similar to Agent Orange, but with a different mixture of 2,4-D and 2,4,5-T.[1-4]

From July to August of 1951, the USDA research station in Brawley, California collaborated with the Army Chemical Corps to test the effectiveness of small droplet sprays of 2,4-D and 2,4,5-T upon small field plots of various crops. From November 1952 to April 1953 at Eglin Air Force base in Florida on test ranges 52 and 57, bomber aircraft tested a large capacity spray system using a mixture of 2,4-D and 2,4,5-T over eighty seven hundred acres. Other tests were undertaken in Bozeman, Montana from July through November 1953 upon the USDA experimental fields in the Gallatin valley, over one hundred and thirty-six acres of wheat crops. In Area B of Fort Detrick, Frederick, Maryland from June to July 1953, US Army Chemical Corps scientists used a tower-based system mounted on a pickup truck to spray plots of soybeans and sweet potatoes with 2,4-D and 2,4,5-T. At Fort Ritchie in Cascade, Maryland from April 1956 to September 1957, the US Army Chemical Corps evaluated five hundred and seventy-seven herbicides which were hand-sprayed upon small field plots.[1-4]

In 1965 Arthur Galston (Yale) and Matthew S. Meselson (Harvard) and others lobbied the US government to stop the use of Agent Orange; and formally requested toxicity studies. Department of Defense scientists validated that the chemicals caused birth defects in laboratory rats. In 1971, information about the toxicity of Agent Orange was provided to former President Richard Nixon, who immediately halted the herbicidal sprays. It seems a bit ironic that Dr. Arthur Galston, one of the original scientists interested in a chemical that would be used in Agent Orange and other rainbow herbicides, died in Hamden, Connecticut, just north of New Haven, on the western edge of Cockaponset State Forest not far from the first reported cluster of Lyme disease cases in the US.[1,2,5,6]

The kinds of chemicals that were released into the US and elsewhere (even experimentally or agriculturally), have the potential to cause mutational changes in the microbes of the soils and waters where they were deployed. As we will learn from an outbreak at Camp Bullis, Texas in 1942-1943, and in Malaysia, such chemicals could be responsible for the development of animal and human infections that might not have arisen had such chemicals never been deployed.[1,2,5,6]

The Institute of Medicine (IOM) has published reports on the topics of Agent Orange and the Gulf War. The institute also published a book titled *Improving the Presumptive Disability Decision-Making Process for Veterans.* The book includes IOM statements and conclusions about Agent Orange and the Gulf War; and the health effects of the herbicides used in Vietnam. The agency provided reports which evaluated the strength of evidence linking herbicides to public health concerns. The current model for IOM presumptions followed the Agent Orange Act of 1991 (public law 102-4, 102d Congress, 2nd session). The IOM also held a special October 11-12, 2010 conference on Lyme disease in Washington, DC. The IOM was charged by the NIH and specifically the NIAID to establish a committee which would examine the state of science concerning Lyme disease. The NIH/NIAID provides the majority of federal funding for scientific research including for Lyme and other tickborne diseases.[5,6]

The final report by the IOM from the conference on Lyme disease was supposed to address the gaps in the prevention and treatment of Lyme and other tickborne diseases. What came out of the IOM conference was somewhat confusing with respect to acknowledging Lyme disease, especially given the evidence in my books. When we consider government agencies that are partly funded by pharmaceutical or agricultural interests including patent royalies, we may see potential conflicts of interest that could color the results of scientific studies and conference reports, either directly or indirectly. If the results of government studies reveal adverse findings, such revelations might significantly impact important industries. Whether this affects the objectivity or outcomes of such meetings is anyone's guess. As a casual observer however, the idea that chronic Lyme "doesn't" exist seems to be the most pervasive sentiment among those who support, or were involved with the formation of the IDSA Lyme disease guidelines. Such lack of acknowledgement may include promoting the party line of scientific consensus to protect important tools and to prevent liability issues.[5,6]

NIH scientists from Texas and California have explored the genes of experimental fruit flies that were genetically engineered with mutant genes (transgenes). A study attempted to analyze how flies with genetically inserted Familial Amyotrophic Lateral Sclerosis (FALS or ALS) genes compared to humans who had the same disease and who exhibited mutations in a gene that deals with oxidative stress. Human ALS is a serious disease that has been hypothesized as being caused by the spirochetes of Lyme disease. Organophosphate chemicals have also been implicated in some research as potential contributing agents to neurologic diseases including Alzheimer's and ALS. In the case of infections caused by aggregate spirochetes, the mutagenic activities of herbicides may have something to do with the development of these kinds of microbes. Maybe that is why French scientists in 1966 studied thirty-five hundred elderly patients who demonstrated a decline in brain function when drinking water that contained fluoride, calcium, and aluminum. If an aggregate Bb spirochete contains mutated pathogens that are Tween, fluoride, chloride, aluminum, and herbicide resistant, then the development of aggregate microbes that cause animal and human diseases makes a lot more sense.[7-15]

Persisting Pollutants

Another source of potential microbial mutators are the residual chemical compounds which remain after the mining and processing of phosphate rocks, bauxite, metals, and mineral ores. Since toxic metals and fluorides are present in the extraction and processing of aluminum from bauxite, some may remain in wastewaters and groundwaters. Bauxite remember is an important aggregate rock that is mined for its alumina content but it has many other uses and is highly valuable especially to the fertilizer and wastewater industries. Fluorides and other potentially mutagenic chemicals are therefore present in products used for wastewater treatment, sugar refining, fertilizers, pesticides, herbicides, and other applications.

Various components that are input during the aluminum and other metal smelting and refining processes include bauxite, sodium hydroxide, alumina slurry, starch, aluminum hydrate, and cryolite. (Since 1957, cryolite in the form of sodium hexafluoroaluminate has also been used as an insecticide on fruits and vegetables.) The waste byproducts from these processes include caustic vapors and particulates; fluorides, fluorine gas, carbon dioxide, sulfur dioxide, carbon monoxide, and perfluorinated carbons (PFCs) in the form of gases and particulates. The solid and liquid wastes from processing may also contain starches, sands, dyes, and/or caustic residues including silicon, iron, titanium, calcium oxides; chemicals, heavy metals, radioactive minerals, and acids. The mining process also requires the use of various nitrated (explosive) chemicals whose byproducts remain in the soil, and which will likewise migrate into water tables.[1,2]

Potassium fluoride is a toxic (alkaline halide) metal fluoride and key reagent used in the refining process of alumina from bauxite ore. During the reduction process, there is a discharge of fluoride and alumina dusts and gases. The bauxite is crushed and mixed with caustic soda solutions, which dissolves the alumina. Potassium fluoride helps determine the level of dissolved alumina in solutions. The finished aluminum becomes the basic feedstock for all aluminum based metals and chemicals. The chemical compound potassium fluoride is the primary source of fluoride ions for manufacturing and chemical applications. In the latter it is used to convert chlorocarbons into fluorocarbons, usually by applying a solvent.[1,2]

Perfluorinated acids are hydrophobic, which means they repel water and oil. These acids are also resistant to heat and chemical stress. Perfluorinated acids and salts include the ammonium salts, and have emerged as an important class of globally persistent environmental pollutants. Biological monitoring surveys analyzed tissue samples from marine organisms (i.e. fish, mussels, birds, seals). Samples demonstrated the presence of PFOS. Both compounds have been found in marine life from many regions around the world.[3,4]

The EPA began investigating perfluorinated chemicals (PFCs) in 1999 after receiving data on a key ingredient, perfluoro-octanesulfonic acid (PFOS); a fluorosurfactant and persistent organic pollutant. This chemical compound was reportedly used in Scotchgard™, a 3M Company fabric protectant. Following EPA investigations, the 3M Company announced it would phase out PFOS, PFOA (perfluorooctanoic acid or "C8"), and related salts and products. PFOAs have been found to be toxicants and carcinogens, and have been detected in human blood samples. PFOAs are associated with thyroid disease, birth defects, increased cancers (i.e. prostate, colon), high cholesterol, strokes, infertility, and changes to lipid levels in the liver and immune systems.[3,5-13]

PFOAs have been found in industrial wastes, stain resistant carpets, microwave popcorn bags, carpet cleaners, and house dust. Fluorinated tolomers and polytetrafluoroethylene (PTFE), have been used on non-stick cook and bakeware products. In animal studies, developmental toxicities from some of these chemicals have ranged from birth size alterations, developmental delays, endocrine disruption, neonatal mortality; to liver, pancreatic, testicular cancers in rats; and liver cancers in rainbow trout. PFOAs also contribute to oxidative stress and are likely to be mutagenic to microbes.[3,5-13]

According to an EPA document, PFOA is liver toxic to animals and persists in the environment. These toxins bioaccumulate in humans, and have an estimated half-life of 4.4 years. PFOAs are thought to be present in the general population of all US geographic regions. PFOA is not a naturally occurring compound, and therefore can be attributed in all human exposures to industrial exposures. In filed legal documents pertaining to the DuPont Washington Works Facility in West Virginia, the EPA alleged there were gender differences found in the way that rats eliminated PFOA. Accusations alleged that the DuPont Company failed to submit data concerning human serum sampling for twelve individuals who lived near the Washington Works facility. When those results were finally obtained, serum samples showed that PFOA levels in the twelve persons sampled ranged from 15.7 ppb (parts per billion) to 128 ppb. The average level of PFOA in typically exposed persons is estimated to be only about 5 ppb.[14-17]

The 3M company began producing PFOA in 1947. In 1951 DuPont began using PFOA to manufacture fluoropolymers for its products including non-stick cookware, or coatings for nuclear reactor components. There are also other similar products sold under various trade names by other companies. Fluoropolymers including perfluorinated acids are used in a wide variety of applications from automotive to aviation, fire protection, defense applications, cable and wire insulations, mobile phones, textiles, plastics, paints, adhesives, inks, sandblasting and etching materials, safety glass, carpeting and flooring, fire extinguishers, propellants, refrigerants, foams, and pharmaceuticals. They are also used in semiconductors, Tyvek®, oil, fuel, and other tank liners, and *fluorinated colored plastic containers that house herbicides and insecticides.* Herbicide containers are made of HDPE plastics because of the interactions between metal containers and the solvents or hydrocarbons contained in these chemical formulas. The plastic containers are *fluorinated* (fluorotainers) to prevent product leakage, corrosion, and package destruction. Now we can see one route that microbes may take to become aggregate spirochetes – from the recombinant insecticides that are stored in fluorinated plastic containers and which donate recombinant microbes, fluorides, plastic polymers, and mutagenic chemicals and dyes to soils and wastewaters upon industrial or agricultural use.[17,18,21-22]

Approximately 90,000 tons of fluoropolymers are marketed globally each year with about 70% of the demand used for PTFE. Some of the most common forms of fluoropolymer plastics are PVC (polyvinyl chloride), PFA (perfluoroalkoxy), and ETFE (ethylene tetrafluorethylene). PVC is used for pipes, clothing, upholstery, cable insulation, inflatable plastics, and drinking water bottles which contain plasticizers as *phthalates.* PFA is used in injection molding, non-stick polymer coatings, as flexible tubing, or scrubbers. PFA can be lined with carbon steel or fibers as reinforced plastics; and used in reactors and pipes that are exposed to halogens or corrosives (i.e. hydrochloric or hydrofluoric acid). ETFE is used to line storage tanks, pipes, as a mold release agent, and to cover electrical wiring or cable wrap because of its thermoplastic properties under high temperatures. ETFE is particularly useful to the aviation, space, and nuclear industries. Thermoplastics have also been engineered to contain pesticides.[17,18,21-22,44,45,87]

Automotive fuel tanks are another example of containers that may be lined with perfluorinated compounds. Fluorinated polymer fibers can be used as stabilizers for dyes, drugs, explosives (nanopowders), and lattices. Lattices may be found in soil treatments of bentonite and other expanding lattice clays that are combined with ammonium salts. A patent assigned to the National Aniline & Chemical Company, Inc. describes the use of these compounds in dyes, germicides, insecticides, fungicides, and other parasiticides. Lattice clay soil liners have been used to control dust and to contain water and toxic chemicals for many decades (i.e. wastewaters, landfills, effluents, petroleum, mining, radioactive nuclear wastes). Petroleum-based soil sealants which contain lattices have been used to line golf course and wastewater ponds, lakes, and fish hatcheries.[22-27]

It is most interesting that *Borrelia burgdorferi* has been found to invade, bind to, and colonize collagen lattices in the human body. This is not difficult to imagine since at least one component of an aggregate Bb spirochete is detectable by a diagnostic test owned by a polymer manufacturer. These bacteria probably have an affinity for collagenous lattices regardless of their origin (insect, animal, human, synthetic). When we realize that collagen is found in the bones, skin, connective tissues, cartilage, intervertebral discs, blood vessels, corneas, and gut tissues; it makes sense that Bb spirochetes are found in these locations. Whatever binds to collagenous materials in the environment, will likely bind with similar lattices in the human body.[39-43]

The kinds of collagenous materials found in wastewaters are numerous and include biodegradable polymers for clinical use (i.e. collagens, bone, skin grafts); drugs, polysaccharides, gelatins, polyesters, elastomers, cyanoacrylates, ceramics, and of course keratins from animal and human hair, feathers, and skin. Since keratin has a high glycine content, and so does collagen, bacteriae that are attracted to the glycine and keratin in wastewaters would also be attracted to these substances in the human host. Glycine is used to create the cell wall polymers of most bacteriae, and is found in the Bb spirochete's plasma membrane (cell wall).[39-43]

Fluoropolymers are highly chemical and heat-resistant, and are not known to degrade by any natural process due to the strength of their carbon-fluorine (fluoride) bonds. Remember that fluorides are taken up by the body and become bound to teeth, bones, and soft tissues. If synthetic polymers are bound to the fluorides and chlorides of wastewaters, be assured that they may also be taken up by microbes, and may likewise bind to the structures in our bodies including teeth and bones. The 3M Company is assignee to a patent for a diagnostic test that detects Bb spirochetes in aqueous solutions and urine (i.e. wastewaters or rodent or human urine), and this would seem strange if we did not understand that there may be a connection between persisting industrial pollutants and the creation of mutant spirochetes that are infectious to animals and humans.[17,18]

In 2000 the scientific community first became aware that perfluorooctanyl sulfonate (PFOS), the key ingredient in fabric stain repellent was being detected at low levels throughout the environment, including within sampled human populations. Since then, environmental scientists and toxicologists have paid more attention to PFOS, and related compounds perfluorooctanoic acid (PFOA), polytetrafluoroethylene (PTFE), and other members of the perfluoroalkyl acid family (PFAA). In 2005 PFOAs were shown in a German drinking water study to be at least indirectly genotoxic. This means these chemicals induce or suppress a broad range of genes. Many of the affected genes control fat, carbohydrate, and protein metabolism; cell communication and adhesion; hormone regulation, growth, immunity, and apoptosis (cell death). These chemicals were shown to inhibit the release of fat metabolizing enzymes which can lead to obesity in affected persons.[6,16]

In 2006, scientists found remarkably high concentrations of perfluorinated surfactants in the Moehne tributary of the Ruhr River in Germany. Perfluorinated surfactants were found in the German water, which is used as a source of drinking water. Reports blamed the contamination on an agricultural area close to the Moehne River where wastes were incorporated into soil amendments and applied to the area. Analyses of local drinking water sources showed it was also contaminated, mainly by PFOA fluorosurfactants. This is interesting because we will learn about another river in the region that was also heavily polluted during the 1950s, and from which a novel, mutated leptospira (leptonema) spirochete was isolated.[3,4,16,18]

A presentation by the Zoology Department & National Food Safety and Toxicology Center of Michigan State University, showed toxicology results for PFOA, PFDA (perfluorodecanoate), PFBA (perfluorobutyric acid), and PFOS. Studies revealed the toxic activities of these compounds in the human body. Undesirable effects include inhibited intercellular communication and organ-specific DNA damage. Additional problems include altered liver enzymes (i.e. cytochrome P450, phospholipase C), reduced T3 and T4 concentrations, decreased serum cholesterol, and increased fatty acids. In short, these compounds affect cellular membrane and mitochondrial function, protein binding, hormone displacement, and gene expression. These chemicals are also associated with anorexia and weight loss, bradycardia, hypothermia, and reduced motor activity. Alterations in p450 cytochromes also affect glutathione levels which are important antioxidants that assist with DNA synthesis and repair. They also assist with enzyme activation and amino acid transport; and are essential for proper human nerve and organ function. Lyme patients who have high levels of perfluorinated compounds in their body may have their disease state significantly complicated by persisting chemicals that alter proper hormone, enzyme, DNA repair, organ function, and/or gene expression.[19,20]

As early as 1961, the DuPont Company was aware that liver enlargement occurred in laboratory mice that consumed PFOA. As a result of the 3M phase-out of PFOA and related chemicals, DuPont constructed a manufacturing plant in Fayetteville, North Carolina in 2002 to manufacture its own ammonium perfluorooctanoate (APFO). Sources say that APFO had been supplied to the company by 3M since 1951. Both the 3M and DuPont companies have been parties to legal actions for chemically contributing to the contamination of groundwater and water streams. Millions of dollars in EPA fines were ordered including a $16.5 million settlement with the EPA against DuPont without admission of liability. DuPont has also been sued for chemical contamination of a river in Ohio and for contaminations to persons living near a West Virginia plant according to reports.[14-16,28,29]

The 3M Company has been accused of contributing toxic pollutants to the Mississippi River and negatively affecting waters along a five-state area. There is now a voluntary EPA program in place to encourage fluoropolymer manufacturers to eliminate these compounds from emissions and from their products by 2015. In 2007, the Minnesota Department of Health lowered its allowable PFOA drinking water limits, according to a source, due to "landfilled industrial wastes from a 3M manufacturing plant."[12,15,30-35]

While municipal water and wastewater treatment plants use activated carbon and/or ionic filters to remove contaminants such as PFCs from groundwater, some toxic compounds escape filtration processes. In addition, some additives to the water treatment process like bauxite exert activity upon remaining microbes. Some perfluorinated surfactants are also ineffectively removed from drinking water supplies. Chemicals may remain after filtered wastewater is discharged into water streams or when concentrated from wastewater sludge and used as soil fertilizers. For example, PFOA contaminated wastes were incorporated into soil amendments and spread upon agricultural land in Germany, which led to drinking water contamination. Water treatment plants can also serve as a source for PFOA, which can be created by the microbial degradation of perfluorinated compounds (PFCs). The end stage compounds from PFAAs are PFOS and PFOA. Regardless of the source of these toxins, they leach into soils and wastewaters and affect resident microbes. They also have the potential to bind to, and affect the human body in an adverse manner.[16,36-38]

During the 1940s, the synthethic herbicide 2,4,5-*Trichlorophenoxyacetic acid* (2,4,5-T) was widely used as an agricultural herbicide and plant growth regulator. The pesticide *dichlorodiphenyltrichloroethane* or DDT with the chemical formula 1,1,1-trichloro-2,2-di(4-chlorophenyl)ethane was a synthetic pesticide that was also being widely applied around the world including in the US at the time of a 1942-1943 (Camp Bullis, Texas) outbreak of a new tickborne infection. Another chemical herbicide, 2,4-Dichlorophenoxyacetic acid, or "2,4-D" was a common herbicide that was also widely deployed around the globe, but especially in North America. It was a major ingredient to the chemical herbicide *Agent Orange*. It was not released for *commercial* use until 1946, but 2,4-D would increase crop yields by enhancing weed control. The herbicide was tested in numerous locations around the US prior to its release. A 50:50 mixture of 2,4,5-T and 2,4-D creates the chemical Agent Orange.[46,47]

Whether this chemical compound is created by man or through the applications of individual herbicides or chemicals that are applied to soils (or which become airborne pollution) and *which combine and degrade naturally under environmental conditions*; these chemicals are *highly mutagenic and exert actions upon microbes including those of insects*. We may wonder if they created the various strains of *Ehrlichiosis* and other infectious diseases (i.e. Bb) that are found today in animals and humans.

The herbicides 2,4-D and 2,4,5-T were contaminated with the highly mutagenic *dioxins.* The group of dioxins includes eighty-seven chlorinated dioxins (polychlorodibenzodioxins) or PCDDs; and forty-nine *furans* (polychlorodibenzofurans) or PCDFs. The toxicity of dioxin and furan formulas is directly dependant upon the number and placement of chlorine atoms in the molecular structure of the compositions. Dioxin-like chemicals including PCBs are sometimes lumped under the general term dioxins because they exert similar activity upon microbes and higher animals. Dioxins in general cause deformities, birth defects, fetal deaths, cancers, endocrine disorders, infertility, wasting syndromes, endometriosis, altered glucose and fat metabolism, impaired neurological function, cognitive deficits, and other health issues. They are known to be the most toxic pollutants on the planet, and they are found in numerous industrial and agricultural chemicals.[46-51]

The main exposures to dioxins occur from consuming foods grown in dioxin-contaminated soils, from dioxin-containing water and food animals, and from airborne contaminants (i.e. coal fly ash, which also may contain chromium VI), burned mixed wastes, wood pulp, and plastics. Dioxins are stored in body fats and are expressed in milk, which may be one reason why public health officials are beginning to force organic raw milk producers to stop selling raw milk and milk products to the public. Remember that Ft. Detrick scientists by 1968 were meeting in Chicago to discuss the progress of aerosolized microbes. Their studies may have been aimed at evaluating the effects of airborne dioxin contaminants upon microbes that may have begun to be detected in animals, and eventually a cluster of patients in Connecticut.[46-51]

Dioxins are by-products of molding, burning, or manufacturing *organic chemicals and plastics that contain chlorine.* The Love Canal (Niagara Falls, New York [Hooker Chemical dump site]), and Times Beach,* Missouri (on the Meramec River near St. Louis), are examples of communities that had to be abandoned in whole or in part as a result of dioxin contaminations.[46,47]

**Times Beach had been sprayed with waste oil by the Russell Bliss Company during the summers of 1972 and 1973 to control dust. It was discovered later that the waste oil may have contained dioxins.*

Chlorinated products (and dioxins) are of course found in thousands of products including plastics, bleach, personal care products, pesticides, fertilizers, and swimming pool chemicals. Chlorinated chemicals plus an organic material (i.e. pulp, wood, paper, natural fibers) plus a catalytic agent (i.e. fire, chemicals) will create dioxins after a chemical reaction. The EPA considers incinerators to be the largest source of dioxin emissions, including military incinerators. Paper, pulp, lumber, textile and crop wastes, plastics industries; coal-fired industries and power plants; metal smelters, cement kilns, automobiles that use leaded gasoline, wood burning; gas and oil industries; and municipal, medical, industrial, private waste burning (garbage, cremation), and bonfires are all sources of dioxins. Nuclear production facilities and nuclear plants have also been known to emit dioxins through airborne and other routes along with other important persisting pollutants.[48-59]

Chlorinated chemicals and dioxins are a common constituent to fertilizers and pesticides. Soil samples were analyzed for the presence of heavy metals and chlorinated compounds in the state of Washington. Results of the surveys revealed that soil conditions and pH affected the bioavailability of heavy metals and dioxins. These conditions are altered by clay content, organic materials, and concentrations of aluminum, manganese, and iron oxides in soils. Phosphate fertilizers, soil amendments, and industrial byproducts typically lack organic matter. Therefore there is a limited protective effect of organic residues in these formulas that would otherwise limit the amount of metals and POPs that are bioavailable to plants and insects. A 1997 report found that the EPA regulations for biosolids were insufficient to protect soils and plants from the adverse effects of metal and toxin accumulations from fertilizer formulas. Most of the dioxin contaminants found in soils are felt to be *long-term transport and deposits of aerial particles from various combustion activities.* But they are also present in soils and wastewaters as a result of applied agricultural and industrial products and processes.[60-63]

Another report described the first nationwide food sampling study to analze the levels of dioxins, dibenzofurans, and polychlorinated biphenyls (PCBs). One hundred and ten food samples were collected in 1995 from supermarkets in Atlanta, GA; Binghamton, NY; Chicago, IL; Louisville, KY; and San Diego, CA. The scientists also collected human milk samples to estimate the levels of contaminants in nursing infants. The food category which revealed the highest levels of dioxins was farm-grown freshwater fish fillets. Levels were compared to World Health Organization (WHO) dioxin toxic equivalent (TEQ) concentrations. The study was undertaken by scientists from the University of Texas-Houston, the UT Southwestern Medical Center (Dallas), the Midwest Research Institute (Kansas City, MO), ERGO Forschungsgesellschaft mbH (Hamburg, Germany), the Department of Pharmacology and Toxicology, SUNY-Buffalo (NY), and the Department of Preventative Medicine, State University of New York (SUNY), Binghamton.[60]

The report revealed that in Belgium, animal feeds that had been made using PCB and dibenzofuran-contaminated animal fats were found to have contaminated chickens, eggs, dairy products, and some pork and beef. Most of the products were removed from shelves and destroyed. Similar chemicals had been found to contaminate rice in Japan in 1968. The report also analyzed food samples including meats (beef, chicken, pork, freshwater and ocean fish, shellfish, and sandwich meats); dairy (butter, cheese, milk, ice cream, eggs); and fruits and vegetables including legumes and cereals. Human breast milk samples were collected from nursing women in Binghamton, New York in 1996 and shipped frozen to Hamburg, Germany where they were analyzed at ERGO laboratory which is certified by the WHO to analyze dioxins in biological samples.[60-63]

The freshwater fish had the highest dioxin levels, followed by butter, ocean fish, meats, poultry and luncheon meats. Next were eggs and dairy products. Last was human breast milk, where total toxins were higher than most of the individual foods when comparing overall dioxin, dibenzofuran, and PCB TEQ levels. For adults, the meats and dairy foods contributed the highest share of overall toxins, followed by vegetables. Nursing infants have a higher level of dioxin intake than adult populations. These results and other reports clearly indicate that the levels of dioxins and persisting pollutants play a key role in the development of many human diseases. This underscores the need to remove such chemicals from the human diet as possible. *We might note the toxic effects of dioxins and other mutagenic chemicals upon poultry and other vaccinated livestock, and what this may mean in terms of their ability to mutate genes including latent retroviral genes or vaccine viruses in animals or humans.* One report reveals that the TCDDs from paper pulp and the combustion of chlorine-containing organic materials causes endocrine disruption, developmental toxicity, liver toxicity, and immunotoxicity in animals. Birds are particularly sensitive to dioxin-type chemicals. Environmental dioxin levels in North America are sufficient to cause biochemical and embryotoxic effects in wild birds. Dioxins probably also adversely affect their insect, arthropod, and microbial passengers, and may have been a contributing factor to the new encephalitis or rickettsialpox outbreaks that emerged in pheasant, equine, and human populations during the mid-20th century.[60-70]

Another study undertaken in 2011 revealed that *quail, pheasants,* and *domestic chickens are particularly sensitive to TCDD, PeCDF, TCDF, and other dioxins and dioxin-like compounds.* We will remember that the first case of Lyme disease to be reported in the US came from a patient who was hunting grouse in northern Wisconsin. We will learn shortly that some of the epidemics that emerged in the northeast included human rickettsialpox infections as transmitted by mites; and rickettsialpox and encephalitis infections in pheasants and horses. We know also that Connecticut had a large poultry industry, which supplied domestic stock and eggs around the world for human food and for laboratory and industrial use. The effects of dioxins and other pollutants upon the viruses and retroviruses that are found in chickens and their embryos may play an important role in the development of animal and human diseases, especially if latent infections are reactivated by an external factor (i.e. microbial insecticides, toxic chemicals).[69]

There are many studies which reveal the relationships between organophosphate/organochloride pesticide resistance in insects and arthopods (i.e. ticks), and the increase in intracellular animal diseases, including *anaplasmosis, ehrlichiosis,* and *rickettsiosis* infections. Even USDA patents describe the activity of organophosphate pesticides (acaricides) upon livestock and their ticks including "cattle fever" ticks (*Boophilus annulatus, B. microplus*) and brown dog ticks (*Rhipicephalus sanguineus*). Cattle fever is *Theileriosis* or *Babesiosis.* Many Lyme patients test positive for babesia infections, and we might assume these infections first had animal origins. There are many different strains of babesia (piroplasmosis), including the most common, *Babesia microti,* and *B. bovis, B. divergens, B. bigemina, B. duncani,* and others, many of which are found in Lyme patients. These organisms may have canine, bovine, feline, rodent, sheep, bird, or monkey origins including from animals that are routinely used for animal or human vaccines. A similar intracellular infection that is found in domestic poultry (chickens, turkey); livestock herbivores (sheep, cattle, goats); rodents (rats, mice, rabbits); and wild birds, bats, and turtles, is *Eimeria,* which causes coccidiosis. This is an important intracellular *Apicomplexan* parasite that may be missed in humans who have other insect and tickborne infections. Lyme patients may need to be screened for these infections as well as other co-infections.[71-74]

The most important note to take away from this section is that *dioxins* and dioxin-like compounds *including anilines* were used agriculturally and industrially as insecticides for decades, according to many patent inventions which describe their use to control insects upon livestock and crops. Dioxins and related compounds also appeared in a number of other products including wood and paper preservatives, fungicides, disinfectants, plasticizers, and *ketonitriles* for herbicides. The mutagenic actions of dioxins, anilines, Tweens, and persisting pollutants upon insects, animals, and their microbial parasites is key to understanding the development of novel microbes that are tick and insect-transmissible, and which become animal or human infections.[75-86]

Mustard Wastes Do Catch Up

Another topic that applies to the story of microbes and mutations is what happens to chemical weapons when they have been banned from use and discarded. The disposal of chemical mutagens in the environment can absolutely influence resident microbes. Perhaps the most well-known chemical warfare agents are the *mustard* agents. Sulfur mustard is a liquid blistering nerve agent that evaporates and can persist in water or soil for months, even in temperatures well below freezing. Sulfur mustard has a distinctive odor that resembles the sweet odor of mustard, garlic, or horseradish.[1-3]

Mustard agents were designed to be deployed as a spray or dropped as bombs or artillery shells. Nerve agents are a class of phosphorus-containing organic chemicals, also known as *organophosphates*. These chemicals interfere with nerve signal transmissions through the blockage of the enzyme *acetylcholinesterase*, which controls the activity of the neurotransmitter acetylcholine. Nitrogen and sulfur mustard gases are not only toxic, they are carcinogenic and also highly mutagenic, so their presence in soil and water could easily facilitate the mutation of microbes. They are classified as *weapons of mass destruction* according to United Nations Resolution 687. They were banned by the Chemical Weapons Convention of 1993, (effective April 29, 1997). Nitrogen, ammonia, and phosphate fertilizers and agrochemicals may exert similar mutagenic effects upon soil and water-borne microbes as their weapons-grade chemical relatives because they are from a similar class of nerve agents.[1-3]

While past weapons deployments are historically significant, past accidental deployments and the deliberate disposal of obsolete nerve agents remains a problem in many parts of the world. The improper disposal of military and industrial wastes particularly impacts marine environments; and the soils and groundwaters where chemical weapons are buried or housed (i.e. military or other storage depots). With the enforcement of the Chemical Weapons Convention, the US military was left with the problem of the disposal of decommissioned chemical weapons. One solution was to dump unspent munitions and nerve agents at sea. Such disposals were undertaken from May 1964 until the early 1970s.[4-6]

One multi-phase Department Of Defense program was called *Operation CHASE* (Cut Holes And Sink 'Em). The program involved loading old munitions and chemical weapons onto ships which were scuttled up to two hundred and fifty miles off-shore, including off the coast of the Atlantic between the state of Florida and the Bahamas. According to a 1998 US Army Chemical Materials Agency report, twenty-six sites off the coast of eleven states on both the western and eastern US coastlines became chemical, munitions, and radioactive waste dumping grounds for the military. Even worse, the agency's poor recordkeeping history means that only about one-half of these locations are known in the present day, with the remaining sites largely forgotten.[4-6]

The US Army admitted to secretly dumping sixty-four million pounds of nerve and mustard agents into ocean sites, along with four hundred thousand chemical-filled bombs, land mines, and rockets; and five hundred tons of radioactive wastes from 1944 to 1970. A number of chemical agents were dumped close to American shores, including off the coasts of Virginia Beach (1957); Atlantic City, New Jersey (CHASE); San Francisco, California (1950s); and four dump sites near Chincoteague (VA) and Assateague (Maryland) islands. These dumps included mustard-filled mortar shells, munitions, and radioactive wastes.[1,2,5,7-10]

Through the CHASE program, the US military disposed of at least eight thousand tons of mustard and chemical warfare gases and other munitions. Some of their dumping exercises included the detonation of cargo once it was submerged. Project CHASE 8 marked the first recorded chemical weapons disposal in 1967. The program involved the sea burial of mustard gas and nerve agent-filled M-55 rockets which were encased in concrete vaults. Other nerve agents were sealed in tin (GB, VX) and were sunk in 1968. There were at least a dozen CHASE operations that were widely reported in major media sources. These activities raised public concerns over environmental safety and led to the enactment of legislation called the *Marine Protection, Research, and Sanctuaries Act* of 1972. The Act prohibited further chemical and weapons disposals into oceanic waters. The Act was not only implemented due to concerns over the program's effects upon marine and wild life, but also because of the possibility that chemical weapons could wash onto shorelines; a fear that was apparently well-founded.[1,2,5,7-10]

Overseas dumping has presented similar problems which have recently emerged in the Skagerrak Strait, between Sweden, Norway, and Denmark. In 2002, several ships that were loaded with German chemical weapons and that had been scuttled since post-WWII; were discovered to be leaking some of their chemical cargo into surrounding waters. Indiscriminate chemical and weapons dumping was carried out on a global scale in places such as the North Sea; off the coasts of Italy, France, Pakistan, the Philippines, the Bay of Bengal, the Arabian Sea, the Coral Sea off the coast of Australia; in the Pacific off the coast of Japan; off the eastern and western US coasts, and by other countries. Many sites have whereabouts which remain classified by the US Army to this day.[1,2,5,7-13]

According to a risk analysis report on the carcinogenic potency of vesicant agents (including sulfur mustards) that were scheduled for destruction by the chemical stockpile disposal program, sulfur mustard is carcinogenic and mutagenic. It also provides evidence that other alkylating compounds other than mustard agents will display similar attributes.[6]

> "...sulfur mustard possesses a carcinogenic potency similar to that of benzo [a] pyrene. Because mustard agents are *alkylating compounds,* they *destroy individual cells by reaction with cellular proteins, enzymes, RNA, and DNA.* Once begun, tissue reaction is irreversible. Mustard agents are mutagenic..."

A revealing paper reported that sixty-seven strains of *Borrelia burgdorferi* sensu lato were isolated by scientists from Finnish *Ixodes ricinus* ticks that were collected in 1992. (Finland is bordered by the Baltic Sea). Scientists were studying the pathogenic differences between *Borrelia burgdorferi* species found on the Åland Islands, at the Finnish southeastern coastal area, and from the southeastern inland territory. According to a paper published in 1995, the study's objectives were to characterize the isolates found; identify them to the species level; and to obtain information on the occurrence and distribution of the three Bb species in Finland: *Bb sensu stricto, Borrelia garinii,* and *Borrelia afzelii.*[14-20]

Only *B. burgdorferi* sensu stricto was found on the Åland Islands in the Baltic Sea southwest of the mainland. However the other two species were found in the remaining areas surveyed. According to sources, ship wrecks in the Baltic Sea during World War II included a number of German war boats, submarines, and battleships. The post-WWII burial of chemical weapons in the Baltic Sea was substantial in scope; especially with regard to disposals that were undertaken by members of the German military. We might also need to consider that ship builders are located along coastal areas; and the metals and processes that are used in the fabrication process (i.e. aluminum, steel, copper) contribute significantly to the toxic pollutants in the waters surrounding such facilities.[14-20]

Agriculturally speaking, Finnish scientists were among those who treated pine sawfly infestations using *borrelina* viruses (like those released in Connecticut during the 1950s). Were scientists simply classifying *Borrelia burgdorferi* strains from a "random" area of the world, or were their interests in the Finnish Islands of the Baltic Sea geared more toward analyzing the mutagenic effects of discarded toxic chemical weapons and a particular group of reoviruses upon the marine and terrestrial leptospires found in the areas studied?[14-20]

Borrelia Mining

In the US by the early 1900s, bauxite production was a booming business. By World War I there was a marked increase in the amount of bauxite and alumina being produced. By the 1920s, production increased to around a half million tons – roughly half the world's production. Not until World War II did demands for aluminum significantly increase. By then only one company still mined bauxite in Arkansas; an ALCOA Aluminum subsidiary. Other companies would subsequently enter the bauxite market, including Dulin, Dixie, General Abrasive, Norton, Kaiser Aluminum, and American Cyanamid & Chemical Corporation. During WWII it was difficult to import bauxite since South American and Caribbean shipments risked attack by German submarines and U-boats roaming the Gulf of Mexico. In response the US government built up a large stockpile of Arkansas bauxite, and also of the equally critical fluoride-containing mineral fluorspar.[5-7]

From 1942 to 1944, about ten million long tons of bauxite were mined in the US. A large portion was used for war-related products and vehicles. Some bauxite was added to the military's defense national stockpile. After the war, reduced government demand caused mining companies to close. For the most part this left ALCOA, American Cyanamid, and Reynolds as the three main bauxite and aluminum producers. Since 1996, the McGeorge Contracting Company has mined Arkansas bauxite where it is processed for proppants (i.e. resin-coated sand), and to create high-density granules useful to the oil and gasoline industries. Bauxite is also used as a catalyst, and in abrasives, chemicals, cements, absorbants, and for refractories (i.e. kilns, crucibles, reactors, incinerators). For example, the Dow Chemical Company is assignee on a patent for a hydraulic cement composition that contains aluminum derived from bauxite. The Defense National Stockpile Center sells tons of refractory-grade bauxite from its stockpiles.[5-8]

The mineral corundum is a crystallized aluminum oxide-iron-titanium-chromium mineral aggregate. Corundum for abrasive use is manufactured out of the mineral rock bauxite. In 1963, the 3M Company founded a biochemical research group to create pharmaceutical products. The company dabbled in agricultural herbicides during this period. The 3M Company uses mined materials and chemicals to manufacture industrial abrasives (i.e. sandpapers, grinding wheels), and polymer products (i.e. adhesives, plastics). The company also has a history in pharmaceuticals. During the 1970s and 1980s, 3M diversified into *radiology* and *energy control*. We can see important connections which may help explain why the company is a patent assignee for a *Borrelia burgdorferi* diagnostic test.[1-4,10-13]

A news report from 2006 revealed that according to 3M Company research, tissue samples taken from fish in the Mississippi River near the company's Cottage Grove plant contained high levels of the industrial compounds PFOA and PFOS. Both chemicals, which are in the perfluorinated compound (PFC) family of persisting chemicals, were reportedly dumped by the manufacturer into the river over many years. I may remind you that Minnesota Mining and Manufacturing Co. (3M) is listed as assignee to a patent invention that describes a diagnostic test for Lyme disease. The patent was filed in 1986 and describes the ability to detect multiple strains of *Borrelia burgdorferi* and leptospires from samples of either human or animal urine.[1-4]

Clues from sworn patent applications relate the very real possibility that chemical pollutants are mutating soil and water-borne spirochetes to cause human diseases. It is also a clue that some manufacturers of products that involve commonly mined products and/or toxic chemical pollutants used in their processes (i.e. chromic or picric acids, dioxins, akylating agents, Tweens) may be aware of a cause-and-effect relationship between discharged wastes and infectious diseases such as *Borrelia burgdorferi*. A 3M patent suggests that rodent urine may be a vehicle for non-tick transmission of Bb spirochetes, and we might ask why a mining company might hold a Bb-related patent. Does the holding of Bb-related patents implicate a company's products in the development of this pathogen? The 3M patent also suggests that human urine and/or other body fluids may also be transmission routes for Bb infections. The patent was filed just four years after the causative agent of Lyme disease was officially announced. The patent also refers to another spirochete from the leptospira family. This could be an admission that there is a *leptospira* component to an aggregate Bb spirochete.[10-15]

During the 1970s, I remember my father driving over an Aurora, Illinois branch of the Fox River after our family visited friends. I asked a question about a small windmill I had seen, and after answering me, I overheard him talking to my mother about the levels of pollution in the Fox River. I was always conscious about pollution, and in high school I even made an 8mm film on the topic. I recently found a 1973 study from that period which discussed pollutants found in the Illinois Fox River. The Fox River system begins northwest of Milwaukee in Waukesha, Wisconsin from underground streams and reportedly draws water from Lake Superior. It flows south and southeast and joins the Illinois River at Ottawa, Illinois; interconnecting with a series of lakes along the way.[16]

The length of the Fox River is roughly 172 miles through the Chicago suburbs where I grew up. Water samples over a one-year period in 1970 analyzed pollutants including commercial cleaners, fuel oils, solvents, factory wastes, oil by-products, insecticides, and herbicides. Of the chemicals found, most were known to persist between six months and two years. Twenty-one hundred fish from the Fox River watershed, and forty-three hundred fish from Canada's Lake Superior were compared for pollutants and tumors. The Fox River samples showed significantly higher levels of persisting pollutants. Samples revealed arsenic, lead, mercury, crude oil, gasoline, toluene, benzanthracene, chlorinated hydrocarbons, phosphates, sulphates, and coliform bacteriae. The study concluded that the pollutants had caused the fish tumors. Studies were underway regarding "fish viruses" and as the paper called them, "those enteric viruses that one might expect in a river system that is termed a 'floating sewer.'" Our freshwater lakes and rivers have for all intents and purposes, largely become floating sewers as a result of all the toxic wastes that have been cast into our environment. We should expect that the result of irresponsible waste disposals over the past century and a half on a global basis would eventually produce globally important diseases.[16]

It is interesting that a 3M patent reveals that Bb infections are transmitted by rodents and dogs (or other canines). These animals are found around humans, waterways, farms, waste dumps; and in the military (i.e. mine-sweeping dogs). The patent identifies nine *Borrelia burgdorferi* strains that were isolated from humans, two strains from animals, and one from a tick. The 3M patent uses the LPS (lipopolysaccharide or toxin) of the Bb's bacterial cell wall, or its outer surface proteins of the cell membrane as antigens in the test. The patent also refers to a hybridoma cell line (hybrid) with a culture database number of HB9126. Hybridoma cells are made using antibody-producing B-lymphocyte cells and myeloma cells, which are oncogenic (cancer-causing), and which come from B-cell cancers. Lyme patients may have hyperactive B-cell responses during infection with Bb spirochetes.[11,17]

When searching through a culture database, I found nothing listed under "HB9126" although I did find two organisms listed under accession number "9126" without the prefix "HB" which I assume represents "hybridoma." The first organism I found was *Sporolactobacillus laevolacticus,* a freeze-dried *Bacillus laevolacticus.* The culture was isolated from a ditch crowfoot (or celery-leaf buttercup, a toxic plant). The second organism I found was *Emericellopsis terricola* van Beyma teleomorph, *an air-borne fungal spore* from Texas. This organism belongs to the *Ascomycota* division of fungi, which is *the same group where we find the Coccidioides immitus (coccidioidomycosis) fungi.* What an interesting coincidence to find a wild fungus strain indirectly mentioned in a Bb diagnostic test. Remember that patent inventions sometimes reference an organism's family members instead of revealing the actual organism being described in the patent, so we don't know if the patent was referring specifically to this fungus in particular or to other fungal family members.[18,19]

Bacillus laevolacticus refers to a group of bacillus strains that are useful for *lactic acid fermentation.* Regardless of the strains in this family, these are *fermentable bacillus strains.* Remember that soil bacteriae are fermented to create the agricultural pesticide B.t.. If we consider the 3M patent information, we may find clues to the idea that the Lyme disease spirochete could be an aggregate, "hybrid" organism that includes a fermented yeast, a sporulating fungus, and possibly a bacillus strain that is fermented (B.t.). At the very least these agents may cross-react with the test probes, and at most may describe one part of an aggregate Bb spirochete.[17]

I looked for other mining companies that might hold borreliae-related patents, and found one assigned to the American Cyanamid & Chemical Corporation. With the discovery of a second mining company that had Bb-related interests, I began to see a pattern. American Cyanamid makes products including fertilizers and agricultural chemicals, surgical appliances and supplies, plastics, biological products, diagnostics, and chemical and pharmaceutical preparations. For example *cyanamid* is a compound made from carbide, lime, and nitrogen; and is suitable for fertilizers. Cyanamid is also useful in the extraction of gold and silver from mined ores. Metal extraction uses alkyloidal reagents which may be capable of driving mutations in bacteria, especially if they contain dioxins or dioxin-like compounds.[20]

From World War II forward, the American Cyanamid Company supplied typhus vaccines and surgical sutures to the Armed Forces. Later the company invented antibiotics to treat pneumonia, and its scientists at Lederle Laboratories developed the first *polio* vaccine. During the early 1960s the company and several major chemical companies were charged with conspiring to monopolize the marketing and manufacturing of the drug *tetracycline.* This is a drug that in the form of doxycycline is now highly recommended for the treatment of *Borrelia burgdorferi* infections. Was there something that the company knew about spirochetes in relation to mined materials and human disease? The chemical companies involved in the scandal paid heavy fines. American Cyanamid's spin-off chemical business is Cytec Industries of West Paterson, New Jersey. Cytec is a specialty chemical and materials company for the aerospace, adhesive, ink, plastics, industrial coating, automotive, and mining industries. It also produces surfactants, microbeads, and other chemicals that are used in insecticidal formulas. The company claims to be the largest supplier of mining reagents in the world. Mines of all kinds recover minerals, elements, oils, and more, often using the wellbore *in situ* process which injects chemical solvents or bacterial leachers into the ground. In situ mining is the most popular form of mining across the globe in both terrestrial and marine environments. The company also provided benzene-derived chemicals that are used in plastics and metal coating processes according to sources.[21-24,33-35]

Another mining company of interest to the Lyme disease story is the Kaiser Aluminum & Chemical Corporation (California). The company produces aluminum products and has operations in the US and Canada. In 1933 Dr. Sidney Garfield opened a hospital east of Los Angeles in the Mojave Desert to provide medical care for workers of the metropolitan water district of southern California's aqueduct system. The company was founded in 1945 by industrialist Henry John Kaiser, the "Father of American shipbuilding," and physician Sidney Garfield. Henry Kaiser's company *Kaiser Shipyard* built Liberty ships during World War II. Following the war, the companies *Kaiser Steel* and *Kaiser Aluminum* were established. Kaiser's industries use important chemicals in metal processing and manufacturing that may have included persisting organic pollutants and dioxin or dioxin-like compounds. We also know that industrially important metals were mined and recovered using chemicals that are capable of mutating bacteria or viruses.[25,26]

The Kaiser Permanente Health Care system, originally created for employees and their families, was the precursor to modern contracted medical care and the origin of the structured prepayment financing plan. Kaiser Permanente is now a non-profit insurance company and the largest managed health care organization in the US. The company is based in Oakland, California as a consortium of three groups, the Kaiser Foundation Health Plan and its subsidiaries; the regional Permanente Medical Groups; and the Kaiser Foundation Hospitals. Kaiser's influence is not limited to insurance or steel. A Kaiser-owned cement company assisted in the construction of civic centers and other large projects such as coal-fired dams. (Cement and asphalt are created out of aggregate rock such as bauxite). In 2005 Kaiser sold commodity interests related to its Jamaican bauxite company.[25,26]

In 2008 the CDC awarded a $338,000 grant to the Kaiser Permanente health care giant to test and interview up to 500 patients who were suffering from a Lyme-like illness called *Morgellon's disease.* The CDC has called the disease "unexplained dermopathy." Some Lyme-Morgellon's patients have anecdotally stated that their Kaiser Permanente physicians have been very vocal about classifying patients who claim to have Morgellon's disease with "delusional parasitosis." With Lyme disease, patients are often called "delusional," or are told their symptoms are "all in their head." Imagine if it could be proven that a link between metal ore mining, the chemicals used in industrial processes, and Bb and Morgellon's diseases actually exists.[27,28]

The CDC-Kaiser Morgellon studies were undertaken in the bay area of northern California, where the majority of Morgellon's patients reside. The study involved a collaborative effort between Kaiser Permanente's Northern California Division of Research, and the US Armed Forces Institute of Pathology. The study was designed to be "careful, objective," and "scientific." The results of these studies were released as I was finishing this book, and basically suggested that the syndrome was not caused by infection; that the fibers found in the skin lesions were "not alive" but were pieces of clothing debris; and that the unsightly sores which sometimes fully cover a Morgellon's patient's body are the result of people picking their own skin. Such conclusions are entirely disappointing from so-called experts. From the perspective of this book however, they are hardly unexpected findings.[29-34,98]

Something in the Water

In 1971, a few years before the offical announcement of "juvenile arthritis" in Connecticut, Rhode Island University's Kingston Narragansett Marine Laboratory was under military contract to analyze fluoride levels of the northwest Atlantic ocean. Scientists were studying the fluoride chlorinity ratios in seawater samples to determine *if there was a high concentration of fluoride near the seafloor* which might be associated with resuspended sediment (i.e. from hydrothermal vents).[1-10]

The studies were carried out at varying depths near the mid-Atlantic ridge, and on the southeast flank of the grand banks. Perhaps it was a geological survey for natural fluoride levels, or it had something to do with determining the extent by which abandoned chemical, nuclear, (or even bacteriological) wastes had contaminated sea waters. Note that the studies were undertaken in the Atlantic, which are the waters adjacent to the eastern US coastline where an emerging epidemic was about to be made public.[1-10]

Echoed across the US (i.e. Mississippi River and the Great Lakes) is the dumping of 900 billion gallons of raw sewage into fresh water sources every year. This is roughly the equivalent of the amount of water that falls over Niagara Falls during a three-week period. The presence of raw sewage and other toxic wastes in water supplies presents a myriad of problems for water filtration systems, nonetheleast of which are bacteria and viruses, biocides, and persisting organic pollutants. Similar releases of industrial wastewaters into Lake Michigan for example have happened on more than one occasion by industries in at least three Great Lakes states. The region of Lake Superior that borders the northern part of Michigan is an area that is also rich in copper deposits, and has been home to important chemical and metal industries.[11-18]

I thought about Kaiser Aluminum's history in mined ores and the idea that some industries might be aware that their wastes could adversely affect microbes. I also wondered how objective could researchers be when undertaking a Morgellon's study, since the disease may be related to an industry that produces products and wastes that may mutate microbes. It seemed curious that the pathology lab of the US Armed Forces was selected for a Morgellon's study as opposed to a private laboratory. However, the aluminum industry, the US military, and the CDC are interested in the outcome of studies which might affect the disposal and management of nuclear and other toxic wastes, or patents or other financial interests of many industries. The organisms which cause Morgellon's and Lyme disease may have been created with the help of toxic chemicals including fluorides, metals, and military, agricultural, and nuclear wastes. Fluoride is another chemical for which toxicity studies were and remain highly classified under "national security" from WWII forward, due to the chemical's connection to the Manhattan Project and the disposal of nuclear or industrial wastes (i.e. solid or liquid wastes, underground storage, airborne exhausts).[11-15]

The CDC previously studied strange mutated leptospires isolated from animals near their Atlanta, Georgia laboratory and wastewater treatment plants beginning in the 1950s. The CDC, which sponsored the 1994 Dearborn conference to standardize Lyme disease testing and surveillance case definitions, has one or more leptospira strains which bear the agency's initials in the strain names. The US Armed Forces has played a key role in nuclear and biological warfare history that involved insects, crops, fluorides, nuclear energy, and nuclear weapons research and development. We might question these somewhat coincidental connections and wonder about the true objectivity of a Morgellon's study.[16,19-21]

I examined a US geological survey from 1960 to 1991 which targeted the Apalachicola-Chattahoochee-Flint river basin (ACF) through Georgia, Alabama, and Florida. The area was one of the first sites selected in 1991 for the national water quality assessment program (NAWQA). Under this nationwide program, scientists evaluated pesticide contaminations of ground and surface waters. In the initial study, about one-third of the area observed was noted under agricultural use. About five percent covered urban and suburban habitats, and the remainder was forested. Pesticide use data is stored in the US Geological Survey National Water Information System (NWIS) and the US EPA Storage and Retrieval System (STOREET). These regions could also have been selected to analyze subsurface leaching of toxic wastes and minerals from mined geologic deposits, or toxic waste dump sites.[22]

In about five percent of roughly twenty-thousand analyses performed on the ACF basin, pesticide concentrations were at or above minimum reporting levels. The majority of toxins detected were organochlorine insecticides (dioxins or dioxin-like compounds). This class of insecticides was subsequently banned in the US, although the chemicals persist in the environment. The samples also detected large amounts of DDT, DDD, and DDE in the aquatic biota and soil sediments. Pesticides in bottom sediments are typically highly persistent, and are hydrophobic compounds. Fish analyzed in the studies showed persisting levels of many chemicals including some that were banned. They also demonstrated four chemicals that were in use at the time of the study; and which registered above minimum reporting levels. Four chemicals were found in the fish, including the pesticides malathion, lindane, chlorpyrifos, and 2,4-D.[22]

DDT was used in the US to control mosquitoes until the end of 1973. DDT was also applied to foods and other crops. Dieldrin, heptachlor, and chlordane were used agriculturally through 1974; with continued use through the late 1980s as a termiticide. These chemicals were employed in commercial and residential pesticides and many are highly mutagenic. All of these chemicals were found within tributary streams which drained from the Atlanta metropolitan area into the main lines of the Chattahoochee River; downstream of the metropolitan areas of Atlanta and Columbus, Georgia. The Savannah River system, which is influenced by the wastewaters of the Savannah River nuclear site, is one of the major watersheds in the areas studied.[23]

Most of the surface waters sampled in the Atlanta metropolitan area displayed detectable levels of the herbicide 2,4-D. In urban and suburban areas; turf, lawn, and roadside pesticides routinely included 2,4-D, dicamba, 2,4-DP, atrazine, mecoprop (MCPP); glyphosate, sulfometuron, bensulide, acifluorfen, and benfluralin. (Some of these chemicals are now banned.) The most prevalent insecticides found in the ACF river basin were aldicarb, acephate, chlorpyrifos, diazinon, dimethoate, malathion, methomyl, parathion-methyl, phorate; fungicides (chlorothalonil); and nematocides (fenamiphos). The Stockholm

Convention, a 2001 global treaty designed to protect human health from persisting toxic chemicals, was entered into force in 2004, and banned a long list of pesticides. However bans have not prevented these chemicals from persisting or affecting resident microbes which may mutate and bring about new microbial species.[22,23]

Pesticides are not the only persisting chemicals of interest to the story. Nuclear wastewaters and other materials must be properly disposed of because they contain radioactive elements which exert mutagenic action toward all life forms, no matter how microscopic in size. The Savannah River Site (SRS) in South Carolina was built during the 1950s to refine radioactive materials for nuclear weapons. The site is owned by the US Department of Energy (DOE). The plant's liquid wastes are now disposed of through a contract with a Savannah River remediation company. There is also a nuclear waste policy Act (NWPA) which supports the use of deep geologic repositories to "safely" store radioactive waste materials. The Act requires Congressional approval for new sites, and directs the DOE regarding storage methods. Before stiffer water pollution standards were enacted in 1972 however (right before the Connecticut outbreak), radioactive wastes were routinely discharged into watersheds by many nuclear plants around the world (and by aerosolized steam from roof vents or evaporative cooling towers). The Savannah River Site (SRS) is also home to the Savannah River National Laboratory.[22-34,31a]

The only source of US tritium comes from the SRS. Tritium is a radioactive form of hydrogen. There is also a mixed oxide fuel (MOX)* fabrication facility on the South Carolina site, which sits on top of a geological fault line. A future objective is to convert legacy weapons-grade plutonium into fuel that is useful for commercial power reactors. During the 1950s, heavy water production began at SRS, and the world's first full-scale PUREX separation plant began radioactive operations November 4, 1954. (PUREX stands for plutonium and uranium extraction.) Nuclear wastes from such sites contaminated rivers, soils, and atmospheres in many areas of the world.[23-27,34-41]

**Mox or mixed oxide fuel is mixed uranium and plutonium oxide.*

The first batch of refined plutonium was received by Los Alamos Laboratory in New Mexico in February of 1945; and many more shipments were made during the 1950s. The Los Alamos lab was built in 1943 and is owned by the DOE. It was established as a laboratory to coordinate top-secret research for the Manhattan Project; and to coordinate the development of the first nuclear weapons under one roof (previously scientists at academic laboratories were scattered across the country). The first nuclear test was undertaken July 16, 1945 near Alamogordo, New Mexico; code named "Trinity." Wherever nuclear tests were undertaken, the residual chemicals and persisting wastes will have affected resident microbes including sporulating soil bacteriae and the inhabitants of aquatic sediments.[23-27,34-41]

The current trend seems to be to dredge up hazardous waste materials including nuclear wastes; and to treat them and discharge them as crop fertilizers. Sewage sludge has for many years been sold as a commercial fertilizer by wastewater facilities across the US. The former Lowry landfill superfund site in Colorado is where Lowry groundwater will be incorporated into the plant's sewage sludge. The former Lowry site is said to have received millions of gallons of hazardous waste materials which were pumped into shallow, unlined pits between 1950 and 1980. These kinds of "fertilizers" have long been controversial since PCBs, pesticides, heavy metals, nuclear wastes, and other chemicals have been found within them. Plutonium, one of the most toxic radioactive chemicals on the planet, may make its way not only into farm fertilizers, but also into foods that may wind up on the dinner table. When we think about the mixture of mined radioactive elements, and the mutation of microbes by these materials, we can only imagine what the outcome will be the more these wastes are recycled.[42-46]

Los Alamos is one of a few laboratories in the US where classified nuclear weapons research was undertaken. Another was the University of California's Lawrence Livermore National Laboratory, founded in 1952. The facility is located in San Joaquin County, in the San Joaquin valley. The Lawrence Livermore National Laboratory is funded mainly by the DOE, and is managed and operated by Lawrence Livermore National Security LLC (LLNS), a partnership that includes Bechtel, the University of California, Babcock and Wilcox, the Washington Division of URS Corporation, and Battelle Memorial Institute; with the Texas A&M University System as an affiliate. The Lawrence Livermore plant was formerly managed by the University of California until 2006 when LLNS assumed control. Sandia National Laboratories are owned by the Sandia Corporation, a subsidiary of Lockheed Martin Corp. The main campus is in Albuquerque, New Mexico, and the other is next to the Lawrence Livermore National Laboratory.[47,48]

Babcock and Wilcox designs and manufactures heavy nuclear components for nuclear power. The company designed and fabricated components for the first nuclear submarine, the USS Nautilus; and for aircraft carriers, power plants, and other nuclear reactors. It also manages Y-12, a national security complex in Tennessee that performs services for the US nuclear program, for reactors and nuclear waste storage; and operates and manages the Pantex plant in Amarillo, Texas which formerly assembled nuclear weapons. The plant now handles security, weapons dismantling, repairs, storage, and recycling of stockpiled nuclear and other weapons. B&W's subsidiary Idaho Treatment Group LLC (ITG) received a half billion dollar mixed waste treatment project management and operations contract for the DOE's Idaho National Laboratory in June, 2011.[91]

Los Alamos National Laboratory is a partner in the Joint Genome Institute (JGI), another DOE institution whose scientists map genomes (genes); and perform DNA sequencing. Their research includes microorganisms which thrive under extreme temperatures and conditions, the *extremophiles*, including those that are radiation and metal-tolerant. The DOE's Joint Genomic Institute group also worked on the Human Genome Project, which focused on understanding human genes. They also undertake bioenergy research, and have comprehensive programs in fungal, microbial, plant, and metagenomics. (Metagenomics refers to the study of microbes that live in communities.)[47-51]

For example a recent *mite genome* project was undertaken at the Walnut Creek, Berkeley location. The project mapped the genes of the *two-spotted spider mite, a silk-producing mite* that is a common and destructive agricultural crop pest. The DOE JGI team chose this mite because of its increasing resistance to insecticides and because economically speaking, it is the most devastating crop pest around the world. JGI scientists also identified *microbial and fungal genes that have become incorporated into the mite's genome. This describes the transfer of genes (DNA) from dissimilar species into a mite's genome.* It is also an example of how *arthropod genes* can be permanently changed by infections and possibly by agricultural or industrial chemicals through permanent mutations that are passed onto their offspring. Such genes may also be transmissible to other species including other insects; or to plants, animals, or even humans. As we have seen from at least one patent, the ability to design genes that provide pesticide resistance, even in humans is not an imaginary process. What occurs with recombinant genes in arthropods and insects may likewise occur in higher animals under similar influences.[47-51]

The J.G.I. institute has also sequenced the complete genome of *"spirochaeta sp. Grapes"* which likely means spirochetes of grapes or grapevines, and may represent the spiroplasmas. Scientists at JGI have also sequenced salt-loving bacteria; and acidophilic (acid-loving), *polymer-degrading bacteriae*; and *a new species of thermophile cyanobacteria* called *Desulfurella acetivorans.* This one comes from New Zealand and is an acetate-oxidizing, sulfur-reducing bacterium. Acetates include salts and esters of acetic acid, which are used as copper acetate, in cellulose, in the food and fermentation industry (i.e. beer, wines, insecticides), as bleaching or descaling agents, as a petroleum feedstock, and as mining regents.[47-51,97]

A side note is that copper and sulfur were used in viticulture (wine making) as fungicides. When chemical fungicides came along, (i.e. dithiocarbammates, mancozeb), they proved toxic to beneficial mites (phytoseiids), while phytophagous mites like the two-spotted spider mite developed OP pesticide resistance. These are mites that feed upon flowers, vegetables, fruits (i.e. grapes, citrus), and forest trees (i.e. poplar, maple, spruce, oak). Beneficial predatory mites normally eat harmful plant-eating mites. Once chemical insecticides were deployed, the beneficial mite populations were killed, allowing harmful species to flourish. This problem also occurred on the east coast and in the south; and contributed to the outbreak of mite-transmited rickettsialpox and other infections in animals and humans during the mid-20th century. Scientists began used beneficial (phytoseiid) mites *Metaseiulus occidentalis* to lower pest mite populations in California vineyards during the 1960s. By 1972, scientists were already aware that harmful mite species had developed resistance to the organophosphate chemicals used in agriculture and began studying why.[92-96]

The Lawrence Livermore Lab "Site 300" has been used as a high-explosives test facility for research, development, and testing of non-nuclear weapons. Due to the level of contaminants found in the site's groundwater and the tons of contaminants deposited in landfills used by the site, Site 300 was added to the US EPA's superfund national priorities list on August 30, 1990. Among the contaminants found in fifty-seven release areas (soil, water, subsurface soils, groundwater), were volatile organic compounds (VOCs), HMX and RDX (explosives), tritium, uranium-238, nitrates, and perchlorate.[47,48]

The laboratory claims to have a program that can "meet the challenges of mitigating the evolving biological threat." This refers to *biosecurity*, which is the rapid detection of unknown biological threats. Such threats may come from *agricultural insecticides including those that are genetically engineered into plants and animals, and those that may be created under the mutagenic action of nuclear or chemical wastes. These threats may cause disease outbreaks and/or permanently change the genomes of living organisms.*[52,52a]

The facility also established a global disease surveillance system; participates in the development of biological threat "countermeasures" (i.e. drugs, vaccines); and provides biological risk analyses and intelligence. Since 2000, LLNL has collaborated with the University of California-Davis cancer center, and we can see how important this relationship would be if nuclear and agricultural wastes and genetically engineered tools can activate bacteria or virus oncogenes (genes that cause cancer). Then again, maybe this is why Fort Detrick was headquarters to the National Cancer Institute – because the activities of chemical, nuclear, and biological weapons of warfare (even as insecticides) are perfectly capable of promoting cancers in more than just the insect population. The question is did scientists know this at the 1942 onset of the War Research Service?[52,52a]

While on the subject, remember the University of California's Lawrence Livermore National laboratory in the San Joaquin valley? San Joaquin valley fever a/k/a coccidiodoidomycosis is caused by the fungus *Coccidioides immitis.* Remember the Fort Detrick scientists who met in 1968 at the Illinois Institute of Technology in Chicago to discuss progress on aerosolized biowarfare agents? Those agents included tularemia (rabbit fever), Venezuelan equine encephalitis (flavivirus), Rocky Mountain spotted fever, yellow fever, and experimental San Joaquin valley fever. Did Ft. Detrick scientists really study aerosolizing these agents for use as biowarfare weapons? Or were their studies evaluating the effects of nuclear radiation and/or OP chemicals upon microbes that had already mutated to form an aggregate agent that was emerging in mites, ticks, and animals; and which would soon emerge as "juvenile arthritis"?[53-55]

Dr. Alan Barbour is listed on approximately one hundred *Borrelia burgdorferi*-related collaborative patents under the University of California and Texas A&M University systems. Uranium mining has been undertaken on the Texas Gulf coast. From 1952 through 1989, plutonium that had been created at Hanford, Washington and the Savannah River site was shipped to the Rocky Flats plant near Denver to make components for nuclear weapons. Rocky Flats workers made "pits" or triggers for weapons which were shipped to Texas at the country's only nuclear weapons assembly site during the Cold War, the Pantex plant near Amarillo. The Department of Energy initiated an investigation into safety at the plant after an anonymous letter was sent in 2006 to the President of BWX Technologies Inc., which operates the plant under a DOE contract. BWX is a member of the Los Alamos National Security Company collaboration (with the Univ. of TX, Univ. of California, and others); and the group that operates the Los Alamos National Laboratory).[53-55,59,91]

Today the Pantex plant's "core missions" are stockpile stewardship, nonproliferation, and the safeguard and security of nuclear weapons in the nation's stockpile. Weapons are evaluated, repaired, dismantled, stored, and monitored. Weapons are stored in monitored *plutonium* pits. Part of the security duties described by the facility's web site includes efforts to: "protect the plant personnel, facilities, materials, and information." Some people wonder if such information includes the ability of nuclear components or chemicals relating to their processes to mutate microbes and to cause human diseases.[55]

The Texas University System has campuses in several locations, including San Antonio. This is a short drive from Camp Bullis where the first *Ehrlichiosis*-like human infections emerged in 1942 and 1943. Camp Bullis has an operational target and training range. Explosives collected during sampling showed elevated levels of thallium, copper, and other "anomalies" in the areas tested from June to July of 2005. One report declared that thallium was "not a contaminant of concern by stakeholders." This does not necessarily mean however that thallium is not a public health concern, especially if it leaches into groundwater or subsurface aquifers. The very toxic thallium was used as a rodenticide until 1972. Whatever was stored at the Texas base in the 1940s, including chemical herbicides, could have contaminated soils and exposed resident insects to mutagenic chemicals to cause a novel human disease.[56]

The thought of proper nuclear and toxic waste disposals and its connections to the development of human infectious diseases such as Ehrlichiosis, STARI, Lyme, Morgellon's, or others is not one to dismiss. Remember that Dr. Alan Barbour, who has worked in both the University of Texas and the University of California Systems, attended the Dearborn Conference in October 1994 where surveillance criteria for case definitions and laboratory testing for Lyme disease was standardized. This was just one year after the 1993 publication of a US Army Corps of Engineers report that described the feasibility of capping "industrial" wastes with *dredged* materials (this could include buried nuclear or chemical wastes). The study discussed capping and industrial waste disposal sites at Texas A&M University. There was also a related report published in May of 1994, five months before the Dearborn conference, that carries access that is restricted only to members of the Army Corps of Engineers.[60]

The Texas Agricultural Experiment Station and the Southern Plains Agricultural Research Center in College Station are also near Camp Bullis. The latter two agencies are the most likely candidates to have tested novel insecticides/herbicides/rodenticides in the area – controls that were just hitting the scene by 1942, including some that were mutagenic chemicals or that held radioactive components. Texas A&M and the Texas University System are assignees to a significant number of patents related to *Borrelia burgdorferi,* and also to biological control agents for agricultural use.[57,58]

A Texas A&M University patent describes peptide and nucleic acids that are genetically engineered to be used as delivery agents (vectors) to treat animal and human diseases. They are also considered to be useful formulas for insecticidal use. According to the patent, herpes or sindbis viruses may be combined with insect baculoviruses. This relationship is important if recombinant insecticides contribute to human diseases when or if those designs fail. The patent speaks to genetically engineered viruses which fuse to the gut walls of insects. The question of course is whether similar gut-binding mechanisms can occur with microbial insecticides to cause human infections as well.[61]

> "As important, beneficial insects that are natural predators of insect pests are not hosts for baculoviruses. Baculovirus AcMNPV has undergone five controlled release trials and these trials indicate that when the virus is genetically modified by deletion of a single gene, it does not persist in the environment...Thus, genetically engineered baculoviruses can be used safely as a "one pass" insecticide that will kill the insect pest and not persist in the environment."
>
> "The host range of insect baculoviruses has been extensively studied and no evidence of infection or pathogenic responses have been identified in non-host insects, plants, vertebrates and man...This feature may make baculoviruses

> an ideal agent to be modified and used for the delivery of drugs, genes, or therapeutics."
>
> "The occlusion derived virus (ODV) is the primary infectious agent to the insect host. *The ODV envelope fuses with the plasma membrane of the gut cell*, thus releasing the nucleocapsid and viral DNA into the cell...In this process, viral envelope proteins are incorporated into the gut cell plasma membrane. Elucidation of the mechanism by which virus expressed genes are targeted to the viral envelope would represent a significant advance in the art."

Another patent assigned to Texas A&M University describes how to make a baculovirus shuttle vector. Genes from an NPV baculovirus such as *Autographa californica, Trichoplusia ni, Rachiplusia ou,* or *Galleria mellonella* can be inserted into an insect as a delivery vehicle to cause a superinfection. An older patent from 1995 describes how insect cells are infected with scorpion toxins and with the AcNPV baculovirus, and then are combined with fungi and bacteria as a toxic insecticide.[62-64]

A 1983 Texas A&M University System patent describes baculovirus vectors which express recombinant genes inside cells that contain wild and engineered baculoviruses. For nearly a century vaccines have contained many of the same microbes that are used as insecticides. Perhaps the vaccines are designed to treat diseases that may be caused by recombinant insecticides. An example of this dual role is revealed in any number of recombinant baculovirus patents: "The recombinant occlusion bodies produced in accordance with the present invention have uses in *vaccine* formulations, immunoassays, immobilized enzyme reactions, as *biological insecticides*, and as expression vectors." Animal or human vaccines may also be engineered to contain built-in insecticides.[65]

Multi-use pathogens described in one patent include *influenza, polyhedron* promoters and proteins, *Hepatitis A* virus, *Heliothis zea* NPV, baculoviruses, and other organisms. We might consider whether the presence of influenza genes in recombinant insecticides is a driving force behind certain influenza or "flu" vaccines recently promoted to the public. A push for an influenza vaccine makes sense even in the absence of an epidemic if scientists know or discovered post-deployment of an insecticide that influenza viruses from the formulas could mutate in the human body to cause or reactivate infections; and that such infections will be more potent because they involve genetically engineered microbes. To use a previous example, we may imagine that recombinant insecticides might accidentally bind to the human gut, and could be affected by GM insecticides that remain on foods as residues. Once introduced into the human body, B.t. and other toxins might mutate with resident gut bacteria to cause systemic diseases. This would mean that genetically engineered insecticides could in fact, fail in their role to attack only targeted populations (insects) and instead, affect non-targeted animals and humans. Some of the bacteria that might become mutated in the human body include an important gut resident, *E. coli*.[65]

Sulfate reducing bacteriae were discovered as early as the mid-1950s. They are felt to be important to the production of petroleum in underground reservoirs but they are also found in many other environments including acid mine wastes, industrial wastewaters, and soils. Several patents pertain to the treatment of oil-bearing sands and shales using bacterial preparations (mining or bioremediation). At least one patent was part of a research project that studied the role of microbes in the genesis of petroleum. That study was sponsored by a grant from the American Petroleum Institute.[66-70]

Studies have shown that bacteriae produce *detergents* which help release the oil by oxidizing its hydrocarbons. Some of the bacteriae that can be used to extract oil are the *Clostridium* and *Pseudomonas* species, as well as *E. coli, Salmonella enteritidis, Aerobacter aerogenes, Proteus vulgaris,* and algae including *Scenedesmus.* The essential food for most of these bacteriae is *phosphate* (as in organophosphates and fertilizers). Many of these bacteriae are found naturally in wastewater, groundwater, and in the soil; or are present due to applications of agrochemicals, biological controls, fertilizers, construction, industrial, nuclear, or mining wastes.[66-70]

A US Army Corps of Engineers report published May 1994 (just five months before the Dearborn Conference that Dr. Alan Barbour attended), described the feasibility of capping industrial waste disposal sites using dredged materials which included clays. It also discussed the necessity of testing such processes before the sites were permanently capped. The study revealed there was no capping of bauxite disposal sites at Texas A&M University during 1992. The feasibility studies were completed in 1993, one year before the Dearborn conference; and a separate report was published in 1994.[71]

Once again for emphasis, Texas A&M is one of the university systems that participated in the early international exchanges with respect to biological controls. It is also an affiliate group member of the team that operates the DOE-funded Lawrence Livermore National Laboratory. The lab's scientists work on classified nuclear research. The facility has a high-explosive testing range, and is where "biosecurity" and genetic engineering studies of microbes important to insecticides are undertaken. Nuclear and mining waste disposals have been a global problem for decades, and many US sites have been identified as superfund sites by the EPA for their persisting radioactive compounds and other toxic chemicals. It is interesting that studies regarding toxic waste disposal were performed just before the Dearborn conference; and that those studies involved Texas A&M University-related waste disposal sites.[72-74]

The Texas A&M University System is assignee to many of Dr. Alan Barbour's *Borrelia burgdorferi*-related patents, which number around one hundred. We have already seen petroleum and mining companies as patent holders of Bb diagnostic tests. We may wonder whether Dr. Barbour's attendance at the 1994 Dearborn conference was some kind of "insurance policy" that Lyme disease surveillance case definitions, or testing standards would be implemented in a manner favorable for important industries, especially as they might concern the detection of an infection possibly caused by improper waste disposal methods. We may further wonder about Dr. Barbour's involvement at Rocky Mountain Labs during the 1980s where he modified a culture medium to enable the identification of the Lyme disease "agent."

Academic scientists from institutions such as the State University of New York; Universities of Pennsylvania, Wisconsin, Minnesota, Missouri, California, Connecticut; and Yale, Harvard, and the North and South Carolina University Systems and some of their spin-off companies hold the majority of Bb-related patents. The US government holds certain rights to some of these inventions as well as those that are agriculturally-related (i.e. insecticides and agriculturally-applicable chemicals). Some of these institutions also have key infectious disease researchers who have been present since the announcement of Lyme disease. Lyme disease, according to the theories in this book, may have important connections to multiple industries and their toxic, persisting pollutants.[71,75-91]

Perhaps the relationships between valuable natural resources, waste management, and the mutagenic effects of persisting (and sometimes radioactive) wastes upon soil and water-borne microbes including those derived from mined and manufactured materials will now shift more clearly into focus. We must remember that these materials and their byproducts, as well as recombinant insecticides (and other "weapons") have been globally deployed. We may also observe who is patenting all things Bb-related, and which state medical boards seem to have specifically targeted physicians who treat Lyme-infected patients outside of infectious disease-recommended "standards of care." Such standards may be dictated by experts whose interests lie not only in defending public health, but also highly profitable industries that may prove to have powerful connections to globally important infectious diseases.

As a result of the intricate relationships that are now more clearly defined, we may wonder whether the protection of incredibly valuable natural resources worth untold trillions of dollars, and the industries which profit upon same, are some of the largest contributing factors to the silencing of epidemics such as Lyme disease – a disease that may yet prove to be the natural offspring of the industrial-agricultural revolution and the biotech industry. ❑

See No Evil.

Six: Tracking Insects and Epidemics

Mites and Rickettsialpox

During the early insect biological warfare (biowarfare) studies of the WWII era, Dr. Edward A. Steinhaus and colleagues were cataloging bacteria associated with ticks and other insects. Their work was revealed in a 1942 publication by Dr. R.R. Parker, then Director of the National Institutes of Health's (NIH) Rocky Mountain Laboratories, in Hamilton, Montana. There were at least two hundred and fifty clearly identified bacterial species that were known to be associated with disease-transmitting insects and arthropods including ticks by the early 20th century. In those early decades, many kinds of parasitizing insects (parasitoids) were being released to naturally control pests that were destroying agriculture and landscapes.[1]

Parasitoid releases were undertaken not only in the field, but also within commercial greenhouses to control many pests. For example scientists used predatory mite species to control pest mite species. Introductions of predatory mites took place in the field through *inoculative* releases. These typically were low volume releases that were designed to establish predatory mite species within a specific area as a natural control. The predatory mites would feed upon pest mites in a cannibalistic manner, thereby eliminating them.[2-7]

What were referred to as *inundative* releases were deployed when large numbers of predatory mites were desired within a regional area. Many of the predatory mite species preyed not only upon other mites, but also upon the larvae and adults of lepidoptera species. This included the gypsy moths which by then were an enormous economic and environmental concern. The multi-pest diet of the predatory mites solved more than one pest problem and was a welcome convenience. Predatory mites were also employed in vineyards to control pest mites such as the borealis spider mite (*Eotetranychus carpini*) that is common to France, Germany, Switzerland, Italy, and The Netherlands.[2-7]

Another pest is the two-spotted spider mite (*Tetranychus urticae*). Both of these predatory mite species attack citrus crops including wine and table grapes in the US. Could the 1920-1940 releases of predatory insects including predatory mites have contributed to regional outbreaks of animal and human diseases? The indiscriminate use of chemical pesticides including DDT (first commercially available in 1940), truly upset the balance of the predatory mite populations in favor of pest mites. Such an imbalance could very well have contributed to the emergence of novel animal and human infections carried by these mites and by their animal hosts including rodents and birds.[2-7]

By 1951, areas of New York and West Hartford, Connecticut were considered to be endemic for *Allodermanyssus sanguineus* mites, which are rodent parasites. Reports of this mite species were also recorded in Washington, DC; Champaign, Illinois; Tucson, Arizona; New York City; Philadelphia, Pennsylvania; Salt Lake City, Utah; Indianapolis, Indiana; Boston, Massachusetts; West Hartford, Connecticut; and Brookline, Massachusetts. Abroad they are found in Egypt, the Ukraine, and Armenia. The mites had been isolated as early as 1909 forward with increased levels reported in the US from 1940 to 1950. This is a period when the organofluoride and organochloride pesticides were first applied agriculturally in many parts of the world.[8]

A 1950 symposium on viral and rickettsial diseases was held by the Society of American Bacteriologists in Baltimore, Maryland. Scientists attended from the US Army Medical Department Research and Graduate School (Washington, DC); the University of Chicago School of Medicine (Chicago IL); the Hospital of the Rockefeller Institute (New York, NY); the Children's Hospital Research Foundation (Cincinnati, OH); Yale University (New Haven, CT); the National Institutes of Health (Bethesda, MD); and the State of California Department of Public Health. Dr. Edwin H. Lennette from the California Department of Public Health gave a presentation where he discussed the New York City Health Department's involvement in the investigation of an outbreak of a new human disease called *Rickettsialpox* that had suddenly emerged in 1946 in New York.[2,9,10]

Dr. Lennette reported that the causative organism was isolated, and was named *Rickettsia akari* since it appeared similar to other rickettsiae, and was isolated from a mite (*akari*). The organism was however noted to be distinctly different from the spotted fever group of rickettsial bacteria. A paper claimed that "unusual" mites were discovered in the households of people who had become infected with rickettsialpox during the New York outbreak. The mites were identified as *Allodermanyssus sanguineus* mites. These are blood feeders that are found on birds and mice; their main amplifying hosts. (An amplifying host is any host that will circulate a transmitted infection, allowing it to multiply and to reassort).[2,9,10-13]

The agent of rickettsialpox is related to the *Poxviruses,* a group that contains not only mammalian, but also insect-infecting viruses. (Today scientists know that rickettsiae are similar to viruses.) In 1983 a scientist proposed that *Lymphocytic choriomeningitis virus* (LCMV, or Armstrong's disease), which is a virus common to house mice, could force human rickettsialpox infections. LCMV is an old world *Arenavirus.* This group includes the lassa fever virus of African rodents. The arenaviruses are not considered to be insect-borne, but they are transmissible to humans through mites or exposure to rodent urine, feces, or saliva. They may also be transmitted through contaminated foods or by inhalation of aerosolized particles.[11-13]

At the time of the New York health department's investigation, basement storerooms and incinerators of apartment houses were found to be heavily infested with mice, and deemed to be the source of the 1946 human rickettsialpox outbreak. Although there was no physical evidence that infected patients were bitten by mites, significant numbers of mites were discovered in the buildings of infected patients. Serologic (blood) examinations of patients revealed they had developed antibodies to the rickettsialpox agent. If a large number of mites were found near garbage incinerators, it is entirely possible that incinerating garbage that was contaminated with virus-infected rodent excrement may have aerosolized virus particles as airborne particulates. People in the surrounding area could have inhaled the virus without being bitten by mites. This could explain a human disease outbreak, the presence of antibodies in patients, and the lack of mice or mites in infected people's homes.[3-6]

Dr. Lennette's symposium presentation also described another rickettsial organism that had begun to surface at the time of the New York rickettsialpox outbreak. The agent's name was *Rickettsia popilliae* or *Coxiella popilliae.* This is a bacterial (rickettsial) infection that causes the fatal "blue disease" of Japanese beetle larvae. The infection was first noted in Japanese beetle larvae collected from Nottingham, Pennsylvania in October 1940 by a scientist named P.S. Clarke. This is the very same year that the pesticide DDT was first commercialized. In 1951, scientists S.R. Dutky and E.L. Gooden attempted to determine the origins of blue disease. The organism's shape was described as similar to *Vibrio* species of bacteria, but its small size and intracellular growth ruled out that particular bacteriae. Nevertheless it had characteristics similar to the *polyhedrosis* viruses of the *lepidoptera* (moths/butterflies). Dr. Steinhaus considered the organism to be a novel rickettsial infection. Remember that microbial insecticides were already in use at this time, which included insect polyhedrosis viruses and soil bacteriae.[3,4,14,15]

Unbeknownst to scientists at the time, there was a novel insect symbiont (latent infection) which would emerge in deer and sheep tick populations. It would not be noted until 1970 by scientists Yamataka and Hayashi. Later it would be determined to be similar to infections caused by protozoan *ciliates*; and the predatory gram-negative *Bdellovibrio* bacteriae. This tick symbiont infection was later identified as *IricES1* or *Ixodes ricinus* EndoSymbiont 1. This parasite is an intracellular (mitochondria) infection that was found in about one half of the male, and nearly all the female deer and sheep ticks analyzed.[16-20]

IricES1 is more prevalent in female ticks because it is found primarily in the ovarian tissues. The organism was found to be closely related to a bacterium from the bird tick *Haemaphysalis wellingtoni.** IricES1 belongs to the alpha-proteobacteria species group (clade) which has a sister clade that includes the following tickborne infections: *Anaplasma, Ehrlichia, Neorickettsia,* and *Wolbachia.* IricES1 represents a new family of rickettsial infections that are largely latent tick infections. *The prevalence of IricES1 in ticks as a symbiont is very high.* It has been isolated from sheep ticks in a dozen countries including Great Britain, Italy, Germany, Switzerland, the Ukraine, and Africa. This may be another intracellular infection that may or may not have been recently renamed, but one that *has been seen* by scientists since at least the early 1950s. It should be considered as a possible co-infection in patients who suffer from tick-borne diseases.[16-20]

**The H. wellingtoni bird tick is also a carrier of Kyasanur Forest disease virus, a flavivirus from a group that includes yellow fever, tickborne encephalitis, dengue fever, St. Louis encephalitis, and West Nile. All of these viruses cause encephalitic syndromes and neurologic disease.*

The prevalence of the IricES1 tick symbiont has been studied in sheep ticks from Algeria, Austria, Czech Republic, England, Germany, Ireland, Italy, Russia, Sweden, Switzerland, Turkey, and Tunisia. In 1971, four years before the Lyme disease outbreak was reported in Connecticut, Brinton and Oliver studied the fine structure of cells during egg production in Rocky Mountain wood ticks. They concluded in essence that IricES1 may become part of the egg yolk cells when present. This means that in birds (i.e. poultry) this symbiont is intrinsically present, and therefore could be a latent contaminant in cell lines if they were grown using infected insect cells and/or chicken embryos. It may also indicate that this symbiont may become a reactivated latent infection when presented with a live virus such as from a recombinant insecticide. Such reactivation may occur not only in insects, but also in animals or humans who have been inoculated with contaminated chicken embryo-grown vaccines.[20,21]

Scientist Dr. Willy Burgdorfer, after whom the Lyme disease agent was named in 1982, was among those studying the "non-pathogenic" rickettsiae in Rocky Mountain wood ticks in 1979 and 1980. Dr. Burgdorfer was also a colleague of L.P. Brinton, who studied the IricES1 tick symbiont. Dr. Burgdorfer also co-authored a paper with other colleagues including Entomologist Dr. Louis A. Magnarelli from the Connecticut Agricultural Experiment Station in 1981, the year before the Lyme disease agent was official declared. The paper discusses the endemicity (high prevalence) of the spotted fever group of rickettsial bacteriae in Connecticut, the source of the Lyme disease outbreak reported in 1975.

These scientists were studying the pathogens found in Rocky Mountain wood ticks, American dog ticks, clinical data from suspected or diagnosed human cases from 1965 to 1977; and the presence of RMSF antibodies in mice and deer. I find it odd that Drs. Burgdorfer, Magnarelli, and others have not spoken out about the presence of important tick symbiont infections including wolbachia, spiroplasmas, IricES1, and other pathogens commonly found in the ticks that transmit Lyme disease. It is even more curious when we understand that Dr. Magnarelli's name is listed on Bb-related patents, including for a Lyme disease vaccine. Was 1981 the year that certain scientists first made a connection between recombinant insecticides and the reactivation of tick symbionts which were being transmitted to the human population?[22-25]

The patent describes methods of creating borrelia antigens, and is assigned to company Symbicom. The exclusive world-wide patent rights to Symbicom's outer surface protein A (OspA)-based Lyme disease vaccine were licensed to vaccine manufacturer Pasteur-Merieux subsidiary Connaught Laboratories in 1991 according to sources. This would have been the competing vaccine to SmithKline Beecham's Lyme vaccine, although the Connaught vaccine never came to market. The patent describes a vaccine to prevent Lyme disease, but the organisms it discusses include bacteriophages, soil bacteria (i.e. *Bacillus subtilis*), and other microbes such as those that are used in recombinant insecticides.[26-33]

The Connecticut Agricultural research station which employs Dr. Magnarelli indicates on its web site that it tests ticks for Lyme disease. The station also manages research and oversees insect controls and plant diseases. The station registers bee keepers, performs inspections on honey bees and nursery stock; and performs town surveys for gypsy moth infestations. Dr. Magnarelli's other patents include Bb-related diagnostic and vaccine processes. Some of these patents were filed just weeks before, or a few months after the Dearborn Conference of October 27-29, 1994 which standardized tests and surveillance criteria for Lyme disease.[26-33]

The Emergence of Ehrlichiosis

During my research into military aspects of biowarfare, I discovered that field studies were undertaken in the form of outdoor experiments using insect-vectored agents. The literature does not always reveal the nature of the experiments, but we might assume their objectives based upon the dates the experiments were undertaken. For example outdoor testing during the 1940s may have involved biological weapons research for military purposes; especially when performed on a military base with an outdoor test area designed for this purpose. Whether the biological weapons being tested were for offensive or defensive purposes for warfare or agriculture probably depended upon the agents under study. Even covert human experiments (i.e. using white coats or prison inmates) could have studied human disease transmission and the effects of military or agriculturally important agents.

One peculiar infectious disease outbreak at a Texas military base may reveal clues to experimentation with chemical or biological warfare agents during the years preceding the declaration of WWII. What is intriguing was the equally sudden appearance and disappearance of an infectious disease and its vector, the Lone Star tick, *Amblyomma americanum*. This tick is a known host and transmitter (vector) of STARI infections, a Lyme-like illness. For two summers (1942-1943), sudden outbreaks of a strange, new tickborne illness erupted at Camp Bullis. Camp Bullis is a Ft. Sam Houston sub-post located roughly eighteen miles north of San Antonio, Texas where about one thousand soldiers were suddenly infected with a tickborne disease. Each patient had a history of tick bite while training at Camp Bullis, and some patients had Lone Star ticks still attached to them at the time of hospitalization. The illness, which was dubbed "Bullis fever," defied identification and caused at least one death. The main clinical symptoms were fever lasting four to fourteen days, a low white blood cell count, severe headaches, and enlarged lymph nodes (lymphadenopathy).[1]

Other symptoms were similar to those of what we know of today as an *Ehrlichiosis* infection. It was presumed that the infections came from the Lone Star ticks due to their unusually high concentration in the area. For example four servicemen collected over four thousand adult Lone Star ticks from beneath a single tree. Incredibly, more than eleven hundred ticks were removed from one soldier who sat in a tick-infested thicket for just two hours. In July 1942, members of a board for "the control of influenza and other epidemic diseases in the Army" arrived at Brooke General hospital at Ft. Sam Houston to examine the patients and their medical records.[1]

Epidemiologic studies were performed at Camp Bullis, during which time thousands of ticks and chiggers were collected from birds and mammals in the area. The predominant blood-feeding arthropod at the base was indeed the Lone Star tick. A human and tick strain of the infectious pathogen was isolated, but the identity of the causative agent was not determined at the time. What is perhaps significant is that academic university laboratories are located in San Antonio, Austin, and Houston; a short distance from the Army base. This could arguably have made Camp Bullis a convenient test site for a novel chemical or biological control agent, whether the intended use was military or agricultural. An application of a novel control on or in the vicinity of the base could certainly have attracted unusually high numbers of ticks if, for example, the deployed agent involved applications of chemicals and/or insect pheromones.

The Texas A&M University campus is a short drive from Camp Bullis, and so are the Texas Agricultural Experiment Station, and the Southern Plains Agricultural Research Center in College Station. The latter two agencies are the most likely candidates to have tested novel control agents for insect pests in the area – controls that were beginning to be explored in 1942. Scientists from, and some institutions within the Texas A&M and the University of Texas Systems are assignees to a significant number of *Borrelia burgdorferi*-related patents; and to microbial insecticide formulas for agricultural or industrial use. It is therefore not difficult to imagine that experimentally tested controls, especially those containing novel chemical pheromones or other chemical compounds, may have attracted a significantly greater number of ticks to the Camp Bullis area.[2]

Early in 1942, the USDA's Laboratory of the Bureau of Entomology and Plant Quarantine in Orlando, Florida began explorations into insecticides and repellants for the Armed Forces. The first discussions of these explorations were prepared in 1944 in two reports which were unpublished. I reviewed a second revision of these reports, published August, 1946. The laboratory had the assistance of the US Army and Navy in executing early DDT pesticidal studies. The research was supported by funding from the Office of Scientific Research and Development, the Rockefeller Foundation, the Arkansas State Board of Health, the Tennessee Valley Authority, and several commercial entities. It is interesting to note that the USDA had this to say about DDT at the time: "DDT is poisonous and all recommendations for its use should be followed carefully." If this chemical was known to be poisonous, we may wonder why it was allowed to be used as a pesticide against insects and upon agricultural crops that would be fed to livestock and to people.[3]

> *"It should be clearly kept in mind that most of the substances under consideration are poisonous. If they were not, they would probably be useless against the insects for which they are recommended. Therefore, the recommendations for the proper use of these substances should be followed. Careless, unnecessary exposure and misuse is fraught with hazard. It should be further kept in mind that probably no chemical is safe for every individual, even when properly used...It is our opinion that at present the justification for the use of the preparations recommended in this bulletin far outweighs any hazard involved."*
>
> —From an August 1946 USDA report by the Laboratory of the Bureau of Entomology and Plant Quarantine about DDT and other insecticides and repellents developed for the US Armed Forces.

DDT contains a number of harmful chemicals such as naphthalene, petroleum oils, coal-tar distillate fractions, aromatic petroleum, and benzene. Some of these and other chemicals in the products are highly mutagenic to microorganisms. DDT was used as a powder, aerosol spray, and as an emulsion in a wide variety of forestry, agricultural, military, and livestock applications. DDT was first synthesized in 1874, but it was not until 1939 that it was felt to be a useful insecticide, as reported by the Swiss J.R. Geigy, A.A. Co., which had a New York subsidiary.[4-6]

Airplanes were deployed as early as 1923 to control mosquito larvae in Louisiana by aerial spray. The earliest patent for the pesticide DDT was issued in 1943. As early as the summer of 1923, aerial deployments of DDT were underway although other sprays and insecticidal powders were already in use agriculturally, for sylviculture (forests), and for military applications. DDT has been used to control fleas, silverfish, bedbugs, lices, cockroaches, flies, mosquitoes, and sand flies. Ticks were not mentioned in the 1946 USDA report, although this pesticide has been used to control ticks and other insects. It is easy to guess that DDT could have been deployed near the Camp Bullis installation. This could have adversely affected the microbes lying otherwise dormant within the bodies of resident Lone Star ticks to force an outbreak of human disease at the base.[4-6]

A number of surface-active agents (surfactants, emulsifiers) were mentioned in the report. These included Duponol C, Triton X-100, Spans, and Tweens. DDT is a chlorinated hydrocarbon-containing pesticide and as such, is a nerve and stomach toxin. DDT, benzene hexachloride, and other related insecticidal compounds are secreted in the milk of dairy animals; and insecticides will persist in a stable manner in soils and marine sediments where they are in contact with insects, larvae, and microbes. *Triton X-100 and other alkylphenols, as well as DDT, lindane, atrazine, PCBs, phthalates (plasticizers), styrenes, and dioxins are among chemicals that are known to be, or are considered to be possible endocrine disrupters and carcinogens.*[4-6,19]

It is also easy to imagine that ticks could have been deployed en masse at Camp Bullis specifically for DDT or other chemical testing purposes in an area of the base that probably would have been chemically treated post-test. It is possible that some of the test "subjects" if deployed or naturally attracted, may have escaped pesticidal applications to cause an unexpected outbreak at the base. We know that Lone Star tick infested test areas were bombed with insecticides according to reports. The Bullis fever outbreak mysteriously vanished the following year with no additional cases reported. This means that the tick vectors were probably destroyed by DDT or another acaracide. The incident was not mentioned publicly until a report was finally issued a decade later in 1952. A much later report published in 1988 included a letter suggesting that the clinical presentation of Bullis fever was consistent with that of *Ehrlichiosis*.[1,2]

A separate study of the Bullis fever outbreak was undertaken in 1943 at the US Army's Eighth Service Command laboratory. The blood of two hundred sixty-one soldiers who had been stationed at Camp Bullis during the 1942-1943 outbreaks was analyzed. Samples had been collected two months after the end of the outbreak from patients with tick bite, and who had severe headache, lymph node involvement, and leukopenia. At the same time many animals around the base were captured, killed, and studied for evidence of similar infections. Scientists examined forty deer, seven rabbits, two raccoons, and an armadillo for the presence of "Bullis fever," typhus, Rocky Mountain spotted fever, and Q fever. The studies concluded that there was no immunological relationship between Bullis fever and RMSF; but rickettsia was observed in patients from the base. It was also noted that Bullis fever was not a strain of typhus or Q fever. Scientists also concluded that animals had contributed to the propagation of the insects that were carrying Bullis fever. An agent was isolated from ticks on the base which seemed to bear a similarity to the agent that was isolated from service personnel who had Bullis fever.[3]

The latter finding was vague and inconclusive considering that scientists studied large numbers of blood samples and several viruses. Were they truly unsure of the agent's origin, or did they simply not wish to reveal it, or how it came to infect personnel? Military scientists concluded that Bullis fever was more severe in 1943 than it was in 1942. They felt that either the agent was increasing in virulence, or else the population of new troops were somehow more susceptible to the agent. From the evidence in this book, we can see that either idea may have been accurate. According to the report:

> "The latest exposures, and those in whom the disease has been rather severe and highly prevalent, are new troops, for the most part originating in relatively tick-free parts of the country such as Chicago or New York."[8]

Were these new personnel exposed to toxic chemicals or infectious microbes that remained latent in their bodies? Here is a clue that an epidemic could have erupted in 1942 simply because agricultural chemicals and microbial controls were being newly applied across the eastern and midwestern United States – chemicals to which service personnel were now being exposed as aerial pollutants. New York and Chicago were among the first areas of the country where new agricultural tools were being attempted, most assuredly near agricultural research stations and military bases. If new chemical or biological controls (or other chemical agents) were applied/stored on or near Camp Bullis prior to the outbreaks of Bullis fever, then resident Lone Star ticks could very well have become affected by the agents two years in a row since such chemicals persist in the environment.

Ticks that transmitted novel infections (i.e. microbes that mutated upon pesticide exposure) to the newly vaccinated troops may have made the Camp Bullis outbreak more severe in 1943, especially if the viruses co-mingled and reassorted with animal pathogens first, only to be transmitted to the military personnel. The other possibility is that a chemical pesticide not only could have mutated pathogens in the tick bodies; it could have caused the reactivation of military vaccine viruses in newly vaccinated troops.[8-11]

On the other hand, there have been recent allegations of water and soil contaminations by mustard gas and other buried weapons that have surfaced in the media, and which concerned a nearby subpost of the San Antonio Arsenal, Camp Stanley (briefly called Camp Funston). The base was operated as an ammunition storage depot. In 1933 it was transferred to the Ordnance Department, and insects could have come into contact with mutated soil pathogens from buried or "leaking" stored weapons. Camp Stanley was also reportedly a subpost of nearby Camp Bullis.[12]

If leaking mustard or other agents led to the mutation of tick pathogens and the military learned of this connection, it may have alerted experiment stations or public health officials that chemical pesticides or military chemicals were not only causing human infections, but that over time the infections were becoming more virulent. It is doubtful had this been known whether public health officials would have broadcast such relationships to the media or to the public, because to do so may have jeopardized any novel agents being attempted for agricultural or military purposes. We have seen how data related to other WWII activities (i.e. Manhattan Project) was sequestered under "national security" claims. It could be expected that operations which concerned the military use of chemical pesticides would have fallen under the same protections. After all, any negative ramifications of their use would have caused an investigation into the safety of weapons storage, use, or disposal. The early agricultural chemicals were on the cusp of a highly profitable future for agrochemical companies and their partners or assignees,* and their future success would have been important to protect, especially for their expected or upcoming use in various war theatres.[8,10-12]

**Patent interests in agricultural chemicals and microbial pesticides are often held by government agencies in many countries, including the United States and Canada.*

When we study the history of chemical warfare, we find clues from the early Camp Bullis outbreaks to help us understand modern day tickborne diseases. The outbreaks may have been an indication there was a problem with the chemical agents being deployed, and the insects being exposed to them. Despite this early alarm, chemical pesticides were promoted from the 1940s into the early 1970s when DDT was finally banned because they were the most effective controls. Before the Camp Bullis outbreak, scientists were deploying chemical as well as microbial controls, and studying their effects. Was the outbreak at Camp Bullis related to the testing of new *chemical warfare agents* meant to be deployed in periods of conflict? Did agricultural chemicals mutate microbes in the environment or insects, allowing ticks to transmit novel infections to military personnel? And would the ban on DDT or other chemical pesticides in favor of biological controls, in time reveal the full spectrum of human infections to be transmitted by insects thanks to the action of mutagenic chemicals? Is a "chemicals-and-recombinant-genes-mutate-microbes-and-degrade-insect-gut-cells-to cause disease" model the reason there is a veil of secrecy around vector-borne diseases and other illnesses with so-called "unknown" causes?

From a pest management study undertaken in 1990, we learn that Army personnel from Ft. McPherson, Georgia collected ticks at Ft. Jackson, South Carolina over a four-day period. Ticks were collected from tick drags and CO_2 traps set in areas where troops trained, and the tick mid-gut contents were examined. From the three hundred and forty-five adult and nymph Lone Star ticks collected, eighteen or 5.2% tested positive for *Borrelia burgdorferi*. A USDA document from 1989 also discussed evidence of Lyme disease transmission by Lone Star ticks. The document revealed that these ticks can also transmit *Theileria cervi* to white-tailed deer. *Theileria* are protozoan infections from cattle and other ruminants that are pathogenic to man. Theileria are similar to, and sometimes identified as *Babesia*. These papers indicate that *Lone Star ticks can indeed transmit Lyme disease.* Reports also emphasize that Lone Star ticks are not limited to the transmission of STARI infections, as is typically advised by public health experts including some whom deny the existence of chronic Lyme disease.[13-18]

So-called "Polio"

From the earliest days of polio outbreaks we may find links which appear strikingly coincidental with the viruses of gypsy moths and Japanese beetles, and the early chemical and microbial controls of agriculture and industry. The earliest recorded outbreak of polio in the US emerged in Vermont in 1894, just twenty-five years after Trouvelot's gypsy moths escaped from their Massachusetts home. In areas where gypsys caused mass defoliation, agencies were attempting to eradicate infestations using microbial insecticides which included *Bacillus popilliae, Bacillus lentimorbus,* and *Bacillus thuringiensis.* Since at least the mid-1880s forward, mutagenic chemicals were also being used in many industries. Some of these chemicals included black powder or dynamite, anilines, chlorides, nitrophenyls, bleaching powders, Bordeaux mixtures, fluorides, and various chemical amines. Any of these may have contributed to the emergence of polio or other epidemic diseases through the activation of latent insect, animal, or human infections.

Additional epidemics of polio occurred in 1907 in New York City; and in Nebraska and Massachusetts in 1909. From a 1910 report we learn that physicians suggested that toxins with an affinity for nervous tissues may have played a role in "polio" patients who showed early paralysis but who recovered. Some fatal cases had an extremely short duration from first symptom to expiration – only seven hours in one case. Could early phosphates of lime (an alkylating agent) be responsible for causing an infective virus to reassort in mosquito guts to cause a fatal encephalitis that was generically named "polio?" *Remember that alkylating agents destroy individual cells by reacting with cellular proteins, enzymes, RNA, and DNA. The effect is irreversible and leads to mutation.*[1-10]

At the turn of the 20th century, Nebraska's dominant crops were corn, wheat, and sugar beets for the sugar industry. Sugar production began in 1890 with the first factory in Grand Island; only the second sugar production factory to operate in the US (after the first in Albany, CA). Sugar beets were processed using boiling water, into which *lime* was added. The slurry was filtered and heated. We might consider the sugar beet pests (and their latent infections), including aphids, leaf hoppers, cutworms, whiteflies, armyworms, and nematodes. The common diseases of beet crops include the yellows viruses, and the curly top and beet mosaic viruses, any of which are known to be degraded by certain clays and surfactants, and which also regularly and easily reassort because they are segmented viruses (i.e. *geminiviruses*). What ended up in factory wastewaters could have easily donated infectious agents that could reassort with polio viruses found in these waters.[1-9]

In 1921 when President Franklin Delano Roosevelt contracted polio, applied chemical and microbial pesticides were already being applied to large areas of the US and abroad. Indeed what would become the most common global agricultural pesticide (*Bacillus thuringiensis*), has been utilized since the earliest days of the 20th century; and some form of lime (potash) has been around since the earliest disease epidemics. By the 1930s in the US, there were more outbreaks of polio in Connecticut and Los Angeles. Since President Roosevelt was himself a victim of "polio," it makes sense that he would receive a letter about "biowarfare" from Secretary of War Henry Stimson, whom Roosevelt had appointed to the position in July of 1940.*[1-5]

**The President may have contracted polio from a Bear Mountain camp (New York on the Hudson River), or from swimming in the waters of Campobello, New Brunswick, Canada (off the tip of Maine), in 1921. Either location would have exposed him to insects that were likewise exposed to important viruses and pesticides.*

The letter Stimson sent to Roosevelt is often quoted as "evidence" by those who claim that Lyme disease is a biowarfare weapon that was developed by the military to make people ill. The letter says: "we must be prepared…and the matter must be handled with great secrecy and as well as great vigor." At the time his letter was written, Stimson sought Presidential approval for a group of advisors who might coordinate and direct all government biowarfare research. These duties would have included overseeing agricultural insecticides, as well as any that might be useful for military purposes. We cannot know the entirety of the discussions between Roosevelt and Stimson, but we may guess that since the President had been recently infected with polio, that any agriculturally applied chemicals or microbes which might cause polio outbreaks would have been a worthwhile and expected topic of discussion; and one that would undoubtedly have been met with the President's utmost enthusiasm.[1-5,14-16]

We can also look at older research papers that discussed the emergence of polio and other outbreaks to see if there is a connection between applied biological controls and livestock animals that came into contact with same. A 1961 paper discussed human cases of Q fever in Idaho that had been recorded from 1951 to June of 1958. Q fever infections were typically found in goats, sheep, and cattle. Outbreaks occurred in California and Idaho. Sheep were the primary source of Q fever infections for humans, with most infections occurring during lambing season. Agricultural workers who came into contact with dairy cattle during calving, and individuals who drank raw milk from Q fever-infected animals were most at risk for the disease. Could a Q fever agent mutate with an insect virus to cause infectious "polio"? Would such mutation come about through the ingestion of a ruminant animal, or chemical herbicides that contained dioxins or other mutagenic agents?[17,18]

Scientists began working on polio vaccines beginning in 1952. This was the same year that the *Sindbis* arbovirus, a parent virus to Old and New World viruses, was isolated from an Egyptian mosquito. Unfortunately there were problems with contaminated polio vaccines during the early days of polio vaccine development. A public health report published in 1958 revealed that seventeen Idaho children from a group of 32,000 aged six to eight, who were inoculated with a live polio vaccine suffered paralytic poliomyelitis infections. Two lots of poliovirus vaccine were associated with the outbreak, which took place in 1955.[19]

Poliovirus lots that were suspected to have caused the children's infections were studied in rhesus, African green, and cynomolgus monkeys. The virus was isolated from cortisone-treated animals that were known to be capable of supporting virus growth. Some of the vaccines were treated with merthiolate (thimerosal), a mercury-containing preservative. Others were treated with merthiolate and versene, a chelating agent that neutralizes harmful metal ions; and some remained untreated. (Merthiolate added to vaccines increased the yield of poliovirus from the infected animals, according to a paper). The preservatives were an attempt to determine whether they would inactivate residual poliovirus in vaccines. Monkeys are said to be about 500 times more susceptible to poliovirus infection than humans. Post-vaccination some monkeys developed seizures and paralysis. Others showed no paralysis, but tremors or other symptoms. Most or all were sacrificed and their tissues studied. The polio monkey experiments revealed that the preservatives affected the antibody response in monkeys, however poliovirus was nevertheless isolated from monkeys that received the treated vaccines.[19,20]

Monkey kidney cells were used in all isolations, and in most cases, human KB carcinoma cells were also used in parallel tests to determine human susceptibility. KB cells are a cell line that was derived from a human carcinoma (cancer) of the nasopharynx. *KB cell lines were offered as stock cultures by Rocky Mountain Laboratory* since they were cost effective and they easily supported the growth of polio and other viruses. What is curious from the paper are these conclusions:

> "With both lots of vaccine, the incidence of paralysis was so much greater in monkeys than in children that a vaccine producing no paralysis in monkeys would be unlikely to have [a] deleterious effect on children. If, along with absence of paralysis, no virus can be detected in blood, brown fat, or lymphoid tissue of monkeys, any chance of harmful effects on children appears remote."

However when the studies are closely examined, we find they also involved the direct inoculation of monkey spinal cords with poliovirus. There was no conclusion in the paper that stated anything with respect to whether poliovirus could be detected from the cerebral spinal fluid of inoculated monkeys, which was a likely place for the poliovirus to hide.[19,20]

Conclusions such as those portrayed in this paper were probably key to supporting the ongoing use of live poliovirus vaccines in humans, despite the Idaho outbreaks – a use of live virus vaccines that continued into future generations. The question of course is whether a Q fever agent could have played a role in the emergence of infectious poliomyelitis epidemics in the US or any other country. When we remember that Q fever is transmitted by goats and cattle, animals that supply fresh milk to children in particular, we may assume some connection. If plant pathogens mutate under the application of agricultural chemicals and/or microbes and scientists know this, then a race to develop "polio" vaccines makes sense. The longer an agricultural chemical or microbial formula is used as a pesticide or herbicide, the greater the chance that humans will be affected by any microbes which mutate in the presenec of such applications.[19,20]

Scientists determined that since KB cells were easy to propagate serially and because they were less expensive and more readily available than monkey kidney cells commonly used to isolate and purify polioviruses, that the KB cells were a good substitute for monkey kidney cells to make vaccines. But if stock cell lines for vaccines were contaminated with infectious agents that were unknown and undetectable to scientists as of the 1950s, such cell lines would have contaminated every vaccine or other tool created by their use in the years to come. The question then becomes whether contaminated cell lines used for animal or human vaccines contained latent infectious agents which may reactivate upon exposure to vectoring insects that have wild or laboratory-derived recombinant infections. Once inside the body, an active insect virus may reactivate a latent virus. Remember this may occur if an insect-introduced virus donates genes to the latent virus. We know that the agricultural agent *Bacillus thuringiensis* is capable of reactivating latent infections in insects. Can the viruses of recombinant insecticides reactivate latent animal and human infections and/or or vaccine viruses to cause diseases with "unknown" cause?[19,20]

Lone Star Virus and Asian Outbreaks

In a 1971 report published by the Navy and Marine Corps, I learned of a pre-service test of an ultra low volume aerial spray system for rotary winged aircraft (helicopters). The unit was developed by the Army Medical Equipment Laboratory at Fort Totten in Flushing, New York. A test was conducted the summer of 1970 whereby pilots treated a five-hundred acre plot that was infested with Lone Star ticks (*Amblyomma americanum*). The chemical used was the mosquito agent Dibrom 14®. The spray system proved adequate for test purposes, and the chemical reduced the tick population 50% over twenty-four hours. I wondered how this large plot became infested with ticks, and what became of the 50% of ticks that survived the test. Some evidence of outdoor tickborne research studies is available. From a paper:[1]

> "The life cycle of ticks reared experimentally under outdoor conditions took 2-3 months in Cairo area summer weather. In winter oviposition ceased (laying eggs), fed larvae failed to molt, and nymphal premolting periods increased significantly....Survival of the tick population depends on the prompt return of host birds to their regular breeding colony in the spring."[2,3]

Another report indicated that tickborne virus studies took place in the Ohio-Mississippi Basin from 1964 to 1970, and which involved the *Lone Star virus.* This virus was called a "hitherto unknown agent" and was isolated from Lone Star ticks according to a paper from the University of Illinois-Urbana. The virus was isolated from ticks that were removed from woodchucks which were captured in western Kentucky in 1966 and 1967. Three other arbovirus infections were also discussed, including sawgrass, hughes, and silverwater. The latter was isolated from a rabbit tick, and hughes virus from a Florida soft tick in 1962. Testing against known US arbovirus strains was performed by Yale scientist Dr. Jordi Casals of the WHO international arbovirus reference center of the Yale Arbovirus Research Unit (YARU).[2,3]

Human serum samples were also tested that had been collected from people living in western Kentucky. All were negative for antibodies to Lone Star virus. The virus was considered to be a new arbovirus, and was believed to be unrelated to other known North American types. Lone Star (LS) virus strain TMA 1381 was discussed in a separate 1970 paper from R.H. Kokernot* while at the University of Texas. The virus found within the Lone Star ticks has been known by researchers from the mid-1960s forward. We may wonder if infectious disease researchers who are familiar with Lyme disease including those from the University of Texas System or the American Lyme Disease Foundation (ALDF), and those among whom claim that Lone Star ticks cannot transmit Lyme disease, are aware of this particular tick virus.[2,3]

**R.H. Kokernot also published while at the University of Illinois at Urbana.*

Dr. Alan Barbour is a patent inventor of a diagnostic test for a "new" spirochete, *Borrelia lone stari* that was filed in May 1995, seven months after the Dearborn conference which Dr. Barbour attended. The patent is assigned to the Board of Regents of the University of Texas System in Austin. The patent refers to older patents assigned to the US Department of Health (PCR assay and cloned DNA); a patent for a PCR test and Bb flagellin (tail) genes assigned to the Research Foundation of State University of New York (SUNY); and a flagellin-based protein and antibody patent assigned to Yale University. The Regents of the UT system are the University of Texas's governing body. One of the duties of such a board might include fundraising for the institution.[5-8]

In 1913 the University of Texas at El Paso created the Texas School of Mines and Metallurgy, which became part of the UT System in 1919. By 1923, a well named "Santa Rita No. 1" struck oil. The first *oil royalty* payment was made into the permanent university fund on August 24, 1923. If mining processes or products were contributing to important infectious disease outbreaks, we might expect institutions that have been made profitable in part from mining and disease-related patent royalties to be somewhat protective of their income earning interests. Could such a scenario produce a scientist who would become part of a core group of individuals from partnering institutions; and whom may have been appointed to keep such relationships tightly under wraps? Could such relationships affect the outcome of legislation, medical treatment guidelines, public health policies, or even laboratory standards? Dr. Alan Barbour was listed on nearly one hundred *Borrelia burgdorferi*-related patents while working within the University of Texas and University of California Systems.[5-8]

A paper reveals that the agent of bovine borreliosis (*Borrelia theileri*) belongs to a distinct group of spirochetes. The group also includes "the *Amblyomma* agent" that causes Southern Tick-Associated Rash Illness (STARI) and the relapsing fever agent *Borrelia miyamotoi* that is also tick-transmitted. *Borrelia miyamotoi* does not cause Lyme disease, but it may be introduced as a co-infection by Bb-infected ticks. Like the Lyme disease agent, *B. miyamotoi* produces very Lyme-like symptoms. We will take a much closer look at *Borrelia miyamotoi* in an upcoming chapter.[9]

The insistence of some scientists that Lyme infections in persons bitten by Lone Star ticks are somehow different than Lyme infections from other tick species may be based upon their knowledge of the Lone Star virus. I wonder why the *Lone Star virus* to date has never been "audibly" discussed by public health experts as having any relationship to Lyme disease. Such individuals may include those who set public health policy, or who have written medical guidelines for Lyme disease. Could there be an important relationship to Lyme disease, viruses, and chemicals or other agents that certain scientists do not want publicly revealed?

In order to fully appreciate the possible links between what emerged in US Lone Star ticks during the 1940s and the agricultural use of herbicides, we might study the history of the outbreak at Camp Bullis, Texas where an ehrlichiosis-like infection erupted due to Lone Star ticks. The first case of human *Ehrlichiosis* that was recorded in the US was said to have been detected in 1986 in a Detroit man who was exposed to ticks while visiting rural Arkansas. In 1990 the CDC isolated a new strain of ehrlichia from the blood of a US Army reservist at Fort Chaffee, Arkansas. The agent was then named *Ehrlichia chaffeensis.* Human ehrlichiosis more likely has an earlier history however, and the Arkansas (military) location provides clues that the short-lived (1942-43) ehrlichosis-like epidemic at Camp Bullis may have had origins in either agricultural herbicides, or in the early *tactical* herbicides.[10]

When we analyze military reports from the 1960s, we find interesting information that may indicate that the military had interests in the effects of airborne pollutants far more than they had in the role of microbes to create military biowarfare weapons. A key statement from a report discussed the three toxins of *Bacillus anthracis,* or anthrax: protective antigen (PA), lethal factor (LF), and edema factor (EF). The report tells us there is a process by which enzymes from this fermented soil bacillus cause infection in higher animals: *"The most surprising and interesting information from this program is that edema factor was proved to be an adenylate cyclase.* Because EF is an enzyme (like cholera and diptheria toxins) it derives its potency by catalytically altering essential molecules in animal cells*." The pesticide B.t. may use the exact same process to alter the cellular membranes of insect, animal, and human gut tissues to cause infections.[14]

**Adenylate cyclase is part of the G protein signaling cascade that transmits chemical signals from outside a cell through the membrane to the inside of the cell, or cytoplasm. These signalers are also found in neurons, near calcium ion channels. Since we know that insecticides disrupt ion channels and signaling as neurotoxicants, similar mechanisms may be at work in B.t. insecticides as are found in the anthrax agent, especially since the two bacteria are closely related.*

The report covered the period immediately after the identification of, and subsequent announcement of the causative agent of Lyme disease, from October 1981 to September 1982. The report included studies of pathogens that *might* be components of an aggregate spirochete called *Borrelia burgdorferi,* the agent of Lyme disease.[14]

The agents studied by military scientists were focused on the "medical defense against biological warfare agents." This is peculiar since there were no active threats as far as bioagents, except for the *very real threat of biological insecticidal agents* that may have already created an emerging human epidemic called Lyme disease. The document noted that "both natural and infectious diseases and potential biological warfare threats exist." No doubt some of those natural infections could be derived from dioxins in the applied chemical or microbial pesticides or herbicides that were used militarily, agriculturally, and industrially. Such threats might include unexpected microbial mutations such as may have caused the ehrlichiosis outbreaks in military personnel or animals. The studies focused on the pathogenesis, diagnosis, prevention, treatment, and epidemiology of infections, among which included these pathogens:

Bacteria: *Bacillus anthracis, Francisella tularensis* (tularemia)
Viruses: Dengue, yellow, rift valley fevers; eastern/western/Japanese B/Venezuelan fevers; chikungunya, and influenza
Rickettsial: *Coxiella burnetii*
Parasite: *Plasmodium falciparum* (malaria)
Toxins: *Pseudomonas A, Diptheria, Botulinum A-G, Anthrax toxins, Mycotoxin T-2, Saxitoxin, Tetrodotoxin, Staphylococcal enterotoxin*

If we look at these lists carefully, we may be able to see close parallels between military studies and the pathogens of an aggregate Bb. Another military report from 1968 reveals environmental microbiology studies by scientists of leading academic institutions, including studies of microbes and mutagenic agents that may have created a Bb aggregate organism:

Sulfur bacteria
Halophlic bacteria (salt-tolerant)
Thiobacilli (terrestrial and marine)
Marine bacteria
Algae
Benthic bacteria

Viral nucleic acids
Actinophages
Host-virus relationships
Arbovirus serologic cross-reactivity and epidemiology
Genetics of *Coxiella Burnetii*
(Aero)biology of Mycoplasmas
Immunity and pathogenesis of Mycoses (fungi)
T3 coliphages
Spore survival in *disinfectants*
Bacteriophages, transformation, and *Bacillus subtilis*
Host-parasite relationships of Nematodes
Combined action of *antibacterials and polyamines* on infections
Biochemical and transformation studies of pleuropneumoniae-like organisms
Fission of *benzene* nucleus in microorganisms
Regulation of growth and division by *benzene derivatives*[14,15]
Isotrichia
Salmonella Bacteriophages
Role of *polyphosphates* in cells
Virus interference
Spore ultrastructure
Pdseudomonas aeruginosa vaccines
Fleas and ticks of medical importance
Detection of airborne microorganisms
Clostridium toxins
L-forms of Group 4 *Streptococci*
Factors affecting behavior of *airborne* microorganisms

We remember that benzene is highly mutagenic. Another military report from 1943 to 1953 describes the kind of work undertaken by Camp Detrick scientists (before it was renamed Ft. Detrick). Most of the early work with infectious agents was aimed at the study of aerobiology (aerosolization of particles and microbes) and the development of vaccines for anthrax, brucellosis, plague, pig tularemia, malleomyces/actinobacillus (spore-formers), San Joaquin valley fever, Q fever, tuberculosis, typhus, Venezuelan/eastern/western equine encephalomyelitis, botulinum toxoid types A-E, blastomycosis, histoplasmosis, *Serratia marcescens, Bacillus globigii,* molds, and *Escherechia coli* bacteriophage T-3. The report indicated there were a total of 340 laboratory accidents at Camp Detrick from 1943 to 1953, which exposed personnel to a number of pathogens. The most frequent exposures were to *B. anthracis, Brucella, P. tularense, C. burnetti, Psittacosis virus,* and *Venezuelan equine encephalitis.*[16]

Today we find new diseases that have only emerged during the latter half of the 20th century, and we must ask why this is so. *Human Monocytic Ehrlichiosis* (HME) and *Human Granulocytic Ehrlichiosis* (HGE) are among the diseases of the modern age of chemical and microbial pesticides. HGE was formerly known as *phagocytophila* and is a common disease of sheep and cattle. It is now called *Anaplasmosis* and its agent is *Anaplasma phagocytophilum*. The very first strain of a human ehrlichiosis ever identified was *Ehrlichiosis sennetsu,* the agent of *Sennetsu rickettsiosis,* or Sennetsu fever, a rickettsial disease. Human cases of Sennetsu fever were reported in *Japan* and *Malaysia* in 1954. *Ehrlichiosis canis*, also called canine ehrlichiosis, a disease of dogs, was reported as early as 1935 in Algeria,* Africa.[11-13,17-20]

**Algeria is a source of important oil reserves (fossil fuels), and has a strong agricultural base, including cereal, citrus, vegetables, and cork.*

New animal strains have emerged since the 1950s including *Ehrlichiosis ewingii,* which is a canine granulocytic ehrlichiosis. Human granulocytic ehrlichiosis first appeared in Duluth, Minnesota from 1990-1993. The location of this infection might be noted as the southwestern tip of Lake Superior where Minnesota meets Wisconsin. Both areas are highly endemic for Lyme disease. Did sewage, airborne particulates, or toxic chemicals from the Great Lakes (i.e. dioxins) contribute to the emergence of this novel infection? Were agricultural herbicides or other agro/industrial chemicals to blame? Was the mining of ores or petroleum products a contributing factor to the emergence of these novel infections? Was contaminated, recycled wastewater, paper pulp, or animal manure used to irrigate or fertilize agricultural crops?[11-13,17-20]

Military work with herbicides began in England in 1940, and her allies including the US and Canada joined the effort with the intent of using chemicals as anti-crop agents against the Axis powers. This was a military alliance formed mainly between Germany, Italy, and Japan during WWII along with other supporting nations.

The British were the first to deploy the herbicides 2,4,5-T; 2,4-D; and STCA (sodium trichloroacetate) to areas of peninsular Malaysia (Malaya), from 1951 to 1953. These herbicides were sprayed upon crops and roadside vegetation as defoliaters. About 200 tons of STCA were purchased from the US, and 80 tons from Sweden by the Malaysian government for these applications; but other herbicides were also used. The other chemicals were mainly supplied by Imperial Chemical Industries (ICI), a large UK-based chemical company. Multiple records also describe ICI's involvement in spraying Malaysian rubber plantations to control leaf blight. ICI's subsidiary Plant Protection Limited was said to have facilitated the British herbicide exploits in Malaysia. The first experiments used a 50:50 mix of n-butyl esters of 2,4-D and 2,4,5-T. This mixture creates the powerful herbicide *Agent Orange*. These chemicals were known toxicants that contained dioxins, a byproduct of manufacture. STCA production was eventually phased out during the 1970s, with production halted altogether in 1985.[21-23]

The US also reportedly deployed herbicides in Southeast Asia during the Vietnam War. Field tests of herbicides in South

Vietnam in 1961 under *Project AGILE* heralded the US military's official herbicide program from 1962 to 1971, code named *Operation Trail Dust.* The program was said to have been directed against "communist insurgents," and vegetation was cleared to eliminate their hiding places. One of my sources was a 1963 report on *Project AGILE*, written by the Battelle Memorial Institute of Columbus, Ohio. [24,25]

Although the Geneva Convention prohibited the use of chemical weapons, deployments of herbicides did occur and included forest burning operations and defoliant sprays. The herbicides deployed under the *Operation Ranch Hand* program as part of *Operation Trail Dust* have been accused of violating the Geneva Convention by some groups. US officials have continually defended the deployments as outside the scope of the agreement.[24,25]

In 1963, an unusual disease emerged in British military dogs in Singapore and Malaysia. The infection was named TCP or *tropical canine pancytopenia.* In the present day this infection is called canine ehrlichiosis (*Ehrlichiosis canis*). In 1967 during the Vietnam War, several military laborador retrievers that had been trained in Malaysia suddenly became ill with a new infection. The following year a number of American German shepherds were infected in Vietnam with what was now considered to be a new epidemic among military dogs. Reports of the day indicated that ticks were most likely the vectors of this lethal infection, and in particular, affected dogs that were heavily tick-infested. It is possible that the deployments of herbicides and defoliants in Malaysia and Vietnam led to mutations in plant and/or soil-borne microbes; infecting ticks and leading to the eruption of a new canine illness.[26-29]

A similar problem may have emerged in the US during early tactical or agricultural herbicide experiments performed on American soils. More simply, the agricultural use of herbicides upon Arkansas or Texas field test plots could have played a role in the emergence of human epidemics of ehrlichiosis. If individual or combined herbicides were sprayed in the vicinity of military bases, then a novel tickborne ehrlichiosis-like infection might have emerged if the chemicals contracted by resident ticks mutated microbes in the tick's bodies. Obviously something was creating new infections during the period that the new chemical herbicides and microbial pesticides were being deployed.[26-33]

It is obvious from the research that scientists were using chemical tactical and agricultural controls over test plots in the US decades before the Geneva Convention. The chemicals deployed included those that when combined, could create the herbicide Agent Orange, a chemical that among others, has proven to be highly mutagenic, carcinogenic, and toxic. During periods of conflict, chemical herbicides that also had agricultural applications were studied or employed for military use. After their deployment, novel diseases emerged in animal and human populations. The evolution of agricultural products both chemical and biological for crop and insect use have not been without their share of environmental issues as we have learned and will study further. The question to ask is whether the early chemical herbicides were capable of forcing insect-borne animal and human diseases after their deployment. While the circumstantial evidence appears to be compelling and favorable for the creation of new disease agents at the hands of mutagenic chemicals, the truth in the final analysis has yet to be definitively and scientifically proven, and publicly acknowledged.

Agricultural Agents and Encephalitis Outbreaks

Other insects besides moths and beetles became environmentally and agriculturally destructive pests from the 1920s to the 1940s. We have learned that in pursuit of new methods of controlling pests, scientists tested and applied natural insecticides which contained *Bacillus popilliae* and *Bacillus lentimorbus*, the agents of "milky spore" disease. By the 1940s the milky spore agents were already being commercially mass-produced and were available for use as agricultural insecticides.

One of the oldest patents for *Bacillus popilliae* and for *Bacillus lentimorbus* was filed in 1940, invented by S.R. Dutky of Moorestown, New Jersey. The patent was assigned to the US Secretary of Agriculture and successors. Before their commercial release, these new natural insecticides were field tested during the late 1930s in small plots on the US northeastern seaboard. Abroad, a soil bacterium called *Bacillus thuringiensis* (B.t.) was also being applied as an agricultural insecticide.[6]

Just a short time after these initial tests, in 1938 there was a sudden outbreak of what was considered to be *eastern equine encephalitis* (EEE) in a flock of Connecticut ring-necked pheasants. In 1953, the EEE agent was again isolated from the brain of a dead rat found near a pen of pheasants during a subsequent Connecticut outbreak. Additional epizootics (insect/animal epidemics) were reported in Connecticut pheasants several times from 1951 to 1959. The area was also endemic for *Allodermanyssus sanguineus* mites, the same mites that had been responsible for the 1946 human rickettsialpox outbreak that emerged in New York and which was linked to incinerated garbage.[1-12]

Ring-neck pheasants are birds of Chinese origin. Their favorite diets are seeds, waste crop grains, fruits, leaves, and insects. They consume large quantities of grasshoppers, crickets, potato beetles, cutworms, tentworms, and the caterpillars of gypsy and brown-tailed moths. Areas defoliated by gypsy moths directly impact pheasant nesting environments. Horses (equines) are among grazing animals that inadvertently eat insect larvae and their eggs; and assist in clearing ground cover. They are also hosts to insects which bite, sting, and suck blood. It seems possible that field manipulations of insects using novel microbial insecticides that contained *B. popilliae, B. lentimorbus,* or *Bacillus thuringiensis* (B.t.), were beginning to force infections in non-targeted animals. These infections were erupting as novel EEE infections in horses and pheasants.[9-12]

We can see that the Connecticut animal EEE outbreaks of 1938 and 1951 emerged around the same time that scientists began field trials with new chemical and microbial pesticides. Other EEE outbreaks surfacced in Massachusetts, New York, and New Jersey, where early microbial insecticides were also initially deployed. Outbreaks of disease also began to emerge in animals and humans beginning in 1951 just as field trials of small and large RNA (and possibly DNA) viruses were deployed as insecticidal enhancers. Although EEE is principally an acute encephalomyelitis that affects pheasants and horses, the question to ask is whether there was a connection between the deployments of novel insecticides; the endemic mite infestations (we know DDT offset mite populations); and animal and human infections caused by mite-transmitted EEE or other agents.[7-12]

According to a 1951 report, outbreaks of human rickettsialpox were recorded in Boston, Massachusetts in 1951; in Connecticut and Pennsylvania in 1952; and in Massachusetts in 1953. Around the world, rickettsialpox was reported in the Ukraine in 1950; Central Africa in 1952; South Africa in 1954; and Bosnia-Herzegovina in 1956. I might remind readers that limited field trials that deployed small and large insect viruses as insecticidal enhancers began in 1951 at the New Haven Forest Experiment Station in Connecticut. These techniques were used as a model for other countries around the world. The USDA and experiment stations were actively investigating useful pesticides from 1930-1940 for field and sweet corn applications. Abroad, similar attempts were made, likely through participating experiment stations that had cooperative programs with US universities, or agricultural or forest experiment stations.[13-23]

It is entirely possible that the 1946 human rickettsialpox outbreak in New York City was related to the early applications of either chemical or biological pesticides. Since mites feed off of lepidoptera and beetles, the mites could have contracted the bacteriae or viruses of the microbial insecticides that could have mutated from chemical herbicides or other pollutants. The bacillus-based insecticides deliberately cause degradation of the insect gut, where latent infections are released from their intracellular spaces to cause bacteremia in insects. In the case of the 1946 outbreak, when the mites subsequently fed upon rodents which carried an *Arenavirus,* the rodents exposed humans to their infectious agents by urinating upon the garbage, which when burned, aerosolized these pathogens.[17-23]

At least a half dozen or more arenaviruses are known to be pathogenic to humans. Insects and animals harbor many infections which are capable of mutating and recombining with other bacteria and viruses within their guts, and which remain infectious in their excrement and salivary glands. Chemicals and recombinant microbes may drive genetic changes to produce infectious diseases which can cross species barriers to infect humans through many transmission routes.[17-23]

Rickettsial agents are common in sewage, lakes, and rivers; and are found in rodents and insects that inhabit these polluted areas. *Vibrio cholera,* a common sewage pathogen, also happens to closely resemble the rickettsialpox agent, *Rickettsia akari.* In a pattern that is repeated countless times in nature, a novel insect pathogen seemed to emerge during the late 1940s and was assigned the name "blue disease." This new insect infection surfaced when new microbial insecticides were first applied to the environment; along with chemical pesticides and herbicides that have the ability to mutate genes. Such mutations may not only affect the genes of insects, animals, humans, and plants, but also the microbes lying within their hosts. On the heels of these deployments, we saw the emergence of new animal and human rickettsialpox, polio, and ehrlichiosis infections.

Another outbreak of EEE emerged in Connecticut in 1972, the very same year that the chemical pesticide DDT was banned within the US for being highly toxic. At the time of this outbreak, a sample infected bird was sent to the Storrs Agricultural Experiment Station at the University of Connecticut for evaluation. There were roughly two dozen outbreaks of EEE in Connecticut in the years between 1938 and 1956. Is this evidence that early controls that were deployed in this area were triggering outbreaks of infectious diseases in animal populations? If we include the human rickettsialpox outbreaks during this period and later outbreaks during the 1960s and 1970s when the epidemic of Lyme disease first emerged, we may see that human epidemics could also be driven by the mutagenic properties of chemicals and recombinant microbes.

We must also remember that the east coast, while the apparent epicenter for certain initially deployed microbial controls, was not the only place in the world that was deploying chemical and microbial controls. Other countries abroad were simultaneously studying and deploying similar formulas. Remember that these techniques were shared through international scientific collaborations. If we were to closely examine the history of similar deployments in other countries, we may find that Connecticut was not the disease's epicenter, but only one area of the world where Lyme disease was emerging.

The deployment of biological controls over wider areas of the globe and which took place at the same time would have created increased incidents of animal and human diseases in those regions as well. This probably occurred in pocketed areas wherever microbial controls were applied. However the easy way to control accidental disease outbreaks in animal or human populations would have been to apply powerful chemical pesticides to areas where such outbreaks might emerge, as soon as they appeared. This would have eliminated the possibility of an outbreak growing into a larger epidemic as long as these chemicals remained available.

When we examine the history of applied biological and chemical controls, we see that a similar situation may have occurred with various outbreaks of "poliomyelitis." We can understand how the use of chemical pesticides in a given area would more than likely eliminate large populations of infection-carrying insects. The eradication of polio was historically attributed to the anti-polio vaccine programs. But if we scrutinize world history we may learn that the greater impact upon polio and other infectious diseases was probably the use of chemical pesticides and the modernization of water sanitation. What happened once powerful pesticides like DDT were eliminated from the picture? The world saw the resurgence of many "polio"-like, neurologic, arthritic, and paralytic diseases including Lyme disease – diseases given fancy new names, but which in earlier days may have simply been called "polio."

A scientific report dated 1951 discussed the 1946 New York rickettsialpox outbreak. This particular study was funded by the Lederle Laboratories Division of the American Cyanamid Company. The work was also supported by an NIH research grant, and was sponsored by the Commission on Virus and Rickettsial Diseases of the Armed Forces Epidemiological Board partly under contract with the Army Office of the Surgeon General, in Washington, DC.[25-28]

American Cyanamid Company is a chemical manufacturer and among its products at the time of these disease outbreaks were phosphate-based fertilizers and pest control products, including the pesticide *malathion* in 1950. Phosphates are mined from deep within the earth, where they are found in the presence of uranium, fluorine (fluoride), bauxite, clays, oxides, and minerals and ores from which copper, aluminum, and other metals are derived. Bauxite is the main source of *alumina* which is commercially processed to make aluminum products. Phosphate rocks typically contain uranium, which is extracted.[28-30]

Lederle Labs was acquired by the American Cyanamid Company in 1930. American Cyanamid's pharmaceutical division was a huge vaccine supplier to the military. By 1954 the company had manufactured the first *oral polio* vaccine. Were the outbreaks of rickettsialpox and polio related to the application of biological controls, chemical pesticides, and phosphate fertilizers after all? If so, was the subsequent development of "polio" vaccines designed to treat the effects of the first deployments of agricultural and industrially important chemicals and microbes that although intended for insects and crop production, were absolutely and entirely capable of initiating human infections? As we are about to learn, disease outbreaks of the past may have had very different origins than what has been announced to the public, and also recorded historically.[24-30]

What is to be done if the arrival of the novel chemical and microbial tools of agriculture and industry caused the mutation of the ubiquitous insect viruses, bacteria, and other infections already present in ticks and other insects as symbionts? The effects of such reassortments might be traced as far back as the first introductions of *Bacillus popilliae, Bacillus thuringiensis* (B.t.) and other applied insecticides. Such applications may have infected mites to manifest as pheasant or horse EEE infections, or human rickettsialpox outbreaks. In a similar manner, modern day "polio" could have emerged after the introduction of parasitoid insects which harbored infectious symbionts, and which were reactivated from latency by chemicals or microbes.

In a similar manner, the presence of mutagenic chemicals in the environment from agricultural, nuclear, industrial, or other uses and from military warfare weapons or wastes could certainly drive novel epidemics in any populations. Such new epidemics could be fostered by vectoring insects whose symbiont infections no longer remained safe within the insect bodies. Instead, through the catalytic action of "pollutants," especially microbial cocktails or wastes that contained phagic microbes (*phages*), these pathogens were released to become transmissible agents once ticks and other vectoring insects took a blood meal.

We might review the history of the millions of chemically (pheromones, insecticides), genetically (radiation, genetic engineering), and microbe-altered mosquitoes and other insects that have been released around the world. When we do, the possibility of mutated symbiont infections does not seem like a far-fetched fantasy, but a full-blown reality. It may be an unintended consequence of the manipulation of insects and our environment for military, industrial, veterinary, medical, and agricultural purposes. It would be absolutely possible for insect-carried pathogens to mutate with the RNA, DNA *baculoviruses*, and other agents and chemicals found in our environment. This likelihood was not a surprise to scientists who were studying these interactions from about the 1940s forward. Chemical and industrial pollutants as happenstances of modern technologies absolutely have the power to create pathogenic organisms which can become public health concerns.[31]

An Outbreak in the Pacific

According to a 1971 textbook, the World Health Organization and the New Zealand government jointly sponsored the first intercountry biological control pilot program. In 1958 they introduced a *Coelomomyces* fungus from Singapore into a Polynesian tiger mosquito (*Aedes polynesiensis*) in an experimental release program on the small Pacific Island of Tokelau. In 1966 another pilot project was undertaken on the island of Nauru. This time *Aedes aegypti* and *Culex pipens fatigans* mosquitoes were released. While public health experts experimented with mosquito releases, various biological control agents were already being released in agricultural and forestry applications in other areas of the world. These techniques were reaching greenhouses by 1967.[1]

In a paper from a 1960 two-day conference that discussed biological controls of the day, we learn about scientific expeditions to the South Pacific islands, and field tests in Hawaii, Fiji, other Pacific islands, and Puerto Rico. There was also a 1959 WHO program in the South Pacific Tokelau Island atolls (Nukunono, Atafu, with Fakaofo as an untreated control) to test the usefulness of the *Coelomomyces* fungi to control mosquito populations. Scientists were attempting to establish mosquito populations and to study biological controls and disease transmission on several remote, but populated islands. It was noted by scientists that the "benefits" of these studies would not be immediate. These locations were carefully selected supposedly because they were "virgin" territory, meaning the experimental insects to be introduced were not already established there. Therefore human inhabitants had no previous immunity to any infections that the insects were designed to carry. But these islands were also either near, or part of the Pacific Proving Grounds, where nuclear weapons were tested between 1946 and 1962. Could scientists have also been studying the effects of nuclear radiation upon the microbes in insects such as mosquitoes?[2-9]

Epidemics of insect arboviruses have occurred in various areas of the world, but in 1979 there was an explosive epidemic of Ross River virus in the South Pacific Islands (Fiji, Cook Islands, and Samoa). This was the largest epidemic in recorded history, with over 50,000 cases reported. Whether this epidemic had anything to do with the 1959 mosquito experiments in the atolls or not, or nuclear fallout for that matter, is open to speculation. Although the early studies discussed a fungal infection, we have no data on what other kinds of biological experiments were attempted in the South Pacific since 1959. We also do not know if scientists had created recombinant constructs using the Ross River virus, or its parent Sindbis virus, but we know that recombinant techniques using either of these viruses were possible during this period. If scientists used either of these viruses, did something trigger a recombinant construct to "fail"? If so, did a failed chimera kick out a virus which soon became transmissible to the human population through vectoring insects?[2,6-9]

If a mosquito population that harbored a particular virus infection and which led to the 1979 epidemic was not found on the islands before the 1958-1959 mosquito control experiments began, then circumstances are favorable for the assumption that these experiments may have triggerd the human epidemic that emerged two decades later. The lapse in time may have been necessary for the mosquito population to grow large enough to drive a human epidemic. Or an epidemic could have been triggered by an external force. Could that force have been the application of herbicides, chemicals, or B.t. to island crops (i.e. GM papaya)? Or could an epidemic have been caused by mutations formed after exposure to nuclear fallout from tests in the area?[2,6-9]

A 2010 paper described the emergence of an ECM-rash-like illness among Caribbean Islanders. One of the patients was a student who grew up in St. Lucia but who travelled to Trinidad, Tobago, and New York. Another young patient and an adult from Trinidad and Tobago; and a woman from Grenada were also discussed in the paper. Each patient displayed an ECM-rash illness. The authors concluded there was an ECM rash illness but could not identify the insect vector because none of the patients were said to have had "foreign exposure to ticks." This is a curious statement since one student had visited New York, a state known to be endemic for Lyme disease.[2,6-9]

What seems disturbing to me is a recent interest of agrochemical giants to have 2,4-D deregulated by the US government so that it can be engineered directly into GM food crops. 2,4-D of course is DDT, one half of the formula that created Agent Orange. The argument that is likely to be pursued in defense of these interests may be that there will be "no dioxins present" in genetically modified plants. However as we have already learned, enzymes are catalytic, and chloride-based chemicals can contribute to the formation of dioxins. Regulators must be told and made to understand that chemicals readily combine in the environment to create novel neurotoxic formulas that will impact microbes, insects, animals, and humans. The lessons of the past which have so far not been heeded very well by many industries, may deliver far harsher lessons in the future if we do not begin to pay attention. These lessons will not only make themselves loud and clear, but may become those which we entirely regret for many generations to come.[10] ❑

Seven: The Origin of a Human Epidemic?

The CDC calls borrelia: "A genus of bacteria with numerous species that cause disease in humans. The diseases associated with these organisms are typically relapsing fevers." Although technically correct, this does not explain how the Lyme disease organism *Borrelia burgdorferi* came to be defined in the manner in which it has to date. In spite of all that we think we know about the origins of Lyme disease, there seems to be a completely different side to the story that has not yet been told to the public. From my perspective, Bb is not what we have been led to believe it is over several decades, and that is perhaps the good news. Perhaps with a fresh new perspective on its history, we may finally move a stalled belief system forward – one that clearly lacks answers for scientists, physicians, and patients. It is also unfortunate that the publicity spotlight has never shone its entire light on certain events that appear to be incredibly important to Lyme history. Once illuminated however, people may wonder why this information was not brought into the open decades ago. I couldn't agree more, so let's jump into the dirty water along with the spirochetes that live there, and see what else was happening while everyone was busy looking the other way.

What does the name *Borrelia burgdorferi* mean? Borrelia means "tick transmitted." Burgdorferi is some kind of agent that was identified by Dr. Willy Burgdorfer. The agent of Lyme was placed into the spirochete class of the genus borrelia. We have already learned about the other organisms that share this genus, and only a few of them are actually known to cause Lyme disease. Most descriptions of *Borrelia burgdorferi* have led the public to believe that the spirochete is a single bacterial spirochete with characteristics in common with its supposed "dumb cousin," another spirochete that is the treponema of Syphilis (*Treponema pallidum*). We must look closely at the history of borrelia organisms, at the other spirochetes within the same phylum, and at the parties and processes involved with the research and patenting of Bb. When we do, we may find important clues that Bb is not exactly "as advertised," and also that what we have been told since the mid-1970s may be a lot farther from the truth than we are expected to believe.

We have seen that Australian beetles were imported to protect California citrus crops during the 1880s. We now know about the release of wasp-parasitized nymph ticks and the mass-rearings and releases of parasitic wasps and flies beginning in the 1920s. These insects harbored a number of viruses which probably spread into the insect and animal populations at large. With the deployment of parasitizing insects, whatever infections they carried were beginning to spread among other populations.

In the interests of finding ways to make pesticides more effective, scientists began exploring the use of insect viruses and bacteria, procured from diseased insects. The most promising bacteriae were from the bacillus family, and included strains *Bacillus popilliae, B. lentimorbus, B. sphaericus*, and *Bacillus thuringiensis* (B.t.). Whatever could be commercially produced on a massive scale and that could be applied by spray to agricultural fields would prove to the best choice. Regional deployments of these early microbial pesticides in addition to the new phosphate fertilizers began during the late 19th century and early part of the 20th century. However the microbial applications were not economical and the products were not easily mass-produced. We know that B.t. was first widely deployed in Hungary and Yugoslavia during the late 1920s. Field tests in Europe and the US were underway by the 1930s for B.t., while commercial production began in 1938 in France when *Sporine* came along. Synthetic chemical pesticides were developed and proved to be more effective and economical and these were globally applied. After WWII B.t. began to gain global popularity, as insects rapidly became immune to chemical pesticides.[1]

B.t. would take its rightful place in global pesticide history during the late 1940s. In a parallel fashion, outbreaks of disease in animals and humans began to appear with the release of the earliest parasitoid insects and the use of the chemical and microbial-based insecticides. Diseases were typically explained as sudden outbreaks with "unknown" origin. Once 1951 came along, the further augmentation of applied microbial insecticides was undertaken using borrelina viruses. Mysterious new animal and human infections began to emerge with equally perplexing origins. Perhaps the unknown origin was simply because public health experts had no idea what scientists who were developing microbial insecticides were unleashing into the environment.[2-4]

From 1947 to 1973, the insect gut bacteria *Bacillus popilliae* was commercially produced by only one laboratory in the United States; Fairfax Biological Laboratory in Clinton Corners, New York. This microbial pesticide was initially sold under the trade name "DOOM." It is no coincidence perhaps that the name of one of the strains of "borrelia" is *Borrelia japonica*, a relapsing fever agent that was isolated from ticks, mice, and shrews from Japan. This infection also carries a name similar to one of the insects against which the earliest pesticides were first deployed: *Popillia japonica*, the Japanese beetle. A 1995 paper discussed Japanese studies of *Borrelia japonica* spirochetes that were collected from ticks and small mammals. Researchers were characterizing bacterial strains and comparing them to European and American strains of *Borrelia burgdorferi*. Antibodies and Bb strains used in these studies were supplied by Lyme notables Drs. Russell C. Johnson (Univ. MN), and Alan G. Barbour (Univ. TX).[5,6]

The year 1947 is when the first milky spore agents were commerically available. This was just three years before borrelina viruses were released in New Haven, Connecticut by scientists to test the ability of the viruses to augment the current microbial insecticides. Sample stocks and information on collecting and processing small and large viruses were offered by New Haven scientists to globally interested parties during the early 1950s. Once these events occurred, the world of microbe-augmented insecticides began to change. All of a sudden new outbreaks of animal and human infections began to emerge, and so did unusual spirochetes. When cultured, they revealed they were mutated, intermediate forms that had never before been seen. With the commercialization and global use of microbial pesticides and the further genetic manipulation of same, disease incidences in animal and human populations skyrocketed. Are these events merely coincidences in timing or something more?[5,6]

Historical accounts which discuss the relapsing fever spirochetes typically fail to venture anywhere near the events of the day that surrounded the outbreak of "juvenile arthritis" which were announced in 1975 as a new outbreak (after which the causative agent was announced in 1982). For this reason I began to look at other spirochetal families to see if something other than "borrelia" might be at the heart of "*Borrelia" burgdorferi*. Naming the organism as a "borrelia" species is technically correct as the agent is tick-transmitted. It appears also to be a relative of the relapsing fever spirochetes in the borrelia category as well. It may be a closer relative to relapsing fever agents than it is to Syphilis spirochetes. But the "burgdorferi" name is a bit more mysterious, and to get to the heart of that name we might examine the history of a very different group of spirochetes.

What is somewhat unique about *Borrelia burgdorferi* strains are their segmented genome. It is said to contain a linear chromosome and at least seventeen plasmids (cellular engines or mini-chromosomes) that are either circular or linear in form. The Bb organism also appears to have a relatively small chromosome (853 genes) as compared to other bacteriae, although the organism itself is complex. Bb is felt to be distantly related to the eubacteria, a large group of gram-positive and gram-negative bacteria that includes many species. Among these are the *Actinobacteria, Firmicutes, Spirochaetes, Thermodesulfobacteria* (sulfate reducers), and the *Deinococcus-Thermus* (thermophiles). The latter bacteriae are highly tolerant of environmental hazards (i.e. radiation, temperature extremes, salts, acids).[7]

The Bb organism is thought to be missing many genes that are considered to be important for metabolism and synthesis. Its dependence upon a host for nutrients is facilitated by porins, which are membrane-spanning channels that allow nutrients to pass through spirochetal membranes. The dependence upon a host for nutrients is a characteristic of saprophytes/saprotrophs.[7]

An analysis of the outer membranes of the Bb spirochete reveals important differences between the porin activities of Bb and those belonging to the relapsing fever spirochetes. This provides another clue that these are two different organisms. *Borrelia burgdorferi* have several porins, while relapsing fever borreliae appear to have only one. I should point out that like Bb, the leptospira spirochetes also have a segmented genome. Certain soil bacteriae including *Bacillus cereus, Agrobacterium tumefaciens, E. coli*, and *Bacillus anthracis* also have segmented genomes. This allows them the ability to reassort genes under the right circumstances. Like the Bb spirochete, the pesticide agent *B. thuringiensis* (B.t.) has a circular chromosome.[8-16]

Another spirochete, the *Spiroplasmas* have special genetic sequences which enable viruses, bacteria, or fungi to be inserted. This facilitates mutations and bonding with compatible organisms including microbes with segmented genomes. This means that a spiroplasma, a B.t. bacterium, and a leptospira spirochete for example may physically combine their genes to make a mutant spirochete the likes of *Borrelia burgdorferi*. Furthermore like Bb spirochetes, many species of *saprotrophic* bacteria including leptospires and spiroplasmas lack metabolic capabilities and therefore must rely upon a host for their nutrients.[8-16]

In 1998 Drs. Alan Barbour and colleague Diego Cadavid published an article discussing the neurologic symptoms (neuroborreliosis) of relapsing fevers. The paper revealed that the spirochetes of relapsing fever are from the genus borrelia. Again this simply means that relapsing fevers are tick-transmitted. They also said, "*...other Borrelia species* cause Lyme disease, avian spirochetosis and possibly epidemic bovine abortion." The distinction between spirochetes of "relapsing fever" and "other" spirochetes that cause Lyme disease acknowledges that Lyme disease is not caused by relapsing fever spirochetes. However this does not rule out the possibility that they may be mutations of relapsing fever spirochetes, or more simply that the two organisms have a leptospira spirochete as a common ancestor. Another paper supports the separation of relapsing fever spirochetes from those which cause Lyme disease.[17-19]

> "Spirochetes of the genus *Borrelia* are known to cause *2 major types of human disease, Lyme disease*, which occurs primarily in temperate regions, *and relapsing fever* (RF), which occurs in both temperate and tropical regions. Many vertebrates serve as enzootic hosts for the bacteria, and borreliosis is related to climatic and other environmental parameters required for the vectors and reservoir hosts."

Dr. Barbour's paper also said this:

> "*Borrelia burgdorferi* is closely related to several other tickborne borreliae which are causative agents for the very serious and debilitating disease, such as relapsing fever. Relapsing fever, although rare in the United States, is endemic in Central America and Africa. Lyme Disease is quite common in the United States; in fact, it is the fastest growing vector-borne disease."

I think it should be very clear by now that relapsing fever borrelia and the borrelia of Lyme disease are entirely different spirochetes. However those differences do not mean that Bb are not related to relapsing fevers since again they may share a common leptospira ancestor, but it does mean that Bb may be an aggregate organism that is comprised of multiple pathogens.[17-19]

Novel Spirochetes Emerge

Public health experts and scientists around the world have long been aware that infections with leptospira spirochetes (leptospirosis) are transmissible from urine-contaminated soil and water. They are also aware that leptospires are especially common in the polluted waters of rivers, lakes, ponds, and streams. Leptospirosis is also a particularly common livestock infection, and millions of people around the world harbor leptospirosis infections but are unaware they are infected. From 1954 to 1966 there were several new leptospiral forms that suddenly emerged in various regions of the world. We must study the events of the day when these strains emerged to see what might have contributed to the creation of such novel organisms; and also why they were being studied.

In 1951, American scientists at the Forest Insect Laboratory in New Haven, Connecticut began conducting biological control field trials whereby they introduced large and small RNA viruses as enhancers to existing insecticides. Shortly thereafter, the laboratory offered samples and information on how to collect and process viruses to interested parties around the world for use within the applied insecticides. The use of these viruses not only significantly enhanced the toxic activity of B.t. insecticides, it allowed the viruses to bind with wild and insecticidal yeast strains to create toxic killing formulas. Just two years after these introductions, in 1953 a new and most unusual strain of spirochete emerged in Romania. It remains to be seen whether an American laboratory provided virus samples or information to Romanian scientists including how to propagate and use these viruses within biological controls. However this could have occurred since the two countries had long established cooperative agricultural and scientific exchanges, especially where crop science was concerned.[1-7]

The new Romanian spirochete was a unique leptospira-like organism that was isolated from a water sample taken from the Dâmboviţa (Dimbovitza) River. The Dimbovitza flows from the Făgăras Mountains of the Transylvanian Alps in the north. It passes through Bucharest and goes southward to the Argeş River. The Argeş eventually meets the Danube River. The Danube is one of the most polluted rivers in Romania because it has endured the direct dumping of hundreds of millions of cubic meters of raw sewage annually. Its waters are so toxic that only the most resilient life forms survive its elevated nitrate, ammonia, phosphorus, and other chemical-laden environment. These waters are home to important bacteriae including not only *E. coli* and leptospires, but also other organisms typically found in heavily polluted waters, including cyanobacteria and extremophiles. We could also expect to find a proliferation of insect and plant viruses, fungi, and organic matter in these waters.[1,8]

The Danube River originates in the Black Forest mountain range in Germany and flows southward through Germany, Austria, Slovakia, Hungary, Croatia, Serbia, Bulgaria, Moldova, Ukraine, and Romania and empties into the Black Sea. Romania is home to nuclear research centers since 1949; heavy water fuel factories, and nuclear power plants, as well as uranium mines. Nuclear medicine and industrial uses of nuclear energy were also employed in the early decades of nuclear technology.[9,10]

In 1995, nearly a year after the Dearborn conference, scientists examined two uranium mine waste heaps that contained leftover uranium mining wastes from the former Soviet-East German company Wismut AG. The heaps were located near Ronnenburg, Thuringia, Germany. They found bacteria which included sulfur, acidophiles, iron-oxiding, and manganese-reducing strains as well as those that metabolized nitrates, to a depth of 5 meters. The most dominant form was *Thiobacillus ferrooxidans*. The Thuringia, Germany area was noted to be a region with "severe environmental problems" and an area that because of radon gas and acid mine drainage, "threatens the health of creatures living in the neighborhood of the heaps." An in situ leach experiment (mining) in Mina Ilba, Romania was also analyzed for similar bacterial forms as those found in Germany.[9,10]

Other bacteria found in similar waste heaps include *Thiobacillus neapolitanus, T. novellus, T. intermedius*, and *Leptospirillum ferrooxidans.* A strain was found that was similar to those from the extremophile group sulfolobus/acidianus. The strain grew in sulfur and pyrite (i.e. found in volcanic springs). Sulfolobus bacteria oxidize sulfur and are infected with lysogenic viruses (DNA bacteriophages or virophages). The phages enter the bacteria as a self-protective measure against the elements. Examples of bacteria that have similar phages are *Vibrio cholerae* (cholera), *Corynebacterium diphtheriae* (diphtheria), *Streptococcus pyogenes* (scarlet fever) and *Shigella dysenteriae* (dysentery). Each of these bacteria produce toxins which are sometimes produced by the active form of these phages, which when latent are called *prophages*.[9,10]

Prophages are latent bacteriophages that become part of the host's DNA (genome) until they are reactivated. Prophages are important aspects of horizontal gene transfer. Gram-positive bacteria that are infected with prophages include *Lactobacillus, Clostridium,* and *Bacillus* strains. Other gram-negative bacteria which contain prophages are *Streptomyces, Bifidobacterium*, and *Mycobacterium*. Of the proteobacteria that affect plants, we find prophages in *E. coli, Xanthomonas, Yersinia, Haemophilus,*

Pseudomonas, Shewanella, and *Salmonella* species. *Bacillus subtilis* is noted to contain nearly a dozen phage forms. This means that related soil bacteria (i.e. B.t.) also contain prophages as well.[9,10]

The odd Romanian leptospira strain discovered in the Dimbovitza River was the first known isolate of its kind, and was named *Leptospira dimbovitza* after its river origin. It was also the very first leptospira isolate from Europe that had the characteristics of what in 1983 (the year after Bb was announced) would eventually become a family of mutated leptospires, the *Leptonema.*[1,8]

This area of Europe from the mid-1940s through 1989 was one of the world's most important sites for uranium mining. The region's mines supplied the Soviet Union with about 300,000 tons of uranium for military use. The mines were located in the Central European Ore Mountains (Erzgebirge) in southern East Germany. There were also mines in Bavaria, Bohemia (now Czech Republic), Romania (Banat, Crucea, others); and in Thuringia, where in 1915 German scientist Ernst Berliner first identified a soil bacteria in flour moth caterpillars which was named *Bacillus thuringiensis*, or B.t.[11-13]

By the way, very high radon levels are found in uranium and non-uranium mines (i.e. mineral, metal, coal). Radioactivity from decaying wastes and the nitrous gases and chemicals from blasting increases the number of extremophile bacteria in the area, and also the likelihood that resident microbes will mutate. We must remember that uranium and thorium mining are integral parts of the production of nuclear power, nuclear research, heavy water fuel production, and the manufacture of nuclear weapons. Their byproducts are extremely important to the story of Lyme disease. These industries began to proliferate across the world beginning in the 1930s. However the use of uranium began during the 1920s when it was used medically; and industrially when incorporated into a paint by US Radium, a factory that produced glow-in-the-dark watch dials.[11-13]

Agriculturally speaking, experimental work in Romanian corn cultivation formally began during the 1840s in Bucharest. An early agricultural research station was established in 1884 in Cluj, Transylvania; followed in 1927 with the first agricultural research institute in Bucharest. By the late 1920s, one of the more impactful Agronomists to Romanian agriculture, Marin Chiritescu-Arva, had already studied genetics and crop improvement in Berlin and at Königsberg, (former Prussia). He completed his studies in Rothamsted, England. Arva's interests were crop production, water plants, fertilizers, and soil microbiology; and such was the legacy he and other scientists of his day would bring to the Romanian landscape.[1-3]

During the first part of the 20th century, a number of scientists including Arva travelled to the US to study agriculture, animal sciences, horticulture, and genetics. At the time, corn was already a major agricultural commodity for Romania. By the late 1920s, Romanian scientists were seriously studying soil fertilizers and incorporating American ideas into agricultural production. Romanian research stations had for a long time focused their interests on corn, but began exchanging information, plants, and other materials with American research stations on a regular basis. In the early part of the last century, Romania was the third largest corn-producing country, running close behind the US. By the 1930s, Romanian scientists had already developed inbred lines of corn. An Iowa State College of Agriculture Professor was invited to teach Romanian scientists how to grow corn using American methods, but another "corn specialist" and Chemist performed the task. Here is evidence there were close collaborations between the US and Romania over mutual agricultural interests by the 1930s.[2,3]

Another point of interest is that the Romanian countryside is peppered with forests that are predominantly spruce and pine in content (with natural parasites such as sawflies and their viruses). The principal resources besides agriculture for the area include rich mineral deposits of petroleum and natural gas as well as coal and lignite (brown coal); and iron ores, bauxite, copper, lead, zinc, manganese, and uranium. Each of the industries that pertain to these resources may be implicated as contributors to the toxic pollutants that become air, soil, and water-borne. These toxins include a number of chemicals including sulfur dioxide, ammonia, and fluorides that make their way into the Danube River and each of its tributaries. This could explain how a mutated leptonema might emerge in the highly polluted waters of the Dimbovitza River.

Romania's nuclear research (medical) program was well established by 1949. What happened to those wastes is anyone's guess. At this time organophosphates and other industrial chemicals were making their way into the agricultural and war arenas, and the rest shall we say, is history. By 1951 we may assume that agricultural collaborations continued between Romanian and American scientists. We might also assume that Romanian scientists would have been intrigued by the proposition of the New Haven Experiment Station scientists regarding new methods of cultivating insect viruses to be used as agricultural pesticides. By 1953, "something" could have facilitated a new strain of mutated leptospira under influence of viral factors and the agricultural, industrial, or atomic chemicals found in the extremely polluted Romanian waters. We might study the history of nuclear energy development (i.e. medicine, atomic energy/weaponry), whether in the former Soviet Union, other European countries, the US, or Canada. When we do, we may find that the locations of "heavy water," chromium, and other nuclear pollutants which largely came into being from the 1930s forward; and the agricultural "biowarfare" chemicals and microbes deployed in these areas provide striking clues to the eruption of novel organisms and subsequent animal and human epidemic diseases.[1]

By the 1940s, the first transposons, or "jumping genes" were discovered. Transposons are segments of mobile DNA (segmented genes) that can move around the genome of a cell and cause mutations. These were discovered in maize (corn) by Barbara McClintock, a Nobel Laureate and one of the first Cytogeneticists (cell science). Transposons were also found in the fruit fly, and these were named the "P-element." Transposons are also found in bacteria, for example inside their plasmids which are like mini-chromosomes. There are also retrotransposons, which copy and paste RNA, not DNA, under a reverse transcriptase (RT) process. The presence of "RT" activity in cells or cell lines may refer to the presence of some kind of bacterial or virus retrotransposons, or segmented genes (transposons) that may be present and which may help to reassort genes.

HIV-1 and other human retroviruses (i.e. HTLV-1 or Human T-cell Lymphotropic Virus-I) behave like retrotransposons. All transposons cause "junk DNA" to form as a result of mutation. In a world where organisms have the ability to mutate and gene jump, especially between species, it is not difficult to imagine that a certain number of natural recombinant events occur under polluted conditions. This can be expected more so when aggregating and growth-enhancing chemicals of industrial, agricultural, or nuclear wastes are included; or if natural or applied viruses facilitate gene-jumping to create novel mutant aggregate bacteriae.

Agricultural agents such as chemical herbicides, antifungals, nematicides, pesticides, soil fumigants, growth enhancers; and industrial, laboratory, mining, or atomic pollutants can and do wash into local soils and waterways to create a toxic soup enriched by organic matter and fermentation. Such heavily polluted environments contribute to the process of eutrophication (pollution) in watersheds. The application of viruses and bacteria and the chemicals found in soils or irrigative waters may redirect the transposons of plants and microbes to mutate. The local flora and fauna are first to succumb to the percolating brews of toxically polluted soil and waters. This includes the insects that live on or near these areas, and their resident microbes. Under such conditions, mutated bacteriae in any region of the world can be expected to emerge, considering the volume of pollutants that have been manufactured, deployed, or otherwise dumped into the environment over the last century and a half.

Animal Trapping in *Georgia*

In 1950 the US government hired the E.I. du Pont Company as contractor for a large nuclear facility to be built by the Savannah River in Aiken, South Carolina. The company had prior experience building the plutonium production plant at Hanford, in southcentral Washington state during WWII as part of the Manhattan Project. The Hanford Works site built near the Columbia River, delivered the first refined batch of plutonium to the Los Alamos Laboratory in New Mexico in February, 1945. The Hanford site's B-reactor was the first large-scale plutonium production reactor in the world. It was designed and built based on a design by Enrico Fermi, of Fermi Laboratory fame. In 1946 the General Electric Company assumed management of the Hanford Works facility under the newly formed Atomic Energy Commission. Canada (and the UK) contributed to the Manhattan Project, constructing North American plants in Nova Scotia; in Trail, British Columbia; and in Ontario on Lake Huron of the Great Lakes.[1-3]

In 1953, the US began to operate the Savannah River nuclear plant in Aiken, South Carolina. The Savannah River Site (SRS) is the US Department of Energy's nuclear complex located twenty-five miles southeast of Augusta, Georgia; and which spans three counties. SRS began operation in its R-reactor in 1953, and P-reactor in 1954. Both reactors produced plutonium and tritium for the US nuclear weapons program (and fluoride and nuclear wastes). Beginning in 1953 the reactors created heavy water in their plutonium production reactors. Heavy water is deuterated water or HDO; water that contains the heavy hydrogen isotope deuterium, which is used to derive plutonium from uranium or to drive atomic reactors for commercial power plants. Heavy water can also be processed to form deuterium fluoride, which is then physically separated.[1-8]

A side note is that when this kind of uranium makes its way into the body, it concentrates in the teeth and bones, and has a half life of 1,600 years. There is no way to remediate it from the body, and therefore it contributes to the destruction of the skeletal structures, and also to cellular mutation (i.e. cancers). It is interesting to note that in the human body we can also find a small quantity of deuterium. This small amount is considered harmless unless one consumes heavy water to the point where it exceeds a certain percentage in the body. This makes me question whether increased levels of radioactive particles when deposited into the body, may increase the amount of "heavy water" that is produced inside the human body, which may lead to human diseases including cancers.[1-8]

A 1960 paper reported that under an Atomic Energy Commission research grant, Columbia University scientists found that deuterium oxide could be mutagenic to some genotypes of bacteria including *E. coli* and *B. subtilis*. This is an incredibly important idea which suggests that a radioactive product can mutate bacteriae found in the soil and water. We already know that uranium is mined from deep within the earth. We must understand the relationship between the viruses and bacteria found among mined phosphates, bauxites, clays, other fertilizer ingredients, as well as uranium and tritium (the latter mined for nuclear fuels). We already know that soil and water microbes are indigenous to these areas. So it should be no surprise to learn that radioactive and chemical catalysts contribute to the mutation of agriculturally or industrially important microbes to produce novel organisms such as a Romanian leptonema.[1-10]

In 2002, a new gram-positive radiation and desiccation-resistant bacterium was isolated from one of the nuclear reactors at the Savannah River Site. It was named *Kineococcus radiotolerans* species novel, and was noted to be a new extremophile bacterium. Quite simply, extremophiles survive extreme conditions including nuclear radiation. This organism appeared to be 96% similar to another extremophile named *Kineococcus aurantiacus*. Compared to another extremophile *Deinococcus radiodurans*, the novel bacterium was not quite as radiation or desiccation resistant. This is just one example of a mutated bacterium that came about in the presence of highly mutagenic nuclear radiation *inside a nuclear reactor*. Genetically engineered radiation-resistant bacteria were in fact developed in a laboratory and applied to acid mine wastes to reduce wastes and to leach metal ores. Such recombinant extremophiles may remain in the uranium or tritium that is used as nuclear fuels. These lab-manipulated organisms could mutate inside nuclear reactors and wind up as wastewater contaminants. A research paper says this:[1-9]

"The toxicity of uranium is exacerbated in the presence of organophosphorous compounds."

These compounds also include the agricultural and industrial chemical and microbial biocides (i.e. pesticides, herbicides, rodenticides, etc.) or even the phosphates found in fertilizers and in animal feed additives, or in persisting industrial chemical wastes. We can understand how radioactive isotopes and chemicals end up in biocide-treated water, possibly exposing mutagenic agents to resident microbes. A 1960 paper reported that under an Atomic Energy Commission research grant, Columbia University scientists found that deuterium oxide could be mutagenic to bacteria including *E. coli* and *Bacillus subtilis*. This same effect may also mutate the important agricultural soil bacillus, *Bacillus thuringiensis,* or B.t.[1-10]

We might also be concerned about *caulobacter,* which are metal-binding, biofilm-forming bacteria that are found in ground waters and fresh water rivers, ponds, and streams. These bacteriae are useful in treating industrial wastewater flows (in biofilters and compounds). They are also useful as plant growth stimulators, in B.t insecticides, for vaccines, and bioreactors. They are particularly useful for nuclear wastewater treatment since caulobacter are able to remove the reactor-created radioactive *Americium* and *Plutonium* isotopes from aqueous flows. If caulobacter mutate in the presence of certain nuclear and chemical wastes, *this could explain why the bacteriophage capsid viruses that have been found within the B31 strain of Borrelia burgdorferi resemble caulobacter.* This would imply that nuclear reactors are helping to create mutant organisms which become Bb strains.[11-20]

Caulobacter and *Bdellovibrio* are members of the proteobacteria *phage* family. While caulobacter may resemble a phage in the B31 strain of *Borrelia burgdorferi*, bdellovibrio may be more strikingly similar than the caulobacter. *Bdellovibrio* bacteria are well known for their ability to open up (lyse) other bacteria, including leptospira spirochetes. In fact there was a grant to scientists at the University of Massachusetts (Amherst) that was awarded for a project which began in 1972 and ended in 1974, just before "Lyme arthritis" would become public knowledge. The project's abstract claimed that the studies would examine various spirochetal strains.[11-20]

> "For these studies, spirochetes will be isolated from diverse natural environments. The pathways of amino acid fermentation in *Treponema denticola* and in <u>other</u> spirochetes will be investigated." No doubt those "other" spirochetes included water-borne leptospires from sewage, nuclear plants, mine wastes, or other water flows that might also contain organophosphate chemicals or related compounds.

For this project scientists also studied spirochetal chemotaxis and motility (movement), the spirochetal shape, and predatory bacteriae such as "bacteriophage or bdellovibrio capable of lysing spirochetes." Scientists were studying how to manipulate spirochetes using a bacteriophage for a "Syphilis" vaccine, just before the "juvenile arthritis" outbreak of 1975. Although grant abstracts readily used the term "Syphilis," studies could have included animal infections caused by leptonema, or the creation of a new or revised livestock vaccine for leptospirosis. The scientific interests in bdellovibrio phages could have been related to the presence of these phages in the environment and how they might open and degrade leptospires to create novel mutant leptonema including some that were isolated from the 1950s forward.[11-20]

The year after the Romanian *Leptospira dimbovitza* was isolated CDC scientists began to trap over one thousand mammals from southwestern Georgia. We might wonder whether the nearby Savannah River nuclear site and the discovery of a Romanian leptospira mutant had anything to do with these investigations. The animal collections took place from November 1954 to March 1956. Animals were tested for the presence of leptospirosis infections. Roughly forty-four percent tested positive for leptospira strains including *Leptospira ballum, L. pomona, L. australis, L. grippotyphosa, L. hebdomadis,* and *L. mitis-hyos* strains. It is possible that the CDC learned of the novel Romanian spirochete and decided to sweep the area around the SRS to see if a similar mutated leptonema might also be detected. About 44% of the animals tested positive for leptospira strains.[21-25]

If the novel Romanian spirochete was felt to be a product of agricultural, industrial, or atomic energy-related pollutants, it would make sense that the CDC might search for any evidence of similar bacteriae in the US. Since the CDC had a laboratory with its own wastewater facility, analyzing water and fauna samples downstream of the SRS nuclear plant would be a useful model to study nuclear wastes in a manner similar to the heavily polluted Dimbovitza River where the novel leptonema emerged in Romania three years earlier. It would only be five more years whereby the University of Georgia would establish the Savannah River Ecology Laboratory to *specifically study the effects of radiation upon microorganisms at the South Carolina nuclear facility.* (The Savannah River flows along the state lines between South Carolina and Georgia). The program was run by Ecologist Eugene Odum, a University of Illinois scientist who joined the University of Georgia in 1940.[21-25]

In 1958, a report was published by the CDC and Emory University Field Station in Newton, Georgia, that described the incidence of leptospirosis in wild mammals from southwestern Georgia. The paper included a report of new hosts for six serotypes of leptospires. Investigations into wildlife reservoirs of leptospirosis were initiated by the CDC in 1953 at the Newton Field Station in Newton, Georgia. Note this was just two years after the introduction of viruses for agricultural use by the New Haven Experiment Station (Connecticut), and the very same year that the novel Romanian leptonema was isolated. If nothing else, it appears an interesting coincidence in timing between what was found in a Romanian river and the CDC's sudden interest in animal leptospirosis in the states.[25]

Was the emergence of a novel, mutated Romanian spirochete the reason that CDC scientists began analyzing leptospira species in the US? Government scientists were actively studying the extent of domestic and wild animal leptospirosis infections. This is because certain leptospira strains are also pathogenic to humans. According to the CDC report, there was an increase in animal leptospirosis infections in Georgian animals due to what a report called "recent expansions in the cattle industry." Along with such expansions came preventative animal vaccines including those for leptospirosis; as well as insect controls, feed supplements, and antibiotics. It is possible that if cattle were the source of a problem that infectious microbes from their excrement may have been making their way into the soil and/or groundwater. We don't know if the origins of the novel infections were the soil and plant microbes that had been treated with insecticides, or whether the leptospires could have come from animals that were vaccinated and treated with applied insecticides but either could have been a contributing factor to the emergence of new leptospira strains.[25]

"Cattle expansion" may not have been the sole reason for the CDC studies. Cattle herds were acquiring leptospirosis infections, and experts thought that the origin of these infections were feral animals. Naturally scientists would want to know what was facilitating such outbreaks. If feral animals were the cause, then they could have picked up infections from the insects and plants in their environment; both of which were being targeted by the new microbial insecticides. Various additional animals were trapped from 1953 until 1956 in southwestern Georgia, and examined for evidence of leptospirosis. A modified culture medium was recommended by scientists at Rocky Mountain Laboratories to facilitate culturing the leptospira strains that were detected from one-thousand and ninety-one animals trapped. (This is the NIH laboratory where Dr. Burgdorfer was working at the time). Specimens came from foxes, dogs, cats, raccoons, skunks, otters, rabbits, opossums, and squirrels. Obviously CDC scientists were keenly interested in the spread of leptospirosis to cattle and other agriculturally important livestock. An additional goal could have been to determine whether mutated leptospires were contaminating American wastewaters, animal vaccines, or feed supplements to cause animal diseases. No mutated leptospiras were found during the massive sweep during the mid-to-late 1950s, but very soon mutated forms would begin to emerge.[25]

To illustrate ongoing concerns over livestock wastes, we look to a nearby state for clues. Texas A&M University's Water Resources Institute published a study about the effects of "cattle expansion" upon water quality and waste management for open lot dairies. The report covered the period September 1988 to August 1991, just prior to a waste disposal feasibility study that was undertaken at Texas A&M University by the Army Corps of Engineers and published in 1993. Topics of discussion included a comparison of open lot runoff and milking parlor wastewater concentrations of solid and liquid wastes; and wastewater concentrations of nitrogen, phosphorus, and potassium at sampled dairies. An area of particular interest was the upper north Bosque River watershed in Erath and Hamilton counties. There is an outcropping called the Paluxy Formation that is an area of concern because it acts as a "recharge" zone for an underground acquifer (Trinity). Scientists were studying the ground water in the watershed.[26,27]

The Bosque River enters a municipal water supply before meeting the Brazos River in Waco, Texas. Remember that Waco, Texas has a quarry where the Tennessee Valley Authority built two of its nitrate fertilizer plants. According to the A&M report, this particular site has been a main problem area for nonpoint source water quality. This means it is a major thorn in the side of those who are monitoring water quality from agriculturally-related runoff pollutants (including fertilizer nitrates and nitrites), and wastes from open lot dairies. Perhaps what was also being studied were the effects of the government's fertilizer plant upon the local water tables. Waco is downstream in the Brazos River watershed from the original Pantex Ordnance Plant that was located in Amarillo, and which assembled nuclear weapons since 1942. The land is now owned by Texas Tech University, an institution that researches cyclodextrins (cellulosine), which are used in various forms in insecticides, mold inhibitors, fabric softeners, drugs, and plastics.[26-28]

In 1987 the Texas Water Commission adopted a regulation that stated the following with respect to the discharge of animal wastes: "there shall be no discharge of waste and/or wastewater from concentrated animal feeding operations into the waters in the state, but rather that these materials shall be collected and disposed of on agricultural land." This means that any feedlot or concentrated animal feeding operation wastes are to be disposed of into fields that grow crops for human or animal consumption. The TWC mandates that manure and wastewaters are disposed of upon land surfaces. Of course this presents an enormous problem in any feedlot areas in any part of the country that become flooded by natural disasters (i.e. hurricanes, torrential rains, etc.). It is obvious also that fertilizer nitrates have become a problem in Texas, but the state is also home to significant petroleum (oil), natural gas, and uranium deposits, and mining operations.[26,27]

As a side note, the cyclodextrins of insecticides, plastics, mold inhibitors, etc. complex with heavy metals, sewage sludge, and organophosphate chemicals such as those found in industrial and agricultural wastewaters. Bacteria such as the *Bacilli* have cyclodextrin glycosyltransferase enzymes (CGTase) which cause chemical reactions and which synthesize and bind sugars that are useful to the organisms. These enzymes are also involved in cholesterol synthesis and storage. Inside the plasma membrane of cells are enzymes and protein receptors that are called lipid rafts. The lipid rafts of organisms are held together by cholesterol. These lipid rafts remain untouched when exposed to surfactants and detergents including Tweens (i.e. Triton X-100). When cells come into contact with chemicals, the cellular membranes degrade, which releases the insoluble lipid rafts. These rafts may then donate genes to other organisms, including toxins or virulence factors which enable infections. In the insect gut, lipid rafts from gut epithelial cells become disrupted by B.t. insecticidal Cry-toxins which bind to the insect's gut and create pores or holes in the gut membranes through enzymatic action. This releases the intracellular infections in the insect which are then free to reassort with the other organisms present, including the insecticide microbes, toxins, and recombinant genes.[28-30]

Bull-Turtle Studies

There are six nuclear plants in Illinois including Braidwood, Byron, Clinton, Dresden, LaSalle County and Quad cities. Of these, the Clinton station is closest to the Urbana-Champaign area, but none of these plants were in operation during the 1950s. The Quad cities location was built years later near the home of the Bettendorf, Iowa ALCOA aluminum plant. The ALCOA plant was built on the Iowa-Illinois border and Mississippi River in 1948. Besides nuclear reactors, there are nuclear power plants and nuclear research facilities in Illinois. Some industrial companies were hired as subcontractors for the Manhattan Project, and their nuclear fuel-processing activities played an active role in contributing pollutants to nearby soils and water sources in the state. Southern Illinois also has coal mining operations which may contribute important extremophile bacteria to the region.[13-15]

In 1940 scientists at the University of Illinois-Urbana fired the first "free beam of electrons" (super X-rays) from the world's first magnetic induction accelerator (particle accelerator), the *Betatron*. In 1950 a new more powerful betatron replaced the older unit (now housed at the Smithsonian Institute in Washington, DC). It is entirely possible that nuclear wastes pertaining to particle physics research undertaken at this and other laboratories contaminated wastewaters and in turn the microbes, insects, and animals found in the surrounding area.[13-15]

The Dixon Springs Agricultural Center is a large outdoor laboratory and experiment station that is operated by the University of Illinois at Urbana near Champaign (twin cities in southeastern Illinois). It was established in 1938 after US Congress passed the Hatch Act on March 2, 1887. The Act allowed land-grant universities to conduct research that may prove beneficial to agriculture and to the public. Dixon Springs originally opened as a field unit of the Illinois Agricultural Experiment Station. The center coordinates research programs with the University's College of Agriculture and other research sites in the state. It also coordinates research projects with local farmers in southern Illinois. It is perhaps the largest animal and agricultural laboratory east of the Mississippi River. The center conducts beef cattle research on the topics of genetics, nutrition, reproduction, and pest management. In addition to horticultural and agricultural crop production research; crop and soil fertility, breeding, and management research is conducted there, as are veterinary investigations of cattle and hog diseases.[1,2]

In March of 1965, scientists were performing routine health evaluations upon a herd of sixty hereford bulls at Dixon station in Dixon Springs, Illinois. Dixon Springs is supported by the University of Illinois-Urbana campus. The station is located southeast of the university campus at the edge of the Shawnee National Forest in Pope County. It is also near the mouth of the Wabash River and along a geologic fault line. (The area also had a grist mill and mineral salt baths/geothermal springs.) The examinations on the two-year-old bulls were undertaken due to a recent outbreak of a pathogenic animal leptospira strain called *Leptospira interrogans pomona*. Scientists attempted to isolate leptospires from the urine of several bulls under examination. During these efforts, a new leptospira strain was isolated from the urine of bull number 3055. The isolate was found to be antigenically unrelated to any known "pathogenic" *Leptospira interrogans* species, or to any "non-pathogenic" (saprotrophic) *Leptospira biflexa* strain which the isolate resembled. The new spirochete appeared to be an intermediate form (mutant) that was part pathogenic, and part saprotrophic leptospira. The new strain was named *Leptospira illini* strain #3055 after its animal origin. Its distinctive genetic characteristics would warrant further examination.[16,17]

To that end, a semen sample from bull #3055 was sent to the WHO/FAO leptospirosis reference laboratory at the Walter Reed Army Institute of Research (WRAIR). This laboratory falls under the administration of the US Department of Defense, and has a research division for bacterial and rickettsial diseases. While there is a WRAIR laboratory located in Silver Spring, Maryland, there is also a specialized detachment in Texas, and one in Illinois. (A source document did not specifically state which location received the bull semen sample.) We might wonder why a bull semen sample with a new leptospira strain would be sent to a research laboratory belonging to the Department of Defense. One reason the sample was sent to WRAIR was simply because it was a good quality laboratory. Another may be that an emerging animal infection could be considered a matter of "national security" if it was somehow associated with global agricultural, industrial, or military tools. A third idea worth considering is whether a novel leptospira strain was isolated from a laboratory where nuclear science was undertaken (i.e. particle physics); and nuclear or agricultural research wastes were suspected to be contributing to the mutation of bacteria.[16,17]

In July of 1965, just four months after the novel bull strain was isolated, sixty-two turtles were collected from sixteen Illinois locations. They were gathered from area ponds, streams, and rivers in Pope, Massac, Saline, Champaign, Piatt, and Kane counties. Obviously scientists were wondering if "something in the water" might be contributing to the emergence of the novel bull leptospira strain. Water and sediment samples were also collected and studied from all but three of the sites where the turtles were collected. Some of the water samples were sent to the Illinois state water survey division in Urbana, and those samples yielded leptospires. The turtles were also examined for leptospirosis infections through blood draws, urine cultures, and by kidney examination upon sacrifice. Just as the bull semen had been sent to the WHO/FAO lab at Walter Reed for identification, the turtle leptospira isolates were also sent to the same lab.[18]

The turtles were found to be positive for several strains of leptospires, and to have antibodies to strains *Leptospira hyos* (later renamed tarassovi), *L. biflexa*, the new *L. illini* strain #3055, and another novel turtle isolate called "A-177." Apparently the bull strain had made its way into area turtles or vice versa, possibly through contaminated water or insects. The A-177 strain was cultured from a male turtle that had been collected from Phelps pond, a family farm pond located in Pope County, Illinois in 1965. Remember that the university held cooperative programs with area farmers through Dixon Springs. This means that farmers participating in crop or livestock research would have practiced novel techniques or products on their family farms. This could have included testing new fertilizers, chemical pesticides, animal feeds, vaccines, or microbial insecticides.[18]

Pope County and Shawnee National Forest are close to the intersection of five states including Illinois, Indiana, Kentucky, Missouri, and Tennessee. The reason this area was selected to analyze turtle infections was probably because it would serve as a reasonable model of turtle populations from the five-state region. Another novel turtle isolate named A-183 was also found in a female turtle near the Embarrass River at this time. Now there were two new turtle leptospira strains, and a new bull strain that had suddenly emerged by 1965.[18,19]

The Embarrass River is a tributary in the southeastern part of the state which runs from Champaign, Illinois through the Shawnee National Forest and Pope County into the Wabash River. The Wabash is a tributary that joins the Ohio River just below Evansville, Illinois. The Ohio River is the largest tributary of the Mississippi River. Were scientists attempting to determine if industrial chemical wastes that were dumped into the Mississippi River were contaminating the watersheds downstream?

Pope County is also close to the fluorspar mines of Kentucky and Illinois, which is referred to as the Illinois-Kentucky Mining District. In 1965, fluorspar (a source of fluoride) became the Illinois state mineral. Fluorspar has been mined from southeastern Illinois since the early 1800s, primarily in Hardin and Pope Counties, and there was a fluorspar mine in Pope County in Rosiclair. Pope County is of course where the two new turtle strains and the new bull leptospira mutant were isolated at Dixon Springs Agricultural Center. The southern tip of Illinois is also home to a large coal deposit and several coal mines. Coal has a naturally high sulfur content, and sulfur-reducing bacteriae and other extremophiles are found among these deposits and mined materials.[18-20]

Fluorite or fluorspar is a halide mineral that is composed of the element fluorine. The mineral fluorite is used in metallurgy, smelting, glass and enamel production, and is a source of fluoride for hydrofluoric acid. Hydrofluoric acid is used to manufacture pharmaceutical drugs such as Fluoxetine (Prozac), and non-stick coatings such as polytetrafluoroethylene (PTFE). The most common form of PTFE is DuPont's Teflon.® DuPont and 3M had plants upstream on the Mississippi River in Minnesota. Industries were cited decades later for dumping or leaching persisting organic pollutants including PFOS and PFCs into the river. Non-stick coatings are of course used in a wide variety of products from textiles to nuclear reactor components. Nuclear facilities also use biocides which may include fluorosurfactants, fungicides, herbicides, or insecticides to treat water flows. These biocides and chemicals, when mixed with nuclear wastewaters are then discharged into fresh water sources.[18,19,21]

These wastewaters can also contain fluorides, chromium, radioactive trace elements, and bacteriae and viruses that are highly resistant to dessication and radiation since they are thermophiles that can withstand the high temperatures in nuclear reactors. Since fluorite is found near geothermal veins and ore deposits, we may guess how certain extremophilic bacteriae and the reoviruses which associate with them may interact below or above ground. By the mid-1960s, were scientists suspecting connections between mined minerals, industrial or nuclear wastes, and extremophiles and reoviruses? Did they understand that polluted soils and waters were harboring mutated bacteriae that were now infecting aquatic turtles and livestock? Were they also aware that this firey combination could potentially cause human disease including one that was quietly smoldering on the east coast?

There are two other points that need to be made. In 1954, the Illinois conservation department of natural resources headed a deer repopulation program. The areas of the state targeted for deer repopulation were along certain rivers in the northwestern, western, and southern regions of the state. The department began releasing white-tailed deer outside of the Shawnee National Forest in Pope County during the early to mid-1950s. We can wonder whether the deer that were intended as replacement herd stock received (contaminated) animal vaccines or chemical pest controls prior to their release. Other eastern US states undertook similar deer repopulation programs at this time.[22]

It was discovered later that tick cell lines used for biological controls or possibly for animal vaccines were contaminated with adventitious agents. Even if the deer were not vaccinated, their diet and exposure to polluted water sources and the insects that surround same, would have made them first among the larger animals to become infected with whatever was mutating in the environment and suddenly infecting Illinois turtles and bulls.[22]

There may have been a very good reason why the state of Illinois and the CDC were so interested in capturing and examining turtles for novel leptospirosis infections. A typical turtle diet includes vegetation, animal matter, small birds, and insects including cutworms, beetles, ants, flies, sawflies, moths, and butterflies. Each of these insects was a target of the insecticides being deployed in the years before the isolation of the new leptospira strains. The microbial insecticides of the day included *Bacillus popilliae, B. lentimorbus, B. sphaericus, B. thuringiensis*, and at least two borrelina sawfly viruses. Remember the borrelina viruses were initially deployed by scientists at the Forest Experiment Station in New Haven, Connecticut during 1951 field tests. Two years later novel spirochetes were isolated from a Romanian river, and a few years later from Illinois bulls and turtles.[18]

In 1965 scientists began a separate collection of one hundred and forty-five turtles from sixteen Illinois locations, and studied the animals for evidence of leptospirosis infections. Scientists were hoping to cultivate leptospires that might represent an "intermediate state between saprophytism and parasitism." This is an important statement since it acknowledges not only forms similar to those found at Dixon Springs and other Illinois locations, but it also supports my hypothesis that leptospires were mutating in the environment under direction of external factors. These spirochetes were available in an intermediate, mutated form that was clearly infecting animals, and probably insects as well. These same leptospira mutants might go on to become human pathogens when introduced by an insect vector, and they were obviously not isolated forms since they had also been detected in Romania. We will soon see how in just a few years the mutated animal strains would migrate into the human population. A strain would even be isolated from a human patient in Connecticut who was suffering from a newly emerging human infection called "juvenile arthritis."[18,23-27]

Meanwhile at the WRAIR laboratory, the #3055 bull semen samples that had been sent in by the Dixon Springs lab underwent typing and serologic testing. The novel bull leptospire was cloned and tested against all known leptospira antisera and against eight unidentified aquatic "biflexa-like" (saprophytic) isolates. One of these, the recent turtle isolate A-177 from the Pope county farm was found to be antigenically similar to the #3055 bull strain. The similarities between the two strains also included genetics, growth, physiological, and phage characteristics. WRAIR scientists were able to confirm that bull strain #3055 was not serologically related to any other known pathogenic or biflexa leptospira serotypes. It is important to state that some of the so-called "non-pathogenic" or saprophytic leptospires are actually pathogenic strains, including some of the aquatic and soil strains.[18,23-27]

Scientists also determined that bull #3055 and A-177 turtle leptospires were the only two known strains that contained a phage-like entity (bacteriophage). Where did the prophage come from, the polluted water or soils where the phage-like B.t. insecticide was applied? Could it have come from the mined phosphate fertilizers or the acid mine wastes of nearby coal, fluorspar, or other mineral mines; or leachates from subsurface uranium veins? The evidence shows that both #3055 and A-177 were entirely new organisms, just as the Romanian dimbovitza leptospira was a unique spirochete. Each of the newly discovered isolates appeared to be mutated leptospires that had settled into an intermediate form somewhere between saprophyte and pathogenic parasite.[18,23-28]

It should be stated again that the #3055 strain was isolated at an agricultural research center where animal, crop, and insect controls are studied and where related genetic experiments took place, including the likely administration of experimental animal vaccines. The new bull and turtle strains did not fit into either species category for pathogenic *Leptospira interrogans* or the so-called "non-pathogenic" (saprophyte) *Leptospira biflexa* groups. Therefore scientists placed these strains into a brand new group called *Leptospira illini*, so-named after the Illinois animals from which they were first isolated.[18,23-31]

From a 1966 paper we learn that some "pathogenic" leptospires have been reclassified as saprophytes. Although saprophytic leptospires are serologically distinct from the so-called pathogenic strains, they are so antigenically complex due to their host adaptations, that they are difficult to classify into distinctive (sero)groups. The saprophytic strains of leptospires have also proven to be much more resistant to the presence of metals (i.e. mercury, copper, lead, iron, brass) than the pathogenic strains, with the exception of two strains (*L. semeranga, L. andamani*). Such metal resistance probably makes the saprophytic leptospires more readily available in waters and soils that contain metallic contaminants.[32-34]

Researchers analyzed the two new illini strains using samples obtained from Dr. Ellinghausen at the National Animal Disease Center in Ames, Iowa. (This is reportedly the same location where the Ames strain of anthrax is housed.) When compared side-by-side, cells from bull strain #3055 and turtle strain A-177 showed they were identical in structure and form. Another study demonstrated that *the two illini strains were found to be similar to the Romanian dimbovitza strain that was discovered in 1953.* This is curious since the strains were located on two different continents, but they emerged during the same decade. This could mean simply that they shared a similar origin which drove the mutation of each leptospira strain in a similar fashion regardless of location. Was a mutagenic chemical waste and/or an agriculturally applied microbial formula responsible for the mutations on two continents?[24,33,37]

From a chapter in a book written by A.E. Ritchie from the Ames National Animal Disease Center we may learn that leptospires typically lack external flagella. (Flagellin/flagellum are "tails" which help bacteria move.) However leptospira cells contain internal axial filaments or flagella, and what are called "body fibrils." Similar structures were found in the illini #3055 bull strain. The illini strains also produced straight cells, and those with hook-shaped ends, similar to the spirochetes of *Borrelia burgdorferi*, which by that time had not yet been identified.[24,37-43]

A single flagellum was observed to be inserted at either end of the illini cells, and wrapped around its helical (spiral) body four or five times. Damaged cells revealed cytoplasmic tubules. The manner in which the illini flagella were inserted was similar to gram-positive bacteriae. Similar structures on other leptospira strains typically resemble gram-negative bacteriae. When the Illini flagella were detached they were not helical, and coiled into spirals. *Borrelia burgdorferi's* flagella are inserted in a manner similar to those of the *L. illini* strains, and they too adopt a coiled shape when detached.[24,37-43]

Cytoplasmic tubules such as those found in the illini strains had never been observed in other leptospira strains, although they were observed in treponemes and other spirochetes. Similar cytoplasmic tubules are found in *Borrelia burgdorferi* strains. This supports my contention that Bb is an aggregate composed in part with a mutated leptospira (leptonema).[24,38,43,44]

The structures at the end of the flagellin of the illini strains (hook-basal body complex) were compared to those of *E. coli* and the soil bacteria *Bacillus subtilis*. The *E. coli* flagellin were similar in structure as those of other gram-negative bacteria. But the flagellin of the illini strains and those belonging to Bb are more similar to gram-positive bacteria. The gram-positive group includes the soil bacteria *Bacillus subtilis*, and the microbial insecticide *Bacillus thuringiensis* (B.t.). While *Borrelia burgdorferi* is considered to be a gram-negative bacterium, in cultures it stains only *weakly* gram-negative. This suggests that the Bb organism contains *gram-positive* components, and quite possibly genes from gram-positive B.t. strains.[30,40,45-47]

According to a paper co-authored by Yale's Paul Duray et al., there is insufficient evidence that the Bb spirochete is truly gram negative, although many scientific papers refer to it as such, probably because of its weak gram-negative staining characteristics. Changing the culture conditions can affect spirochetal morphology (structure, form), as will the age of the cultures. Bb gram-staining is said to be "generally unsuccessful." Indeed the difficulties culturing and staining Bb, and in detecting human antibodies to the Bb spirochete are well known. Photographs of spirochete isolates from the illini strains #3055 and A-177 appear strikingly similar to those of the Bb spirochete when visually compared.[1,25,37,42,44,47,48]

The *Leptospira dimbovitza* strain was reexamined three decades after it was first discovered. When compared to the two *L. illini strains,* dimbovitza was found to be biologically similar to both. The illini and dimbovitza strains were later found to be similar to other saprophytic leptospires with the exception that unlike saprophytes, the dimbovitza and illini strains were able to grow in a special medium called trypticase soy broth. A phagic organism (prophage) was isolated from illini strain #3055. Now there was a group of leptospires that were unique; with at least one strain harboring a bacteriophage. *Borrelia burgdorferi* strain "B31" has also been identified as harboring some kind of bacteriophage.[24-27,37]

There is a bacteriophage that forms stable infections (lysogens) in *E. coli,* a bacterium common to feces, soils, and polluted wastewaters. This bacteriophage is named "N15" and it contains a mixture of phage and plasmid-derived genes. Among its genes are those that enable plasmid duplication, and others which assist with beginning and ending gene transcription processes. We see a tiny phagic bacterium that infects *E. coli*, and that can cause genetic transcription to occur (reassortment of genes). What is also noteworthy about this particular phage is that it has an odd structure on the end of its chromosome called a *telomere.* This structure is similar to the odd telomeric structure found on the linear plasmid of *Borrelia burgdorferi* spirochetes.

This telomere is called a "hairpin" loop and is shaped kind of like a dumbbell. This structure is found in only a few bacteriae;

and in the insect *Iridescent* viruses (Iridopoxviruses). The iridescent viruses are large DNA viruses which replicate intracellularly. This group includes "PjIV," the virus that contributes to milky spore disease in Japanese beetles. This is interesting because some B.t. patents for genetically-engineered or transgenic crops refer to the process of identifying and eliminating genetic sequences (insect viruses) that may give rise to hairpins, repeats, or other sequences. These hairpin loops are considered to be undesirable in recombinant constructs (i.e. for insecticides). The transgenic plants described in this patent are designed to more fully express B.t. Cry-toxin genes. Under normal circumstances, B.t. insecticide toxins are poorly expressed in GM plants without adding manipulated genes to ramp up B.t. Cry toxin gene expression. Did scientists determine that B.t. phages were contributing to the reassortment of bacteria? Does a B.t. phage include an important insect virus that is commonly found in Japanese beetles, and in the early applied *bacillus-based* microbial insecticides?[24-27,37,49-61]

Remember that two kinds of milky spore agents were applied as insecticides, Type A *Bacillius popilliae*, and Type B *Bacillus lentimorbus*. These bacteriae belong to the *Paenibacillus* group. This is the same group that includes *Paenibacillus larvae*, which causes American foulbrood disease in honey bees. This group also contains the *Thermobacillus*, thermophilic bacteria that are found in hydrothermal veins/springs; and in mined minerals, ores, and acid mine wastes. The thermobacilli are also used to leach metals and during mining extraction, recovery, and/or bioremediation processes.[24-27,37,49-61]

Thermophiles are typically infected by *prophages*, including viruses which could include the "Pj" virus. As spore-forming bacteriae, thermophiles are related to the soil bacteriae *B. cereus, B. spaericus, B. anthracis* (anthrax), *B. subtilis*, and *Bacillus thuringiensis* (B.t.). *Borrelia burgdorferi* has linear plasmids that are similar to those found in bacteriophage N15. Is this further evidence that *Borrelia burgdorferi* also contains an N15-like phage derived from an important agriculturally applied insecticide? It is interesting that no such linear plasmids have been detected in *E. coli.*[24-27,37,49-61]

There is another spirochete that was discussed in a 1969 paper from scientists at the University of Massachusetts. That spirochete is called *Spirochaeta aurantia*. This spirochete was isolated from mud from a duck pond near Urbana, Illinois (where the bull and turtle leptospires were found). Although this spirochete came from a similar source as the novel leptospires, the strain was not found to be closely related to either the leptospires or *Borrelia burgdorferi* spirochetes. Therefore we may safely rule *Spirochaeta aurantia* out as a co-factor to our novel mutant animal pathogens.[62-64]

The *Borrelia burgdorferi* strain B31 that was originally isolated from New York ticks in 1981, has DNA with a G+C content that is slightly reduced in size (27.5-30.5 mol%) compared to the DNA content of the *Leptospira illini* strains (51.2%). Other spirochetes from the treponema species range in size from 35-53.0 mol% while unmutated leptospires range in size from 35-40.4 mol%. If Bb are related to the leptospires, then Bb's reduced DNA content may demonstrate that these spirochetes undergo a gene reduction process during mutation. It is known that bacterial mutants undergo a similar reduction of genes, since the genes that are lost are not required for the survival of the new mutant organism. This kind of gene loss can occur in a nutrient rich environment; by infection with viral or bacterial agents which contain transcriptional elements (i.e. phages); or under influence of chemical pollutants including surfactants or other mutagenic or degrading agents.[24-27,37]

Around 1973, scientists collected fifty-six different leptospira isolates from animals trapped in a woody southern Illinois location which spanned five thousand acres and was dotted with about thirty ponds. Animals that were kept on the property included cattle, sheep, and swine. The land is part of the Dixon Springs Agricultural Center in Simpson; on the edge of the Shawnee National Forest. Antibodies to a number of leptospira species were found in the deer, reptiles, and amphibians surveyed; including antibodies to *L. illini* strains. This means that new leptospira strains were spreading throughout the area. Contaminated water can act as the principal vector for leptospirosis infections from wild to domestic animals or vice versa, and rodents are commonly blamed for transmissions since they are a primary host. The question to ask is where do rodents acquire such infections? They might obtain them from soil, water, from vectoring insects, or from the insects they eat and which are the targets of the biological controls which harbor powerful microbial cocktails meant to activate latent insect infections.[65]

Since the 1950s, researchers were also comparing leptospira strains to understand their antigenic relationships (immune stimulation). What they discovered was that some of the water-borne saprophytes were cross-reactive with some of the pathogenic strains. It became apparent that some of the isolates represented intermediate forms that fell somewhere between pathogenic and non-pathogenic types. In other words scientists had isolated novel mutated leptospires. These mutants were known to exist in Romania and the US from the 1950s forward – up to two decades before the 1975 Connecticut outbreak of juvenile arthritis was reported. Similar strains were also being detected in other Illinois animals from the 1960s forward. It is clearly evident that academic and government scientists were well aware of the presence of mutant spirochetes and their ability to infect insects and animals. Furthermore, scientists seemed to be actively defining the origins of these agents for more than two decades by the time the human outbreak of "juvenile arthritis" (Lyme) disease emerged in Connecticut.[65]

At the University of Illinois from 1960 to 1964, eighty-four amphibians and reptiles were collected near the Dixon Springs Agricultural Center in western Pope County (a few animals came from nearby Johnson and Massac counties). Among the animals collected in this survey were salamanders, tree frogs, snapping turtles, eastern box turtles, fence lizards, race runners, skinks, and a number of terrestrial and water snakes. The animals were examined for leptospirosis infections.[66,67]

Aquatic turtles were collected in August 1964 from three Illinois counties including from Cullom pond at the agricultural center. The center's pond was described as "characteristic" of artificial impoundments that are used as stock ponds in southern Illinois (fish ponds). It was noted that about seventy-percent of the pond was covered with yellow water lilies. We might also take into consideration the known viruses and bacteria of aquatic plants, including the cyanobacteria, and plant and water spirochetes.[66,67]

All of the animals were checked for leptospirosis infections. All cultures were negative but some animals exhibited serum antibodies to several leptospira strains. The highest percentage of serum positive reactions was found in red-eared turtles. Leptospire antibodies were also found in some of the lizards collected. There was a relatively large number of serum antibodies to the *Leptospira ballum* (mouse strain) found in the snake sera (blood), possibly because rodents are their prey of choice. This parasite is also typically found in the wild house mouse (*Mus musculus*), which is a smaller relative of the white-footed mouse, and a known host of Lyme disease spirochetes.[66,67]

Fence lizards collected during the Illinois studies were also negative for leptospires, but they were not tested for agglutinins (antibodies), which is unfortunate as it would have been nice to know the results. (The western fence lizard found in the American southwest demonstrates resistance to natural and experimental *Borrelia burgdorferi* infections.) Serum from some of the turtles, and a frog species from Illinois were shown to possess bactericidal activity against leptospires. While *L. biflexa* leptospires are typically killed by mammalian antibodies, pathogenic leptospira strains are known to be more resistant to animal immune systems.[66-72]

The agglutination studies of the Illinois aquatic turtles mirrored studies undertaken in 1959 by Romanian scientist Combiesco. They also mirrored studies of turtles that were removed from Georgia settling ponds in 1960; and studies by van der Hoeden in 1961 in Israel. In each of these studies, aquatic turtles showed higher antibody sensitivity to leptospires than did the land turtles. Aquatic turtles had more antibodies than their terrestrial counterparts probably because they more frequently encounter leptospires in their natural aquatic environment.[66-73]

By 1964, the CDC already had in its possession, leptospira strains biflexa ("CDC" strain); a saprophyte strain "A-183" from a turtle, and a strain called "Wa Rieden." The fact that these infections including *L. tarassovi* were found in turtles from 1959 to the mid-1960s suggests that the infections were probably present in other animal species for several years. One paper reveals that *L. tarassovi* infections are typically not screened in animals except by the CDC. Perhaps if they had been properly surveyed, they may have been shown to cause leptospirosis in other animals as well as aquatic turtles.[73-84]

One study described a human urine sample that was examined under darkfield microscopy. Both leptospira and treponema spirochetes were identified. The sample came from a patient who was suspected of having an acute spirochetal infection. Routine serologic tests for leptospirosis and Syphilis were inconclusive and had led to a diagnosis of an "unidentified" leptospirosis infection. The diagnosis was made based on an absent antibody reaction to Syphilis serology, and a weak reaction to *Treponema calligyrum*. This is an intermediate form (mutant) Syphilis-relapsing fever spirochete that was discovered by Hideyo Noguchi in 1912.[85-88]

Yale scientists have indicated that patients who have antibodies to Bb may also have a positive treponema (Syphilis) antibody test. This is interesting because it may indicate that the Lyme disease organism may have a *relapsing fever component* to it, or in other words, it is a distant relative of relapsing fever, or the leptospiral organism that makes up both the relapsing fever and Bb spirochetes. At least one person I know who was diagnosed with Rheumatoid Arthritis returned positive on a military Syphilis test, but did not have Syphilis. The patient has a Lyme-like arthritis in the knee and hand joints. If Rheumatoid Arthritis is ever found to be caused by Bb, it could explain this patient's symptoms as well as a *false positive* Syphilis test.[85-88]

The combination of a leptospira-treponema infection might be identified as a *Leptonema* infection. This is the same name that was eventually assigned to a human genital spirochete in 1917 (*Leptospira Noguchi 1917*). This unusual spirochete was identified by Rockefeller Institute Bacteriologist Hideyo Noguchi. Dr. Noguchi discovered the agent of Syphilis in 1911; and he also isolated the polio virus in 1917, the same year he discovered a novel human leptonema spirochete. We might also consider that if a leptospira and a bacterionema were combined as an aggregate organism in the environment, that the combination could also be called a leptonema. (Bacterionema are mosquito-borne pathogens.) In the same sense, a *Leptospirillum* extremophile and any bacterial form such as a leptospira and a bacterionema might combine to form an intermediate leptonema.[25,86,89]

It is interesting that the authors of another paper openly anticipated that other strains of leptonema would emerge in the future. It seems clear that scientists understood the probable origins of the novel leptonema strains illini and dimbovitza. The question is whether the mutated leptonema could have emerged with help from an agricultural bacterium named B.t. Perhaps it came about from a water or soil-borne phage with a special talent of opening leptospira spirochetes (i.e. bdellovibrio or Pj virus). The globally applied B.t. is an aggregator, growth enhancer and prophage that activates latent infections. It not only may attach to insect gut membranes, but also in a piggyback fashion to other bacteria including spirochetes. Once introduced into an animal or human, the digestive process may allow this hitchhiker to degrade gut membranes whereby an attached spirochete may enter.[25,86]

Each of the three novel leptonema strains was found to be very similar yet unique to other previously identified leptospires. In each case polluted water sources were present in highly agricultural areas. There was an agricultural laboratory and mining industries near where the Illinois strains were isolated. In such polluted environments, leptospires may mutate and be carried into local animal herds through mosquito inoculations, aquatic turtles, rodents, or other fauna which enter grazing areas and contaminate soils and water with their excrement. Another aspect to consider is that livestock and sometimes feral animals are vaccinated against pathogens, and their wastes donate pathogenic organisms to soils and waters. Finally, the agrochemicals and biological controls that farmers use upon or within GM crops may contribute chemical and microbial pollutants to the environment. These may be especially concentrated at agricultural research stations or field test sites which are among the first areas where new products are experimentally tested.[90-93]

In 1983, two years after the Bb agent was identified by Burgdorfer et al., and one year after the agent of Lyme was formally announced, scientists finally proposed that the two illini strains and the dimbovitza strain should be placed into a separate genus. It is most curious that this took three decades to achieve. There was some dispute among scientific circles about the "proper" naming of these unique organisms. In 1965 at the University of Paris (France), J. Pillot proposed that leptospires should comprise a unique genera called *Leptospiraceae*. The name wasn't formally adopted until 1983, the year after the Lyme disease agent was announced, at which time the type species *Leptonema* was adopted for a group which would thereafter include the human pathogen *Leptospira Noguchi* from 1917; the two illini animal strains #3055 and A-177; and the serologically distinct dimbovitza strain that was found in a polluted Romanian river.[37,94-97]

This group of intermediate (mutant) leptonema spirochetes now included "Noguchi," a human genital treponema-leptospira form; two animal leptospira strains that might have been a cross between an animal genital, oral, or intestinal pathogen and an environmental spirochete; and a third mutant leptospira that was isolated from a highly polluted European river. Remember that leptospires can transfer their genetic information and virulence factors between strains, and between other compatible bacteria or viruses by way of mobile plasmids.[90-93,98-102]

When searching for "leptonema" in a patent database, thirteen results returned. The oldest patent was filed in 1993 and is assigned to petroleum giant, the Amoco Corporation. The patent is for nucleic acid probes that are useful to detect Lyme disease spirochetes (for diagnostic tests). What are the possible reasons why a petroleum company would desire to own a diagnostic test patent to detect Bb strains? Perhaps industrial oils, chemicals, processes, products, or mining wastes are helping to create these unique human pathogens after all.[102]

According to the Amoco patent, the diagnostic probes of the invention can detect organisms including but not limited to *E. coli, Haemophilus influenza, Brucella abortus, Clostridium perfringens, Staphylococcus aureus,* and *Bifidobacterium dentium*. Most of these organisms can be found inside the human body, but also deep underground. Some like *C. perfringens* may be found in decaying vegetation, marine sediments, soils, waters, or in the guts of insects or animals. While some of these agents may be part of a test to rule out human pathogens, another point to consider is whether "Bb" infections may involve a spirochetal aggregate that is created in part from animals and the environment. The test probes for the 1993 Amoco patent invention are capable of detecting the following borrelia and leptospira strains:[102]

B31 type-NY	P/Gu German	Czech Bb	MN mouse Bb
CONN Veery bird	CONN PI2699	TX human TH GW	CRT Dogontick
MN Bb	CT Sparo #5,9789	MI Charlietick	M1J ECH (LINY)
20047P2	Fr.tick	IP-2 (Fr.CSF)	N40 tick NY
M1001 *Borrelia hermsii*	*Borrelia turicatae*	*Treponema bryantii*	*Leptonema biflexa* (Patoc-Patoc)
Leptonema biflexa (illini)	*Leptospira interrogans* (pomona)		

These probes are able to detect most of the known Bb strain groups. They can also detect other organisms including two treponema periodontal strains, and several others including *T. hyodysenteriae*, the agent of swine dysentery. The probes can also detect *Bactercides fragilis*, normal stool RNA, wheat germ RNA, RNA from a human cell line, *Candida albicans*, and *Cryptococcus neoformans,* a yeast which lives in plants and animals. The test also detects *recombinant* organisms including the following: cloned Lambda phage DNA; cloned *Treponema pallidum**; cloned *Rickettsia prowazekii**; and cloned *Ehrlichia risticii.** Last, the probes of this invention may be arranged in such a way as to facilitate the identification of potential waterborne pathogens that cause human or animal disease. Obviously this patent, which was filed in 1993, was looking for something in wastewater or laboratory samples that could cause human infections, including the spirochetes of Lyme disease.[102]

**These organisms contain cloned, (lab created) or recombinant DNA. The first is a recombinant Syphilis agent; the second a recombinant*

Rocky Mountain spotted fever; the third a recombinant Potomac horse fever. Each of these agents affects animals.

If microbes can recombine in the human body with externally introduced pathogens to create the full complex of Lyme disease, then it would be important to identify which microbes are present. Judging by the probes used within various Bb diagnostic tests, we may get a general idea of what the tests are actually trying to detect. This may lend important clues to the different kinds of Bb infections that exist, and the microbes which physicians may wish to target to cure Lyme infections.

Like *Leptospira interrogans*, *Borrelia burgdorferi* has a wide genotypic variation. How interesting that this leptospira strain was mentioned in another research paper as well as the Amoco patent. The antigenic variation in the genus leptospira is felt to be "considerable" in importance. Borreliae and leptospirae strains exhibit significant genotypic variations. Perhaps this is possible because Bb is created from a leptospira strain and other organisms through gene-influencing environmental and microbial factors. According to a publication, the minor banding differences between virulent and avirulent Bb strain "297" are the result of a lost plasmid in the avirulent strain. This represents gene reduction as previously discussed. Despite their differences, the two Bb 297 strains examined were otherwise considered to be the same. They probably mutated differently, with one strain losing an important plasmid whose genes code for virulence. Therefore one strain was probably not as virulent as the other one.[103]

Three separate patent inventions describe how there are ten genetic groups to the *Leptospiraceae* family. These groups include the following, and please pay close attention to their names ("serovar" means "type").[104-106]

- *Leptonema illini* serovar illini (bull and turtle strains)
- *Leptospira biflexa* serovars patoc, semaranga, and codice (aquatic saprophytes)
- *Leptospira interrogans* serovars icterohaemorrhagiae, fort bragg, ballum, celledoni, and borincana (animal pathogens)
- *Leptospira interrogans serovar Lyme* (A pathogenic leptospira strain classified as "Lyme")

The ten samples of chromosomal DNA used in the aforementioned patents were provided by R.L. Zuerner of the National Pig Disease Center in Ames, Iowa. The three patents each describe diagnostic tests capable of detecting *Serpulina hyodysenteriae*, the agent of swine dysentery. This of course is a swine enterobacteria, and what some reports have labeled as a "swine flu." These important patents also indicate there is a pathogenic leptospira that has been named "Lyme." Is this an admission that "Lyme" disease is caused by a leptospira that mutated from an animal pathogen called *Leptospira interrogans*? If so, it may also be a loose admission that Lyme disease is related to the "swine flu." Does this mean that "swine flu" vaccines might also be targeting Lyme patients? Why would a pathogenic leptospira be assigned the same name as a human infection caused by the "borrelia" of Lyme disease? Is this because there is a Lyme disease agent that is transmitted by other insects in addition to ticks? Those that are transmitted by ticks are called "borrelia." Those that are found in the environment before they are reassorted inside the bodies of ticks or other blood-feeders go by another name, which in some cases become Bb or mutant leptonema, depending on the total number of microbes with which it aggregates inside the insect or animal host.[104-107]

Other patents under the name "leptonema" describe leptospira membrane proteins. One patent makes important statements about Lyme infections that not every public health expert in the current medical arena will openly admit. According to the patent:[108-110]

> "Both syphilis and Lyme borreliosis are characterized by widespread dissemination early in the course of disease, including invasion of the central nervous system. Leptospira share this ability with other pathogenic spirochetes such that *meningitis is a common manifestation of leptospirosis*. Another feature of spirochetal infections is the ability to *persist chronically* in the host, as manifested in cases of tertiary Syphilis and *chronic Lyme arthritis*."

This speaks to persistence and to chronic, systemic infections for both leptospirosis and Lyme disease alike. The patent also indicates that leptospirosis infections cause neurologic disease such as is experienced by Lyme patients.[108-110]

A spirochete named *Leptospira tarassovi* (previously *hyos* strain) was isolated in 1960 and again in 1972 from sewage settling ponds at the CDC Lawrenceville, Georgia wastewater facility, just northeast of Atlanta. The ponds receive and process sewage wastes from the CDC's laboratory. Based on the number of turtle kidney cultures that were pooled together and which tested positive for leptospires, it was predicted that the infection rate of *L. tarassovi* in turtles at the facility was between thirty-three and sixty-six percent by 1972. The source of the leptospira infections were unknown, but scientists felt that either the turtles had introduced them into the ponds and served as an amplifying host; or that contaminated urine from other infected animals including wildlife or *laboratory animals at the CDC's Lawrenceville facility* were responsible for the turtle infections. The Lawrenceville facility was originally designed and used as an animal breeding laboratory.[109,110]

Although the *Leptospira tarassovi* infections were considered to be "exotic," they are a *pig-adapted strain* that causes reproductive problems similar to those caused by *L. pomona*. A British web site says there are few reports of *L. tarassovi* in pigs except in Europe, Australia, New Zealand, Hungary, and western Russia. Please note that the source may not know that the CDC found *L. tarassovi* in its sewage settling ponds and resident turtles as early as 1960. This means the infection is present in the US; in particular in the southeast where commercial pig farms proliferate near an important nuclear plant, the Savannah River Site.[111-117]

In a 1976 book edited by Dr. Russell Johnson of the University of Minnesota, there is a photograph of an unclassified leptospira that was isolated from a CDC turtle. The image reveals intracellular phage development and signs of disintegration including bulbous projections and cysts. This means that the turtle leptospira in the photograph was probably harboring a bacteriophage, and that it formed blebs and cysts – just as occurs with the degrading form of a Bb spirochete.[116]

There was a brief discussion in a paper about the Dixon Springs Agricultural Center illini turtle strain named A-177, and the bull strain #3055. Although the relationships between the two organisms could not be fully examined at the time of the report, their similarities were stunning because what was considered to be the same strain of saprophytic leptospira had been isolated from two taxonomically different animal species (turtle, bovine). The paper called it "of special interest" that certain strains of saprophytic leptospires were able to infect both warm and cold-blooded animals.[116,118]

Comparisons of the enzyme activities of each of the turtle-isolated leptospira strains revealed lipase, except for strains A-177 and #3055. Lipase when produced by bacteria or viruses allows the break down and penetration of lipids (fatty acids) and cholesterol in host organisms. Lipases can also cause a reverse chemical reaction called "esterification" which creates ester bonds. In this way lipases act as chemical catalysts. Esters are compounds that contain a hydroxyl (alcohol or phenol) and an oxoacid (oxygenated acid). The nomenclature of esters extends to inorganic acids, especially phosphoric, sulfuric, and nitric acids. Esters are used in fragrances, flavoring agents, and polymers (i.e. Teflon®). Bacteriae which have lipase enzymes may be present in waters polluted by industrial chemicals and polymer compounds.[16,102,119-122]

Different bacteriae secrete different lipases that are measured in kilodaltons (kDa). *Bacillus thuringiensis* for example produces a 38-kDa phospholipase. According to a paper co-authored by spirochetologist Russell C. Johnson, all of the *Leptospira biflexa*, the leptonema; (some) *L. interrogans* and the *Leptospira inadai* Lyme strains produce lipases; while *L. interrogans, L. borgpetersenii, L. noguchi, L. santarosai* and *L. weilii* strains do not. This should help narrow down the species which may comprise an aggregate Bb if it proves to be from a leptospiral source. While it is clear that strains A-177 and #3055 do not produce lipase enzymes, we might note that this may be because they have yet to reassort with a component that will provide these genes. Once this occurs inside the body of an insect for example, the new aggregate may finally become a human pathogen called the Bb spirochete.[16,102,119-122]

How leptospires gain or lose a key enzyme such as lipase is a curious thing. Perhaps the loss in the illini strains was achieved through genetic engineering in a laboratory; or under influence of chemicals from industrial, nuclear pollutants, or agricultural chemicals. Phages may also cause the loss of lipase by helping to degrade bacteria or viruses to the point that key enzyme genes are lost or become otherwise inactive.[117,123-125]

A 1971 patent assigned to Merck & Co., Inc. (Rahway, NJ) describes the use of various compositions as antimicrobials for agricultural purposes. These compositions contain organic carboxylic esters, and bauxite and clays as diluting agents. Remember these materials can contain residual fluorides and can aggregate microbes. If these enzyme-degrading formulas are used within agricultural products, it is not difficult to imagine that they and other chemicals present in sewage treatment plants or in the environment help bacteria including leptospires to mutate (and gain or lose lipases). Through the resulting mutation caused by enzymes and chemicals, novel leptonemas and human pathogenic spirochetes could certainly be created.[125,126]

What we find in mines, mined materials, and acid mine wastes is important to our story. For example we find *Thiobacillus* and *Leptospirillum* bacteriae in uranium and other mines. *Leptospirillum ferrooxidans* is naturally abundant in iron-rich, low pH environments, and can be found in slime layers as many extremophiles are slime/biofilm-formers. It is also an iron and sulfur-oxidizer/reducer and plays an important role in reducing acid mine wastes and in degrading ores. This makes it an exceptional candidate for contributing genes to a mutated soil or water leptospira strain that may be found in a pollutated river or even a farm pond (as fertilizers are mined from phophates).[127-142]

These and other similar reducing extremophile bacteriae have been used industrially in bioreactors, *and to leach oil and metals from ore deposits* (i.e. copper from chalcopyrite, manganese from manganese ores, etc.). They have also been used for decades to bioremediate acid mine and other wastes, to recover silver from photographic film, to remove heavy metals from wastewaters, and to recover other metals from aqueous solutions. These formulas not only employ multiple forms of extremophile bacteria and their clones, they also use chemical surfactants, quaternary amines, and chloride, ammonium, and other chemical compounds in their processes, including some that are known mutagens. Any of these can easily adversely affect the microbes found naturally in wastewaters and soils.[127-142]

Thiobacillus feroxidans seems to have been the most widely deployed microbe during the 20th century, although other reducers have been used including: *Leptospirillum ferrooxidans, Thiobacillus thiooxidans, Ferrobacillus ferrooxidans, Thiobacillus thioparus,* and a recombinant clone (#8158). When I looked up this number in a culture database, it returned with a *Paenibacillus polymyxa* spore-forming bacillus, a fungus *Aspergillus microcysticus,* and *Salmonella enterica* subspecies *bongori.* Other known reducers include *Sulfolobus acideocoldarius, Sulfobacillus thermosulfidooxidans, Sulfolobus acidophilus, Metallogenium* species, and *Gallionella ferruginea.* There may also be other species that have been employed industrially, or that will be found naturally. At least one new strain has been recently discovered, *Mariprofundus ferrooxydans.* I suspect because of their connections to important industries, that these may be among the most important bacteria to the Lyme disease story. When we think about their presence in the mined materials of so many industries, and the fact that they are employed to aid in the extraction of important minerals and other resources, we may understand why they are so valuable.

Something to think about is that any extremophile genes that may be part of an aggregate Bb organism could be derived from one of these metal-reducers. If so, the most likely candidates are those which reduce manganese, since the Bb organism has replaced all of its iron-sulfur cluster enzymes with those that use manganese.[143-146]

Among the bacteria that are known reducers of iron and manganese are these, although this is probably not a complete list:

Alternaria *Bacillus* *Clostridium* *Desulfovibrio* *E. coli*
Ferribacterium *Fusarium* *Geobacter* *Geothrix* *Lactobacillus*
Pelobacter *Pseudomonas* *Sulfolobus* *Shewanella* *Thiobacillus*

Many of these bacteriae are used in agricultural insecticides, and others are found naturally in the environment, or have been used industrially in mining or leaching formulas. When we consider what makes up a mutated leptospira that might have infected bulls, turtles, and eventually humans, we might carefully consider any of these bacterial donors.

Rocky Mountain Leptospires

Leptospires are gram-negative, finely coiled spirochetes that thrive in water and soils around the world. They are most prevalent in the spring and fall when there is ample wet soil and moderate temperatures. They prefer habitats with high humidity and a neutral pH (6.9-7.4) such as may be found in shallow lakes, ponds, bogs, puddles, and polluted waters (i.e. sewers, retention ponds, some mine pits). Their optimal growth pH is 7.2-7.6, roughly the same as the human intestine. There are pathogenic and saprotrophic strains. Generally the pathogenic strains include those considered to be enterobacteria (gut). Leptospires can survive in water for several weeks.[1]

A leptospirosis infection begins with a high fever, chills, severe headache, and muscle pains in the back and legs. There may be a burning sensation in the eyes and conjunctivitis, iritis, or other ophthalmic symptoms. In the 1950s, the treatment of choice for leptospirosis infections included the antibiotics chloramphenicol, aureomycin, penicillin, and streptomycin. According to a publication, leptospires are far more common than first realized and often lead to an inaccurate diagnosis of "viral encephalitis" since they are able to invade the central nervous system.[2-7]

Leptospires that were isolated from New Jersey dairy cattle in 1948 were of the species *Leptospira pomona.* This strain was also isolated in 1950 from cattle in New York, New Jersey, Pennsylvania, Georgia, and California. According to a patent that discusses leptospires:[2-7]

> "There is a large spectrum of animal species which serve as reservoirs for the bacteria. As a result, *human leptospirosis* is found throughout the world, and is considered to be *the most widespread zoonotic disease.* High risk groups include *military personnel, farmers, miners, sewage and waste removal workers, veterinarians, and abattoir* [slaughterhouse] *workers.*"

Leptospires are spread through contact with the urine of an infected animal; from urine contaminated water (i.e. ponds, raw sewage); or by contact or consumption of contaminated plants or soils. Other modes of infection include abrasions or wounds; eye or mucous membrane contact; contact or ingestion of contaminated meats from domestic or wild animals (i.e. deer, raccoon, rabbit, fowl, etc.) or reptiles (i.e. snakes, turtles); or through sexual reproduction. Leptospires were first observed in kidney tissues from a human patient who died as a result of what was considered to be *yellow fever* in 1907. This may be our first clue that leptospires and their mutants, and the mollicutes of "yellows" diseases together cause human infections.[1,8-10]

This is an interesting point since yellow fever is transmitted by mosquitoes, and so are arboviruses and other pathogens we have explored that are related to the yellows diseases of plants. For example the agent of aster yellows is a phytoplasma mollicute that is transmitted by leafhoppers. Leptospires are transmitted by any number of vectoring insects including mosquitoes, mites, and ticks. The kidneys, spleen, intestines, and liver are considered to be optimal breeding grounds for leptospires in mammals. These are the same organs that are commonly found to be significantly infected in Lyme disease patients.[1,8-10]

One source described an outbreak of human leptospirosis in nine children who became infected after swimming in a stream that ran through pastures where swine and cattle were kept. Another source described a Florida man who owned rodents and snakes and was putatively infected with a leptospira strain. In another source, two Florida men were infected after swimming in a contaminated Illinois lake (Lake Springfield) while participating in a triathalon. According to a CDC report, leptospires were the etiologic agent for these illnesses in "athletes and in persons with occupational or recreational exposure to Lake Springfield, where the [triathlon] event was held in Illinois."[11,12]

A CDC update also reported with regard to leptospirosis infections that "recreational exposure to natural water sources is a common route of transmission." It is obvious the CDC is aware that leptospires can be transmitted via contaminated water sources to cause human infections. I cannot understand however why I have lived five decades before I discovered this important information which I did not learn from any public service announcement or clinical materials, but from my own intensive research.[11,12]

Leptospires are generally divided into two species, the largely "non-pathogenic" *Leptospira biflexa*, and the "pathogenic" *Leptospira interrogans*. Both groups contain strains that are considered to be pathogenic to animals and humans. In animals, some of the most commonly isolated leptospira strains are *L. icterohaemorrhagiae, L. pomona,* and *L. canicola.* The latter causes leptospirosis in dogs. *L. interrogans* is further divided into strains based on antigen differences, much in the same manner that Bb spirochetes are divided. Antigens are cell-surface markers that stimulate antibody production in a host. Antigens do not produce antibodies that will protect across multiple strains, but they can cause laboratory tests to cross-react. This may make it difficult to discern which leptospira strain is present in an infected host. Cross-reactions may result in "false positive" laboratory tests. A similar problem may cause a false positive in some Lyme disease diagnostic tests if the patient is infected not with a true Lyme disease, but with a leptospira strain that produces very Lyme-like symptoms.[1,13]

Leptospires have a cellular envelope that is composed of a cytoplasmic membrane and an outer membrane. They also have two flagella (tails) that attach to the cytoplasmic membrane in what is called the periplasmic space at each end of the bacterium. When faced with adverse conditions (i.e. increased saline in brackish water); or when the organism is undergoing a growth phase, leptospires can detach their outer envelope. This allows them to form spherical blebs on the cell surface.[14-16]

The outer surface of a leptospire is composed of lipoproteins and outer membrane proteins, just as are found in *Borrelia burgdorferi* spirochetes. The outer surface proteins of leptospires can vary in form depending upon whether the organism was isolated in a culture dish or from an infected host. The same thing occurs with the Bb organism where its outer surface proteins and form varies depending upon insect or animal host, or culture conditions.[14-16]

Like leptospires, Bb spirochetes have a proplasmic cylinder and cytoplasmic tubules. In the leptospira strain *interrogans*, the three major antibody (immunoblot) protein bands have a molecular weight of 25, 32, and 41-kDa. Two scientists who were present at the 1994 Dearborn conference studied Bb plasmids and those of pathogenic and saprotrophic leptospires. Their studies indicated they probably knew important information about the similarities between the plasmids of both kinds of spirochetes before attending the Dearborn conference. Their studies also covered the multiple and mini-chromosomes of Bb; those of the proteobacterium *Rhodobacter sphaeroides*, and various yeasts and protozoans. They could have been studying various organisms to determine which might comprise an aggregate Bb spirochete. Their research also seems to conclude that a linear molecule from Bb may have come from a pathogenic leptospira.[14-16]

Efforts to identify *leptospira* strains for potential vaccine use have identified the organisms' outer membrane (surface) proteins. It is interesting that they have molecular weights of 31, 32, 36, and 41-kDa. These are identical to the outer surface proteins of the Bb spirochete (numbers vary 1-2 digits depending on strain). Indeed the 31-kDa protein of Bb represents the outer surface protein A (OspA) used in the first generation Lyme vaccine. Two of the most prominent leptospira proteins at 31 and 41-kDa, appear to provide protection against leptospirosis infections in hamsters. The 41-kDa protein may represent not "just" a flagellin gene, but an outer surface protein of a leptonema or Bb spirochete that has a surface-exposed Osp protein located on the top-most part of its flagellin or tail. Therefore a positive 41-kDa diagnostic band may be specific for either a leptospirosis infection, a Bb/leptonema infection, or any other mutated leptospira-based infection (i.e. relapsing fever).[17-23]

A patent identifies *pathogenic* leptospira outer membrane proteins including one at <u>93-kDa.</u> The patent is for a diagnostic test and vaccine for leptospirosis infections. The patent refers to scientific papers which describe the outer membrane proteins of the Bb spirochete (revealing they are similar). *An important Bb outer membrane protein that has been identified in recent years is in fact, the 93-kDa protein.* Often in chronically infected Lyme patients, this is the only diagnostic band that will register positive on Western blot IgM* tests. The 93 band is excluded from the CDC's IgM standardized banding pattern, but is included on the IgG test.[24-27]

**IgM is immunoglobulin M, the first antibody produced during infection. Western blot tests for Lyme disease check for IgM and IgG. IgG is immunoglobulin G, an abundant antibody produced during secondary stages of infection. Antibodies may persist over time or be entirely absent in seronegative patients who are infected with Bb.*

Leptospira outer surface proteins are similar in molecular weight as those found in Bb strains. A University of California patent identifies novel leptospira surface proteins named LipL1 (35-kDa) and LipL2 (41-kDa), and its flagellin, also at 41-kDa. The most important outer surface proteins of Bb are OspA (31-kDa) and OspB (34-kDa); and its flagellin (41-kDa). We now may question whether there is also a 41-kDa surface protein in Bb strains about which we have not been told. From two 1989 papers, we read that according to Lyme notables Benjamin Luft, Raymond Dattwyler, and Jorge Benach at the State University of New York at Stony Brook (SUNY), the 41-kDa protein of Bb strains (endoflagellin) may be a *surface* protein or have a surface exposure. The major leptospira protein bands are found in zones 21 to 31-kDa; in particular at 25-31, 32-34, and 45-kDa in pathogenic strains. The zone that differentiates the pathogenic leptospires from saprotrophic species lies between 21 and 45-kDa, although the proteins can migrate during testing. In short, important leptospira proteins are identical in molecular weight to those that are found in the Bb organism. This may support the idea that Bb spirochetes have a mutated leptospira component.[28,86,87]

Although the Dearborn conference standardized the Bb protein band numbers detectable in tests, it excluded the important OspA and OspB bands, which vary slightly in number among Bb strains. These numbers also vary between leptospira species, and it may be difficult to pinpoint specific strains when there are so many. For example leptospira strain *L. icterohaemorrhagiae* is found in swine, while strains *L. pomona* and *L. hebdomadis* are associated with cattle. If a leptospira protein is included in Bb diagnostic test probes, it would have to be a protein that is found in nearly all leptospira strains either pathogenic or saprotrophic; and one that is also common among the majority of Bb strains. That protein would probably be assocated with a virulence factor, and one that would maintain infections in insects, arthropods, animals, and humans alike.[1,28,29-39]

In the Bb spirochete, OspC is a 23-kDa protein that is expressed when spirochetes are transmitted to insects, animals, and humans. In patients with leptospirosis, IgM immunoblot tests typically produce antigens at bands 14-18, 19-23, 24-30, 32, 35/36, 37, and 41-42. It is possible that the 23-kDa band that was chosen for the Bb Western blot is the most commonly produced band between Bb and leptospira strains. If so, this is likely because Bb is first and foremost a mutated leptospira in origin. The OspC protein is in fact, a virulence protein that is necessary to maintain infections.[1,28,29-39]

There is a high prevalence of leptospirosis in mice and sewer rats, as well as wild animals and marine animals (i.e. California sea lions). Strains such as *L. pomona* and *L. grippotyphosa* became more prevalent in the environment in part because animals have been vaccinated with leptospirosis vaccines for a long time. These two strains emerged as dominant wild strains because they were excluded from preventative animal vaccines. This may be another valid reason why the OspA and OspB strains for the Bb organism were excluded from the diagnostic tests at Dearborn if one of them belongs to a leptospira protein, and there was another leptospira protein already included in the Dearborn tests – the 23-kDa (OspC) protein that remains during infection.[1,28,29-39]

There are interesting statements in another patent text that may address why the 41-kDa band was permitted to remain in the standardized Bb diagnostic tests. The patent is for an animal leptospirosis vaccine formula but compares antibody responses from human Lyme patients to the formula, including human Lyme serum samples from the Pasteur Institute in Paris. Does the 41-kDa band in Bb tests represent a pathogenic leptospira surface exposed protein from its endoflagellin? It certainly appears to be so from these patent statements:[40]

> "Priya et al (2003) reported that immunoreactive antigens of 15-20, 23-24, and 27 kDa were the lipopoly-saccharides of the organisms and associated with uveitis [eye infections] in leptospirosis patients…The immunoreactive antigen of 41 kDa was reported to be a *leptospiral lipoprotein*, present in both cytoplasmic and outer membranes…and *found only in pathogenic leptospire* species…that were recognized by leptospirosis sera."
>
> "...serum 153272 from the case confirmed to be Lyme-positive shows a significant IgM serological response against the recombinant PPL protein...The results show that, for confirmed cases of Lyme disease that are free of leptospirosis... the IgM and IgG response against the PP peptide is of the same order as that of the control (pool of sera)."

This seems to say that people with Lyme disease do not have a leptospirosis infection, but they may have an aggregate Bb organism that is *composed in part by a mutated leptospira. It may also reveal that a mutated leptospira that Dr. Steere et al. found in a Lyme patient in 1981 before Bb was announced was probably part leptospira and the causative agent of Lyme disease.*

What is unique to unmutated leptospires and to Bb spirochetes is that both activate toll-like receptors (TLR2) of the human immune system. These are signaling gateways that alert the immune system to the presence of foreign invaders. In leptospirosis, this activation is caused by the unique structure of the lipid A lipopolysaccharide (LPS) molecule of the spirochete. The very same mechanism that triggers the human immune response during leptospirosis infection does the same during Bb infection.[30,41-45]

According to genetic taxonomy browsers (which describes organisms and their relationship to other organisms), *Borrelia burgdorferi* strains are clearly offshoots or mutated versions of pathogenic and saprophytic *leptospires.* Despite the overwhelming evidence of such a link that is readily available within the research, scientists have failed to make this audible connection at any time from the discovery of the Bb organism to the present day. A refusal to mention mutated leptospires (leptonema) may have seriously undermined the ability of physicians to identify human diseases and to treat patients. We have to wonder why there is so much silence around an epidemic human disease. We may imagine that if the contents of this book are accurate, that the answers are obvious. According to phylogenic trees, the leptospires that are related to the Bb spirochetes include but are not limited to these strains:

Leptospira interrogans serovar Copenhageni (canine)
Leptospira interrogans serovar Lai (China 1966)
Leptospira interrogans serovar Djasiman (Slovakia 1972)
Leptospira interrograns serovar Pomona (pigs)
Leptospira interrogans serovar Grippotyphosa (livestock)
Leptospira interrogans serovar Canicola (canine)
Leptospira interrogans serovar Bulgarica (Australia)
Leptospira interrogans serovar Zanoni (Australia dairy cattle)
Leptospira Noguchi (this is the 1917 leptonema)
Leptospira weilii (Weil's disease [rodents])
Leptospira borgpetersenii serovar Hardjo-bovis (causes livestock abortions)
Leptospira santarosai (USA, Denmark, Central and South America, Trinidad, Sri Lanka)
Leptospira licerasiae serovar Varillal (Amazon rodents)
Leptospira biflexa serovar Patoc 1 Ames (stream water, maintained at Pasteur Institute, France)
Leptospira biflexa serovar Patoc 1 Paris (stream water, maintained at Pasteur Institute, France)
Leptospira interrogans miscellaneous serovars

Of course the other serotypes not listed in the taxonomy browser as related to Bb strains include the leptonemas from a group that includes *Leptospira Noguchi*; the *leptonemas* found in the Romanian river, in the Illinois turtles and bulls, and another human *leptonema strain that was found in a Lyme patient in 1981* but which never really made Lyme disease "headlines."[46]

At the same time that animal trappings were taking place in 1954 in southwest Georgia; at the Rocky Mountain Laboratories in Hamilton, Montana, Dr. Willy Burgdorfer and colleague E.G. Pickens were experimentally infecting relapsing fever (*Argasid*) ticks* using embryonated chicken eggs that were infected with Q fever, tularemia, pathogenic leptospires (*L. icterohaemorrhagiae*), and western equine encephalitis virus. The experiments demonstrated that the ticks could be infected with these organisms, which grew well in the chicken egg cultures.[47,48]

**Ornithodoros turicata and O. moubata are soft-bodied relapsing fever-transmitting <u>livestock</u> ticks found in the US midwest and southwest.*

Unpublished data according to the article demonstrated that leptospires persisted in the tick tissues for up to three-hundred and fifty days. The results of the studies led to a series of investigations involving soft-bodied *Argasid* and hard-bodied *Ixodes* ticks as possible vectors of leptospirosis. It is perhaps no coincidence then that at the same time that a novel leptonema was discovered in Romania and subsequent strains uncovered in the US in Illinois and Georgia, that Dr. Burgdorfer and his colleagues at RML were busy studying what were essentially the very same organisms. Three decades later Dr. Steere et al. would find a similar organism in a Lyme patient's ECM skin rash culture but this spirochete's name never really came to the public's attention.[47,48]

Besides the obvious interest in animal leptospirosis, one possible study objective was to determine whether ticks could infect embryonated cell lines used to create animal vaccines. As it was 1954 and the Korean conflict was technically over, it is unlikely these studies were for any military-style biological warfare experiments. Perhaps Burgdorfer et al. were instead investigating a newly emerging pathogen that included pathogenic leptospires or intermediate leptonema forms – strains that may have been surfacing in Romania and possibly also in the US before the Illinois strains emerged, for which scientists may have already been working on a useful vaccine. Perhaps their concerns were that animal vaccine cell lines were contaminated with an agent that was being excreted in animal wastes. If so they would have rightfully worried that the agent(s) could be transmitted by vectoring insects into the human population.[47,48]

In 1956, Dr. Burgdorfer was again studying leptospires and relapsing fever ticks as spirochetal vectors. We might assume that by now the novel leptonema strains had peaked scientific interest and the vector of these agents was actively being studied. In the Burgdorfer studies, nymph and adult soft ticks were engorged on embryonated chicken eggs that were inoculated with a tenth passage of animal leptospira strain *L. pomona* which came from Illinois swine in 1953. This was the same year that the dimbovitza (river) strain of an odd leptospira first surfaced in Romania.[48-54]

This was also just before novel illini strains first appeared in Illinois animals. Dr. Burgdorfer would continue to study ticks as vectors of leptospirosis well into the 1960s, and he published several papers during the late 1950s on the topic. Dr. Burgdorfer's studies seem entirely possible that he was made aware of a connection between the spirochete found in the Romanian river and a connection to those which would also soon emerge in Illinois animals.[48-54]

Since Dr. Burgdorfer was studying whether chicken embryos could be infected with livestock pathogens, it seems highly likely that he was trying to ascertain whether livestock vaccines (which may be grown in chicken embryos) could have been contaminated with specific pathogens. In other words were livestock vaccines contaminated with important infections that could have led to the creation of a mutated leptonema the likes of those found in Romania and the Illinois bulls and turtles? Another explanation for the studies is that a combination animal vaccine could have been attempted at some point that eventually failed, only to combine its recombinant pathogens with the microbial insecticides ingested as animal feed supplements (or applied insecticides) to create an aggregate organism which could be excreted in animal wastes.[48-54]

It is noteworthy that one of the references in a Burgdorfer paper from this period denotes a publication by Japanese researchers Inada and Ito. Dr. Inada identified the leptospira agent of Weil's disease.* Inada is the scientist after whom a novel leptospira strain was named in 1981 by a colleague of Dr. Burgdorfer, Dr. Allen Steere, as *Leptospira inadai Lyme*. However Dr. Steere and his team did not make this spirochete public for some time after the event. Even when this occurred, almost no one in the Lyme community noticed the publication, or if they did, they failed to discuss it publicly. Dr. Burgdorfer was the scientist after whom the Bb spirochete would be named the following year (1982). Perhaps one reason was because he would discover not only that a key component of the Bb spirochete may be a spiroplasma, but also that Bb included a mutated leptospira. Such leptospire may have come from a natural infection, a contaminated leptospirosis animal vaccine, or the microbes of recombinant insecticides.[48-57,85]

**Weil's disease is a rodent leptospirosis infection that was first identified in 1908. It is highly prevalent in coal miners, fish cleaners, and sewage workers.*

Dr. Willy Burgdorfer, the scientist credited with isolating the Bb spirochete, has long studied pathogenic agents of ticks. His earlier work included various strains of leptospires, including an *L. pomona* strain that he discovered in hard-shelled Gulf coast ticks (*Amblyomma maculatum*), Rocky Mt. wood ticks (*Dermacentor andersoni*), and relapsing fever ticks (*Ornithodoros turicata*). He studied these species along with soft-bodied ticks as early as 1954. Dr. Burgdorfer wrote that *he had also isolated Leptospira ballum and L. pomona from some of these tick species.* These leptospira strains are pathogenic to humans and animals and are commonly found on cattle, pigs, mice, deer, horses, dogs, and other animals.[58,59]

From 1940 to the late 1950s tick transmission of leptospirosis was being studied at Rocky Mountain Labs. Dr. Burgdorfer was studying the persistence of leptospires in tick tissues during this period, and published at least two papers discussing persisting leptospirosis infections in ticks. He detected leptospires from tick salivary glands, coxal organs, the central ganglion, and tissues of the genital and excretory systems. Mice and guinea pigs developed infections within four days of inoculation; and leptospires were recoverable from blood cultures. Nine days after feeding ticks an infectious blood meal, thirty-eight of seventy-one guinea pigs were found to be infected with leptospires. In another experiment, seventy-five soft ticks fed upon infected, inoculated chicken embryos. Within twenty-four days, eighteen emitted leptospires from their coxal fluid (feces).[49,60-63]

Fifty of the remaining ticks were used in guinea pig leptospirosis transmission experiments. In another experiment, eighty ticks were fed inoculated chicken embryos. In some instances, leptospires could be cultured from pig blood. The experiments showed that ticks feeding upon even mildly infected guinea pigs would contract leptospirosis.[49,60-63]

In one paper Dr. Burgdorfer discussed how strains of *Leptospira grippotyphosa* were cultured from *Dermacentor marginatus* ticks that were removed from *cattle* in the Union of Soviet Socialist Republics; and from a brown dog tick found on an Israeli hedgehog. *Leptospira pomona* could also be transmitted by *Ixodes* Rocky Mt. wood ticks and Gulf coast ticks which are common *livestock parasites*. However *Leptospira pomona* could not be maintained as a permanent infection during the experiments. Colorado tick fever virus in mouse tissues was also studied by Dr. Burgdorfer during the late 1950s. This is important because Colorado tick fever is caused by a reovirus such as those found deep in the ground where mined phosphates and ores are found.[49,60-63]

A key finding of Dr. Burgdorfer's experiments was that infections persisted in ticks where spirochetes had penetrated the gut wall and entered the body cavity. Dr. Burgdorfer observed that "practically all organs of the tick" became infected with leptospires. However the article stated with respect to soft ticks, that those which fed on hamsters became infected and transmitted leptospirosis to other animals. The authors stated it was not their intent to infer that these ticks were natural vectors of leptospirosis.[60,61]

What the results also suggested were that some mechanism may allow leptospires access through the midgut tissues into the body cavity. It is possible that the microbes which degrade gut tissues to create pores (holes), allow leptospires entry along with other pathogens and toxins. If scientists had determined that chemicals or microbial insecticides were creating persistently infected ticks and animals, they might be expected to contact or visit private or academic laboratories with industry ties to share such findings. Perhaps this explains an historic visit by Russian scientists to key US universities including one in Missouri, an arguable hub of agrochemical research by 1957. Such visits would have been important if scientists understood that vectoring insects had the potential to spread novel pathogens to the human population (i.e. biological controls), and they wished to determine how best to handle the situation if it became a global public health concern.[60,61]

In June of 1956, Dr. Burgdorfer published another paper on the artificial feeding of *Ixodes* ticks to study disease transmission of *Leptospira pomona,* a pathogenic animal strain. In these studies, Rocky Mt. wood ticks and Gulf coast ticks were fed using techniques from his earlier studies. Transmission experiments were undertaken using infected ticks that were allowed to feed upon weanling guinea pigs, thus infecting the ticks with *L. pomona* spirochetes. Dr. Burgdorfer observed that ticks could become infected within a few hours of feeding on the infected chicken embryos. Although no mention of a rabies virus was specifically made in the article, there was a notation that the technique proved suitable for experimental infections of Rocky Mt. wood ticks and Gulf coast ticks with *L. pomona*; and for experimental infections of Rocky Mt. wood ticks with rabies virus.[64]

Although Dr. Burgdorfer did not elaborate on this aspect of study in his paper, he may have been speculating on rabies transmission, or he undertook such studies directly but simply omitted those results from the article. The question to ask is why would he be studying rabies and leptospires? Perhaps scientists of the day were concerned that mutated tickborne spirochetes, when combined with an insect arbovirus could fabricate a human infection that might cause an encephalomyelitis, or Multiple Sclerosis-like syndrome. This may have been the same model which Russian scientists (who would come to the US) were studying. The Russian scientists were using a rabies-related virus in an attempt to create a curative mouse-brain derived encephalitis/Multiple Sclerosis vaccine.[64]

Another article by Dr. Burgdorfer and RML colleagues revealed that the rabies virus was studied during the late 1950s. Over the past three years (1953-1956) rabies virus was frequently isolated from insect-eating bats. The studies focused on two strains of rabies virus that included a Pasteur strain and a bat strain. Ticks used in the experiments included soft tick species; brown dog ticks, and Rocky Mt. wood ticks from the insectary at Rocky Mountain Labs. During transmission experiments rabies virus could only be detected for up to three days in *Ixodid* ticks; two weeks in nymphs, and twenty days in adult *Argasids*. This rather limited artificial transmission of rabies in ticks nevertheless occurred, although the studies found transmission rates to be low. (What occurs in the lab may differ in nature.)[65]

On the other side of the world in the Republic of Slovenia, outbreaks of human meningo-encephalitis were erupting from 1946 to the early 1960s. Remember that during the mid-1940s the biological controls *Bacillus popilliae* and B.t. were making their way around the world. Just a few years later outbreaks of meningo-encephalitis were suddenly emerging in the human population. According to a paper, a "special form of meningitis of unknown origin" was observed. In 1953 (the year the Romanian dimbovitza leptonema was isolated), there was one such meningo-encephalitis outbreak. The paper detailed case histories of two-hundred and eight patients. The agent was found to be indistinguishable from Czech encephalitis, Russian spring-summer encephalitis,* Australian encephalitis (a/k/a Murray valley), or Louping-ill viruses. The sheep tick was found to be the main vector of these infections. These are all flaviviruses which can infect and replicate inside cells (intracellular infection). Flaviviruses may be degraded reoviruses in the sense that they may have mutated and lost some of their genes as compared to an intact reovirus that has not reassorted in an insect's body.[66-68]

**Russian Spring-Summer Encephalitis (RSSE) is also called Taiga encephalitis (think Taiga tick).*

In June of 1955, a Yugoslavian railway signalman contracted a case of meningo-encephalitis. He recalled having many tick bites. In July of the year, one-hundred and forty ticks were collected from the forest area where the man had worked. The virus strain isolated belonged to the RSSE and Louping ill group of arboviruses. It is possible that among the insect viruses collected and processed to augment early microbial insecticides in Europe were rabies and its sindbis relatives which are common infections in insects and animals. The question is if these kinds of viruses were collected and used in this manner, were they now leading to human encephalitis cases?[66,67]

It is interesting that scientists on both sides of the globe were busy studying members of the encephalitis group of viruses. These viruses have a close kinship with the African sindbis virus, and the plant and insect reoviruses. The sindbis virus has been used in recombinant constructs since the 1950s. The sindbis virus was determined by Russian scientists Shubladze and colleague Margulis to be antigenically identical to the rabies virus.[68-70]

Drs. Margulis and Shubladze were developing a vaccine for Multiple Sclerosis/tickborne encephalitis at the time, and were using an "S.V." strain of acute encephalomyelitis. This was probably a street virus strain of rabies, or could have been its ancestor, sindbis. It is noteworthy to state that in 1965 Russian scientists had investigated a fatal case of RSSE in the village of Aleksee-Nikol'sk that had occurred two years earlier in 1963. Cases of leptospirosis had also been found in that region of the outbreak. What was this curious correlation between insect viruses and leptospira bacteriae? What I should point out is that the village is located in the Kavalerovo *mining* district in the Primorskiy Kray (region).[68-73]

By 1972, three years before the outbreak of Lyme arthritis in the US, Russian scientists were studying the antigenic features of alphaviruses including West Nile (a mosquito-borne flavivirus) and sindbis. Were scientists concerned that genetically engineered chimera were failing in the presence of mixed infections transmitted by mosquitoes and ticks? In 1968 and 1970, a new tickborne group B viral agent that is related to the RSSE virus was isolated from African bird ticks (*Argas hermanni*) collected from pigeon pet shops in Kabul City, Afghanistan; and from pigeon houses on the Royal Farm near Kabul. The new virus was named royal farm virus, and was found to be closely related to powassan and langat viruses, two arboviruses found in the US. While all of these viruses are closely related to one another, they are also closely related to the sindbis virus and the rabies virus (rabies is antigenically identical to sindbis). According to a WHO bulletin from 1960, there is a large group of tick-transmissible arboviruses that on the surface appear to be considerably variable, however they are so closely related that they are felt to be variant strains of the sindbis virus.[69,70,74,75]

We may question the objectives of the Burgdorfer et al. studies of rabies, WEE, and tickborne leptospirosis when undertaken. Was there a novel organism that was already appearing in Eastern Europe (i.e. Russia, Romania, Slovenia) as well as the US (i.e. Georgia, Illinois)? Were scientists of the day already aware of, and attempting to identify these novel agents and how they were spreading among animal and possibly human populations? Were there concerns that these agents would soon be vectored into global human populations since they were showing up in Europe?

In 1957 in an historic event, a half dozen female Russian scientists including Dr. Shubladze (who was working on the vaccine for tickborne encephalitis/Multiple Sclerosis), made an unprecedented visit to the US to several universities including Washington University School of Medicine in St. Louis, Missouri. The institution has a close working relationship with agrochemical companies. Indeed in a recent announcement, the university partnered with AstraZeneca to study Alzheimer's disease, an illness that may be caused by Lyme spirochetes. Was the 1957 visit, which was the first time Russian scientists had entered the states since WWII, an indication that a serious agricultural problem had been detected, and that it was responsible for the creation of mutated leptospires? Were scientists brainstorming about how to solve a problem that was expected to become a major public health issue in the decades to come? Or was their visit merely a coincidence in timing, and quite possibly, subject matter?[76-84]

Spiroplasma 277F

Years ago I began second-guessing whether *Borrelia burgdorferi,* the Lyme disease agent was exactly as it has been described to be. I knew what I had experienced as a patient, and my experiences simply did not reconcile with the image that public health experts painted for this illness. That was my first clue that something was not quite right. The logic behind the scientific comparisons of an extremely complex Bb spirochete to its supposed "dumb cousin" Syphilis (which by the way shares few remarkable genes in common with Bb) simply did not make sense to me. Knowing that a case of "mistaken identity" was unlikely, I began to search for answers to what lie behind the mask of Lyme disease – an organism that for decades has been surrounded by hidden agendas and conspiracy theories. As patient, all I wanted were answers. Why wouldn't my doctors say the words "Lyme disease?" Why couldn't I get medications to treat this thing? Why was I still sick after oral, intramuscular, and intravenous medicines and a list of "other" therapies? What was to become of my life and my family when I could no longer function?

I became more concerned about what appeared to me to be the "hidden truths" concerning Lyme disease after reading a paper by Dr. Willy Burgdorfer and two colleagues from 1968. The paper described the discovery and identification of a novel spirochete isolated by Dr. Burgdorfer and colleagues. According to their account, an unidentified spirochete which they named the 277F agent was isolated in 1967 from western Montana rabbit ticks. The agent was found fourteen years before the Lyme disease organism would subsequently be identified by, and named after Dr. Burgdorfer. It is entirely possible that the Bb spirochete of Lyme disease was named after Dr. Burgdorfer specifically because of these early studies, and also because the Bb organism may be composed in part by the genes of the spiroplasmas; such as those from the 277F agent that Dr. Burgdorfer's team isolated.[1]

Spiroplasmas are essentially plant fungi, and under darkfield microscopy they appear corkscrew-like and tightly coiled. Experiments were undertaken which involved the inoculation of chicken embryos with the 277F agent. The organisms were maintained in non-fertile eggs and in an enriched culture media. The 277F agent was filterable at smaller sizes, was heat and antibiotic resistant, and noted to be markedly inhibited by streptomycin and broad-spectrum antibiotics. The 277F spiroplasma demonstrated both granules and spherical bodies which elongated into curved rods (divisional forms). These forms are characteristic of fungi and some bacteria. The 277F agent also exhibited motile spirochetes just as is seen with the agent of Lyme disease that Dr. Burgdorfer helped identify more than a dozen years later.[1]

Colonies of the 277F agent exhibited granular centers and were surrounded by satellite colonies that were smaller in size (biofilms or slime aggregates). The granular forms were felt to either represent localized detachments from the spirochetal envelope, or else they were products of self-propagation (autolysis). The researchers felt that the granular forms of 277F might remain infectious and fully capable of producing viable spirochetes, much like the granules found in some fungi and in Bb spirochetes. The 277F agent was not thought to be a derivative of the relapsing fever spirochetes *Borrelia recurrentis, B.*

duttonii, or *B. anserina* according to another source, and this is important because this indicates that spiroplasmas are different spirochetes than the relapsing fever strains.[1,2]

The 277F tick strain of spiroplasma is said to have a system of 3 nm thread-like filaments on the exterior layer of its outer membrane, similar to those found in filamentous fungi. In a research paper from 1978, two distinct phages were cultivated from the 277F agent. These phages were said to be similar to viruses that typically associate with *Spiroplasma citri. S. citri* causes "stubborn disease" of citrus plants, and brittle root disease in horseradish plants. In a 1978 citrus industry textbook, photographs of *Spiroplasma citri* cells at x13,000 magnification show sack-like blebs, and spiral filaments that look much like the spirochete of *Borrelia burgdorferi.* The *Spiroplasma citri* organism at x36,000 magnification displays typical spherical or rounded cells. Citrus spiroplasmas are said to be completely inhibited by the antibiotics erythromycin, neomycin, tetracycline, and thallium acetate.[1-8]

One Yale paper reported that the 277F spiroplasma may not be a natural inhabitant of the rabbit tick, and also that it probably did not originate from an arthropod source. The 277F spiroplasma was thought to be a parasite of hares and rabbits, with ticks acting only as a mechanical vector. This would imply that the 277F spiroplasma may have originated from the soil, a plant, animal, or even a laboratory. Spiroplasmas are plant parasites that are transmitted by the insects which feed and/or walk upon them. Spiroplasmas have possibly also inadvertently become cell culture contaminants. Since several kinds of mollicutes have been deployed to control mosquito populations, their distribution is by now probably ubiquitous. However it has become clear to me that the spiroplasmas only emerged on the scene since the early 1940s when they were first isolated. Therefore they are probably a novel mutated form of plant pathogens that came about from the deployment of chemical, nuclear, microbial, or other "pollutants." However they have arrived, the problem for us now is they are present in ticks that bite humans, and which transmit Lyme disease and other tickborne infections.[9-12]

A Yale paper commented about the effectiveness of the antibiotics chloramphenicol and streptomycin against the 277F spiroplasma, with the former as the most effective. Twenty-two years later Drs. Barbour and Hayes would write that *Borrelia burgdorferi* are also sensitive to chloramphenicol. Additional antibiotics penicillin and sodium sulfadiazine were shown not to be effective against 277F in one study. Chloramphenicol because of its toxicity to human bone marrow, is not a commonly used antibiotic.[13,14]

A 1978 article described how spiroplasma 277F was a helical, motile mycoplasma. Despite the name, mycoplasmas are fungi-like bacteria. The paper described Burgdorfer's 1967 find and detailed how *digitonin* (derived from *Digitalis purpurea*) *inhibited growth of the 277F organism.* Colonies of 277F revealed granular centers surrounded by smaller "satellite" colonies. This seems to describe biofilms which the Bb spirochete is said to either form or utilize in the body to protect itself. I realized that the 277F agent could be an organism that aggregates with other microbes, or a pathogen that may be mistaken for another spirochete. In fact one publication from 1982 also indicates that the 277F agent could be easily mistaken for another spirochete. According to the paper, "helical forms were recognized earlier but could not be cultured and were thought to be spirochetes." The references cited in the paper include Burgdorfer et al.'s 1967 spirochete from the rabbit tick, and a 1961 sex-ratio spiroplasma agent that had been isolated from fruit flies.[15-18]

In another paper, a cloned 277F agent was found to be antigenically different from the suckling mouse cataract agent, the corn stunt, and the citrus spiroplasmas. The 277F agent was also weakly cross-reactive with *S. citri,* and exhibited threadlike filaments (flagella) in the exterior layer of its membrane covering. Drs. Burgdorfer and Brinton demonstrated that the 277F agent's structure and form was similar to other spiroplasmas. Dr. Burgdorfer placed the 277F spiroplasma in the *Actinomycetes* class of gram-positive bacteria. This is an interesting choice as this class contains organisms that are both mold- and bacteria-like.[19-23]

The most mold-like forms resemble *Fungi imperfecti* (imperfect fungi) more so than they do the bacteria-like *Actinobacteridae,* which has several subclasses including *Actinomycetes* and *Bifidobacteriales.* Many of the actinomycetes bacteriae reproduce by segmenting and sporulating. These organisms can break apart into spiral-shapes (spirillum), rods (bacillary), or round granular (coccoid) forms. All forms are very fragile and capable of producing new organisms. Similar forms are created by Bb spirochetes. Indeed the Bb organism may be composed in part by spiroplasmas that have mutated with a member of the actinomycetes subclass of fungal bacteria. We know that spiroplasmas are found within the guts of Lyme-transmitting ticks, but so are the *Fungi imperfecti.* It should be noted that the Bb genome, just like fungi imperfecti, contains multiple plasmids. If Bb plasmids were examined genetically, they may have proven in part to be of spiroplasma and fungal origins. Perhaps each component of an aggregate Bb spirochete is "inconvenient" for the world to know.[19-23]

In 1982 after Burgdorfer et al. announced the discovery of the causative agent of Lyme disease, scientists at the mycoplasma section of the laboratory of molecular microbiology of the NIAID in Frederick, Maryland were studying mycoplasmas and acholeplasmas (mollicutes) of plants and insects. Their studies were published in a Yale journal. The paper makes reference to "newly developed culture mediums" which it says "should be applied to those situations where one suspects involvement of mycoplasmas or other mollicutes."[24]

This paper seems to be referring to a culture medium that Dr. Barbour specifically modified to isolate the Bb spirochete in 1981. Scientists were long aware that spiroplasmas were present within insect bodies, and so the search for the pathogenic agent of Lyme disease should have included the screening of culture samples for spiroplasmas, especially since Dr. Burgdorfer was personally familiar with tick spiroplasmas for at least two decades. We might assume that scientists including Dr. Barbour would have used any culture medium capable of isolating any mollicutes that might be present. Yet I found no mention of screening for any mollicutes in the Yale article when I read the description of the Bb culture techniques used.[10]

In another paper we see evidence that in 1981 there was a culture medium that was newly developed for newly isolated plant and insect mycoplasmas (i.e. spiroplasmas). According to the paper, this medium is called "SP-4" and it "markedly improved" the recovery of *Mycoplasma pneumonia* from human clinical materials. The paper was published July of 1981, the period when Dr. Alan Barbour modified the BSK-II medium to better culture the possible agent of Lyme disease. I happen to be a Lyme patient who was bitten by ticks, and like many Lyme patients, I have antibodies to *Mycoplasma pneumonia*.[25]

The report also described potential reasons why it might be difficult to recover mycoplasmas from hosts and from cultures. Some of those reasons are due to the presence of antibiotics or drugs in fluids or tissues; the presence of inhibitors or enzymes in tissues; the presence of antibodies in samples; or too low of antibody levels in samples. The report described new mycoplasmas including spiroplasma strains G-37 and M-30; as well as a new mycoplasma from laboratory mice, *Mycoplasma muris*. The paper also discussed the tick spiroplasma strains including some "Y32" strains that were cultured from *Ixodes pacificus* and *Dermacentor variabilis* ticks – ticks that transmit Lyme disease to humans.[25]

The paper says that the discovery of spiroplasmas as important inhabitants and pathogens of plant and insect hosts has had a "profound" effect on the study of prokaryotes.* It cites the SP-4 culture medium as an important tool in screening for these pathogens. The document said that some organisms with properties similar to *Mycoplasma genitalium* or *Mycoplasma muris* may escape detection under conventional culture techniques. Is this why Dr. Barbour modified the culture medium to the new BSK-II formula – to better culture these particular organisms when analyzing tick cultures for the Bb spirochete?[24,26,27]

**Cells that lack a membrane are the prokaryotes.*

If so, we can certainly ask whether the scientists who studied these tick cultures in their search for a causative agent of Bb found any spiroplasmas or other mollicutes in the process. By the way, two later publications discuss the presence of various mycoplasma strains that were isolated from desert tortoises and gopher tortoises in the western United States. Could scientists in Romania and the US have also been looking for spiroplasmas when screening turtle sera, bull semen, and other wildlife during the 1950s and 1960s? When they discovered mutated leptospires (leptonema), we can wonder if they also found spiroplasmas as well.[26,27]

Will the Real Bb Stand Up?

A 1967 World Health Organization document described the difficulty of classifying leptospires into two groups, the saprophytic "non-pathogenic" and the "pathogenic" strains. A group of experts from Italy, Denmark, USSR, USA, Hungary, Japan, France, Israel, The Netherlands, and Czechoslovakia met July 18-21, 1966 at the WHO leptospirosis reference laboratory at the Gamaleja Institute of Epidemiology and Microbiology in Moscow. There experts discussed leptospirosis research and the reclassification of these spirochetes.[1]

What came out of the discussions was a recommendation that the current practice of linking *Leptospira interrogans* strains with parasitism, and *Leptospira biflexa* strains with saprophytism be discontinued. The group suggested instead that the genus *Leptospira* be considered monospecific until individual species could be identified with greater confidence. The group gave the name *Leptospira interrogans* to all leptospires, whether saprophytic or pathogenic, yet they still classified the strains by their serological differences. Regardless of how the strains are classified, the WHO group preferred to think of them as one collective genotype. Scientists felt that leptospira serogroups could not be clearly defined at the time. The article indicated that the current arrangement of serogroups had limitations; specifically since some strains might be allocated to either group.[1]

This is an interesting observation because what it does for the story I tell is to legitimize the idea that so-called saprophyte/saprotrophs can be pathogenic to humans. If we consider that water-borne leptospires can mutate and aggregate with other bacteriae and viruses to become an important human pathogen, we can stop playing the taxonomic "name game." Instead we may embrace the idea that the leptospires of soil or water origin may be at the heart of an organism that causes Lyme disease. At the time of the WHO report in 1967, the only leptospira strains identified as "parasitic" were these:[1]

L. ictohaemorrhagiae	*L. javanica*	*L. canicola*	*L. castellonis*	*L. pyrogenes*
L. butembo	*L. autumnalis*	*L. bratislava*	*L. pomona*	*L. grippotyphosa*
L. wolffii	*L. borincana*	*L. bataviae*	*L. tarassovi**	*L. patoc*

**Formerly named hyos*

Notice there was no mention of leptonema strains in this 1967 WHO report, even though these were already detected in Romania by 1953; and by the CDC in Atlanta, Georgia, and Dixon Springs, Illinois, beginning in 1965. Each of these dates occurred prior to this WHO meeting. Did the WHO not have the information about the new leptonema strains? The document noted under the *Leptospira autumnalis* group, types "Fort-bragg Fort Bragg" (isolated from a human in 1942); "Louisiana LSU 1945" (US armadillo); and "Orleans LSU 2580" (US coypu or nutria – a semiaquatic otter-like rodent). (Fort Bragg is located in North Carolina). In the *tarassovi group* we find "Atlantae reference strain LT 81" (US opossum-1955). Rodents, birds, insectivores, reptiles, carnivores, ruminants, and other mammals were determined to be hosts of leptospirosis. The report also noted that animals could carry more than one leptospirosis strain at a time. We now know they can also carry mutated *leptonema.*[1]

What exactly are the leptonemas? Obviously they are a mutated, intermediate form of spirochete, most likely a leptospira. While we know there are unmutated leptospires in the environment, what exactly may have mutated with the leptospires of soil and water to create the new, intermediate forms? When we remember that borrelia are simply some kind of spirochete that is tick-transmitted, we might also think about the tick-transmitted relapsing fevers.

According to the older literature, *Spironema* and *Treponema* are groups of parasitic spirochetes that cause human diseases including Syphilis, Yaws, and the relapsing fevers of animals and humans. There are also non-pathogenic strains that can be found on or near the oral, alimentary, and genital mucous membranes.[2-4]

In the earlier literature there was division between the two groups spironema and treponema, based largely upon their different forms (rigid vs. flexible). Eventually they were lumped into a single group *Treponemes*. There is little difficulty distinguishing the treponemes and spironemas from the leptospiras or other spirochetes. The literature also clearly refers to the spironema which cause relapsing fevers in animals and humans. Examples include *Spironema recurrentis,* and *Spironema duttoni.* We may recognize these today as *Borrelia recurrentis* and *Borrelia duttoni,* or the relapsing fever spirochetes. Remember that "borrelia" only denotes that an organism is tick-transmitted. Therefore a leptonema spirochete that is an intermediate form of a leptospira could be called a borrelia strain if transmitted by a tick.[2,4,5]

We also know there was a human spirochete discovered in 1917 by Hideyo Noguchi which was named *Leptospira Noguchi* 1917, which was later added to a novel leptonema family. This is the same family where we find the leptonema that were discovered in a Romanian river, and in Illinois bulls and turtles. In the case of the Noguchi leptonema, the organism was probably formed from a pathogenic "infectious jaundice" (yellow fever) leptospira that mutated with a spirochete (treponema) normally found in human flora.[3]

The possible candidates for the mutant *Leptospira Noguchi* that were identified at the time of discovery included the so-called non-pathogenic *Spironema refringens, Treponema calligyrum,* and *Treponema minutum* (a novel species). *T. calligyrum* was said to stand somewhere between a Syphilis spirochete and *Spironema refringens*, a relapsing fever. Remember that the agents of "yellows" diseases of plants include spiroplasmas and their satellite viruses. Did Noguchi's agent include a non-mutated plant spirillum? Are those plant spirillum one half of the spirillum-fungi mutants we find as spiroplasmas today?[2-7]

We may imagine that the Romanian river and the Illinois bull and turtle leptonema strains also involved a pathogenic yellows agent (spiroplasma) as well as a mutated soil or water-borne leptospira to create the animal leptonemas. These were similar to those found in 1917 by Dr. Noguchi. Remember also that in 1917 the agent of polio was isolated by Dr. Noguchi. Was the leptonema that he found responsible for polio outbreaks of his day? Did that leptonema include a natural extremophile bacterium? Did the early applied agricultural insecticides or virus-carrying parasitoid insects transmit viruses that were able to create a mutant leptonema in Noguchi's day? Was Noguchi's strain the result of the earliest chemical or agricultural pollutants?

What is the difference between the odd leptospira from 1917 that may have caused polio, and the odd spirochetes of today which cause polio-like symptoms? Furthermore, why did it take so long for another leptonema strain to be identified after the initial 1917 Noguchi strain? Many of the same chemical pollutants that were used industrially in Noguchi's day are still in use today. Perhaps the only difference between the leptonema of Noguchi's era and those of today are the far more virulent insecticides and newer chemical formulas now found as pollutants. Today's leptonemas probably contain recombinant microbes and other contaminants than were available in the environment of Noguchi's day.

Connecticut Rheumatologist Dr. Allen Steere and colleagues from the University of Minnesota, the CDC, and a veterinary lab in Denmark published a scientific paper in 1986 which revealed the discovery of an important novel human pathogenic leptospira. Their paper described the discovery in August 1981 of a novel leptospira that was cultured from the skin of a 69-year-old man. The man had been bitten by an *Ixodes dammini* tick on May 1, 1981, and developed all the acute symptoms of Lyme disease. The Steere et al. group isolated from a culture of the patient's ECM rash, a new leptospira strain that they temporarily named *Leptospira strain 10.*[8]

Steere et al. performed antibody testing upon strain 10. The scientists did not consider it to be a member of an existing group because it did not react strongly to other members of the group against which it was tested. Using hyperimmune rabbit antiserum, the strain was tested against *L. interrogans* celledoni, a "straight" spirochetal strain that was isolated in 1952 from an Australian man. *L. celledoni** was the only leptospira strain that strain 10 reacted to serologically, although the reaction was at a low titer (1:400).[8]

**L. celledoni is also a serogroup of the species L. borgpetersenii, which includes L. tarassovi, a turtle strain. The novel Leptospira inadai*

Lyme is from the species Leptospira inadai icterohaemorrhagiae, serogroup Ictero, which describes an animal pathogen that was part rodent (inadai), part cattle agent (icterohaemorrhagiae). The new L. inadai lyme strain was placed into a pathogenic leptospira group (genera).

The paper said that strain 10 did not react to 6% of the same (homologous) titer of any recognized *Leptospira interrogans* groups. This 6% rate is required in order to be considered as a new serovar within an existing serogroup. This means that the new strain 10 was probably a unique leptospira organism, a novel mutant, or an intermediate form. It is interesting also that human serum that was used came from an Australian as opposed to an American patient. Perhaps this is because a fungal infection that may be part of a novel Bb spirochete is more common among Australian citizens than Americans (coccidioidomycosis). Scientists may have been attempting to determine whether strain 10 contained this important fungal component as well as a leptospira agent. Animal testing was performed with strain 10 on an African green and a spider monkey; and upon hamsters and guinea pigs. The new strain caused animal infections in each species tested. Next the scientists compared the fatty acid content of the spirochete with known pathogenic leptospires. Strain 10 was similar to, but outside the range of known saprophytic and pathogenic leptospires.[8,9]

The DNA relatedness of strain 10 was next compared to thirty-nine pathogenic leptospires including *L. interrogans, L. parva,* and *Leptonema illini;* and five *L. biflexa* saprophytes. The new strain 10 had less than a 10% relationship to any of the strains studied. The sample was also tested to ensure that it was not a culture contaminant. The organism was determined to be "intrinsically present" and not a contaminant. The paper claims that no leptospires were found in any other cultures that day. This may simply have been because spirochetes are extremely fragile and difficult to culture.[2]

Most significant is that the culture medium used was wholly inadequate in 1981 when scientists including Drs. Steere, Barbour, Burgdorfer, and others were attempting to culture the Bb agent and the novel leptospira strain 10. As a result of these difficulties, Dr. Barbour developed a modified culture medium that was subsequently named BSK-II. By August 1981, the new leptospira strain 10 that Steere et al. cultured from the Lyme patient's skin just three months earlier was either never retested in the newly modified BSK-II medium; or if it was, the results of those tests remained conspicuously unpublished. *The new Leptospira strain #10 was subsequently renamed by Steere et al. to be Leptospira inadai serovar Lyme.*[2,10]

The authors of the Steere et al. paper published comments that could have allowed a very different conclusion than what was offered. First, the wavelength of the "strain 10" leptospira organism was declared to be comparable to that of other leptonema. This of course refers to the Noguchi, illini, and dimbovitza strains which are the other members of the leptonema group, to which this strain would eventually be added. Other physical characteristics were described as compatible with other leptospires. What they were looking at from the Lyme patient's skin biopsy was probably a mutated, intermediate form of leptospira that was similar to, or identical to one or more previously discovered leptonema strains (i.e. dimbovitza, bull, turtle).[2,10]

Furthermore, antibodies to leptospira strain 10 and Bb were found in serum samples from the Lyme patient who provided the skin biopsy that produced strain 10. Yet the antibody levels for strain 10 were "considerably lower" than those "typically detected" in other leptospirosis patients. This may be so because the mutated strain 10 did not provoke as strong an antibody response as expected from a normal non-mutated leptospirosis infection. A reduced response would not be odd for a mutated leptospira, and we know strain 10 was probably a mutant. If we read the paper carefully we find that the antibodies to strain 10 and Bb are described as if they are the very same antibodies; not as if they are produced by two different organisms. Finally, the antibody titers produced by Bb were "consistent" with the serologic diagnostic criteria for Lyme disease.[2,10]

To Steere et al, the novel leptospira was probably similar to other leptonema. It also provoked a weak cross-reactive response to unmutated leptospires, and an expected reaction to Bb antibodies. The writers may have been indirectly stating that the novel agent was in fact a leptonema. They may have also indirectly revealed that *the leptonema agent is the causative agent of Lyme disease* that was renamed *Borrelia burgdorferi.* However they seem to have carefully avoided this specific statement within the publication. Instead their conclusions appear to entirely minimize the leptonema's presence. The only conclusions they published are:

- that leptospira strain 10 was "intrinsically" present in the skin biopsy sample (everywhere).
- that based on morphology (shape, form), strain 10 was a mutant leptospira or leptonema.
- that despite animal pathogenicity, they did not feel the "available evidence" supported an etiologic role for the organism in the culture-positive patient's Lyme infection. (This means the leptonema was not considered part of the patient's infection!)

The culture medium could have been directly responsible for the lack of "available evidence." Remember the culture medium used to detect spirochete 10 was of a kind before Dr. Barbour modified the medium to better detect spirochetes. We may assume that strain 10 was retested in the modified Barbour medium. If it was, the results have gone conspicuously unreported unless after modification strain 10 was simply renamed as the Bb agent. If it was not, new evidence could have been gathered during a retest in the new culture medium at any time from 1981 to the present day. It would appear strange that with the advent of a new culture medium at Rocky Mountain Labs, that no one would have retested strain 10. The discovery of an important new leptonema in a Lyme patient was certainly nothing to dismiss.

Steere et al. named the new strain 10 mutant *Leptospira inadai Lyme* after Japanese physician Ryokichi Inada, who studied the etiologic agent of Weil's disease. The name "Lyme" should appear obvious since the name originated from the Lyme patient sample that came from the area of the Connecticut "juvenile arthritis" outbreak.[8,10]

If we look up the agent of Weil's disease, we find it is a leptospirosis infection that is also called rat catcher's *yellows,* Fort

Bragg fever, 7-day fever, or canicola fever. The agent of Weil's is a rodent leptospira according to modern literature. This pathogen causes acute infections which present with an enlarged spleen, jaundice, and nephritis. If we look up the "Fort Bragg" serotype of the serogroup *Leptospira autumnalis,* we find other serotypes listed, including rachmati, sumatrana, bulgarica, bangkinang, erinacei-auriti, morris, sentot, Louisiana, Orleans, djasiman and gurungi. These are all classified in the *Leptospira interrogans* pathogenic group. Perhaps this is why the three patents I described earlier listed a *Leptospira interrogans serovar Lyme,* or a pathogenic leptospira strain.[8,10,11]

In the older literature Weil's disease is said to be caused by a member of the proteus group (protozoans). Why this could be interesting is if the strain 10 discovered by Dr. Steere et al. included a protozoan-like spiroplasma, and a leptospira. Remember that plant, insect, and animal guts harbor plant spirillum. Since spiroplasmas appear to be a recent emergence, a mutated spirillum could have met up with a leptospira strain and a fungus to create a mutant, intermediate leptonema. This sounds complex but it really isn't when we consider that all kinds of bacteria/fungi/protozoans etc. will reassort in the presence of mutagenic chemicals or microbes that promote these activities. If we think about the *leptospirillum* that are found deep in the ground; the plant spirillum-fungi, and the water or soil-borne leptospires, we can see how a mutant organism may be formed in a highly polluted environment.[8,10-12]

The carefully selected name "inadai" after the Japanese physician who studied an agent of rodent leptospirosis (i.e. sewer rats) provides an important clue to the idea that those who carefully selected this spirochete's name may have understood the origins of the Bb agent about to be officially identified and announced to the world. However the leptospira relationship to the Lyme patient's ECM rash was never effectively and publicly communicated at the time, nor any time since, for over three decades as I write this book. What caused this important connection to fall between the cracks of the scientific, clinical, and public arenas?[8,11]

While we wonder why no one declared a connection between the rash-cultured leptonema and the human infection known as Lyme disease, I did find an important comment made by Steere et al. in a 2006 article:

> "Bb strains vary in their capacity to disseminate, but almost all strains isolated from EM lesions sometimes cause disseminated disease."

If this is true, then it would seem pertinent for scientists to have spoken up about the odd spirochete they cultured from the Lyme patient's rash in 1981 since it could very well have been directly involved in the Lyme patient's disease![8,11,13]

The Lyme patient from whom the new leptonema was isolated, was reportedly bitten by an *Ixodes* nymph tick on **May 1, 1981.** The discovery of the new strain 10 was made by Steere et al. in **August of the same year.** Suddenly in **September and October,** tick collections were extensively undertaken at Shelter Island, New York, where Lyme disease was already known to be endemic. Obviously the discovery of a novel spirochete flagged the attention of these scientists to cause a sudden and intense interest in tick specimens. Since Dr. Burgdorfer was studying leptospires and relapsing fever ticks during the early 1950s, we may now understand that his role in the identification of the Bb agent was no coincidence.[8,10,11]

Dr. Burgdorfer was probably already aware of the animal *illini* leptonema mutants since he was given a 1953 swine strain from Illinois during *L. pomona* studies soft ticks in 1956. He was aware of the novel 277F rabbit tick spiroplasmas because he first isolated them in 1967. Dr. Burgdorfer was therefore a good candidate to be charged with the identification of the Lyme disease agent since he was well versed in the novel agents emerging in ticks and animals over the previous three decades. Some of these same agents were probably now present in the body of at least one important Lyme patient.[8,10,11,38,39]

Just three months after the discovery of *Leptospira inadai Lyme,* adult *Ixodes* ticks were collected on Shelter Island by Dr. Jorge Benach and co-workers. The ticks were sent to Drs. Burgdorfer, Barbour, and colleagues at Rocky Mountain Labs. Dr. Burgdorfer provided the Shelter Island tick midgut tissue pools to Dr. Barbour on **November 13, 1981** to culture in his brand new, specially modified, mutant-spirochete-friendly BSK-II culture medium. In the process of examining the Shelter Island ticks, Dr. Barbour uncovered gram-positive rod-like bacteria (B.t.?) and an *Actinomycete*-like organism (spiroplasma?) along with nematodes and novel "Bb" (leptonema?) spirochetes from the tick midgut pools. Still no mention of these critical discoveries hit the ears of the interested public except to say they found a causative agent of Lyme disease they named Bb.[8,10,11]

Dr. Barbour's new medium did reveal the causative agent of Lyme, which was named *Borrelia burgdorferi* strain "B31." The question is whether the midgut pools from the Shelter Island ticks produced the very same leptonema that Dr. Steere et al. had isolated from the Lyme patient's skin culture. If so, it is possible that at least one scientist realized the possible origins of an emerging human epidemic.[14-16]

If this occurred, it could explain the events of the day including the later "standardization" of surveillance criteria and laboratory diagnostic tests for Lyme disease, the alleged confiscation of an NIH scientist's laboratory notes; what appeared to be retaliatory measures taken against physicians/researchers who attempted to tell the truth about Lyme disease, or doctors who treat patients outside the "standards of care" established by a core group. It may also explain verbal attacks against Lyme patients or advocates; the media or scientific spin-doctoring of Lyme disease; and the political backlash surrounding all things Lyme-related.[14-16]

It is extremely important to examine the connections between a leptonema from a Lyme patient's rash and the Bb agent. If scientists recognized the connections between the Bb agent and animals, they may have suspected that agricultural, industrial, medical, and/or nuclear "wastes" may have had something to do with the spirochete's origins, and an upcoming human epidemic that was emerging in many parts of the world, not just Connecticut. If this is what happened, we might expect to see a flurry of research grants and studies aimed at investigating the origins of these novel human pathogens. Copious research on each of these aspects did subsequently follow in what appears to have been a mad dash for research funding to determine the "origins" of Lyme disease. At the same time, Lyme disease and its patients were strategically dismissed, probably in the hope that the epidemic would remain regional, or that no one would figure out the source(s) of what would become a global epidemic.

We can also guess that when Steere et al. cultivated the new spirochete fourteen years after Burgdorfer first isolated the 277F rabbit tick spiroplasma, whether the novel spirochete named "inadai Lyme" was quietly renamed *Borrelia burgdorferi* in honor of Dr. Burgdorfer's earlier discovery. If so, why would the spiroplasma and the leptonema connections (and whatever other pathogens were found inside Lyme-transmitting ticks remain "unannounced" to the public?[38,39]

Is this because scientists were following "evidence-based" logic and there was no "conclusive" evidence yet that each of the pathogens found were contributing to Lyme disease? Did the scientists fully comprehend what they were studying? Or as some people may speculate, was the reason for the "silence" about certain aspects of study because there was a relationship between the pathogens found in the Shelter Island ticks, in the Lyme patient's ECM rash, and in the biocides or chemicals of the day that demanded further study? Would such studies be left up to Dr. Steere and his colleagues to pursue? Was there a public health directive issued to EIS employees which mandated silence about any relationships between tick pathogens, human illness, and industrial or agricultural "wastes"?[8,10,11,15]

The Shelter Island tick collections which took place immediately on the heels of Dr. Steere et al.'s discovery of the leptonema they named "inadai Lyme" appears to have been ordered specifically to determine whether or not the patient's infection was an isolated incident. Indeed it was not as the Lyme disease "agent" would be isolated from the Shelter Island tick pools. Dr. Burgdorfer was bestowed the honor of having the organisms named after him since he was the first to identify the "agent" of Lyme disease, or so we have been told. This ability probably came easily to him since he was well versed in the spiroplasmas, reoviruses, insect symbionts, and animal leptospires he and his colleagues had been studying for nearly three decades. Just because the agent of Lyme disease was called something other than the leptonema discovered by Steere et al., does not mean that strain 10, *Leptospira inadai Lyme,* and "Bb" are not the same, or similar organisms capable of causing Lyme disease.[8,10,11,38,39]

Note also that the nymph tick that bit the Lyme patient with the new strain was the same species of tick (*Ixodes dammini*) collected at Shelter Island, and from which the Bb agent would be isolated. This is not how "the story" usually goes when told by the scientists. Sources claim that "other" ticks were the original target of study but were somehow seasonally "unavailable" and other tidbits which don't seem to reconcile with the published research.[2,8,10]

By the way, a photograph in a *Science* article shows an electron micrograph of Bb spirochetes in the vicinity of the microvilli brush border membranes of a tick's midgut. This is the main infection entry point in insects, arthropods, animals, and humans which involve Bb, leptospirosis, and the applied insecticide *Bacillus thuringiensis* (B.t.).[2,8,10]

To date Steere et al.'s important findings of a novel leptospira's probable connections to Lyme disease have never really been discussed in a manner that would properly present the event to the public. We may ask why this is so even though the scientists had claimed that the new leptospira strain was "intrinsically present" in the Lyme patient's skin sample at the time of discovery. The lack of "public" discussion is curious, especially by a key scientist who first isolated and helped name the novel strain. This individual was perhaps the most influential voice at the Dearborn conference. His recommendations influenced the Lyme disease diagnostic testing process, and medical guidelines for decades to come. His recommendations would also significantly impact an upcoming Lyme vaccine for which he would run clinical trials.[8,17,18]

Such highly significant information and clues to important connections remained unpublished until five years after the announcement of the causative agent of Lyme disease. By then the public was not paying close attention to the published research because Lyme was still a newly emerging disease, and not yet considered to be a global epidemic. Was such a delay in publication because certain circles did not desire that connections be made between a human infection caused by the Bb agent, and a novel "Lyme" leptonema – a pathogen that may have had agriculturally and industrially important origins?[8]

Most people do not realize that Bb spirochetes are considered to be distinctly different than other borrelia spirochetes. If they are proven to contain a mutated leptonema, this would clearly make them different. The provision of the name "borrelia" as we have seen simply indicates that the agents are tick-transmitted. We know that "burgdorferi" represents Dr. Burgdorfer's last name. If the name "leptonema" or "spiroplasma" had been used to identify the Bb organism from the beginning of its identification forward, it is doubtful whether the huge paradigm of denial about Lyme disease could exist today.

However under another name, a novel organism may have provided a huge opportunity to research and patent the dickens out of everything Bb-related for years to come. Had the organism been categorized differently, perhaps valuable agricultural and industrial tools might have been called into question. If so, this could have caused a potential problem in terms of liability as well as product availability – but only if Bb is ever proven to have the kinds of relationships such as those described in this book. Remember the conclusions I make are speculative, and could be partly or entirely wrong.

Regardless of the name that was ultimately used to identify the agent of Lyme disease, it is not difficult to believe that soil, water, plant, or insect spirochetes of any kind are at the heart of an organism that through a process of mutational change and aggregation with other microbes, created a human epidemic. The combinations of mutating microbes that are formed as aggregates will determine the final number of "Bb" strains that ultimately exist; just as scientists have predicted will emerge over time.

When we look at the history of spirochetal research from 1951 to 1981, we see important events surrounding the discovery of the pathogen(s) of Lyme disease, and also the strikingly different, publicly-promoted interpretations of the events of the day. Typically these accounts exclude any mention of some of the most important events and discoveries by key persons in the scientific community. This failure to discuss the events completely may be due to an intentional effort to keep the origins of Lyme from public scrutiny. Upon close examination, the actual events when viewed along a timeline and from an untarnished, innocent perspective seem to paint a very different picture than what borrelia patent holders, researchers, and those with strong ties to government, academia, and important industries portray in personal interviews, consensus papers, sworn or other testimonials, or even in clinical practice guidelines for Lyme disease.

Shortly before the agent of Lyme disease was announced, the Steere et al. paper seemed to summarily dismiss the new leptonema strain as neither a causative nor a contributing factor to the Lyme patient's infection. We have yet to see this novel leptonema surface in any other source in connection to Lyme disease since these early studies. The organism was also not mentioned in another report co-authored by Drs. Steere, Barbour, and colleagues written in 1984, just three years after the Bb agent was first identified. The paper characterized the Lyme disease spirochete, but wasn't published until 1986; five years after its studies were performed and after the announcement of the Bb agent. Over a decade later one paper would finally reference the *Leptospira inadai* species, naming two strains: N10 (the original strain No. 10) and another, identified as EMJH 86.[8,19-22,38,39]

Although references were made in another study to the original ECM rash cultured in Steere et al.'s 1981 studies, there appears to be no mention of the name *Leptospira inadai Lyme;* not in the 1984 paper, and certainly not in an earlier 1983 paper cited by the 1984 paper, even though the earlier one was co-authored by Drs. Steere, Barbour, and Burgdorfer. "Nobody" cared to openly discuss either strain of a novel spirochete called *Leptospira inadai "Lyme"* in publications when discussing the etiologic agent of Lyme disease. We must ask why there was and continues to be such "silence" by three of the most influential scientists of the day or by their colleagues.[8,19-22,28]

The stunningly brief appearance and equally rapid disappearance of a link between a novel leptospira called *Leptospira inadai Lyme* and a patient with an ECM rash has been completely overlooked by just about everyone for decades. Was this an accident or was the novel leptospira simply renamed *Borrelia burgdorferi* and its connections to leptospires and other tick pathogens discretely hidden under its new name? After studying the research and the controversy surrounding the Lyme disease organism and the possible denial of illness in thousands of persons around the world, it might seem that while everyone was looking the other way, any known association between leptospires, spiroplasmas, (other tick pathogens) and the agent of Lyme disease slipped quietly out the laboratory door to disappear off into the sunset.[21]

In later years many new species of leptospires would be discovered, including seven isolates from rats, buffalo, and contaminated media. Each of these demonstrated DNA sequences similar to *Leptospira inadai Lyme.* One paper mentioned a type strain L60T. I looked up this strain in a culture database and found *Harposporium leptospira* drechsler, a soil fungal spirochete that is an internal pathogenic parasite of *nematodes.*[23-25]

Perhaps Dr. Steere et al's leptonema really was felt to be related to the biological controls of the day. At the time nematodes were widely deployed in agriculture, and Dr. Burgdorfer had already discovered nematodes (filaria) inside the bodies of ticks, years earlier. Perhaps the Steere group believed that the leptonema was present in the ECM culture simply because the Lyme-transmitting tick was co-infected with a nematode; so they chose to ignore its presence. Did they also realize its possible insect "biowarfare" connections?

In 1981 another novel leptospira strain was identified as a contaminant in a laboratory culture. This organism came from a bottle of bovine albumin medium (cattle blood protein). The novel organism was named *Leptospira parva* strain HT. It was shown to have characteristics in common with saprophytic and pathogenic leptospires. A similar strain was discovered in a sow in Ireland, and was identical to the bovine albumin contaminant. In 1982 (the year the Bb agent was announced), the *Leptospira parva* mutant was reclassified into a new genus called *Turneriella*, as *Turneriella parva.* It was reclassified by scientists from the meningitis and special pathogens branch of the bacterial and mycotic diseases center at the CDC in Atlanta, Georgia. The new strain is interesting because at the 1990 ICSB subcommittee on the taxonomy of leptospira, it was proposed to transfer *L. parva* from a leptospira genus into a new genus called *Turneria.*[23-28]

I wondered why scientists from the meningitis branch of mycotic (fungal) disease center were worried about the name of the new organism. Perhaps this leptospira mutant was found to be a fungal pathogen of cattle or ruminant deer. If so, it would have been disconcerting to scientists if it was believed to have anything to do with fungicides or other applied agricultural agents such as insecticides used on fungally-infected livestock feeds or their insect vectors.[23-28]

This novel species was also found to be distinctively different from other known leptospires, and the *Leptospira illini* strains (bulls, turtles). The name *Turneria* is the name of the genera of plants (*Dicotyledones: Turneraceae*) and animals (*Formicidae, Hymenoptera;* and *Sauroptergia, Reptilia*). Therefore the name may describe a unique leptospira with an intermediate mutant form that lies somewhere between a pathogenic and a saprophytic leptospire found in plants, animals, and aquatic reptiles.[28]

The organism may have mutated from pathogens found in animals and plants; or perhaps from insects, plants, and animals, if the name hymenoptera bears any weight. (Hymenoptera are sawflies, bees, wasps, ants.) "Turneria" comes from English Microbiologist Leslie Turner who contributed to the scientific knowledge of leptospirosis. It is possible that the Bb organism could be another example of a similarly mutated leptonema (intermediate form) that has aggregated with pathogens collected from plants, insects, and animals. If so we must question what is causing the leptospires to mutate and to form new intermediate species. The obvious answers are industrial and agricultural "wastes," and other matters of public health concern.[28]

In a paper published in 1984 by Dr. Willy Burgdorfer, it is stated that early hypotheses suggested that the ECM rash of Lyme disease was an allergic reaction to a tick toxin. This theory was abandoned once penicillin proved beneficial in treating the ECM rash. Since the ECM rash is a known aspect of Lyme infection, it is perplexing that the *Leptospira inadai Lyme* spirochete that Dr. Allen Steere et al. cultured from a Lyme patient's rash was dismissed as either inconsequential or unrelated to the patient's illness. Some may argue that Dr. Steere et al. had no idea what they cultured, or that they were simply following evidence-based science at the time. Since more than three decades have passed, there is no excuse for any scientist to remain silent about the early history of Lyme disease. There is also no reason to remain silent about the organisms that were cultured from ticks from the 1950s until the present day. Such disclosures may help scientists and physicians provide better diagnostic and treatment options for Lyme patients.[8,29]

After learning about the *Leptonema inadai Lyme* strain found in the Lyme patient's rash, I felt the following was of interest. The leptospira component of at least one Bb strain may be a strain of *Leptospira meyeri*, which is a pathogenic leptospirosis infection that was isolated from a leopard frog kidney (*Rana pipiens*) from Iowa. This is interesting because another component of the spirochete appears to involve a hybrid soybean plant that is adapted to the eastern plains states (of which Iowa is a member). Recombinent genes from animals and reptiles are cultivated using kidney tissues, and cells or cell lines are grown in them to create chimera for insecticides and vaccines.[30]

If a strain of "Lyme" spirochete was derived from recombinant chimera, then we might find clues in related patent inventions to how it might come about. One patent for a B.t. insecticide for agricultural use describes a recombinant soybean cultivar that is adapated to eastern plains states. The design of the insecticidal formula includes genes for various toxins. Some of the toxins designed for the patent include wasp, snake, spider, or scorpion toxin; *animal enzymes*, viral toxins, insect hormones and antibodies, hormone antagonists, channel blockers, a tobacco protein inhibitor, a rapeseed (canola) structural gene, amino acid promoters (ALS)* as soybean rust resistance genes; gene development arresting proteins, bacteria including *Agrobacterium tumefaciens*, and mouse or other enzyme marker genes such as those from any animal or *reptile* that can metabolically detoxify a select chemical agent or herbicide. The recombinant construct is engineered to be multiply antibiotic resistant. According to another patent, *Rana pipiens* or leopard frog embryos are grown and their endotoxins are removed. They are then used in an antibiotic to treat tumors. If a recombinant soybean strain contains frog toxin enzymes, we can see how the enzymes might be used to create antibiotic resistance in transgenic soybeans or other crops.[30-36]

If a leptonema contained a mouse marker gene, it would certainly have been detectable in a laboratory that was analyzing the isolate, and which may explain why a novel strain would be named after Dr. Inada. However just because a leptonema strain appears to be a recombinant, does not prove it was designed in a laboratory; but it is a likely possibility. Similar recombinant constructs may be created by nature herself using the very tools used in the laboratory. However mutations can also occur when driven by nuclear or chemical wastes. If we study chemical pesticide patents, we may find clues to understanding how such recombinant events might occur (i.e. mutagenic herbicides, quats, Tweens, benzenes, etc.). If recombinant chimera from genetically engineered crops or insecticides are falling apart inside the insect or arthropod gut, we can see how reassorted components may donate genes to make up the highly complex Bb organisms that are found around the world. The question is of course, what was discovered about the leptonemas that would have been important to keep out of any announcement of the causative agent of Lyme disease?[30-36]

**The ALS gene is a gene that encodes an enzyme called acetolactate synthase. Plants and bacteria have this gene, animals do not. When expressed, it allows the production of amino acids necessary for plant growth.*

If the entire truth about Lyme disease has never been revealed (until perhaps now), we might ask what could motivate scientists or public health experts to "hide" the origins of important human pathogens for decades. Why haven't the leptonemas, spiroplasmas, nematodes, intracellular pathogens, natural toxins, or other factors been divulged in relation to Lyme infections until now? Issues of liability are a tremendous motivator for silence. But so too are threats against a scientist's career or reputation, or the loss of federal funding or key academic positions if one dares reveal all that is known in the high stakes environment of industrial and academic politics. Unfortunately in such a game, over the long haul, absolutely no one wins, except perhaps the microorganisms themselves which happily proliferate in the environment while patients suffer.

If revelations showed that well-known industrial pollutants or agrochemicals were causing human diseases, this may be an enormous motivator for decades of silence. While we have no answers at present, they may become painfully evident if the circumstances described within this book are ever proven to be accurate. While it may be possible to justify the concealment of important pathogens on an order of "national security" or some other interest, it is an entirely different matter to deny medical care to thousands of patients suffering and dying from diseases that may be caused by something "no one" cares to discuss.

The Secret Agent

In 1983, a year after the Bb agent was announced, a paper was published in a Yale journal by NIAID, USDA, and French scientists. The paper described the spiroplasmas of Group I, the *Spiroplasma citri* cluster. The paper proposed that the group which includes *S. citri*, the honeybee, and the corn stunt agents, be further divided into seven subgroups, determined by DNA. The paper described the first international congress on mycoplasmas. The event was held in Bordeaux, France in 1974, one year before the declaration of a juvenile arthritis outbreak in Connecticut. We might wonder why this conference was held. Perhaps it had to do with the French "May" disease of honey bees and their spiroplasmas, since strains were surfacing in insects (but so too were mutated leptonemas in animals). Perhaps scientists decided to put their heads together to determine how best to cope with what would prove to be a globally emerging public health issue.[1,2]

At the time of the mycoplasma conference, only three helical mycoplasma-like organisms (spiroplasmas) had been identified. These were the agents of citrus stubborn, corn stunt, and the Drosophila (fruit fly) sex ratio agent. According to a Yale paper, during the 1960s the agents of citrus stubborn and corn stunt had not yet been identified; although another spiroplasma (277F) had already been isolated by Dr. Burgdorfer in 1967. (This agent was later declared to be similar to *Spiroplasma citri*). Two additional agents were isolated from rabbit ticks and were grown in chicken embryos. These were described as viruses or mycoplasmas by the early 1970s. These agents turned out to be the SMCA and the GT-48 spiroplasmas. In 1980 after all currently known spiroplasma strains were analyzed, the organisms were finally reclassified, just one year before the "discovery" of the causative agent of Lyme disease; and the isolation of a novel leptonema in a Lyme patient's ECM rash.[3-7]

Another paper published in 1982 described the reclassification of, and recommendations for serotyping spiroplasma isolates. It was written by scientists from the following institutions:

ARS/USDA (Beltsville, Maryland)
Mycoplasma Section Lab, NIAID Frederick Cancer Research Center (Frederick, Maryland)
Department of Anatomical Sciences at the State University of New York at Stony Brook (SUNY)
University of Bordeaux, (Pont de la Maye, France)

By the time the Lyme disease agent was announced to the world (but not that it may have a spiroplasma or a leptonema component); many spiroplasma strains were known, including new strains from the syrphid fly and the North American potter wasp. The latter feeds on pollen and small caterpillar larvae. This wasp is widely distributed from Mexico through Kansas into Wisconsin; to the eastern seaboard, and into Canada. The paper described the known spiroplasma strains as of 1982. Among them are the 277F agent, and strains isolated from tulip trees from Maryland and Connecticut. There was also an entire category of strains that were "not known" to cause disease and it is these strains that we should examine closely. These strains are:[8]

277F spiroplasma (rabbit tick, flowers)
PP81 spiroplasma (flowers)
Ixodes spiroplasma (hard-shell ticks)
Cocos spiroplasma (Cocos)
Maryland flower spiroplasma (*Spiroplasma brevi*, tulip tree)
Spiroplasma floricola (BNR1 tulip tree, insects)
SR-3 spiroplasma *Spiroplasma apis* (Connecticut tulip tree)[8]
Green leaf bug spiroplasma
L89 spiroplasma (spittlebug)
Monobia spiroplasma (potter wasp)
Syrphid spiroplasma (syrphid fly)

The tulip tree strains of spiroplasmas are highly important because tulip trees (*Liriodendron tulipifera*) are yellow poplars, also called cottonwoods. Poplar wood is used in many industries but most notably in the paper and paper pulp industry. It is also used in leather tanning since the wood has a high tannin content. We know that tannery wastes are used as agricultural fertilizers, but they are also used as livestock feed additives. Poplar is also used for furniture, musical instruments and construction materials such as timber and flooring. The western balsam poplar was the very first tree to have its DNA sequenced by scientists. Perhaps this was because it plays an integral role in human Lyme disease. Cottonwood leaves are also a favored food of deer and rodents.[9,10]

There is an early plant growth regulator patent that uses alkyl phosphonic acids and related derivatives to retard growth. This is an early herbicide patent that is assigned to the FMC Corporation. The company serves many industries including those in agriculture. It manufactures soda ash, silicates, hydrogen peroxide, biopolymers, pharmaceutical additives, lithium for batteries, and industrial chemicals including specialty polymers. The company also acquired two fungicide companies from Bayer CropScience in December 2011. This patent refers to other older herbicide patents by Monsanto, Bayer, Stauffer Chemical, Virginia-Carolina Chemical, and Esso for alkyl ester and related chemical herbicides. When I read the patents it became clear that very toxic chemicals are mixed together. The chemicals clearly have the potential to mutate microbes, and are far from inert since phosphoesters are the backbone of DNA molecules. Polyesters are used in plastics, and nitrate esters are those which have expolosive properties. Each has formed the basis of agricultural and industrial chemicals (which contain surfactants by the way), for the better part of a century.[11-20]

While spiroplasmas have been isolated from Connecticut and Maryland; the tulip tree or yellow poplar is the state tree of Kentucky, Tennessee, and Indiana. This species is found all along the eastern seaboard. Related species are found in the Midwest and northwest into Canada. Indiana state is also home to the Wabash River, a tributary of the Ohio River which flows southward into the southern half of Illinois where it meets the Embarrass River. That area is Pope County, where turtles were trapped and surveyed for the presence of leptonema spirochetes. It is also near the Shawnee National Forest where herds of deer were released in repopulation efforts during the 1950s. It is also downstream from the University of Illinois-Urbana campus, home of the first betatron particle accelerator. The river also flows past the Dixon Springs agricultural station. If Bb spirochetes have nothing to do with the mutated leptonemas found in the Illinois bulls and turtles from this area, then it is interesting how such connections keep turning up at every corner.[9,10,21]

The Coco or cocos spiroplasma was probably isolated from one or more of the Cocos (Keeling) Islands. This is a group of more than two dozen islands and atolls in the eastern Indian Ocean between Australia and Sri Lanka. The islands were formed by volcanoes and are home to a unique variety of birds and flora, including *Pandanus tectorius* variety cocosensis B.C. Stone, a native (Tahitian) screwpine (evergreen shrub). Pest insects of this shrub are scale insects. These insects are polyphagic, and have been found to destroy over one hundred plant families (i.e. crops, palms, cut flowers, woody ornamentals). We know that ladybird beetles were imported from Australia into the US during the late 1880s to treat scale insects on citrus crops.

A few important hosts to scale insects are gooseberry, ferns, coconut, mulberry, plantain, oleander, olive, peach, pear, and wine grapes. Each of these has been important to the story in this book. What is also interesting about the screwpine's name is that it has also been called *Pandanus tectorius Parkinson ex Du Roi.* Panadus palms are neither palms nor pines, but are evergreens native to Malaysia, Australia, and the Pacific Islands. Its fruits and seeds are eaten, the latter as flour to make bread. Similar seeds are eaten from the related cycad palms. These are also evergreen, sporulating, nitrogen-fixing trees that not only have cyanobacteria (blue-green algae) living in their root systems, these bacteria produce neurotoxins that are implicated in Alzheimer's, Parkinson's, and other neurodegenerative diseases in humans who consume these seeds. There may be a connection between the plant parasites of these trees, which could be a mutated cyanobacterium-fungus-spirillum spirochete called the Coco spiroplasma. Bb spirochetes have been found in the brain tissues of deceased Alzheimer's patients, and spiroplasmas have also been implicated in prion diseases.[22-31]

On August 18, 1856, the US Congress passed federal legislation called the Guano Islands Act. The government decided that on behalf of the federal government, it would allow citizens to take possession of any unclaimed islands which had large deposits of bat guano (poop). This was prized not only for its phosphate content as a fertilizer, but also because it was useful to make saltpeter for gunpowder. Approximately one hundred islands have been claimed under this Act. Most are in the Pacific, among the world's largest coral reefs, roughly in the center of the volcanic "Ring of Fire." The bacteria and viruses that are located in deep sea sediments include the cyanobacteria, the paenibacillus, and the thermophiles or extremophiles, the sulfur-reducers (sulfidophiles), and the salt-tolerant species (halophiles). Those that exist in marine sediments are the thermohalophiles, which are highly salt and temperature resistant. The viruses that associate with these sediments under the ocean floor are the same as those found in mined areas, including the CPVs of the reovirus family.

Among the islands claimed under the Guano Act are those located in what was known as the US military's Pacific Proving Grounds. This is the area of the Pacific Ocean where hydrogen and atomic bombs were exploded by British, French, and US militaries from 1946 to 1958. The islands in this area are owned by the US, France, and New Zealand governments. Among the US-owned islands are the Johnston Islands (Johnston atoll) and Midway atoll. The PPC also included the infamous Bikini atoll in the Marshall Islands, and Kiritimati (Christmas) Island. Ballistic missle tests and nuclear bombs were detonated at Johnson and Christmas Islands in 1962.[32-34]

Christmas Island is roughly twelve hundred miles southeast of Johnston Island, which is roughly seven hundred miles southwest of Honolulu, Hawaii. While many nuclear bombs were exploded in the air, other detonations took place on land. Fallout from these events has been tracked for decades, and hundreds of millions of dollars have already been paid to civilians and service personnel who were exposed to radiation and genetic damage which included cancers and birth defects in offspring. The marine sediments and the islands themselves are remnants of volcanic activity that formed these islands. Naturally they were severely impacted by the nuclear blasts that took place over a decade, even obliterating an island in the process.[35,36]

The force of the atomic blasts had the ability to throw not only soil and sea sediments into the air, but which irradiated same along with the microbes, plants, and insects in the surrounding area of the blast zones. This would have included the extremophiles, cyanobacteria, viruse, bacteriae, and plant spirillum. The question is what kind of microbes might thereafter become airborne to spread across the world in the form of nuclear fallout that first hit the coastlines by air and seawaters?

Of course nuclear energy had an earlier history in medicine before it was used as a weapon of warfare. Remember also that the US dropped atomic bombs on Japan in August, 1945; and the hydrogen bomb "Ivy Mike" was exploded in 1952. Abroad the largest hydrogen bomb ever detonated was Tsar Bomba in 1961. Most of the Soviet bombs were detonated near the Barents Sea, just upwind of the region where scientists surveyed the sixty-seven strains of *Borrelia burgdorferi* from Finnish sheep ticks in 1992. Scientists were studying the pathogenic differences between the three Bb serogroups (*B. burgdorferi* sensu stricto, *B. afzelii, B. garinii*). Each was found in the ticks from the Åland Islands and southeastern Finnish territories.[35,36,42-47]

According to a 1983 Yale report, among newly discovered spiroplasma strains were some "unclassified" serovars, including the Coco spiroplasma, the green leaf bug spiroplasma, and the Maryland flower spiroplasma. When the report was published, none of the unclassified serovars or the 277F spiroplasma were identified as agents of any particular disease, even though it was known that spiroplasmas were found in disease-transmitting ticks.[37,38]

A chart in the paper indicated their role as pathogen was "unknown." In France, a well-known honeybee May disease had already been associated with spiroplasmas from Group IV. By the conclusion of the Yale study, it seems clear that spiroplasmas *S. citri* and those of the honeybee and corn stunt groups were considered to be pathogenic. Other members of various subgroups were remarkably similar. We must consider whether they are also pathogenic, including the 277F agent isolated from rabbit ticks by Dr. Burgdorfer in 1967.[37,38]

Another paper published in 1981 suggested that vertically transmitted spiroplasmas may be more widespread in insects than was previously believed. Researchers cited the fruit fly population in Ito, Japan which was believed to be forty percent infected with spiroplasmas. Leafhoppers in Florida were also found with high numbers of spiroplasmas. Spiroplasmas are largely observed in the insect circulation. Spiroplasmas must pass through and multiply within at least two cell types including gut epithelial cells and the salivary glands for a full life cycle.[39-41]

This process could be completed in two separate hosts to complete a life cycle – a situation we also find with Bb spirochetes. Rabbit ticks have yielded both the 277F and the SMCA spiroplasma agents. According to a 1981 study, although SMCA was not yet isolated from vertebrates, an association was assumed likely. In contrast, the 277F agent which had been cultured from Burgdorfer's rabbit ticks in 1967 was not yet associated with vertebrate infections. Another report published in 1981 described spiroplasmas that were isolated from *Ixodes* ticks. These were referred to as "helical mycoplasmas." The Bb organism is also helical in shape. According to the paper:[39-41]

> "...the vertebrate pathogenicity of spiroplasmas raises questions about their potential pathogenicity for man. Spiroplasmas recovered from rabbit ticks may have limited potential for transmission to humans, since these arthropods infrequently bite man."

This last comment is a bit short-sighted since rabbit ticks are not the only species that either harbors spiroplasmas or that bites humans. A possible association of pathogenicity toward humans was proposed for spiroplasmas just before the announcement that the Bb agent had been isolated; and yet *spiroplasmas were not, and have never been openly mentioned in association with the agent of Lyme disease*. The article goes on to say that other North American tick species including *Amblyomma, Dermacentor,* and *Ixodes* species represented a "more serious pathogenic potential" due to the presence of spiroplasmas in these human-biting ticks. The paper also refers to a "human disease of unknown etiology, the so-called 'Lyme disease' [which] directed our attention to the possibility that spiroplasmas may occur in this tick genus. We now report the discovery of a new spiroplasma from *Ixodes*."[48]

It is obvious that scientists have known about spiroplasmas for the past half century. We must wonder why those with this knowledge have failed to discuss the spiroplasmas found in ticks as being associated with Lyme disease infections even though it has been nearly three decades since the Bb agent was first isolated by Burgdorfer et al. Why aren't spiroplasmas discussed?

According to one paper, thirty pools of *Ixodes pacificus* ticks were analyzed. *Spiroplasmas were recovered from seven pools of ticks that were collected between March and May 1980.* This time period was just one year before the May 1981 tick bite patient was seen by Dr. Allen Steere et al., and wherefrom his team isolated a novel leptonema from the patient's ECM rash, which they named *Leptospira inadai serovar Lyme.* Thereafter, these scientists promptly dismissed the leptospira as insignificant to the ECM rash and to the Lyme patient's illness.[48]

Spiroplasmas could also be cultured from laboratory-maintained dog/wood tick cell lines. None of the isolates grew in conventional mycoplasma broth media (SP-4). It was noted that the media required further modification to support spiroplasma growth. All seven tick pool isolates were found to be serologically similar, although the tick cell line isolates were "clearly distinct" from all other spiroplasma groups studied.[48]

The 1981 paper described the symptoms of Lyme disease and noted three distinct areas of the US where the disease was known to occur: the northeastern coast, Wisconsin in the Midwest, and California and Oregon in the northwest. The paper also claimed that while there was "no evidence" to relate spiroplasmas to Lyme disease, the isolation of a new spiroplasma from

Ixodes pacificus ticks provided scientists the ability to analyze how pathogenic spiroplasmas might be to vertebrates. It also provided the opportunity to determine whether human or animal serum generated specific antibodies to these organisms. The article was written by scientists from the NIAID (Bethesda, MD), Rocky Mountain Laboratories (Hamilton, MT), the USDA (Beltsville, MD) and the State University of New York at Stony Brook (SUNY). These are curious statements considering they were published in 1981, just before the public announcement of the "causative" agent of Lyme disease, *Borrelia burgdorferi. It is also curious why nothing was said at the time of the announcement of Bb about the spiroplasmas* – either that they were found in Lyme disease-transmitting ticks, or that they could potentially be a factor in Lyme disease infections.[48]

Perhaps there was "no evidence" available to link spiroplasmas to Lyme disease because the scientific objectives at the time were merely to identify which pathogens were found inside the bodies of ticks. Scientists may not have even studied spiroplasma associations to Lyme disease. The paper fails to mention any studies pertaining to human antibodies or sera which might have elucidated this critical link. We can certainly ask why this information to date *still has not been made known* to the general public, especially since there are such obvious links between Bb strains and spiroplasmas.[48]

While scientists seem to be on the same page that there are spiroplasmas, leptospires, leptonemas, nematodes and other important organisms in ticks, absolutely no one seems willing to publish or broadcast any connections between them and the agent of Lyme disease. Just because this link does not directly appear in print does not mean there is no evidence of a link. Indeed, it would hardly be possible to believe that scientists would simply isolate these pathogens from ticks or patients and then never investigate their possible links to an important human epidemic.[49-52]

Is the tragic "denial" of an epidemic for decades based upon a "lack of evidence" or something more? In 1983, the year after the Bb agent was announced; Yale and other academic scientists were suddenly intently studying tick spiroplasmas as evidenced by their research grants. If spiroplasmas were cultured from the same tick pools as the Bb organism, was someone responsible for making a decision not to openly report the presence of the nematodes, spiroplasmas, or leptonemas in relation to Lyme? Research grants reveal that scientists adopted a keen interest in leptospires and other agents. Despite Dr. Steere et al's discovery of a novel leptonema in a Lyme patient's ECM rash, no real audible mention of this discovery or any related leptonemas have been made publicy in association with Lyme disease when Bb was first announced, nor any time since.[49-52]

A publication claims that spiroplasmas were first noted in ticks beginning in 1976, the year after the public announcement of the "juvenile arthritis" outbreak in Connecticut. But we know this is untrue because they were first isolated in 1944 in citrus trees. Another scientific paper showed that SMCA spiroplasmas were recovered from pooled extracts of Georgia rabbit ticks in 1964. The 277F agent was isolated from Montana rabbit ticks by Burgdorfer in 1967. A later paper detailed the collection of six hundred adult *Ixodes pacificus* ticks from southern Oregon between December 1979 and July 1980, from which eight new spiroplasma strains were found. *Again spiroplasmas were found in Lyme-transmitting ticks.* If these spirochetes were known to be important from the 1960s forward, how and why is it that scientists have failed to mention their presence in ticks and their possible role in animal and human diseases?[49-52]

Many spiroplasma isolates were collected and maintained as individual reference collections in the laboratories of Beltsville, Frederick, and State University of New York at Stony Brook (SUNY). By 1995, eight serologically related spiroplasmas from western black-legged ticks were the only spirochetes found except for those associated with rabbits. The western black-legged tick (*Ixodes pacificus*) is a principal host and transmission vector of western Bb strains. Other tick species examined by then had not revealed spiroplasmas. Reptiles or other animals were thought to be more important hosts to spiroplasmas than birds. The extent of spiroplasma infections in ticks was "unknown" at the time because epidemiological surveys had never been performed. Why haven't such studies been performed to date? If they have, why haven't the results been published? The answers may be simply because to reveal the origins of Lyme disease may mean the end of federal research dollars, and/or the exposure of important agricultural/nuclear/industrial links to a human epidemic, which may mean liability or an end to profitable biotech tools.[49-53]

Neither Bb nor spiroplasmas are easily differentiated under darkfield microscopy. Therefore (says a paper) assessments should not be based upon direct observations. This suggests that either the two organisms are so similar they are easily mistaken, or that Bb contains a spiroplasma component. The paper describes the presence of spiroplasmas in different blood-feeding insects including deerflies and mosquitoes. Patent inventions have also revealed that Bb is found within these insects although Lyme experts continually fail to communicate that Lyme may be transmitted by any other insects other than ticks.[49-53]

Oddly enough the paper also suggests that spiroplasmas may have the potential to become human disease agents. It emphasized the ability to *use current knowledge for future infections*. Why not retroactively apply this same tidbit of knowledge to past epidemics of formerly "unknown" etiology (i.e. Lyme)? The answer may be that because Lyme is already defined, it is no longer of "unknown etiology." According to the paper, "...however, descriptions of the biologic and serologic properties of microbial agents such as the Y32T group [tick spiroplasma] may provide the basis for a useful detection system if in the future tick-derived diseases of unknown etiology appear."[49-53]

As we have learned, Bb, spiroplasmas, and leptospiras are found in the guts of many blood-sucking insects including ticks, mosquitoes, and deerflies. Why is there an acknowledgement of spiroplasmas in ticks for *future* diseases with unknown etiology, but not for *past or current* tickborne diseases that have already been named? In a separate 1981 paper, Dr. Gerold Stanek, co-author of the 2006 IDSA medical guidelines for Lyme disease, was cited as a reference on the topic of spiroplasmas. He co-authored a paper on spiroplasmas in 1980, one year before the Bb agent was identified by colleagues Burgdorfer et al. Dr. Stanek previously reported on the 1941 studies of Alfred Bannwarth (Munich) who described patients who had intense nerve root pain; and who described how to treat Lyme borreliosis.[53-56]

The "Y32T group" (T = type strain) mentioned in the previous paper refers to the *Spiroplasma ixodetis* which was first isolated from tick pools of western black-legged ticks from Oregon between December 1979 and July 1980. This is a novel *Ixodes* tick spiroplasma that was collected a year before the Bb organism was identified! It is interesting that *the paper which details this isolation during these 1979-1980 studies remained unpublished until January 1995, three months after the Dearborn Conference,* and we may wonder why the fifteen year delay in publication. The paper was co-authored by scientists from the State University of New York (SUNY), the NIH Rocky Mt. Labs; the USDA in Beltsville, MD; the NIAID's Infectious disease research facility in Frederick, Maryland; and curiously enough, a French laboratory.[55,57]

The fact that ticks carry unique spiroplasmas, leptonemas, and nematodes was known by scientists at these laboratories long before the Dearborn Conference, even before the announcement of the causative agent of Lyme disease. Still there was never any "audible" mention of spiroplasmas, leptospires, or leptonemas by anyone attending the Dearborn conference according to transcripts or the official conference booklet. And there has never been any audible connections made between spiroplasmas and Lyme disease from 1967 forward, even though spiroplasmas are known pathogens of insects and animals.[57]

No one mentioned these pathogens from the CDC, NIH, or from the Dearborn planning committee members during important Lyme-related public events. Individuals who attended the Dearborn conference include Drs. Duane Gubler, Barbara Johnson, and David Dennis (CDC); Raymond Dattwyler (SUNY-Stony Brook), Russell Johnson (MN), Raymond Ryan (Univ. CT), Allen Steere (Tufts NEMC), Arthur Weinstein (NYMC), and Alan Barbour (Univ TX). None of the investigators who supplied antibodies for the immunoblot tests studied by the Dearborn work group mentioned these important tick pathogens. The Dearborn work group included Drs. Benjamin Luft (SUNY), Alan Barbour, Thomas Schwan (NIH/Rocky Mt.), Denée Thomas (Univ. TX), Steven Padula (Univ CT), and Jorge Benach, (SUNY Stony Brook).[57]

Nothing appears to have been said by Drs. Edward McSweegan (NIAID, Bethesda, MD); by Frank Dressler (Hannover, Germany); or colleague IDSA Lyme disease guidelines co-author Gerold Stanek (Vienna, Austria) who published a paper on spiroplasmas, about the possibility that spiroplasmas may be a factor during Lyme disease. There was no discussion of spiroplasmas or leptospires by any vaccine manufacturer representatives attending the Dearborn conference, including those whose upcoming Lyme vaccines would be affected by Dearborn's outcome.[57]

The state public health departments that had representatives at Dearborn included AR, CT, DE, IA, IL, MA, MI, MN, MO, NC, NH, NJ, NY, OH, SC, TX, WI; and abroad from Canada, Vienna, and the UK. There was even a representative from the Alfred I. du Pont Institute* Research Department (Wilmington, DE) listed as a Dearborn attendee. I found no evidence that spiroplasmas, leptonemas, thermophiles, or nematodes were mentioned during the standardization of the surveillance and diagnostic test criteria for Lyme disease. The noticeable absense of these pathogens in the historical events surrounding Lyme disease is interesting. Is this because Bb spirochetes are comprised of pathogens whose presence is largely due to industrial and agricultural practices for which no one wants to be held accountable?[55,57-59]

**According to their web site, the institute is part of the Alfred I. duPont testamentary trust; established by the Nemours Foundation at the bequest of Alfred I. duPont in 1935. Alfred I. duPont was the grandson of Eleuthère Iréné duPont, founder of the duPont gun powder dynasty, founded in July 1802 as a gunpowder mill. The company became the largest supplier of gunpowder to the US military. Later the company was ordered under the Sherman Antitrust Act to divest, which created the Hercules Powder Company (now Hercules, Inc.) and the Atlas Powder Company (now AstraZeneca), and established its industrial laboratories. Atlas Powder Company created the Tweens that are used in the applied agricultural controls.*

Mollicutes or possible mollicutes (members of the spiroplasma family) are mentioned in Monsanto patents for transgenic corn and other crops. Du Pont's mylar polyester films (aluminum or gold coated on one side) are used by Monsanto scientists to bombard transgenic plants with genetically engineered **circular plasmids** of transfected genes. These genes may include plant infection resistance genes (i.e. maize red leaf and stripe, cereal tillering disease, mottle and chlorotic diseases, yellow striata, dwarf mosaic, stunt, and other viruses). *The Bb agent contains circular plasmids that may provide similar resistance genes to the organism. Bb's OspC virulence genes are located on a circular plasmid called cp26.* The OspC outer surface protein is required for tick to mammal transmission. Bb could be an aggregate organism (i.e. leptospira) that becomes infected with spiroplasma and other genes from recombinant formulas. Resistance genes may enable pathogens to thrive within other bacteriae where they may be transmitted by an insect vector.[78-80]

Some Monsanto patents describe resistance genes that may be transfected into GM crops including from these sources:[78,79]

Pseudomonas species (leaf blight)
Erwinia species (stalk and top rot)
Corynebacterium (leaf freckles)
Colletotrichum (anthracnose leaf blight)
Curvularis/Cochliobolus (leaf spot)
Sclreophthora (downy mildew)
Helminthosporium (rot)
Bacillus subtilis (seedling blight)
Spiroplasma kunkelii (maize stunt spiroplasma)
Xanthomonas species (stalk rot)
Clavibacter species (bacterial wilt)
Cephalosporium species (kernel rot)
Aspergillus (ear and kernel rot)
Diplodia (ear rot, leaf streak)
Botrytis, Fusarium (ear rots, wilts)
Nematode parasite resistance genes
Puccinia (rust blights)
Mesa central or Rio Grande (maize stunt)

Imagine what could happen if genetically engineered corn, soybean, cottonseed or other crops that are fed to vaccinated livestock and poultry cause recombinant "accidents" through the reassortment of genes. If such a problem occurred in livestock that were vaccinated with leptospirosis vaccines and in poultry that were vaccinated with chicken cholera or other important vaccines, we can see how unexpected recombinant accidents might contribute to the reassortment of genes. Vaccinated livestock could then transfer "damaged" genes and broken chimera into animal wastes and products for fertilizers and foods. As animal wastes, reassorted feed and vaccine genes may be picked up by insects and arthropods (ticks) in the environment, where they may be transmitted to larger animals including humans by vectoring insects and arthropods.

In a 1978 paper written by Yale colleagues Drs. Allen C. Steere, Thomas F. Broderick, and Stephen E. Malawista, we learn about a retrospective analysis from December 1975 through April 1976 of fifty-one residents from three Connecticut communities (Old Lyme, Lyme, East Haddam) who presented with arthritis-like symptoms. The paper also discussed the prospective study of thirty-two patients with acute onset of ECM and/or arthritis. The patients came from Connecticut, Cape Cod, Massachusetts; Rhode Island; and Long Island, New York; and were among the first patients connected to the emerging Connecticut cluster of "juvenile arthritis" (Lyme).[60]

The paper described how skin biopsies, and throat and rectal swabs were examined and tested against a variety of agents including more than two hundred *arboviruses*, twenty-two *leptospirae*, four *rickettsiae*, the *spiroplasma* suckling mouse cataract agent (SMCA), and *Babesia microti*. However the tests did not suggest infection with any of the agents. Note that testing for one spiroplasma strain does not mean no spiroplasmas were present. Even if present, the culture medium may have been inadequate to properly detect spiroplasmas at the time of the tests. No details of the arboviruses or the leptospira strains that were evaluated were described in the paper. There is no evidence one way or the other if other leptospires, leptonema, or spiroplasmas could have been present and causing infections in any of these patients. It is however interesting to note which agents were tested against the patient samples.[60]

The paper does however mention that cryoprecipitates (cryoimmunoglobulins) were associated with clinical involvement of skin and joints. The finding of, and interest in cryoimmunoglobulins (serum antibodies) by these scientists who were investigating the causative agent of Lyme disease may have something to do with the possibility that viruses and bacteria are possible co-factors in rheumatic diseases including Lyme. If the scientists were concerned that infectious agents were causing Lyme arthritis, it may explain why they tested Connecticut patient samples against these infectious agents. Each of the agents they tested for are found in the bodies of ticks and other insects which transmit the Lyme disease agent.[60]

In other papers which describe Lyme arthritis studies, Dr. Steere and colleagues wrote that cryoprecipitates or cryoimmunoglobulins are associated with the skin and joint symptoms of Lyme disease. Cryoprecipitates also appear in a frozen blood product that is prepared from human plasma (and bovine albumin*) and used as a clotting agent for hemophiliacs. This is also called cryoprecipitated antihemophilic factor, or "cryo." The reference in the Dr. Steere et al. article may mean there was evidence of serum antibodies in the patients studied. However it could mean that samples were studied to detect a contaminating virus such as one that led to HIV/AIDS infections in hemophiliacs who used blood clotting agents during the 1960-1970s. Scientists may have suspected a link between what led to HIV blood contaminations and the agent that causes Lyme disease. Remember that the beginning of the HIV/AIDS story revolved around contaminated blood supplies, including products that may have been made using nematode proteins and/or bovine albumin. Could either product have been infected by leptospires, spiroplasmas, or an extremophile bacteria?[60-63]

**We learned previously that bovine albumin samples have been found to be contaminated by leptospires.*

A 1968 study of rabbit cry-immunology discusses immunoglobulin (antibody) production during the antibody response. The paper tells us that the material injected into test rabbits came from bacteria, viruses, or other animal species. In all cases the studies involved the production of *heteroantibodies*, not *autoantibodies*. The studies led to the identification of specific antibodies that were produced by the rabbits to the injected stimuli. The paper refers to studies on the production of autoantibodies after intravenous injection of adjuvants (i.e. vaccines).[64]

I should ask if the presence of heteroantibodies, which are antibodies to foreign proteins, can be mistaken as "autoantibodies" in patients who have infections. Furthermore, are heteroantibodies sometimes made in response to reactivated vaccine virus proteins – proteins that are foreign (heterologous) in origin, but native (homologous) once incorporated into the human genome? Can the insistence by Steere et al. that persistent Lyme disease is an "autoimmune" disorder be the result of a misinterpretation of what the "autoimmune" antibody factors actually represent? Are "autoimmune" diseases really a proper reaction to foreign proteins that have lodged in the human genome of cells? According to a patent:[64,65]

> "Late stage Lyme Disease is characterized by both circulating anti-spirochetal immunoglobulins and PBL [peripheral blood lymphocytes] T-cell responsiveness to spirochetal antigens. The spirochetal antigens detected by the humoral immune response have been determined and most are cell surface antigens. With few exceptions, the epitopes recognized by the T-cell immune response remain unknown."

The patent speaks to the presence of foreign proteins which cause T-cell immune responses. Epitopes are antigen sites which bind antibodies. Scientists don't seem to know specifically what causes our immune system to recognize or overlook Bb. But when we study the spiroplasma spirochetes we find they are fully capable of immune modulation.[65]

> "Immune response in humans has been studied primarily involving the humoral immune response. Characteristic antibodies develop in most patients as a function of disease progression and it is this immune response that is used clinically to diagnose infection and efficacy of therapy. The cellular immune response is less well studied and understood."

The patent speaks to persistence of the Bb organism:[65]

> "Since the spirochete apparently contains multiple antigens capable of eliciting an immune response, the question arises from the prior art research as to why the anti-spirochetal immune response *fails to clear the organism from the body*. No answer is presently clear. The present invention, however, attempts to address the limitation in the art by presenting multiple antigens of *Borrelia burgdorferi* in a sonicated cell mixture in such a way to produce prevention of Lyme disease in laboratory test animals which serve as useful and accurate models of the human system."

In the later stages of Lyme disease, antibodies are sometimes made and may be detectable by laboratory tests, but only if the correct strain probes are present. During early infection the spirochetes avoid detection by the immune system:[65]

> "Because the spirochete is so unabundant that it avoids detection by direct methods in infected patients, the humoral immune response of patients is used diagnostically to detect infection. The disease course as revealed by specific changes in immune response may be important in disease progression."
>
> "The immune response in the early stage disease is characterized by infiltration of the ECM lesion by macrophage and neutrophils (PMN). PBL derived T-cells are unresponsive to spirochetal antigens and serum does not contain circulating antibodies. Activity of Natural Killer (NK) cells in both the early and late stage Lyme Disease patients is inhibited but NK function is normal in patients that are in remission. Analysis in vitro has shown that NK cells are actually inhibited by spirochetes. There is a characteristic B-cell hyperactivity displayed by patients in various stages of Lyme Disease."[65]

Remember that spiroplasma spiralin proteins can stimulate this kind of B-cell response. It seems this hyperactivity is directed at the antigens of the Bb organism which may have spiroplasma components. The patent does not discuss any sort of "autoimmune" process taking place, but rather a proper immune response to *foreign antigens*.

Another paper indicates that regardless of the antigenic stimuli, the antibody response is exactly the same. This means that no matter what substance enters the body, the immune response is simply reactive and will try to produce antibodies. This may hold equally true for reactivated vaccine virus proteins. Antibodies directed against "non-self" proteins that have been incorporated into our genome as "self" may be what Dr. Steere et al. describes as an "autoimmune" process – a process that may actually represent proper immune activation against heterologous, or *foreign* vaccine proteins (or infections) and not those of "self." This would seem to imply that there is a direct cause and effect relationship between foreign proteins and autoimmune disease (diseases that once the foreign proteins are identified, may or may not be treatable).[65,66]

We can see evidence of cryoimmunoglobulin antibody production in synovial (joint) tissues of patients who suffer from a plant-induced arthritis. This effect seems to mirror the antibody production found in synovial tissues of patients with Lyme arthritis. One helpful paper describes how five children with an inflammatory arthritis became afflicted after a joint was penetrated by a plant thorn. Curiously the pattern of illness in the children reflected that of Lyme arthritis; a transient, acute joint inflammation with an asymptomatic period, but later eruption of a chronic arthritis. Polarized light microscopy revealed the presence of plant tissue within the childrens' joint tissues.[65]

Surgical excision of the affected joint returned function to the affected joints. This form of arthritis and surgical treatment is reflected in reports about the removal of arthritis-affected synovial tissues in Lyme patients which is also "curative" for the affected joint. Perhaps the arthritis was caused by a plant spiroplasma that was transmitted by the thorn. And perhaps the spirochetes of Lyme disease, which are commonly found in the synovial tissues of patients afflicted with Lyme arthritis, may have a similar spiroplasma component. If Lyme arthritis was simply an autoimmune response to self, then the arthritis should not be cured by surgery alone. Rather, the removal of the offending heterologous (foreign) proteins seems to resolve the localized arthritis issue, while antibiotics and a restoration of the patient's vitamin D levels (hormones) and elimination of dietary fluorides often alleviates arthritis-like symptoms.[67,68]

Another study showed that chromosomal DNA (foreign or heterologous proteins) from a variety of bacterial species may be found in joint tissues from patients with various kinds of arthritis. Some of the bacterial species associated with arthritis are:[68-74]

Neisseria	*Acinetobacter*	*Moraxella*	*Salmonella*
Pseudomonas	*Chlamydia*	*Trachomatis*	*Yersinia*
Campylobacter	*Chlamydia pneumonia*	*Mycobacteria*	*Haemophilus*
Clostridia	*Borrelia*	*Tropheryma whippelii*	*Mycoplasma*

The presence of "Bb" bacteria as an aggregate with a spiroplasma component (or lack thereof) may help determine whether patients suffer from arthritic symptoms during Lyme infections. This may explain why some patients not only manifest the arthritic form of the illness, but also the cardiac and neurologic forms; and many test positive for one or more mollicutes (mycoplasmas). While some genetic factors may play a role in the manifestation of Lyme symptoms, symptom presentation may be more dependent upon the combination of pathogens present in an infectious aggregate pathogen.

These individualized infections which may be highly varied between patients, speaks to the necessity of treating patients with individualized and not standardized treatment therapies. By the way, one reference from 1985 with Dr. Allen Steere as co-author indicates that Bb spirochetes may survive for years in affected synovium and may be responsible for microvascular injury. This means that according to Dr. Steere, Bb may be persistent and continue to cause tissue injury for years; which describes a chronic disease state.[67,67]

Among the known spiroplasma strains listed in a Yale article (written by scientists from the NIAID, USDA, SUNY Stony Brook, NY and a French laboratory) were these:

beetle strains	corn stunt	honeybees	syrphid fly
green leaf bug	coconut palm	flower	wasp
Spiroplasma floricola	Bee-flower (B31)	tick (Y32)	tick (277F)
Spiroplasma citri	sex ratio organism (WSRO/Wolbachia)		*Spiroplasma mirum* (SMCA)

There is a "B31" strain of *Borrelia burgdorferi* that was the very first Lyme disease-causing "Bb" strain to be identified. There is also a "B31" bee-flower spiroplasma. Naturally we must ask whether the Bb strain "B31" is named this way because it contains a "B31" bee-flower spiroplasma. Is this name another hint that Bb is an aggregate organism that is part plant, part insect, and part animal pathogen?[75]

In 1975 and 1977, soon after the sudden announcement of a "Lyme arthritis" outbreak, the NIAID awarded two grants to Dr. L.P. Brinton, co-author of nearly a dozen articles from 1970-1975 with colleagues including Dr. Willy Burgdorfer. Brinton's studies under these grants included Colorado tick fever virus development (a reovirus) in Rocky Mountain wood ticks, and the structure of the gut from normal and Rocky Mountain spotted fever-infected ticks.[76,77]

The two grants also funded comparative work on the fine structure of wolbachia-like organisms in various tick species; the structure of RMSF and other rickettsiae in brown dog ticks from Mississippi as grown in vero cells; and the investigation of the spiroplasma 277F agent in cotton tail rabbit ticks. If tick-carried spiroplasmas had absolutely nothing to do with Lyme disease, then it is curious that "everybody" was so fascinated with them at the time of the Connecticut outbreak, including colleagues of Dr. Burgdorfer. It is also rather curious that nothing whatsoever was publicly declared about the relationship between spiroplasmas and Lyme disease when its causative agent made its debut in 1982; or any time since for that matter.[76,77]

It would be most interesting to determine scientifically and independently whether spiroplasmas and their satellite viruses were present in the Romanian dimbovitza; the Illinois illini strains; the CDC turtle strains; and the Lyme patient by Dr. Steere et al. – all leptonemas considered to be novel organisms. Each emerged before the Connecticut cluster of Lyme disease was announced. If compared to *Leptonema Noguchi* from the early part of the last century, it may be found that the Noguchi strain lacks a spiroplasma component found in the modern strains. If so, this may lend validation to the emergence of novel spiroplasmas during the latter part of the twentieth century. This would therefore be in alignment with the development and implementation of agricultural, industrial, and nuclear technologies. This may also support the contention that Bb may have its origins in the modern "weapons" of insect (or other) warfare. Perhaps the term "biowarfare" describes the natural formation of novel microbes from the remnants of insect, nuclear, and industrial "warfare."

Drink To Our Health

The most perplexing aspect of the story is that "everybody" seems to know about the causative agents of Lyme disease, except those who are directly affected by it; the patients and their treating physicians. To understand how this assumption might be made, we have only to look at the past history of Lyme and the biological warfare that has been practiced against insect pests for over a century. Our story began with the early fertilizers and fungicides which used special formulas to control pest insects of many kinds. We have also learned about the application of phosphate fertilizers and agricultural chemicals. We know that many agricultural and industrial tools include metals and radioactive elements. What I haven't really addressed yet is why France, a country that is extremely dependent upon nuclear energy; and one that is practically the birthplace of medicine, agriculture, and other industries, might be important to our story. In the chapter titled "The Secret Agent," I mentioned a 1983 paper that was published in the *Yale Journal of Biology and Medicine* by US, NIAID, and French scientists. It described the spiroplasmas of Group I, which is the *Spiroplasma citri* group.[1,2]

The paper described the first international congress on mycoplasmas that was held in Bordeaux, France in 1974. This was the year before scientists declared an outbreak of an arthritis-like illness in Connecticut. The reason for the conference was due to the scientific interest in the French "May" disease of honey bees, caused by group IV spiroplasmas. However the 1967 emergence of the 277F novel tick spiroplasmas in the US was probably also discussed at the event.[1,2]

The Yale paper described at length the kinds of spiroplasmas that had been identified to date, including the citrus spiroplasmas and Burgdorfer's 277F spiroplasma that was found in rabbit ticks; and which resembled *S. citri*. In 1980 a year before the agent of Lyme disease was announced to the world, all known spiroplasma strains were suddenly reclassified. The Yale report mentioned there were still unclassified agents including M55, the Maryland flower spiroplasma, the Coco spiroplasma N525, the green leaf bug spiroplasma LB-12, and others. The Yale paper is clear that many spiroplasma strains were considered pathogenic. Other spiroplasmas (i.e. 277F) were found to be remarkably similar. Were they also noted to be pathogenic?[1-6]

This is significant because the Montana rabbit ticks that had 277F spiroplasma infections came from an area that has a huge copper deposit, and a history of mining and copper smelting. In Bordeaux, France where the mycoplasma conference was held, we find a century of history in wine-making that is clearly part of the Lyme disease story. If we use Bordeaux, France as a model for our story, we learn that wine is affected by a number of pest insects as well as fungal pathogens. The most significant of the fungi is the species *Phoma exigua variety heteromorpha*, a common fungus of oleander. Oleander is a flowering ornamental shrub that is common to France, Italy, the Netherlands, Spain, and the US (Texas, California, Florida, Virginia). Oleander is an ancient plant, having been found in images uncovered at Pompeii. It was cultivated in Basil, Switzerland as early as 1560. The Dutch and the French established botanical centers in Italy, The Netherlands, the Caribbean Islands, and in England by 1760 to spread oleander cultivars. The plant also grows naturally in Africa, the Middle East, and Mediterranean countries.[7,8]

The fungi *Phoma exigua* can be found in the USDA's mycology and microbiology database, where strains were isolated as early as 1847. It was formerly known as *Boeremia exigua*. This fungus is very important to viticulturists. A bacterium that is extremely deadly to grapevines is *Xylella fastidiosa* (Xf), or Pierce's disease. Xylella is a *gammaproteobacterium* that is an important grape, citrus, peach, and ornamental pathogen. It is introduced into citrus groves and vineyards by leafhoppers known as the sharpshooters (spittle bugs). This bacterial infection blocks water uptake in the xylem of plants, dehydrating them, and causing *wilt disease*. Pierce's disease was first discovered in the *San Joaquin* valley in Anaheim, California grapes in 1892 by Newton B. Pierce, a plant Pathologist. Glassy-winged sharpshooters are highly endemic in California, particularly in the south.[15]

Xylella is a bacterium that causes phoney peach disease; and in South America, citrus variegated chlorosis disease. In the US, Connecticut had peach groves before it was known for its poultry industry. Georgia of course is renowned for its peaches, but so are Alabama, Arkansas, California, Florida, Indiana, Oregon, South Carolina, Michigan, Texas, Washington, and Ontario (Canada). California exports the most peaches according to records, so by 2000 the California Department of Agriculture, several extensions of the University of California, and the University of Houston began studying this pest at length. There is currently no cure for *Xylella fastidiosa*, at least not in plants.

Leaf hoppers are the vector of this infection, and they spread other infections including spiroplasmas and fungi. Therefore this gammaproteobacteria and other pathogens may infect Bb spirochetes, and probably already have in some strains, or a Los

Alamos patent would probably not mention Bb spirochetes. Whether Xylella are actually part of a Bb spirochete is speculative, but seems a reasonable assumption. The gammaproteobacteria are largely enterobacteria, and include many orders, a few of which we have already explored:

- *Vibrionales* (Vibrio) these are flagellated, capable of fermentation, and produce a powerful neurotoxin that is a sodium (Na+) pump inhibitor, called TTX, or tetrodotoxin.*[9-14,31-33]
- *Enterobacteriales* (*E. coli, Yersinia pestis, Klebsiella, Shigella, Salmonella*)
- *Pseudomonadales* (*Pseudomonas, Azotobacter, Rhizobacter*)
- *Coxiellaceae* (Q fever)
- *Francisellaceae* (Tularemia)
- *Xanthomonadales* (*Xanthomonas*)
- *Chromatiales* (purple sulfur bacteria)
- *Pasteurellaceae* (*Haemophilus influenzae*)
- *Acidithiobacillales* (*Acidithiobacillus ferrooxidans, Thiobacillus ferrooxidans*) acid-tolerant extremophiles

**TTX is a toxin that is also found in Japanese blowfish. There is no known antidote for this toxin, although fampridine has been shown to reverse toxicity in animals. Dalfampridine has also been shown to improve neurologic function in patients diagnosed with Multiple Sclerosis. Perhaps this is because MS is caused by bacterial neurotoxins from organisms such as gammaproteobacteriae or other extremophiles.*

The gammaproteobacteria are found in areas where there are fault lines (earthquake zones); and in hydrothermal and geothermal veins because they are extremophiles. Some are sulfur reducers, acidophiles or halophiles; and some oxidize methane. There are also some that are *marine* in origin. The extremophiles may have their origins first and foremost from soil bacteria, including from mined minerals such as metal ores or phosphates that have been used as fertilizers. Insect larvae pick up these bacteriae through a variety of methods including direct contact and from parental transmission. The presence of these bacteriae in the environment has probably been helped along by the industrially and agriculturally applied pesticides.

One method of controlling fungal infections on grape vines was introduced during the mid-19th century. It was known as the Millardet-David treatment after French Botany Professor Pierre-Marie-Alexis Millardet from the University of Bordeaux. He studied vineyard diseases in the region, and discovered that vines near roadsides were sprayed with a mixture of copper sulfate and lime (phosphates) to keep passersby from eating the grapes. He conducted field trials of the mixture with the help of then Technical Director Ernest David of a vineyard at Château Dauzac. Their findings were published in 1885, and recommended the use of "Bordeaux mixture" to treat downy mildew of grapes. Bordeaux mixture has been used since the mid-1880s to treat vineyards all over the world, including in the United States. Although it is still used today, Bordeaux mixture has been found to harm fish, livestock, and earthworms because the copper and lime leaches into the soils and watersheds.[15]

The great wine blight of France took place from the late 1850s to the mid-1870s. It was caused by an aphid called the North American grape *phylloxera,* which injects a toxic poison into plants while feeding. These pests were the cause of crop damage to European grape vines which were grown by French colonists in Florida during the 16th century. European vines would not grow on American soils because of these pests. However during the mid-1800s when French horticulturists were experimenting with American vines, many species were imported and probably accidentally introduced the American pest into France between 1858 and 1862.[16]

The first known vineyard attack by phylloxera took place in the French province of *Languedoc,* in the southeastern part of the country. Wine growers in Pujualt in the Gard, a small Languedoc department, did not notice aphid infestations, and this led to a loss of roughly 40% of French grape vines over a fifteen-year period. Another region badly hit by the blight was *Lyon,* a region north of *Languedoc*; a region best known for wine (i.e. Beaujolais), and which was then the silk processing hub of the country.*[16]

**The Languedoc region also had a large book printing industry. The discharge of paper pulp wastes, wood viruses; and printing or textile dyes contributed to pollutants and possibly to disease outbreaks such as an earlier Morgellon's-like infection in children.*

The cause of the blight was finally discovered in 1868 by French Biologist Jules-Emile Planchon and two colleagues who detected aphids sucking on the roots of a plant they had exhumed. In 1870 American Entomologist Charles Valentine Riley confirmed Planchon's theory about the aphid-blight connection. Riley was the first chief of the USDA Entomology division, and who initiated the USDA programs that were the beginning of *insect biowarfare* effforts in the US.[16]

Today aphids and other pests continue to devastate crops including citrus groves and vineyards. The glassy-winged sharpshooter, the vector of Pierce's disease, is controlled not only by chemical pesticides, but also by techniques which genetically engineer Pierce's disease resistance genes directly into grape cultivars. These techniques are possible because of the effect a particular bacteria (*Xylella fastidiosa*) has upon grape plant cell signaling. A topical application of what are called neonicotinoid insecticides are useful to control sharpshooter populations in vineyards and citrus groves.[17-21]

The most common insecticide from this group is *Imidacloprid*; a Bayer CropScience product sold as Admire, Merit, or Goucho. Common weeds are known to host sharpshooters, so chemical herbicides are another way to control them on important crops. Scientists in the San Joaquin valley are monitoring sharpshooter and aphid populations to ensure they are successfully controlled. The *neonicotinoid* insecticides have been implicated in colony collapse disorder of honey bees. These insectical residues accumulate in pollen and nectar for several years after use, and act upon the central nervous system of the bees; binding at the nicotinic acetylcholine receptors. These insecticides are not only useful against aphids, but also beetles, weevils, and moths. Seed treatments that contain these agents are globally applied upon agricultural crops including potatoes, cereals, soybeans, rapeseed, corn, cotton, and other fruits and vegetables. Bayer and Syngenta hold patents on neonicotinoid insecticides.[17-21]

Genetically engineered chimera have also been developed to include spider, sea urchin, and other natural toxins that are used in a manner analogous to that of tetrodotoxin or TTX. These toxins are used as sodium-channel blockers to paralyze insects, according to an insecticide patent assigned to the FMC Corporation. It seems reasonable to believe that if "natural" neurotoxins are introduced as insecticides and are engineered into plants; that patients with neurologic illnesses (i.e. MS, ALS, Lyme, Parkinson's), may be affected in part by microbes that have acquired neurotoxin-producing genes from agricultural and industrial insecticides to which they have been exposed.[34-36]

When we look at a patent that is assigned to the Los Alamos National Security Company for the treatment of Pierce's disease of grapevines, we may see a clear connection between the diseases of citrus plants and *Borrelia burgdorferi*. Remember that the company is a consortium of four organizations (Bechtel, Babcock & Wilcox, URS Energy and Construction, and the University of California). The group runs the Los Alamos National Laboratory and the National Nuclear Security Administration for the US DOE. As we analyze historical events, we may be able to detect seemingly common denominators: herbicides, insecticides, and nuclear wastes. This is because nuclear energy is used "peaceably" for agricultural and industrial techniques, including the irradiation of seeds, plants, plastics, and the creation of radiotracer labels. Nuclear reactors require radioactive fuels that must first be mined or recycled from stockpiled weapons. What is unearthed from the soil may end up in finished products or wastewaters whether that means as agricultural, industrial, or nuclear wastes. We may also see more clearly that as an aggregate spirochete, Bb probably has an agent or two in common with grapevines and other citrus plants, such as a gammaproteobacteria, a fungi, and a spiroplasma. Otherwise why would a patent for Pierce's disease in grapevines also be useful to combat the Bb spirochete?[22,23]

The Los Alamos patent describes a method of using human elastase, which is expressed by genes, to kill the aphids of Pierce's disease and the spirochetes of Lyme disease. An older Italian paper from 1998 reveals that scientists have been studying the effects of human elastase for over a decade. The study describes how Bb spirochetes from European *Borrelia garinii* species were isolated from sheep ticks and cultured. In addition, a virulent Bb strain called *Borrelia tirelli* was isolated from an infected patient and cultured in the same medium. The results proved that human elastase was efficient at killing Bb spirochetes, at least in the laboratory (in vitro).[22-29]

We have already studied the history of the emergence of Lyme disease in the US. We watched those who tracked the emergence of novel spirochetes from Romania to the US. We discovered that Russian scientists were engineering vaccines to treat Multiple Sclerosis and encephalitis which may be caused by bacteria that are extremophiles and which may infect viruses. We also saw them come to the United States during a period when unusual animal spirochetes were also surfacing in Europe. We saw animals and water samples being analyzed from the 1950 to 1960s for strange leptonema and other pathogens that are carried by ticks. We learned about NIH scientists who studied ticks from copper mining areas in the northeast (Connecticut), and from the Rocky Mountains (Montana). And we have seen a glimpse of the history of agricultural and nuclear "warfare," including the peaceful nuclear techniques of industry and agriculture, and their relationship to mined nuclear and other materials, and the microbes which live deep underground. We can see there are definite connections between industry, agriculture, pollutants, and Lyme disease. There is another human disease which may help us to understand the full impact of modern day tickborne illnesses. This emerging infection also has important historical connections to early French industries.

Morgellon's: Another Multi-Factored Infection

Another significant aspect of the Lyme disease story is Morgellon's disease. The name neurocutaneous syndrome is sometimes used interchangeably with "Morgellon's," which is a Lyme-like infection. Morgellon's has the additional burden of producing strange multi-colored "fibers" which grow out of hideous skin lesions in patients with the affliction. I think of Morgellon's as "Lyme-plus." The peculiar hair-like fibers come in several colors, including red, white, black, brown, purple, and blue – all colors which can be produced by keratin, the fibrous protein substance in the body that produces skin, hair, and nails. The wounds are devastating, disfiguring, and painful, and the fibers can produce pain upon removal. Like Lyme patients, those with Morgellon's have been called "delusional," and have been diagnosed with "delusional parasitosis" by some doctors. This essentially calls patients crazy for believing they are infected with an as yet undefined disease with some very obvious skin manifestations.[1-6]

An American woman named Mary Leitao is credited with being the first to bring Morgellon's into the spotlight when she noticed an ulcerative lesion on her then two-year old son's lip which produced strange "fibers." Her discovery was made in 2001, and a year later the Morgellon's Research Foundation was founded in honor of Mary's son. The name Morgellon's disease was coined by Mary after what appeared to be a description of a similar illness in French children from the 1600's that also produced strange hairs. It was noticed from a monograph by physician Thomas Browne, titled "A Letter to a Friend." The letter was written between 1656 and 1672, and published in 1690 after his death. He described what appeared to be an unusual illness as follows:[7-10]

> "Hairs which have amused me have not been in the face or head, but on the back, and not in men but children, as I long ago observed in that endemial distemper of little children in Languedock, called the Morgellons, wherein they critically break out with harsh hairs on their backs, which takes off the unquiet symptoms of disease and delivers them from coughs and convulsions."

As a physician, Browne was well versed in diseases of the seventeenth century, which included malaria, plague, and smallpox. He was also credited with being the first to suggest that rabies could be transmitted between two animals. Centuries later, physician C.E. Kellett from Newcastle-on-Tyne, England (think Newcastle disease) criticized Browne's monograph, but noted a reference to Browne's stay at Montpellier in Languedoc, France (southeast coastline) while he was a young student. According to Kellett, the arrival of Thomas Browne at Montpellier was around the period that the King (in Lyons at the time) fell critically ill. Other references are cited by Kellett in his own 1935 commentary when describing Browne's letter. References in Kellett's work also reported similar hair-like "worms":[11]

> "Worms or, as others will have it, hairs, which are wont to infest the muscles of the arms, calves, and back in infants and children, and which are unknown to the old authorities..."

He follows with a quote from Leonellus Faventinus de Victoriis:[11-13]

> "There exists in little children certain living principles having the appearance of worms, that are called by the common folk Dracontia...these little creatures have this property that, unless they are extirpated by the appropriate remedies, they lead either to a hurtful separation, or else forthwith cause the child to waste."

This sounds a bit like a nematode parasitic infection. Nematodes come in different sizes from the microscopic to those which may be plainly seen as they are several inches in length. Since they live in soil, fresh and salt water, hot springs, plants, insects, animals, and even other nematodes; these worms are perhaps the most abundant creatures on the planet. Nematodes are particularly common around rotting timbers, *among various species of fungi,* especially in heavily forested regions. They are also found *in wood products* of all kinds, and are typically transmitted by bark beetles, gypsy moths, and other wood-dwelling larvae.[11-13]

What would make something seemingly so benign and rare in terms of an infectious agent suddenly appear inside the bodies of ticks and able to infect people? We know that nematodes were first observed in 1912 in southern California orange groves, followed by detection in citrus groves in the southeast. Glaser and Fox investigated them in 1929 when studying Japanese beetle grubs on a New Jersey golf course. The USDA however reports that the pinewood nematode was first detected in 1934 and was associated with the fungi found in timber, but it wasn't until 1979 when the nematode was known to cause pine wilt in non-native Missouri pines. This seems to skate over the truth about the agricultural use of nematodes by the USDA from 1933 forward.[12-19]

Indeed it was a USDA scientist (Oldham) who was the first to suggest the use of nematodes for biological control of pest insects. From about 1935 forward, field tests at ten locations in New Jersey were undertaken for this purpose. Soon another four dozen tests were undertaken. By 1939 a statewide colonization program began for nematodes when they were released at five hundred and sixty-three locations in New Jersey, followed by releases in other New England states. The US was not the only country deploying nematodes agriculturally, as other countries were following the same trends overseas.[12-19]

A book published in 1544 appears to have been the first to describe the worm or hair-like Morgellons fibers. Indeed Lyon, France began its silk industry in 1466 when King Louis XI established silk manufacturing in the city (including textile dyes). By 1540 the region held a monopoly on silk manufacturing. So it is not surprising that "Morgellon's" emerged in this area, if it was related to silkworms because these insects harbor nematode parasites.[11]

Another author named Schenckius described worms in the skin that only partly exited the pores, but which had tiny heads with little black points or spots. Symptoms of profuse itching, insomnia, and restlessness were described in the publication. These symptoms appear to be similar to those experienced by modern day Morgellon's patients. Four other authors described "worms" or "hairs," including a doctor from Lyon, our silk textile hub. In Provence, the condition was known as "Masclous;" and in Haute-Provence, "Soyes" (bristles). These regions are due south of Lyon, and happen to be adjacent to the ports where textiles both entered and exited France. The Rhône River passes through these parts from the northern Netherlands through Germany along the Swiss-Austrian border into France past Lyon to the Mediterranean Sea – dragging textile, dye, paper pulp, chemical, and other important industrial wastes along the way.[11,20]

In an older book is a drawing of the "parasites" of the tiny worms that have been found on silkworm caterpillars. In 1776 these worms were referred to as crinons, crinones, cridones, or comedones (black heads). The worms that protruded from the silkworm caterpillars had black spots on their tip. In 1791, J.G. Wolf prepared a thesis on the comedones for his doctoral degree, which was reviewed in the *Journal of Medicine.* According to the publication:[11]

> "With the help of the microscope these cinder-coloured animals may be made out, having two hair. These worms are terrible to look at."

In 1843 Simon described the *Demodex folliculorum,* a common inhabitant of comedones (which are blackheads found on the face and body), and which may well have been the mite-like parasites seen on silkworms. In April 1884, Radcliffe Crocker published a series of cases describing children with a Morgellon's-like illness.[11]

Demodex is a worm-like mite that is found on everyone's skin and eyebrows, and which lives within hair follicles. Where these symbiont mites are found in large numbers, skin conditions emerge (i.e. blackheads, acne, rosacea). Those who suffer from hair loss and thinning hair have been shown to have an extraordinary large number of demodex in their scalp follicles. Such hair loss is a frequent manifestation of Lyme disease. Herbal shampoos and dietary adjustments can help reduce mite numbers to normal levels. The mite has been known since the 1840s to cause mange (hair loss) in animals. A Parasitologist communicated that his patients use soaps and creams which contain the essential oil sea buckthorn (*Hippophae rhamnoides*), and which is thought to be effective against these mites.[21]

When we think about the "worms" that were seen in the French children, we might remember that nematodes can be very large in size. They are in fact worms, however the hair-like manifestations of modern day Morgellon's lesions may or may not be nematodal in origin. Some persons report that the "hairs" retreat when trying to remove them. Therefore there may be nematodes involved in some Morgellon's cases, but not others.[11]

When Morgellon's patients discuss their neurologic symptoms, they describe biting, stinging, or crawling sensations which feel as if there are insects or worms crawling under their skin. Similar sensations are felt during skin mite or nematodal infestations. Additional Morgellon's symptoms are neurologically very "Lyme-like." These may include confusion, short-term memory loss, fatigue, joint pain, mood issues, insomnia, and vision changes. Lyme patients are often co-infected with nematodes and mites, so it would not be surprising if Morgellon's patients are as well. However the horrible skin lesions of Morgellon's are not associated with Lyme disease. The ulcerative, weeping sores of Morgellon's are red, painful, and disfiguring. The lesions may yield strange worm-like hairs or fibers, as well as colored specks, clumps of cotton-like material, and other debris.[22]

I learned of many silkworm diseases from an 1860's horticultural journal. These infections often produce various colored pigments upon the larval body, silk, or adult moth's wings. For example one infection creates a black tar-like substance, while another produces crystal-like formations or other debris. One infection in particular is called "the spot." This appears after the fourth "sleep." This describes the fifth instar larva, which is a mature caterpillar. (Each stage of sleep/molt is called an instar.)[23]

The spot malady produces various colored spots including white, transparent, red, yellow, black, "livid" or blue to purplish-black, or rose/red or cinnamon colors. Remember that the "reds" disease of silkworms is caused by the fungus *Beauveria bassiana.* This fungus was widely deployed in the US and Europe for centuries. These colors are rather coincidentally the same colors seen in the strange "fibers" which are produced by Morgellon's lesions. In the 19th century description of infected silkworm larvae, the "most minute lice" could be seen covering the affected silkworms. When Morgellon's lesions are seen at high magnification, worm-like mites or funny looking insect-like creatures may sometimes be seen.[23]

We have an idea that the tiny worm-like creatures may be nematodes and their parasites; the very worm-like demodex mites. Both of these are parasites of silkworms. Parasites plausibly explain the creepy crawly and biting sensations, and the presence of each of these creatures on some, but not necessarily all Morgellon's patients. Fairly recent texts also describe what may be *collembola* as sometimes associated with Morgellon's sores. Some collembola are flea-sized, while others are microscopic in size. These are part of a family of *hexapods* or *springtails*, which are not true insects.[24-26]

Collembola feed upon algae and bacteria. Some species are *parasites of nematodes,* including those used agriculturally upon citrus and other crops, and which infest silkworms and other insects. These parasites may appear in lesions of patients bitten by ticks that were exposed to nematodes, mites, and other parasites. It is not difficult to imagine that parasites hitching a ride upon vectoring insects may drop onto human skin to initiate infections and to breed and proliferate on the very hospitable environment of human skin, even though it is not a typical parasitic home. Collembola are not considered by the CDC to be known human parasites, so humans may be accidental hosts. Regardless of whether collembola are properly acknowledged by the public health sector, their accidental introduction onto the human species by insect vectors nevertheless facilitates human infections, and extends their normal host range. Some Morgellon's patients have complained of contracting their infections after being bitten by bird mites, so here is another interesting mite-Morgellon's connection. Like ticks, mites are blood-feeding parasites that are extremely small – so small that their human hosts are unaware of their presence.[24,25]

The idea that microscopic parasites may be found in or on skin lesions in patients with insect-borne infections should not be dismissed. Proper scientific investigation by those without ties to industries which are related to agricultural controls could be undertaken. Researchers from the Oklahoma State Department of Health and the National Pediculosis Association found collembola present on eighteen out of twenty Morgellon's patient skin lesions that were microscopically examined.[24-26]

The most striking manifestation of Morgellon's infections are the red, ulcerative skin lesions which produce the strange hairs or fibers and other debris. This debris may consist of cotton-like clumps or lint; black spotted granules, or crystals. Some but not all of this debris will fluoresce under UV (black) light. Some people have attempted to explain these fibers as cotton, perhaps derived from the patient's clothing. However there is evidence that a fluorescent bacterium may be the reason for these glow-in-the-dark like artifacts.

Pseudomonas fluorescens, Pseudomonas aeruginosa, and other members of this *gammaproteobacteria* family are gram-negative bacteriae common to soil and water, and true plant parasites. They are also routinely used within genetic engineering processes, including as "reporter" genes or fluorescent markers. These genes tell scientists by fluorescence whether a genetic construct has taken up the desired engineered genes. These bacteriae are also found naturally in the environment, so there is no telling from where they truly originate, although since they are more frequently found than years past, it might be assumed their increased presence is related to genetically engineered crops. The crown gall disease bacterium *Agrobacterium tumefaciens* for example is engineered using a fluorescent marker gene from a *Pseudomonas* bacterial strain, for transgenic crops.[27-29]

In my last book *God Science,* I discussed the role that *Agrobacterium tumefaciens* may play in Morgellon's disease. This bacterium is routinely engineered into insecticides for citrus and other crops. *Agrobacterium tumefaciens* is the agent of *crown gall disease*. Its scientific name is *Rhizobium radiobacter.* It is a soil-based bacterium that belongs to the family of nitrogen-fixing legume bacteriae that are commonly found in plant root systems.[30]

In the US, the coastlines and the Gulf of Mexico are where the bulk of Morgellon's patients are found, although a few families reside in other states. These regions are known for their citrus crops, grapes, stone fruits, and nut trees. *A. tumefaciens* also naturally infects rhubarb and *horseradish* plants – plants that are also affected by an important spirochete, the spiroplasmas. It makes sense if recently designed genetic engineering tools that are highly useful as insecticides are accidentally contributing to the equation of a novel Lyme-like human disease called Morgellon's.[30]

Agrobacterium tumefaciens has been extensively used within genetically engineered "chimera" (formulas) because it naturally inserts a small segment of its DNA from its mobile *plasmid* into infected plant cells. Think of plasmids as little chromosome islands that contain important virulence genes. This insertion of DNA causes tumors or galls to form upon the infected plants. *A. tumefaciens* is highly useful to scientists to control the transcription process during genetic engineering. (This is the duplication of cells.) *A. tumefaciens* bacteriae create *cellulose fibrils* (strands) which anchor themselves to the cells of infected plants. After these fibrils are produced, they are covered with a calcium outer membrane protein. *Cellulose* is the most abundant "biopolymer" on earth, and is a component of plant cell walls. The soil bacteria *Cytophaga hutchinsonii* is able to digest cellulose. This organism has been sequenced by scientists, and is genetically engineered into insecticides. The organism is part of the *Cytophaga-Flavobacterium* extremophile family of microbes found deep underground and inside insect bodies. An early DuPont patent describes how natural and synthetic fibers may be formulated:[31-32]

> "Structural polypeptides may also be synthesized by either *recombinant DNA* or, in some cases, by classical organic synthetic methods."

These fibers can be dissolved in acids that contain chlorides, fluorides, and acetic acid, which is vinegar or ethanoic acid. Acetic acid is a chemical reagent used to produce many chemical compounds. It is used in dyes (as trichloroacetic acid), photographic film, descaling agents, wood glue, paint (i.e. verdigris [copper acetate]), and vinyl acetate to make polymers and adhesives. Acetic acid can also be made from petroleum-based chemicals. Synthetic acetic acid was first produced in 1847. Organic acetic acid is made from distilling wood with lime and sulfuric acid.[33,34]

Natural and synthetic acetic acid are produced by bacterial fermentation, typically by *Clostridium* or *Acetobacter* bacteriae. When changed to an ester, acetic acid becomes a solvent for inks, paints, aniline dyes (aluminum acetate), pesticides (silver acetate), and coatings. Copper acetate is used as a preservative and antifungal agent upon livestock silage (food). Other important chemicals that dissolve natural or synthetic fibers include surfactants and quaternary compounds, which are halogen-containing acids. Fibers that are dissoved by chemicals (even in wastewaters) may release proteins that may be taken up by other microbes, including those which produce hair-like projections or fibrils.[33,34]

What is interesting is that Morgellon's patients may complain of pain if their skin fibers are disturbed or removed. This may represent the attachment of *A. tumefaciens* or other bacterial fibrils to nerve endings or capillaries under the skin. The fibers that are produced in Morgellon's lesions are of "unknown" composition. One explanation is that they may be of keratin or cellulose origin since as far as we know the body cannot manufacture synthetic fibers of its own accord. The human body however does produce soft vellus hairs which fit the description of the Morgellon's "fibers" or hairs, and which hurt to remove.[35-38]

Natural vegetable fibers are typically cellulose in origin. These come from *cotton,* hemp, flax, and other plants. There are also seed and other fibers from plants including cotton, leaves, and fruits. We are already familiar with animal fibers, which include *wool,* alpaca, goat hair, the *silk from silkworms, spiders, mites,* and other silk-producing insects; and avian fibers in the form of feathers. Natural fibers are used in construction, automotive, plastics, and other industries to strengthen products. Over the past decades, *synthetic fibers* (polymers) have been created out of *cellulose, minerals,* and *synthetic polymers*. These may include silk, rayon, acetate, glass, metallic acrylic, Kevlar,® nylon, polyester, polyethylene, spandex, and Gore-Tex.® Biopolymers and synthetic polymers in wastewaters and soils can also be degraded by bacteriae that have this ability. Once degraded, these proteins may once again be taken up by any microbes that are present.

Some Morgellon's patients say their hair has fallen out, and that they have lost finger or toe nails. Nails and hair are made of fibrous structural proteins called *keratin.* Clusters of filaments form bundles which are very strong and insoluble in water. Another biological material that is approximately as tough as human or animal hair is a special keratinized tissue found in insects, called *chitin* (pronounced "kite-in"). This is the hard exterior shell that forms the insect body. Scientists have engineered genetic constructs that can degrade insect chitin. Some chemical agents and natural bacteriae may do the same. Although *chitinase* enzymes are absent in most bacteriae, scientists have figured out a way to genetically engineer B.t., *Bacillus popilliae,* or *Bacillus moritai* insecticides to degrade insect chitin using NPV viruses, entomopathogenic fungi, microsporidiae, or poxviruses. The degraded insect chitin thus becomes part of the loose proteins that may be taken up by other microbes in soils or wastewaters.[40-43]

Certain tick species display a level of resistance to chitinase enzymes, including American dog ticks and Lone Star ticks. One way around this is to engineer chitinase enzymes into insecticides to gain access to the tick body so toxic spores and other insecticidal microbes may enter. One patent invention says the following (remember that the fungi *B. bassiana* is the cause of "reds" disease in silkworms):[39-48]

> "It was found that the activity of *B. thuringiensis* was considerably increased when chitinase was added to the preparation; larval mortality provoked by commercial preparations of *B. thuringiensis* was advanced by from 4 to 6 or more days for the various temperatures."

> "In accordance with this invention, it has now been found that the combination of or the concurrent use of the enzyme chitinase is able to increase the insecticidal effectiveness of these enteric microorganisms (including viruses) ...Chitinase is produced extracellularly by certain bacteria and fungi. Material can be obtained from various strains of *Beauveria* e.g., *B. bassiana*..."

We know about the probability that chickens and chicken products have been contaminated with retroviruses and other viruses that for the most part cannot be separated from the tissues or eggs of vaccinated birds. What is also important to understand is that there are important bacillus bacteriae that are related to the insecticidal bacteria "B.t." that have been isolated from poultry (i.e. *Bacillus fastidiosus*). Chicken entrails have been used in the testing of chitin and B.t.-containing insecticides. With such experiments scientists may have also tried to ascertain if B.t. could cause a *transfer of genes between B.t. formulas and symbiont poultry bacteria.* One patent described such aerial sprays:[49]

> "In the aerial spraying tests a semi-purified material obtained from chicken entrails was used (about 890-950 nephelometric units)... Applications of *Bacillus thuringiensis* by airplane or ground equipment have been used with little success in the control of [Spruce budworm]."

Remember that poultry and their offspring are inherently infected with bacteria, viruses, and retroviruses simply because they have long been vaccinated. Anything made using poultry products could potentially cause disease if activated from latency since B.t. products are specifically designed to cause microbes to reactivate. What happens if microbes found in the environment or within *poultry or other vaccinated animals* become infected with the microbes found in recombinant B.t. formulas? The answer is they may become toxic facilitators of infections for any organisms that come into contact with them. The patent continues:[49]

> "Experimental sprayings with commercial preparations of *B. thuringiensis* alone, and with chitinase, were carried out in balsam fir stands severely infested by spruce budworm. Three 100-acre plots were established in these stands: Plot 1 was sprayed with Thuricide HPC plus chitinase, Plot 2 with Thuricide HPC alone, and Plot 3 served as control. Spraying was done by a Steerman aircraft equipped with micron-aire sprayers, which permitted an even and good coverage..."

> "An extensive field trial was made on 10,000 acres of budworm-infested fir stands. Aerial spraying was carried out using the following unit formula...The number of insects killed and the foliage saved were as good as that obtainable by the commercial application of chemical insecticides and better than obtainable from the application of Thuricide alone. This biological insecticide would have a minimal effect on the ecology..."[49]

Insect chitin is a natural polymer that is composed of N-acetylglucosamine, a glucose derivative. It is biocompatible with human tissue and is used in surgical applications to promote wound healing. The EPA also approved the use of chitinase enzymes to *treat drinking water and sewage* because they separate organic compounds and heavy metals, precipitate anionic wastes, reduce phosphates, and capture pollutants including DDT and PCBs. Chitinase in its deacetylated form *aggressively binds to mammalian and microbial cells.* (This means it may also bind persisting chemicals to human cells.) It is because of these properties that chitin is also used as a *skin substitute*.[41-43,50]

It is interesting to note that the Lyme disease spirochetes contain enzymes which degrade chitin (HMG-CoA). The only other known bacterium with a similar enzyme is *Pseudomonas mevalonii.* This is a gram-negative *proteobacteria* that is found in the soil and water, and which forms biofilms. Are there *Pseudomonas* species genes in Bb spirochetes? According to research, *Pseudomonas* species carry genes which allow them to create biofilms, and which provide antibiotic resistance.[41-43,50]

I should mention that when I had a dermoid cyst removed from my reproductive tract, I realized anything is possible in the human body as far as growing weird hairs or other structures where they are not supposed to grow. The cyst contained strange fibers that also resembled hairs. There are several genetic disorders that will affect the growth of connective tissues. The question remains, what exactly are the Morgellon's fibers made of, and what causes the ulcerative skin lesions found on these patients?[51]

Since our model silkworms and some mites create silk, and silk is a *cellulose* fiber, it makes sense that similar fibers might be found among Morgellon's lesions. It is tough to decide whether such fibers would be of plant, insect, bacterial, or synthetic origin without analysis. We have already accounted for the various colors found in the hairs or fibers as caused by silkworm infections. But these colors are also found in human hair which is largely keratin-based. Hair color is regulated by melanin, so the composition of the Morgellon's hairs should provide vital clues to their natural or synthetic origins.

There are a number of *bacillus* bacteriae that are classified as *Flavobacterium* (extremophiles). This group includes the *paenibacillus* family that is found in insect guts including silkworms. Many strains degrade natural and synthetic polymers (fibers), and they are found in industrial wastewaters and soils. Some of these bacteriae fluoresce while others produce colored filaments. The colors range from transparent, cream, grey, white, and yellow; to orange, red, pink, blue, brown, and black hues depending on strain. Of course yellow and blue could make green as well. These bacteriae may explain why silkworms and Morgellon's patients have colored filament-producing infections. Of the color-producing bacillus strains that are spore-formers we find these (including the insecticide B.t. because it is a fermented *Bacillus cereus*):[52]

Bacillus cereus	*B. subtilis*	*B. aquimaris*	*B. carboniphilus*
B. arseniciselenatis	*B. clarkii*	*B. endophyticus*	*B. fastidiosus*
B. firmus	*B. gibsonii*	*B. hwajinpoensis*	*B. indicus*
B. jeotgali	*B. marisflavi*	*B. megaterium*	*B. pseudofirmus*
B. sonorensis	*B. atrophaeus*	*B. agicola*	

Whether the mysterious Morgellon's fibers are derived from cellulose or keratin; from natural fibers such as silk, cotton, wool, or flax; or synthetic polymer fibers that have been degraded has yet to be scientifically proven. It is possible that bacterial plasmids changed in wastewaters or soils by chemicals or surfactants could have picked up recombinant polymer genes if the genes were derived from natural fiber producing plants or insects. It is also possible that B.t. insecticides that contain pigment-producing bacteria are able to become part of an insect-transmissible infection which because of its recombinant genes, causes human skin to manifest lesions which produce colored hairs. The hairs may be as simple as vellus hairs that are changed in color by bacterial infection of the hair follicles. Or the hairs may be produced by pigmented bacteria that are able to genetically direct the follicles to produce hair-like filaments from bacterial genes that contain chitin enzymes which act upon human keratin in the follicles.

It may also be possible for bacteria to excrete nanofibers that were airborne (thus landing upon soils); and inhaled or ingested by the infected patient. These nanofibers are genetically engineered into food crops, and may be dissolved in the human gut when we eat genetically modified foods (i.e. corn, soy). The nanofiber proteins could hypothetically migrate into the microbes which infect the patients. There the nanofiber protein genes may contribute genetic information to the bacteria to produce filaments in human skin. Or the bacteria may simply invade human tissues and the genes donate instructions to human hair follicles to produce bacteria and nanofiber-influenced hairs. It is probably highly likely that the Morgellon's fibers are human vellus hair that has received the "wrong" genetic information from foreign genes that have become part of an infectious microbe. Follicles produce hairs according to the genetic instructions supplied, whether by human cells or those from pigmented bacteria. I studied many patent inventions for genetically engineered cotton, human "skin," artificial silks, and other textile (polymer) fibers to understand how this may be possible.[53,54]

Scientists have managed to genetically engineer spider silk, which is made of simple proteins, into transgenic goats, to excrete these recombinant silk proteins into their milk. The protein fibers are then recoverable and may be used as a human skin substitute. Because of their strength and flexibility, spider proteins can also be woven into bullet-proof garments. There are about four dozen patents on the topic of goat and spider silks, proving that the technology is moving forward. Some of the patents describe how spider silk proteins are recoverable from the milk or urine of transgenic animals. These fibers are the microfibers or nanofibers. What can be created using spider silk applies also to silkworm or mite silks. Patent inventions will not always list the *exact* formulas for an invention, but may instead substitute a related product or organism that lies within the same family or product line to conceal the actual intended agent while permitting it to remain part of an invention.[53-58]

Scientists have also managed to identify bacterial and fungal genes that have *become incorporated into the genes (genome) of the two-spotted spider mite, which is a silk-producing mite.* Perhaps these or other related mite species can be found on the skin of persons who have Morgellon's disease. If so, then their silk-producing talents when combined with the bacteria which produce filaments may significantly affect the color, texture, and production of human vellus hairs. If the hairs are first human in origin, it could explain why they hurt to pull them from the skin.[53-58]

In a similar sense, perhaps the demodex mites found upon normal human skin can incorporate the bacterial and fungal genes of a bacterial infection to influence hair production. Demodex mites naturally harbor *Bacillus oleronius,* which produces highly antigenic (immune stimulating) proteins that cause inflammation in the skin. These bacteriae are among a group of endospore-formers that are found in the hind guts of termites, roaches, and mites. As *thermophiles,* these bacteria can withstand high temperatures. These bacteria are also found in milk, and can withstand pasteurization.[82,83]

Related bacteria are *Bacillus sporothermodurans, B. licheniformis, Geobacillus pallidus* and *Anoxybacillus* species. *These thermophiles are closely related to other bacilli so we might expect them to reassort with the applied bacillus-based (B.t.) insecticides.* People who have suppressed immune systems (i.e. infections) are unable to keep demodex mites under control, and therefore they proliferate to cause skin infections and hair (and nail) loss. One of the more effective antibiotic treatments for these mites is *metronidazole cream.*[82,83]

Recombinant or natural genes from spider, silkworm, or plant fibers that were first dissolved by chemical wastes are acquired by microbes in our polluted environment. We know that mites can incorporate bacterial and fungal genes into their cells. Environmental microbes and the thermophilic bacteria found in milk-producing animals may be transferred to vectoring insects. We know there are transgenic crops and animals that are used to produce artificial fibers from insect silk-producing genes. We also know that transgenic animals can produce fibers in their milk or urine. Is it hard to believe that wastes can make their way into fish in coastal areas, crops, or timber; any of which are used as animal feeds? Microbes in an animal's body either natural or recombinant in origin, may be transmitted to the microbes in vectoring insects and then to humans.[53-58]

The US Secretary of the Army is assignee on a recombinant silk patent that describes how spider silks may be engineered to be soluble, and are recovered for use in products including military textiles and ballistic materials. This process involves a roughly 50:50 mix of hydrochloric acid and propionic acid to dissolve the silk proteins. A patent from 1939 relates to the manufacturing of proteins from fibroin (i.e. silk), *casein*, gelatin, wool, or alginic acid. (Casein is a milk protein.) The patent describes the extraction of fibrous proteins by a solution using *quaternary benzyl substituted ammonium base.* These are the quaternary-ammonia amines that we discussed earlier.[59,60]

Propionic acid is derived from propane and is a component of sugar degradation. In one form it is a soapy potassium salt. Propanoic acids are byproducts of the manufacture of acetic acid. It also inhibits the growth of mold and some bacteria. Propionic acid is used as an *animal feed supplement* in the form of the antibiotic *Monensin*; and as an animal and human food preservative. It is also useful as an intermediate chemical especially in the manufacturing of polymers, thermoplastics, pharmaceuticals, and pesticides. The *thermoplastics* include the *fluoroplastics* PTFE, PFA and other polymers, many of which have already been targeted as persisting environmental pollutants. Bacteria in the guts of ruminant animals and those found in human sweat glands (skin) are *propionibacterium* which use this acid in their metabolic processes.

Propionibacterium cause the skin condition *Acne vulgaris*, and this is interesting because these bacteria, which are found on skin in pre-pubescent children, are said to fully colonize the skin from one to three years before the age of sexual maturity. This is the same timeframe where demodex mites populate human skin. An overpopulation of mites can cause intense itching, and reminds us of the child-affecting French illness of the 17th century. The "classic" Morgellon's in that century did not involve the modern genetically engineered bacteria or viruses from insecticides or vaccines. But similar chemicals which exert negative influences upon fibers and microbes were present in the industrial wastes and in finished textiles of that era. The triggering agents for such an odd skin disease are probably the very same chemicals and natural contaminants found in modern watersheds today, just as they were present long ago. In previous centuries, pollutants came from industrial wastes of agriculture (i.e. viticulture), glassmaking, metalworking, textile processing, paper mills, printing inks, papermaking, and textile dyes. Today we have the addition of industrial chemicals, surfactants, agrochemicals and recombinant insecticides, vaccines, and antibiotics.[11,20,21]

In earlier centuries after processing silk, remnants of pierced empty coccoons (which contained viruses, fungi and bacterial spores); and leftover silk, floss, and wastes were carded, spun, and mixed with wool, cotton, or flax, for durability. Then they were woven into inexpensive, everyday wearable products. Clothing made from parasite-contaminated discards in conjunction with the natural colonization of demodex mites on pre-pubescent children's skin; and exposures to manufacturing wastes could bring forth the "Morgellons" affliction as well as the strange hairs or fibers found on the French children.[11,20,24]

The modern version of Morgellon's may be attributed to similar mechanisms caused by the exposure of vectoring insects to the same bacteriae, viruses, and nematodes of yesterday; plus those that are genetically engineered into today's insecticides. Industrial chemicals that are now ubiquitous to the soil and water as environmental pollutants also contain recombinant fibers that contain genes which may be acquired by bacteria. These fibers include the various polymers that are part of many industrial products nonetheleast of which are textile, plastic, or agricultural in origin. Where there are recombinant fibers, there are lab-maniuplated genes to create them, including insect viruses and bacteria such as *Agrobacterium tumefaciens*, or other family members including *Flavobacterium*.

The emergence of Morgellon's in the 21st century as opposed to the 20th century when modern Lyme disease first emerged is also explainable. The addition of genetically engineered fibers and/or fiber-producing crops which were introduced during the late 1990s; and the 20th century textile and other polymers which use recombinant genes may be the final contributing factors to the emergence of today's Morgellon's disease – an infection that is truly "Lyme-plus."

We have seen how spider and silkworm silks may be dissolved using industrial or agricultural chemicals. Synthetic fibers are created using similar processes and any of these important proteins and their recombinant genes can be incorporated into bacteriae found in wastewaters or soils. These genes are introduced into plants, and make their way into insects, animals, and now humans as accidental hosts. We know that genes control the expression or formation of skin, hair, nails, and other processes. We can only imagine what happens when these worlds collide to create natural or partly synthetic fibers that may be expressed in human skin cells during a mixed infection introduced by a vectoring insect. While we can see that this is entirely possible, it may be far harder to accept as a matter of reality.

In short, industrial and agricultural chemicals are fully capable of dissolving spider, silkworm, mite, cotton, wool, cornsilk, and other natural fibers (fibroins) as well as synthetic polymer fibers. Any of these proteins or genes including those from recombinant insecticides, crops, or products become free-floating proteins in polluted soils and wastewaters. Such proteins are taken up by microbes that are transmitted by vectoring insects. We *know* this happens because patent inventions tell us so, and because scientists exploit gene-swapping in order to create recombinant crops, polymers, and insecticides.

Some manufacturers have created recombinant spider silk dragline using the bacteriae *E. coli* and *Bacillus subtilis,* a soil bacteria related to *Bacillus thuringiensis* (B.t.) and to *Bacillus anthracis* (anthrax). We can see that recombinant silks can be created by bacteria in the laboratory, just as they are naturally created. It is not hard to imagine that a soil bacteria like B.t. and an infected bacterium got together to create the lesions and hairs of Morgellon's disease. The colored aspect could of course come from insect viruses, and the "lint" or cotton-like materials from recombinant cotton, trees, or other plants or microbes which produce cellulose. These proteins may be incorporated into human keratin to produce the tiny clumps of lint, and the other remnants found in Morgellon's lesions. Mites and nematodes may be inconsequential to the hairs or fibers, except that they live on and within the follicles and skin during infestations, and contribute to the biting and crawling sensations felt by patients.[53-63]

A patent from E. I. du Pont de Nemours and Company describes the creation of a host cell that has been transformed using a bacterial plasmid (mini chromosome) which makes the cells *secrete spider silk proteins.* We now see that bacterial plasmids can transport and contribute spider, silkworm, cotton or other fibrous proteins to the microbes of insects, animals, or humans to cause infectious diseases which might in turn express these proteins, even within human skin.[63]

According to the patent, host cells may be selected from a group which includes *E. coli, Bacillus subtilis,* the yeast *Saccharomyces cerevisiae* (used to create B.t.), *Schizosaccharomyces pombe,* Pichia pastoris,*† and molds *Aspergillus* or *Streptomyces*. The patent also mentions how the cloning and expression of silk-like proteins are described in other patents. One such patent cloned the silk fibroin gene complete with gene sequences from the silkworm moth *Bombyx mori,* and introduced them into *E. coli* cells. A 1987 European patent (EP 230702) by Petty-Saphon et al. disclosed the recombinant production of silk fibroin and silk sericin from host cells which included *E. coli, Saccharomyces cerevisiae, Pseudomonas* species, *Rhodopseudomonas, Bacillus,* and *Streptomyces*. The inventors of the E.I. du Pont de Nemours Company patent had this to say in their invention: "In the preferred embodiments the expression of silk proteins derived from *Bombyx mori* is discussed." Folks this is our friend the silkworm. These explanations plausibly explain why we may find natural or recombinant proteins from cotton, spiders, silkworm moths, or even chemical polymers helping to create the odd "hairs" or "fibers" found in Morgellon's skin lesions.[53-67]

**Schizosaccharomyces pombe is a fission yeast of millet beers, and is common to citrus crops including apples and grapes. †Pichia pastoris is a model yeast to genetic engineering, and is used as an expression vector system (chimera) in genetically engineered products including insecticides. These vectors are called "pPICZα" A, B, and C.*

It seems clear that silkworm silks (or other proteins) may be expressed within Morgellon's lesions by bacteria such as the Bb spirochete, if the agent has taken up those genes from the environment. The silkworm *Bombyx mori* produces huge amounts of silk proteins during the final stage of larval development, the fifth instar. This is the mature caterpillar stage that is affected by the multi-colored "spot" infections. The silk proteins are stored inside the middle silk gland of the larvae. The proteins are *fibroin* and *sericin* (an adhesive for making silk coccoons). In addition, prostaglandins are locally active hormones which alter silk synthesis by controlling silk gene expression.[68-71]

During bacterial infections, prostaglandins are rapidly synthesized in animal and human cells. Prostaglandins change resting hair follicles to an active growth phase; enlarge the hair follicles, and change the quality of hair produced. These chemicals also control the quality and growth of human hair even if the hair contains foreign proteins. We already know that human hair stores foreign proteins from drugs and heavy metals, so foreign proteins are expressed through hair follicles. When cells are infected with bacteria that carry natural or genetically engineered plasmids, those genes insert the "wrong" instructions into follicle cells, which could force them to produce the mysterious colored fibers seen in Morgellon's lesions.[68-71]

Scientists have designed ways to create *human fibrous proteins* using spider or other silk and genetic engineering techniques. The same inventions that can create these products are also applicable for *treating disorders that are associated with the expression of these same proteins*. Another patent describes the use of silkworm or other silk-producing arthropod proteins from *insect silk glands,* for use as feedstocks for various industrial products.[72,73]

This leaves us with just one question. What causes the ulcerating skin lesions of Morgellon's disease? These lesions range from red irritations to streaks, and ulcerating, weeping sores with craters. *Cutaneous anthrax,* also called "wool sorter's disease" because it is found among people who work in textile or animal hide processing, is a form of contact anthrax infection. We know that anthrax is caused by the soil bacteria *Bacillus anthracis*, and we also know that agricultural insecticides contain an anthrax-related *Bacillus thuringiensis*. B.t. insecticidal proteins or related bacteria may be part of the Morgellon's disease complex. We also know that certain livestock antibiotics are fed to ruminant animals where they ferment along with feed supplements hemp, flax, and cottonseed (the remaining plant portion of cotton crops after the lint has been removed).

It is not difficult to understand that B.t. insecticides that use *Agrobacterium tumefaciens* are applied or engineered into genetically modified (GM) crops. Using the silkworm model, modified plant or insect fibers may become part of the Morgellon's equation. Cotton has been genetically engineered not only to contain B.t. insecticides, but also to contain genetically altered fibers. As well, the crown gall disease *Agrobacterium tumefaciens* promotes the expression of *foreign structural genes* in bacteria including *E. coli* found in the bovine gut. Under gut fermentation, recombinant insecticides, vaccines, and GM feeds may be able to create a complex microbe the likes of Bb that produces Lyme disease, and in Morgellon's patients a cutaneous form of anthrax.[74-79]

Remember that livestock have been vaccinated against infections including leptospirosis. The vaccines don't always protect against all leptospirosis strains. The vaccines also typically contain Tweens and other chemicals that may be mutagenic, or which may affect latent microbes. We already know that vaccine cell lines can contain viruses, retroviruses, or bacterial contaminants. The potential for the development of a Morgellon's, Lyme, or a mutated leptonema is now more easily understood as an unintentional and uncontrollable byproduct of genetic engineering techniques.

The CDC describes Morgellon's as "unexplained dermopathy." In an earlier chapter I mentioned studies regarding Morgellon's disease origins that are sponsored by the CDC under a \$338,000 grant to Kaiser Permanente and US military scientists. We can see perhaps why these entities may be involved in these studies. Past and current industrial, military, and/or agricultural products and processes may be causing human infectious diseases. As a result, we can expect to see the kind of medical paradigms of denial we find today with Lyme and Morgellon's diseases.[80,81]

Trouble Ahead for Biocides and Animal Vaccines

Two cell lines have been described as useful for replicating viruses and bacteriae, including arboviruses, chlamydiae, rickettsiae, spiroplasmas, and protozoans. Pathogens that easily replicate in cell lines according to the patents allow scientists to produce antibodies and antitoxins. One such cell line is useful for animal vaccines and insecticides:[1-4]

> "...for producing biological control agents for ticks, such as arthropod directed pathogens, e.g. Nosema, or microsporidia (which are pathogenic to ticks)."

What if cell lines that are used to create vaccines or applied insecticides were found to be contaminated? What if such a discovery occurred long after products were manufactured and deployed? What if the contaminants contributed to animal or human diseases? What if upon the identification of the causative agents of an emerging human infection, that new tick or other cell lines had to be fabricated *to replace older contaminated cell lines?*

A *tick cell line* patent was filed January 22, 1981 by NIH scientists at Rocky Mountain Laboratories in Hamilton, Montana. This is the same laboratory where Dr. Willy Burgdorfer et al. would declare the identification of the causative agent of Lyme disease only a few months later. The patent is assigned to the US Department of Health. This means that manufacturers of biological controls or vaccines which utilize these cell lines are paying patent royalties to the US government.[4]

According to the patent *six new Ixodes cell lines* were created; four from the embryonic tissues of American dog ticks (*Dermacentor variabilis*); and two from rabbit ticks (*D. parumapertus*). The patent refers to older patents that are suitable for animal vaccines. The new tick cell lines also use arboviruses from a group which includes *Powassan, Colorado Tick Fever, Sawgrass, Cascade, St. Louis encephalitis,* and others. These are viruses that are found in some Lyme patients. The patent describes a selection of a number of rickettsial species including Rocky Mountain spotted fever; rickettsialpox, typhus, and a soft tick-isolated microbe (#113704-14). One patent describes a monkey kidney cell line that is used as a substrate for other vaccines. If any cell lines are contaminated, then anything made from them will likely be contaminated as well.[1,4-10]

The soft tick isolate #113704-14 is interesting to us because research refers to this number in a discussion of *polycyclic and cyclic products which involve a manganese oxidation process.* The tick isolate may contain a Bb spirochetal strain, or component of Bb that (like Bb) uses *manganese enzyme sets.* Is one of the new cell lines designed to protect animals from Bb spirochetal infections? Is it disguised as "soft-tick" (think livestock) isolate #113704-14? Only a few bacteria actually use manganese enzymes. Those which do are *capable of degrading persisting organic pollutants including polycyclic aromatic hydrocarbons, or PAHs. These are persisting organic pollutants (POPs) that are derived from burning fossil fuels, garbage, factory wastes, and organic matter (i.e. wood pulp).*[38]

The new cell line patent from 1981 uses viruses from a group that includes the *Reoviruses* and possible degraded reoviruses in the form of insect arboviruses to grow cells for the new cell lines. Once again this new cell line can be used for animal (or human) vaccines, and for recombinant insecticides or transgenic crops. According to the patent, the few tick cell lines that were formerly established:[6-15]

> "...are difficult to manage because of slow growth and the fastidious nature of the cells."

The patent claims that the established cell line, which came from 1977 cultures:

> "...has accidentally been extinguished by toxic culture medium and bacterial contamination of frozen stocks."

Perhaps the contamination came from non-sterile dionized water that could have contained filterable *leptospira spirochetes.* The establishment of new cell lines for animal vaccines and for insecticides is most curious in timing since the patent was filed just a few months before the declaration of a "juvenile arthritis" outbreak in Connecticut. The previous cell lines were reportedly infected with viruses including West Nile, Louping Ill, Langat, and Quaranfil (an orthomyxovirus or poxvirus). Looping Ill and Langat are members of the Russian spring-summer encephalitis virus family. Like the other members of this family (i.e. Powassan, RSSE, Central European encephalitis etc.), Langat and Louping Ill produce very similar symptoms to Lyme disease. Did someone destroy earlier cell lines to "fix" a contaminated cell line problem that would soon have global consequences? Or was this rather convenient "destruction" of key cell lines truly a coincidence in timing to the Lyme-related events of the day? If globally important insecticides and animal vaccines were made using contaminated cell lines, we can see how the problem would affect every country that used these products over decades. Such a disastrous thing would be difficult for scientists and public health officials to admit publicly. It could absolutely explain the events of the day such as we have seen in the highly contentious world of Lyme, Morgellon's and other infectious diseases including those with "unknown" origins.[6-15]

The new tick cell line patent goes on to discuss cell lines that are unable to propagate mosquito cells, corn earworm moth cells, or certain viruses or rickettsiae; and the necessity of having *tick cell lines* that can do this. This refers to the desire for new and improved cell lines for biological insecticide and animal vaccines. The tick cell line patent stresses the ability of cell lines to grow arboviruses from blood-feeding insects. This is of course important because insect viruses are widely used in recombinant genes for GM crops, and because they can reassort in the bodies of insects and animals. According to the patent:[16]

> "The cell lines for this invention may be used for replicating viruses, rickettsias, chlamydias, *spiroplasmas,* and protozoans. These replicated pathogens can probably be utilized for the production of *vaccines,* antibodies, antitoxins, and the like. Additional possible uses of replicated pathogens would be to produce antigens for allergic sensitivity testing and *for producing biological control agents for ticks,* such as arthropod directed pathogens, e.g. Nosema, or microsporidian (which are pathogenic to ticks)."

"The cell lines of this invention are *particularly useful for the replication of pathogens which infect livestock* and are arthropod vectored."[16]

Did NIH scientists find it necessary to replace "destroyed" tick cell lines that were found to have been contaminated with agents that created Bb spirochetes? Did they intend to replace them with new tick cell lines that were better designed for livestock vaccines and applied insecticides that were especially useful against ticks? Did the former cell line(s) contain spiroplasmas, arboviruses, leptospires, and other contaminants? Were those contaminants traced back from the leptonema found in the environment and from vaccinated animals to the tick cell lines that had been used to create global vaccines and insecticides?

It is most curious that this new tick cell line patent was filed the very same year that NIH scientists at the very same lab would work (less than six months later) to identify the causative agent of a new human epidemic called Lyme disease. This actually fits very neatly into the story's timeline because the juvenile arthritis outbreak came about in the late 1960s. This is the same timeframe that scientists began studying mutated leptonema. It might take some time to trace an animal pathogen all the way back to continuous insect cell lines for insecticides and animal vaccines. If they did this and were successful as described, we can expect enormous concern over the scope of a now emerging human epidemic. We can also expect there would be an announcement a short while after the agent's origins were discovered, that scientists had found the causative agent of the emerging human infection called Lyme disease. We would also expect patents for new revised cell lines to be filed – and they were.[16]

If infected cell lines were used to create early animal vaccines and insecticides for industrial and agricultural purposes then such vaccines could have transmitted infections to livestock animals in a number of ways. First, insecticides were added to animal feeds before they were fed to livestock. Second, livestock are routinely vaccinated before slaughter. Cell cultures and even the laboratory water used to make vaccines are routinely contaminated with leptospire spirochetes and other agents.[17-23]

Contaminated feeds or animal vaccines could certainly explain the emergence of an immune deficiency virus which also began to emerge in the US cattle population beginning around 1969, especially among feedlot livestock. According to a *New York Times* article, USDA scientists isolated an immune-suppressing virus they had collected from cow serum in Louisiana. The USDA scientist credited with isolating the causative agent was Dr. Martin J. Van Der Maaten, a veterinarian from the Ames, Iowa National Animal Disease Center. At the time the article was published, beef and dairy cattle comprised a $55 *billion* dollar industry that was already plagued by millions in annual losses due to diseases. This was the "recent cattle expansion" mentioned by the CDC scientists who were analyzing leptospirosis infections in animals around the time that mutated leptonema first emerged during the 1950s and 1960s.[17-23]

The FDA had already been cracking down on antibiotic use in livestock animals due to carcinogenic ingredients and residues that were found lurking in consumer products and foods. Unfortunately this new virus, which was named *Bovine Immunodeficiency Virus* (BIV), did not receive heavy scrutiny for two more decades, and very little fanfare in the media. Finally in 1987, Dr. Van Der Maaten and colleagues took an interest in the virus and began studying it. Among their objectives were to determine if there was a human risk from exposure to BIV virus. No such risk was reported, and we may wonder whether a completely independent laboratory would have arrived at a similar conclusion. Government agencies claimed that the risk of human infection from BIV was "zero." But that certainly does not account for the ability of an animal virus to be reassorted within the gut of a biting fly or blood-sucking tick where through host amplification and gene-swapping, a new virus may be created, including one that *could* pose a health risk to humans. That new virus could have been an HIV virus that emerged at the same time in blood products that used bovine albumin and/or nematodal proteins.[17-23]

Microbial gene reassortment is a fact of nature. Scientists discovered that fruit flies, corn (maize), and the potato-like tuber *cassava* (as examples) contain genes with transposable elements (transposons). These special genes allow gene swapping to occur between organisms including microbes like the *cassava latent virus,* a *geminivirus* that frequently mutates. Scientists have learned there are close structual resemblances between the transposons of the fruit fly and the Moloney mouse leukemia virus, a virus that is similar to human adult T-cell Leukemia (HTLV). HTLV viruses are part of the HTLV/HIV-AIDS virus family. Similarities were also discovered between the Hepatitis B virus and those of the cauliflower mosaic virus, a plant-infecting *baculovirus.* We know that baculoviruses are used in recombinant insecticides. Structural similarities between cowpea mosaic virus and picornaviruses as examples which enable viruses to horizontally transfer genes across a wide host range including insects, animals, or humans. Several patents are designed for vaccines and diagnostic tests for diseases caused by microbes that are used in recombinant insecticides. The cell lines are said in patents to be:[17-26]

"...particularly useful for the replication of *pathogens which infect livestock and are arthropod vectored.* This is because *mammalian cell lines may not produce a high enough titer when infected with arthropod-borne pathogens,* possibly because the pathogens require arthropod hosts at some point in their life cycle. Thus, a more potent pathogen strain may be obtained using the cell lines of this invention, which will afford a better vaccine, etc."

This appears to hint that *human* infections with arthropod-borne diseases (i.e. Lyme) might also fail to produce a high enough titer for antibodies to be accurately detected using diagnostic tests such as those standardized for Lyme disease. A lack of a high titer in Lyme patients may be caused by a leptospira/spiroplasma component of an aggregate Bb organism, "if" Bb contains spiroplasma and/or leptospira proteins. This lack of a high titer may also be a legitimate reason why many patients who are infected with Lyme disease will have a negative or equivocal test result (seronegative). Human beings quite simply are not insects; and pathogens vary in antigenicity between insect, animal, and human hosts. Outer surface proteins of leptospires and spiroplasmas are also able to escape immune detection in humans or animals so no antibodies may be created during infections with these pathogens.

A related patent was filed in 1969, a period preceding the Connecticut Lyme outbreak. This patent is for heteroploid (continuous) cell lines, and has a Great Britain claims priority from October 8, 1968. The heterploid cell lines were derived from cat embryo cells. These cells support pathogenic virus growth from feline infectious enteritis, feline distemper (*panleucopoenia* virus); feline herpesvirus 1 (*rhinotracheitis*); bovine (herpes) mammalitis; cat leukemia virus, and feline picornavirus (polio). If these cell lines were used to make animal or human vaccines and they were contaminated with transmissible agents, it could explain the emergence of certain illnesses of today with "unknown cause" (i.e. XMRV retrovirus, MS).[27-30]

Livestock have been the target of insecticides for decades. In modern times scientists have directed their attentions toward making cattle, chickens, and other food and medically useful animals more "antigenically friendly." This means that the human immune system should react in a less hostile manner toward the tissues and cells of *transgenic* animals or those that have been vaccinated with recombinant microbes. Scientists have also been working to reduce the potential for human exposures to *foreign proteins* when animal tissues or cells are used in recombinant vaccines, foods, or human biological products.

For example a patent is assigned to a Japanese company for transgenic cattle which have *reduced prion protein production.* The patent is for genetically engineered cattle that produce fewer prion proteins in their tissues. The transgenically altered cattle are a "...safer source of human antibodies for pharmaceutical use and a safer source of agricultural products."[31]

The patent describes animals that are safer for pharmaceuticals (i.e. antibodies, collagen), or are safer to eat. The transgenic animals carry a gene mutation which allows them to express (create proteins) called *xenogenous* antibodies (outside the species). This is a clue that the cattle have antibodies to an infectious agent that is recombinantly engineered into their genes. This makes the cows resistant to the specific infective or foreign agent. The inventors described a cloned transgenic cow with prion protein activity that is reduced thanks to the marvels of genetic engineering. The cattle in turn genetically pass this prion "knockout" gene onto their offspring.[31]

Although the science of transgenics is relatively new, there are a large number of patents with this technology that have been designed for insecticides, vaccines, cancer research, transgenic plants, and other purposes. The University of Massachusetts is assignee to a transgenic mouse patent for example. Another patent assigned to a Japanese company refers to transgenic animals including cows with reduced levels of "...endogenous IgM heavy chain and/or prion protein" (foreign prion-disease causing proteins).[32]

A patent titled *Peptides for discrimination of prions* describes a method of monitoring *Transmissible Spongiform Encephalopathies* (TSE) or "prion" disease proteins. According to the patent:

> "Human prion disease is known as Creutzfeldt-Jakob disease (CJD), which usually affects elderly persons. Depending on disease phenotype, sporadic (sCJD) accounts for most of CJD, while about 10% are familial CJD (fCJD)."

Familial refers to genetically inherited prion disease agents. The patent continues:[32]

> "Only recently, a new variant of CJD (vCJD) has emerged which occurs in young adults. *Since 1995, more than 100 cases have been reported.* Prion diseases affect many species of domestic and wild animals, manifestations of which are often given unique names, for example, scrapie in sheep and goats...chronic wasting disease (CWD) in cervids and bovine spongiform encephalopathy (BSE, or "mad cow" disease) in cattle."[32]

Is this "new CJD variant" disease from about 1995 forward a result of *contaminants* that were discovered to be present in animal vaccines or insecticides made from insect cell lines? Were contaminated insect cell lines used in insecticides that were applied to human and livestock feeds (i.e. corn, soy, cottonseed)? This sounds like the new human CJD variant that is described on the CDC's web site. It would appear that a new variant of CJD has recently emerged *since around 1995.* We must ask what significant events took place around this period which may have contributed to a new variant disease in beef cattle, in deer, and in humans. Perhaps the answer lies within a *novel feedstuff or biological control agent (insecticides, vaccines, antigens, cell lines) that contained contaminants.* Such contaminants would be among those found in insect cell lines that were suddenly replaced in favor of new animal vaccines and insecticides that would protect against reoviruses, spiroplasmas, and other important agents just as we examined earlier.

Let's take a look at an Australian-assigned patent titled *DNA encoding a cell membrane glycoprotein of a tick gut.* The patent describes *antigens that are derived from tick guts, and which are purified for use within cattle vaccines to protect them from tick infestations.* This vaccine would be a form of biological insecticide for agriculturally important livestock. The invention also allows for the creation of *tick cell lines* to be used for *human* vaccines, for example against tickborne diseases including Lyme. Alternatively such tick cell lines are useful for applied insecticides or for GM crops. We might question whether these new and improved cell lines were used within the first generation Lyme vaccine. If not, were older contaminated cell lines used for a human vaccine, and which may have led to a "treatment-resistant" form of arthritis in some Lyme vaccine recipients? Either way, could the official explanation of "molecular mimicry" as the cause of treatment-resistant arthritis have been caused by a cell line contaminant? Of note is the statement in the patent that during purification techniques with the product:

> "...a contaminant of lower molecular weight was observed...This *contaminant could be partially, though not entirely removed*...The amounts of this impurity are variable from preparation to preparation."[33]

A contaminant *is* present, and *could not* be entirely removed from the formula. Is the contaminant an arbovirus, a reovirus, spiroplasma, thermophile, or some other agent? Is the contaminant the same agent that may be responsible for the human prion disease (CJD variant)? What happens if from the mid-1990s forward, cattle and other livestock have been inoculated with a genetically engineered "anti-tick" vaccine that contained "contaminants" – agents that could only be partly removed? What if the older tick cell lines were contaminated with agents that likewise could not be removed? Were animals immunized using vaccines made from contaminated tick cell lines? Were these same cell lines used to create insecticides that were applied to animals, and to animal and human feed crops?

What if a new vaccine/insecticide formula was invented to "fix" an emerging tick-related problem not only in animals but also within the human population? What if cell line contaminants caused the "new variant" CJD that suddenly emerged within a year of the new patent's filing? Did tainted cell lines *cause prion diseases* and *immune deficiency diseases* in humans, cattle, and deer? Could vaccinated animals have passively transferred contaminants to their offspring in the form of a genetic vaccine, thereby tainting the commercial meat supply? Were deer inoculations taking place before their release during the 1950s using a contaminated cell line-created vaccine which caused a new variant chronic wasting (prion) disease of deer? Are prion diseases transmissible to humans who consume animal meats? Are older contaminated cell lines the key to understanding the origins of many of the modern diseases of our day? Or are such contaminants really "no big deal"? If contaminated cell lines were part of a comedy of biotech blunders which contributed to animal and human epidemics, do you think that scientists and their industrial partners would necessarily inform the global public of such devastating revelations? Or would they simply attempt to correct such a grievous error through the destruction of old cell lines, the redesign of new cell lines, and quietly move forward?

According to an Australian patent, scientists used purified antigens collected from the midgut of ticks for the *new cattle vaccine.* The vaccine could also be used for domestic animals. The premise of the patent was this:[33]

> "...the animal host produces an immune response capable of damaging the plasma membrane of the gut cells of ticks feeding on said host to such an extent that the majority of said ticks fail to survive to adult stage or surviving ticks become red in colour and the reproductive capacity of said surviving ticks is substantially decreased..."

This sounds quite a bit like the premise of the first generation Lyme vaccine. Immunize people against the Bb spirochete so that when infected ticks feed upon us, our bodies create an immediate immune response, thereby thwarting an infection. Was the standardization of Lyme disease testing and surveillance cases at the 1994 Dearborn conference done in response to an emerging human infection? Or was it a preemptive strike related to an emerging human epidemic caused by the application of insecticides and animal vaccines that were made from contaminated insect cell lines? Were the Dearborn conference, the Australian animal vaccine, the new tick cell lines, and the eruption of a new variant CJD all merely unrelated coincidences in timing?

The cattle vaccine patent claims its antigens are derived from *agriculturally significant tick species Boophilus microplus,* (southern cattle ticks), or from *Haemaphysalis, Otobius, Rhiphicephalus, Amblyomma, Dermacentor, Ixodes, and Hyalomma* tick species. These ticks are quite coincidentally vectors of animal and human Lyme disease. According to the cattle vaccine patent:[33]

> "By protecting against infestation with ticks, the antigen may also provide protection against diseases caused by agents such as *Babesia bovis, Babesia bigemina, Anaplasma marginale, Cowdria ruminantium, Theileria parva parva, T. parva lawrencii, T. annulata and T. hirci*."

Notice the mention of several intracellular infections that can be detected in livestock, but also as co-infections in many Lyme disease patients! Are blood-feeding parasites able to take up recombinant genes from vaccinated animals which may reassort inside the insect gut with the recombinant insecticides that are applied agriculturally or industrially?[33]

Recombinant products of many kinds have been used in the environment for years as chemical and microbial pesticides and other products. If genetic engineering techniques are ever proven to be unsafe for humans either directly or indirectly, we might expect to see "cover-our-butt" techniques developed before any adverse information becomes publicly known. Such techniques might be deployed to mask the effects of recombinant accidents with the goal of indefinitely extending the useful life of unsafe agricultural or industrially important tools. This is a process I labeled "snowball science," which includes the creation of medical means to offset the effects of biotech processes that are neither entirely safe nor effective. The sole objective of their use would be to preserve the pipeline of profits and processes that lack feasible alternatives; despite any inherent health risks to the human population.

Consider a recent patent that was granted to inventors Drs. Raymond J. Dattwyler and Maria Gomes-Solecki, for an *oral vaccine for borrelia.* Dr. Dattwyler has been an important figure to the history of Lyme disease. The device describes the use of vaccines to *control borrelia infections in animal and human populations*. Note it does not say to "prevent," but to "control." The product is designed to target populations that are already infected, or are in the process of becoming infected with Bb. The products would contain recombinant bacteria that are engineered to express immune-stimulating antigens of *Borrelia burgdorferi.* (This creates an antibody response.) Such agents could be added to food products or freeze-dried and placed into beverages such as coffee.[34-36]

The invention also describes the use of *E. coli* and *lactobacilli.* The preferred strain appears to be *Lactobacillus plantarum.* This is a widespread bacterium found in many fermented foods. It is also present in anaerobic plant matter and human saliva. *Lactobacillus plantarum* is a *firmicute* from the *bacilli* class. The addition of *E. coli,* an iron user to *L. plantarum,* a manganese user, allows them to work together as catalysts. *L. plantarum* consumes oxygen *in a reaction that ultimately produces hydrogen peroxide.* Some physicians have used hydrogen peroxide IVs to treat Lyme patients, and hydrogen peroxide is added as a detoxification aid in epsom salt baths by Lyme patients.[34-36]

Meanwhile individuals who support the idea that Lyme disease is an easy-to-treat infection also commonly frown upon the use of hydrogen peroxide IVs to treat Lyme disease. In the IDSA guidelines for Lyme disease which were co-authored by patent inventor Dr. Dattwyler, we find under a section marked "therapeutic modalities not recommended," that:[36]

> "Because of a lack of biologic plausibility, lack of efficacy, absence of supporting data, or the potential for harm to the patient"...[that a number of therapies are]..."not recommended for treatment of patients with any manifestation of Lyme disease."

Such therapies include "intravenous hydrogen peroxide." And yet here we find a patent that may in effect, *help to create hydrogen peroxide inside the human body to treat Bb infections as an oral vaccine!* Again this patent was co-invented by one of the IDSA Lyme disease guidelines authors, Dr. Raymond J. Dattwyler, who in consensus guidelines contraindicated the use of hydrogen peroxide to treat Bb infections. What readers do not know is that *Lactobacillus plantarum is also the most common bacterium found within silage.* Silage is a fermented high-moisture food that is fed to animals such as cattle, pigs, and sheep. Silage is also useful as a biofuel. It is made from corn, sorghum, other cereal crops, and grass. There is also haylate from alfalfa and oatlage from oats.[35,36]

Dr. Dattwyler and associates' new patent also describes the use of the outer surface proteins A and C (OspA, OspC) of the Bb spirochete within a food or medicine. What if one of more of these proteins actually came from an applied biological control agent such as B.t., and a spiroplasma protein that may be found in infected grain crops – crops meant for animal and human consumption?[34]

Among the food products described in the patent are dairy products such as milk, yogurt, or cheese; or grains including seeds, breads, or cereals. In addition this "oral vaccine" could be added to animal chows (pet foods) or used as a rodent or other animal vaccine. Here are examples of the intended targets of the invention:[34]

> "The method of claim 25, wherein said mammal is a domesticated animal comprising one or more of a dog, a cat, a cow, and a horse...The method of claim 25, wherein said mammal is a feral animal comprising one or more of a mouse, a chipmunk, a squirrel, a shrew, a vole, a rat, a raccoon, an opossum, a skunk, a rabbit, and a *deer*...The method of claim 25, wherein said mammal is a *human.*"
>
> "Additionally, an oral Lyme disease vaccine for human consumption would be a pleasing alternative to traditional intramuscular or intradermal vaccines, for preventing human morbidity associated with bites from *B. burgdorferi*-infected ticks."[34]

Do you think that we will be told ahead of time that the dairy, bread, cereal product, or cup of coffee we ingest will contain oral vaccines that we may not wish to ingest? Do you think the public would be pleased to learn that foods will be fabricated to contain oral vaccines that may attempt to abrogate a genetic engineering, industrial, or agricultural "accident" that has gotten vastly out of control? There are few if any labeling requirements for genetically engineered foods. There are certainly inadequate requirements for foods that contain genetically engineered *medicines or microbes* including any substances intended for use as vaccines, or which may be used *in conjunction with vaccines.*

We have recently witnessed the production of yogurts which claim to help "regulate" our digestive systems. (This is essentially our immune system which begins in the gut). We may soon be facing *the new secret inoculations of snowball science.* Scientists will not only create products that are useful to industry that may cause disease, but they may also create products that are designed to *erase any evidence of such illnesses*, whether we know about them or not. Without the strict ability to determine exactly what goes into our bodies by way of proper food labeling, we may become no different than the other laboratory animals that are already being experimented upon by the scientists of recombinant genetics. By the way, the Dattwyler et al. patent had this to say about Lyme disease:[34]

> "Lyme disease has rapidly emerged as the most prevalent zoonotic vector-borne infectious disease in the United States, and its geographical range is expanding...In 2002, nearly 24,000 cases of Lyme disease were reported to the Centers for Disease Control and Prevention (MMWR, 52:741-750, 2003), and more than 150,000 cases have been reported to U.S. health authorities since 1982, when a systematic national surveillance was initiated...The regrowth of natural forests from farmland in the northeastern United States in the twentieth century has created conditions conducive to the spread of human Lyme disease."

This redeveloped agricultural land (formerly sprayed with chemical and microbial pesticides) has been converted to suburban habitat, and this process has created ideal conditions for the spread of Lyme disease. The patent continues:[34]

> "Suburban communities are now often adjacent to forested areas where *Ixodes scapularis* populations thrive along with deer (*Odocoileus virginianus*) and white-footed mice (*Peromyscus leucopus*), known to be the major natural reservoir for *B. burgdorferi*. Methods to control *B. burgdorferi* through acaricide or antimicrobial agents are limited and many, such as *organochlorine pesticides,* have had negative environmental and human health effects sufficient to outlaw their use."

Scientists including Dr. Dattwyler seem to be aware of the problems associated with chemical pesticides, but they also seem to carefully dodge any reference to the words "organophosphates" or "B.t." within their patents. And yet these same scientists are inventing medical devices that are probably meant to abrogate the effects of chemical and microbial applications or perhaps the diseases that may come about because of their use. There appears to be sufficient evidence among patents, research grants, and published research papers of a huge paradigm of denial about emerging human diseases, and a purposeful protection of industry "secrets." Does such a cause and effect relationship exist? If so, is it the driving force behind the silencing of epidemics including the flagship infection called Lyme disease?[37]

From one US patent titled *Chimeric Alphavirus replicon particles*, we may read an important statement:

> "Vaccine strains that have undergone multiple in vivo passages *should not be considered avirulent simply because they are vaccine strains*."

In vivo passages means to infect an animal with an agent, culture cells from the animal, and inject the cells into another animal and reculture and repeat any number of times before collecting the finished cells for vaccine use. Such in vivo passage can render an infectious agent far less, or far more virulent than its original natural, or wild-type infection. This process is used routinely in biotechnology processes for vaccines. Discovering how to work with viruses is just one part of the puzzle for scientists intending to use them to provoke immune responses through vaccination or other processes. Unfortunately there is no way to predict what may happen once recombinant microbes enter the human body, especially over time after exposure to pollutants with an ability to adversely affect genes of hosts and pathogens alike.

When Good Ideas Turn Bad

From a 1998 *Federal Register* notice I learned of a group called the International Conference on Harmonisation of Technical Requirements for Registration of Pharmaceuticals for Human Use (ICH). This is a really long name for a group that provides industry guidance for the testing and evaluation of the viral safety of biotechnology products which originate from human and animal cell lines. The ICH was designed with input from federal regulatory agencies, and industry and consumer representatives. The ICH's jurisdiction covers policy guidance for the US, the European Union, and Japan.[1]

The sponsors of the ICH include the European Commission, the European Federation of Pharmaceutical Industries Associations, the Japanese Ministry of Health and Welfare, the Japanese Pharmaceutical Manufacturers Association, the Centers for Drug Evaluation and Research and Biologics Evaluation and Research, the Food and Drug Administration, and the Pharmaceutical Research and Manufacturers of America. The ICH allowed members of the following on the steering committee: ICH sponsors, the International Federation of Pharmaceutical Manufacturers Association (IFPMA), the WHO, the Canadian Health Protection Branch, and the European Free Trade Area.[1]

There is also an FDA document which addresses the testing, evaluation, and safety of mammal, bird, and insect cell line products. The covered products include anything derived from cell lines, cell banks, in vitro (lab) cell cultures, (i.e. interferons, recombinant DNA, monoclonal antibodies); or any products derived from recombinant subunit vaccines. It also includes products derived from *hybridoma cells* that are grown in the body. Exclusions appear to be inactivated vaccines, live vaccines that contain self-replicating agents, and genetically engineered live vectors. This is a bit disconcerting because many of the insecticide and vaccine agents in use today should be regulated, but do not always seem to be.[1]

> "The *risk of viral contamination* is a feature common to all biotechnology products *derived from cell lines*. Such contamination could have serious clinical consequences and *can arise from the contamination of the source cell lines* themselves (cell substrates) or from adventitious introduction of virus during production."

The document provides three approaches to virus removal and inactivation. It clearly outlines the risks of using cell lines, including how cells may have "latent" or "persistent" infections, or an "endogenous retrovirus" that can be transmitted between cell generations. These are ancient viruses that are part of a host insect, animal, or human's DNA. The document also acknowledges that there are other possible viral contaminants.[1]

> "Cell lines derived from *rodents usually contain endogenous retrovirus* particles or retrovirus-like particles, which may be infectious (C-type particles) or noninfectious (cytoplasmic A- and R-type particles)."

Rodents of course can become infected with any number of arboviruses and parasites including leptospires and leptonema. Rodents are found in all areas of the world, in particular around mines, sewage systems, dumps, and other industrial and agricultural sources. There is no mention of monkey cell lines or chicken embryos in this patent however, which scientists and patent holders have openly acknowledged as being contaminated by disease-causing viruses. We must realize that recombinant vaccine or insecticidal formulas which harbor retroviruses and other viruses can cause the reactivation of latent human pathogens and retroviral genes because of the unpredictability of the microbes in the genetically engineered formulas. The FDA document also stated:[1]

> "Viral clearance studies are useful for contributing to the assurance that an acceptable level of safety in the final product is achieved but do not by themselves establish safety…a number of factors in the design and execution of viral clearance studies may lead to an incorrect estimate of the ability of the process to remove virus infectivity..."
>
> "...it is possible that virus escaping a first inactivation step may be more resistant to subsequent steps…for example, if the resistant fraction takes the form of virus aggregates, infectivity may be resistant to a range of different chemical treatments and to heating."[1]

A mathematical algorithm is used to determine virus reduction levels. This technique seems problematic. If manufacturers use algorithms to reduce viral loads, what assurance does the population have that the end products are non-infective? What assurance does anyone have that viruses, even when inactive, remain so inside the animal or human body? I have already shown that vaccines and biological products contain viruses with the potential to become infectious or oncogenic (cancer-causing). The bottom line is there are *no* guarantees that vaccines or any other recombinant products used in the environment, in or on our foods, or within our bodies are completely safe, nor that they will remain so under all conditions, in perpetuity.

History has already revealed that the use of live viruses within vaccine preparations and other products has sometimes proven to be hazardous. While the antibody response is more favorable with live virus vaccines, there are inherent risks that such vaccines can (and do) transmit infections to recipients. An example of this transmission occurred with early polio vaccines.[2]

According to a 1993 publication from scientists at the State University of New York (SUNY), **recombination within the bodies of polio virus vaccine recipients is the result of artificial conditions; and recombination between wild-type polio virus strains is expected within natural settings**. This means that the polio virus can reassort inside the bodies of insects, animals, or humans under certain conditions, both natural and artificial; and may also do so in the external environment. Artificial conditions may include the reactivation of live or neutralized polio vaccine viruses in the human body upon exposure to an insect which harbors a compatible virus capable of donating its genes to the latent virus. Are humans who have been inoculated with polio (or other) vaccines, sitting ducks for the reactivation of old vaccine viruses once they meet up with an infective insect vector?[2]

Of the poxviruses that infect humans, the most common are variola, monkeypox, smallpox, cowpox, and vaccinia. Vaccinia has been used within human vaccines for many years. In addition, fowlpox, swinepox, sheep pox, and a few others are also poxviruses. Insect entomopoxviruses that are part of the larger poxvirus group are Type A: *Melolontha melolontha entomopoxvirus* of the European cockchafer beetle (May bug); Type B: *Amsacta moorei entomopoxvirus* (gypsy moth); an NPV found in mosquitoes, flies, midges, grasshoppers, and locusts; and Type C: *Chironomus luridus entomopoxvirus* of the Israeli benthic midge. This is significant because two research papers from 1960 reveal that **heat-inactivated poxviruses can be reactivated by any other active (live) poxvirus.**[2-5]

This reactivation can occur in one of two ways, through *homoreactivation* or *heteroreactivation.* Homoreactivation describes the reactivation of an inactive poxvirus by a closely related active virus. Reactivation may be accomplished by a mutant of the inactivated strain, or by a natural virus from the same poxvirus subgroup. *Heteroreactivation* describes the reactivation of an inactive poxvirus by an active poxvirus from some other subgroup (i.e. reactivation of vaccinia by type B entomopoxvirus *Amsacta moorei*). Once again the reactivation of older vaccine viruses in the animal or human body may be possible upon exposure to a live, compatible or related insect virus that donates the genes necessary to reactivate latent vaccine viruses. This is actually a process that recombinant microbial insecticides *are designed to do within the insect body.* Unfortunately such reactivations may likewise occur inside the human body.[2-5]

When we find diseases with symptoms similar to those of infectious poliomyelitis, we may wonder about the possibility of dormant vaccine viruses being reactivated to cause disease, especially in patients whose symptoms fail to subside after antibiotic treatment. From a SUNY publication we read a comment that may apply not only to insects, but to vaccinted animals or humans as well:[2-5]

> "Recombination, together with the high rate of spontaneous point mutations, can lead to the evolution of highly virulent polio virus strains in vaccine recipients."

Similar problems may arise with attenuated vaccines. These contain viruses that have been made less virulent than their live counterparts, but which remain infectious. The viruses of attenuated vaccines may not be quite as virulent as live viruses, but that doesn't matter if a live insect infection provides the missing component to reactivate the virus into an infective state.

When live or attenuated viruses are introduced into the human body, the recipient may run the risk of having the vaccine viruses reassort with other viruses or bacteria already present in the recipient's body. A reactivated vaccine component or latent virus is one way that the post-vaccine syndrome Guillain-Barré might occur. The recipient may also run the risk of a virus undergoing a natural mutation, either at the time of inoculation or years later when reactivated by some genetic change caused by another virus, chemical exposure, radiation, a vectored insect infection, or another factor.

A textbook published in 1998 includes a chapter about RNA viruses. A key idea from the book is that viruses can recombine with other related viruses during mixed infections. This reassortment allows the viruses to mix up their genes to form new mutants. This process of *natural recombination* eliminates genes that are defective or unnecessary to the new mutant organism. RNA or DNA viruses can naturally recombine within insect or animal cells, including humans. This natural recombinant process can backfire in the external environment or within our bodies when microbial insecticides, vaccines, insect-delivered microbes, or genetically engineered foodstuffs form unexpected, infective chimera.

There are many scientific techniques when preparing recombinant genes to render infectious agents *for the most part* neutralized. There are also definite and long-standing problems when neutralizing infectious agents. Scientists are only beginning to understand the nuances of the functions and susceptibilities of microbes; and how to make them less infective while still using their proteins to achieve a desired goal. The unpredictable nature of microbes and the human body makes the process of fabricating useful controls and medicaments that much more difficult.

Unfortunately techniques that were formerly used to filter and neutralize viruses and bacteria have been repeatedly found to be far less effective than once believed. As a result it would appear that viral and/or bacterial contaminations may have had an opportunity to wreak havoc on virtually all vaccine preparations, whether for animal or human use. This is because scientists believed that former virus neutralization techniques were sufficient. There has been no entirely reliable method of ensuring that neutralized agents *will remain neutralized forever or that they won't be capable of being incorporated into other chimera, or of ever being reactivated.* There appears to be no reliable means by which any recombinant formulas are completely purified of contaminants. Even so-called "killed" or neutralized vaccine preparations may contain dead or neutralized viruses which may be resurrected inside the human body to initiate active latent diseases, even at a later date.

In 1937, it was agreed by attendees of a *League of Nations* conference that live virus vaccines offered greater protection than those with killed viruses. Some committee members expressed a feeling that **when epidemics arise, the risks involved in the use of live virus vaccines could be disregarded.** However there were also those who felt that ignoring the risks was unwise and premature with respect to live vaccines. One scientist referred to an experience in Chile where a typhus-inoculated guinea pig vaccine caused vaccine-related human deaths. Eventually scientists learned that live virus vaccines, although better at soliciting an immune antibody response, were not without serious risks to vaccine recipients.[6]

One of the risks associated with vaccines and insecticides that contain live viruses, is that microbes, even when neutralized or attenuated, can spring back to life with *increased virulence* under the right conditions, in the external environment or inside the body. There is much evidence of this problem within the research and registered scientific patents. There is also evidence that the most commonly used agricultural insecticide *Bacillus thuringiensis* may be helping to promote infections in more than just insects. From an important scientific textbook we find:

> "A consequence of mixed infections of pathogens in vivo or in vitro are *recombinations of genetic factors*, which may give rise to new types. Especially, the origin of strains of increased virulence from moderately virulent ones could be expected...*Bacteriophages also may cause genetic conversion* or transduction. This is possible because the genetic material of phages and that of their host bacteria are derived from common ancestors of lysogenic bacteria... Commercial preparations of *B. thuringiensis* [B.t.] often contain lysogenic bacteria or are contaminated by phages."

In short, bacteriophages or other agents contaminate B.t. insecticides and can readily cause genes to reassort. This helps microbes to spring back to life through the donation of essential genes during mixed infections with compatible donor organisms.[7]

> "Latent viroses [viruses] may also be activated by non-viral pathogens such as *B. thuringiensis* [B.t.]. For example, Vasiljevic (1957) reported that up to 90% of larvae of *Hyphantria cunea*, (fall webworm moth) which had ingested *B. thuringiensis*, died of a nuclear polyhedrosis instead of bacteriosis. Only 10-15% of untreated caterpillars, however, died of polyhedrosis."

These statements are admissions that bacteriophages and other agents can infect the very bacteriae that are used as insecticides; and also that these bacteria can modify genes in other organisms to create new mutant strains! It also appears that B.t. can become contaminated by other microbes, and its phages and other contaminants help reactivate latent (previously inactive) infections. We must understand also that the infections that are reactivated and which reassort will be *far more virulent*. Similar mutations may occur in the human body through the introduction of phages and lysogenic bacteria from insecticidal formulas, or as delivered by a vectoring insect that harbors mixed infections.[7,8]

In 1928 Fred Griffith of the British Ministry of Health studied the bacteria *pneumococcus* by injecting it into mice. In the process he learned that when two viruses were combined (one virulent and one heat-killed), that the two viruses *combine to form a new, virulent mutant.* If this occurs in animals and insects for which recombinant insecticides are designed; then the same process is capable of occuring in the human body as well.[7,8]

In insect populations, reactivation of latent virus infections occurs naturally under various environmental stressors. Weather, overpopulation, lack of food, predators, chemical pesticides, or super-infections with other microbes can disrupt host homeostasis to cause diseases. Other stressors are biological controls which induce activation of latent viruses such as the granulosis virus (GV) of the fall webworm moth. This baculovirus can be reactivated from latency upon exposure to B.t. according to a text that has been extremely important to microbiologists. This reactivation concern has been known by scientists for decades, and has been deliberately exploited to kill insect pests.[7]

Reactivation may also occur in humans who harbor subclinical or latent viral infections. It might even cause a live virus vaccine to contribute genes during a mixed infection that is introduced by an insect vector to cause neurologic illness that can be very "polio," "vaccinia," or "rubella"-like (or whatever live or attenuated virus may be present and able to reassort). Various forms of environmental, physical, or emotional stressors including vaccines, chemical toxins, surgery, heavy metals, pharmaceuticals, accidents, and exposures to recombinant microbes overtax the human immune system. The introduction of pathogenic microbes and lysogenic bacteria (phages) by vectoring insects becomes the straw that breaks the camel's back. At some point the immune system cannot surmount the number of infections, toxins, and other issues that arise, and disease ensues. If old vaccine viruses are caused to reactivate, the end result can be devastating for the patient who now has a disease complex of mixed infections that require a multi-tiered approach to treatment.[7]

On November 19-20, 1998, there was an advisory meeting of the FDA/HHS Center for Biologics Evaluation and Research held in Bethesda, Maryland for vaccines and related biological products. Attendees included representatives from the FDA, University of Minnesota, Stanford (Palo Alto CA, VA Hospital), Vanderbilt (Nashville, TN), CDC, Mayo Clinic (Rochester, MN), Children's Hospital (Los Angeles, CA), University of Rochester (NY), University of California (San Francisco), University of Chicago, University of Colorado, University of California (San Diego) and the San Diego VA Hospital. Others came from St. Louis University, Chapel Hill (NC), National Vaccine Program Office, Office of AIDS Research, Public Citizens Health Research Group, NCI, NIAID, and the Frederick Cancer Research and Development Center. Most of these names appear frequently within vaccine patents and grants. Reported conflicts of interest with some of the attendees included collaborations with vaccine manufacturers Immunex, Merck, or SmithKline Beecham.[1]

One of the topics of discussion at the event was the discovery of reverse transcriptase (RT) activity in chicken cell-derived vaccines. The initial findings were reported to the World Health Organization (WHO). Studies were performed in the US and Europe by CDC, FDA, and NIBSC scientists to confirm these startling findings. The results of those studies were published in 1997 and 1998.[1]

The document confirmed that the **RT activity was found in all chicken cell-derived vaccines.** The focus then became whether RT activity was associated with a retrovirus. If it was, scientists wondered if a retrovirus could infect and replicate within human cells, **"and therefore be a public health concern."** There was also a discussion about **how twenty years earlier,**

similar RT activity had also been reported. Those studies were reviewed by the WHO and the FDA at the time, but the use of RT-contaminated cell lines was nevertheless advised and allowed to continue for decades despite the risks. An important statement was made at this meeting:[1]

> "Okay, because there were retroviral particles associated with the RT activity, there was still a theoretical possibility that the virus could enter the cell and infect the cell and the sequences integrate into the human body."

This was apparent acknowledgement by the scientific sector that reverse transcriptase activity remained in vaccines that were grown using chicken embryo cell lines. This RT component had the potential to cause genetic changes in the human body, with unknown effects. Such effects included the very real possibility of human diseases at a later date after some triggering event. Could such an event include the administration of an experimental vaccine, exposure to recombinant insecticides, contaminated animal products, or by transmission of infectious diseases by vectoring insects?[1]

These startling statements indicate that some scientists and regulators knew that all chicken-cell derived vaccines likely contained reverse transcriptase activity at least from the 1950s forward, and quite likely also into the present day.

The document also indicated that the RT contaminants could possibly infect human cells and *become integrated into the human genome as a new retrovirus.* An example of chicken-cell derived vaccines, are *polio* vaccines. This means that vaccines grown in these cell lines may have contained viruses that were capable of activating and initiating polio or other virus replication. Therefore they may be capable of creating new retroviruses within the human body. They are also quite possibly capable of causing cancer if viral oncogenes ever become activated. They may even be able to spring back to life in the event that a vectoring insect introduced a compatible picorna, entomopox, or other virus into the human body to produce the very polio-like symptoms displayed in persons suffering from Multiple Sclerosis or Lyme disease. From the same document we read:[1,9]

> "The concern was because, for retroviruses, there are examples in which retroviral-induced oncogenesis can occur by insertional mutagenesis. And I've listed some examples here in which case some retroviruses can activate protooncogenes and, in more rare cases, inactivation of tumor suppressor gene can occur."

Again this means that a contaminant could possibly incorporate into the human genome of our cells, and trigger cancer at a later date. Such events could also possibly lead to serious and novel human infectious diseases when activated by some external factor, such as a tickborne infection.

A slide presentation at the 1998 advisory meeting indicated that high levels of reverse transcription activity had been found within chicken embryo fibroblast supernatants.* There was discussion of the processes in an effort to determine if any "integrated" viral DNA could be incorporated into human cells. The attendees felt there was "no evidence" to support this idea according to the studies performed. A lack of evidence does not mean this could not of course occur, especially if studies are flawed; the effects of contaminants are completely unknown; or some other factors come into play at a later date.[1]

**Supernatants are the remaining floating particles after settling, precipitation, or centrifugation*

There was a discussion of whether "unintegrated" viral DNA might "slip through" the process and remain present in the final vaccine products. This means that scientists wondered whether some virus particles might still contaminate chicken embryo cell lines, and be capable of incorporation into our bodies after receipt of a vaccine to cause disease.[1]

This same problem could occur with other cell lines if there were similar contaminants. There was much banter over viral activity and how to test for it under then current methods. Here we see evidence that genetic engineering processes can sometimes harbor unexpected contaminants that can run uncontrollably rampant in the body. These agents may be able to activate illnesses or cancers; especially when triggered by an external factor such as the bite of a blood-sucking insect or arthropod that is infected with microbes from recombinant insecticides that were agriculturally or industrially applied.[1]

Cell lines that are contaminated with adventitious or other viruses and oncogenes are acknowledged to be capable of infecting humans via vaccines or other products if the pathogens are unfiltered or improperly neutralized during manufacture. In the case of the chicken embryo cell lines, RT activity could not be neutralized or removed because it was part of the embryo itself. Chickens have long been vaccinated and have incorporated vaccine genes into their genome in a kind of permanent vaccination. An FDA document revealed the following:[1]

> "...human tumor cells have, on very rare occasions, been grafted into allogeneic humans...The formation of recombinants between vaccine virons and adventitious viral agents present in cell substrates occurred in adenovirus vaccines that were prepared in rhesus monkey kidney cells in the 1950s...Before the discovery of SV40 in 1960, humans were immunized with adenovirus vaccines that contained adenovirus SV40 hybrid viruses."

"Allogeneic" or allogenic means between two individuals of the same species with different genetic information. Finally we have admission that vaccines during the 1950s (the early polio era) or later were indeed contaminated with reassorted SV40 (simian #40 virus) mutants. We also know that cell line contaminations very likely continued at least into the 1990s if not the present day within certain cell lines (i.e. chicken, tick). The FDA does not admit in this document to any knowledge of the rate of the recombination of SV40 and adenovirus, or any other viruses in monkey cells. It also does not admit to any knowledge of the ratio of hybrid or non-hybrid adenoviruses that may have been present in vaccines used at any time. Other concerns expressed about these cell lines however were that **"...viruses, especially retroviruses, can parasitize the genome of large DNA viruses such as herpes viruses."**[1]

This means that vaccine contaminants could act as virophages (virus phages) and enter and infect other viruses and retroviruses when they are contaminants of vaccines and other recombinant tools. *Introduced viruses, even recombinant ones, can also parasitize the latent human retroviruses or those of our resident gut bacteria.* When exposed to live recombinant microbes, any viruses may revert to a living form, or any bacteria infected with viruses can cause disease.[1]

> "More concerning is the potential for exposure to adventitious oncogenic viruses. The primary reasons for this concern are that screening methods for these viruses are difficult or relatively insensitive, and that there may exist currently unknown or occult agents that have never before been detected despite use of current technology."

Scientists admitted there may still be unknown agents which remain in cell lines, vaccines, or biological controls that are as yet unknown. This is troubling not only to us, but it was also troubling to the scientists at the 1998 meeting. The participants were attempting to weigh benefits v. risk, and economic advantage before pressing forward with cell lines known to contain contaminants. It is clear that the use of viruses, vaccines, cell lines, and recombinant processes are not without serious risks – some of which may be unavoidable and inherent to the processes. The transcripts demonstrate that some scientists and manufacturers of the day may be acutely aware of the risks and flaws associated with the use of recombinant products. Sometimes the risks were noted and discussed but nothing more; and the technologies planning to use them pressed resolutely forward despite them. Unfortunately such risks may not have been effectively communicated to the global population who was and will continue to be subjected to vaccines, insecticides, and other recombinant products.

Some patent inventions describe the use of arboviruses such as Semliki forest, the Sendai strain of parainfluenza; and Newcastle and fowl plague. A patent from 1965 refers to the use of sindbis virus in chicken embryos. Perhaps a recombinant sindbis virus or one of its relatives are responsible for activating the reverse transcriptase (RT) contaminant found in cell lines. We already learned that sindbis is problematic when used as genetic constructs, and that chicken embryo cell lines were found to contain "RT" activity. Sindbis virus can be reactivated even after neutralization, and can be kicked out of genetically engineered constructs. But what factor causes a virus to be ejected from a construct in the first place? Would this occur upon exposure to genetically engineered insecticides either applied or ingested in the form of GM foods?[10-16]

Viral contamination of vaccines has happened before, and this information was made public. A 1965 patent was co-invented by Merck pharmaceutical scientist Maurice R. Hilleman. The patent is for a *rubella* vaccine that was grown in monkey kidney cells. The patent was assigned to vaccine manufacturer Merck & Co., Inc. (Rahway, NJ). Dr. Maurice Hilleman is the scientist who coined the phrase "detecting the undetectable viruses." He was shown in videos allegedly declaring that SV40 originated from infected monkey kidney tissues, and that it is a contaminant in a number of vaccines.[17,18]

Evidence from a number of patents and historic records confirms that the SV40 (simian #40) virus is in fact, commonly found in monkey kidney cells; and that it has contaminated human vaccines. In recent years, the SV40 virus is deliberately being used within genetic engineering processes of all kinds. Like another monkey virus (sindbis); once identified, viruses once seen as contaminants are deliberately put to work in vaccines and microbial insecticides. In fact the sindbis virus and its clones are some of the most heavily used and widely patented recombinant tools. We can see multiple sindbis-related patents held by North Carolina academic institutions and privately owned companies for example.[17,18]

Another patent filed in June 1967 is assigned to the US Secretary of the Department of Health, Education, and Welfare (now the Department of Health and Human Services). The patent is for a diagnostic test to detect *rubella* infections. Another rubella-related patent was filed in 1968 and assigned to the Wistar Institute in Philadelphia, PA. The patent is for an attenuated intranasal rubella vaccine that was passaged through human diploid lung tissues. According to the 1967 patent, researchers were already aware that animal viruses were contaminating vaccine formulas. From the patent we read:[19,20]

> "The use of this cell line for the propagation of the virus minimizes the likelihood of latent animal viruses being transmitted to a vaccinee by means of the vaccine."

Subacute Sclerosing Panencephalitis (SSPE) is a neurodegenerative disease that according to research is caused by a persistent rubella virus infection. Some researchers have the hypothesis that Multiple Sclerosis is caused by a measles virus since this infection provokes a similar immune response when patients are infected with the virus. In one paper scientists warned that *Rubella infections may present with polyarthritis.* Rubella is related to the sindbis virus, a virus that has been used within recombinant constructs. In an earlier chapter I proposed that the bull's-eye rash of Lyme disease may be a reactivated rubella virus. But rubella may not be the only latent virus that may be reactivated to cause an aspect of a complex disease.[18-27]

History shows that *chicken cholera* and *vibrio cholera* vaccines were attempted at the Pasteur Institute a century and a half ago. If we trace the history of vaccines and poultry farms, some interesting facts emerge. Chickens have been an important part of the human diet for centuries. There are a number of infectious diseases that are important to the poultry indutry. Those more well-known are Newcastle disease, chicken cholera, and Marek's disease. Newcastle was first seen in 1926 in northeast England at Newcastle upon Tyne, although other slightly different strains were found in other parts of the world. Human exposures to this agent usually involve poultry farm or laboratory workers. In humans the illness causes flu-like symptoms and conjunctivitis. It is usually contracted through bird feces or contaminated food, water, clothing, or equipment. The virus is from the paramyxovirus family, the same family where we find the "polio" viruses. Since insecticides are engineered in the laboratory to use viruses, they may be capable of reactivating latent paramyxoviruses. Is the reactivation of human viruses by insecticide viruses at the core of "avian flu" epidemics as well as Lyme disease or other disorders?

What was once thought of as *poliomyelitis* may have had something to do with avian viruses that could have reassorted with mosquito or other viruses to cause human polio outbreaks. *Newcastle disease* was studied as a potential biowarfare weapon by the US military, although it is unclear if it was ever weaponized. The virus is able to survive in the air for a time, and *indefinitely within frozen tissues.** In birds, this infection causes muscle and nervous system symptoms, swollen facial tissues, twisted neck, and droppy wings; and thin shells and reduced egg production. It is interesting to note that Newcastle upon Tyne was an area that was known for its coal mining, wool, and shipbuilding industries. Newcastle disease is also called *Avian parainfluenza,* or *"Avian flu."* We should be familiar with this agent, as in recent years there has been a global "threat" of this flu, and a push for preventative vaccines by public health agencies around the world.[28]

**We will learn about "Frozen Fritz" in an upcoming chapter.*

Fowl cholera is also called *avian cholera, avian hemorrhagic septicemia,* or *avian pasteurellosis.* It is caused by *Pasteurella multocida,* a *gammaproteobacteria* that affects birds, mainly fowl; but also humans. Indeed some Lyme patients have tested positive for this infection. This infection affects the nervous, respiratory, digestive, and reproductive systems, and can be isolated from lung, liver, spleen, kidney, and brain tissues. It was first discovered in 1878 in birds suffering from a cholera-like illness. Louis Pasteur isolated it in 1880, and the agent was named after him as *Pasteurella.* Pasteur felt that the agent of fowl cholera reacts in the manner that the cow pox virus does for smallpox. That is, people who suffered from cow pox became immune to the smallpox virus. Antibodies to fowl cholera might therefore provide birds protection from other infections.[28]

The group *gammaproteobacteria* in the *Pasteurellaceae* family includes these genera, with *Actinobacillus, Aggregatibacter,* and *Pasteurella* perhaps the most important to our story:

Actinobacillus (meningitis, pneumonias)
*Aggregatibacter** (see below)
Haemophilus (sepsis, meningitis)
Lonepinella (tannin degrader)
Pasteurella (bovine respiratory disease)
Mannheimia (bovine respiratory disease)
Phocoenobacter (from *Pasteurella* group)

**Aggregatibacter actinomycetemcomitans* is an *Actinomycete* (fungus) found mainly in the oral cavity. It was first isolated from human fungal lesions in 1912. Remember that Dr. Willy Burgdorfer also classified the 277F tick spiroplasma as an *Actinomycetes,* a group that includes the *Bacterionema.* (The actinomycetes are chitin and cellulose degraders.) When we talk about the spiroplasmas, we may be talking about a plant spirillum that has mutated with a bacterionema, and a fungus which becomes infected with a gammaproteobacterial phage such as any from the aforementioned group, or previously discussed forms (i.e. enterobacteriae, vibrionales, pseudomonadales, acidithiobacillales, etc.). To determine which microbes may comprise a tick spiroplasma, we have only to find out which gammaproteobacteriae are typically found in the bodies of ticks, and these are widely varied. The spiroplasmas may therefore have a bacterionema, a gammaproteobacterium, a fungus, and a plant spirillum; or an acid mine waste, metal-reducing *Leptospirillum* bacteria as part of their makeup.[29-32]

The avian cholera bacterium is found in livestock and domestic animals, especially birds. In pigs, it can lead to a pneumonia-like illness called *atrophic rhinitis,* or in short, "swine flu." In cattle, it can lead to *bovine respiratory* illness. In humans, this agent is the most common cause of infection in people who have been bitten or scratched by livestock or domestic animals. It can cause respiratory illness, inflammation at the site of the injury, cellulitis, and swollen lymph glands. In severe cases, it can lead to bactermia, meningitis, endocarditis, or osteomyelitis. These bacteriae also harbor a bacteriophage which is responsible for producing toxins. The usual treatment is tetracycline or fluoroquinolone antibiotics. Most gammaproteobacteriae produce some kind of toxin. In the *Pasteurellaceae* group we find virulent, pore-forming RTX toxins. In the *Vibrionales* group we find the TTX toxin producers.[32-35]

As for Marek's disease, we find a fowl virus that is similar to a herpes virus. It is common wherever chickens are present, although it infects other birds (i.e. turkeys, pheasants). The infection causes lesions in the nervous system, eyes, viscera, skeletal muscles, and *most importantly the feather follicles of the skin.* Symptoms may include paralysis, polyneuritis, lymphomatoses, acute leukosis, iritis, failure to gain weight, and dehydration. In 1968, thirty-six million broiler chickens were condemned in USDA plants because of Marek's disease.[36-48]

A new *Marek's* disease vaccine patent was filed in 1969, and assigned to pharmaceutical company Eli Lilly. The original vaccine used against Marek's included a live, attenuated *Newcastle disease virus* which was given to young chicks. The vaccine improved their weight gain and reduced the number of processing plant condemnations in chickens exposed to Marek's disease. The gammaproteobacteria or Newcastle virus may be at the heart of the contaminated chicken embryo cells that we learned about and which contained *reverse transcriptase* or RT activity. *This contaminant cannot be removed from chicken embryos including those used to create vaccine or insecticide cell lines.*[36-48]

Cultures of a B1 strain of Newcastle disease were kept at the Newcastle disease virus repository at the University of Wisconsin-Madison according to a patent. The strain was described as a live virus that was first isolated by Beaudette, who studied Newcastle disease at the New Jersey Agricultural Experiment station in 1946. This is just two years after the isolation of the very first spiroplasma strain. The B1 virus strain was weak enough not to produce symptoms, but strong enough to induce antibody production in vaccinated chickens. There is no known cure or protective agent for this virus once birds are infected. One of the bird vaccines used a turkey herpes virus that was nonpathogenic to chickens but which was protective against Marek's disease.[36-48]

The "contamination" of chicken embryo cell lines that was revealed earlier, likely comes from chickens that have been vaccinated against *Marek's disease* or *Avian Sarcoma Leukosis Virus*. The Marek's vaccine is intended to protect against an avian herpes (DNA) virus by introducing a live, non-infectious Newcastle disease virus as a vaccine. The vaccines can be made using "sterile" water and bovine albumin and serum. (We already know that contaminated sterile water and bovine albumin has been a problem in labs.) A 1966 *Avian Leukosis* vaccine patent is assigned to Abbott Laboratories (North Chicago, IL). It uses the *Rous sarcoma virus* to produce a poultry vaccine. This virus causes connective tissue tumors in chickens, turkeys, ducks, geese, and *pheasants.* In 2006, avian leukosis virus was isolated from four lots of Marek's disease vaccines that were produced by two laboratories.[49-52,60]

The *Avian Sarcoma Leukosis Virus* used in poultry vaccines is an RNA retrovirus from the family of alpharetroviruses. It is related to a family of lentiviruses that includes the *bovine immunodeficiency virus* (BIV), the *feline immunodeficiency virus* (FIV), and the *human immunodeficiency virus* (HIV). If this virus is a satellite virus that infects poultry host cells, it may play an integral role in the development of diseases at a later period, including possibly human HIV/AIDS.[49-52]

Vaccines that are grown in chicken embryo cells are used to inoculate chickens against industrially important diseases. These viruses, whether DNA or RNA in origin, become incorporated into the genome of chicken cells, and thus chicken embryo cell lines that are used to create human vaccines. Viral and/or bacterial contaminants remain in the finished vaccine products when present. We can see how a chicken retrovirus could retain its ability to cause RT or reverse transcriptase activity in chicken embryo cell lines. We may imagine that transcriptional events can occur under the right circumstances.[49-52]

We also have seen that shortly after the application of microbial insecticides and parasitoid insects in the environment for agricultural and industrial purposes, there were outbreaks of rickettsialpox and equine encephalitis in animals (i.e. horses, pheasants); and polio and yellow fever in humans. We know also that viruses were released from 1951 forward to purposely infect *baculoviruses* (DNA viruses) with smaller RNA viruses to ramp up the effectiveness of applied insecticides. We also saw the development of *novel immunodeficiency viruses and new retroviruses* emerge within human and animal populations during the period that genetic engineering techniques were being deployed for agriculture and industry.

We have also seen the emergence of novel radiation-resistant viruses, retroviruses, or bacteriae that were employed by, or found within industrial environments including nuclear wastewaters or reactors. The questions are whether these microbes contaminate insect cells lines or animal or human vaccines. If so, will they reactivate upon introduction of insect or arthropod-borne mixed infections in susceptible, vaccinated animals and people? After all, this is what they are designed to do in insects.[49-52]

Besides mining, Connecticut has an interesting poultry and shipbuilding history. (Remember that Newcastle disease was first isolated from a shipbuilding/mining region in the UK in 1926.) From 1785 to about 1823, Roswell Hollister owned a large shipyard at Log Landing in south Glastonbury, Connecticut. After his last ship wrecked off Cape Hatteras, the hub of shipbuilding moved down the Connecticut River to Saybrook and Haddam. This is the area where the first cases of Lyme disease were found in Connecticut (and near the New London submarine base in Groton in 1951). The first nuclear submarine the *Nautilus* which used a pressurized water nuclear reactor, was built at the electric boat division of *General Dynamics,* which was based in Groton. General Dynamics is one of the largest defense contractors in the world. The *Nautilus* was launched in 1954 into the Thames River (but its keel was laid in CT in 1952). This of course was just after the first experiments by New Haven scientists who began field-testing *borrelina* RNA viruses as baculovirus (DNA) insecticidal enhancers.[53-57]

Could microbes have migrated into waterways (and thus birds, fauna, and insects) from Cockaponset or Nehantic State Forests as potential insecticide field test areas to each of the waterside towns first affected by the early Lyme disease outbreaks – Lyme, Old Lyme, East Haddam, Haddam, and also Groton? *Did marine bacteria or viruses become superinfected with the borrelina or baculoviruses that were being used as regional insecticides to cause Lyme?* An old resource described the soil erosion in the region at a rate of twenty feet per year. Whatever washed into Long Island Sound from industries and agricultural applications over a period of the previous century could have contributed to the toxic wastes and microbes found in Long Island Sound over many decades.[53-57]

History shows that Long Island Sound would be tainted not only by the explosions of two million pounds of ammunitions stored at Black Tom Island in 1916; but would also become the unlucky recipient of industrial and toxic wastes dumped into the Sound over a century and a half. Some of those wastes came from upstream, via rivers that were contaminated by nuclear, agricultural, and industrial toxic wastes which made their way into the Sound through natural watersheds.[53-57]

Glastonbury was also home to airplane manufacturers, textiles, leather tanners, and peach growers. Here again are hints to the presence of gammaproteobacteria and other significant bacteriae and insect viruses. Around 1900, Italian Frank Saglio took a job in the J.H. Hale peach orchards and then bought his own farm which he named Arbor Acres. There he raised vegetables and fruits for sale, and a few chickens. His son Henry was interested in breeding chickens, and won a competition to find the "chicken of tomorrow." The company marketed a white rock broiler chicken during the 1950s that was sold globally. By 1958 roughly half the world's chickens carried Arbor Acre genes. The farm was also the largest cauliflower (cruficer) producer in Connecticut.[58,59]

The International Basic Economy Corporation (IBEC), founded by former US Vice-President Nelson Aldrich Rockefeller, purchased Arbor Acres over time, owning a majority share by 1964. A company called Booker PLC bought IBEC by 1985 when Henry Saglio left the company. Arbor Acres remains a global brand although the company has been sold several times. Arbor Acres was not only a supplier of poultry to the world, it also supplied *genetic material for poultry stock.* This could have included fertilized eggs (chicken embryos) for use in laboratory-based products (i.e. insect, animal, or human cell lines). Arbor Acres would become Connecticut's largest agricultural business. Whatever was used to vaccinate poultry over time is probably responsible for the retrovirus or reverse transcriptase activity that remains in all chicken embryo tissues used for food production, laboratory use; and which has been repeatedly discussed as a possible human vaccine concern by scientists and public health experts over decades.[58,59]

While many will disagree with the decision of scientists to continue to use what were clearly identified in scientific reports as *contaminated cell lines to create vaccines,* there is little that can be done about these practices today except to implement oversight and to devise new techniques that will eliminate or minimize such threats in the future. Since the source of the contaminants may be retroviruses which come from the very animals used to make the cell lines, eliminating retroviruses and other contaminants from source tissues may be virtually impossible. Of course scientists should revise current cell lines in use to ensure that they are as free from infectious agents as possible. Those who receive vaccines must be warned that these tools do not come without risks of many kinds – including the reactivation of vaccine viruses by unknown future factors including insect-borne infections or even GM foods.

Perhaps the revision of important, contaminated cell lines is exactly what scientists were attempting to do in 1994 shortly before the Dearborn conference for Lyme disease when tick cell lines were found to be contaminated and new cell lines were created for cattle vaccines. The other consideration with respect to contaminated cell lines is to publicly acknowledge past mistakes, and to acknowledge patients who have become ill from flawed recombinant products. Scientists must also be charged with the task of inventing curative solutions for those who suffer the ill effects of recombinant "accidents" that may arrive in the form of vectoring insects and novel human epidemic diseases.[1]

Our bodies now harbor viruses/retroviruses which may have come from contaminated vaccines, animal products, or insecticides. Now the global presence of illnesses with "no known cause" makes far more sense. The question is whether contaminated cell lines are a major contributing factor to human diseases, including those transmitted by insects. What we may find in the available research are clues that what we are exposed to on many levels may leave us open to the reactivation of diseases by forces beyond our control. When we honestly consider the earliest applications of agricultural and industrial pesticides to the present day; and the emergence of novel animal and human infections during a similar period where recombinant microbes were deployed, we may find evidence that many epidemic diseases have had laboratory as well as natural origins.

Even Microbes Get Sick

We have already learned a bit about the *baculoviruses,* which are a group of large DNA viruses that have been used within recombinant insecticides. These are also found naturally in insects including the parasitoids that were deployed agriculturally. Baculoviruses replicate inside the cell nucleus and the cell cytoplasm. Baculoviruses are divided into subgroups which include the *Eubaculovirinae* (occluded viruses), and the *Nudibaculovirinae* (non-occluded viruses). The latter group are descendants of the *Nudiviruses.* This is a related group of viruses that includes insect viruses that have been used as "expression vectors" (recombinant constructs) in insecticides. The eubaculovirinae infect insects that are important to our story; the larvae of the lepidoptera, coleoptera, diptera, hymenoptera, other insects and crustaceans (i.e. shrimp, crabs). The eubaculoviruses produce crystalline proteins that are called occlusion bodies.[1-2]

(Eu)baculoviruses that are encased in their virus capsid or shell (occlusion body) are protected from ultraviolet light and other environmental degraders. The eubaculoviruses are the larger DNA viruses (NPVs, GVs) we have discussed previously. The nudibaculoviruses are smaller in size, lack an occlusion body, and require protection from UV light. The occluded eubaculoviruses make two kinds of virus particles (virions). These are the occluded polyhedra-derived virion (PDV), and the budded virions (BV). PDVs are found upon contaminated leaves and are eaten by insects. They contain the smaller encapsulated BVs that are released during digestion. Once released, the BVs spread infections between insects. These viruses are commonly found as *contaminants in insect cell lines.* These contaminants may infect the other viruses or bacteria in the cell lines.[1,2]

Scientists discovered that the *transposons* of large DNA viruses may have been influenced by the *Mavirus virophage* eons ago. The Mavirus probably got its transposons from its ancient Maverick/Polinton virus relatives. Scientists believe that although the RNA and DNA viruses have evolved differently, they all seem to have had common ancestors. Therefore viruses such as tobacco mosaic virus, polio virus, herpes, human papilloma, or poxviruses may each have evolved from large DNA viruses. What this means to us is that any of the large DNA viruses may be able to become infected with smaller RNA viruses, and will work together with their viral partners as co-infections which become ultra-infective to insects and vertebrate animals. Remember that we have alreaday learned that *poxviruses may be reactivated in the presence of compatible viruses.*[1-3]

Any DNA or RNA viruses may be reactivated by similar family members that donate compatible, necessary genes to the inactive virus. The viruses that may be compatible partners include the herpes, polio, insect pox and iridescent viruses; and plant viruses such as brome and tobacco mosaic, the yellows disease viruses, and geminiviruses (i.e. cassava latent virus) as examples. Any of these viruses when used as insecticides may be capable of donating genes to vaccinated animals or humans to cause the reactivation of latent viruses to cause diseases.[1-3]

The DNA and RNA viruses can contain RT or *reverse transcriptase activity.* This means they may be capable of initiating virus replication under optimal circumstances. This may also suggest that once the viruses of recombinant insecticides are introduced into animals or humans, they may *reactivate the viruses or retroviruses of vertebrates, including the viral components of previous vaccines!*[1-3]

This appears to have been the exact scenario that scientists were concerned about when they discovered decades ago that chicken embryo cell lines were contaminated with infective agents and RT activity. Those cell lines were left in continued use for animal and human vaccines despite the risks of reactivation. Remember scientists also discovered that insect cell lines were found to have been contaminated, and that early polio vaccines (and others) have admittedly been contaminated with infective agents.

We now know that microbial insecticides have been used in industrial settings (i.e. to treat water flows) and agriculturally (i.e. crop insecticides) over decades. Several suppliers provide baculovirus-containing products including *Novartis Crop Protection, Inc.; Thermo Trilogy Corp., Natural Plant Protection* (France), and the USDA Forest Service (Hamden, CT). The Group I baculoviruses that we have examined so far included the *wilt diseases* of silkworms, Japanese beetles, and other insects. Over time the baculoviruses were used within *insect cell lines* (i.e. Sf 9, Sf 21 from fall armyworm larvae) and within *baculovirus expression vectors* not only to make insecticides, but also *animal and human vaccines.* Scientists at *Texas A&M University* (where Dr. Alan Barbour has worked) established an insect Sf 9 cell line from the fall army worm *Spodoptera frugiperda.* The Sf 9 line was a clone of another (Sf 21) line that was originally developed in the 1970s by the USDA Beltsville Agricultural Research Center in Maryland. It is the largest agricultural reseach complex in the world, and its scientists deal with plant, animal, food, soil, crop, and related diseases and development. Their studies also include the genetic research of plants and animals (i.e. dairy cattle).[2,4]

Beginning in 1951 in the US, scientists began releasing RNA viruses (i.e. borrelinas) into the environment to ramp up the effectiveness of baculovirus-containing insecticides. These techniques were also being deployed in other areas of the world. The RNA viruses which include the *reoviruses* or CPVs (cypoviruses), replicate inside the cell *cytoplasm.* Although the DNA and RNA viruses replicate in different compartments of co-infected host cells, together they produce mixed infections which proved to be far more lethal to co-infected insects. Remember that the early *parasitoid insects harbored polydnaviruses* which include the Group I DNA insect baculoviruses from the groups *Ichnovirus* and *Bracovirus* (wasps). The *segmented* baculoviruses are capable of changing the DNA structure and the immune function of the organisms they infect.[3,6-8,12]

The *Nucleocytoplasmic viruses* (NCLDV) are one group of *large DNA viruses* that are called *virophages. These include the larger group of NPV baculoviruses we have discussed.* Virophages are found in soil and in *marine environments* and are common among algae blooms such as blue-green algae. This may explain the coastal evolution of the Lyme disease spirochete if it involves at least one virophage. These viruses literally "eat" other viruses. There are virophages that infect algae, insects, animals, and humans. The NCLDV group includes the following virus families. Note these families play an integral role in insecticides, human diseases, and vaccine formulas. At least one family, *Asfarvirus* which has only one member called the *African swine fever virus,* was observed by Lyme noteable Dr. Alan Barbour to have structures which resemble those found in the Bb spirochete of Lyme disease. Here are the members of the NCLDV virus families:[3,6-8]

Asfarviridae (i.e. African swine fever virus)	*Irodoviridae* (i.e. insect iridescent viruses [Japanese beetles])
Poxviridae (i.e. cowpox, monkeypox, smallpox)	*Phycodnaviridae* (i.e. freshwater algae viruses)*
Mimiviridae (i.e. CroV, Mamavirus, Mimivirus)†	*Megaviridae* (single species: *Megavirus chilensis*)‡
Marseilleviridae (similar to Mimivirus)	*Dinodnavirus* (i.e. marine plankton [pfiesteria], *coral reefs*)

**Thought to have evolved from the Iridoviridae family. †CroV is the Cafeteria roenbergensis virus that infects marine zooplankton. ‡Includes a single species, Megavirus chilensis, which is related to the Acanthamoeba polyphaga mimivirus. It is sometimes called "Megavirus." It is the virus with the largest virus capsid, and has the most complex genome of all viruses.*

Studies with phages began just before the turn of the 20th century. In 1922 the Pasteur Institute published a book on the role of bacteriophages in immunity. The publication covered bacteriophages that attacked various *Bacillus* species as well as *Staphylococcus, Salmonella,* and *Vibrio cholerae.* By the 1940s, experiments with phages were undertaken at biological laboratories at Cold Spring Harbor (NY), Indiana, Vanderbilt, and Washington Universities (St. Louis, MO).

The discovery of new DNA virophages took place in the late 20th century as new species were found in marine environments including in the waters and microbes of *nuclear reactors*. Virophages are typically found replicating inside of *Amoeba* such as *Acanthamoeba polyphaga,* a common soil and waterborne protozoan. The *Acanthamoeba polyphaga mimivirus* or *Mimivirus* (mimicking microbe), was first isolated from a nuclear cooling tower in the UK in 2003 during research into *Legionellosis,* which causes *Legionnaires' disease* and *Pontiac fever*. Legionnaires' disease was named after a 1976 outbreak at a Philadelphia hotel in people who attended an American Legion convention.[6,8-11]

Other virophages are found in the environment. The 1976 timeline is interesting since this was when the Lyme disease outbreak in Connecticut was first announced. The Delaware River separates Pennsylvania from New Jersey, and dumps into the Delaware Bay which of course is connected to the Atlantic Ocean, just south of Atlantic City, New Jersey. We remember that there were military toxic waste dump sites off the eastern seaboard, including off the cost of Atlantic City. It is probable that toxins infected marine bacteria, algae, and their protozoan parasites only to be carried into coastal sediments and the microbes therein.[6,8-10]

It is also possible that discharged industrial wastes and their microbes were not only discharged in wastewaters, but became aerosolized as evaporative mists that were subsequently released as airborne pathogens able to settle onto the soils around nuclear facilities. The newest virophages that have been discovered in recent decades including those that have been found in nuclear wastewaters and their microbes include a group called *Mimiviridae*. Some of these viruses have their own virophages or satellite viruses. For example the *Sputnik* virophage is a satellite virus of the Mamavirus. These are the *Mimiviridae* group viruses: *Cafeteria roenbergensis virus* (CroV), *Courdovirus, Mamavirus, Mimivirus, Moumouvirus, Terravirus 1, and Terravirus 2.*[6,8-10]

It should be stated that the *Acanthamoeba* protozoae are able to infect humans, and they cause central nervous system diseases and keratitis (inflamed cornea). These protozoans can be inhaled through an airborne route (i.e. nuclear cooling tower or steam vents) or an agricultural route. These amoeba are highly antibiotic-resistant and they produce meningitis, encephalitis, or tuberculosis-like infections; but are considered to be "rare." Still, they are able to create cysts and to cross the blood-brain barrier where they destroy brain cells. These infections can become fatal within days to weeks. These amoeba are able to lyse or open up other bacteria, and to produce enzymes that degrade chitin or cellulose. Acanthamoeba is usually found in patients who have immunodeficiencies, diabetes, cancers, or malnutrition. Can they also play a role in persisting Lyme disease?

We can see important connections between the Bb spirochete, virophage families that seem to have similar genetics, and the location of Lyme disease outbreaks that are coincidentally near areas where important rare earth elements and their nuclear technologies are deployed. Is a protozoan phage responsible for some of the genes in the Lyme disease spirochete? Are the insect viruses and their satellite phages that were deployed agriculturally and industrially as insecticides the key to understanding diseases such as Lyme and Morgellon's? After all, nuclear plants use insecticidal formulas to treat their water flows, and so do various industries. Wherever we look, we return to the same insecticides which seem to be at the heart of the animal and human diseases that have emerged over the past century and a half. ❑

Do No Evil.

> *"...And he shall judge among the nations, and shall rebuke many people: and they shall beat their swords into plowshares, and their spears into pruning hooks: nation shall not lift up sword against nation, neither shall they learn war any more"*

This quote was taken from *The Holy Bible*, King James edition (Micah 4:3; Isaiah 2:4) to name *Project Plowshare,* the US government's program from 1961-1977 to develop "peaceful" nuclear explosions (i.e. build dams, waterways, mines; for agricultural use, etc.). More than two dozen test detonations occurred (mostly at a Nevada site), and which hurled radioactive tritium high into the earth's atmosphere.

This biblical excerpt may be referencing the "last days" or the "end times" wherein the battle of Armageddon is yet to come. Perhaps such a battle will not be fought using nuclear or other weapons of traditional warfare. Rather as a mural in the Denver, Colorado airport depicts, it will arrive as a biological Armageddon the likes of which the world has not yet seen. Maybe Armageddon will come in the form of a recombinant plague or a novel formula created from microbes collected from 25 million year-old fossilized amber. Such weapons may not yet have been developed, but they soon will be; and may be disbursed as industrial or agricultural insecticides.

Could mankind be well on the path of his own destruction through the manipulation of microbes? Is the future of mankind uncertain and highly dependent upon the choices we make today? I for one would be the first to venture a guess...

Eight: If All Else Fails, Play the Red Herring*

Another Look at Dearborn's Elite

At the beginning of this book I provided a brief history of an historic event that was highly important to the history of Lyme disease. It was the 1994 CDC-sponsored Dearborn conference where surveillance case definitions, diagnostic test recommendations, and testing methods were standardized. It has become abundantly clear from numerous sources that certain personnel in attendance at Dearborn were more than vaguely aware that *Borrelia burgdorferi* infections were both persistent and chronic. We can see evidence of this from some of their earlier published research and patent inventions. It is also entirely obvious that some very important facts about Lyme disease were known prior to the 1994 conference.

The Dearborn conference took place nearly *two decades after* the Connecticut Lyme disease outbreak was first formally announced. It was also a dozen years after the causative agent of Lyme disease was announced to be *Borrelia burgdorferi.* What happened at Dearborn has contributed to the grand chasm of dissenting viewpoints about whether Lyme disease is a debilitating, chronic infection; or an easily treated, acute illness. This leads us to question the motivations behind holding the Dearborn conference and the sudden standardization of surveillance case definitions and laboratory tests for the illness.

Several Dearborn conference attendees and a few of their colleagues have played important roles in the patenting of, standardization of, dissemination of information, and/or control of the processes and public opinion of Lyme disease. Several of these individuals are key patent holders for important Bb-related vaccine and diagnostic tools. Three have co-authored medical guidelines for Lyme disease treatment, and one was lead investigator for the first generation Lyme vaccine and who conducted vaccine clinical trials. Several individuals have received federal and/or industry funding to study Lyme disease according to patents, grants, and scientific reports. Patients and physicians wonder why patent holders or academic researchers who do not treat patients within clinical settings are allowed to dictate disease guidelines and standards that define or deny any diseases.

There are several pieces of correspondence from one of the key players in the Lyme disease story, Dr. Allen C. Steere. In a letter from July 30, 1990, Dr. Steere makes clear some concerns about Lyme advocacy groups, and that two Lyme treating physicians have become "major spokesmen" for Lyme disease. The letter's Dr. Steere asks the addressee, the Director of the Department of Health's Medical Division in Milford, CT, for "ideas" regarding "what to do" about the situation. Dr. Steere is an EIS employee of the CDC. As such, his relationship with the public health agency may play a role in his opinions. Part of his duties may include acting as liaison officer for the reporting and dissemination of information about Lyme disease, which by 1990 was a growing epidemic.[1]

A second piece of correspondence is a letter dated June 14, 1990, from Dr. Steere to a New York physician who treats Lyme patients. In the letter Dr. Steere had this to say about an article about *Borrelia burgdorferi,* written by Preac-Mursic:[2]

> "Because they were able to culture the spirochete, they certainly proved that one may have persistent infection after intensive antibiotic therapy and despite seronegativity."

The comments in the second letter clearly acknowledged persistent Bb infection, patient seronegativity (negative test results despite infection), and infection after "intensive" antibiotic treatment. Unfortunately these ideas were apparently not championed by Dr. Steere when he attended the later 1994 Dearborn conference; nor when he co-authored the 2000 and 2006 IDSA medical guidelines for Lyme disease. At the Dearborn conference Dr. Steere would take an opposite opinion that Lyme disease was both "over diagnosed" and "over treated." It is interesting that one point of view might be promoted to another treating physician in private, while the opposite position is promoted during public policymaking. This is especially interesting when we realize that an upcoming Lyme vaccine for which Dr. Steere would become lead investigator and run clinical trials in the days to come, would be significantly impacted by the outcome of the Dearborn conference.[2]

A third piece of correspondence contradicts the recommendations Dr. Steere made at Dearborn. This was a form letter signed by Dr. Steere which was sent to former patients of his clinic. The letter is dated August 11, 1994, just *two months before* the Dearborn conference where Steere presented the Dressler/Steere "Lyme disease is over diagnosed and over treated" paper. The form letter was written on Tufts NEMC letterhead and was received by a former patient who lived in New London, Connecticut at the time.[3]

The letter invited the clinic's former patients to participate in long-term follow-up studies for Lyme disease. The follow up studies mentioned in the letter were funded by the NIH and the CDC. According to the letter's text:

> "It has become increasingly apparent that the Lyme disease spirochete, *Borrelia burgdorferi, may persist in some patients for years.* Of particular concern, recent studies have shown that the spirochete may persist in the nervous

**Red herring: The process of diverting attention away from an item or event of significance*

system in a small percentage of patients and may cause chronic neurologic involvement."

The purpose of the long-term follow up studies according to the letter were to "determine whether past patients may still have evidence of Lyme disease and if so, to offer appropriate treatment."[3]

It is perhaps curious then that CDC representatives and Dr. Steere, who attended and influenced the decisions made at the CDC-sponsored Dearborn conference two months later; failed to address at Dearborn the suspected persistence of the Bb organism, patient seronegativity, or the long-term follow-up studies already underway at the time of the conference. We may also ask why Bb persistence and seronegativity was not addressed when the 2000 and 2006 IDSA guidelines for Lyme disease were co-authored and published by Drs. Steere, Dattwyler (both years), and Luft (2000). Each of these men reportedly attended the Dearborn conference.[4]

The Dearborn planning committee members included Drs. Duane Gubler, Barbara Johnson, and David Dennis (CDC), Raymond Dattwyler (SUNY-Stony Brook), Russell Johnson (Univ. MN), Raymond Ryan (University of CT), Allen Steere (Tufts NEMC), Arthur Weinstein (NYMC), and Alan Barbour (University of TX).[4]

Several of these investigators supplied the monoclonal antibodies for select Bb proteins that were used to calibrate the Immunoblot tests for the Dearborn conference work group studies. The results of those studies would become the model for the diagnostic test standards that would be established for Lyme disease from 1994 to the present day. The unfortunate outcome of the standardization of the Lyme disease tests has resulted in the inability to detect real infections in thousands of patients around the world.

Monoclonal Antibodies at Dearborn

The next section may seem highly technical, but it is necessary for its relevance to the story. The discussion focuses on the antibodies that were supplied to the Dearborn work group to study as a model for the diagnostic test probes to be used in the new standardization process. This model would determine how diagnostic tests would be interpreted, using the antibody markers selected by the work group. Here I mention the antibodies that were supplied, as well as a possible description of what those antibodies represent. The analysis is theoretical, but I provide it to suggest there are alternative reasons why the antibodies were selected for use in the new standardized Lyme tests.

Several investigators supplied monoclonal antibodies for select "Bb" proteins to calibrate the Immunoblot tests for the Dearborn conference work group studies. The investigators who belonged to the work group committee were Drs. Benjamin Luft, Alan Barbour, Thomas Schwan (NIH Rocky Mt. Labs, Hamilton, MT); Denée Thomas (UT Health Sciences Center, San Antonio, TX); Steven Padula (University of Connecticut health center in Farmington), and Jorge Benach (SUNY at Stony Brook, NY). Note that Drs. Barbour and Benach co-published the June 1982 paper along with Drs. Willy Burgdorfer, Stanley Hayes, Jeffrey Davis, and Edgar Grunwaldt that announced the causative agent of Lyme disease to the world.

Drs. Burgdorfer, Barbour, and Hayes worked at Rocky Mt. Labs, while Dr. Benach was at SUNY Stony Brook; Dr. Grunwaldt at Shelter Island, NY; and Dr. Davis at the WI Dept. of Health at the time of the 1982 publication. (Dr. Davis is now Chief Medical Officer and State Epidemiologist for the state of Wisconsin.) The monoclonal antibodies (MAbs) supplied by these investigators at Dearborn are listed below, including the name of the antibody, its molecular weight, and the name of the investigator who supplied the antibody.[1,2]

Antibody	Specificity/molecular weight	Investigator
181.1	93 kDa	Benjamin Luft
8D5	66 kDa	Alan Barbour
149	GroEL, 66 kDa	Benjamin Luft
H9724	Flagella 41 kDa	Alan Barbour
H1141	BmpA, 39 kDa	Thomas Schwan
84C	OspB, 34 kDa	Denée Thomas
H5332	OspA, 31 kDa	Alan Barbour
H1C8*	OspD, 29 kDa	Alan Barbour
4B8F4	OspC, 23 kDa	Steven Padula
CB625	22 kDa	Jorge Benach

**Said to be reactive with Bb strain B31 (NY strain), but not with other important strains 297 (from a neuroborreliosis patient's cerebral spinal fluid) or strain 2591, a Connecticut isolate.*[3,4]

The Bb strain from the NY isolate "B31" that had been isolated from Shelter Island tick pools in 1981 became part of the antibodies used in the newly standardized tests. However according to research, antibodies to two strains isolated from

Connecticut, and from patient cerebrospinal fluid samples were not used in the new tests. The Shelter Island ticks were the same ticks from which the Bb agent was originally isolated. The B31 strain is the most common strain found in patients, and probably the one that Dr. Steere was most familiar. It may or may not have been the same strain from which Dr. Steere et al. originally cultured the novel *Leptospira inadai Lyme.* This was the *leptonema* spirochete that "nobody" has talked about as having any kind of connection to Lyme disease infections (until perhaps now).

The monoclonal antibodies (MAbs) were used to calibrate the immunoblot (lab) tests at Dearborn. The results would establish the diagnostic testing standards for Lyme disease for decades. Once settled, the CDC recommended for Western Immunoblot tests (Western blot), that the following diagnostic bands must test positive in order for patients to be considered as positive for Lyme disease. The CDC requires that *five* of the following *ten* antibody bands for IgG† should register positive: 18, 21*, 28, 30, 39, 41, 45, 58, 66, and 93; and *two* of the following *three* bands for IgM† should register as positive: 24*, 39, 41.

**According to the CDC, the molecular mass of the OspC band varies according to Bb strain tested. The 24 and 21-kDa proteins are considered to be the same despite band number differences. Research tells us that the OspC band ranges from 21 to 25-kDa, depending on strain.*[48]

†IgG is the Immunoglobulin G antibody, and IgM is the Immunoglobulin M antibody.

The Dearborn test bands were established to detect *the body's response* to the antigens of an aggregate Bb spirochete, not necessarily the individual organism, as everyone believes. Each band may correspond to a different microbial component of a Bb aggregate or *a response by the body*. The major protein bands of Bb spirochetes can be detected at band numbers 21-25, 30, and 34-kDa, with flagella at the 41-kDa band. The 30 and 34 bands vary betwen Bb species (i.e. 30-36). These bands also correspond to those that are detectable during leptospirosis infection. Major leptospira outer membrane proteins are detectable at 22, 28, 32, 35, 41, and 67-kDa, although more than a dozen outer membrane proteins are known. Like Bb, leptospira bands are *variable* and strain dependent. The three major protein bands from *Leptospira interrogans* strains are detectable at 25, 32, and 41-kDa. Minor protein bands are detected at 22.5, 36, 77, and 112-kDa. The LPS (bacterial endotoxins) of strain *Leptospira copenhageni* have an "O" antigen at 22-kDa, while *L. interrogans* and *L. biflexa* measure around 20-kDa.[41,49-52]

What if the antibody bands are markers not only for a spirochete, but also for antibodies that are produced to excreted *human proteins* during a Bb infection? From this perspective we'll look for agents with the same molecular weight that may be detected by the test probes. Let's examine the role that *human and microbial agents* together may play in the Lyme infection *process.* In essence Lyme diagnostic tests may be detecting both "self" and "non-self" (foreign) proteins. We will also examine each MAb used in the work group sessions for their hypothetical, alternative use in Lyme diagnostic tests.

Monoclonal Antibody (MAb) 181.1: This 93-kDa antibody is said to be a "p93" minor protein from the Bb spirochete's protoplasmic cylinder. The monoclonal antibody for the test probe appears to have been developed using mice. The antibody may be produced during infection with any of at least four European or American Bb strains. There is also a human MAb that was developed to secrete an *Epstein-Barr* virus-transformed B-cell line. That MAb has a weight of 93-kDa according to a 1991 paper co-authored by Dr. Benjamin Luft. Dr. Luft provided a 181.1 MAb to the Dearborn work group just three years later.

Perhaps this antibody is detecting a recombinant Epstein-Barr virus and not the whole Bb organism. If so, this band may detect the *reactivation* of an Epstein-Barr virus from a natural infection, a recombinant vaccine, or an applied insecticide that used a recombinant EBV virus that is co-infected with a virophage. Viruses that infect host cells may not necessarily cause disease until they are co-infected by a satellite virus or a virophage as we have learned. We have seen that viruses have been genetically engineered into insecticides. EBV or another virus like HTLV is fully capable of growing inside a host cell when co-infected with a satellite or virophage such as those found in insecticides or nature.

The 93-kDa antibody band *is included in the standardized Lyme disease IgM tests,* but not for IgG. This would indicate that the 93-kDa protein is detectable during early infections, and not necessarily during disseminated disease. The 93-kDa protein also has the same molecular weight as an *important outer surface protein of Leptospire spirochetes.* This antibody could be detecting a mutated leptospira spirochete protein or the presence of a recombinant insecticide in a human host.[5,6]

8D5 & 149: As a heat shock response, the 8D5 and 149 MAbs with a molecular weight of 66-kDa may represent an antibody to *beta dystroglycan.* This is an essential element of the neuromuscular junction and proteins from skeletal muscle fibers. A different paper says the molecular weight is 44-kDa, which is the same molecular weight as a B.t. phage. This MAb may also represent a 66-kDa protein found in the neurofilaments of the mammalian brain and spinal cord.[7,8]

The 66-kDa protein could represent a *Leucine* heat shock protein. This essential amino acid is a major component of ferritin and other buffer proteins which work to slow the destruction of muscle proteins. It is used in the liver; is broken down in fat and muscle tissue, and helps form sterols like cholesterol. In excess, *leucine toxicity* causes delirium and neurologic problems that can be life-threatening from *high ammonia levels* (i.e. pellagra). Pellagra is a vitamin deficiency of Vitamin B3 (niacin).

Pellagra causes lesions and thickened skin. A balanced diet or small amount of brewer's yeast prevents pellagra. In yeast genetics, mutants which lack the ability to synthesize leucine are transformed using a leucine plasmid. L-leucine is a food additive and flavor enhancer. Patients with Lyme disease often display deficiencies in the B-vitamin family. Some have high ammonia levels and others are advised by their doctors to consume probiotics or *S. cerevisiae* (brewer's yeast). Others are given vitamin B injections or oral or sublingual vitamins to treat Vitamin B deficiency.[7,8]

H9724: According to a paper co-authored by Drs. Sigal et al. at the Robert Wood Johnson Medical School at the University of Medicine and Dentistry of New Jersey, the "H9724" MAb is an antibody to the Bb flagellin (tail) at 41-kDa that binds to heat shock protein #60 (HSP60) of neuroblastoma cells (nerve cell cancer). This antibody may bind to proteins that are secreted by the Bb organism when the body is under stress, such as during infection. Here we're not necessarily looking at the Bb organism, but rather at an immune response to infection and a stress response in the form of proteins expressed by infected human host cells. This MAb could instead represent an antibody that is created in response to the exposure of the patient to a recombinant insecticide that was first modified in a laboratory using a neuroblastoma cell line to culture recombinant (GM) microbes.[9]

H1141: The H1141 (BmpA) MAb may represent proteins common among *B. afzelii, B. garinii,* and *B. burgdorferi* sensu stricto strains. There is also a 39-kDa human cartilage glycoprotein. Insecticides that contain bioengineered chitin may cause a human to produce this antibody when exposed to natural chitin or to a recombinant chitin-dissolving enzyme in the formula.

There is also a 39-kDa protein that belongs to the organism *Avian Pasteurella multocida,* the agent of *fowl cholera* or *bird anthrax*. (This is caused by a gammaproteobacterium that is probably infected with a virus.) This may be a hint that the 39-kDa protein commonly expressed by most Lyme patients may represent a protein from a B.t. insecticide that contains chitin-degrading enzymes, or proteins from a gammaproteobacterium that may be found in all Bb spirochetal strain groups. Or perhaps the 39-kDa protein is evidence that contaminated chicken embryo-grown vaccines in the body have been brought out of latency upon exposure to a vectoring insect that has been exposed to recombinant pesticides. The 39-kDa protein therefore may represent the reactivated latent components of a chicken embryo-grown human vaccine.

A 39-kDa protein is produced by the *Shigella sonnei* gammaproteobacterium. This agent causes dysentery. Other shigella species promote inflammation in mucous membranes. There are other *Shigella* species, Types A-D. All are lactose-fermenting bacteria. *S. sonnei* thrives in the human gastrointestinal tract during infection and is a major food-borne threat to the public. It is transmitted by contaminated water or wastewater, or improperly cooked foods via the oral-fecal route.

The shigella organism has a circular genome. It uses chromosomal and plasmid-encoded genes to remain infectious and is closely related to *E. coli. Acanthamoeba* protozoans and other microbes are known to take up shigella into their cells where they remain protected from the elements, and in return help to promote growth. We discussed *acanthamoeba* in an earlier section. But to recap they may be found in wastewater streams, sewage, pools, hot tubs, HVAC systems, potable water systems, and nuclear cooling towers or the steam that escapes from vents at pressurized water reactor facilities.[10-16,67]

Virophages like *Sputnik* infect *Acanthamoeba* species. This virophage was first isolated in 2008 in a Parisian water cooling tower. Virophages like sputnik depend on their host cells to become infected with *satellite viruses.* In an acantamoeba that is infected with *Mimivirus,* sputnik is able to replicate. Satellite viruses such as *borrelina* and the baculoviruses are deployed as insecticides. When their hosts are co-infected with a compatible satellite virus, virophages begin replication by hijacking satellite virus proteins that are needed to reproduce. Virophages help DNA viruses like baculoviruses or retroviruses to *reassort* (mutate) and horizontally transfer genes through transposons or retrotransposons (mobile DNA). Sputnik is an example of a virophage that is able to infect bacteria, archaea, and eukaryotes. This includes multiple families from fungi and amoeba to plants, animals, and humans. The application of borrelina, baculoviruses, and other large and small viruses to industrial and agricultural insecticides and metal leaching processes seems to have opened the door for bacteriophages and for virophages to infect far more microbes than they naturally would. The bacterophages and virophages of industrial and agricultural insecticides may have accidentally brought about many new insect, animal, and human diseases.[67]

A number of industrial and agriculturally-related patents describe shigella. Some also describe antibodies that can be engineered into plants as insecticides, using host cells from a number of species including those listed here. Antibodies are used within insecticides that contain B.t.-Cry toxins, or they may be used to produce transgenic plants. Some patents are assigned to Novartis, and were not incidentally filed just a few months after the Dearborn conference, which a Novartis grantee attended.[17-24]

> "...Specific organisms include *Pseudomonas aeurginosa, Pseudomonas fluorescens, Saccharomyces cerevisiae, Bacillus thuringiensis, Escherichia coli, Bacillus subtilis,* and the like."[9-24] These agents are used in insecticides.

Pesticide-containing host cells are treated with the following plant-colonizing bacteria to prolong the activity of B.t. Cry-toxins when applied to crops (or engineered into them). You will probably recognize some of the more useful bacteria:

Enterobacteriaceae: *Escherichia, Erwinia, Shigella, Salmonella, Proteus*

Bacillaceae: *Bacillus* species, *Rhizobiceae*, such as *Rhizobium* and *Rhizobacter; Lactobacillus*

Spirillaceae: *Spirillum, Vibrio, Desulfovibrio, Serratia, Photobacterium, Zymomonas, Aeromonas*
Lactobacillaceae: *Pseudomonadaceae* (*Pseudomonas, Acetobacter*)
Azotobacteraceae: (cyst former) gammaproteobacteria from the *Pseudomonadales* order
Nitrobacteraceae: (soil and water-borne nitrogen fixers) alphaproteobacteriae
Fungi: *Phycomycetes* and *Ascomycetes*, including yeasts (*Saccharomyces* and *Schizosaccharomyces*)
Basidiomycetes yeast: *Rhodotorula, Aureobasidium, Sporobolomyces*
Phylloplane: (found on leaf surface) *Flavobacterium, Pseudomonas*

A patent for *Antigenic proteins of Borrelia burgdorferi* was filed in 1993. Its inventors include Dr. Tom G. Schwan of Hamilton, Montana. The patent uses the "flagella-less" proteins described by a Dr. Alan Barbour patent. This represents the strain-unique Bb proteins that lack the flagellin structures which propel the organism and that are unique to each strain. *This patent probably describes only the surface exposed portion of a key protein of these pathogenic organisms, not the entire tail structure itself, and this is important to differentiate.* Dr. Schwan was a work group member who supplied MAb antibodies to calibrate the immunoblot tests at Dearborn. He was also one of the co-authors (along with Dr. Burgdorfer) of the paper that announced the causative agent of Lyme disease to the world in 1982. From the Schwan patent:

> "The present invention relates to antigenic proteins specific to *Borrelia burgdorferi* which have a molecular weight of 28 kDa or 39 kDa…the proteins, *especially the 39 kDa proteins…*can be used to diagnose mammals previously or currently infected with the Lyme borreliosis causing agent."[25]

Maybe the 39-kDa protein is so helpful because it belongs to a B.t. insecticide Cry toxin gene or another microbe that becomes attached to the Bb organism. Either of the important and Bb-specific 28-kDa or 39-kDa proteins may be cloned into a B.t. insecticide. The 39-kDa protein was cloned according to a foreign patent assigned to the CDC and vaccine manufacturer SmithKline Beecham. This was the company that created the first geneation Lyme disease vaccine.

The 39-kDa protein is an important and specific bacterial membrane protein of *Borrelia burgdorferi.* It also has the same molecular weight of a nonstructural protein (nsp2) of the *sindbis* virus; a virus that is used in recombinant constructs such as insecticides. Nsp2 is an enzyme that is essential for viral replication and maturity. According to patents including one from Texas A&M University, 39-kDa may indeed represent important insect virus enzymes that are used in B.t. insecticides as transcription (gene) promoters.[26,27,68,69]

Insecticidal proteins from B.t. strains have molecular weights that range from 34-kDa to 39-kDa. The molecular weight of a 39-kDa protein may represent Bb proteins that are from a B.t. Cry toxin or the sindbis virus of recombinant insecticides. 39-kDa is one of the diagnostic bands that is frequently detected in Lyme patients. This band is included in the CDC diagnostic test standards for Lyme disease. Is this because it belongs to B.t. Cry toxins or to a recombinant virus of the applied plant insecticides, or GM plant transgenes?[26,27]

The "H1141" BmpA MAb may instead be used to detect bone morphogenetic protein. This is a group of growth factors and cytokines that are related to the repair of damaged bone and cartilage. Antibodies to these proteins are created during infection, especially if a bacterium structurally damages myelin or skeletal structures. The Bb spirochete may be able to physically do this by enzymatic processes, and released myelin may cause antibody production and an "autoimmune" state.[26-31]

Mutations in Bmps and their inhibitors are responsible for disorders that affect the musculoskeletal system. We know that Bb spirochetes adversely affect the musculoskeletal system. A study describes the effects of *fluoride* upon the activities of bone morphogenetic proteins (BMP). We may consider that most people have lifetime exposures to fluorides (fluorosis). The demineralization of stored fluorides from bones by bacterial enzymes actively contributes to elevated circulating fluoride levels and therefore many of the musculoskeletal symptoms associated with Lyme disease, Morgellon's, or other illnesses.[26-31]

According to a study, *fluoride increased the activities of osteoblasts† and accelerated mineralization while inhibiting the activities of osetoclasts.‡* This means that *fluoride can directly and adversely affect the biological activities of BMP,* which leads to disorders affecting the musculoskeletal system. Perhaps this explains the production of such antibodies and why lab tests might be seeking evidence of same.

†Bone osteoblasts are germ cells that form bone. ‡ *Bone osteoclasts are cells responsible for bone resorption*

This antibody might be used to detect the presence of a *gammaproteobacterium,* or B.t. Cry toxin genes. But it may also be used as a marker to detect the effects of released fluorides in the body during Bb infection. There is also a 39-kDa core protein from the *vaccinia* virus that could be detected by this antibody *if a latent vaccinia virus becomes reactivated during Bb infection.* Vaccinia was used in smallpox vaccines, and is a member of the *Orthopox* family. It may also be used in insecticides. Remember that *poxviruses and related viruses may be reactivated* by compatible viruses; including perhaps those provided by an infected vectoring insect or arthropod.[26-35]

84C: These MAb proteins could belong to the *Cytomegalovirus* (CMV), including one with a molecular weight of 34-kDa that is found inside the cell (cytoplasm). CMV has been used to create vaccines and biological controls of all kinds, including insecticides. A B.t. strain also creates Cry toxins with a 34-kDa molecular weight. Other B.t. strains vary in molecular weight depending on strain, from about 30 to 40-kDa.

The MAb in this example is said to be the outer surface protein B (OspB) of the Bb spirochete. Perhaps OspB proteins come from an organism that carries B.t. genes. If so, it may contain a baculovirus that was engineered with CMV genes. The chimera may be able to cause infection or reactivate CMV genes in the presence of a reverse transcriptase (RT) promoter. I wonder if CMV like the sindbis virus is also kicked out of a chimera when bound to a satellite virus or when infected by a virophage?[36,37]

H5332: This is the MAb for the outer surface protein A (OspA) of the Bb spirochete at 31-kDa. In the body, skin keratinocytes produce Interleukin-1 (IL-1) beta precursor proteins at 31-kDa. During immune stimulus and inflammation, IL-1 cytokine production is altered. IL-1 promotes fevers, increases and controls bone marrow cell production, and helps *deteriorate bone joints*. Increased IL-1 beta accelerates the onset of insulin-dependent diabetes and lymphocytic thyroiditis in rats. A study showed that IL-1 beta is a potent modulator of autoimmune diabetes and thyroid diseases.[38-40]

Persistent Bb infections stimulate the release of IL-1 which can be detected in the joints of Lyme patients. A virus that stimulates antibodies at 31-kDa is sindbis (band number varies with strain). The fact that sindbis is used in genetic engineering and is from a family of wild viruses that can be detected by the 31-kDa probe may mean that a recombinant or wild virus is sought by the tests. Perhaps the probe detects IL-1 expression as a result of a failed (broken) recombinant chimera that kicked out its sindbis virus, and which thereafter becomes an active infection. This seems likely when we understand that sindbis causes Lyme-like symptoms and many Lyme patients have new thyroid and insulin-resistance problems.[38-40]

H1C8: Insect polyhedrosis outer surface proteins vary in weight, but are roughly 28-kDa. This MAb may represent an antibody to an insect virus (NPV, GV, CPV/reovirus) or its virophage. Sources list "H1C8" as an *ascites* clone. Ascites is the fluid that accumulates in the abdomen during liver disease or low serum albumin levels. It is also seen in pancreatic cancer, pancreatitis, ovarian cancer, congestive heart failure, tuberculosis, colon cancer, or portal vein thrombosis (clots in liver veins). It is also sometimes seen in Lyme patients who have altered P450 liver enzyme pathways.

Since a number of insecticides have been genetically engineered to specifically alter insect P450 enzyme pathways, humans adversely affected by insecticides could produce ascites fluid from impaired digestive, liver, pancreatic, or other enzymes. Such enzymes may also be created by a bacterium that harbors a mollicute or yellow's disease virus.[41-43]

4B8F4: The insecticide B.t. subspecies *fukuokaensis* produces a 24-kDa Cry toxin. Other B.t. strains encode toxins that have molecular weights which vary from 30 to 40-kDa. Perhaps this MAb detects proteins from specific B.t. strain Cry toxins.[44]

CB625: There are 22-kDa proteins that are secreted by the "Sf 9" fall armyworm (*Spodoptera frugiperda*) which most B.t. insecticides have targeted, because these insects are so prevalent. The Sf 9 and Sf 21 insect cell lines were created by USDA and Texas A&M University scientists for use in insecticides and vaccines.

Fall armyworm and other insect genes are engineered into recombinant B.t. insecticides and GM plants that will carry insecticidal genes. Perhaps this MAb represents important insect proteins from viruses, virophages, or baculoviruses that are found in fall armyworms or their insect cell lines, including those that may have been contaminated. A 1989 article reveals that sindbis virus has been used to genetically engineer Sf 9 or fall armyworm host cells *specifically to express baculoviruses in B.t. insecticides.* Did a failed chimera kick out a sindbis virus because of a cell line contaminant (phage) which infected the chimera and thereafter became infective? Is an insect cell line contaminant part of an aggregate Bb spirochete?[45-47]

The 58-kDa "GroEL" Bb protein is a *chaperonin* protein that is required for proper protein folding in all bacteria. Certain proteins are expressed when an organism is exposed to high temperatures or other stressors. These proteins are called "heat shock" proteins. They typically have a molecular weight of 60, 70, or 90-kDa. In mammals, a mitochondrial heat shock protein is "hsp58" (58-kDa). Mitochondria are the little cellular engines that produce energy. It is unclear whether the band numbered "58" looks for a human mitochondrial heat shock protein or if the protein belongs to the Bb organism or one of its viral components. Viruses are used in vaccines and diagnostic tests as well as insecticides. Hoffmann-La Roche scientist Kenneth Lundstrom published a paper in 2000 discussing the usefulness of viruses including some that were injected into rodent (mouse) brains. The paper reports that a high level of neuron-specific gene expression was detected in brain tissue cultures from the hippocampus. According to the study:[53,54]

> "Traditionally Alphavirus vectors, either attenuated strains or replication-deficient particles, have been used to elicit efficient immune responses in animals…Alphavirus vectors can therefore be considered as potentially promising vectors for vaccine production."

Since alphaviruses like sindbis are used in vaccines and insecticides, they can also be used in diagnostic tests to detect related arbovirus infections (i.e. rabies, encephalitis, reoviruses). After viral infection, ".beta-galactosoidase" genes produce enzymes that are detectable in the neurons of most nervous system tissues. Insect viruses infect the cells of the brain and central nervous system to cause neurologic disease (i.e. encephalitis, meningitis). Bb antibody tests use .beta-galactosidase enzymes to detect antibodies, meaning there are probably insect virus-associated genes that are part of the Bb spirochete.[54-57]

Not only are arboviruses used in genetically engineered products (i.e. insecticides, vaccines); but they can also be used to genetically engineer *spider* or *silkworm* silks. Such recombinant silks can be made using cells from the yeast *Pichia pastoris – a yeast that can be transformed by and which can express .beta-galactosidase enzymes.*

Insecticides have been engineered to contain spider toxins and silkworm genes. Some strains of *Pichia* may be engineered to be antibiotic resistant (Zeocin™). This is a copper-chelated antibiotic that is produced by a recombinant *Streptomyces verticillus.* When we consider that silk spiders (*Nephila clavipes* [golden silk orb weaver]) or other spiders and "natural" insect toxins are engineered into insecticides and GM plants, we can understand how such toxins may lead to neurologic disease states. And we can see the need to detect such toxins in people with tickborne infections that may harbor B.t. and other insecticidal toxins.[54-62]

A Lyme patent revealed that .beta.-galactosidases and other compounds useful to diagnostic tests *must not be a normal constituent of animal or human serum.* That way they remain useful as diagnostic labels or reporter molecules. From a patent:

> "It has been found that labels of non-animal, including non-human origin, are especially useful in the detection of *B. burgdorferi* antibodies, as these labels are not naturally present in the animal or human sera to be tested..."
>
> "When using substances naturally present in animal or human serum as labels, e.g. using alkaline phosphatase as a label, these substances of serum origin may contribute to the signal obtained in the determination employing these substances as a label and thus result in a value which is too high for representing the amount of bound antibody from the sample." (This means it ramps up the proteins to a detectable level, and may contribute to detectable totals.)
>
> "Thus, labels of *plant origin* have been found to be very useful, e.g. labels comprising plant peroxidases, such as *horseradish peroxidase."*

This means it is best to use probes/labels derived from microbes, insects, or plants for animal or human diagnostic tests. The patent specifically names labels of a plant origin such as *horseradish peroxidase.* The horseradish peroxidase enzyme is *widely used* in molecular biology because it amplifies weak molecular signals. It is also of the desired non-human or animal origin. What might not be obvious is that the *imported cabbage worm* larvae, which are targets of B.t. insecticides, and which have *baculoviruses* engineered into them, are an *important and widespread pest insect of horseradish plants.*[57,63-65]

Horseradish plants are also attacked by the fungus *Agrobacterium tumefaciens,* and by *Spiroplasma citri,* which causes brittle root disease in the plant. *A. tumefaciens* is also widely used in genetically engineered B.t. insecticides and GM plants. In addition, the nuclearpolyhedrosis virus *Trichoplusia ni NPV is a baculovirus that commonly infects imported cabbage worm larvae.* The *Trichoplusia ni* baculovirus has also been widely used in B.t. insecticides.[57,63-65]

An aggregate Bb spirochete may harbor B.t. Cry toxin genes, an NPV such as *Trichoplusia ni*, a *spiroplasma,* a bacterium such as *Agrobacterium tumefaciens,* a fungi such as *coccidioides immitus,* a virophage, and other organisms including a mutated leptonema or a gammproteobacterium. Therefore the use of horseradish peroxidase in a Bb diagnostic test may *amplify existing microbial proteins* including any just mentioned that may be part of an aggregate Bb spirochete.[57,63-65]

> *"It is anticipated that such antibodies will remain detectable in a human or an animal for up to one year P.I. or longer because in most cases the spirochete will persist in the host for long periods of time."*[66]

This is an alternative and hypothetical explanation for what the Dearborn standardized diagnostic test probes for Lyme disease might actually be seeking. These explanations present a very different scenario than what the public believes is being sought by the tests. It also feasibly explains how these tests may seek specific pathogens of an aggregate organism that are entirely related to agricultural and industrial insecticides; and human immune markers which may illustrate how the body responds during a Bb infection. Diagnostic tests that are standardized could be highly protective of agricultural tools while detecting only a few infections – possibly just enough so a few patients who succumb to recombinant accidents are acknowledged.Standardized laboratory tests significantly under report the number of Lyme patients. They also foster an atmosphere where ill patients whose diseases are not detected demand acknowledgement and explanations for the industry-wide denial of same.

Silly Rice and the Dearborn Conference

Natural fungal infections of crops were studied during Bassi and Metchnikoff's time; resulting in early attempts to use fungi as insecticides. A natural fungi of rice called *Bakanae* was first described in 1898 by Japanese researcher Shotaro Hori. In 1926 a plant pathologist was studying the "foolish seedling" disease of rice, and recognized the causative agent to be a soilborne fungus called *Gibberella fujikuroi.* This research led to the understanding of what today is known as *Fusarium wilt,* and what we might also consider to be one of the "wilt" diseases of silkworms. Gibberella ear rot of corn is caused by the strain *Gibberella zeae;* also known as *Fusarium graminearum.* Some strains of this fungus can produce mycotoxins (myco means fungi) that are harmful to insects, animals, and humans.[1-3]

Bakanae affects crops in North America, Asia, and Africa. The fungus causes an over-production of gibberellic acid (GA). This is an important growth hormone (phytohormone) of plants. The GA metabolic hormones also detect environmental conditions including temperature extremes, lack of nutrients, water, and other stressors. All living organisms from bacteriae to humans secrete stress-response proteins or *heat shock proteins.* In plants these are known as *gibberillins.* The *gibberillins* are related to the heat shock proteins, the chaperonin proteins, and the "Gro-EL" proteins.[1,2]

Soil fungi are common around the world, and they attack the roots of deciduous (i.e. mulberry) and coniferous trees (i.e. poplar, pine, spruce, junipers, cypress, yews). Early Japanese scientists emphasized that soil conditions of rice crops (i.e. nitrogenous fertilizers, seedling density) determined the development of the *rice blast* fungus, *Magnaporthe grisea.* A Ft. Detrick scientist developed the *rice blast fungus* "LX" for use as an early anti-crop biowarfare weapon. Scientific interest in this fungus began shortly after WWII. Scientists at Camp Detrick (before it became Ft. Detrick) were studying gibberellin production in the nitrogen-fixing broad or fava bean *Vicia faba.* This legume is commonly attacked by the rust and spot diseases, and by spiroplasma-carrying aphids. (Spiroplasmas were first isolated in 1944.) The fava bean is extremely temperature and salt-tolerant and grows in nutrient-poor soils. It is one of the oldest edible legumes, dating back thousands of years.[2]

Fava beans are rich in tyramine, vicine, *tannins,* and L-dopa. The latter is a chemical used to treat Parkinson's disease. The beans are commonly found in areas where malaria is present. They can cause hemolytic anemia when eaten raw by patients who lack specific enzymes called G6PD. This is an interesting connection because patients with tickborne infections such as *Babesia microti,* a malaria-like infection may suffer from hemolytic anemia. In some respects fava beans may be protective in people with normal enzyme profiles, since the malaria protozoa *Plasmodium falcipacrum* is sensitive to the oxidation damage that occurs during infection, and which remains in cells in the absence of effective G6PD enzymes. As a result, people who lack these enzymes are usually resistant or immune to malaria caused by this protozoan parasite. It is possible that GM crops contain formulas meant to target insect G6PD enzymes. This would seem to promote infections not only in insects, but possibly also in higher animals including humans.[1-7,43,44]

G6PD enzymes are glucose 6-phosphate dehydrogenase enzymes which supply energy to red blood cells. They also maintain co-enzymes required for healthy cellular levels of glutathione. Lyme patients are often deficient in glutathione, which deals with free radical damage to cells. Glutathione also regulates nitric oxcide, repairs DNA, metabolizes iron, and assists with amino acid transport. Every system of the body is affected by glutathione levels, especially the brain, nervous system, gastrointestinal system, and lungs. Lyme patients who are low in Vitamin D are probably deficient in calcitrol, which helps produce glutathione. Low glutathione levels contribute to "wasting" seen in AIDS, sepsis, cancers, and Lyme. Low glutathione levels contribute to bipolar disease, depression, schizophrenia, and neurologic symptoms.[1-7,43,44]

Patent inventions describe the treatment of G6PD enzyme deficiencies, as well as the use of these enzymes in plants to detect resistance genes for herbicides, pesticides, and insecticides. Once again, what may target plant and insect enzyme pathways may also adversely affect similar enzyme systems in humans. A Monsanto patent has this to say about G6D enzymes:[1-7,43,44]

> "G6PD may be a preferable target for double stranded RNA mediated inhibition in an invertebrate pest."

This means the enzyme may be manipulated to inhibit unwanted viral replication. Such double stranded RNA viruses are already deployed in B.t. insecticides. These viruses according to the patent include those found in fall armyworms, European corn borers, cotton boll weevils, Colorado potato beetles, red flour beetles, black cutworms, white grubs, wireworms, mosquito larvae, corn rootworms, pea *aphids,* brown *citrus aphids, lepidoptera including silkworms,* or honey bees. Some of these viruses might include the baculovirus NPVs or GVs, the cypovirus (CPVs) and their virophages as we have previously discussed. **Insecticide patents use plasmids that are genetically engineered to overexpress bacteriophage enzymes (i.e. T3 RNA polymerase). These are used as transcription vectors that carry special promoter genes in their plasmid(s).**[43-47]

An example is described in a patent that is assigned to the University of Medicine and Dentistry of New Jersey. The medical school for this institution is in Piscataway, New Jersey where Chief of Rheumatology and Director of the Lyme Disease center Dr. Leonard Sigal is employed.[48]

A Texas A&M patent for recombinant DNA insect viruses describes the use of enzymes from insect baculovirus proteins at 39-kDa including *Autographa californica, Tricoplusia ni, Rachiplusia ou,* or *Galleria mellonella.* Patents readily acknowledge the 39-kDa proteins that are engineered into insecticides as transcription promoters. We know that the 39-kDa protein band is important to detect, and is found in Lyme patients. Is this diagnostic band an indication that Bb spirochetes are carrying recombinant B.t. insecticidal genes?[48]

The Imperial Chemical Industries (ICI) Company developed the earliest *Interferon** and supplied chemical herbicides to British military forces to spray in Malasia during the 1950s. ICI also produced the *quaternary* ammonium herbicide *Paraquat;* a globally applied herbicide (until it was banned in many parts of the world). Paraquat was first synthesized in 1882, but wasn't commercially produced until 1961. ICI is now owned by Syngenta, a division of Monsanto. ICI also developed *gibberellin pathway plant growth inhibitors for use in commercial pesticides.*[8-15]

**Interferons are proteins produced by infected cells. Interferons are used to combat diseases such as Multiple Sclerosis.*

In 1957, Professor of viticulture Robert J. Weaver at the University of California-Davis reported that gibberellin hormones may be useful to grape production; especially for Thompson seedless table grapes. Field research was undertaken that year, and five years later the hormone was being sprayed upon nearly all California grape crops in order to increase the size of the fruits. Eventually the hormone was used on other crops. By the mid-1960s it was one of the most popular plant growth hormones used on agricultural crops around the world. Before this period herbicides were already targeting *gibberellin* pathways to inhibit the hormone in weeds. Eventually gibberellin and other plant growth hormones would be added to insecticidal formulas and genetically engineered plants to increase crop yields. We must not overlook this important hormone because citrus and other crops were also being sprayed with *organophosphate* pesticides that likewise altered these hormones; and quite possibly the genes of microbes lying within the plants and their insect parasites as well.[16-18]

Under modern agricultural techniques, seeds are coated with seed protectants, herbicides, and anti-fungal agents. Plants are engineered to contain growth hormones and herbicide resistance genes. Hormones and heat shock proteins are key factors which provide the plant resistance to stressors such as insect or drought resistance. Patents that are related to these hormones describe how cottonseeds are treated with zinc trichlorophenate (chlorinated phenol), or Dow's "9-B" fungicide and seed protectant. The active ingredient in the formula is zinc 2,4,5-trichlorophenate. This is a metabolite that is produced by degrading a 2,4,5-T herbicide (one half the Agent Orange formula). Chlorophenoxy herbicides are no longer used as either plant growth hormones or herbicides but many herbicidal chemicals persist in the environment.[19-22]

Organophosphorus insecticides including diazinon and chlorpyrifos cause oxidative stress in humans, animals, insects, and plants by disturbing cellular calcium levels. Yale scientists have been studying the gibberellins, heat-shock proteins, and related chaperonin proteins for many years. Patent inventions for chaperonin are covered in the next section. One Yale Professor named Arthur Horwich has published on the topic of heat shock proteins; specifically the heat shock protein #60, also called Hsp60. (The number represents the protein's molecular weight.) Heat shock proteins are also used in vaccine formulas to stimulate an immune response.[23]

Heat shock proteins have been studied by scientists at the University of Medicine and Dentistry of New Jersey-Robert Wood Johnson Medical School in relation to *Borrelia burgdorferi* infections. More specifically they are studied in relation to Bb flagellin genes and the process of molecular mimicry. Molecular mimicry was felt to be a problem in people who received the first generation Lyme vaccine. The monoclonal antibodies supplied at Dearborn by Lyme disease guidelines co-author Benjamin Luft and colleague Alan Barbour involved the Bb "149" (GroEL, 66-kDa); and "8D5" (66-kDa) antibodies.[23-32]

Dr. Luft has also published on the topic of the heat shock protein 70 (Hsp70) response during Lyme infections along with colleague Dr. Raymond J. Dattwyler. (Remember heat shock proteins are typically 60, 70, or 90-kDa in size.) Other Lyme notables Drs. John J Dunn, Gerold Stanek, Erol Fikrig, and Jorge Benach have each published on the topics of Lyme disease and heat shock proteins. Dr. Benach supplied a Bb monoclonal antibody (CB625) to the Dearborn conference work group. Much of the literature on Bb and heat shock proteins was published a year or two before the conference which Drs. Luft, Dattwyler, Benach, and Barbour reportedly attended along with Dr. Allen Steere and other colleagues.[23-32]

Therefore we know that heat shock proteins were understood in response to Lyme disease infections at least by the timeframe of Dearborn. Drs. Benjamin Luft and Raymond Dattwyler claimed in their research that the 66 and 73-kDa proteins from the Bb spirochete are the dominant immune antigens (immunogens) expressed by all Bb strains. They also reported that the (humoral) immune response to these antigens occurs early during Lyme infection. Perhaps this is why the 66-kDa band of a heat shock protein is among the diagnostic bands that were standardized at Dearborn – to detect the human immune response to the presence of the Bb spirochete. This means the band does not necessarily belong to the spirochete, and that some diagnostic bands may as predicted, be seeking *the body's response* to Bb infection.[23-32]

Let's touch on molecular mimicry in patients who received the first generation Lyme vaccine. The H9724 flagellin antibody supplied by Dr. Barbour at Dearborn is specific for Bb flagellin. The antibody cross-reacts with human axons (nerve cells), and may detect a major protein of human neuroblastoma cells (nerve cell cancers). This cross-reactive protein was isolated from calf adrenal cells, an organ tissue often found to be infected with viruses or bacteria; and which is used to make vaccines.[33-42]

It is important to study the individuals who attended the Dearborn conference, especially when many are members of the American Lyme Disease Foundation (ALDF), a group that has criticized a Lyme disease documentary film "Under Our Skin," calling it "deceptive." The group continually defends the IDSA Lyme disease guidelines many of them helped to write; and which were found to be flawed by Connecticut Attorney General Richard Blumenthal's recent anti-trust lawsuit. The group continually perpetuates the same tired party line that chronic Lyme disease is a poorly defined syndrome in patients who have been "properly" treated with antibiotics. They also make other statements which clearly conflict with research evidence published by experts outside their core group, as well as anecdotal evidence gathered from clinical patient and physician experience.

Calling "Doctor Johnson"

> *"How small, of all that human hearts endure, that part which laws or kings can cause or cure!"*
> – Samuel Johnson

Dr. Barbara Johnson of the CDC is a well-known colleague of some of the co-authors of the IDSA guidelines for Lyme disease. She was also a Dearborn conference planning committee member, and is listed as co-inventor on a SmithKline Beecham patent for a Lyme disease vaccine and diagnostic test. The patent was filed before Dearborn (1993) and published five months after the conference that she helped to organize.[1]

The following information from the patent text provides clues that *certain antibody bands that are not part of the tests standardized at Dearborn may be more important than those that were defined at Dearborn and established as important diagnostic criteria to detect Lyme.* The text discusses these "more useful" antigens:

> "A number of bacterial antigens have been identified that may be **more useful in serodiagnosis, including outer surface proteins A and B (OspA and OspB)**, flagellin, and other proteins designated P**21**, P**39**, P**66**, and P**83** according to their *estimated* molecular weights." ("P" signifies protein, and note the kDa bands 21, 39, 66, and 83.)[1]

The two Osp bands mentioned in Dr. Johnson's patent for OspA and OspB were those that were *excluded* from the diagnostic tests standardized at Dearborn. And yet **the Johnson patent admits just five months later that these are among the more useful bands for the serodiagnosis of Lyme disease**. We must ask why if these bands were so important for diagnosis were they excluded from the test standards established at Dearborn. Some people will say that the answer is so that the Lyme vaccine trials, for which Dr. Allen Steere would become lead investigator, could move forward.

Meanwhile diagnostic tests like that patented by Dr. Johnson could be developed. Were the Dearborn standards carefully modified in favor of the upcoming Lyme vaccine and to slow-play an epidemic with agricultural "roots," while scientists capitalized on its agent by patenting "all things" Bb-related? Even worse, since the Lyme vaccine was pulled from the market nearly a decade ago, these two "important" Bb bands have *never been added to the Lyme disease testing standards* even though the bands are *known to be highly significant*. The reason for this continued exclusion might be purposeful if the bands represent B.t. Cry toxin proteins and an outer spiralin protein of a leptospira/leptonema. If they do, they could be cross-reactive, and detectable in nearly anyone exposed to insect vectors; or those who eat foods treated or engineered with B.t. pesticides. This is practically everyone, even people who eat organic foods! Leaving the OspA and OspB proteins out of standardized tests also ensures that future vaccines that are based on these proteins may continue to be produced. If this explanation is valid, omitting Osp proteins would seem to serve industrial interests over patient interests.

A separate patent application lists the name Barbara Johnson on an invention designed to modulate *toll-like receptor* signaling (TLR). This is a key process of the human immune system that controls inflammation levels during Bb infection. Toll-like receptors alert our bodies that pathogens are present, and activate key immune defenses. The invention may be useful for Lyme disease and other neurologic or so-called "autoimmune" diseases which cause TLR signaling dysfunction. The patent is titled *Chaperonin 10-Induced Immunomodulation*. The applicant company is CBio Limited, an Australian company with a global reach that develops products to treat autoimmune and inflammatory diseases including Lyme disease.[2]

Another patent lists the name Barbara Jane Johnson and is titled *Chaperonin 10 Modulation of Toll-like Receptor-Inducible*

Cytokine and Chemokine Secretion. This patent describes the use of "Cpn10" or chaperonin to regulate TLR signaling or immunomodular secretions against pro-inflammatory cytokines and chemokines. These chemicals which cause inflammation, are released as cellular signals in the presence of foreign pathogens.[2-4]

The Cpn10 of the patent properly regulates toll-like receptors. It is designed to treat diseases like Lyme that cause over secretion of pro-inflammatory chemicals. The patent targets bacterial endotoxins like those produced by Bb spirochetes. It could also work to repair TLR receptors that are improperly triggered by synthetic vaccine proteins. This is a problem that arose with the first generation Lyme disease vaccine – one that caused a treatment-resistant form of arthritis to occur in some people who received the Lyme vaccine.[2-4]

Another patent application lists the name Barbara Jane Johnson et al. It too utilizes chaperonin 10. Another important patent describes *novel granules that can be dispersed in water* and which contain a polymer and an oil. The granules include a Cpn10 (chaperonin 10) polypeptide that contains immune modulating activity, but lacks protein folding activity. This means the invention cannot contribute to recombinant gene folding errors which might occur as a result of unanticipated recombinant events or "accidents." Such events may be caused by chemical or microbe-caused mutations for example from industrial wastes or agricultural chemicals, polymers, or oils. Mutated microbes may be found in lakes, rivers, ponds, wastewater plants, industrial water flows, or soils. The granules may be applied to correct a problem causing mutation anywhere toxic or mutagenic chemicals meet bacteria, fungi, or baculoviruses. In the lab, animal vaccine formulas that use chemicals and microbes may have protein folding errors due to contaminants which might also be corrected by this product. Examples of how the product may be used includes as an additive for sterilized laboratory water or for bovine albumin or other vaccine-related solutions.[2-5]

According to the Johnson patent, the product is intended to treat a disease or condition from a group of acute or chronic inflammatory diseases such as asthma, allergies, Multiple Sclerosis, or graft-versus-host-disease. Treatments may also target so-called "autoimmune" disorders such as Lyme disease. We might examine insecticide patents that use transgenic viruses including insect *transcription factors* from developmental hormones which guide molting and metamorphosis, to see how they are used. We may find that insect DNA and viruses from *entomopox* and *baculovirus* families are being used.[2-5]

Remember that *poxviruses can be reactivated upon exposure to other poxviruses which donate needed genes.* This reactivation could cause a protein folding error and a reactivated disease process. Insecticides are designed to specifically do this in pest insects. Problems arise however if this same process causes protein-folding errors in animals or humans, such as occurs in prion diseases. Did prion diseases originate from the application of recombinant insecticides and their activity upon latent viruses or retroviruses that are found in insects, poultry, animals, and humans? One invention has this to say about viral insecticides:[2-5]

> "Occlusion bodies containing virus particles contaminating the foliage are eaten and dissolved by the insect's midgut juices, releasing virus particles. These particles pass through the gut cells and infect tracheal and other body tissues of the host larva. Over a typical period of 15 days, the virus replicates in susceptible tissues eventually causing death."

Since the human body has similar gut and tracheal cells as those targeted by genetically engineered insecticides, we have to wonder if inventions like the chaperonins described previously are designed to "fix" disorders possibly caused by insecticidal tools. We may find these inventions used within oral or injectible vaccines *or perhaps within municipal and industrial water supplies as an additive for "public health."* (The governmental condoning of future "oral" vaccines as potential additives to our municipal water supplies or foods is something about which we should all be thoroughly concerned.)[2-6]

Mammalian chaperonin 10 is also called "heat shock protein 10" or Hsp10. This is a mitochondrial (cellular engine) protein that assists with the protein folding process, and works in tandem with chaperonin 60. Chaperonins 10 and 60 are similar to bacterial proteins "GroES" and "GroEL." Dr. Benjamin Luft of (SUNY-Stony Brook) supplied a 66-kDa GroEL monoclonal antibody to the Dearborn work group that standardized the tests for Lyme disease.[2-6]

We now know that heat-shock proteins serve as toll-like receptor inflammatory mediators. They are expressed in synovial (joint) tissues, something about which Rheumatologist Dr. Allen Steere should be very familiar. "Hsp10" is also said to inhibit the action of the TLRs, such as those that are malfunctioning during Lyme infection. The purpose of the aforementioned chaperonin patents may be to "fix" or to suppress accidental TLR activation in the body. The products may be applied medically or environmentally (i.e. wastewater treatment, insecticides). The products could fix a problem that may have been caused by a Lyme vaccine which triggered TLR pathways into a permanent state of activation. This activation led to a form of treatment-resistant arthritis in some Lyme vaccine recipients.[5-8]

In a study, Cpn10 was provided intravenously to fifty Multiple Sclerosis patients for a short period. According to a research paper co-authored by Barbara Johnson, after treatment leukocytes from treated patients produced significantly lower levels of key proinflammatory cytokines. This means the product lowered inflammation in the patients. Chaperonin 10 has also been shown to be a possible treatment for patients with Rheumatoid Arthritis (and may soon be suggested for treating Lyme patients).[5-8]

Scientists have constructed Cpn10-based protein systems using chaperonins from bacteriae including *Thermus thermophilus.* This bacterium is used as a model organism during gene manipulation. More importantly, the organism is used to degrade organic materials (i.e. compost piles, soil chemical toxins). *It is also used to recover oil from oil reservoirs; and to construct recombinant baculovirus expression vectors that will be used within insecticides or GM plants.*[5,9-21]

The organism is a member of the *extremophile* family, a family that includes *Deinococcus radiodurans,* a bacterium that is mentioned in a *Borrelia burgdorferi* patent that is assigned to the Amoco Company. *This family of extreme bacteriae are radiation resistant and they "eat" nuclear wastes and other chemical toxins.* They can survive extremes in temperature; underground, in hot springs, in acid mine wastes, petroleum reserves, and in some cases, outer space. *They have segmented genomes and are able to horizontally transfer their genes between other compatible organisms.*[5,9-21]

These bacteriae have two cell walls. The outer membrane stains *gram-positive,* but the inner membrane is similar to gram-negative bacteriae. This is the same structure found in Bb spirochetes, which also stain in the same manner. The extremophiles were the first life forms on Earth, and are felt to be responsible for the creation of geological structures and soils (think mined materials, rocks). *Thermus thermophilus* is also used to construct recombinant vectors and to transform host cells to produce a *recombinant thermostable enzyme.* **Genetically engineered constructs made from *T. thermophilus* are efficient reverse transcriptase activators in the presence of manganese.** This means it can cause cells to replicate in the presence of manganese.[5,9-21]

Proteobacteriae are also extremophiles and they can infect other soil bacteriae. The important extremophiles include the spore-forming *paenibacillus.* Indeed *Bacillus popilliae* is also called *Paenibacillus popilliae;* the agents of milky spore disease that have been used for nearly a century as an insecticide.[5,9-21]

Imagine how the combination of thermostable bacterial enzymes (i.e. from thermophiles) which contain efficient RNA promoters may reactivate latent viruses in an insect, animal, or a human host to cause infections including quite possibly, Lyme disease. Is this the mechanism of "accidental" recombinant events that takes place in patients with Lyme disease – the reactivation of viruses by a recombinant insecticide that contains transcription promoters and other agents that were supposed to only target insects?

If so, a recombinant construct such as that described in the Johnson chapeonin patents might be created to correct or turn off the activity of a *wild or recombinant thermophile enzyme* that has become incorporated into a bacterium including the Bb spirochete. Perhaps an enzyme improperly activates a phage or a virus to begin transcription, and therefore reactivates infections in humans (i.e. an insect encephalitis virus, human polio or vaccinia virus, or latent retrovirus).

Borrelia burgdorferi spirochetes have replaced all of their iron-sulfur enzymes with those that use *manganese.* This is a similar behavior in *Thermus thermophilus,* an agent of milky spore disease and which may be found in other bacillus strains. It would be interesting to know if Bb contains genes from a thermophile/paenibacillus or a B.t. bacterium with manganese-friendly enzymes. I say this because there are industry patents for Lyme disease that can detect both thermophile bacteriae and Bb spirochetes and we can see how this makes perfect sense under this scenario.[5,9-17,21]

Another extremophile that is used to reduce metal oxides (bioreduction) is *Rhodobacter sphaeroides.* It might be employed for example to *deliberately reduce acid mine wastes, during bioremediation of in situ or other mines.* The Board of Regents of the University of Texas is assignee to such recombinant patents including one that was published just *weeks before the Dearborn conference* which University of Texas scientist Dr. Alan Barbour attended. The conference of course determined the outcome of the diagnostic test standards and surveillance case criteria for Lyme disease.[5,9-24]

Another member of the extremophile family is *Thermus aquaticus* from which *Taq polymerase* (Taq Pol) is derived. This is a most useful enzyme for PCR tests. The enzyme helps read and translate DNA. Taq from *T. aquaticus* replaced an older version that was created using *E. coli* because the new bacteriae are more resistant to higher temperatures (thermostable). *E. coli* strains are also engineered to express B.t.-Cry toxin proteins.[5,9-21]

Bacillus thuringiensis (B.t.) contains a calcium-salt, thermostable toxin that can be precipitated from fermentation broths. This is probably because B.t. contains thermophile enzymes like Taq Pol. There have been patent disputes over the *billion dollar royalty-producing Taq polymerase* enzymes, including patents owned by Hoffmann-La Roche. In the natural world, *T. aquaticus* lives in *geothermal veins and hot springs* where fluorides are found. It is useful for practically any recombinant constructs including vaccines, human biologicals, insecticides, and bioremediation tools as well as industrial products that require genetically engineered DNA.[5,9-26]

An interesting patent is assigned to the Amoco Corporation. It can be used to detect organisms including bacillus soil bacteriae (i.e. B.t.); enteric (gut) bacteriae such as gammaproteobacteriae, and *Borrelia burgdorferi* spirochetes. The test probes described in the patent are identified by number and discussed in the next section. The test is designed to detect bacteriae from clinical samples including blood, urine, cerebrospinal fluid, biopsies, synovial fluid, or other tissue or fluid samples from animals or humans. It is an interesting patent for many reasons, nonetheleast of which is because the company that it is assigned to is located in the town where I grew up – right between Fermi and Argonne National (nuclear) laboratories.[27]

The probes can also be used to test substances that are presumed to be sterile (i.e. pharmaceutical products, filtered water). If other diagnostic tests to detect human Lyme disease are designed in a similar manner as this invention, then *those probes might be detecting more than one bacterium as well*. This could support my theory that Lyme disease is caused by an aggregate organism that involves more than one microbe. The probes from the Amoco patent are designed to detect *Borrelia burgdorferi* and other bacteriae including these listed here:[27]

Probe 1638: Detects most eubacteria (rod-shaped gram-negative bacteriae)

Probe 1642: Detects enteric microbes and their relatives found in soil, water, rocks, and living organisms, including *Chlamydiae*, *Firmicutes*, *Actinobacteria,* and others. This probe may detect *mollicutes, clostridiae,* or *bacilli* including those which produce endospores; and those of B.t. insecticides. Remember that spiroplasmas may be descended from *clostridium* species. Clostridium has been found within the bodies of western tent caterpillars and other moth species.

Probe 1643: Detects *Borrelia* spirochetes (This represents a 16SMF primer/probe of Bb sensu lato nucleotides #1529-1510, from the 5'-3' end)[28]†

Probe 1637: Detects most eubacteria (i.e. gram-negatives like *E. coli* from water, soil, human flora)

Probe 1639: Detects enteric bacteria; and *Deinococcus** and *Campylobacter.* (The latter is a gram-negative spiral, food-borne bacterium). Other bacteriae in this group include *Thermus thermophilus,* an *extremophile* (survives to 65°C, 149°F).**

Probe 1640: Detects most eubacteria

Probe 1641: Detects *Fusobacteria* and some *Bacilli. Fusobacteria contribute to periodontal disease and topical skin ulcers like those seen in Morgellon's disease.* Fusobacteria have toxic LPS. This probe may also detect B.t. spores, or *Streptobacillus moniliformis* (Haverhill fever/rat-bite fever) which causes similar tuberculin-like skin lesions.[27,28]

It is interesting that the Amoco patent attempts to detect pathogens that should have no relationship to the human body. These include the extremophiles found in association with mining or petroleum industry activities; or those found in sewage, nuclear, agricultural, or other wastewaters; or in the animals that may be found around these areas.[27,28]

†The gram-positive and gram-negative probes in the invention include those which detect *Borrelia burgdorferi; Borrelia turicatae* (relapsing fever of soft ticks); *Leptospira interrogans-pomona, Leptospira biflexa* (Patoc-Patoc); *Leptospira biflexa* (CDC) strain; *Spirochaeta aurantia* (pigmented mud bacterium); and a long list including *Mycoplasma* species, *Bacillus subtilis, Bacillus brevis, Pseudomonas* species, as well as *extremophile* bacteriae.[27,28]

****Deinococcus radiodurans*** is a large, spherical, radiation-resistant bacterium. As an *extremophile* it survives extreme cold, dehydration, vacuums, and acid environments (i.e. acid mine drainage). Its cell walls are similar to gram-negative bacteria; but the organism stains gram-positive (like Bb). *D. radiodurans* does not form endospores. It is found in habitats rich in organic material (i.e. soil, polluted water, feces, meat, sewage). It has also been found in dust, textiles, dried foods, and on medical instruments. *Deinococcus* has been nicknamed "Conan the bacterium" and is known in the *Guinness Book of World Records* as the world's toughest bacterium. It is closely related to the *Thermus* strains. It was first found in 1956. All family members of the Deinococcus-Thermus family are radiation-resistant, and some strains are thermophiles (temperature resistant).[29-32]

****Extremophiles** include bacteriae that are used in recombinant genetics; to bioremediate oil spills; and are *found naturally in thermal veins* (i.e. Yellowstone park); and in mined phosphates (i.e. fertilizers) where the mineral fluorite (fluoride) is also found. They are also employed industrially within concrete formulas to naturally "repair" structural cracks. Deep within the earth these bacteriae associate not only with fluorite but among rocks where the sindbis virus-like reoviruses (CPVs) and other bacteria live. Like Bb, some extremophiles are cork-screw shaped spirochetes.[33-36]

Extremophiles are so powerful they can degrade organic material, toxic chemicals, and nuclear wastes. They are nearly impossible to kill, even under high temperatures or radiation levels normally lethal to animals and bacteriae. They are extremely small; they form biofilms, and calcify into plaques. In the human body they are extremely resistant to antibiotics and they invade red blood cells and vessels. These bacteriae also have the ability to indefinitely lie dormant in hostile environments, and can hide out in areas of the body that other bacteriae cannot (i.e. kidney stones). There they grow slowly, neatly sequestered from the immune system.[33-36]

The only "effective" antibiotic against some of these bacteriae, which some sources have labeled are *nanobacteria,* is said to be **tetracycline hydrochloride**, at least in vitro (in the lab). Perhaps if Bb is composed in part by an extremophile, this is why the IDSA recommends treating Lyme patients with a tetracycline drug like doxycycline. However Lyme infections, even when treated with "doxy" are said to persist; by patients and doctors alike. Perhaps the persistence of Lyme disease is partly due to the presence of a calcified, persistent extremophile that cannot be easily killed. Nanobacteriae can also be found within the dental pulp and other skeletal structures of the human body. These structures also happen to incorporate ingested fluorides. It is possible that skeletal fluorides assist the survival of Bb organisms that contain extremophile genes. Even if the other components of a Bb spirochete are killed by antibiotics, an extremophile component that is bound to skeletal structures may be alive and well and causing diseases that cannot be detected using standard laboratory tests.[33-36]

A novel strain of *Deinococcus radiodurans* was isolated in 1956 from irradiated canned animal meat by A.W. Anderson at the Oregon Agricultural Experiment Station in Corvallis. Scientists were trying to determine whether canned foods could be sterilized using high dose gamma radiation. A can of food was irradiated at a dose thought to kill all life forms. The food reportedly spoiled, yet *D. radiodurans* survived.[29]

This bacterium is also highly resistant to ultraviolet light, desiccation, oxidizing, and electrophilic agents, such as those used in refining processes. Its genome contains two circular chromosomes, a megaplasmid, a plasmid; and almost 4,000 genes. Other bacteriae that are radiation resistant are the *Cyanobacteria* (blue-green algae), some *Actinobacteriae*, and *Thermococcus.* Scientists have proposed that *D. radiodurans* uses *manganese* as an antioxidant to protect itself from radiation damage, because the organism has high levels of intracellular manganese. Since the Bb spirochete has replaced all of its important enzymes with those that use manganese, this is another argument to support the existance of thermophile genes in Bb spirochetes.[29]

Scientists have cloned a *mercuric reductase gene* (reduces mercury) from *E. coli* into *D. radiodurans.* It is useful to bioremediate or to detoxify mercury residues in radioactive wastes, such as those generated from nuclear weapons manufacturing or nuclear power plants. This recombinant strain can detoxify mercury and toluene from radioactive wastes. This could allow the organism to remain in wastewaters where it may reassort with other bacteriae under the right conditions.[37-40]

The recombinant *D. radiodurans* was also genetically engineered to produce a synthetic organism called *Mycoplasma laboratorium.* This synthetic mycoplasma has been used as a *microbial-based basic data storage and retrieval system.* This describes a future technology where personal information may be inserted into our bodies as a *microbial microchip* which might be delivered by an oral or an injectible vaccine![37-40]

Mycoplasma laboratorium is a lab-created synthetic bacterium that was derived from the genes of *Mycoplasma genitalium.** Some scientists have suggested that *M. laboratorium is directly related to Borrelia burgdorferi.* This may prove to be an interesting clue when we see patents that are owned by mining or petroleum companies which detect Bb and extremophiles. We know that extremophiles have been cloned as bioremediation tools, including to reduce wastes at nuclear weapons manufacturing sites or nuclear power plants. *But they are also used to leach ores during mining processes.* If recombinant extremophiles play a key role in important human diseases, then their presence in the environment can be assumed to have been entirely influenced by humankind. Such involvement could also force scientists to remain absolutely silent about highly political "industrial" disease origins. This is more important when certain thermophile organisms may save governments *hundreds of billions of dollars* in atomic waste remediation costs when employed for those purposes because of their ability to change nuclear wastes into less harmful forms. Likewise, the use of important extremophiles for metal and other ore recovery could be jeopardized if they are linked to human disease epidemics. Do Bb spirochetes contain recombinant or natural extremophiles that are important to aluminum, copper, uranium, or other ore mining industries?[41-47]

**Azithromycin is the preferred treatment for this infection, although Moxifloxacin has shown effectiveness. Moxifloxacin is not used to treat patients with Lyme disease, although Azithromycin is used to treat Lyme.*

The work on *M. laboratorium* was undertaken at the J. Craig Venter Institute (Rockville, MD) under the *Minimal Genome Project.* The goal was to remove or knock out genes to create the smallest working set of genes for an organism to live and successfully reproduce. One of the laboratories that supplies mycoplasma strains to other researchers is the mycoplasma lab at the College of Veterinary Medicine at North Carolina State University according to patents. It is interesting that some physicians who treat Lyme disease outside the IDSA "standards of care" have been heavily targeted by medical boards in several states, including physicians who have practiced in the Carolinas.

The genome for *Mycoplasma laboratorium* has been synthesized and a patent application has been filed. Its patent holders intend to use the chimeric construct to create a future source of *ethanol biofuel.* This would constitute the first synthetically created species, and patent holders could hold a monopoly on the tools that normally allow other scientists open access to genetic processes – including the creation of novel "life forms." [41-47]

Mycoplasma genitalium is a close relative of *Mycoplasma pneumonia,* both of which are pathogenic to humans and animals. The consequences of such man-made life forms through genetic engineering techniques should be pondered very carefully as they may have far-reaching consequences if allowed to move forward. The "parent" organisms of recombinant microbes may already have contributed to global outbreaks of human disease, and some scientists may already be aware of this. Man-made recombinant constructs using these same bacteriae may thereby contribute to future epidemics yet to be realized – some of which may become airborne as a result of being used as biofuels.[41-47]

What is important to note is that *Thermus* or heat-resistant extremophiles are in the same class as the *Mollicutes* (mycoplasmas, spiroplasmas). Thermophiles such as *D. radiodurans* have *segmented genomes* and can horizontally transfer genes to other compatible organisms. This includes the transfer of genes to spiroplasmas, mycoplasmas, and spirillum.[47-49]

The Bb organism is a member of a family that utilizes *metallopeptidases*, which are enzymes whose catalytic mechanism involves metals. Most of the members of this class are zinc-dependent, although some use cobalt. The enzyme that digests proteins (aminopeptidase) from Bb appears to be both thermophilic and zinc-dependent. According to an article **the Bb aminopeptidase is sensitive to Bestatin,** which is a powerful enzyme inhibitor. *Bestatin* (Ubenimex) was tested against human leukemic cells and was shown to inhibit growth by inducing apoptosis. To my knowledge, Bestatin is not typically used to treat patients with Lyme disease.[47-49]

Another patent of interest is assigned to the Amoco Corporation to detect Lyme disease spirochetes. This patent lists the following among the spirochete strains it can detect: *Leptospira biflexa illini, L. interrogans pomona,* CDC *L. biflexa, L. biflexa Patoc-Patoc,* and *Treponema* species. According to the patent, various borreliae tested positive or weakly positive to the probes in the Amoco invention. Two strains of leptospires were also tested against the probes, *L. biflexa* (Patoc-Patoc), and the *L. biflexa* CDC strain. They both tested weakly positive to probe #1616. If we analyze the probes used to detect Bb in the patent, we may find precisely what kind of hybrid organism is sought.[50]

The patent suggests using probe #1617 in addition to one of the other probes numbered #1616; and probes #1617 to #1619 to detect Lyme disease in serologic samples. Probe #1616 represents the US and European strains of Bb; and probe #1617 detects these strains: *Leptospira biflexa* (Patoc-Patoc), *Leptospira biflexa* (CDC); relapsing fevers *Borrelia hermsii, Borrelia turicatae;* oral spirochetes *Treponema denticola, Treponema pectinovorum; Treponema succinifaciens* (swine intestinal spirochetes); and *Treponema pallidum* (Syphilis spirochetes). It appears that the test detects US and European Lyme strains, and spirochetes that cross-breed (hybridize) with these organisms:[50]

Leptospires	Relapsing fever borreliae	Oral spirochetes
Syphilis (genital) spirochetes	Spirochetes of swine intestines which might cause "swine flu"	

Is the Amoco patent *direct* evidence that what has been called "Bb" or the "Lyme disease spirochete" is actually a complex of intermediate form mutant spirochetes from any of the aforementioned species? Can these species mutate or aggregate with soil or water-borne microbes under direction of fluorides, phosphates, animal wastes, radioactive wastes, radiation, or other chemicals? Can they likewise mutate in the body to produce an aggregate spirochete? One of the most important comments from the Amoco patent describes the site where tissues were cultured from an ECM rash of a Lyme patient in 1981 and where an intermediate form of leptospira was isolated. The new spirochete was named *Leptospira inadai Lyme* by CDC/EIS employee Dr. Allen C. Steere and colleagues. We know that this leptospira was eventually named a *Leptonema* and placed into the same group as novel spirochetes found in Romania, in Illinois bulls and turtles, and in the earlier Noguchi form. According to the patent:[50]

> "Skin is one of the better sites to visualize spirochetes, particularly during stage one Lyme disease."

The idea that mining, manufacturing, or oil companies are assignees on patents that are capable of detecting pathogenic leptospires and Bb spirochetes might seem peculiar unless we consider that these companies utilize bauxite, ammonia, fluoride, phosphates, metals, rare earth elements, chemicals and salts; or produce some of these compounds in their refining, mining, manufacturing, construction, and/or remediation processes or products. Remember that these industries sell products to fertilizer, pesticide, textile, paper, chemical, food, metal, and nuclear industries; and some of these chemicals or compounds have important mutagenic properties. Obviously scientists in industries are aware of the mutagenic characteristics of their products. That is the strongest argument as to why they are patent holders on diagnostic tests that may be used to detect human pathogenic spirochetes. If we consider whether Bb is an aggregate organism, we can understand why Lyme diagnostic tests may be seeking something more than "just" borreliae proteins. It is also easier to understand why a spirochete that may have been formed in the presence of industrial products or processes, may become one of the most highly protected and politically denied illnesses in history.

Another Use for Chaperonin

The Chaperonin 10 (Cpn10) described in the Barbara Johnson et al. patents *has been shown to have immunosuppressive activity in experimental autoimmune encephalomyelitis (EAE)*; and in delayed hypersensitivity reactions in allograft disease (graft vs. host) rejection. Autoimmune encephalomyelitis is considered to be an attack by the immune system upon "self." However this problem has only been known since the days of the earliest vaccine formulas.

During EAE, the human immune system may be attacking "self" proteins which contain foreign DNA/RNA or "non-self" proteins such as those that incorporate into our cells once we are vaccinated. It seems to me that autoimmune encephalitis (AE) is a complication that could potentially occur with any vaccine.

Vaccines are immunosuppressive, and may be designed to suppress a process that would naturally occur in the body upon vaccination since vaccines present foreign antigens to the body over time. (Antigens are proteins that stimulate an immune response). The immune system is designed to identify and remove all foreign or damaged proteins. It would therefore respond to vaccine proteins the way it responds to other invaders in a seek-and-destroy mission.

Vaccines are an attempt to fool the immune system into recognizing foreign proteins, and establishing antibodies to same without triggering illness or the destruction of the vaccine formula proteins. Something in the vaccine adjuvant or formula is designed to partly suppress the immune response (immunosuppressive). Without such design, autoimmune encephalitis could occur once the vaccine viral antigens incorporate into the genome of our cells.

There are viral, bacterial, and amoebic forms of encephalitis. What if the viral proteins or a contaminant in a vaccine preparation are responsible for cases of so-called "autoimmune" encephalitis? We know that viruses allow penetration of pathogens across the blood-brain barrier to cause encephalitis and meningitis. What if vaccine proteins which "fail" to remain where they are supposed to (inside the cell) instead manage to infect other microorganisms in the body (or themselves become infected and are ejected from vaccine chimera) only to cross into the brain and central nervous system to cause disease?

From patent inventions we learn that Cpn10 helps suppress the problem of autoimmune encephalitis. This problem may have accidentally occurred with the first generation Lyme vaccine. If so, it could also occur with any other human vaccine. It may be possible for recombinant vaccine designs to fail in the presence of a virus or bacterium that binds with the viral components of recombinant constructs that lie latent in the body. Such infections may be introduced by vectoring insects that have been exposed to environmental microbes including those from recombinant insecticides or the genes of GM plants.

Such viral escapees could cause an "autoimmune"-like disease which is basically an infection with immune activation that continually attacks the foreign virus proteins which remain in our cells. Since not all chimerae will fail, those which remain in the body may become a target for the immune system to attack. This is because it now recognizes the presence of the foreign proteins it failed to eliminate before the immune system was suppressed. Of course this is only speculative theory, but from what I have seen and read, such events appear to not only be logical, but a very real possibility.

Scientists know that experimental autoimmune encephalitis can be prevented by pretreating newborn or adult animals with vaccines that contain whole brain tissue that is infected with encephalitis, or tubercule bacilli. In human vaccines, *Freund's incomplete* adjuvant is used instead of *Freund's complete* formula. Adjuvants are substances that help alert the immune system to the presence of foreign materials; and which help deliver viral antigens to the body over a long period of time. This allows the body to create long-term antibodies to the antigens being released. My question is whether human vaccines are designed to block the phenomenon of autoimmune encephalitis. If this is done, the process may be flawed due to the unpredictability of chimeric constructs, and what happens when phages of bacterial or viral origin come into contact with the latent vaccine viruses.

If vaccine formulas can fail due to some recombinant problem upon exposure to phagic bacteria or viruses by vectoring insects, then the vaccinated populations are at risk for the reactivation of a disease state. A latent vaccine virus reactivation may cause a polio-like encephalomyelitis, rubella-like rash, influenza-like illness, Lyme disease, Morgellon's, or any other related poxvirus-caused illness. Perhaps what is seen in some Lyme disease cases is the reactivation of former vaccine virus proteins by way of insect-introduced mixed infections. If so, this problem could represent a serious *biological conflict of interest* between the animal and human vaccinated populations and the applied insecticides and recombinant microbes important to industries and agriculture. The severity of illness may be entirely dependent upon the microbes which trigger vaccine virus reactivation.

Factors such as viral interference and body toxin burdens may help determine the final outcome of mixed infections that carry the additional burden of a vaccine virus that gets kicked out of its chimera to become a reactivated infection. After all, recombinant insecticides are designed to reactivate latent infections in insects. The problem is that it looks as if the same process is occurring in the animal and human populations as well. If this is what occurs, then autoimmune encephalitis that is a potential threat with any vaccine is a serious complication of an immune system that becomes overburdened with active mixed infections and toxins.

The failure of vaccine formulas to suppress autoimmune encephalitis may be simply because once certain microbes enter the body, "all bets are off" and viruses and bacteria become infected with phages and reassort. Even stored toxins are released in conjunction with bacterial toxins and enzymes to create highly complex chronic diseases including Lyme disease.[1,2]

Out of curiosity I briefly examined old rabies patents, including one assigned to Eli Lily and Company (Indianapolis, IN). To the immune system, rabies is antigenically the same as sindbis virus, which is commonly used to manipulate genes. The preferred virus for the patent is an *inactivated mouse brain strain* that was obtained from the NIH. The patent describes the Russian (Margulis-Shubladze) mouse-brain strain and the "S.V." strain of acute encephalomyelitis. This virus was written about in 1946 by Shubladze when discussing formalin-inactivated vaccines from 1942. From the Eli Lily patent we learn that up until the time of the patent, vaccines were:

> "...characterized by the presence of some factor or agent which all too frequently produces in the person treated with the vaccine a *post-vaccinal, neurolytic paralysis*, often with fatal consequences."[3,4]

At the time of the 1953 Eli Lily patent, the causative factor of this paralysis was unknown, but thought to be derived from some constituent of mammalian nerve tissue which, according to the patent:[3,4]

"...because of the method of preparation, is inevitably present in the vaccine."

This refers to a contaminant, a sensitized animal tissue, a virus, or a retrovirus – one of a size and type that may include the sindbis virus. After all, this virus causes an acute encephalomyelitis, and is antigenically the same as, and is related to the rabies virus. Both viruses infect monkeys and birds. These animals are routinely used to propagate viruses for vaccines. This could also refer to chicken embryo cells that contain a retrovirus. Recombinant insecticides can reactivate latent rabies or other insect or animal infections which may be transmitted to humans. In an insect exposed to a recombiant chimera made with sindbis virus, perhaps a wild animal rabies virus reassorts to cause one form of a rabies-like disease that can cause neurologic Lyme disease once trasmitted to a human.[3,4]

A 1963 research paper described how *paraffin oil* and killed *mycobacteriae* are used in Freund's adjuvants to help stimulate antibody production. Paraffin wax/oil is found on petroleum fractions (gas oils); and contains straight chain hydrocarbons. This is then converted into a useful product for animal vaccines. The remaining hydrocarbons that are not removed from the product may contribute to a contamination problem in vaccine adjuvants, and hypersensitivity issues in animal tissues. Animal vaccines also typically use *Mycobacterium tuberculosis* as a stimulating bacterium to flag the immune system to pay attention to the vaccine formula, and to create antibodies in the vaccinated animal. Scientists pursued the use of paraffin oil and mycobacteriae in livestock, veterinary, and human vaccines despite the fact that these substances are known to:

> "...induce delayed-type hypersensitivity and organ-specific 'auto-immune' diseases."[5,6]

Multiple Sclerosis researcher Dr. Byron Waksman (Harvard and Massachusetts General Hospital) experimentally reproduced "auto-allergic" lesions in laboratory animals by sensitizing them with tissue constituents using adjuvants that contained mycobacteriae. According to Dr. Waksman:

> "Adequate evidence is available to prove beyond question that these are actually hypersensitive responses to autologous tissue antigens...the auto-allergic lesions are similar histologically to well-recognized delayed allergic responses (tuberculin reaction, contact allergy) and *can be passively transferred with living lymphoid cells from sensitized donors.*"[5]

This means that cell lines that are used to produce animal or human vaccines may contain not only viral, retroviral, bacterial, protozoal, or other contaminants; but also proteins that are pre-sensitized to adjuvants and mycobacteriae. It also suggests that such pre-sensitized proteins can be passively transferred into cells used to create human vaccines. This may leave us wide open for the reactivation of diseases upon introduction of recombinant insecticides that are designed to do this.

The so-called "auto-allergic" lesions described by Dr. Waksman affected the eyes, thyroid, adrenals, testes, and central and peripheral nervous systems of sensitized animals. He also said that the lesions were not the same as those caused by anaphylactic or vasculitis-necrosis type allergic responses. They are instead very similar to delayed allergic responses such as those caused by contact allergies or tuberculin reactions. In other words, adjuvant or mycobacterium-sensitized animals *pass their tuberculin or mycobacterium-sensitized tissues onto the host cells that are used in cell lines* for animal and human vaccines.[5,7-9]

Are reactivated latent viruses part of the cause of "autoimmune" diseases of today? Are humans exposed to pre-sensitized host cells from animal vaccine adjuvants which transfer their sensitivities to us? Are mycobacterium or tuberculin-sensitized cell lines or their hydrocarbon contaminants responsible for allergies, arthritis, or autoimmune disorders in generations of vaccinated humans? Could failed or contaminated *leptospirosis* or other animal vaccines have caused *Mycobacterium tuberculosis adjuvants in animal vaccines to fail and to produce a mutated leptonema in animals?* Did such a recombinant organism that was reassorted in the bodies of livestock contaminate soils and wastewaters in the areas where the animals lived? Do the genes of recombinant insecticides similarly pollute plant and environmental microbes to create similar leptonema that are transmissible by vectoring insects and arthropods?[5,7-9]

E-coli bacteriae also produce chaperonin 60 (groEL) and chaperonin 10 (groES) proteins. GroEL is a ubiquitous protein that is stress and heat-inducible in activated sludge. It is used as a standard biological process in wastewater treatment. For those who are working to degrade biofuels and other toxic chemicals from wastewater or other sources, the chaperonins can be applied in granular form in a method described by Barbara Johnson et al.'s chaperonin patent(s). These formulas help to control the reassortment of microbes and their sometimes improper gene-folding activities.

The chaperonins may also be used in pharmaceutical compositions; applied to standing water to reduce pollutants (i.e. rivers, ponds); or within agricultural fertilizers as soil amendments. Their use could possibly offset the effects of certain bacteriae (B.t.) and related agricultural tools which in one form or another seem to have been adversely affecting the "non-targeted" human species for the better part of a century and a half.[10,11]

Since many insects including flies, mosquitoes, and ticks have developed resistance to *organophosphate* pesticides, we can imagine that the spirochetes living inside of them as symbionts or parasites are also of keen interest to scientists for their ability to thrive despite the effects of pesticides. The University of Minnesota St. Paul is where we may find a number of renowned bacteriologists and spirochetologists including Dr. Russell C. Johnson. Dr. Johnson is listed as an inventor on a number of Bb-related patents. Minnesota is also home to the Mayo Clinic, whose current laboratory director is Dr. Franklin R. Cockerill, III.

Dr. Cockerill is listed on patents for diagnostic tests for tuberculosis, streptococcus, legionella, antibiotic-resistant enterococcus, and group B streptococci. He published papers on genetic methods to assess antimicrobial resistance, and a *biopesticide* (microbial insecticide) that contains an antibiotic resistance gene. Dr. Cockerill has consulted for a number of companies with interesting ties to the Lyme disease story.[13-18]

The Mayo Foundation for Medical Education and Research (MN) is co-assignee with Roche Molecular Systems, Inc. (NJ) on a patent to detect antibiotic-resistant genes (rifampin) in mycobacterial cultures and clinical specimens. The patent is used to detect the presence of *Mycobacterium tuberculosis* or its mutants. *Mycobacterium tuberculosis* is used within Freund's adjuvants as components of animal vaccines; including some that may have been developed in part from contaminated insect cell lines. Dr. Cockerill has consulted for several companies including a fertilizer company with the same (sur)name:[13-18]

Cockerill Fertilizer Co. (Nebraska)	bio-Merieux-Vitek, (France)
COMBACT Diagnostics, Inc., (Israel)	bio-Merieux Scientific Advisory Board (Missouri)
Molecular Systems (Indiana)	Roche Applied Science/Roche Wampole Labs, (New Jersey)

Dr. Cockerill was also listed as a member of an ad hoc NIH/NIAID study section for tuberculosis (1994); a member of the infectious diseases work group of the negotiated rulemaking committee on clinical diagnostic laboratory tests; and the healthcare financing agency representing the American Medical Group Association (AMA) in 1998. He also serves as a consultant to the FDA on the advisory committee for microbiology devices panel; has been a laboratory response network member since 2003; and since 2001 has served on the NIH/NIAID study section for infectious diseases and microbiology.[14-16]

Dr. Cockerill has also licensed ten of his inventions to Roche Diagnostics GmbH and has written many peer-reviewed articles on HIV, fungemia, bacteremia, antibiotics, decontamination of the digestive tract; and the gut bacteriae *Helicobacter pylori* and *E. coli* and their adherence to epithelial cells. This kind of adherence to gut epithelial cells is important to understand when studying the biological effects of microbial insecticides that contain B.t. upon human intestinal tissues. At the very least we might note the interests of a major Midwest medical clinic that conducts serosurveys of patients with suspected arbovirus infections; and at least one fertilizer manufacturer. Arboviruses of course are any infectious viruses that are transmitted by insects and arthropods. This includes those related to reoviruses, sindbis, and rabies; and which may reassort with those introduced into insects through insecticides or genetic manipulations of insect genes by scientists who then release GM bugs into the environment as population replacers.[14-16]

Dr. Cockerill co-authored a paper on the detection of DNA from the *Orthopox** Dryvax vaccine strain, herpes simplex, and varicella zoster. The article begins by announcing that smallpox virus is a "major threat as an agent of bioterrorism." At present only biosafety level 4 (BSL-4) laboratories are allowed to handle agents as infectious as smallpox, anthrax, botulism, tularemia, or plague. Since smallpox as a human infection was essentially eliminated from the planet, it is curious that it should remain so disconcerting unless we understand that smallpox and other viruses are useful to microbial insecticide formulas.[17,18]

**Orthopox viruses include smallpox, vaccinia, monkeypox, cowpox.*

The fact that *poxviruses can be reactivated by other compatible poxviruses should not escape our notice.* The term "bioterrorism" may thus take on a very different meaning including one that doesn't necessarily involve the deployment of microbes by extremist human terrorists. Instead, bioterrorism may represent the hidden hazards of the scientific deployments of microbes that are useful as biological controls and vaccines; and which may accidentally cause diseases through recombinant "accidents."

Mycobacterium bovis, which is the agent of bovine tubercle bacillus (cattle tuberculosis) and a microbe for which Dr. Cockerill also holds a patent interest, is discussed in the text of a recombinant vaccine patent for *Borrelia burgdorferi.* Cattle tuberculosis is related to human tuberculosis. The most common animals that harbor this infection are cattle, badgers, and white-tailed deer. A resource shows that this infection enters the human body through the ingestion of contaminated milk, meats, or by inhalation.[19-25]

A *Mycoplasma bovis* infection can enter the bones and joints to cause joint tuberculosis and the well-known pulmonary (respiratory) form. A publication from July 1993 co-authored by Dr. Alan Barbour describes a recombinant, attenuated bovine tubercle bacillus called *Bacille Calmette-Guerin* or BCG. This agent was developed as a vaccine "vehicle" for human pathogens, including for *Borrelia burgdorferi.* According to the paper, scientists have developed *Salmonella* and *E. coli* vaccine vehicles which target antigens or other sites on the bacterial surface of the Bb spirochete by using flagella, the OspA protein, the major outer membrane protein A (OmpA), or a lambda phage receptor (bacteriophage). Of course when such formulas fail, we may see the chaperonins coming to the rescue.[19-25]

Were some of the key attendees at the Dearborn conference aware of the origins of Lyme disease, and did some of them hold patent or vaccine interests meant to "fix" recombinant "accidents" on a global scale? Did the Dearborn conference yield standardized laboratory tests to avoid the embarrassment of failed genetic engineering techniques? Were animal and human vaccines found to be conflicting with recombinant insecticides and chemical and nuclear wastes? Is Lyme disease the Pandora's box of the biotech industry? Environmental contamination is one of the Achilles heels of genetic engineering techniques. The other is undoubtedly the common reassortments which take place outside the laboratory, and which are influenced by many factors including environmental pollutants of many kinds.[26,27]

We may postulate about the formulas used to create vaccines and biological controls using insect and animal cell lines that are repeatedly described as contaminated. We know that transposons and genes jump between their own chromosomes as well as those of other species. We know that recombinant science is unpredictable in the insect, the environment, and in higher animals. We may imagine what happens when animals and humans are vaccinated with genetically engineered formulas that may fail upon exposure to reassorted microbes from insects that have been exposed to recombinant insecticides. We now see the perfect storm that has probably produced a superbug called *Borrelia burgdorferi.* This supermicrobe is part genetic accident, part natural recombinant; and multi-host dependent, needing an insect and higher animal in order to proliferate.

Cooking the Red Herring

In October 2007 on the heels of the Connecticut Attorney General's investigation into the IDSA guidelines for Lyme disease, a cohort of researchers with interesting ties to industry published a paper titled *A Critical Appraisal of "Chronic Lyme Disease."* Out of the six lead authors and the twenty-five ad hoc committee member co-authors, were researchers who have important ties to the story in this book. Many of the co-authors of the 2006 IDSA Lyme disease guidelines that were under investigation by the Connecticut Attorney General participated in writing this 2007 critical appraisal paper. If you look closely at the co-authors, you will see a tightly knit group of infectious disease and public health officials with long ties to industry and great influence over the politics and history of Lyme disease around the world.[1,2]

The appraisal paper argued against the chronic nature of Lyme disease; declaring that infections beyond six months are a "post-Lyme syndrome," a term first proposed by Dr. Allen Steere. It also contraindicates long-term antibiotics; promotes a belief there is "public confusion" about the disease; and claims that chronic Lyme is:

> "...the latest in a series of syndromes that have been postulated in an attempt to attribute medically unexplained symptoms to particular infections."

Lyme disease is hardly an unexplained infection. The article's lead authors include those whom agree that the very serious chronic Lyme disease either "does not exist," or does, but perhaps for only a brief period after which recovery without treatment is inevitable. Lead author Dr. Henry M. Feder Jr. of the University of Connecticut disclosed that he receives lecture fees from pharmaceutical company Merck; and serves as an expert witness in medical malpractice cases related to Lyme disease. Dr. Barbara J.B. Johnson of the CDC in Fort Collins, Colorado reportedly holds patents on diagnostic antigens for Lyme disease. There was no mention of chaperonins unless those are the patents to which she refers.[1]

Dr. Susan O'Connell from the Health Protection Agency of Southampton, UK reported that she has served as an expert witness on Lyme disease issues in English civil and criminal suits. Dr. Eugene Shapiro from Yale University reported that he served as an expert witness in medical malpractice cases relating to Lyme; he reviews Lyme disability claims for Metropolitan Life Insurance Company; and he receives speaker fees from pharmaceutical companies Merck and Sanofi-Aventis.[1]

Dr. Allen Steere from Massachusetts General Hospital, Harvard Medical School, and New York Medical College reported that he received a research grant from Viramed, and (consulting) fees from Novartis. We have already covered the "Steere letters" showing Lyme persistence and seronegativity.[1]

Dr. Gary Wormser revealed that he received research grants related to Lyme disease from Immunetics, Bio-Rad, and Biopeptides as well as "education grants" from Merck and AstraZeneca "to New York Medical College for visiting lectures for infectious disease grand rounds." He reports that he is part owner of the biotech company Diaspex; is an equity owner in pharmaceutical company Abbott; has served as an expert witness in a medical malpractice case; and is "being retained" in other medical malpractice cases for Lyme disease. He also indicated that he "may" become a consultant to Biopeptides, a company that develops vaccines and laboratory diagnostics including those to detect Lyme infections. Among the individuals of the ad hoc committee are scientists from these academic centers:[1]

Johns Hopkins, Baltimore and Crofton
Yale University, New Haven, Connecticut
Danbury Hospital, Danbury, CT
New York University School of Medicine
St. Luke's Hospital, Duluth, Minnesota
New York Medical College, Valhalla, New York
Atlantic Neuroscience Institute, Summit, NJ
Boston University

University of Connecticut
University of British Columbia, Vancouver
University of Medicine and Dentistry, New Jersey-Robert Wood Johnson Med. School, Piscataway, NJ
Gundersen Lutheran Medical Foundation, La Crosse, Wisconsin
National Microbiology Laboratory, Health Canada, Winnipeg, Manitoba
Schneider Children's Hospital at North Shore, Manhasset, New York
Washington Hospital Center and Georgetown University Medical Center, Washington, DC
New York State Department of Health, Albany
Connecticut Children's Medical Center, University of Connecticut, Hartford.[1]
Centers for Disease Control (CDC)
Main Medical Center, Portland, ME

Despite the academic and public health denials, in the background "all" things Bb-related are researched and patented in the name of vaccines, diagnostic tests, research, and occasionally in connection with agricultural or industrial products. It is curious to know that there are accurate tests which can detect Bb spirochetes in the laboratory or in industry. However Bb tests intended for public use are for some reason far less able to detect clinical cases of Lyme disease. Meanwhile, some of the co-authors of the Feder Jr. et al. paper and their associates are key patent holders to borrelia-related inventions.

Might the reason for the "denial" of aspects of Lyme disease have something to do with the profitability of the Lyme disease organism? Or could the reason for the apparent "denial" of the chronicity of Lyme disease and the idea that there are significantly more patients than are acknowledged, be the *origins* of the organisms? Would those origins have been influenced by genetic engineering, chemical pollutants, nuclear and mining wastes, and the deployment of microbes in agriculture and other industries?

There is a 1999 patent for a recombinant outer surface protein C (OspC)-based Lyme disease vaccine and diagnostic test. The patent is assigned to the Gundersen Lutheran Medical Foundation in La Crosse, Wisconsin. Dr. W.A. Agger, also from Gundersen was a member of the ad hoc committee that co-authored the previous Feder Jr. et al. paper *"A Critical Appraisal of 'Chronic Lyme Disease."*[1,3]

The paper's co-authors collectively described the chronic symptoms of Lyme disease as "post-Lyme disease symptoms," which the paper called "usually mild and self-limiting." The group also called the symptoms described by Lyme patients as:

> "a broad array of illness or symptom complexes for which there is no reproducible or convincing scientific evidence of any relationship to *B. burgdorferi* infection."

This statement is flatly misleading as there is both convincing and reproducible evidence for Bb infections. I have photographic evidence of my own Bb spirochetes that were recently cultured using a new laboratory technique. I have had Lyme disease for most of my life, and have been rebitten as recently as 2000. This would at the very least provide evidence of Bb infection for a minimum of a dozen years, despite being treated with antibiotics.[1]

The group appears to describe patient symptoms as little more than broad or non-specific, with no legitimate connection to active Lyme infections. The authors describe how the term "chronic Lyme disease" is used in the US and Europe as a diagnosis for patients with some or all of the following symptoms: persistent pain, neurocognitive symptoms, and fatigue. They also claim that the diagnosis is given to patients *without clinical or serologic evidence of previous Lyme disease infection*, which they describe as "previous early" or "late" infection. The paper's authors also appear to criticize patients who claim to have Lyme symptoms. The paper classifies patients into categories numbered 1 through 4. The categories are described in summary, based upon my interpretation of them, which may or may not be accurate:[1]

> Category 1: People who lack objective clinical manifestations or laboratory evidence of Bb infection, but who have a diagnosis based on "nonspecific" symptoms which the paper's authors claim are found in only 10% of patients including in areas where Lyme disease is not considered to be endemic.
>
> Category 2: People with identifiable illnesses or syndromes that are not Lyme disease whether the patients have a history of Lyme or not; which the paper claims may be a misdiagnosis or a diagnosis for "some other disease" that the patients are "reluctant to accept" and so have sought out a doctor willing to treat them specifically for Lyme.
>
> Category 3: Patients without history of objective clinical findings consistent with Lyme disease, although their serum contains antibodies to Bb as determined by standardized assays that were ordered to investigate some illness with "unknown cause." The paper claims people in this group have at best, equivocal evidence of Bb infection since the predictive ability of the tests are "low." The paper's authors recommend that doctors tell patients in this category that their diagnosis is "uncertain" and that a benefit from treatment is "unlikely."
>
> Category 4: Patients in this category have symptoms consistent with "post-Lyme disease syndrome;" a term that Dr. Allen Steere created years ago to explain people who "still" have symptoms of Lyme after a prescribed period of time.

At the time Steere called this a *possible* but not a definite syndrome, although this qualifier is frequently missing when quoted by academics, research papers, or clinicians.[1]

According to my interpretation of the Feder Jr. et al. paper, *there appears to be no such thing as an active Lyme infection.* There are only Bb antibodies in some patients for an illness with "unknown cause" since the paper appears to categorize virtually *no patients with any actual symptoms or active disease states* considered to legitimately be Lyme disease. Although probably not their intent, if this is the case, then why have tens of millions of dollars been spent researching Bb and developing patents for diagnostic tests and vaccines (including the patent for an OspC-based vaccine and diagnostic test)? Why are researchers actively studying the possibility of chronic Lyme disease if it truly does not exist? Let's see if the Gunderson Lutheran patent contains statements in agreement with the Feder Jr. et al. group's appraisal of chronic Lyme disease. According to the Gunderson patent, the following important statements about Bb may need to be reviewed by the Feder Jr. et al. team:[1,3]

> "Lyme disease is caused by the spirochete *Borrelia burgdorferi* (B.b.), which is primarily transmitted during the blood feeding of *Ixodes* ssp. ticks. Initially, spirochetes infect the skin and, in the majority of early cases, cause an erythema migrans lesion (2)."
>
> "Those stricken may not become ill for weeks, and nervous system symptoms (headaches, dizziness, hearing problems, tingling and trouble concentrating) may not occur for weeks or months."
>
> "It is now known that *infection can spread to the nervous system or joints, and the risk of neurological or joint complications increases the longer the disease goes untreated. Infection can be asymptomatic, or have a range of clinical presentations*, depending on the tissues affected, the duration of infection, host factors such as the vulnerability of the immune system and immunogenetic factors which could predispose a patient to the development of certain complications."
>
> "The treatment of symptomatic patients is currently with a range of antibiotics, e.g., tetracyclines, penicillin and cephalosporins, but studies show mixed results. *Left untreated, the bacteria can spread to the central nervous system, heart, brain, or joints, causing arthritis, cardiac infections and neurologic problems, and in rare cases, death (3-6).*"

This hardly sounds like the highly minimized chronic Lyme disease described by the Feder Jr. et al. bunch who appear to define "chronic Lyme disease" as perhaps an imaginary or non-specific illness that is neither easy to detect nor one that manifests in clinical symptoms that can be diagnosed by a competent medical professional.[3]

Also from the Gunderson patent we find what appears to be referrals to the first generation Lyme vaccine that was pulled from the market:[3]

> "The applicants recently demonstrated the inability of a commercial OspA vaccination to sustain adequate levels of anti-OspA borreliacidal antibodies in humans (23)...In support, infection with B.b. has been documented in OspA-vaccinated humans and dogs (26,27). These results highlight the need to evaluate other Lyme borreliosis vaccine components."
>
> "In addition, Lyme disease is ordinarily diagnosed by detecting antibodies in the blood or cerebral spinal fluid, but **the most commonly used tests are often inaccurate.** False-negative, and more commonly, false-positive results continue to plague the serodiagnosis of Lyme disease. Unfortunately, little improvement has occurred and **misdiagnosis continues to cause significant economic and health effects**..."
>
> "If OspC truly induces an early B.b. borreliacidal antibody response, then it follows that detection of this highly specific antibody response can be used to detect Lyme disease more accurately and to monitor elimination of the organism after therapy than with other diagnostic assays that do not detect anti-OspC borreliacidal antibodies."

The Gunderson patent cites these specific references to support the existence of "chronic" Lyme disease – a stage of Lyme infection that the Feder Jr. et al. bunch seems to discount:

- Fikrig, E. et al., Sera from Patients with Chronic Lyme Disease Protect Mice from Lyme Borreliosis. *The Journal of Infectious Diseases*. 1994:169:568-574.
- Zhong, W. et al., Therapeutic Passive Vaccination Against Chronic Lyme Disease in Mice. *Proc. Natl. Acad. Sci. USA*. 1997:94:12533-12539.

I suppose mice are permitted to have chronic Lyme disease, but people are not. It seems that some of Gunderson's own scientists are unaware of the facility's patent which states the following:

> "Lyme disease (Lyme borreliosis) is spread by a bite from an infected tick, and is the most commonly reported tickborne infection in Europe and North America (1). This multi-system disorder has caused significant morbidity worldwide."

If Lyme disease doesn't exist except as an acute, easily treated infection, or a vague description of delusional patients who suffer from "something else," then how can it cause significant economic, health effects, and morbidity worldwide?[3]

The Gunderson Lutheran patent belongs to a La Crosse, Wisconsin medical institution. Three states* in the region are highly endemic for Lyme disease (WI, IL, IA), and yet patients are routinely told by doctors in these states that there is "no Lyme disease" in their state. Someone may want to inform midwest physicians that not only is Lyme disease a reality, but that one or more of its medical centers holds patent interests in vaccines and/or diagnostic kits to detect the disease.[3-5]

**William Wallace Cargill founded the Cargill Empire (corn/grain and other businesses) and eventually settled in Austin, Minnesota in 1868. By 1875 the company's headquarters and family home were in La Crosse. Cargill's grain operations spanned several states that became endemic for Lyme disease; but its hub was in the Midwest. La Crosse borders the heavily polluted Mississippi River and the Minnesota and Iowa state lines, and is downstream of major chemical companies that manufacture products with persisting organic pollutants (POPs).*

The Gunderson patent explains that an OspA-based vaccine for Bb probably won't work when using "conventional" (standardized) diagnostic tests. This is precisely why the OspA and OspB proteins were excluded from the standardized laboratory tests at Dearborn – to benefit a (then) upcoming Lyme disease vaccine based on OspA/B antigens. According to the Gunderson patent:[3-5]

> "Several schemes using conventional diagnostic assays have been developed to more accurately detect Lyme disease. Unfortunately, little improvement has occurred and misdiagnosis continues to cause significant economic and health effects. In addition, *the recent approval of an OspA Lyme disease vaccine will further confound conventional diagnostic testing*. Thus, a sensitive and specific Lyme disease test which can be made widely available as a commercial kit and can discriminate between vaccinated individuals and patients with Lyme disease is still needed."

Scientific patents openly acknowledge that an OspA-based Lyme vaccine will cause problems when using standardized diagnostic tests to detect Lyme. Patents explain that important OspA and OspB bands were excluded from diagnostic tests at Dearborn. Were these proteins cross-reactive with other agents found in nearly everyone's body? OspA and B may represent agricultural microbes including B.t. Cry toxins and fungal toxins to which most people are exposed every day.[3]

The CDC-recommended diagnostic tests for Lyme which the 1999 Gunderson patent suggests are insensitive and confounding, remain in use today. Better tests are available and are more frequently being used by physicians in the US and abroad. Despite this, better diagnostic tools are dismissed and contraindicated by public health experts in the US (CDC/IDSA) and abroad (UK/Health Protection Agency) since European physicians often follow CDC or IDSA recommendations. It is curious that patents and older research papers routinely identify "chronic Lyme disease" while academic researchers who promote public health "consensus" statements increasingly do not want to call it by this name. However difficult the disease is to acknowledge in public, in private Lyme disease is easily pronounced in order to secure federal research dollars to study its chronic form![3]

The UK Health Protection Agency's web site refers to "unorthodox" and "unvalidated" tests that are "proven not to be of value," and that are available "mainly in the USA." These refer to non-standardized, non-CDC or IDSA-recommended specialty diagnostic tests that are better able to detect Bb infections. The reason they are useful is because they contain more varieties of Bb antigens to detect a wider group of pathogens than the standardized tests.[1,6-14]

These better tests are described in a report written by the inspector of microbiology and infection control at the UK Department of Health in what seems an attempt to dismiss valuable diagnostic tools which differ from those recommended by the CDC. What is happening overseas may be the promotion by public health agencies of a global partyline based on CDC-recommended standardized tests. Unfortunately these less sensitive tests are failing Lyme patients around the world for many reasons. This happens because the tests were not designed to detect European Bb strains nor the majority of American strains.[1,6-14]

The UK scientists cite CDC reports, the IDSA guidelines for Lyme disease, and research articles that were published by Lyme guidelines co-authors Klempner, Halperin, Steere, Stanek, Dattwyler, Strle, and colleagues including Shapiro, Finkel, and Sigal. We can see the long arm of a collective few US academic colleagues who seem to be at the helm of the ship that is working to control all aspects of public information about Lyme disease across the globe.[1,6-15]

It is obvious also that these parties' collective influence has set sail across the Atlantic from the US to dock in the port of the European Union of scientific opinion. Such influence is easy to understand if the Bb organism has direct connections to globally applied insecticides, vaccines, or industrial processes. Since each are globally important, it is necessary to reach global consensus if an epidemic is caused by recombinant accidents or the use of profitable tools. Right or wrong, consensus opinion may also serve to protect global industrial and agricultural interests, including those which significantly fund academic institutions and research laboratories around the world with grant monies, patent earnings, and more.[1,6-15]

A Yale University patent describes a method to detect Lyme disease. The patent was invented by Richard Flavell, Erol Fikrig, and Robert Berland, and was filed December 1993, just ten months before the Dearborn conference. The conference work group did not select this diagnostic test for standardization. It is interesting that the patent does not seem to have ever been developed as a useful diagnostic tool despite the fact that the Bb flagella (tails) are distinctly different between species. This recombinant patent could have been a useful diagnostic test to standardize at Dearborn. However as a new Lyme vaccine was about to be marketed, this test probably would also have confounded the results of the upcoming vaccine's clinical trials.[16]

Another patent describes the various stages of Lyme disease, including an advanced stage of severe disability that is the result of Bb persistence. From the patent we read:

> "Stage three, or late infection, is defined as *persistent infection*, and can be *severely disabling. Chronic* arthritis, and syndromes of the central and peripheral nervous system appear during this stage, as a result of the *ongoing infection* and *perhaps* a resulting auto-immune disease…"
>
> "Early in human infection, antibodies are generated primarily against the 41-kDa flagellar protein. In later stages, antibodies to the outer surface proteins OspA and OspB, among others, appear..."
>
> "Further, the sera from patients with neurologic manifestations of Lyme disease have IgM antibodies that bind human axons; *binding is weak or absent* in patients without neurologic disease…"
>
> "Treatment of early disease is usually effective, *however the cardiac, arthritis and nervous system disorders associated with the later stages often do not respond to therapy* [A.C. Steere, "Lyme Disease," N. Engl. J. Med., 321, pp. 586-96 (1989)]."

Dr. Allen Steere is quoted stating that patients often do not respond to antibiotic therapy. The patent continues:

> "However, serologic testing is not yet standardized, and results may vary between laboratories and commercial kits, causing false negative and, more commonly, false positive results…in addition, *available serologic tests have limited usefulness early in infection prior to the development of a measurable antibody response...*"[16]

These comments are a far cry from some infectious disease experts' claims that Lyme disease is not a serious infection. An older publication contained an interesting description by Dr. Allen Steere of the three distinct stages of Lyme disease. These stages are said to occasionally overlap in some patients. The paper claims that the ECM rash is the "hallmark" of early infection; that approximately 20% of patients do not develop a rash; and that it is common for patients to experience headaches, chills, fever, fatigue, muscle aches, and nausea.[17-19]

The second stage of Lyme disease according to Dr. Steere, develops weeks or months later. The list of possible symptoms is described as "long." Second stage symptoms commonly seen are skin, nervous system and musculoskeletal problems, and debilitating fatigue and malaise. Cardiac issues (inflammation of heart muscles and membranes, irregular beats), and fainting spells if they occur, may last days to weeks. There are also a variety of neurological symptoms including Bell's palsy (paralysis of facial nerves), meningitis, or encephalitis.[17-19]

The third stage says Dr. Steere, manifests as painful swollen joints, inflamed tendons, and muscle aches. These are arthritic problems which may occur "intermittently at first but [which] eventually become chronic." In another resource, Dr. Alan Barbour is quoted stating that patients in the early stage of infection "may prove seronegative because it can take several weeks after exposure for antibodies to be detected."[17-19]

A patent that was filed just three weeks before the Dearborn conference had this to say about Lyme disease: "Lyme disease may be missed or misdiagnosed when it does appear." The patent was Yale's invention for a Lyme vaccine and corresponding diagnostic test to detect the outer surface proteins A and B (OspA, OspB) of the Bb spirochete. The vaccine was based on these two outer surface proteins; and would be summarily excluded from CDC standardized diagnostic tests. Another patent from 2002 lists Dr. Alan Barbour as an inventor, and says:[20-23]

> "The infection, if untreated, commonly *persists for months to years* despite the occurrence of host antibody and cellular responses; this observation indicates effective evasion of the immune response. Lyme disease may be disabling (particularly in its *chronic form*), and thus there is a need for effective therapeutic and prophylactic treatment...animal studies indicate that *OspA vaccination may not be effective against all strains of Lyme disease Borreliae.*"

An Amoco Corporation patent describes nucleic acid probes that are useful to detect Bb spirochetes. The patent provides supportive statements which affirm that Lyme diagnostic tests may be inaccurate. The patent was applied for on October 27, 1993. This was exactly one year to the day before the historic Lyme disease Dearborn conference which established CDC surveillance case definitions and diagnostic test criteria for the disease. The Amoco patent has key statements that do not reflect the decisions made at Dearborn one year later, including these:

> "Lyme disease is a *serious chronic borrelial infection* characterized by a diversity of symptoms at various stages…The combination of low numbers of spirochetes and antigenically bland outer membrane yields [a] weak host immune

response..."

This means that people will not make sufficient antibodies to the organism sought by the test. The patent also says:

"Seroconversion takes some period of time after infection. During the height of spirochetemia, within weeks of the initial tick bite, a patient presenting with fever and ECM *may fail to evince antibody...*"

"The antibody response is transitory. During Stage two or Stage three, when circulating bacteria are fewest, *antibody titers may be very low*...Cell mediated immunity may detract from circulating antibody signal, that is, *classical host IgG and IgM response is decreased or absent due to masked antigens*."

How is it that the scientists who attended the Dearborn conference "did not have" this important information while a petroleum company knew all about these highly important aspects of Lyme disease a full year before the Dearborn event?[24]

In 2004, agricultural giants BASF, Bayer CropScience, Cerexagri Inc., Crompton Corporation, Dow AgroSciences, DuPont Agricultural Products, Syngenta, and others sponsored a New Haven, Connecticut Entomological Society of America annual meeting. Dr. Peter Krause (IDSA guidelines co-author) provided a presentation on *Human Babesiosis: Surveillance from the clinical side*. Dr. Durland Fish, a 2000 IDSA guidelines co-author was co-moderator of the event. Posters on display throughout the meeting covered diverse topics, and symposiums that were held discussed these seemingly Lyme-related subjects:

- Strain analysis of *Wolbachia* in plum curculio (tree fruit pest) populations in five northern states
- Habitat specificity and potential for non-targeted effects of the introduced biological control agent *Trichogramma ostriniae* (*Hymenoptera: Trichogrammatidae*)
- Termites vs. nematodes
- Resistance monitoring in the corn earworm
- Effects of transgenic field corn that expresses leptidopteran-specific insecticidal proteins on the invertebrate community
- Performance of insecticidal seed treatments for field corn in Virginia
- West Nile surveillance in Connecticut
- Mapping *Ixodes* vectors
- Inactivation and stabilization of RNA viruses (US Army Virology Div. Ft. Detrick)
- African swine fever virus: endemic vs. epidemic (USDHS Plum Island Animal Disease Center)
- Regulatory issues in biological controls
- Biological controls and entomopathogens
- GMO technology in vegetable pest management
- Sprayable pheromones (hormones)
- Managing resistance in B.t. crops and biotechnology and pest management in the Northeast[25]

It may be easy to conclude from the event that some infectious disease experts who are key to the Lyme disease story have interesting connections to biological control research. That connection may be as simple as entomology, or as complex as a relationship with a crop science corporation or laboratory; or the control of information pertaining to diseases possibly caused by recombinant insecticides.

When I mentioned earlier that Dr. Allen Steere has reported receiving at least one grant from Novartis, I felt it important to illustrate some of the agricultural patents which relate to B.t. insecticides and which list Novartis as patent assignee. We have already seen by the evidence that Bb spirochetes could be created in part from the applied or genetically engineered insecticides. If persons attending the Dearborn conference had first-hand information that a number of new agriculturally important patents were about to be filed within six months of the conference; such information could have influenced recommendations made at the event. We haven't yet considered whether the establishment of surveillance and diagnostic criteria decided upon at Dearborn was critically important to the success of B.t.-containing insecticides; especially if Lyme disease is the flagship illness caused or influenced by such products.

Just for review are some of the Novartis patents which may have connections to the history of Lyme disease. Each of these patents is assigned to the Novartis Corporation or to the Novartis Finance Corporation (NY). These primarily list North Carolina inventors, although some are additionally assigned to other parties (i.e. Ohio State University or the US Secretary of Agriculture). It is interesting that most of the patents were filed within one year of the Dearborn conference attended by a Novartis grant recipient, Dr. Allen Steere. The Dearborn conference took place on October 27-29, 1994. A flurry of new Novartis patents for B.t. were filed beginning just seven months after the Dearborn conference. Remember that Cry toxins are the crystal endotoxins of *Bacillus thuringiensis* (B.t.) insecticides.

US Patent #	Title of patent	Date filed
5,650,505	Chemically regulatable and anti-pathogenic DNA sequences and uses thereof	05/24/95
5,654,414	Chemically inducible promoter of a cucumber chitinase/lysozyme gene	05/19/95
5,686,600	Antibodies which bind to insect gut proteins and their use	05/15/95
5,689,044	Chemically inducible promoter of a plant PR-1 gene	05/24/95
5,767,369	DNA sequences encoding SAR8.2 proteins and uses thereof	05/31/95
5,770,696	Auxiliary proteins for enhancing the insecticidal activity of pesticidal proteins	06/06/95
5,777,200	Chemically regulatable and anti-pathogenic DNA sequences and uses thereof	05/31/95
5,789,214	Method of inducing gene transcription in a plant	05/31/95
5,804,693	Chemically regulatable and anti-pathogenic DNA sequences and uses thereof	05/31/95
5,840,868	Pesticidal proteins and strains (uses Cry toxins)	06/06/95
5,847,258	DNA encoding .beta.-1,3-glucanases	05/31/95
5,849,870	Pesticidal proteins and strains (uses Cry toxins)	06/05/95
5,851,766	Process for isolating chemically regulatable DNA sequences	05/31/95
5,856,154	Method of protecting plants from oomycete pathogens	05/31/95
5,859,336	Synthetic DNA sequence having enhanced activity in maize	06/02/95
5,866,326	Method for isolating vegetative insecticidal protein genes (uses Cry toxins)	06/06/95
5,872,212	Pesticidal proteins and strains (uses Cry toxins)	06/06/95
5,880,328	DNA encoding plant chitinases (enzymes to degrade insect cuticles)	05/31/95
5,888,801	Pesticidal strains of bacillus (uses Cry toxins)	06/06/95
5,889,174	Nucleotide sequences encoding pesticidal proteins. (uses Cry toxins)	06/06/95
5,990,383	Stably transformed plants comprising novel insecticidal proteins. (Cry toxins)	06/06/95
6,018,104	Nucleic acid promoter fragment isolated from a plant tryptophan synthase alpha subunit (trpA) gene	06/02/95
6,051,760	Synthetic DNA sequence having enhanced insecticidal activity in maize	06/02/95
6,069,301	Antibodies which bind to insect gut proteins and their use	06/20/95
6,075,185	Synthetic DNA sequence having enhanced insecticidal activity in maize	06/02/95
6,121,014	Method for producing a plant-optimized nucleic acid coding sequence	06/02/95
6,002,068	Methods for conferring insect resistance to a monocot using a perioxidase coding sequence	12/19/96
5,942,662	Inducible herbicide resistance	11/14/97
5,877,012	Class of proteins for the control of plant pests (Cry toxins)	04/03/97
5,885,603	Insecticidal matrix and process for preparation thereof (Cry toxins, baculoviruses)	08/07/97
6,204,246	Hybrid toxin	12/31/97
6,121,521	Chimeric insecticidal protein and DNA coding therefor	04/01/98
6,162,965	Plant transformation methods	06/02/98
6,066,783	Genes encoding insecticidal proteins (uses Cry toxins)	04/27/99
6,137,033	Class of proteins for the control of plant pests	01/20/99
6,262,342	DNA sequences encoding polypeptides having .beta.-1,3-glucanase activity	07/09/99
6,107,279	Class of proteins for the control of plant pests (uses Cry toxins)	08/22/00
6,632,981	DNA sequences encoding polypeptides having .beta.-1,3-glucanase activity	07/16/01

Again the bulk of these patents were filed within a year of the Dearborn conference, while others were filed later. Scientists will sometimes admit they have received funding from companies. But it is critical to grasp the scope of the relationships between scientists and the companies who fund them to fully appreciate what is and is not revealed as possible conflicts of interest. There is simply not enough space to accommodate the thousands of borrelia, alphavirus, B.t., and other recombinant patents that have been registered in the name of biotech, medicine, or agriculture.

The patents included here provide a glimpse of some of the kinds of inventions that could play a role in a slow-played epidemic with virtually unlimited research potential the longer adverse events remain hidden. For those who ask why anyone might wish for patients to remain ill with any disease, the answer is simply that the stronger motivator for any industry is always profit. After all, just about any chemicals or recombinant microbes deployed industrially or agriculturally carry risks of disease. The name of the biotech game may be described as *risk vs. reward.* Risks will be assessed and taken by industry and public health officials who oversee global health concerns; and will often lean toward solving industrial problems that are not necessarily clearly linked to human disease epidemics.

Choices simply must be made in order to protect our foods and other resources. However without the public's active input, the choices made will not necessarily be in the public's best interests. They will however undoubtedly benefit the industries and representatives of the world economies advocating for them as well as the objectives of the problems to be solved. Higher animals including humans thus become the innocent recipients of biotech problem-solving. The least that scientists can offer at this point in time are solutions to recombinant "accidents" when and if they are created. Those solutions however imperfect, will be antibiotics, vaccines, stem cell replacement, and other medical therapies; with the most important being acknowledgement.

I find it extremely difficult to imagine why so little progress has been made with respect to Lyme disease over the span of nearly four decades since 1975 when the disease was first publicly announced. It is harder to grasp after seeing the proliferation of medical texts, patents, and millions of dollars in grant awards; that very little progress has moved the Lyme community forward in terms of diagnostic and treatment options or meaningful cures. Insitutions generally fund only vaccine research which churns out more of the same experimental vaccines which do nothing to prevent or cure Lyme disease.

A recent database search for "Lyme disease" revealed that the NIAID alone awarded $17.3 million in grants for fiscal year 2009 for Lyme disease, and this is a small drop in the bucket. With all of the federal dollars being earmarked for research on an infection that is supposedly "over diagnosed" and "over treated," why have so few advances been made? The answer may simply be that those in receipt of the funds do not know what Lyme disease is. If they do, then they may not wish to tell the entire truth about an organism that now has a global presence. Stepping outside of consensus science leads to demotions, denied grant applications, personal threats, lawsuits, and scientific ostracization.

I studied a number of grant awards to various institutions and spin-off companies. They revealed funding awards for interests in new diagnostic tools, studies on Bb's effects on the immune system, and new vaccines. For an illness said by experts not to be chronic, but one that is "all in our heads," it is perplexing to see the subject matter of some of the current studies receiving federal research dollars. The truth is that these grants help validate decades of patient and physician claims that Bb is a serious, chronic infectious disease. The grants also provide hints that Bb may have origins as described in the pages of this book. Here are a few interesting studies that are funded by federal research dollars:

FY2009 Grant #	Awarded to	Primary Investigator	Title	Award
1R43AI081339-01	Ventria Bioscience, CO	Huang, Ning	Production of OspA in Rice for the Control of Lyme Disease	$126,530

This grant may be studying the addition of Bb lipoproteins to food crops for animal or human consumption as an oral vaccine and/or it may be studying how to bioengineer rice crops to control Lyme disease at its source, a plant. Notice the rice reference here (i.e. rice blast fungus or Magnaporthe grisea).

5R01AR040445-19	UNY Stony Brook	Benach, Jorge	*Borrelia burgdorferi*: Invasion & Chronicity	$400,577

This grant to the State University of New York, Stony Brook scientists are studying "chronic" Bb which has been argued by both sides of the debate for years. Dr. Benjamin Luft narrated a CME videotape on Lyme disease back in 1997; stating then that Lyme disease was a multi-systemic disease, and that when disseminated, could be severe and chronic.[26]

1R15AI082515-01	Humboldt State, CA	Zhong, Jianmin	A Rickettsial Symbiont Model for the Control of Tickborne Diseases	$209,795

This grant is studying rickettsial symbionts such as wolbachia, cardinium, or spiroplasmas. These are plant pathogens that are transmitted by mites, aphids, leafhoppers, and other insects (i.e. ticks, mosquitoes, bees, wasps, beetles). If Lyme patients were screened for these pathogens, the results may confirm their presence in patients. These agents are also found in nematodes.

Last we review a patent filed June 1994 for cloned Bb virulence protein(s). It was assigned to the Regents of the University of California, and created under an NIH grant. The patent represents a Bb "sample" that can be isolated from humans, cattle, or swine. The patent also discusses virulence determinant studies and a system that was used for *Treponema pallidum* and *Leptospira alstoni.* Signal peptides that contained proteins from both organisms were exported into *E. coli.* Of interest is a possible acknowledgement of a leptospiral component to Bb spirochetes. According to the patent:

> "The dosage ranges for the administration of monoclonal antibodies of the invention are those large enough to produce the desired effect in which the onset symptoms of the *leptospiral disease* are ameliorated. The dosage should not be so large as to cause adverse side effects, such as unwanted cross-reactions, anaphylactic reactions, and the like."[27]

The patent describes antigens for animal or human Lyme disease vaccines and diagnostic tests. In case you think the above "leptospiral" reference pertains to a *leptospirosis* infection, read this from the patent to clarify that it refers to Bb:

"1. Field of the Invention: This invention relates generally to an antigenic preparation and *specifically to a Borrelia*

> *burgdorferi protein* (EppA) which is used to induce a protective immune response in animals. This protein can be used immunologically *as a vaccine for Lyme disease* caused by this organism. Alternatively, diagnosis of Lyme disease can be performed by detecting the presence of the protein, antibody to the protein, or polynucleotide which encodes the protein."
>
> "2. Description of Related Art: Lyme disease is an infection with world-wide distribution caused by the spirochete *Borrelia burgdorferi*, and is the most commonly reported arthropod-borne disease in the United States. About 10,000 reported cases of Lyme disease occur every year in the United States, caused by deer-tick bites that transmit the *Borrelia burgdorferi* organism. If not identified early, by flu-like symptoms and the bull's-eye rash that usually appears at the site of infection, untreated Lyme disease can cause heart problems, arthritis, and neurological symptoms. *A large group of patients suffer from lasting neurological symptoms, including vision loss, that can recur for years as a result of Lyme disease.*"[27]

The patent acknowledges a large group of patients who suffer from lasting symptoms. This patent also appears to acknowledge that Bb is a *leptospiral* infection. Remember that Dr. Allen Steere et al. found a mutated spirochete in a Lyme patient's ECM rash culture in 1981. At that time scientists isolated a new spirochete which they named *Leptospira inadai Lyme.* The organism was eventually added to the *Leptonema* group. For some reason however, scientists have never seemed to "audibly" inform the public about the relationship of the intermediate forms of leptospira spirochetes to a human epidemic called Lyme disease. This patent was filed in June 1994, *just four months before the Dearborn conference that Dr. Steere and other experts attended.*[27]

Some Very Real Threats Lurk on the Horizon

Dr. Julie Gerberding is the former Director of the CDC. She became the new President of Merck Vaccines effective January 25, 2010. At the CDC, Dr. Gerberding was responsible for leading the CDC response to the 2001 anthrax "bioterrorism" threat. Remember that anthrax is a biological weapon of warfare and is closely related to the widely used insecticide *Bacillus thuringiensis* (B.t.). Since *B. anthracis* and *B. thuringiensis* are both created through a fermentation process using what is essentially the same soil bacterium, the agricultural pesticide B.t. might essentially be a "dumbed down" version of anthrax. The real secret to a bioterrorism "threat" for anthrax may actually be derived from agricultural applications of an anthrax-related insecticide, and not necessarily for its availability to extremist human "terrorists." It may be possible for an agricultural product to be refermented into a virulent anthrax bioweapon. If so this admittedly could be an international security threat. However the idea that anthrax is a potentially huge global threat makes far more sense when we consider that B.t. has been globally applied; and that recombinant insecticides have a greater potential to cause natural reassortments and accidental "anthrax"-like disease outbreaks.

Dr. Gerberding was previously a faculty member at the University of California-San Francisco. She was also acting Deputy Director of the NCID (National Center for Infectious Diseases). It is not surprising that she would take a position with a vaccine company. The CDC, as the government's public health agency responsible for the control of infectious diseases, has among its chief interests, the promotion of vaccines including for diseases possibly caused by the microbes of agricultural and industrial insecticides.

A co-author of the IDSA Lyme disease medical guidelines is Dr. Gerold Stanek, Professor at the Klinisches Institut für Hygiene und Medizinische Mikrobiologie der Medizinischen Univesität Wien in Austria, and member of the European Union Concerted Action on Lyme Borreliosis (EUCALB). Dr. Stanek has published alongside colleagues Drs. Gary Wormser, Franc Strle, and others. Topics of discussion have been borrelia and co-infections including *Mycoplasma pneumoniae* (a possible vaccine contaminant), babesia, anaplasma; and *Chlamydia trachomatis* infections in infertile patients. Dr. Stanek also published a paper about a leptospirosis infection which presented as carpal tunnel syndrome, and which produced IgG and IgM antibody persistence for three years.[1-5]

Oddly enough, some of the reported symptoms and pathology of Lyme disease outlined by Dr. Stanek's articles do not correlate with those described in the IDSA guidelines for Lyme disease that Dr. Stanek co-authored. Yet some comments, such as the idea that Lyme arthritis is "more prevalent" in the US than in Europe; and the mention of a "post-Lyme syndrome" do parrot the IDSA Lyme disease guidelines co-author party line. For example, the pages on the UK Health Protection Agency's web site which discuss Lyme disease quote Stanek's colleagues including Franc Strle, Allen Steere, J.J. Halperin, Gary Wormser, and Raymond Dattwyler. In the UK, public health officials follow the American IDSA guidelines edict for Lyme disease. This may be one reason why Lyme patients in the EU find themselves ignored by public health agencies, just as US patients are often dismissed by physicians after treatment according to IDSA guidelines recommendations.[6-10]

A colleague of Dr. Stanek is Dr. Raymond Dattwyler. Like Stanek, Dattwyler is a co-author of the IDSA medical guidelines for Lyme disease. Dr. Dattwyler is also listed on an important new US patent for a live bacterial vaccine. The patent describes a *Lactobacillus bacterium* (strain *L. plantarum* 256). The bacterium is genetically engineered to express Bb OspA proteins. This may be a B.t., fungal, or spiroplasma protein; and makes sense since we are exposed to B.t. pesticides in raw and processed foods.[11]

Lactobacillus is used as a starter culture for lactic acid fermentation. Soil bacteriae create lactic acid, including a strain called *Bacillus laevolacticus.* The invention may include proteins (polypeptides) from the *Yersinia pestis* bacterium. This is a gut bacterium (enterobacteria) that is the very same **bubonic plague** bacterium (Black Death) that in the mid-1300s killed roughly one-third of the European population or roughly 50-75 million people. The bubonic plague comes in three forms, pneumonic, bubonic, and septicemic. If there is anyone with a mindset of reducing the world's total population numbers, then a plague bacterium would certainly be the tool to do so. This is of course not the same as saying that anyone plans such a terrible thing. But imagine if a recombinant accident occurs after deploying this microbe in a recombinant insecticide. The global population would be left to fend for themselves against a deadly pathogen for which humans have no natural immunity.[11]

Why would a Lyme disease medical guidelines co-author and infectious disease scientist design a patent for vaccines and diagnostic tests useful against bubonic plague? **Perhaps it is because novel biological controls are about to be genetically engineered to contain the plague microbe; and the consequence for its use within insecticides will be a necessary human vaccine and diagnostic test.** Are scientists such as Dr. Dattwyler anticipating a plague-type human epidemic that will come about due to the very same vectoring insects that already transmit *Borrelia burgdorferi*? Will insects and arthropods soon transmit a recombinant insecticide that contains a genetically manipulated bubonic plague virus? What might become of human health if such a construct were to fail? Remember that "failure" refers to entering the animal and human populations, not the insect populations. And over time, what enters the insect world also enters the greater "animal" kingdom.

When searching for the answers to these very sensitive questions in a US patent database, no less than 600 patent applications returned under the terms "*Yersinia pestis*" and "insect." One of the patent applications was another Dattwyler et al. application for an oral vaccine for *Borrelia burgdorferi.* This vaccine patent described a *lactobacillus* to be used in combination with OspA and OspC proteins from Bb; and which may be used with *E. coli* or *Yersinia pestis* (bubonic plague).

This describes designs for *an oral vaccine for a tick or other insect-borne bubonic plague*. Such a vaccine might be implemented in a two-step process. First people would ingest the lactobacillus as a digestive bacterium meant to be "good for us" (i.e. yogurt). The second step might involve the separate ingestion of another recombinant product that contains an engineered oral vaccine with microbes including bubonic plague. Perhaps the intent is to engineer such microbes directly into plants so humans no longer need "bother" themselves with any vaccines. The engineering of vaccines, insecticides, and microbes directly into our foods not only eliminates freedom of choice as to what enters our bodies; the techniques may be in violation of the Hague agreement (or its intent) against the use of weapons of biological warfare. They also make the human species not too far removed from the laboratory mice upon which most of these processes are first tested. What happens if recombinant oral vaccines are also contaminated with adventitious agents; or worse, become reactivated through a natural recombinant accident in the years to come, to cause a global human epidemic?[12]

Another patent application describes the creation of antibody-directed insecticides that will specifically target microbes inside the bodies of animals, humans, or insects. The formulas could be applied as bactericidal enzymes, as IgA, IgE, IgG, or IgM receptor molecules (antibodies), insecticides, or other formulas. The patent discusses food contamination issues with *E. coli* or *Listeriosis* but fails to define the "national defense" reference. These proteins may be used in transgenic animals, transgenic plants, transgenic microbes (insecticides), or animal or human vaccines. We may guess this represents protection against recombinant microbes or toxins which accidentally reassort and cause disease. The patent describes the use of encephalomyocarditis virus, simian [monkey] cytomegalovirus, and Rous sarcoma virus in combination with other microbes to target pathogens which might include Bb, plague, or even prion disease agents.[13]

Eleven US patent applications are listed in a database search under "*Yersinia pestis*" and "biological control." It appears that scientists are targeting insects with an historically dangerous microbe, to kill moths and other insects. This means that applied and transgenic insecticides *are* possible and may use a recombinant plague microbe. The chimera could then be released into the environment with unknown consequences to the non-target animal and human species, where Lyme notable Dr. Dattwyler's patent might prove to be not only useful, but highly profitable.

One patent application describes the use of nematodes as trojan horses to deliver bacteriae into the body of targeted insects through defecation. The released bacteriae will kill the insect, and nematodes will parasitize the dead insects. Thereafter they will reproduce and kill more insects. Among the bacteriae carried by the nematodes will be *Yersinia pestis*, the plague bacterium. Dr. Dattwyler et al. seem to be anticipating the need for a plague vaccine and corresponding diagnostic test because the very same insects which transmit current human diseases *may soon transmit the worst epidemics in human history*.[14,15]

To illustrate this valid concern we should look at the recent manipulation of the plague virus for vaccine constructs. In

September 2009 Molecular Geneticist Malcolm Casadaban of the University of Chicago died as a result of his work with a "weakened laboratory strain" of *Yersinia pestis.* The strain was in development as a vaccine. According to a news article, the CDC had approved the weakened strain for laboratory studies. The new Dattwyler et al. patent for a recombinant plague was filed on December 31, 2009, just three months after Dr. Casadaban's death.[14]

We can imagine the consequences of another failed OspA-based invention, this time a Bb-lactobacillus-plague vaccine that may not only have the potential to cause a treatment-resistant form of arthritis in susceptible people much like the first generation OspA Lyme vaccine probably did, but far worse. Will we see a treatment-resistant plague bacterium that will cause untold sickness and death tolls? Worse, any adventitious agents that might be present in cell lines used to create such a vaccine might have the potential to cause the reactivation of one of the most deadly pathogens on the planet, with unimaginable consequences.

I really don't want to think about a biological Armageddon of this magnitude. The problem may not be simply the development of a recombinant plague. Plague is a *naturally occurring infection of rodents* and other feral animals. As such, it is already present in the environment and fully capable of reassorting with any of the recombinant microbes that have already been deployed in B.t. and other insecticides. The advent of a plague vaccine may be a necessity and not a whim because recombinant agricultural and industrial tools may already be causing most of the disease epidemics of our day. The introduction of recombinant plague may cause a reassortment of a natural plague to cause any of the known, or an unknown plague. The biggest secret of the biotech industries may be simply that genetic engineering techniques are flawed, and there is no way to predict or control what happens once engineered microbes enter the environment. What is created in the laboratory to reactivate insect infections may do the same in higher animals, and this process *is not able to be controlled by laboratory scientists, except in theory.*

Another disturbing patent reveals the recovery of ancient organisms and biological materials from fossilized amber sources that are *tens of millions of years old.* One such patent was granted in 1997 to a San Francisco company. The ancient organisms are isolated from amber fossils that are recovered anywhere in the world. These unpredictabe organisms could be useful in agricultural and industrial processes as well as medicines. As described in the patent:

> "The present invention relates to the recovery of ancient organisms and biological materials from sources capable of preserving such biological materials and organisms for many millions of years…more specifically…from amber and similar naturally-occurring resins."
>
> "Various uses for these ancient microorganisms are envisioned, including their use in *agriculture, industrial processes, bioremediation, diagnostic and disease treatment*...Such microorganisms include but are not limited to bacteria, fungi, protozoa, viruses and microalgae...the present invention is directed to the recovery of ancient organisms and biological matter from amber and similar naturally occurring resins, including pollen, plants, arthropods of different groups and nematodes."[16]

The logic behind the search for, and recovery of these materials is explained within the patent:

> "Changing patterns in animal and human health, *agricultural, industrial and environmental processes* demand a search for new sources of microbial by-products for medical, diagnostic and industrial applications. For example, numerous pathogenic microorganisms have become resistant to antibiotics currently derived from modern microorganisms…"[16]

Please note that the antibiotic-resistance problem has been created largely by the methods to create genetically engineered insecticides and other microbes useful to industries.

> "Similarly, many widely used *agrochemicals* have been shown to be toxic to flora and fauna and to cause *contamination to water resources.* Growing resistance to traditional antimicrobial compounds, new demands created by modern industrial processes, the need to develop alternatives to chemical pesticides and herbicides, and the need to eliminate environmental contaminants create opportunities for using novel microbes and their by-products."[16]

Note the references which admit to polluted water, toxic chemicals, and the flora and fauna including microbes that are adversely affected by same. These tools may be used to bioremediate acid mine and industrial wastes; for agricultural and industrial insecticides; and as vaccines, gene therapy tools, or antibiotics. Ancient microbes will make their way not only into the insect populations, but also into the human food chain and the human body by vectoring insects and contaminated animal products. The patent describes how ancient microorganisms may be *recovered and revived to a viable state even after being fossilized in amber or other resins for twenty-five to forty million years!*[16]

This once again speaks to the **reanimation of extinct microbes upon exposure to and donation of live, compatible genetic material.** We can't even begin to understand what caused the extinction of dinosaurs, or what kinds of pathogenic organisms lived during the periods surrounding their extinction. Imagine the extremophiles and cyanobacteriae that thrived in the acidic volcanic environment of eons ago. Do we really want unknown and very ancient organisms in our bodies in the form of vaccines, human biologicals, or agricultural or industrial insecticides? It seems that with this kind of microbial prospecting, that logic and reasoning have already flown out the laboratory window.

What we do know about ancient organisms comes from German amber specimens. From these, soil and insect debris have been recovered that contained *Bacillus subtilis*-like gram-positive bacteria. According to the patent,

> "In a particular embodiment of the invention, described more fully below, *more than a dozen viable strains of ancient Bacillus bacteria* were isolated from the preserved *abdominal cavity tissues of four ancient stingless bees*, Proplebeia dominicana, fossilized in Dominican amber some 25 to 40 million years ago."[16]

What lies within the midgut tissues and intracellular spaces of ancient insects can only be imagined. Keep in mind that known and unknown viruses, microsporidiae, bacteriae and other parasites are already present in modern day insects. These organisms appear to be mutating at the hands of genetically engineered microbes of the present day. Imagine what will happen when ancient organisms meet modern diseases?

Unknown life forms from insects, arthropods, and plants that are millions of years old may unleash indescribable epidemics within our lifetime if current GM trends continue unchecked.

On the flip side, such microbes might offer renewed hope for curative therapies for some of the ills of our modern day. On the other hand, they may also be capable of causing a global epidemic that will herald the extinction of mankind. While this seems an extremist viewpoint, we must ask ourselves who can accurately predict the manner in which the biological scales will be tipped? Should scientists be allowed to manipulate current or future organisms that are tens of millions of years old in a quest for ever more powerful insecticides and vaccines *just because they can*? Should ancient microbes that are for all intents and purposes extinct, be tampered with for any reason; or are these best left entirely alone?

The longer the biotech industry is allowed to practice unregulated or loosely regulated techniques without serious restraint and oversight, the greater the potential will be for the accidental deployment of microbes and unimaginable diseases. Even with the best intent, recombinant "accidents" as they are described in scientific patents can, have, and will continue to emerge and may cause novel diseases. When we consider the possibility that future "weapons of mass destruction" may be derived from recombinant tools developed from ancient or synthetic organisms with unknown potential (including the ability to drive mass extinctions), then such explorations must be carefully considered before they lead to a biological Armageddon of global and permanent proportions.

Time and again the connections between the various biological controls that have been deployed require the invention of "curative" vaccines. The creation of vaccines is supposed to be driven by diseases which already exist; not by those that have yet to be realized, created by triggers that are first created in a laboratory and then released into the environment as insecticides.

We repeatedly find direct evidence that industries, their academic partners, and genetically engineered products seem to be the driving force behind many human diseases of our day. This is blatantly obvious from numerous patents for transgenes and other biological controls which also include methods for vaccines and diagnostic tools that become necessary upon a product's deployment. The scientists who invent these tools are the first to admit that the technologies are inherently flawed. The problem is that the public and legislators seem to be largely unaware of the risks and the benefits of using recombinant tools.

Whatever the original hopes or intent, the unfortunate reality is that not only have scientists created insect epizootics that have failed to control pests throughout the world; they also seem to have helped insects proliferate, and have created antibiotic-resistant and mutated microbes as well as new animal and human epidemics. If allowed to continue along the same trends that have been deployed over the past century, the future biowarfare and related tools will, as they probably have done in the past, generate novel diseases (and biotech profits) for generations to come.

Arsenic and Old Lace

During the late 1700s, President of Yale University Dr. Ezra Stiles wore official silk robes made from his own silkworms. I found this interesting as I studied the history of the textile industry. Ornate lace and braids in silk, flax, cotton, or gold plate (or other metals) were and are used to trim the robes and uniforms of academic, clergy, and military officials. The history of lace goes back at least to the 14th century in *Flanders,* an area between France and Belgium. Eventually it made its way across Europe and elsewhere. We have already learned about the history of silk manufacturing, and the *paenibacillus* and other extremophile microbes that live in insects including silkworms and Japanese beetles. Centuries later, Yale scientists would publish papers on important extremophiles including those that affect silkworms.

Drs. Lennette and Spaulding knew about the *Flavobacterium* extremophiles in 1974, but they were first described by Bergey et al. in 1923. This was the period when the early parasitoid insects were being imported into the US as natural biological controls. Dr. Edwin H. Lennette was an Army Epidemiologist who worked at the Rockefeller Foundation on viral diseases from the 1930s to the 1940s. He went to Ft. Detrick for a time, and by 1973 he was Chief of the Viral and Rickettsial laboratory at the California State Department of Health. Dr. Lennette also gave a presentation on the New York rickettsialpox outbreak of 1946. This was the human outbreak caused by the aerosolized microbes from rodent mites and urine-soaked garbage. Lennette also discussed the new "blue" disease of Japanese beetles (*Coxiella popilliae*).

Flavobacterium are found in acid mine wastes, by mining areas, near metal smelters, geothermal veins and springs, and in environments where blasting, nuclear, fireworks, and military munitions are manufactured, tested, stored (if leaking), or deployed. These bacteriae are among the few that are able to utilize arsenic compounds as well as phosphates.

Mulberry trees which silkworms (and sheep) use for food; produce berries with trace levels of organic arsenic compounds. Mulberry trees grow well when flavobacterium and other nitrogen-fixing bacteriae are present. Mulberry trees are among the few plants which produce *phenolic* compounds (phenols). This stimulates the bacteriae to degrade organic and inorganic polyphenols (i.e. PCBs, PHA) in the environment. This means that mulberry trees produce compounds that help bacteriae bioremediate toxic metals, metalloids, and other materials. This is important because not only do the trees take up toxic materials, their bacteriae also feed off same. Insects or animals that consume mulberry tree leaves are on the receiving end of mulberry-beneficial microbes. Unfortunately in the case of sheep, the combination of soil bacteria plus extremophiles under fermentation of the sheep gut creates *Bacillus anthracis* or anthrax. Microbes commonly beneficial to mulberry trees include these, many of which are deployed as recombinant insecticides and GM crops:[1-17]

Pseudomonas (gammaproteobacteria)
Flavobacterium (extremophiles)
Micrococcus (saprotrophic bacteria)
Arthrobacter (Actinomycetes bacteria)
Azotospirillum (nitrogen fixer bacteria)
Biejerinckia (nitrogen fixer bacteria)
Acetobacter (bacteria, converts ethanol to acetic acid)
Achromobacter (proteobacteria)
Bacillus megaterium (and other bacilli species)
Azotobacter (slime bacteria)
Aspergillus (mold)
Glomus (fungi)

In 1926 scientists fed mature, fifth instar silkworm larvae droplets of arsenic to study the uptake and speed of toxic action of arsenic in the insects. Studies were probably aimed at methods of controlling the pests, which were widespread in the northeast at the time. The paper referenced older papers including a 1917 study of goldfish by Urbana, Illinois scientists. In that text we find that citrus crops and tomatoes that were fumigated with *hydrocyanic acid* (HCN) produced larger fruit than non-treated crops. This acid is extremely toxic to insects, animals, and humans.[18,19]

HCN also increases germination in treated seeds; and causes *scale* insect eggs to hatch earlier than normal. The protoplasm or *cytoplasm* holds the contents of a cell and is surrounded by a plasma membrane. Cystine, an amino acid that is an organosulfur compound, and the protoplasm become contaminated by arsenic and other toxins. Cystine is linked to cellular respiration. Remember the CPVs, or *cytoplasmic polyhedrosis viruses*? These include the *reoviruses that infect the cytoplasm of insect and plant cells*. When bothered by oxidative stress, infections, or chemical toxins, the cellular membrane is damaged and the contents spill out of the cell to cause bacteremia (systemic infection). This also enables any intracellular co-infections to be spread through the bite of a vectoring insect.[18,19]

The *Cypo-Flavobacterium* family are phagic bacteriae that invade the *cytoplasm* of cells. They have many family members, and belong to the *Paenibacillus* group of extremophiles. For example we find the infection *Paenibacillus larvae,* which causes American foulbrood disease in honey bees. In this same family we find the milky spore agents *Bacillus popilliae, B. lentimorbus* (and others). The flavobacterium are relatives of other important soil bacteria, namely *Bacillus thuringiensis* (B.t.), and *Bacillus anthracis* (anthrax). This group of spore-forming bacteriae also include other extremophiles, thermophiles; acidophiles such as *Deinococcus radiodurans,* and other radiation-resistant bacteriae.

Flavobacterium are known sulfur and nitrogen reducers. They are found in extreme conditions including water (i.e. polluted wastewaters, industrial flows, acid mine wastes); and soils (i.e. agricutural, industrial, mines, munitions). These bacteriae are supported in conditions where sulfur, nitrates, nitrites, arsenic, copper, uranium, and phosphorus compounds are found. The denitrifying soil bacteriae produce nitrous oxide and they have pro-inflammatory properties. *Borrelia burgdorferi* spirochetes are also known to stimulate nitric oxide production in the human body, which releases pro-inflammatory hormones (cytokines). Among the soil denitrifiers are *Brucella, Flavobacterium, Pseudomonas, Ralstonia,* and other species.[20-24]

Some of the flavobacterium produce a *yellow* pigment. These could be our "yellows" disease agents. These bacteriae are from the *Cytophaga* group, which means they are phages (phagic) to other bacteria and will damage the cytoplasm of cells.

They literally eat their way into the inside to infect cells. Any cells that become infected with these bacteriae will spill their co-infected cell contents (viruses, bacteria) into the blood stream. Cytophages are known to cause meningitis and bacteremia (septicemia) in insects (i.e. silkworms, Japanese beetles), animals (i.e. rodents, birds, horses), and humans.

Flavobacterium have also been attributed to *moon blindness*, an eye problem (uveitis) in horses and cattle that was identified as early as 1929. Perhaps this is why *equine encephalitis viruses* came about in 1938 in Connecticut ring-neck pheasants shortly after the first applications of *Bacillus popilliae* and *Bacillus lentimorbus* spores as early applied insecticides. These bacteriae may have been infected (or affected) by soil phages; causing an animal EEE infection.[25-31]

Once again in 1953, two years after the 1951 introduction of *Borrelina reoviruses* in Connecticut, (which are cypoviruses), there was another outbreak of EEE in Connecticut ring-neck pheasants. This occurred in an area endemic for the same kind of mites that would be associated with a 1946 outbreak of human rickettsialpox in New York. I think we are beginning to see a possible relationship between applied insecticides and animal and human outbreaks with phagic bacteria and viruses; or *intra-cellular* viruses and bacteria that infect the cytoplasm of cells and the microbes that enter them.[25-31]

Flavobacterium are gram-negative and can be found in water and soils, in foods, plants, fish, birds, humans, livestock including pigs; and wild animals (i.e. rodents and deer). I found an incredibly revealing 2005 paper from the University of Connecticut and Rutgers University which discussed intracellular symbionts and other bacteriae associated with deer ticks. The paper described symbionts found in *Ixodes scapularis* ticks that were collected from Nantucket, and Wellfleet, Cape Cod, Massachusetts from June to July of 2002. Among the many symbionts found in the ticks were the *Cytophaga-Flavobacterium-Bacteroides* soil bacillus bacteriae (phages).[32,33]

The paper's authors noted that these bacteriae "recently have been implicated in parthenogenesis of parasitoid wasps and phytophagous mites." Parthenogenesis is the ability to reproduce without need of a male. This may also mean that scientists are aware that the same mites that were implicated in the rickettsialpox, and EEE outbreaks (NY-humans, CT-pheasants); and the parasitoid wasps (i.e. those released on Naushon Island, etc. during the 1920s), also harbor the same *flavobacterium* that may be found in Lyme disease-transmitting *Ixodes scapularis* ticks collected from these areas. Remember that these wasps also harbored *polydna viruses* that have the ability to *alter the genes of the host cells they invade.*[34]

> *It is incredibly odd however that the intracellular cypoviruses and the flavobacterium of insects are always "over-looked" as possible contributing infections in Lyme disease or any other illnesses.*

The paper very carefully acknowledges the presence of "CFB," the *Cytophaga-Flavobacterium-Bacteroides,* yet appears to minimize its name by abbreviation, and by referring to it as an "endosymbiont" instead of identifying it by strain as all the other bacteriae listed in the paper. This distinctive handling of such an apparently important group of pathogens seems most peculiar. By the time of this 2004 paper, there were many strains of *Flavobacterium* that had been identified. Perhaps these bacteriae are never "audibly" mentioned because they are known to be part of an aggregate spirochete called *Borrelia burgdorferi.* If so, this is important because B.t. strains are members of the Cytophaga-Flavobacterium-Bacteroides family. Not only can B.t. strains be isolated from the human gut, most likely from dietary exposures; but these globally important agricultural tools are making their way into the human body by insects that also transmit Lyme disease.[35,36,39]

When I researched the strain numbers for the "CFB" flavobacterium provided by the 2004 paper, I found one hundred and sixty species listed. The results could not have been more vague. However it is easy to look at the list and decipher what could be of interest for insecticidal purposes. I located seven *clones* which included *Bacillus thuringiensis* subspecies *kurstaki.* The kurstaki strains target only needle and leaf-eating caterpillars.[37,38]

The B.t. clones I examined were deposited by the Monsanto Company. Other clones in the list were *Flavobacterium okea-nokoites* (Zobell and Upham 1944) deposited by New England Biolabs Inc.; and *Deinococcus radiodurans* (ex Raj et al. 1960) Brooks and Murray strains (1981). This latter strain is an important extremophile. Deinococcus as we know is detectable using a 1993 Amoco patent invention that also detects *Borrelia burgdorferi.* Note the dates of isolation of these organisms are 1960 and 1981 respectively. The latter strain could represent an extremophile that was isolated from the Lyme disease agent *Borrelia burgdorferi* and then was cloned and deposited into the culture database, while scientists were attempting to decipher exactly what comprised the Bb organism – studies that were undertaken in 1981 by Burgdorfer, Barbour, et al.[37,38]

Another clone listed was *Elizabethkingia miricola,* a strain that was formerly known as *Flavobacterium meningosepticum.* This is a strain that causes meningitis and encephalitis in animals and humans. It could represent a strain that causes encephali-tis outbreaks such as EEE or the encephalitis of deer. One of the B.t. strains (kurstaki) that were deposited by Monsanto, hints at the purpose of the culture. The organisms that can be specifically infected with B.t. clones include these, which are found in soil, plants, and insects:

Pseudomonas *Agrobacterium* *Rhizobium*
Erwinia *Azotobacter* *Azospirillum*
Klebsiella *Alcaligenes* *Flavobacterium*

These are members of the flavobacterium family, and **so is B.t. and the milky spore agents.** Patents referenced by the clones include: Monsanto B.t. clones: #5,229,112; New England Biolabs, Inc. clone *Flavobacterium okeanokoites:* #4,999,294; Genzyme Corp. *Elizabethkingia miricola* clone: #5,238,821 (f/k/a *Flavobacterium meningosepticum*). The three *Deinococcus radiodurans* clones from the Institute for Genomic Research also use flavobacterium including *F. meningosepticum.* This means that the radiation-resistant *Deinococcus radiodurans* that can be detected by the Amoco "Bb" patent probably also contains a *Flavobacterium meningosepticum,* <u>which is a strain that causes meningitis and encephalitis in animals and humans</u>. If *Deinococcus radiodurans* is a recombinant thermophile, it is a mutant that could be "contaminated" with B.t. spores or another extremophile.[40,41]

The presence of B.t., a *Leptospire,* and a *Flavobacterium* in an aggregate Bb spirochete could explain why I was according to the doctor, an hour or two from death in a hospital emergency room in 2002 when I had septicemia. It also explains why I responded so well to treatment using high-dose intravenous Keflex (cephalexin). According to a 1972 Japanese patent, this drug can be derived from bacterial enzymes of *Alcaligenes, Achromobacter, Bacillus, Beneckea,* or *Flavobacterium.* Keflex is a first-generation cephalosporin antibiotic first introduced in 1967 by Eli Lilly and Company. This of course is the very same year that Dr. Burgdorfer identified the "277F" rabbit tick agent – and rabbit dung was the scurce of *Flavobacterium meningosepticum* discussed previously. [42-45]

Keflex is a drug that physicians might wish to evaluate for its clinical usefulness in treating Lyme disease. Other cephalosporins are used to treat Lyme patients, but their effectiveness varies. Since Keflex is also useful to treat some pathogenic *Leptospira* strains, it appears interesting that it worked so well in myself.[42-45]

We might also note that members of the cytophaga-flavobacterium-bacteroides group have been found to be intracellular symbiont infections of the *Acanthamoebae.* This is key if these amoeba are part of some Bb strains, because not only are the amoeba antibiotic resistant and rapidly fatal, their intracellular infections, as extremophiles are also hard to kill. The difference between a disseminated case of Lyme, CJD, or another neurologic illness that is unresponsive to antibiotics and rapidly fatal may be the absence or presence of an acanthamoeba strain. Most if not all Bb strains probably harbor a flavobacterium (i.e. B.t., milky spore agent). Those that are infrequently fatal (or that cause prion diseases) may carry a flavobacterium-infected acanthamoeba or its genes.[110]

We see now that several important *Flavobacterium* strains are widely used in genetic engineering processes, especially insecticides. Several strains have been isolated from Lyme disease-transmitting ticks (i.e. deer and wood ticks). According to a gene database, the plasmids (mini chromosomes) which belong to the Monsanto B.t. clones we discussed previously are useful to combat plant pests using plant-colonizing microorganisms that contain B.t. toxin genes "*as a chromosomal insertion.*" I think we can all imagine the consequences of B.t. plasmids that reassort with other bacteria and viruses that are found in co-infected plants and insects. We can see how airborne spores from applied insecticides or acanthamoeba may contaminate other important bacteriae including those in acid mines, wastewaters, soils, or water flows. After all the sporulating B.t. is designed to infect insects, and to introduce and reactivate diseases. There is only a problem if microbes from insecticides and other recombinant products enter the human body by ingestion, inhalation, or by vectoring insects to cause diseases.[46-48]

Some of the *Flavobacterium* that were identified by 1959, two years after Dr. Burgdorfer first identified a rabbit tick spiroplasma 277F agent, include these:

Flavobacterium arborescens *F. aquatile* (from a water sample)
F. aurantiacum *F. denitrificans*
F. esteroaromaticum *F. flavescens*
F. suaveolens *F. suphureum*
F. resinovorum (degrades rosin; sample from Paris, France)
Pseudomonas putrificans (formerly classified as *Flavobacterium*)
An unidentified *Flavobacterium* species from Bloomington, Indiana
Erwinia carotovora and *Xanthomonas campestris* (from ICI and Akers Lab, England)
Flavobacterium meningosepticum (serologic strains A-C, which caused neonatal meningitis)

By 1961, a new strain that causes neonatal meningitis was isolated from human cerebrospinal fluid and classified as *Flavobacterium meningosepticum.* Novel species of *Flavobacterium multivorum* and *F. spiritivorum* were isolated in 1981 and 1982 respectively, from human clinical samples. This of course is the same period of time when Bb was first identified and then announced as the causative agent of Lyme disease. Several strains were isolated from clinical specimens during the late 1970s, and were reclassified, perhaps as part of a retrospective survey of "Lyme" patient serum. There was in fact, a retrospective study of Lyme patients undertaken during the late 1970s by Yale's Dr. Allen Steere and colleagues. They reexamined the research from fifty-one of the original Connecticut patients who presented with "juvenile arthritis." At the time they also compared samples against other important agents which included arboviruses, leptospires, spiroplasmas, rickettsias, and *Babesia microti,* an intracellular malaria-like infection. Malaria is caused by a *Flavobacterium* strain, and it would appear that intracellular symbionts including flavobacterium are well-known by scientists. We can see the link between some common Lyme co-infections and members of the cytophaga-flavobacterium-bacteroides group.[49-57]

There is evidence for horizontal gene transfers (gene swapping) between *Bacteroidetes* bacteriae and dinoflagellates. We already discussed "CFB," the tick-isolated *Cytophaga-Flavobacterium-Bacteroides* bacterium. The *Bacteroidetes* are a subclass of the CFB group (phylum). The dinoflagellates are the tiny bacteriae that are found in marine algae blooms and that are responsible for red tides. What is interesting is that the CFB's resemble long uncoiled spirochetes. The dinoflagellates have cellulose plates that act like armor and flagella which propel them. Some dinoflagellates produce neurotoxins, and have been noted during natural fish kills (i.e. *Pfiesteria*).[58-62]

In 1989 scientists from the Pasteur Institute in Paris were studying the gene patterns or "fingerprints" of bacteriae including (gut) enterobacteria; and *Pseudomonas, Acinetobacter, Brucella,* and *Leptospires.* Another paper described gene sequencing to study surface receptors of bacteria. Scientists were keenly studying the very same bacterial combinations that appear to be part of an aggregate Bb spirochete. This includes *Leptospira* (spirochetes), *Coxiella* (*Cytophaga*), and *Bacillus anthracis* (or the closely related B.t. which are *Flavobacterium*).[61-66]

Scientists have been trying to determine how bacterial genes are horizontally or laterally exchanged. One paper studied the *Bacillus anthracis* (anthrax) strain "Ames Ancestor;" *Bacillus cereus,* and *B. thuringiensis* serovar konkukian; as well as *Cytophaga hutchinsonii,* and the pathogenic *Leptospira interrogans.* (This is the exact model for Bb: leptospira-B.t.-Cytophaga/ Flavobacterium). A more recent study examined the ability of leptospires to survive in the company of *Flavobacterium* species. The scientists also studied persistence in biofilms of the pathogenic *Leptospira interrogans* strains. Since the *Paenibacillus* and *Flavobacterium* are slime formers, we can see where the biofilms might come from. Flavobacterium are sensitive to tetracyclines and rifampicin. However according to research, B.t. clones are commonly engineered to be antibiotic resistant. If they become part of an aggregate organism, this resistance could make them much harder to treat.[61-66,92,93]

Dr. Alan Barbour is listed on about one hundred Bb-related patents. He also published a paper with colleagues in 2007 that described a "*Coxiella* species" bacterial endosymbiont that was highly prevalent in laboratory-reared and field-collected Lone Star ticks (*Amblyomma americanum*). These ticks transmit a Lyme-like infection that is said to be "different" than Lyme disease; and is identified as "STARI" or Southern Tick-Associated Rash Illness. Dr. Barbour consistently identifies the agent as "Coxiella sp." (sp. means species) It appears that Lone Star ticks harbor a flavobacterium the likes of *Coxiella popilliae.* In modern times it is known as *Bacillus popilliae,* the famed "blue" disease of Japanese beetle larvae which is caused by an agent of "milky spore" disease.[67-69]

Since the STARI infections are said to be similar but not identical to Lyme, we can see how the difference between *Bacillus popilliae* and *Bacillus thuringiensis* might cause similar, but not exactly identical infections. It may also mean that the *Ehrlichiosis*-like infections which first surfaced in the US in 1942 and 1943 at Camp Bullis may have been caused by the flavobacterium *Bacillus popilliae.* Other human *Ehrlichiosis* infections may be assisted by another flavobacterium strain such as *Bacillus thuringiensis* or *Bacillus sphaericus* for example.[67-69]

A 2002 Yale University study described the amino acid activation of various bacteria. Among those studied were: *Saccharomyces cerevisiae, Borrelia burgdorferi, Cytophaga hutchinsonii, Deinococcus radiodurans,* and *Thermus thermophilus.* If you have paid attention to the names of the microbes in this book, you may see which may be part of an aggregate Bb spirochete, and why scientists are studying them. We can see hints at extremophiles from many Bb-related patents.[70]

A 1955 study revealed that a strain of *Myxobacterium* was classified in the genus *Cytophaga* under the name *Cytophaga fermentans* novel species. The myxobacteriae are not true bacteria, since they lack flagella and a rigid cell wall (wall-less). The cytophaga were assembled into a single genus in 1942 at the start of the War Research Service and "biological warfare" studies. There are various strains which degrade cellulose, chitin, or agar (marine). Perhaps the soil version of one bacterium is *Cytophaga fermentens,* while the version that infects plants, animals, and humans is the well-known *Mycoplasma fermentens.* The name of a microbe changes based on the host from which it was isolated. For example, a soil bacteria may have a different name when cultured from an insect, than the name assigned when isolated from a human being. Another paper similarly discusses the *Mycobacterium, Cytophaga,* and *Borrelia burgdorferi.* If there were no connections between these bacteriae, then we might not expect them to be discussed together in so many sources.[71,72]

The bacterium *Agrobacterium tumefaciens* is used in genetic engineering, and to deliver B.t. insecticide genes to GM plants. It is a yeast-like bacterium that can degrade simple aromatic compounds that are related to wood, called *lignins*. Examples are phenols, corn cobs, and the chemical nitrobenzene which is used to manufacture aniline (and is a flavoring or perfume additive). Other denitrifying bacteriae also share this same "remediation" talent. We might expect to see deer, rodents, and "wood" ticks capable of contracting flavobacterium or other denitrifying bacteriae from the habitats they share. We might also expect to find *Pseudomonas, Agrobacterium, Flavobacterium, phages, leptospires,* and other microbes in a Bb aggregate bacterium that causes Lyme and the related Mogellon's disease.[73-78]

Flavobacterium can synthesize sulfite liquors and other wastes. After treating wood chips with sulfuric acid salts, sulfite liquors are produced. This creates wood pulp that has been converted to cellulose fibers. The cellulose is used for paper (i.e. tissues, newsprint); textiles (i.e. rayon, acetate); cellophane tape; acetate film or tapes; and methylcellulose (i.e. adhesives, pharmaceuticals, baked goods). Sulfite byproducts include mannose, which can be fermented for ethanol; and lignosulfonates. These are used to tan leather hides, to create a water soluble transport vehicle for insoluble materials, to produce artificial vanilla for baking, artificial flavors for foods and beverages, and for concrete, drilling, drywall, and fertilizers or soil amendments. The sulfite liquor process was invented in 1840 by F.G. Keller in Germany. The very first commercial sulfite pulp mill was built in Sweden in 1874. In 1909 the first ECM rash illnesses would be reported by Swedish Dermatologist Arvid Afzelius.[79-84]

Herbicides and other agricultural products promote the growth of flavobacterium species, especially under the influence of phosphates and certain heavy metals. Agent blue, a rainbow herbicide used by the US military during the Vietnam War, is a mixture of two arsenic-containing compounds, cacodylic acid and sodium cacodylate. Cacodylic acid and its compounds are known teratogens (cause birth defects). Over a million gallons were sprayed in Vietnam, including on rice paddies as an anti-crop agent.[86]

Chemical herbicides are used on lawns and crops today, including golf courses and private lawns. They are also sprayed on cotton before harvest to remove the leaves and allow cleaner processing. The EPA listed Agent blue as one of the top ten toxic herbicides, insecticides, and fungicides – chemicals that have been partly deregulated. Chemical herbicidal residues are found in meat, milk, poultry, and eggs; and may be detected in cooking oils or cattle and poultry feed additives. Agent blue is an arsenic-containing herbicide that supports the growth of bacteriae which utilize arsenic in their cellular processes. When arsenic is unavailable, it seems these bacteriae can substitute phosphates and vice versa.[86]

Other arsenic compounds are also used as feed additives for poultry, including arsonic acid (4-hydroxy-3-nitrobenzenearsonic acid or "3-Nitro") under the name *Roxarsone*. Recently the FDA allowed a Pfizer subsidiary to continue selling the product for a month before pulling the product from the market. It was discontinued due to high levels of inorganic arsenic that were detected in chickens fed arsenic acid-containing feeds. The additive has been used for many years to help poultry gain weight and to protect them from *Coccidiosis* infections. Other similar arsenic-containing feed additives are used in pigs.[87-90]

There appears to be evidence that toxic arsenic can replace the essential nutrient phosphorus in the biomolecules of bacteriae. This means that instead of using phosphorus to function, that certain bacteriae including the flavobacterium and other sulfur and nitrogen reducers can use arsenic in their cellular processes, depending upon the environment. It makes sense then why Lyme patients often have high levels of arsenic in their body. Not only is arsenic making its way into the air we breathe, but it is a known toxicant found in drinking water, and it appears on fruits and vegetables since it is a component of herbicides and other pesticides. If arsenic-loving bacteriae are present in the body in the form of a spirochete such as Bb, and they can take up arsenic from the residues in the foods we eat, it makes sense why a heavy metal (metalloid) like arsenic may stay in the body instead of being excreted by the kidneys or digestive process. In a sense the bacteria may become little metal retrieval vehicles and storage vessels.[87-91]

In a similar manner, if bacteria are utilizing the phosphorus stored in our teeth, bones, and soft tissues, they are in effect causing the release of stored phosphorus and whatever is bound to the phophorus ions in the body. Because the fluoride-phosphorus bond is one of the strongest in chemistry, we can see how a spirochete that is fluoride-tolerant may be able to utilize the phosphorus and ignore or eliminate the fluoride components as bacterial wastes into the body. There circulating fluoride levels may increase during bacterial infection, which of course helps produce a significant number of fluoride-toxicity related symptoms. These symptoms are found in many chronic illnesses including fluorosis, Lyme disease, Morgellon's, chronic fatigue, and a number of other illnesses. An interesting note is that children who have been treated for copper and arsenic toxicity and who were formerly labelled as having ADD or ADHD behavior disorders, were significantly improved following treatment. Microbes not only take up arsenic, but copper, aluminum, and other heavy metals from any environment where they are found, including the human body. People who have imbalances in their ability to metabolize copper are more likely to suffer from chronic *Candida albicans* infections, and this yeast is common among Lyme and other patients with chronic illnesses.

German and American uranium mines have produced important bacteriae that thrive in mine (and weapons) wastes. In the uranium mill tailings* of Schlema/Alberoda, Germany, wastes were dominated by *Nitrospina*-like bacteria. These are nitrite-oxidizing, nitrate producing, and ammonia-oxidizing extremophile bacteriae that live in soil and waters where high levels of ammonia are found. Other examples include sewage, wastewaters, metal-leaching mines, nuclear production plants, and fertilized agricultural fields. The nitrospinia are proteobacteria. Depending on the family, they may be rods, motile, helical, or cocci in form, and can resemble spirochetes with flagella, tubules; or be vibroid-shaped (Vibrio-like).

**Uranium mill tailings are radioactive remnants, usually from production of nuclear weapons or fuel ingots. They contain radium, which decays to radon gas, an important airborne radioactive environmental pollutant. The disposal of nuclear wastes remains an ongoing problem since radium has a long half-life, and disposal sites are few and nearly full of spent nuclear fuel wastes.*

Uranium mill tailings of Shiprock, New Mexico revealed mostly *Fruteria* and *gamma-Pseudomonas* bacteriae. However there were also bacteriae from the *Cytophaga-Flavobacterium-Bacteroides* group, and a few *delta-Proteobacteriae* found. The latter group was also found in tailings from Gittersee/Coschütz, Germany, and Steinsee Deponie B1, Germany. The latter group produced a large number of *Acinetobacter*. This is interesting when we examine the kinds of bacteriae for which infectious disease researchers currently apply for federal grant funding, and we see some of these extremophiles mentioned.[94-96]

Wastewaters in rivers from South Wales (UK) were analyzed and demonstrated *Cyanobacteria, Proteobacteria,* and *Cytophaga-Flexibacter-Bacteroides* strains. Uranium waste dump sites produced several groups of bacteriae including these that are commonly found associating with metals, ores, metal leaching wastes, and radioactive wastes (i.e. test sites, nuclear plants):

Holophaga/Acidobacterium	*Cytophaga/Flavobacterium/Bacteroides*
Cyanobacteria (green non-sulfur bacteria)	*Nitrospira/Leptospirillum*

Some of these bacterial groups are currently of great interest to scientists connected to Lyme disease history. These bacteriae are related to the gene-swapping *Agrobacterium tumefaciens.* Any of these family members may become infected with viruses and bacteria from applied insecticides, and may be capable of swapping genes in the process, including with *leptospires*. Insecticides are delivered to the environment by numerous industries. Bacterial, mold, and fungal spores easily become airborne contaminants that are not only highly resistant to dessication, but are small enough to drift far and wide and to infect bacteria and viruses in many environments.[97,98]

Agricultural areas also reveal gram-positive nitrogen and ammonia-oxidizing soil bacteriae including the *Paenibacillus, Bacillus sphaericus, Bacillus megaterium, Bacillus subtilis,* and *Bacillus circulans* families. These bacteriae happen to be subgroups of *Escherichia coli* (*E. coli*). Each of these groups have been used as applied insecticides, and were also present in the early parasitoid insects. *Bacillus megaterium* was studied as early as the 1940s during early *bacteriophage* research, and is used as a soil innoculant. *B. megaterium* is the largest of the bacteriophages. *B. sphaericus* is a larvicide used to control mosquitoes. *B. subtilis* of course is a soil bacterium. This group is further divided into *fifteen* strains:

Paenibacillus amylolyticus	*Paenibacillus alginolyticus*	*Paenibacillus alvei*
Paenibacillus apiarius	*Paenibacillus azotofixans*	*Paenibacillus chondroitinus*
Paenibacillus curdlanolyticus	*Paenibacillus glucanolyticus*	*Paenibacillus kobensis*
Paenibacillus larvae subsp. Pulvifaciens	*Paenibacillus lautus*	*Paenibacillus macerans*
Paenibacillus macquariensis	*Paenibacillus pabuli*	*Paenibacillus peoriae*
Paenibacillus polymyxa	*Paenibacillus thiaminolyticus*	*Paenibacillus validus*[99-101]

Many of these strains in 1986 were identified as "*Bacillus*" but were renamed by 2004 as "*Paenibacillus*." For example *Bacillus amylolyticus* is now known as *Paenibacillus amylolyticus*; and *Bacillus polymyxa* is now called *Paenibacillus polymyxa.* Also *Bacillus lentimorbus,* a "milky spore" agent is now called *Paenibacillus lentimorbus. Bacillus amyloliquefacients* is a bacterium that is the source of a restriction enzyme called "BamH1." Restriction enzymes cut foreign DNA at a specific point and are useful in genetic engineering techniques to create many products including vaccines and insecticides. Are the paenibacillus of recombinant genetics themselves becoming infected with the reactivated latent infections of insects, animals, and humans?[102-105]

The *Firmicutes* group contains not only the mollicutes (i.e. mycoplasmas, spiroplasmas) but also the *Selenomonadales*. These are motile, flagellated, and crescent-shaped clostridia-like bacteria that stain gram-negative unlike other members of their group. *Selenomonas* were first described by van Leeuwenhoek in 1683. Those that infect animals were described by Certes in 1889; and in 1906 by Hoffman and von Prowazek. There are multiple genus including *Selenomonas sputigena,* and *Selenomonas ruminantium.* These subgroups include *Spirillum* strains of gut parasites that can be cultured from humans, rodents, or ruminant animals. It is interesting that spirillum keep surfacing in our story.[106-108]

Perhaps the spirillum of plants mutate with another plant pathogen to make a *Spiroplasma.* In the same way, spirillum in the animal gut may mutate to create a pathogenic animal *spiroplasma* or *leptonema* strain. We know that sheep have these bacteriae in their gut (and so do mice, rats, rabbits, shrews). We can see how under the action of fermentation with soil bacteria (i.e. *Bacillis subtilis*), that gut spirillum may mutate to create an animal (and human) pathogen called *Anthrax.* In the insect gut, early literature reveals that relapsing fever (a/k/a famine fever), was once called *Spirillum Obermeieri.* It was also called *Spironema recurrentis* of Obermeier. So is a leptonema a relapsing fever spirillum and a leptospira? And could this agent include a plant spirillum? Since spirillum are found in insects, it is not impossible to believe they mutate under influence of chemicals and recombinant microbes to form the animal and human infecting *spiroplasmas* or *leptonemas.* This may help to explain why spiroplasma strain "B31" has the same name as the "B31" strain of *Borrelia burgdorferi;* as well as the many other spiroplasma and leptospira connections that seem to run rampant throughout Lyme disease history.[106-109]

The Iceman Cometh Bearing News of Borrelia

A 2011 article discussed "Ötzi" the iceman, who has been nicknamed "Frozen Fritz." This is a frozen mummy that was originally found by German tourists in September 1991 in the Ötztal Alps (between Austria and Italy). The roughly 45-year old man's body was frozen in the permafrost approximately 3,300 years ago. Scientists recently thawed enough ice from the mummy to collect multiple biological samples. During the examination scientists determined the DNA of the man's stomach contents. They found bits of wheat grain and red meat. The meat came from an alpine ibex, a kind of mountain goat. (We might want to examine the diet of the Ibex which includes twigs, grass, moss, leaves, and flowers; all hosts to mollicute infections.) Based on the elevated copper and arsenic levels found in the man's hair samples, scientists speculated that Fritz may have been a copper smelter.[1]

The iceman's body also revealed DNA evidence of "the genetic footprint" of the bacteria that has in modern times been identified as *Borrelia burgdorferi*; the spirochete of Lyme disease. Since we are now aware of the *Flavobacterium* and the *Cyphophaga* bacteriae, it is not hard to imagine that the scientists may be referring to *an extremophile or a soil bacterium of an aggregate Bb spirochete*; not that they discovered the actual Bb spirochete per sea. The article's author went so far as to suggest that Fritz is perhaps the oldest known victim of Lyme disease.[1]

This comment from the article struck me as peculiar in a scientific culture that has repeatedly denied the Lyme disease organism. The information also seems to be a thinly disguised attempt to describe the connections between metals, the food remnants found in the man's gut, and the parasites with which he was also found to be infected. I wondered also why scientists bothered to test the mummy for Lyme disease. If they discovered one or more organisms as we have discussed in this book, then Bb is an aggregate organism. It may also mean that scientists well know the makeup of the spirochete that causes Lyme disease, although they have not yet made any public admissions of such. The discovery could of course simply have been the result of a soil bacterium that was in contact with, or that contaminated the mummy. What was the organism that they detected, a leptospira, flavobacterium, relapsing fever bacterium, poxvirus, soil bacteriae, or something else?[1]

It is also interesting that the man was found to have a whipworm infection (intestinal round worms). These worms are nematodes. Many Lyme patients are co-infected with various nematodes and/or flukes. The man also lived during the Chalcolithic or Copper Age, which was a transitional period between the Stone and Bronze Ages. This was an era where mined ores were smelted to fabricate weapons and other artifacts. It was also a period where glass and clay beads that were colored with copper were being made using potash. People from this age were thought to be early farmers or pastoralists. Their diets included meats and grains such as sorghum (millets). The reason that the iceman is a valuable clue to us is because of the man's connections to parasites, copper smelting, farming, the use of clays, potash, and the same elements (potassium/phosphates) that are mined today for their agricultural and industrial value.[2,3]

The oldest archaeological site to show evidence of copper smelting is located in southeastern Europe (Serbia), although other sites in Turkey and Iran may date back 7,000 to 10,000 years. During the time of the Egyptians, copper smelting was also popular. Egyptian stone tablets recorded the presence of a polio-like illness during this period. This is most interesting to the history of the origins of certain insect pathogens which may contribute to an aggregate Lyme spirochete and to other disease outbreaks such as polio (i.e. *pox or myxoviruses*) in the modern world.[1-4]

Was the curious mention of the Lyme disease agent an attempt by spindoctors of public health reports to distance the causative agent of Lyme disease from any possible connection to current agricultural controls? If people think that Bb spirochetes have simply been around for thousands of years, then there is no perceived liability for their emergence in the modern human population. What possessed scientists to look for the "genetic footprint" of Bb in the iceman in the first place? It seems rather unlikely that scientists would simply stumble upon a Bb spirochete and announce it to the world. Then again, the article never stated that an intact Bb spirochete was actually isolated. Rather it refers to the "DNA footprint" of the agent, which could in theory represent any component of an aggregate organism that comprises the highly political *Borrelia burgdorferi.*

The Russian Model of an Agricultural Agent

Recently Yale researchers reported that they had received an NIH grant to develop a novel diagnostic test for a "new" strain of borrelia, called *Borrelia miyamotoi.* The "new" bacterium causes a high fever, and is said to be a "distant relative" of the pathogen that causes Lyme disease. This strain causes a relapsing fever infection, which is distinctively different than a Lyme disease infection. Because this infection is transmitted by ticks that can also transmit Lyme disease, this infection could be included as a co-infection in a small number of patients.[1,2]

According to Dr. Gary Wormser from New York Medical College who is a co-author of past Lyme disease medical guidelines; roughly four percent of the adult deer ticks surveyed in Westchester County, New York were found to have this infection. More recently researchers have found this agent in ill Russian patients according to a study published in November of 2011.[1,2]

Russian and Yale scientists reported that the relapsing fever *Borrelia miyamotoi* was detected in forty-six patients, although no such laboratory test is commercially available for public use. According to these scientists, *Borrelia miyamotoi* is supposedly not life-threatening. Just as some public health experts continue to claim about Lyme disease, *B. miyamotoi* infections appear to "clear" with antibiotics.[1,2]

An article posted on the CDC's Emerging Infectious Diseases web site and which includes Yale's Drs. Durland Fish and P.J. Krause as co-authors says that the organism "may cause relapsing fever and Lyme disease-like symptoms" because its vector is the *Ixodes* tick. According to the article, the illness is "more distantly related" to *B. burgdorferi.* The scientists are inferring that this relapsing fever agent isn't Lyme disease, but "something else." The idea that *Borrelia myamotoi* is distantly related to Bb, is actually accurate if you believe the contents of this book. *Borrelia miyamotoi* is a non-mutated relapsing fever agent, while Bb is likely to be a *mutated relapsing fever agent that includes other microbes;* although both organisms may include a mutated leptospira.[1-3]

It may be that Lyme notables will attempt to say that Lyme patients who have been treated "properly" with antibiotics and whom remain infected with "something else" will be told their infections must be *Borrelia miyamotoi.* But this is simply not possible and I will tell you why as we go along. I will use myself as an "anecdotal" patient with Lyme disease just to make a point. My infections began back in 1969 when I had my first bull's-eye rash. I have been infected ever since, although I have been rebitten at least twice, and treated many times with antibiotics (orals, IV, intramuscular). I have had the IDSA recommended treatment of doxycycline but now I'm apparently "sick with something else" according to certain IDSA guidelines authors.

Recently I was lucky enough to be a participant in the development of a novel diagnostic test for Bb that is just now available to physicians. The test holds enormous promise for patients who have long tested seronegative according to CDC standardized tests. What is that "something else" that causes infections in my case, is a spirochete that persists, not one that is a *Borrelia miyamotoi* infection.

The new *Borrelia burgdorferi* test, which was developed by an independent US laboratory in Pennsylvania, was able to culture Bb spirochetes from my blood in an amazingly short period of less than a week. Typical Bb tests take up to four weeks or longer to culture spirochetes. The organisms were identified by DNA PCR and by DNA sequencing as good old fashioned *Borrelia burgdorferi* sensu stricto, with sequences nearly identical to the east coast strain of B31; and I have never been to Connecticut. "B31" is the Bb strain that was found within Shelter Island New York ticks collected at the eastern end of Long Island in 1981. These are the ticks from which the Bb organism was originally identified, but I live in the Midwest. However it is possible that I could have been infected during the late 1960s when we briefly lived in southwestern Pennsylvania.

I now have *digital images* of the spirochetes that were recently cultured from my blood. This is clear evidence to me along with my ongoing symptoms that I have a bona fide Bb strain that is not *Borrelia miyamotoi.* The majority of American Lyme patients whose symptoms remain after antibiotic treatments such as those recommended by IDSA Lyme disease guidelines co-authors, may also not have a *Borrelia miyamotoi* infection. It is interesting however to see the generous research grants that were recently awarded to Lyme notables to "investigate" the organism's "possible" link to Lyme disease. It is also interesting that this is occurring a full sixteen years after the organism was first discovered in Japan and a decade after it was detected in the US.[2]

According to a CDC publication, *B. miyamotoi* is found only "in a small percentage of all species of *Ixodid* tick vectors" of Bb. This means that the "something else" that Dr. Steere et al. claim that Lyme patients suffer from is probably not the relapsing fever *B. miyamotoi.* After all, it was Dr. Willy Burgdorfer who clearly indicated that relapsing fever spirochetes are *not the same* as *Borrelia burgdorferi.* Dr. Burgdorfer felt that the various strains of relapsing fever borrelia were probably derived from a single taxonomic entity, *Borrelia recurrentis.* Although Bb is not a true relapsing fever, it is distantly related. All one has to do is to read the available research to discern this fact. It certainly does not require large sums of federal grant dollars. Scientists performed huge studies on tickborne infections in Asia and in Russia and knew since the 1930s that there were ticks infected with relapsing fevers. Such studies were undertaken in Turkmen SSR, Uzbek SSR, and Azerbaidghan SSR as well as other regions across the continents from the 1930s forward.[2]

Let's look for a moment at the older research concerning *B. miyamotoi*. In 1996, Japanese and French scientists analyzed known borrelia species and reported their findings based upon flagellin and other gene sequences.* The Genus borrelia (the relapsing fevers) was divided into three clusters. These included "New World" relapsing fevers: *Borrelia turicatae, B. parkeri,* and *B. hermsii*; The "Old World" relapsing fevers: *B. crocidurae, B. duttonii,* and *B. hispanica;* and the group of Lyme disease borreliae which includes *B. burgdorferi sensu stricto*, *B. garinii,* and *B. afzelii.*[1-7]

**Dr. Alan Barbour filed three patents for "flagella-less" borreliae diagnostic tests – two prior to this publication, and one five years later. The patents are assigned to the University of Texas System in Austin.*

The infectious animal spirochetoses were listed as: *B. coriaceae* and *B. anserina,* according to Japanese scientists. The French scientists divided the groups differently, and assigned *B. crocidurae, B. duttonii, B. recurrentis,* and *B. hispanica* to the first branch of a second cluster. They also assigned *B. coriaceae,* <u>*Borrelia lonestari*</u>, and <u>*Borrelia miyamotoi*</u> to a second cluster; and *B. parkeri, B. turicatae,* and *B. hersmii* to the second branch of the second cluster. *Borrelia anserina* a bird pathogen, was the only member of a third cluster. *Borrelia persica,* a human tickborne relapsing fever, was not placed into any cluster.[1-7]

We might think about how rice is the most important staple food in Japan. Remember that the rice blast fungus (*Magnaporthe grisea*) was formulated into "LX" as a biological warfare weapon. If LX had ever been deployed during the Korean War, then a relapsing fever bacterium the likes of *Borrelia miyamotoi* in the Far East could become highly interesting. Perhaps it came about naturally by way of agricultural chemicals which mutated an insect relapsing fever (*Borrelia japonica*) and a natural rice fungi (rice blast) to form a mutant *Borrelia miyamotoi.* Perhaps this mutant even has the potential to cause Lyme disease if further combined with an extremophile soil bacteria, a spiroplasma, cyanobacteria, and/or other agents.

In Japan, the problem of nuclear wastes has recently been compounded after major earthquakes devastated the island's nuclear plants. If *Borrelia miyamotoi* does combine in a manner similar to those that formed Bb spirochetes, we may in time find a new member of the *Borrelia burgdorferi* sensu lato (broad sense) group. This group will include a new member that mainly infects people in Japan and the Russian Far East, and that will be based on *B. miyamotoi.*[8-19,86]

Since rice blast was experimented upon in the US during the 1960s, we would expect to see strains of *Borrelia miyamotoi* emerge in the US as well. And from the available research, it would appear that this has in fact sporadically occurred. *B. miyamotoi* is indeed found in Lyme disease-transmitting ticks in the US. It was also isolated in Japan in 1994, the year of the Dearborn conference. Japan has a sizable nuclear power industry, and there were several nuclear accidents that occurred there during the 1990s, about the time that the new relapsing fever strain was first isolated.[8-19,86]

A 1995 Japanese-American collaborative paper that was published just months after the Dearborn conference reported on the discovery of a new species of relapsing fever which was detected in *Ixodes persulcatus* (Taiga) ticks in Japan. This tick species is the most important vector of Lyme disease for Japan. Analysis revealed that *Borrelia miyamotoi* was only 8-13% related to the DNA of previously described Lyme disease borreliae (*B. burgdorferi, B. garinii, B. afzelii*). Therefore the agent was considered to be a "new" species that was distinctively different from, but distantly related to the relapsing fever borreliae and to the Lyme disease borreliae strains. This is not hard to believe, since *B. miyamotoi* is probably also a mutated relapsing fever.[16]

The following year in 1996, other Japanese scientists established that relapsing fevers *B. miyamotoi* and *B.turicatae* had genes that were "quite similar" to those found in *Borrelia burgdorferi* sensu lato strains. However their conclusion was that *B. miyamotoi* was "neither the same as nor related to any of the Lyme disease borrelia species" based on genetic and biological characteristics. Their findings are an important commentary as to the evolution of borrelia species and their adaptation to various tick species. This also means that relapsing fevers and those that cause Lyme disease infections in humans are quite possibly mutating in adaptation to their hosts. In short, while there are differences between organisms, those differences are probably caused by the differing host environments, and mutated strains will vary between geographic regions. As environmental chemicals and other mutagenic catalysts cause bacteria to mutate, we will see new species emerge and colonize new hosts.[20,21]

The French scientists also included *Borrelia burgdorferi* as part of the relapsing fever group. This separation is important to note because American scientists support the separation of the Bb cluster from relapsing fevers. Borrelia species that are considered to be "unknown" in terms of whether they are specifically animal or human pathogens include *B. miyamotoi* and *Borrelia lonestari,* although both cause human disease. These two agents are thought to be more closely related to the relapsing fevers than are the Bb strains. *Borrelia lonestari* is the agent found in hard-shelled *Amblyomma americanum* (Lone Star) ticks.[16-23]

In very general terms, relapsing fevers are transmitted by soft-bodied ticks, and Lyme borreliosis is transmitted by hard-shelled *Ixodes* ticks. Therein lies the main difference between the two groups. If we were to assume that all relapsing fevers and Lyme disease spirochetes were at one time established from a single species, then we may suspect that something in the hard-tick species maintains or increases Bb virulence; while the soft-tick species may not amplify in virulence or may even lose some virulence genes during host adaptation. There is little evidence to suggest these groups were one and the same, but even so host adaptation plays an important role in the difference between spirochetal species and strains.[17,22-23]

From one publication we learn that the Lyme disease borreliae; two additional species that are related, (*B. japonica, B. andersonii*); and a few other newly described groups are closely related. However each are said to have been formed on independent branches of the phylogenetic tree. These differences could be caused by slightly different evolutionary paths in different host animals. Dr. Alan Barbour published a paper in 2005 that emphasized that *Borrelia miyamotoi* was a relapsing fever and not a Lyme disease-causing borrelia. As I said, it probably has not yet mutated or accumulated the additional pathogens that are necessary to become a full-fledged Bb strain.[17,22-23]

In 2001 scientists including those from Tufts, Harvard, and the University of Illinois-Urbana published a paper stating that the Lone Star spirochete *B. lonestari*; the relapsing fever agent *Borrelia miyamotoi,* and the agent of bovine borreliosis *Borrelia theileri,** form a natural, distinct group that are different than, but closely related to the relapsing fever borreliae. The *Borrelia theileri* and *Borrelia lonestari* agents were respectively found to be 98% and 97% genetically similar by analysis of their flagellin genes. Once again we see a livestock connection to the agents that are transmitted to humans.[17,22-23]

**Borrelia theileri causes a Lyme disease-like infection in cattle.*

A 2011 study was undertaken with the assistance of Drs. Fish and Krause from May 19 to August 25, 2009 at a hospital in Yekaterinburg City, Russia. Patients with suspected tickborne infections were enrolled in the study. This is a city that is about twelve hundred miles east of Moscow, at the Asian end of Russia. Viral tickborne encephalitis and borreliosis (relapsing fevers) are common to the region. About one-third of the world's recoverable uranium oxide resources are found in Australia (first), followed by other countries including Kazakhstan, Canada, South Africa, Russia, Brazil, Namibia and the US. Scientists collected ticks from regions across Russia including Yekaterinburg, Kurgan, Chelyabinsk, Izhevsk, Vologda, Yaroslavl, Moscow, Lipetzk, Stavropol; and from Kazakhstan. Let's examine the industries and happenstances of each of the areas from where the tick drags occurred to see if there are any interesting connections to Lyme disease and *Borrelia miyamotoi.*[24]

These regions are located on or near the border of Belarus, the Ukraine, and Kazakhstan. The frequency of *B. garinii, B. afzelii, B. burgdorferi,* and *B. miyamotoi* were studied in *Ixodes ricinus* sheep ticks collected in these regions by tick drags. Once again we see studies of the ticks that bite sheep – a grazing animal commonly associated with natural anthrax outbreaks. During a 2004-2007 study, 0.9% of ticks in Yekaterinburg, and 6.4% of ticks from Izhevsk were found to be infected with *B. miyamotoi*. The number has apparently increased slightly. This region is also one that harbors "TV rock," which is a mineral rock called Ulexite. This rock is known for its optical qualities and is found in association with gypsum, halite, and borax,* which was mined for cosmetics, enamel glazes, detergents, pottery, ceramics, glass, polyvinyl-based putty, adhesives, flame retardants, buffer solutions, fiberglass, flux, fluoride detoxification, insecticides, and soil amendments.[24,25]

**One of the largest borax mines in the world is located in the Great Basin Desert of Nevada; but borax is also found in California, Chile, Turkey, and Romania.*

The city of Yekaterinburg is a curious place for Lyme notables Drs. Fish, Krause, et al. to be studying relapsing fever borreliae. I say this because this city is heavy in many important industries, nonetheleast of which is agriculture. **It was also the site of an April-May, 1979 outbreak of the biological warfare agent Anthrax.** As we have already learned, the agent of anthrax (*Bacillus anthracis*) is an organism that is "closely related" to the globally applied insecticide *Bacillus thuringiensis* (B.t.). The anthrax outbreak in this city was originally blamed on locals who had eaten contaminated meats. However American scientists believed that anthrax spores had been aerosolized and released from a nearby military microbiological laboratory, Sverdlovsk-19 (Compound 19). The accident was called the "biological Chernobyl," and about 100 persons died as a result.[26-29]

Industries in Sverdlovsk at one time produced military tanks, armaments, and nuclear weapons. The Sverdlovsk laboratory was responsible for Russian biowarfare studies. The lab was run by Dr. Kanatjan Alibekov (Ken Alibek), who wrote a book about his work there, and who came to the US to perform biowarfare research. In 1994, a team of American researchers concluded that the 1979 anthrax outbreak had been the result of an anthrax release at the Russian laboratory. But the word "anthrax" could instead disguise another meaning that has a far greater global significance, despite admissions by Boris Yeltsin in 1992 that the 1979 outbreak was caused by the Russian military.[26-29]

The insecticide B.t. is fermented from a soil bacteria that may also naturally ferment an anthrax strain. Is "anthrax" created during the fermentation of soil bacteria to create B.t.? I previously discussed research that indicates that a virulent anthrax can be further fermented in a process to create a less virulent form. Is this less virulent form an "almost anthrax," or what is essentially the widely deployed agricultural agent B.t.?[30-35]

Some reasonable questions we may ask are: Could the Russian laboratory have been re-fermenting former anthrax weapons in order to recycle older weapons into an agricultural insecticide? Was the anthrax outbreak in Russia caused by an accidental release of a fermenting agricultural insecticide? If it was, the fact that spores created a deadly human outbreak could easily jeopardize the use of B.t. insecticides around the world, because *B.t. could be declared dangerously unsafe*.

Have any countries eliminated their past, obsolete anthrax biological warfare weapons by re-fermenting them into a widely applied global insecticide? Or is the concern that in order to create a B.t. insecticide, that soil bacteria must be fermented for a period of time during which time an anthrax, or anthrax-like agent is created? Is the problem as simple as the idea that B.t. crystal (Cry) toxins are among the same toxins which belong to the anthrax agent? If B.t. insecticides are "almost anthrax," then we can understand why militaries, governments, and everyone tied to the story may desire to keep anthrax-B.t. relationships a secret in order to protect B.t.'s highly profitable agricultural and industrial uses.[30-35]

Have B.t. insecticides sometimes been created using recycled anthrax spores? We will learn there are other military weapons that are being recycled. Do the globally applied B.t. insecticides lead to outbreaks of human diseases as well as epizootics in targeted insects? In any event, the ability of globally applied insecticides to reassort with other microbes to create a natural anthrax strain remains a realistic threat. It is perhaps also a threat that agricultural insecticides such as B.t. may be easily acquired by people who wish to create "bioterrorism" weapons, and who have access to laboratories to do so.[30-37]

B.t. is a *phagic* organism that is known to aggregate or attach itself to the outer protein walls of other bacteria, including borrelia strains *B. recurrentis* and *B. hermsii*, both agents of tickborne relapsing fevers. Two scientists who are IDSA Lyme disease guidelines co-authors are studying a relapsing fever organism that is found within the bodies of sheep ticks that can also transmit Lyme disease. We have to ask why are they so interested in Russian ticks? Perhaps the reason has to do with agricultural, military weapons, or other industrial ties, and the kinds of moths that lay their eggs upon the foods these animals eat – silkworms whose pathogens include extremophiles that are ingested by the worms and by grazing animals.[33-42]

If Lyme disease is caused by an aggregate organism that includes an attached B.t. phage, then the Russian studies by American scientists makes sense. If a Russian model of a relapsing fever spirochete has a B.t. phage, then scientists can rather conveniently study the organism and its relationship to a Lyme-like illness that is a global epidemic. Such studies would not raise suspicions or reveal any relationship between Lyme disease and the highly valuable insecticide called "B.t."

If Bb has a B.t. phage attached to it (and we know that Bb has some kind of phage), it makes sense that the presence of the spiroplasmas or the leptonemas found within the bodies of Lyme transmitting ticks are never mentioned. What if someone makes the connection between Bb and agricultural/industrial tools?[38-42]

A peculiar finding was described by Dr. Alan Barbour just three years before he attended the Dearborn conference. Dr. Barbour claimed that the genetic structures and sequences of the linear plasmids of Bb were similar to those found in the African swine fever virus. These genes may belong to an insect virus such as *Tipula* from the common cranefly, or those of the "Pj" iridescent virus. This virus is associated with the milky spore agents, *Bacillus sphaericus, B. megaterium,* and B.t. Does the Bb spirochete contain insect iridescent virus genes? It is curious that Drs. Barbour and Fish have been studying *Borrelia miyamotoi* and Bb in the same tick vectors for several years (Fish at least since 2001; Barbour-Fish since 2009). The 2011 studies were suddenly announced after receipt of a sizeable research grant.[38-44]

There are other curiosities about each of the cities where *Borrelia miyamotoi* infected ticks were collected for the Fish-Krause Russian studies besides the 1979 anthrax outbreak. In Yaroslavl we find oil and gas mining operations and other industries, including a factory that during WWII produced detonators for mines and grenades, and components for anti-tank and other artillery. The area is located in the Russian forests where we find timber processing, oil deposits, gas fields, and mined materials (i.e. sand, gravel, brick earth, haydite), peat, and a huge cache of sapropel. Sapropel in raw form is used as fertilizer, and when processed is useful to rubber, paint, and oil refining industries; and as an animal feed additive.[45]

A quick word about sapropel, which is found as a sedimentary deposit. When consolidated into rock, sapropel becomes oil shale, bituminous shale, or torbanite (boghead coal). This is an intermediate mineral between shale and coal. Torbanite produces paraffinic and olefinic hydrocarbons. These are compounds that are linked to carbon chains. Paraffin and straight chain hydrocarbons have been used within animal vaccines and other products. Torbanite is found in France, New South Wales, South Africa, and the northeastern US.[46-50]

Many organisms are cultivated upon hydrocarbons derived from petroleum (crude oil), and are treated with solvents (i.e. hexane) to be "substantially free" of hydrocarbons. The organisms of insecticides can also be grown on petroleum straight chain hydrocarbons, which by the way, may be mutagenic. The principal components of sapropel are minerals and decomposed fragments of spores, fungi, and bacteria.[46-50]

Most animal feeds are contaminated with mycotoxins. These are toxins that are produced by molds and fungi. Mycotoxins cause chronic poisoning of animals. Sapropel is added to their food to counteract these toxins. Sapropel contains roughly 16% protein, amino acids, and mineral salts. It aids in the fermentation that takes place inside the animal gut. Sapropel also absorbs mycotoxins and has an additional bactericidal effect to help decrease the number of infectious organisms. If this works inside an animal's body, then it certainly works to aggregate bacteria, molds, fungi, and viruses underground where it is mined; or in the soils and wastewaters where it eventually migrates or is applied.

In Vologda, Russia we find salt mines, gold mining operations, textile factories, ironworks, timber processing, mined potash, and charcoal for fertilizers. In Moscow besides the Moscow State Mining University which prepares mining engineers; we find oil, gas, coal, precious metals, and rare earth mineral deposits including uranium. The city of Izhevsk is noted for its military industry. It is also home to Russia's largest munitions enterprise. There military, small arms, and assault rifles (i.e. AK-47) have been produced since 1948.[51,52]

Yekaterinburg is on the east side of the Ural Mountains. It is the administrative center of the heavily industrialized Sverdlovsk Oblast. This was the site of the 1979 Russian anthrax outbreak. Kurgan was named after mounds of earth (tumulus) that cover their ancient graves. Kurgan barrows were characteristic of people from the Bronze Age, and are found throughout the region, and into Romania and Bulgaria. (Was the "iceman" checked for Lyme disease because he came from this area and scientists suspect or know the real origins of the Lyme disease organism but aren't telling?)[51]

Kurgan lies on the banks of the Tobol and Iset rivers. It also borders oil and gas bearing districts in Tyumen and Tomsk Oblasts. Large oil and gas pipelines pass through the region and we find Ural and Siberian oil refineries nearby. The Kurgan Oblast is not known for its mineral reserves, however it has significant food industries including creameries, powdered milk, and meat packing.[51]

The city of Lipetzk has a cast iron factory near iron ore deposits that are mined for the production of artillery shells. The principal industries in the area are metallurgy, machinery, chemicals, food, and textiles. The area is also home to the oldest mud bath (balneological) resorts in Russia (1805). There peat mud and mineral laden springs which contain sulphates and sodium chlorides can be found (geothermal springs). We also find a profitable steel industry, a metallurgical plant, chemical and other factories; and the second largest rapeseed (canola) oil producer in Russia. The kinds of microbial pesticides (i.e. B.t.) that are applied to agricultural crops and mined ores as we know, are significant to the story.[51,53]

The city of Stavropol was founded as a military encampment. There we find furniture, automobile, construction equipment, and agricultural industries. Former Soviet Union leader Nikita Khrushchev ordered that corn be planted all over Russia. Indeed, Stavropol, Moscow, Ryazan and Chuvash represent a major portion of Russian agricultural crop producing regions. The University of Maryland is partnered with Stavropol State Agrarian University (SSAU), and together they are creating a regional distance learning center in southern Russia. Other Russian partners with the university are Kursk Agricultural Academy, Novgorod State University, and Moscow State University of Environmental Engineering (MSUE).[54]

In Chelyabinsk which is just east of the Urals on the Miass River, is a metallurgical plant that was built in the 1930s. There, weapons facilities produced tanks and rocket launchers in the city once known as Tankograd (tank city). It is also home to the Chelyabinsk-70 nuclear facility where top-secret research was undertaken. There was a serious nuclear accident in 1957 at the Mayak nuclear fuel reprocessing plant, about 150 km northwest of the city. The accident caused deaths in the Chelvavinsk Oblast, but none were reported in the city. The region is home to the oldest university, Chelyabinsk State Agroengineering Academy, founded in 1930. It is also home to major industries, especially metallurgy, military machinery, metal forging, and electronics (i.e. semiconductors). The area is home to Mechel OAO, one of Russia's leading coal, steel, iron ore concentrate, heat and electric power, ferroalloys, and rolled product producers. The company has production facilities in thirteen Russian regions, and in Kazakhstan, Romania, Lithania, Bulgaria, and the US.[54,55]

The city of Kazakhstan borders on the Caspian Sea. It is comprised of mountains and rocky canyons. The area was home to several major campaigns including Khrushchev's Virgin Lands campaign; and was the former USSR's primary nuclear weapons testing site. In 1949 a nuclear bomb was tested in Kazakh SSR in Semey. This greatly disturbed the region on many levels. The Virgin Lands program was founded in 1953 when Khrushchev wanted to turn the area pasture lands into a major grain producing region for the Soviet Union. The area is also a leading exporter of uranium, and there are large oil and natural gas stores. If the oil reserves can be developed, the region will become among the top ten oil producing nations in the world.[54]

Agriculturally speaking the region is the seventh largest producer of grain in the world. Its major crops include cotton, wheat, rice, and barley. Livestock is also a booming business as are dairy, leather, meat, and wool. The area holds the largest uranium, chromium, lead, and zinc reserves; and is in the top ten countries for coal, iron, gold, and diamonds. We must scrutinize the industries and past history that may have influenced microbes and the ticks in the regions where they are collected.[54]

Yale Entomologist Dr. Durland Fish claims that *Borrelia miyamotoi* was found in Connecticut deer ticks *a decade ago.* An article quoted Dr. Fish stating that they have for a "long time" known that *B. miyamotoi* is found in ticks. Indeed it was discovered in 1995 by Japanese scientist Fukunaga. Dr. Fish also claimed that this spirochete was found in ticks "wherever there is Lyme disease." Fish's statements are unclear whether he means that the agent is found in Lyme-transmitting ticks collected from specific areas, or something else. The scientific literature reveals that the incidence of *B. miyamotoi* is considerably *lower* than Lyme disease in all areas of the world. Dr. Fish's statements are curious since as co-author of 2000 Lyme disease medical guidelines there was no mention of this pathogen lurking within the bodies of Lyme disease-transmitting ticks. No audible mention of *B. miyamotoi* seems to have been made from 1995 until the present day when a grant was awarded. Neither was it mentioned audibly to the public as a possible co-infection in people who contract Lyme disease.[56-59]

According to a *New York Times* article which announced the recent Russian studies and grant award, Dr. Fish claimed that he tried to get an NIH grant ten years ago, but was "repeatedly refused" since he could not demonstrate that the agent caused human illness. Regardless of any attempts, the words *Borrelia miyamotoi* never hit the "streets" until now, and it would seem so only to publicize a recent grant award. Perhaps the "rediscovery" of the *B. miyamotoi* ticks will be the final scapegoat that will be used by scientists to describe what may be ailing patients who say they are suffering from chronic Lyme disease – a state which Dr. Fish or his colleagues do not seem too willing to acknowledge is genuine.[60-62]

According to the *Times* article, Dr. Fish found *B. miyamotoi* in just 2% of deer ticks in the northeastern US; and in the upper Midwest in 2001 in mice. The press release claims a 4% incidence. However a CDC article claims its prevelance is from 1-16%. From the CDC article:[60-62]

> "In Russia, the rate of *B. miyamotoi* infection in *Ixodes persulcatus* ticks was 1%-16%, similar to rates in *I. ricinus* ticks in western Europe and *I. scapularis* ticks in the United States."

So what is the real rate of this relapsing fever within the US? If it is a mere 16%, it hardly explains the large numbers of chronic Lyme disease patients who have been suffering for decades with "something else."[60-62]

There may be other clues to the interests of scientists in the Russian model. *Borrelia japonica* is a Bb sensu lato strain that was first isolated from *Ixodes ovatus* ticks found on wild mice captured in Honshu, Japan in 1994. What is important about this strain is that there is a mosquito *Aedes japonicus* that is native to eastern Asia, (Japan, Korea) as well as China, Russian, and Taiwan. In recent years it has become widely disbursed in North America and in central Europe (France, Germany, Belgium). This mosquito first appeared in the US in New York, Connecticut, and Illinois in 1998; which is rather curious since these three states always seem to be at the hub of agricultural experiments to control pest insects.[63]

Scientists believe that the *Aedes japonica* mosquitoes were introduced into the US no earlier than 1992. The mosquito rapidly spread, and by 2005 its host range had extended into nineteen northeast states. It is also found in Quebec, Canada; Hawaii, and the western state of Washington. This may represent its spread across Canada into the States, or its presence as an import into Washington upon citrus trees for example. Let's not forget that genetically altered mosquito "population replacers" were released in the millions across the US, and in other parts of the world. Isolated populations of this mosquito were found in France in 2000, and Belgium in 2004. This mosquito has been shown to be a vector of West Nile, eastern equine encephalitis, St. Louis encephalitis, and La Crosse encephalitis viruses.[63]

The year 1998 is well within the "decade ago" time slot that Dr. Fish indicated was when scientists first identified *Borrelia miyamotoi* in the US. Remember that "borrelia" means something that is "tick-transmitted." The word "miyamotoi" could be derived from a 17th century swordsman Miyamoto Musachi who was born in the Harima Province – an area that was a part of Honshu, and that is now the southwestern part of Hyōgo Prefecture in Japan. Isn't it interesting that Honshu is also the area where *Borrelia japonica* was first isolated? Besides being a famous swordsman, Miyamoto wrote a book titled Gorin no shô (The Book of Five Rings), which was popular in the states during the 1980s. If we think about mosquitoes, they are little flying swordsmen in their own right![64-66]

All this is well and good but when we study grant award recipients from the 1980s forward, we find an interesting group of scientists who have been studying the *Aedes japonicus* mosquito for over a decade. Their studies appear to be aimed at **this particular mosquito, a *Flavobacterium,* and its role in the degradation of polymers.** What we find when we study the flavobacterium are that a team of Japanese scientists found a strain which thrives in wastewater ponds at a nylon factory. These bacteriae were found to contain enzymes that differed significantly from enzymes found in any other bacteriae. These enzymes are able to degrade certain byproducts of "Nylon 6." This is a polymer that was developed by Paul Schlack while at I.G. Farben. It was invented as a competitor to "Nylon 6,6" which is a polymer that is used in the textile and plastics industries. The Nylon 6 polymer was named Perlon in 1952.[67-69]

Paul Schlack's patents go back to 1928, where we find several related to the improvement in the manufacture of artificial silk threads, and woolen fibers that are derived from a mixed cellulose of nitric acid and fatty acids. He also holds patents for coloring organic products using aniline dyes. One patent describes the use of his patent on hydrocarbons, nitro-compounds, waxes, fatty acids, cellulose derivatives and threads, varnishes, oil emulsions (i.e. leather industry), candles, soaps, pharmaceuticals, foods, cosmetics, textile lecithins, and more. Another patent describes the sizing of artificial silk. The process can use oils from rape seed, cotton seed, or soy beans; and is made with the aid of a soap or an emulsifier, for example turkey red oil (sulfonated caster oil) and oil-soluble soaps made from amines (amine soaps i.e. triethanol amine); and perboric acid, benzene, or solvent naptha. *Manganese soaps* were used in the mid-to late 1800s forward, and this is important since *Borrelia burgdorferi* spirochetes have enzymes that use manganese, and these enzymes are required for infectivity.[69-74]

Turkey red oil is a sulfonated castor oil (surfactant) made from the *Ricinus communis* castor oil plant. This plant has lepidoptera as pests, including the *Eri silkmoth*. The plants contain the highly toxic ricin, which is a natural nerve agent that was also developed as a nerve agent for military use. Turkey red oil was the first synthetic detergent (soap) and was used in the dye process, and for softeners and lubricants. It is also used as a defoaming agent in the textile and sugar industries. Castor bean plants are perhaps the most poisonous plants in the world. During the First World War, scientists from the USDA and the State officials of Florida collaborated in efforts to eradicate armyworms that were decimating castor bean fields in Florida. Approximately 40,000 acres were planted with castor beans to supply the War Department with fuel oil for military aircraft. Several tons of lead arsenate were used to combat these pests at the time.[75,85]

As far as polymers go, we now know that processes that involved dying, silk, wool, harmful chemicals, "nerve agents," surfactants, and artificial fibers all come together to produce byproducts that end up in wastewaters including at nylon manufacturing and other polymer plants. When we take a look at the microbes in those wastewaters, we find the *Flavobacterium* (i.e. species K172). These bacteriae have developed highly sophisticated and unique enzymes to degrade (man-made) nylon 6 polymers. And these bacteria were first discovered in 1975, the very same year that the Lyme disease outbreak in Connecticut was formally announced. Perhaps this explains why some polymer manufacturers hold patent interests in diagnostic tests that can detect extremophiles from the flavobacterium family, and the leptospires and Bb spirochetes that may become polluted in the industrial wastewaters influenced in part by manufacturing chemicals.[76-79]

These unique enzymes are important because this demonstrates that a bacterium developed an ability that did not exist before the creation of the man-made fiber nylon, which was first synthesized in 1935. As described by the first patent for "artificial silk," which was created in 1855 in England by a Swiss chemist Audemars; the inner bark of the mulberry tree was dissolved by chemicals to produce cellulose. Threads were formed by dipping needles into solutions and drawing them out like taffy. Artificial silk was shown at the Paris Exhibition in 1889, and the first commercial rayon plant was built in Besancon, France, by French Chemist Count Hilaire de Chardonnet. Besancon is located northeast of Lyon, the silk textile hub of the country at the time. We can see the history of textiles and chemicals, especially solvents and surfactants which keep rearing their heads no matter where we turn in Lyme disease history. Even in modern times, we can see how polymers and other important chemicals have been used in many industries connected to the story, including as polymerized coatings of nuclear reactor components.[76-79]

Today under NIAID grants, scientists are studying the interactions between mosquitoes that harbor *Flavobacterium* strains including those which "eat" nylon fibers. These same mosquitoes, which were first isolated by Japanese scientists, can also carry important viruses and borrelia strains in their midguts. Japanese eels (*Anguilla japonica*) were experimentally infected with *Flavobacterium columnare* to produce the same symptoms as those found in eels that are naturally infected with *Flavobacterium psychrophilum* (cold water disease). The *Aedes japonicus* or Asian bush mosquito, which is native to Japan, Korea, Taiwan, and China; was first seen in the US in Connecticut, New York, and New Jersey in 1998. They were subsequently found in Massachusetts, Virginia, Ohio, Illinois, and Minnesota. This mosquito is an important vector of Japanese encephalitis, West Nile, eastern equine encephalitis, La Crosse virus, and St. Louis encephalitis viruses. We can guess this is because of its ability to transmit *Flavobacterium* and the aforementioned flaviviruses that probably infect same. It also suggests that mosquito-borne infections can easily become part of aggreate Bb spirochetes.[80-84]

The Bottom Line?

Uranium and other rare elements are important to the story of Lyme disease since uranium is used as fuel in nuclear power plants; it can be used to make plutonium, is useful for nuclear medicine, and was used in the manufacture of nuclear weapons. Uranium is also found in "trace amounts" in organophosphate fertilizers, insecticides, and herbicides including glyphosate (in the form of phosphorus trichloride or PCl_3). The main suppliers of phosphates for the world besides Florida are Morocco, Jordan, and Kazakhstan. Other suppliers are located in Brazil, Egypt, Saudi Arabia, Israel, Mexico, Syria, and the US. Besides fertilizers, phosphates are also used in soft drinks, when treating fish fillets, potato processing, poultry processing (including eggs), oral health products, cleaning agents and detergents, textiles, carpets (and thus fibers, polymers), flame retardants, and baking mixtures.[1]

Uranium is only part of the equation. Thorium is another radioactive element that is useful for fuelling nuclear reactors, and it can be processed for nuclear weapons. Thorium's radioactive daughter is a form of uranium. Thorium may be used in other applications including high temperature ceramics (crucibles), rocket fuel, glass, petroleum cracking (splitting hydrocarbons); and as thorium dioxide to convert ammonia to the highly corrosive, explosive, and toxic nitric acid.* Thorium powered the first nuclear reactors in the US and Russia during the Cold War, however the element was not a good nuclear weapon due to the kind of radiation it produces, and for other reasons so uraniuim was used instead. However, thorium is far more abundant than uranium, and current natural deposits may be literally inexhaustible. Unlike thorium, uranium requires conversion and enrichment before it can be used. The future of nuclear reactor energy production will probably be derived from thorium rather than uranium.[2-4]

**A dilute form of nitric acid is used in woodworking and to etch metals. It also produces a yellow hue on contact with skin. Could "yellows" diseases be caused in part by a mutation caused by the reaction of nitric acid and its effects upon microbes such as the extremophiles found near radioactive elements?*

Thorium is another rare earth mineral that is a byproduct of refining the phosphate mineral Monazite. This mineral is also a byproduct of processing heavy-mineral rocks (bauxite) which also bear fluorides and alumina (aluminum) among other metals. Mineral rocks that contain rare earth elements are also absorbed by clays. In soils, wastewaters, pond liners, and fertilizers; this means the absorption of nuclear wastes and metals are faciliated by clays including bentonite. According to a US Geological Survey report, thorium mine production in the US decreased at the end of 1994, as demand for same was on the decline since the 1980s. Thorium refinery production and reserves are located in the US, Australia, Brazil, Canada, India, Malaysia, Norway, South Africa, and other countries. India has the largest natural stores. Thorium can also be mined from thorium-bearing quartz. In the US, Idaho, Montana, and Wyoming have veins which yield thorium. In North and South Carolina, there has been great activity in the mining of monazite (thorium-containing) sands since the earliest bauxite/aluminum mines opened in the late 1800s.[5-13]

A US-Russian research consortium was founded in 1993 right before the Dearborn conference for Lyme disease. The purpose was partly to study which experiments would be required to determine safety and fuel performance for nuclear plants that are powered by thorium fuels. The consortium included scientists from the Radkowsky Thorium Power Corporation, Raytheon Nuclear Inc., the *Brookhaven National Laboratory,* and the Kurchatov Institute in Moscow. In 1995, the US DOE approved a $550,000 grant award for the group's research project. Also since 1994, the date of the Dearborn conference for Lyme disease, the US and Russia have had an agreement called Megatons for Megawatts. The program was designed to convert (recycle) highly enriched uranium from obsolete nuclear warhead stockpiles into low enriched uranium that is useful to commercial nuclear power plants in the US. Both countries also agreed to convert a percentage of uranium into mixed oxide fuels (MOX). In the US, the Savannah River Site is home to a new MOX facility.[5-7,9,10-12,14]

The agreement between the two countries ends in 2013, and this is important since uranium stockpiles from Cold War weapons are running extremely low due to the continued recycling efforts upon a limited supply. The recycling of obsolete weapons over mining new ores was a better source for uranium than mining existing stores since mining produces radioactive wastes that are problematic for many reasons. One of them may include the production of Bb spirochetes due to the chemicals and microbes used to leach and recover important ores. Uranium mines are of somewhat limited stores, and the element has a long radioactive half-life; far longer than that of the related thorium. The idea of using thorium as a uranium substitute seems a reasonable alternative when it is roughly three times more abundant, has been used before, and has other attractive qualities.[5-12]

However mining and nuclear wastes remain a huge challenge for those who must dispose of them regardless of their source. Any bacteria and viruses known to associate with these elements will of course also remain clinically important, especially the extremophiles. Any may mutate in the presence of chemicals and radioactive minerals. If they become infected with soil or airborne recombinants, B.t., mold, amoeba, or fungal spores, then they may continue to cause novel infections in animals and humans alike, in a manner that may have been tracked by public health officials ever since the early days of the War Research Service and the Manhattan project. Perhaps now we may understand the possible connections between important industries and the mutated leptonemas that have been followed by public health officials for decades. Isn't it interesting that a leptonema was isolated from a Lyme patient's ECM skin rash in 1981?[5-12]

European precious metal and ore mining has a lengthy history. At the beginning of the 16th century, silver was mined for coins in an area between Bohemia (Czech Republic) and Saxony (Germany) near *Thuringia*, where the first B.t. isolate was originally found. Indeed the first metal rush in European history was not for gold, but for silver in an area that became the town of Sankt Joachimsthal,* or the Valley of Saint Joachim (San Joaquin). Remember the California version of Valley fever (coccidioidomycosis) in the grape wine-rich *San Joaquin valley*? By 1789, German Chemist Martin Klaproth discovered a black pitch ("pech") blend of minerals that would become known as *Uranium,* named after the last planet to have been discovered at the time.[13-16]

**Silver produced large silver coins called "Joachimsthaler"; a name shortened to "Thaler," which was distorted to the word "dollar."*

A decade and a half later, uranium would be discovered in significant quantities in England, Austria, Romania; and in Morvan, a limestone escarpment in Burgundy in the Côte d'Or, the southeastern part of France* and the heart of French wine country. The area is a main watershed from northern to southern Europe to the Mediterranean Sea. Early uranium was used to produce yellow glass that fluoresced green, and for ceramic and porcelain glazes; and later for making sepia tones in photography. Glass making and glass blowing is an ancient art, and it of course involves a mined material, silica (sand). The height of glassmaking was the Italian Renaissance, and Venice and Murano, Italy became the center of the industry. The trade then swept through France, Germany, the Netherlands, Spain, Sweden, and England by the 17th century. In France glassmaking began in Normandy (NW) and Lorraine (SE of Paris, near Zurich, Switzerland). We can see what may have wound up in wastewaters of important rivers and watersheds from several industries.[15-18]

**The Côte d'Or contains limestone, rocks from this current Quaternary period, which of course contains coprolites, or fossilized dinosaur poop that was used for military munitions and fertilizers.*

It appears highly likely that current interests in nuclear science and thorium acquisition may play a role for those who have connections or colleagues from Battelle; and who are currently visiting Russia to study a novel tickborne infection called *Borrelia miyamotoi*. Maybe one reason Dr. Allen Steere who identified a novel mutated leptonema from a Lyme patient's rash in 1981 visited Russia in 1993 to study Lyme borreliosis was due to the "nuclear" element link. When he returned from abroad, the recommendations he made at Dearborn the following year were reflective of his studies abroad. However they may not have been made purely for the reasons that most people think (vaccines), but for other, more industrially impactful reasons.

Southern France has a long history of nuclear energy and waste storage. It is the largest user of nuclear energy in Europe, and the country processes nuclear wastes that are imported from other countries. Nuclear wastes are processed in the Languedoc-Roussillon region at the Centraco nuclear site. Centraco is located on the grounds of another nuclear site called Marcoule – the site of a recent blast in a metallic waste oven. Surface or underground mining of uranium operated from 1975 to 1997 in mines near Montpellier on the southeast coast. Of course Languedoc is the same area where the Morgellon's children danced around during the late 17th century with a strange illness that may have resembled today's Morgellon's disease.[19,20]

We should be able to see more clearly why scientists tied to Lyme disease may be in Russia studying *Borrelia miyamotoi*; especially if it is a tick-transmitted *Borrelia japonica* that has mutated under forces found in the area where it is being studied. Perhaps it truly is a model for how Lyme disease develops from environmental, industrial, and insect-borne factors.

However another reason why there is so much attention on a "new" (old) relapsing fever organism may have to do with the new research grant that Drs. Fish and Krause (Yale) recently acquired. It seems that members of the same small group of individuals who have been "in the know" about the Lyme disease organism for four decades, while arguably "secretive" about what they find inside tick bodies, are nevertheless profiting rather nicely on borrelia-related studies the longer the Bb agent remains a "mystery." The casual observer may feel that scientists who have valuable information about an emerging epidemic as well as what lies inside the bodies of its vectors have a duty to report all they find to public health experts and to the doctors who treat patients so all may benefit from shared knowledge. However sharing important information freely in the world of Lyme disease and patent royalties for recombinant organisms seems to be more wishful thinking than it is a reality.

If scientists have knowingly withheld important evidence of tick symbionts, extremophiles, spiroplasmas, and other microbes and their important connections to Lyme disease, then this probably did not occur because everyone was "unaware" or simply "forgot" to mention their presence. Due to the significant number of "coincidences" throughout Lyme disease history, including who was studying (and tracking) important microbes it seems improbable that scientists whose research is funded by multi-millions of federal dollars would never uncover the information that I have provided in this book. Whatever lurks inside the bodies of Lyme disease-transmitting ticks (and the fact that other insects carry Bb spirochetes) should have been placed upon the examination table for all to see at least as early as 1975. This was a time when most if not all of the agents I discuss in this book were already known to exist, and when the Connecticut outbreak first went public.

It has become painfully obvious over time and from reviewing the information that I have put into my books, that what has *not* been revealed to the public over many decades may be more important to us than what has over time managed to leak out as a result of public pressure. The question remains what else has not yet been revealed? I'm afraid the answers we seek may be clearly outlined by clues found within the pages of this book. These answers may prove to have "roots" in industrial mining and in the biological warfare weapons of mass insect destruction.

I wonder if it was ever predicted that scientific interventions for the world of insecticides might one day collide with the animal and human populations. I wonder also if any of the agriculturally and industrially deployed microbes were ever considered with respect to their possible effects upon populations that were inoculated with vaccines and other recombinant products. Surely scientists must have known that genetically engineered bioagents might create a *biological conflict of interest* capable of causing diseases in non-targeted populations. But then perhaps this is one very strong reason why a pharmaceutical firm partnered with the War Research Service at the onset of chemical, nuclear, and biological warfare weapons research during the 1940s – because such conflicts of interest may have been known to be unavoidably inevitable. ❑

Nine: Now the Story is Told

Dirty Little Bacteria

Spirochetes are not the only bacteriae that are exposed to pollutants including agricultural and industrial wastes. There are hundreds of known bacillus species that have been identified over the last century and a half. We are mainly interested in the spore-forming variety since those are what have been applied to the environment as insecticies; as biowarfare "simulants," and other tools. Approximately twenty-two sporulating bacillus strains were identified before 1983, the year after the Lyme disease causative agent was formally announced. Of these, over a dozen have been agriculturally and industrially important. If we ignore several routine sporulating strains, we are left with roughly <u>fifteen</u> *Bacillus* strains as listed below. Note that exactly fifteen strains of *Bacillus cereus* of the variety *thuringiensis* were isolated from diseased insects to create the "original" fifteen B.t. strains for insecticidal use. There are exactly fifteen strains of *Borrelia burgdorferi* mentioned in a patent invention for a Lyme disease vaccine and diagnostic test. The patent is assigned to lyme notables Drs. Dattwyler, Luft, and colleague Gomes-Solecki. If we assume the original fifteen B.t. strains were fermented from one or more of the "important" strains, then B.t. strains may be derived from any of the following, in chronologic order by date of isolation:[1]

Bacillus subtilis (1835) isolated from soil, dust, vegetation a/k/a *Vibrio subtilis*
Bacillus anthracis (1872) isolated from animal blood, carcasses, animal products, soil
Bacillus megaterium (1884) isolated from foods and cattle feces
Bacillus cereus (1887) isolated from soil, milk, foods
*Bacillus circulans** (1890) isolated from sewage, soil, food, infant bile
Bacillus licheniformis (1898) isolated from soil, foods, milk
Bacillus pumilus (1901) isolated from soil, foods, veterinarian specimens
Bacillus sphaericus (1904) isolated from soil; used as a mosquito larvicide
Bacillus coagulans (1915) from soil, silage, canned foods, milk, medicines, gelatin, tomato juice
Bacillus thuringiensis (1915) isolated from flour moths
Bacillus badius (1919) isolated from feces, dust, marine environments, foods, gelatin factory, antacids
Bacillus fastidiosus (1929) isolated from soil, poultry litter
Bacillus alcalophilus (1934) isolated from soda ash (early fertilizer)
Bacillus psychrosaccharolyticus (1967) cold sugar fermenter from soil, lowlands, marshes
Bacillus schlegelii (1981) isolated from lake sediment, geothermal soils, sugar factory sludge

**The Bacillus circulans group has 7 Bacillus* strains, and 8 *Paenibacillus strains that might instead comprise the original 15 strains from which B.t. insecticides are fermented. There are also fifteen paenibacillus groups.*

Of these strains, we know that *Bacillus anthracis* was fermented as a biowarfare weapon (anthrax). We also know that the name "*Bacillus licheniformis*" is synonymous with *Bacillus globigii.* So-called "harmless" *B. globigii* biowarfare experiments were undertaken beginning in 1962 under the US military's *Project SHAD.* If past biowarfare experiments led to the development of human infections, such revelations could be expected to remain hidden from the public.[2,3]

There is no way to know exactly what is in the original "B.t." insecticides unless we scrutinize manufacturing processes. Since today's B.t. formulas are likely to include recombinant clones, this makes B.t. use problematic because the plasmids (mobile genes) from B.t. strains may migrate into other bacteriae to form new mutants that are capable of causing infectious diseases not only in insects, but higher animals. This is really a problem if B.t. strains have been engineered to include a *flavobacterium* that causes encephalitis and meningitis in animals and humans – as several B.t. formulas with cloned microbes seem to indicate.

We know that any bacillus strains that become infected with viruses (especially CPV/reoviruses), can make already virulent bacterial mutants able to cause serious infections. Since there are many varieties of bacillus bacteriae found in nature, an unlimited number of infectious diseases may emerge from *the contamination of other bacteria by viruses and phagic bacteria.* It makes no difference if the microbes are natural in origin, or whether they are recombinantly created in a laboratory and then applied as insecticides. The use of viruses (i.e. baculoviruses, reoviruses) to assist (infect) the phagic bacteriae of insecticides was the intended purpose of introducing borrelina viruses in 1951.

Certain bacteriae are able to thrive among specific environmental pollutants. Extremophiles are able to withstand conditions that are highly acidic (acidophilic), alkaline (alkaliphilic), neutral (neutrophilic), salty (halophilic), moderate (mesophilic), cold (psychrophilic) or hot-tempered (thermophilic). The kinds of bacteria found in these environments and the kinds of airborne spores that contaminate same, determine the menu of infectious agents that may be picked up by insects and animals.

Since microbial insecticides contain bacterial and fungal spores, these agents remain in the environment as viable infections. Industrial products such as radioactive elements, polymers, or even tannery wastes from animals and insects contribute to the pathogens present in polluted wastewaters. Even the microbes of biowarfare "simulant" experiments have contributed to the possible agents available for reassortment in the environment.

There are a number of spore-forming bacilli that are found in key industrial areas, and these bacteria are being examined with keen interest today. Most strains degrade biopolymers. Some will degrade synthetic polymers, and most utilize nitrogen or ammonia in their cellular processes. Some strains are highly acid and arsenic tolerant; while others feed off of sugar refinery wastes, wood pulp, nuclear or acid mine wastes; or degrade toxic persisting organic pollutants.[3,4]

Bacteriae that are chitin and cellulose degraders are useful in industrial biocides. Strains which oxidize nitrites and ammonia are common in soil and water, especially as toxic mine, tannery, agriculture, and other industrial wastes. Bacillus strains such as *B. licheniformis* or *B. subtilis* accumulate toxins and metals including copper, cobalt, aluminum, cadmium, zinc, iron, and aluminosilicates. *Bacillus megaterium* which was used as an early insecticide, is able to accumulate gold, palladium, platinum, silver, and rhodium. *Pseudomonas* strains are also known to be arsenic tolerant and to bind metals and metalloids.

Bacterial strains which take up radioactive elements, mine wastes, and explosives are important as well. Arsenic and uranium are found in trace amounts in organophosphate fertilizers. Arsenic is found in plastics, textile dyes, and other products. This allows the bacteriae to become important delivery vehicles for environmental toxins and heavy metals.[5-14]

New methods to bioremediate arsenic from drinking water are using plastics and the amino acid cysteine. Scientists at Monmouth University in New Jersey are developing techniques to treat drinking water in this way since cysteine binds arsenic to the plastic polymers. (Some bacteria use cysteine in their metabolic processes.) This suggests that cysteine may also help bind arsenic from humans who have toxic levels in their body.[15-17]

It is possible that spores from past biowarfare "simulants" (*Bacillus globigii*) and insecticides (*B. sphaericus, B. megaterium, B. lentimorbus, B.t.*) have contaminated the bacteria found at copper, aluminum, uranium, and other metal, ore, and smelting sites. If so, we may expect to see similar bacterial contaminations in and around other industries including nuclear, canneries, wastewater treatment, tanneries, paper/lumber mills, and more. We may also find "contaminated" bacteriae that remain in textile wastes. For example *Bacillus endophyticus* is a bacterium found in the inner tissues of cotton plants – cotton that is now genetically engineered to contain B.t. endotoxins. *B. endophyticus* and other paenibacillus family members excrete enzymes and other substances that will mobilize metals from the soil and from fly ash (a byproduct of burning coal).

Fly ash is used in concrete. Like coal it contains radioactive elements including uranium and thorium. When coal is burned, it releases airborne particulates including radioactive elements which become airborne contaminants capable of contributing to human cancers and the mutation of microbes. Where there are fly ash impoundments (i.e. Pennsylvania), elevated cancer cases and contaminated water tables are found due to airborne pollution and soil leaching. This is a serious problem of which the EPA has long been aware. It is also a problem of which the public was poorly informed according to EPA documents. Keep in mind that coal-fired plants and other industries burn not only coal, but other fuels in a process called "co-burning." Up to half of the waste mixtures that are burned for fuel along with coal include the following; any of which harbor bacterial spores. Once these materials are burned, they become infectious airborne contaminants.[18-28]

agricultural refuse	auto shredder fluff	bark and other wood
biomass	boiler cleaning wastes	mill rejects
paper mill sludge	peat	petroleum coke
railroad ties	sewage sludge	straw
contaminated soils	refuse derived fuel	regeneration waste streams
tire-derived fuel	used oil	wastes from manufactures at gas plant sites
acid mine wastes	dried clay	furnace brick
oil combustion wastes	limestone	coal-fuel and non-coal-fuel mixtures

In addition, cement kiln dust is used to cap wastes and to control leachates into ground water. Bentonite clay is used to line retention ponds and waste landfills, and we know about its "leaky" properties under radiation saturation. It is also an efficient collector of bacteria and viruses. This information lends new meaning to what Ft. Detrick scientists were studying with respect to airborne pollutants and certain infectious disease families back in 1968, the progress of which they discussed at the Illinois Institute of Technology conference on aerobiology in Chicago. Perhaps airborne, soil-borne, and water-borne wastes really have contributed to infectious diseases all along.[18-28]

Whatever is thrust into the atmosphere eventually makes its way to the ground and water. Our focus for contaminants is really on the soil, water, and the wastes which contaminate same. There are a number of soil bacteriae other than those we have discussed. Any of these have the potential to become contaminated with mutagenic or radioactive wastes, or phagic bacteria or viruses. For example *Bacillus nealsonii* was isolated from a spacecraft assembly plant. *Bacillus funiculus* and *B. thermocloacae* are found in wastewaters and sludge. *Bacillus mojavensis* is found in desert soil. *Bacillus infirmus* is found in shale; while *B. vedderi* is found in bauxite processing (red mud).

Bacillus methanolicus is a methanol-tolerant strain found in raw milk, and several strains are found in pasteurized milk. *Bacillus cereus, B. fastidiosus, B. halodurans, B. pumilus,* and *B. subtilis* have been found in poultry litter, feathers, and manure. *Bacillus mycoides* has been found in moths. *B. luciferensis* and other strains are found in geothermally heated waters. Silage isolates have produced strains including *B. coagulans* and *B. siralis.* Related *Clostridium* species that are the segmented bacteria of poultry, rodents, and fish may become a problem since they are highly compatible and capable of gene reassortments with bacillus species.

Some B.t. strains are virtually identical to *B. cereus, B. anthracis, B. mycoides, B. pseudomycoides,* and *B. weihenstephanensis* strains. The B.t. strains are divided into groups by their unique flagellar antigens. These immune-stimulating proteins are part of the flagellin or tail of the bacteriae, and are used for locomotion. *Borrelia burgdorferi* is also differentiated by flagellar antigens. Any bacteriae can become infected by sporulating bacteriae from *flavobacterium, paenibacillus,* or *bacillus* families. From the available evidence it seems that the pollution of soil and waterborne bacteriae including the *leptospires* and the spiroplasmas are perhaps the most relevant to the history of Lyme disease and Morgellon's.[29,30]

A scientific textbook reveals that bacterial strains commonly found upon sheep fleece include *Bacillus cereus* and *Bacillus thuringiensis* (B.t.). It also says that *Bacillus anthracis* (anthrax) is *only isolated from sheep hides, blood, or tissues* from infected animals. This might point our attentions in the direction of *tannery wastes* as one culprit of infectious disease outbreaks. The book also says that anthrax is "not" highly contagious; that cutaneous anthrax is "readily treated," and only life-threatening in "exceptional" cases. It also claims that intestinal anthrax is treatable if recognized; and that oral infective doses are quite high at roughly 10,000 spores. However it is a fact that inhaled anthrax is an efficient and virulent route of infection. Airborne spores are the most likely form of transmission, and a route for which infectious disease experts are rightly concerned.[31]

The information in this book should shed new light on efforts by infectious disease experts to warn the public against "anthrax" outbreaks. It would appear that the *real* anthrax threat may not be military, but from the airborne spores of fermented, globally-applied insecticides; and the ability of B.t. strains under influence of viruses and chemicals to donate their infectious plasmids to other microbes. Scientists already know that B.t. parasporal crystals are contained within the mobile plasmids. These plasmids have been found to transfer into soil strains of *Bacillus cereus* (from which anthrax is fermented). They have also been found to migrate into *Bacillus pumilus,* a 1904 strain that was isolated from soil, food, and animal samples.[31]

The random transfer of DNA by B.t. insecticides into other compatible soil or waterborne bacteria would understandably create the necessity of a "homeland security" division of the federal government. It would also explain the sudden push for "anthrax" preparedness, and future vaccines. It might also usher in the trends toward denied illnesses in favor of protecting important biowarfare tools that may be causing human diseases. However the *actual* threat to the *global* population as far as anthrax outbreaks are concerned will probably come from the agricultural and industrial insecticides already in use for the past century and a half.[31]

Thoughts on Bb and Lyme Disease

From a book that discusses cell wall deficient bacterial forms, we may learn clues about the spirochetes of Lyme. Bb forms blebs, granules, cysts, and motile spirochetes, and can produce filaments from which new spirochetes emerge. This of course sounds a lot like some of the sporulating fungi or the *Actinomycetes*, which are fungal-like bacteria we learned about in an earlier chapter on *Spiroplasmas.* The cystic form of Bb differs from the L-forms of other bacteria, because instead of forming numerous spirochetes within a cyst, they will make only a few inside the cyst.[1]

Fluorescent antibody studies have been performed on the 277F rabbit tick spiroplasma, and also on *Leptospira icterohemorrhagiae*, the infectious leptospires of animals and humans. In the L-form laboratory at Wayne State University in Michigan, scientists discovered that fluorescent antibodies to *Borrelia burdorferi* reacted with "both the spirochetal forms and atypical forms of the organism in culture." This means that Bb antibodies reacted to one or both spirochetes, and this is not surprising considering that Bb may be an aggregate organism that includes a leptospiral component.[1]

We must ask ourselves why would Bb antibodies react to the 277F agent and to a pathogenic leptospire? Why also would patent inventions by Lyme-notables be capable of detecting a *Brucellosis* agent, an infection that was not only aerosolized and militarily tested as an agent of biowarfare, but that is also highly prevalent in livestock animals we use for food? Why would registered patents held by mining and petroleum companies that are useful to detect *Borrelia burgdorferi* in human or animal urine samples, also be capable of detecting extremophiles and other bacteriae that are found deep in the earth's crust?

Why would an agricultural insecticide continue to appear in various patents and research papers when there is discussion of the Lyme disease organism? Why are scientists so afraid of "anthrax" outbreaks? Why were scientists screening Lyme patients for antibodies to arboviruses and spiroplasmas? Why would Lyme notables write papers that describe an insect virus that appears similar to the genetic structure of a Bb chromosome or a B.t. phage? Why would insects that are targeted with B.t. insecticides be described within diagnostic tests and vaccine patents for *Borrelia burgdorferi*?

Borrelia burgdorferi is likely to be an aggregate organism that contains a leptospira, spiroplasma, thermophile, an agriculturally applied B.t. phage, an agricultural fungi (natural or applied), bacteriae such as vibrio or flavobacterium, and at least one or more insect poxviruses such as the "Pj" virus. Once again the Pj virus may be found in *Bacillus popilliae* and *Bacillus lentimorbus,* the milky spore agents; and it might also make its home in *Bacillus thuringiensis* strains.

Bb spirochetes may also contain any of a number of phagic bacteria and viruses. The individual components are important and will vary somewhat among Bb strains; causing some patients to become more sick than others. Regardless of their composition, all Bb strains seem to contain several common microbes. These aggregate spirochetes cause human disease, but so do their individual components. Patients who are not infected with leptonema/spiroplasma components may still be infected with other microbes including B.t. phages, thermophiles, bacteria, fungi, and viruses. The mixtures depend upon what lies within the body of the vectoring insect. Any combinations may produce different human diseases (i.e. chronic fatigue, diabetes, etc.). Some of the individual components, with or without the Lyme spirochete, may be able to reactivate latent infections in the human body.

While this sounds like a lot of individual microbes gang up to cause disease; remember that Bb spirochetes are far more complex than other spirochetes from the same family. We must also think about the complex recombinant formulas used as insecticides and which have increased in toxicity over time. Even microbes can become infected with multiple pathogens, and those pathogens are found in the highly polluted agricultural, industrial, and "nuclear" wastes found in soils, waters, and our foods.

We have learned that microbial insecticides are specifically designed to contain viruses, toxins, and bacteria that combine to form gut-deteriorating phages. Once the bacteriae enters the insect's body, any of the insect's bacterial or viral symbionts, even when latent, become tools that are targeted for reactivation inside insects. This means that if an insect is infected with brucella, Q fever, ehrlichia, wolbachia, spiroplasmas, mycoplasmas, chlamydia, Rocky Mt. spotted fever, or other pathogens, whatever is there can and will be used against the insect as an effective killing tool. This is the design and intent of the applied microbial insecticides. Phagic bacteria are used to prepare the way for toxic microbial cocktails to enter an insect, and to reactivate any latent infections that are present, to kill pest insects.

However industrial pollutants abound and are contributing to these infections, especially as antibacterial formulas are applied to industrial polymers; and agricultural biocides contaminate wastewaters and soils where extremophiles, and phages also thrive. Chemical catalysts from industrial and agricultural wastes contribute to the mutation of soil and water-based spirochetes; thereafter infecting the plants and the insects which feed upon, or come into contact with them. The insects transfer highly complex mixed infections that have mutated/reassorted in the presence of chemicals and radioactive elements, into their animal and human hosts. With the advent of genetic engineering came far more virulent pathogens which migrated into the environment and into the bodies of vectoring insects. Together with very toxic, persisting chemicals which permeate and contaminate the air, water, and soils we depend upon for our survival, came a new era of infectious diseases which formerly did not exist.

The World Health Organization and other scientists are keenly aware that microbes are becoming polluted by industrial wastes and other pollutants. The WHO guidelines for recreational water environments speak of the "hazards" of water environments for humans. These hazards include gastroenteritis, acute respiratory infections, and ear infections which arise from *the pollution of water leptospires*, and contact with blooms of toxigenic cyanobacteria (algae) in fresh or marine water and from dinoflagellates (plankton) of marine waters. Pollutants in marine environments also affect the smallest microbes including important *phages.*[2,3]

From September 1978 to September 1979, scientists at the Connecticut University Health Center in Farmington were studying *the effects of low levels of fluoride on bacterial metabolism, bacterial attachment,* and dental caries. These studies may also have been analyzing the release of fluorides from skeletal structures in addition to teeth. The fluoride levels that were detected were felt to be directly influential toward bacterial aggregation and mutation. This hints that fluoridated water and other products may have a direct impact upon the mutation of microbes in *any* environment, including the *human body.*[2,3]

Insects which come into contact with applied insecticides and pollutants in their environment will become infected with the agents, and will transfer the contaminants into animal and human hosts. It is entirely naïve to believe that animals and humans will not at some point become infected with insecticidal agents or the chemicals and microbes that were intended to protect products or food crops from insects and important microbes. When we research the emergence of infectious diseases over the last century and a half, we find there has always been some form of chemical catalyst (i.e. phosphate, fluoride, chloride, radioactivity) in the picture. There is also the very long history of applied pesticides and fertilizers that are also omnipresent. The application of industrial biocides seems to have contributed the most to the development of animal and human disease epidemics.

Infectious diseases may be traced back to the earliest use of industrial chemicals and phosphate fertilizers exhumed from mined materials which also contained radioactive elements, fluorides, and microbes. In later centuries the applied chemicals and microbes of agriculture, and persisting industrial wastes have expanded in their toxic activity and in their global use. The onslaught of genetically engineered formulas has contributed to the kinds of microbes that are available to reassort today. This explains why what centuries ago were only a few scattered cases of an ECM-rash illness became a globally important infectious disease epidemic called Lyme disease (and the "Lyme-plus" Morgellon's).[4-8]

The history of synthetic fertilizers and pesticides has clearly been fraught with safety and toxicity issues. Some of the world history related to industrial chemicals and chemical nerve agents are the most tragic in human history. The development of nuclear energy has heralded some of the most powerful weapons in history, but also invited the proliferation of extremophile organisms which formerly thrived underground. The ongoing use of fertilizers with high phosphate content and the natural and synthetic pesticides and industrial pollutants appear to be the hidden driving forces behind the development of novel pathogens found in plants, insects, animals, and humans over the past century and a half. Microbes, insects, animals, and humans are now contaminated with heavy metals, "plastics," chemical toxins, pollutants, insecticides, herbicides, fungicides, and microbes that have happily mutated in the presence of many of these agents. Some of them were manipulated in the laboratory before being applied as weapons of insect biowarfare and industrial helpers.

It is obvious that over the past century and a half, efforts to improve the world around us for many reasons have not prevented the emergence of novel diseases that were unheard of decades ago; and that have become more virulent the longer the tools which may create them remain in use. While the scientists behind the design and selection of chemical and microbial tools are creating them with good intentions, the bottom line is whatever we put into the environment will eventually make its way into our bodies. Those who diagnose and treat human diseases must become better educated about the various pathogens that are emerging within plants, insects, and animals. What affects the lower inhabitants of the planet ultimately affects the global human population as well.

> *Those who are obviously aware of what causes important human infections have the responsibility not to sequester valuable information necessary to diagnose and treat patients!*

The wildlife, plants, insects, and sea creatures that have already suffered the devastating negative effects of the chemicals and microbes that have been globally applied in the past, were the first to sound the alarm that what man was doing to the environment was probably not a good idea. It took us long enough, but we began to turn our attentions toward these warnings when harmful pesticides like DDT were banned during the 20th century. Now that human infectious disease epidemics have surfaced over a similar period, we see that the concerns expressed by scientists who in the early days of recombinant engineering cautioned against using GM techniques, may not have been without some degree of merit. Unfortunately those who regulate chemical, microbial, and recombinant insecticides and other important tools are failing to heed the subtle whispers of the "non-targeted" insects being killed by current designs.

Centuries of irresponsible waste disposal practices have contributed the most to human disease epidemics. However in the modern era, the purposeful introduction of recombinant microbes including some that never previously existed exponentially elevates the risks of human disease epidemics. Some of the microbial formulas on the horizon will become highly virulent and possibly incurable once they enter the human landscape.

Some scientists continue to ignore the obvious cries of the bird and bee populations that have literally fallen from the skies; or died in their hives as a result of globally disbursed microbes and pollutants. They continue to ignore the loud echoes of oceanic creatures found disoriented and beached upon land; and the numbers of animal species which disappear due to "unknown" causes. We watch helplessly as expansive rain forests and marine coral reefs vanish within a lifetime. All around us life forms of all orders are suffering the effects of man-made pollutants, toxins, agricultural and industrial wastes, and from human and for-profit expansion.

The same agencies, governments, and scientists whom failed to listen to the deafening cries of the ill populations; have barely acknowledged that chronic diseases such as Lyme or Morgellon's are legitimate. Will these individuals also ignore the new diseases on the horizon when they arrive at the hands of newly designed genetic weapons of industrial warfare? What is to become of our world when a new bubonic plague or microbes from the days of the dinosaurs are globally unleashed in the interest of killing pest insects or infectious microbes? What happens to humans when such recombinant cocktails cause another genetic engineering "accident;" or contaminate cell lines to adversely affect everything from insecticides to vaccines?

I wonder if the presentation of real evidence that plausibly links Lyme disease and other important infections of today to industrial wastes and agricultural tools used over the last century and a half will make any difference whatsoever to current biotech trends. Will such revelations cause an outcry among patients and physicians who are forced to deal with the effects of these tools upon the "non-targeted" human species? Are such tools really as "safe" as they are advertised or we are expected to believe? Perhaps "safety" issues are why such endeavors were "undertaken with great secrecy and vigor" all those years ago – because some of the scientists involved in the early War Research Service years were keenly aware that whatever microbes would be used agriculturally, militarily, and industrially, would also covertly inoculate animal and human populations as well. As Dr. MacArthur said in 1969, in five or ten years:[9,10]

> "...it would probably be possible to make a new infective organism...Most important of these is that it might be refractory to the immunological and therapeutic processes upon which we depend to maintain our relative freedom from infectious disease."

Whether such an agent was ever intended for development or not, it seems that such agents have certainly come about, with the Lyme disease agent leading the way. Whether scientists actually ever intentionally created such an organism, or whether it was simply an accident of recombinant processes, by now should be obvious. A number of factors likely converged to create the new epidemics of our day, including Lyme disease. It is interesting that the new agricultural tools of modern times, and also the pursuit of nuclear weapons have managed to live up to another statement made by Dr. MacArthur decades ago:[10]

> "It is a highly controversial issue and there are many who believe such research should not be undertaken lest it lead to yet another method of massive killing of large populations."

Perhaps the first method of killing large populations that was under discussion at the time was the use of nuclear weapons; and the second may have been the use of weapons of insect (and microbial) biowarfare.

I believe that the reason there has never been a *complete Borrelia burgdorferi* spirochete isolated from the environment is because it is "built" as an aggregate organism based upon the pollutants that are found in the environment and what lies within the insect (and animal) hosts. Through *host amplification*, the deterioration of the gut under the action of microbial insecticides allows a complex mixture of infectious agents to reassort and to become pathogenic to insects, animals, and humans.

Therefore people on both sides of the political debate about "Lyme disease" have been right all along – well sort of, anyway. The *classic* ECM rash illness found in people who had the disease before it became the *modern* Lyme disease we see today, was probably far more easily treated than today's version. The early ECM rash illnesses of the 19th and early 20th centuries probably did not involve a spiroplasma component, although it may have involved a radiation-tolerant microbe that was comfortable in uranium or thorium-containing wastes. There were powerful chemicals being used by industires even as early as the 1600s, and those chemicals had mutagenic potential. In the mid-20th century, more powerful chemicals were created as nerve agents and insecticides used in industry and agriculture. These chemicals seem to have afforded the mutation of modern microbes into forms which may be found in blood-feeding parasites. With the application of superphosphate fertilizers which contained surfactants, clays, radioactive elements; and the introduction of recombinant and natural insecticides, the kinds of gene reassortments which may create novel infectious diseases most certainly went to work. Soon they began to emerge not only in insect populations, but also in animal and human populations.

Genetic engineering technologies are imperfect. As scientists and their patents repeatedly describe, recombinant formulas have repeatedly led to "accidents" and "reassortments" – most of which were considered to be "adventitious," "illegitimate," and certainly undesirable. Any insect cell lines that were contaminated with one or more infectious agents affects all insecticides and vaccines or other biological formulas made from them. An example of a livestock vaccine that may be derived from an insect cell line is a leptospirosis vaccine. Whether natural or vaccine-derived, animals were found to be infected with mutated spirochetes in the form of *leptonema.* Animal wastes would pass such infections into nearby soils, wastewaters, and fertilizers that are applied to agricultural crops, or even golf courses. Insecticidal and other formulas that are sprayed upon food crops make their way into the animal, poultry, and human diets. Is it a surprise then that scientists discovered a mutated leptonema strain in the ECM rash of a Lyme disease patient in 1981? We can see why this discovery might become "inconvenient" to discuss in association with Lyme disease.

Manure has been applied as fertilizer for centuries. Along with acid mine wastes, fertilizers leach into rivers and other watersheds; where a mutated leptonema would be isolated. Bulls at an agricultural research station that were inoculated with vaccines (or fed additives) might easily produce a mutated leptonema in their urine or semen. In the wild, animals such as turtles would be among the first creatures to be exposed to nuclear, industrial, and agricultural wastes; and the mutated leptonemas they likely produced in contaminated soils and waters. Many industries use agricultural fungicides, algaecides, and insecticides to treat their wastewaters and/or their products during manufacturing. These chemicals are the same as, or are similar to those in agricultural use.

The initial "ECM-rash illness" agents of Lyme disease from the early 20th century may have been "curable" using short-course antibiotics. But the "other" agents of the late 20th century forward (i.e. spiroplasmas, fungi, extremophiles, phages); the recombinant microbes of "B.t." and related formulas; and the persisting nuclear and chemical pollutants wreak havoc in the human body. They may even reactivate latent retroviruses or vaccine viruses to contribute to disease states. The recombinant microbes and extremophiles which have been brought to the surface and sometimes are engineered into microbial formulas now have antibiotic-resistance genes and the ability to repair their own DNA.

Any of these factors may be the "something else" that some infectious disease researchers seem to know about, and which they claim is the *real* problem with "chronic" Lyme disease patients. To date however, no one has been anything but reluctant to identify what that "something else" might be. Patients such as myself are living proof that the spirochetes of Lyme disease persist in the body even after antibiotics. These microbes can be cultured from the blood to prove they "still" exist. However patients who are ill don't necessarily want to fully understand what lives inside of them, or why. Their only wish is to become well and to recapture their lives to the extent possible.

When we examine the metallic chemical elements in various states of decay in the environment, some have a longer half-life than others (time to non-radioactivity). Degradation varies by element, and its current state of decay when found. Radioactive elements may last from a few hours to millions of years. The elements adhere to skeletal structures of our teeth and bones where they bind with fluorides and other toxins that are part of our physical structures. Over time stored fluorides and other pollutants are released which may produce symptoms common to many "chronic" illnesses. In the presence of microbes which produce enzymes that degrade our skeletal structures, more toxins will be released over time. These will contribute to the bacterial toxins that are created by infectious agents.

Bound chemical and nuclear wastes continually expose our cells to highly mutagenic radicals, and may promote cancers. The development of antibodies to circulating fluorides and the persisting wastes which readily adhere to our body structures are not surprising to find but this concept does not seem to have made its way into medical schools. Many of these elements are able to degrade the protective myelin sheaths of the human nervous system to contribute to diseases such as Multiple Sclerosis. When there is an infectious agent involved that harbors genes which degrade certain chemicals, we can understand how persisting organic pollutants that are stored in the body will become part of complex human diseases.

In addition, vaccinated humans produce antibodies to bacteria, viruses, and substrates of the vaccine formulas used. Any of these ingredients may comprise that "something else" from which we all collectively suffer from one degree to another. Some of the recombinant and natural infections introduced by vectoring insects are not only able to reactivate infections in insects, but they seem also to reactivate latent infections in animal and human bodies. The ever-evolving mixtures of industrial and recombinant pollutants make it more difficult for our bodies to protect us from our highly toxic environment. It is unfortunate that patients who suffer from the illnesses of today (and especially Lyme and Morgellon's patients), are not given the credence they deserve. We all suffer the burden of toxic elements and chemical wastes. But chronically ill patients have the likely additional burdens of recombinant and natural microbes. These pathogens not only develop clever mechanisms to persist in their environment, they are introduced into our bodies by vectoring insects and arthropods.

To these tough microbes, our bodies must appear pristine when compared to the highly toxic and polluted environments from which they came. No wonder they are quite happy to persist inside our bodies. Parts of some microbes were first made in a laboratory to be antibiotic resistant. One way or another they landed in toxic waste sites (soil, water) where the toughest microbes survive in hostile environments and are free to reassort with them. These new mutations become insect, animal, and human parasites. It is hardly realistic to believe these microbes may be killed by short-course antibiotics; after which they magically morph into "something else" that is neither a chronic disease nor something capable of evading the best laboratory tests. When we understand that some of these agents in their natural or recombinant form *are currently undetectable by any laboratory tests but by symptom presentation only*, we can see why some patients are called "crazy" for believing they are ill. Unfortunately for the scientists who are unaware of these "undetectable" microbes, their insistence that patients are crazy is cruel, because the patients are indeed ill with something that evidence-based medicine cannot easily validate at this time.

While to the patient it doesn't really matter what you call this "thing" that makes them devastatingly ill, the name of "Lyme disease" or other diseases seems to excessively matter to those who are entrenched in the medico-political debate. Some of these parties have established guidelines and parameters which supposedly define infectious diseases and defend patients. In the end it may be that the patients, the infectious disease doctors, and people on both sides of the debate are partly right, *but only in some respects.* I hope that we now have some idea of what *Borrelia burgdorferi* sensu lato may really be, at least according to this book. Perhaps with these new revelations, public health experts will finally acknowledge chronically ill patients and their physicians.

It is my hope that after considering the points in my books, that the public can finally take meaningful steps forward. The most critical changes currently necessary are freedoms from restrictive laboratory and surveillance criteria; and for physicians to be allowed to treat Lyme patients *until they are well,* however long this may take. The definitions of certain diseases may need to be written to embrace the realities of toxic pollutants and the effects of same upon not only the human species, but every species down the smallest polluted microbe.

The Aggregate Bb

The evidence appears overwhelmingly real that Lyme disease, Morgellon's, and possibly other infectious agents may have had a history that is markedly different than what the scientific, public health, and world in general currently believes. I'm sorry to say that if the information in this book is accurate, then the history of infectious diseases may need to be rewritten because the origins of infectious diseases have not been fully, or perhaps truthfully revealed.

Unfortunately the ideas and information in this book are long overdue for public scrutiny. The explanations of some researchers and public health experts have fallen far short of being supportive of patients who suffer many diseases. Cures elude despite tens of billions of research dollars spent. Many inexpensive alternative treatments for cancers and other diseases are contraindicated by public health experts despite increasing evidence that many of these therapies are safer and more effective than some mainstream pharmaceuticals. What seems to have appeared over time is not a world where cures are promoted, but pharmaceuticals often meant to mask disease symptoms which may have industrial or agricultural origins. Furthermore, the same tools that may have caused important disease epidemics may continue to be used regardless of the consequences.

Practically every family of organisms described within these pages have at one time or another been part of the scientific search to determine what is a Bb spirochete. None of the agents I discuss should come as a surprise to the scientists who create biocides of military, medical, industrial, or veterinary importance. And none of these will probably come as a surprise to those who have over decades researched the Bb spirochete under federal monetary support.

For those who do not yet grasp the significance of the various chemicals and other agents that have polluted the environment to produce pollution-resistant aggregate microbes, I will recap with an industrial process which embraces many of the elements and processes that we have discussed. In the *leather tanning* industry (tanneries), such as those found in upstate New York, deer hides are processed using organic fungicides and other chemicals. Before 1980 when the Lyme disease organism was really beginning to be studied by scientists, TCMB (i.e. *Busan*) or 2-(thiocyanomethylthio)benzothazole, a benzene chemical; and quicksilver (mercury base) biocides and their derivatives were used in the tanning process. They are said to have been banned for this purpose, although busan has also been used as an anti-fungal agent to treat agricultural seeds (i.e. cereal crops, sugar beets, cotton, vegetables, ornamentals) as well as for processing animal hides.

Other highly mutagenic and toxic chemicals such as *chromium sulfate* are applied to soaked hides to remove hair, fat, skin, blood, and other animal wastes. Deer ticks which remain on the carcasses are picked off of the hides, and sometimes even the tannery workers; and scars are visible on the deer hides where ticks were attached. The hides are then dyed using various dye formulas, and which may contain anilines, benzenes, or other toxic chemicals. Other dehairing agents include sodium hydroxide, sodium sulfide, sodium hydrosulfite, dimethyl amines, calcium hydrosulfide, or sodium sulfhydrate. The hides then go through a *deliming* and pickling process where lime is used. Mineral rock-containing grinding wheels also help remove hair and other substances from the hides during processing.

Vegetable tanning uses tannins from the bark and leaves of chestnut, oak, tanoak, acacia, mulberry, and other woods; or chemical polyphenols. Mineral tanning uses chromium III sulfate or other minerals. Chromium III dissolves to make polychromium compounds. We known that chromium VI is also used in nuclear processes. Later in the tanning process, aluminum salts or alum, potash, and other agents are used. Leftovers from tanning process wastes are used to make glues, animal feeds, and agricultural fertilizers. These and other pollutants are discharged into water sources as wastes. When the waste chemicals from multiple industries contaminate rivers such as those found in our example New York state, we can see how mixed wastes from tanneries, nuclear, chemical, aluminum, and other manufacturers and industries mix in fluoridated waters. Despite water treatment, which adds in other important biocides, wastes are discharged and are available to mix with the microbes that live in these environments.

The pollutants from any number of industries which employ anti-fungals, anti-bacterials, anti-algicides, and other biocides play a key role in the mutation of microbes found in water and soil environments. The more contaminated the environment, the more chemically resistant the microbes become. If we look for common chemicals and recombinant formulas used in any of the industries we discussed in this book, we see several agents that are common denominators. These include the amines, radioactive elements, persisting organic pollutants (i.e. synthetic polymers), phosphates, and toxic minerals and chemicals. The pollution of microbes with these agents and the introduction of recombinant genetics have heralded the major infectious diseases of today; and with the exception of the laboratory recombinants, of centuries past. Novel neurological diseases may be brought forth by the introduction of current microbes to persisting chemical agents. All that is needed to create a new disease epidemic is an infected human who was exposed to contaminated waters, soils, foods, products, or vectoring insect or arthropod. Since pollutants are a global problem, the emergence of related global human epidemics is not surprising to find. One example of this process is the Bb spirochete.

What makes up the four different groups of Borrelia burgdorferi sensu lato? When we examine the reovirus family we find human pathogens including those of the *Influenza* class. We also find those from insects and plants; and encephalitis viruses (i.e.

Russian-Spring-Summer, Eyach). Many of these viruses cause Multiple Sclerosis, polio, or Parkinsonian disorders. There are four classifications of reoviruses and there are four classifications of *Borrelia burgdorferi* – three of which cause Lyme disease.

The four Bb groups might be categorized based on specific reovirus groups. For example, perhaps insect reoviruses are those which make up the *Borrelia burgdorferi* sensu stricto strains. In the second group, we might find plant reoviruses that when reassorted comprise the *Borrelia garinii* strains. In the third group we might see animal reoviruses which reassort to become *Borrelia afzelii* strains. The fourth classification of reoviruses that do not cause Lyme disease and which include the human relapsing fever agent *Borrelia japonica,* when reassorted with a reo- or another virus may cause human influenzas such as "avian" flu, "swine" flu, or another flu not yet announced.

The influenza strain group members are possibly caused by the *rotavirus* group of reoviruses. These influenza strains are commonly genetically engineered into insecticides. With or without a corresponding relapsing fever *B. japonica* spirochete, these microbes may be transmissible by insect vectors. If this is how the various Bb strain groups are defined, it also means that "flu" vaccines are meant to prevent infections that may be caused in part by recombinant insecticides. It also suggests that insecticidal formulas are wrongly targeting human populations when they are only supposed to affect insects and their resident microbes.

We also know that reoviruses are naturally found in association with baculoviruses. Reoviruses thrive in the environment, but sawfly viruses were also imported into the US from Sweden. In 1951 they were released by Connecticut scientists as insecticidal helpers. Thereafter other scientists adopted similar techniques. This significantly increased the presence of these "satellite" viruses in the environment as baculovirus helpers. Insecticides are engineered using baculoviruses, toxins, enzymes, and other genes to promote transcription and insect infections. One of the most profitable for the biotech industry has been *Taq polymerase,* an enzyme derived from a *cyanobacterium,* which is an extremophile blue-green algae. There is evidence that some genetically engineered chimera are faulty in their construction. This appears to allow important insect viruses (i.e. sindbis as a model) to be kicked out of a recombinant construct under the right circumstances, such as exposure to a satellite virus. Once loose in the body, the virus is free to reassort to cause new or reactivated diseases.

Reoviruses are also naturally found among mined materials including fertilizer phosphates. They are also naturally present in plants, animals, and birds that are fed upon by ticks and insects. Mined minerals and ores are important to many industries, including copper, steel, aluminum, and nuclear industries. These industries produce fluorides and other wastes as byproducts of manufacturing, production, or refining. The reoviruses are highly fluoride-tolerant since they inhabit the same areas where fluorides are found. They are also highly tolerant of organofluoride and organochloride chemicals used in agriculture, nuclear, metal, plastics, and other industries. They easily survive in wastewaters as candidates for viral reassortment under the right catalysts. During mixed infections, viruses contribute the genes necessary to reactivate latent microbes into active, infective pathogens. The vaccine components which remain in animal or human bodies may help this process along, because the formulas contain known contaminants capable of initiating gene reassortments inside the body when presented with live genes.

There is probably a leptonema (mutated leptospira) component to an aggregate Bb spirochete. It is a tad difficult to decide which spirochetal strains are involved in this intermediate form, because they may vary. Noguchi's 1917 leptonema came from a patient with infectious jaundice (yellow's disease). The yellows diseases usually involve an insect flavivirus (degraded reovirus) and some kind of pathogenic leptospira. In human yellow fever, a leptospira becomes infected with a flavivirus, or it could become infected with a flavobacterium. However Noguchi's leptonema probably did not involve a mutated spiroplasma like we find today, because the spiroplasmas seem to be a product of late 20th century recombinant tools and chemicals. We do know that Noguchi's leptonema was an intermediate mutant, just like the leptonema found in a Romanian river and the Illinois bulls and turtles. Dr. Allen Steere et al.'s leptonema from the Lyme patient skin rash was also an intermediate leptospira, although "nobody" has talked about this spirochete in relation to Lyme disease, at least not audibly to the public before now.[1-6]

We know that picric acid and other chemical solvents, surfactants, toxins, and persisting chemicals in wastewaters and soils (including radioactive elements); contribute to the erosion and mutation of microbes. We have also been told by the CDC that leptospires become polluted by the microbes that share their homes. Some studies demonstrated that fluorides exert mutagenic activity against spirochetes. Other studies reveal the activity of picric acid upon the xylem of plants. Scientists discuss the conversion of picric acid to a mutagen by the soil bacterium *Pseudomonas aeruginosa.* These bacteriae are found naturally but they are also used in genetic engineering formulas of many kinds including insecticides and as toxic and chemical waste bioremediators. Their presence is a particular problem in the bioremediation of obsolete explosives (i.e. mining, military). It was also discovered that picric acid and other phenols are highly resistant to microbial degradation. This resistance increases as the number of nitro groups in the chemical compounds increase (dinitro- vs. trinitro-).[7-9]

This means that these compounds persist in the environment and that they can be converted into mutagenic agents that continue to persist, and which become more difficult to degrade through the enzyme activity of microbes. Furthermore if picric acid is degraded from trinitrophenol to a lesser form (dinitrophenol), it produces a compound that is potentially more harmful than its parent picrate would be. It is most interesting also that picric acid, like brucellosis and leptospirosis, malaria, and yellow fever each cause a *yellowing of the conjunctiva* – the white portion of the eyeball. Are the "yellow" fever agents influenced by the chemical picric acid including that which was used to make aniline dyes a century and a half ago? To that end, the mutation of microbes seems to be specifically driven by a particular chemical, element, or other mutagen, depending upon the microbe. What accumulates around chromium for example, will mutate differently than microbes found in industrial wastewaters from polymer manufacturers. One example microbe that has probably mutated in the latter environment, are the Bb spirochetes.[7-9]

It is also interesting that Hideyo Noguchi used a picric acid test to check for antibodies in spinal fluid, the same year the Weil-Felix antibody test for typhus fever and infectious jaundice was developed. Infectious jaundice is caused by *Leptospira icterohaemorrhagiae*; the pathogenic spirochete of *slime fever.* The Weil-Felix antibody test has been globally used to test people for the presence of rickettsial infections. The basis of the test is a cross-reaction between certain rickettsiae species and certain non-motile *Proteus vulgaris* bacteria. These bacteriae include the scrub typhus and spotted fever groups. However the test, much like the Bb tests of our time, is not very specific or sensitive. The *Proteus vulgaris* bacteriae are found in the intestinal tracts of animals and humans. They can also be found in soil, water, and wastewaters. The name "proteus" refers to its pleomorphic, or changeable form; a talent that is clearly shared by the Bb spirochete. Does the Bb spirochete also contain genes from this important *gammaproteobacteria?*

Infectious jaundice is also called *slime fever.* There have been Japanese studies on slime fever spirochetes that took place in the 1920s during early biological warfare weapons development. Many people blame the origins of the Lyme disease spirochete on Japanese biological warfare experiments. However the truth is that these spirochetes were first gathered from the environment by the Japanese, because they were already present due to industrial wastes including from the silk and dye industries that had a centuries-old presence in Asia and Japan. The slime factor of course could have been caused by slime-producing *Pseudomonas, Paenibacillus,* or *Flavobacterium* strains which could have contaminated the resident *leptospires* of wastewaters and soils to create the highly infectious slime fever spirochetes.

Leptospira spirochetes cause animal and human infections and may have led to those which surfaced in Europe during the silk processing days of the 1800s; later during World War I as "slime fever," and other human outbreaks, including yellow fever, depending upon what kind of insect virus is transmitted, and which bacteria are infected by same. In the case of slime fever, it is possible that a degraded insect-borne reovirus is involved with a leptospira and probably a "yellows"-causing bacterium, such as one found in nutrient poor soil or the human gut. The difference between pathogens of a similar nature are the specific combinations of microbes which comprise the final infective agent.

Weil's disease was first described in 1886 by German physician Adolf Weil. Its cause was not identified until 1908 by Ryokichi Inada. In 1916 it was identified in rats, which are exposed to industrial wastewaters. This is most curious because slime fever spirochetes include a pathogenic *Leptospira icterohaemorrhagiae,* the main spirochete of rats. But slime fever may also include any number of pathogens, such as relapsing fever borrelia strain; or two diseases discussed in my book *God Science,* the *rat-bite* and *Haverhill fevers*. These two agents are similar rodent-borne pathogens that cause human disease. Either may be mild, persist for years, or be fatal. Symptoms include endocarditis, meningitis, and metastatic abscess formations which resemble granulomas.

Rat-bite fever is caused by a fusobacteria called *Streptobacillus moniliformis*, and haverhill fever is caused by a gram-negative spirochetal bacterium *Spirillum minus.* We know that fusobacteria are sought by an Amoco Bb patent; and they produce skin ulcers of the sort seen in Morgellon's patients. The spirillum are those that may have mutated into spiroplasmas at the hands of toxic wastes and/or DNA-changing microbes.[10-13]

Both infections were highly prevalent in Massachusetts in 1926 when outbreaks were blamed on unpasteurized milk. In haverhill fever, a deep purplish rash may occur during acute infection, and the infection causes arthritic erythema. Rat-bite and haverhill fevers are rodent infections that were not only common to the east coast, but could become part of an aggregate Lyme spirochete today in affected areas. The WHO and CDC are keenly aware that the pollution of leptospire spirochetes is a global problem. We can see the basis for mixed infections that are at the core of important insect-borne diseases caused by industrially-polluted spirochetes.[10-13]

Rat-bite fevers were considered to be endemic in rodents by 1949, but the disease was first described by Carter in 1888. We find several strains of spirillum species described in an 1890 manual on bacteriology, including those found in marsh and brackish water, among organic matter and algae; those found in putrid mouse tissues and stagnant liquids, and those isolated from saliva. If spirillum mutate under pressures from chemicals or pollutants to become spiroplasmas, then we can understand why there are so many different spiroplasma strains that have emerged during the 20th and 21st centuries, and why they may be part of an aggregate Bb spirochete.[14-20]

The first cases of human rat-bite fever in the US were reported in 1931, whereby *Spirillum minus* was isolated. Remember that rats also harbor leptospirosis. If *Spirillum minus* mutated to become the Sucking Mouse Cataract Agent (SMCA) spiroplasma, we can now see the correlation. Larson reported on twenty clinical cases of *Spirillum minus* in 1941. There were also cases identified in Iowa in 1932; and in Idaho, Illinois, California, Montana, and Washington, DC by the late 1930s and 1940s. Abroad, Engle in 1949 reported cases in Belgium, Denmark, France, Germany, Greece, Norway, Spain, Sweden, Switzerland, and the UK. Others reported cases of rat-bite fever in Australia, Brazil, China, India, Italy, Morocco, the Philippines, and Scotland. Cilento reported on rat-bite fever in New Guinea in 1927, and Miyake reported on a case in Japan as early as 1900. This was decades before Japanese scientists began experimenting with "slime fever" spirochetes. In 1948 a 9-year old US girl was bitten on the finger by a mouse she found in her yard on a family farm, ten miles from Bozeman, Montana. She was treated with streptomycin and recovered. It is the *S. moniliformis* that is nonmotile, shows a central swelling, forms filamentous, nonbranching chains (string of beads), and has an L-phase and a transitional phase just like *Borrelia burgdorferi.*[10-20]

During the 1920s and 1930s, **rat-bite fever was induced in five "controlled" epidemics in an attempt to treat Syphilis.** This could be very bad news for scientists if the infection has become part of a global or regional aggregate spirochetal infection. At the time, patients were inoculated with infected rat, guinea pig, or mouse blood because it was felt that pyrotherapy (inducing fevers) was beneficial. This makes me recall an article written in 1986 by Lyme notables Drs. Alan Barbour and Stanley Hayes. In it they discussed the use of relapsing fever borreliae as pyrotherapy for Syphilis (and for rheumatoid and other forms of arthritis). Did these two scientists get this idea from the early rat-bite fever experiments to treat Syphilis patients during the early part of the 20th century? If so, then why haven't rat-bite or haverhill fevers been brought to the conversation coffee table during the Dearborn conference which Dr. Barbour and Connecticut colleague Rheumatologist Dr. Allen Steere attended?[10-26]

This is important because relapsing fevers and rat-bite fever mixed infections have been reported. Wild and domestic animals including cattle, pigs, dogs, cats, and rodents represent the largest pool of carriers, although *Spirillum moniliformis* has been found in a koala. Turkeys but not chickens are susceptible to *Spirillum moniliformis*, and experimental transmissions to sheep using turkey isolates were unsucccessful. The literature suggests that besides animal bite transmission, *S. moniliformis* may spread by an *airborne* route or through contact with an infected animal. Perhaps spiroplasmas travel by airborne route as well. There have been reports of possible tick transmissions of spirillum, although neither haverhill nor rat-bite fevers are known to be spread person-to-person through direct contact. However this appears peculiar as saliva and urine from infected animals may spread spirillum infections. The treatments of choice for these infections include parenteral penicillin, erythromycin, clindamycin, tetracycline, and cephalosporins; or intramuscular penicillin as recommended in some sources. These drugs are also commonly prescribed to treat patients with Lyme disease and Morgellon's infections.[10-20]

Not incidentally when Dr. Allen Steere et al. discovered a mutated leptonema in the ECM skin rash from a Connecticut Lyme patient in 1981, the team named the organism after Japanese scientist Ryokichi Inada in honor of *Weil's disease*. The *Leptospira inadai Lyme* (leptonema) was not reported as being related to the Lyme disease agent, nor was its discovery published until later. It has never been discussed in relation to Lyme disease or to Morgellon's to any audible degree to the public either, at least not before I have published my books. And yet we have seen at least one patent that specifically identified a pathogenic leptospira strain by the name of *Leptospira inadai Lyme.*[27-30]

In the literature we may find clues to the origins of slime fever spirochetes, which we know are caused by *Leptospira icterrohaemorrhagiae*. It seems that the rickettsiael agents and the spirochetes of relapsing fever borreliae create slime layers; and so do Bb spirochetes. *Streptococci* bacteriae that are common to wastewaters and the human body are also slime formers. What aggregates among slime layers (biofilms) in the environment or our bodies, is able to reassort genes with compatible organisms. When we find Dr. Willy Burgdorfer studying Rocky Mountain spotted fever (*Rickettsia rickettsii*), we can imagine he was interested in the slime-layers produced by these bacteriae. RMSF is prevalent in the west and northeast, and may be the dominant rickettsia in the Lyme disease strains found there.

We also find that Drs. Willy Burgdorfer and Louis Magnarelli (from the CT Agricultural Experiment station) studied "nonpathogenic" rickettsiae in Rocky Mt. spotted fever ticks and American dog ticks in 1979 and 1980. They published their paper in 1981 the year before the Lyme agent was announced. The "non-pathogenic" leptospires are of interest to us if they form a leptonema that comprises the Bb spirochete. Their paper also discussed the endemicity of spotted fever rickettsiae in Connecticut; clinical data from human cases from 1965-1977; and the presence of RMSF antibodies in mice and deer. Dr. Magnarelli is named on an OspA-based Lyme vaccine patent, along with Dr. Alan Barbour.[31-35]

When we see other Lyme notables such as Drs. Durland Fish and Peter Krause from Yale studying the relapsing fever rickettsia *Borrelia miyamotoi,* another slime producer, we can see the (Lyme) model they are currently studying in Russia. Their interests probably have a lot to do with figuring out how a relapsing fever borrelia (rickettsia) can mutate with leptospira bacteria such as those found in wastewaters or soils in areas (Russia) where there is uranium, picric acid, metals such as copper (and the use of copper-based regeants [cuprates] for extraction); and other chemicals used in those processes.

Uranium mines and mills use amines (solvents), surfactants (i.e. Tweens) and copper regeants for extraction. Agriculturally speaking, the same components are present in the formulas applied to, or engineered into our food crops and livestock animals; and ditto for the textile, plastics, paper, timber, tanning, and printing trades. So we can see how various aspects of the story are neatly tied together. Each of these industries have likely donated important components of aggregate spirochetes to create the "classic" ECM rash illnesses of yesterday, and the modern Lyme and Morgellon's diseases we find today.[36]

We can imagine that *Borrelia miyamotoi* was probably formed from a relapsing fever *Borrelia japonica* from wild rodents, which mutated with a rodent leptospira. Remember that *Borrelia japonica* was first isolated from *Ixodes ovatus* ticks in Hokkaido, Japan in 1993; from long-clawed shrews (*Sorex unguiculatus*), which are found only in Japan and Russia. Dr. Russell C. Johnson, spirochetologist from the University of Minnesota, and Dr. Alan G. Barbour (University of Texas-San Antonio), provided the borrelia strains and monoclonal antibodies for 1993 studies of *Borrelia japonica*. Dr. Barbour would attend the Dearborn conference the following year. Since both individuals have been intricately involved in Lyme disease research, we can imagine that most of the scientists involved in the history of Lyme are probably well aware of Bb's causative agents, and also how Bb aggregates may be formed from environmental and industrial sources that pollute resident bacteria such as leptospires.[37-45]

There is likely to be a spiroplasma component to a mutanted, aggregate Bb spirochete of modern day Lyme disease. This spirochete may or may not have been present in the Morgellon's disease of 19th century France, depending on whether picric acid, coal tars, or other surfactants are the mutagenic agents to plant or animal spirochetes (i.e. spirillum, bacterionema). The earliest spiroplasmas were described in 1944 from citrus trees; followed by some new strains in 1964 in Maryland, and Atlanta, Georgia. These appeared shortly after important herbicidal chemicals were deployed for agricultural purposes.

We also know of the discovery of Dr. Burgdorfer's 277F tick spiroplasma in 1967, and other strains have been discovered. It is fairly obvious that these spirochetes are recent emergences in the evolutionary wheel. They probably began as spirochetes of plants, insects, and animals in the form of spironema or spirillum strains which mutated under direction of industrial or chemical agents with the help of viruses. For example, the triple superphosphates are known to bind certain nutrients in the soil, and may actually help foster the growth of certain bacteriae and viruses, making them more prevalent within a given area. Chemical herbicides and other chemicals used in agricultural tools (i.e. Tweens); industrial surfactants and other chemicals (picric acid, dioxins) exert pressures upon microbes, causing them to exchange genes. The mutation process is assisted in the presence of radioactive elements either present naturally, or as applied or other "nuclear" wastes.

The emergence of modern day spiroplasmas could also have been assisted by an unstable fungus which arrived in the US during the late 1880s on or in the bodies of the early parasitoid insects used as agricultural controls. These were first applied to California citrus crops where the first spiroplasmas were later isolated. These emerged shortly after the early applications of B.t.-containing insecticides, the triple superphosphate fertilizers, and the highly mutagenic chemical herbicides. Other agriculturally applied fungi could also mutate under similiar pressures to create novel spiroplasma strains. We have seen that the organophosphate chemicals ramp up the mutagenic activity of uranium and other toxic wastes.

In the presence of co-infected citrus trees that were fungally infected by imported Australian beetles and/or applied agricultural fungi; the unstable fungi and plant bacteria could form a novel mutant spirochete (spiroplasma). A satellite virus probably plays a role in this mutation process, because spiroplasmas have satellite viruses. Any compatible RNA virus such as those used as insecticidal helpers could contribute to the formation of the diverse spiroplasma strains that emerged over time.

It is significant that *Spironema obermeieri,* also known as *Spironema recurrentis, Spirillum obermeieri,* or more recently, *Borrelia recurrentis*, was found as early as 1873 in the blood of persons suffering from relapsing fever. *Spironema duttoni* was shown to be the cause of African tick fever in 1905. *Borrelia duttoni* is the name for the tick-transmitted African tick fever spirochete (*Spironema duttoni*). *Spironema galliinarum* is the fowl spirochete. The fowl nematode *Heterakis gallinarum* is found in poultry (i.e. chickens, turkeys) and wild birds including *pheasants*.* This nematode often has its own protozoan parasite called *Histomonas meleagridis,* and causes histomoniasis or "blackhead" disease. This is of course most interesting when we remember that silkworms also suffer from the same protozoan disorder; and the nematodes of Morgellon's disease were once called blackheads.

**Remember the early applied biological control agents that contained B.t., and the sudden outbreaks of encephalitis in pheasant populations in Connecticut?*

Remember also that the relapsing fever spirochetes are distinctively different than Bb spirochetes. This is because Bb contains additional components which comprise a mutated spirochete. These components may include spiroplasmas and agriculturally important bacteria, fungi, and insect viruses. Lyme-transmitting vectors however can also transmit relapsing fevers as co-infections. The very first strain of a Lyme disease causing *Borrelia burgdorferi* spirochete was named "B31." There is a spiroplasma strain with the very same name, the "B31" bee-flower spiroplasma. This may represent a spiroplasma which came about through the mutation of a microsporidian-fungally infected honey bee, and a plant phytoplasma or mycoplasma-like organism (spirillum).

Under the mutagenic actions of OP chemicals or fertilizers, a novel mutant B31 spiroplasma may have emerged. After all, honey bees pollinate flowers including those of citrus trees, and they are exposed to persisting chemicals.[46,47]

Scientists investigated whether Dr. Burgdorfer's 277F spiroplasma was a derivative of relapsing fever spirochetes, *Borrelia recurrentis, Borrelia duttonii*, or *Borrelia anserina* (bird septicemia). We know this is important now because the relapsing fever agents are spirillum or spironemas. What was discovered during these investigations was that spiroplasmas are very different spirochetes. Of course they are, if they are mutated spironemas and leptospires (leptonema). We can imagine the interest in these spirochetes since they are infectious to livestock animals that have been vaccinated using cell lines that have proven over time to contain contaminants and reverse transcription activity. The problem with this is that vaccine agents may reactivate under the right conditions such as when provided with the proper genetic materials which allow them to do so – genes that may be provided by way of a tick or insect-borne disease.[48,49]

There is likely to be an extremophile bacterium to Bb aggregates. Millions of years ago during periods of volcanic activity, sulfur-tolerant bacteriae and viruses proliferated, and remained in the sedimentary layers of centuries past. As atmospheric conditions changed on the planet, the amount of UV solar radiation reduced enough to maintain stable bacterial forms. The extremophiles that were buried long ago have been exhumed through the activity of mining over the past century and a half. These extremophiles include the *Flavobacterium-Cytophaga-Bacteroides* which are cytoplasm-invading bacteriae (i.e. paenibacillus) and which can be found in insects, soil, and water, (i.e. the sulfur-reducers, vibrio, or clostridium).

The group also includes the *proteobacteriae.* These are gram-negative bacteria whose outer membranes are largely made of *lipoproteins* or *lipopolysaccharides.* They move about using flagellum, or by gliding. This group is composed of the *alpha, beta, gamma, delta, epsilon, and zetaproteobacteria.* Most of the tickborne infections are from the related *Rickettsiale* family. This group includes the intracellular infections anaplasmosis, ehrlichiosis, wolbachia, rickettsiosis, and neorickettsiosis. The gammaproteobacteriae group includes *Escherichia coli, vibrio, salmonella, Pseudomonas aeruginosa, klebsiella,* and others that have been used in biocides for decades. The delta group contains the important sulfur and iron-reducers. The epsilon group contains the *Helicobacter pylori* organism that is found in gastric ulcers, cancers, and in the guts of ticks and some Lyme patients.

Soils are also where we find the cypoviruses which are our reoviruses. These are also called CPV or cytoplasmic polyhedrosis viruses. We know these were used to augment the early applied insecticides, and were later lab-engineered to work in tandem with the microbes of recombinant insecticides. We need only to examine the bacteriae and viruses found near mines; hydro/geothermal veins and vents; and marine environments to find the extremophiles. It is also important to remember that global insecticides were created using natural or recombinant strains of flavobacterium including at least one strain that causes encephalitis and meningitis in humans. These tiny bacteriae are found in the bellies of important blood-feeding arthropods and insects, including ticks, lice, and mites; some of which are so small you may never see them. In the case of mites, we know that insects have not only developed resistance to chemical and microbial insecticides, but they have managed to pass on those genes to their offspring, and quite possibly to their human hosts.

Perhaps this is why the thermophile/extremophiles can be found as part of some industrially-owned diagnostic tests that also detect *Borrelia burgdorferi* bacteriae. Extremophiles are highly resistant to radiation and to antibiotics. They are also found within insects that are infected with milky spore and wilt diseases (i.e. silkworms, Japanese beetles, wasps, flies, sawflies). They are left unharmed by radioactive wastes found in uranium or thorium mines, in nuclear plant wastewaters, volcanic regions, or acid mine or industrial soils and wastewaters. Some strains can degrade natural and synthetic polymers, they are encouraged to aggregate and to grow by agricultural chemicals, and they "eat" nuclear wastes, toxic chemicals, and industrial pollutants. They also infect the smallest amoeba and other organisms that may become infectious airborne pollutants. Indeed we saw that in 1968 Ft. Detrick scientists were in Chicago discussing the progress at Dugway with aerosolized microbes that may in fact be part of an aggregate Bb spirochete that was identified a decade before a 1975 declared outbreak in Connecticut.

We can see how the microbes living in the wastewaters and soils around nuclear plants, other industries, and agricultural areas play a role in the formation of complex infectious diseases. These bacteriae are able to take up metals and metalloids that are important toxicants. Bacteriae which carry these "heavy metals," nuclear wastes, and other toxic agents (i.e. POPs); will introduce same into humans when they become infected with these bacteria. And they will not only remediate such wastes from their environment, they may help to chelate similar wastes from sequestered sites in the human body, *which releases toxins into the circulation where they may contribute to disease states and active symptoms.*[50-54]

As the environment has changed with the industrialization and modernation of a global population, so too has the content of our own atmosphere in the form of aerosolized pollutants and particulates. Each contributing pollutant has negatively impacted the planet. Whether trees are eliminated from forests which reduces the oxygen content and habitat of insects and animals; coal-fired furnaces belch particulates into the air, or other atmosphere-destroying processes occur; the ability of the earth's atmosphere to protect us from damaging UV radiation decreases. The rise in microbial mutations is also affected by the increased radiation levels produced by an ozone layer thinned by decades of garbage and coal-burning, and other man-made contributions to our heavily polluted planet. With this situation increasing, sulfobacteria, cyanobacteria, and other radiation-resistant extremophiles proliferate and are available to be taken up by insect vectors, just as they were highly prevalent in the highly acidic ancient ecosystems. As the environment of the human body turns acidic from alkaline because of toxins, GM foods, and recombinant microbes; expect acid-tolerant microbes to thrive and to become increasingly antibiotic resistant.

There may be insect poxvirus genes involved in a mutated Bb spirochete. The end of the Bb chromosome contains an oddly shaped "telomere" that is found in only a few organisms; namely insect poxviruses (Iridescent) viruses. I propose that the "Pj" virus or a similar poxvirus may be present, since it was likely in the insect cell lines that were used to create the original fifteen strains of "B.t." insecticides. These agricultural insecticides have been globally applied, and are more recently being genetically engineered into foods, textiles, and other products. We know that poxviruses can become reactivated in the presence of other poxviruses and this is highly problematic for vaccinated animals and people (including against various poxviruses). More disturbing is the idea that other virus families used in vaccines may be reactivated upon exposure to recombinant viruses from related families as they are attempted in insecticidal formulas.

Global B.t. pesticides were created using dead insects that were culled from the environment. Whatever was inside the insects as latent infections became inherent to the cultures and could not be removed. These include the nematodes, bacteria, fungi, or viruses that contribute to "wilt" and "blue" diseases. We have seen that patent inventions discuss the inability to remove certain components from cell lines, and that these components are considered to be contaminants (i.e. retroviruses). We also know that insect, animal, and human cell lines were found to be contaminated, and that new insect cell lines and cattle vaccines were suddenly created around the period of the Dearborn conference.

Shortly thereafter we saw newly designed B.t. insecticide patents being filed by agricultural industries. We also saw the filing of patents for formulas that contained chaperonin-10. These patents name an individual who was key to the Dearborn event. These products could be applied to soils or wastewaters to abrogate a problem that appears to be related to Lyme disease. Did recombinant biocide patents that utilize B.t. and extremophiles like flavobacterium capitalize on the criteria that were established at the Dearborn conference? If insecticidal formulas are known to be harming animals and humans but are being used anyway, could a conference like Dearborn have been designed to control what was becoming an emerging human epidemic – one that public health experts knew about, but could do "nothing" to prevent? If so, we might expect to see new cell lines created to eliminate some of the problematic agents. We might also expect to see the production of formulas that could treat wastewaters or soils; and the rise of vaccines to prevent the further spread of one or more recombinant (GM) "accidents."

There could also be a mycobacterium or similar bacteria in some aggregate Bb strains. Insect cell lines are also useful for animal vaccines, so contaminants are important, especially if an animal vaccine contains a recombinant construct that can fail (break apart). An applied insecticide may have contaminated animal feeds to cause the failure of an animal vaccine. If so, this would be a huge problem for livestock animals, and for people who eat these products. Remember that certain bacteria and viruses are left untouched after herbicide treatments or other biocides including *Mycobacterium tuberculosis* – a bacterium used in animal vaccines as an immune-stimulating agent.

What if bacteriae from animal vaccines are passively transferred from a vaccinated animal into a human by eating or drinking animal products? *Mycoplasma tuberculosis* was used in livestock vaccines and to possibly vaccinate deer for repopulation programs. A faulty recombinant vaccine or insecticide could have led to the development of the "prion" diseases of deer, cattle, and humans. Likewise either vaccines or insecticides could have contributed to the newly emerging immune deficiency syndromes found in deer, cattle, or humans that also mysteriously surfaced during the latter half of the 20th century.

When we look at how many people harbor *Mycoplasma* infections of varying strains, we have to ask if these are simply natural infections. Were they engineered into or became contaminants of animal or human vaccines, or were they the result of applied biocides upon agricultural crops or industrial products? We know that a percentage of the population is positive for antibodies to *Mycobacterium tuberculosis* (TB), and we know that animal vaccines contained this bacterium. We can find many patent inventions that discuss the ability of vaccines to reactivate and to passively transfer genes into vaccinated animals. Livestock of course are used for our foods, and their byproducts are used in many products and industries. What goes wrong in these animals produces an extended ripple effect. We can read in many scientific papers how vaccine and adjuvant sensitized animal tissues passively transfer these sensitivities into offspring and tissues used for vaccines and human biological products. We can also understand that animal vaccine "accidents" can produce microbes that wind up in livestock manure, and in the polluted wastewaters and soils where bacteria, insects, and animals can become infected.

There are other components involved in the development of the Bb spirochete, among which may include fungi, bacteria such as *Agrobacterium tumefaciens, Pseudomonas aeruginosa, E. coli,* and the viruses of genetically engineered insecticides and/or crops. Depending upon what has been engineered into insecticidal formulas or what is found in industrial wastewaters;

the "ingredients" of Bb strains will be somewhat varied. Many bacteria and viruses from Bb strains are directly related to soil conditions, including the use of applied fertilizers and the copper or other metal contents in the soil or water. As well, insects acquire infectious diseases during blood meals, and those infections are as widely varied in insects as they are when found among Lyme and Morgellon's patients. In the case of the latter, organic or synthetic polymers and recombinant genes as well as insect parasites and plant molds may play a role in the manifestation of physical symptoms.

While there are several basic infectious agents that comprise most Bb spirochetes, others are capable of tagging along for the ride during mixed infections, as "co-infections." This is why we find some Lyme patients with only a few, or several infections. Mutagenic processes and phagic organisms dump intracellular contents into the tick gut where they reassort to become part of a mixed infection. That is why we find tularemia, ehrlichiosis, brucellosis, anaplasma, babesia, bartonella, theleiria, molds, powassan, Q fever, nosema, toxoplasma, enterobacteria, and other infections in some, but not all Lyme patients. We may also find unusual tick symbionts such as IricES1 and others that are primarily animal infections, among many infections whose names are new to our ears. The exact combination of infective agents is dependent upon what the vectoring insect was exposed to from the environment, or from other insects or animals before donating the reassorted mixture to a human host. The strength of the mixture also depends on the ability of viruses to interfere with one another, or toxic chemicals to ramp up the virulence of the mixed infections; and what is reactivated in the body.

There are nuclear, polymer, persisting organic, and other pollutants which seem to be highly prevalent among persons with "chronic" illnesses. Among the Bb strains we find clues to pollutants including PTFE, PPAs, PVB, PBE, C8, and other persisting toxic pollutants that may contaminate these spirochetes. These chemicals bind with fluorides and chlorides, and any of these chemicals may produce symptoms that are highly variable when circulating in the body. When introduced into the human body, flourides, chlorides, dioxins, radioactive (nuclear) wastes and POPs accumulate in the tissues, organs, fat, skin, teeth, and bones. We are exposed to these and other chemicals through water treatment, environmental pollutants, airborne exposures, swimming in chemically treated waters, products that contain radioactive trace elements; and from the chemicals, metals, and radiotracers of vaccines, and biocides on or in animal and plant foods we consume.

The destruction of skeletal tissues by daily doses of radiation, even in "safe" amounts (no levels = safety), causes the degradation of cells (i.e. myelin sheaths) to be released into the body where antibodies will form to cause "autoimmune" diseases. The high levels of circulating fluorides, chemical toxins, and persisting pollutants released by enzymes of bioremediating bacteriae contributes to the damage of cells, leading to host amplified diseases. When we consider the persisting chemicals and elements to which we are routinely exposed, we will find that diseases which develop over time are complicated by the levels of toxins found in our bodies and the environment. We are the products of our environment in every sense of the word. In a toxic world, we are living, breathing, toxic people. The introduction of natural and recombinant mutant genes by insect vectors tips the scales in favor of virulent diseases which overwhelm human immune defenses. The best we can offer to ourselves and to our children is to remediate our bodies and the environment. We must also ask public health experts to admit that the illnesses of the new era are *real*, and that patients have a right to be made well. But then again liability issues are a concern for many industries, and this could prove to be the largest motivating factor that could entice highly paid scientific experts to keep silent about infectious diseases that may be caused by industrial "accidents."

Bb Outer Surface Proteins

Outer Surface Protein A (OspA): The outer surface protein A (OspA) of the Bb spirochete is cast aside upon transmission from insect to animal or human host. OspA may represent a spiroplasma protein. Spiralin is an outer surface protein of spiroplasmas, and may be part spirillum, part fungi. It could be a leptospirillum from deep underground, or one found on plants, or in soils or waters. The spirillin may have mutated with a fungi, and the spiralin-fungal combinations may vary depending on type of fungi or mold acquired. This may explain the wide diversity of spiroplasma strains.

The spiralin/fungal protein is required for infectivity in animals. This OspA protein is found in non-mutated spiroplasmas and in Bb spirochetes. We know that the OspA protein can induce a chronic form of arthritis in patients, and the spiroplasma is a mycoplasma-like organism. Mycoplasmas are known to cause arthritis. The first generation Lyme vaccine was based on an OspA protein, and it triggered a similar treatment-resistant form of arthritis in some vaccine recipients.

The spiroplasma outer surface protein spiralin is highly antigenic, and thus immune and inflammation-provoking, just like the Bb spirochete. If a vaccine OspA protein also contained a fungal component, it would explain the phenomenon of molecular mimicry because fungal cells and human cells are very similar. Therefore spirillin-fungal proteins, even if synthetically made, may induce an "autoimmune" type response that could become permanent (i.e. failed vaccine antigens).

Fungi also produce the same effects in the body that are seen during Bb infection (i.e. decreased tumor necrosis factor, pro-inflammatory cytokines, etc.). A fungal component may also explain the fungal-like infection seen during acute Lyme disease where bull's-eye or atypical rashes are produced in many patients.

It is interesting when we read about a human gastritis that is associated with another Lyme co-infection, *Helicobacter pylori.* These spiral organisms (spirochetes) can be seen under electron microscopy as *Gastrospirillum hominis* or in other words, spirillum of the human (or animal) gut. Similar forms can be seen in humans who do not have gastric inflammation. When they associate with the bacteria *Helicobacter pylori*, they produce ulcers and inflammation. Isn't it curious that spirillum in the presence of other bacteriae may also be responsible for causing the gut-disabling Lyme disease?[1]

Outer Surface Protein B (OspB): The OspB protein of the Bb spirochete may represent a B.t. bacterial gene or Cry toxin since OspB is required for host attachment. We know that B.t. is a phagic bacteria that can attach to other bacteria. For B.t. to become infective, its toxins must be released by digestion. Once released, B.t. toxins attach to the brush border membranes of the insect's gut wall, where they produce holes in the membranes and initiate infection. The Bb spirochete has been found to contain a bacteriophage, and this might come from the applied B.t. agricultural pesticides, soil microbes, or gut bacteria (i.e. *E. coli*) that have become infected by same.

The OspA and OspB diagnostic bands were excluded from the Lyme disease laboratory standards decided upon at Dearborn. This seems to have occurred because an upcoming Lyme vaccine contained OspA and OspB proteins (perhaps as a spiralin-fungal-B.t. toxin linked set). If OspB represents a B.t. protein, it would have been removed since most people have been exposed to B.t. endotoxins on or in foods. They may already make antibodies to B.t. toxins because of prior exposures. Therefore B.t. antigens, or an OspB band would be basically useless in a diagnostic test for Lyme disease. We can have B.t. toxins or antibodies in our bodies and not be infected with Lyme disease, if we eat foods that are contaminated with B.t. toxins.

Actual "Lyme" disease involves the necessary other components of the Bb spirochete, which could be detected at least theoretically using the remaining probes found in the tests standardized at Dearborn. However in the absence of Lyme spirochetes, similar Lyme-like illnesses may still emerge because of common denominators; namely B.t. bacteria, and spiroplasma-fungal infections. These "other" illnesses simply lack the complex leptonema component and its inherent infections found in Bb.

Outer Surface Protein C (OspC): The OspC of a Bb spirochete may represent a mutated leptospira (leptonema) spirochetal protein since OspC is required to maintain infectivity in a host. We know that the leptonema are mutated leptospires that probably have a spiroplasma and rickettsial component. The outer surface protein of a spiroplasma is cast off upon infectivity (OspA). Unmutated leptospires also cast off their outer surface proteins. Both will bind to the same immune regulators as those which bind to Bb spirochetes within the body.

The new generation of OspA-OspC vaccines may contain a spiralin protein and a leptospiral protein, while omitting the B.t. toxin component that may have been present as the OspB protein in the first generation Lyme vaccine. This approach may be attempted in an effort to overcome a problem with the original Lyme vaccine. There "fungal" antigens mimicked human cells (molecular mimicry), and B.t. toxin genes may have established a permanent neurotoxic state. The problem could have been caused by toxic yeast strains from the fermented B.t. insecticides. Thereafter the immune system which was alerted by the vaccine's antigens attacked the patient's own tissues by mistake, because fungi and human cells are similar. This process could have established a chronic "autoimmune" illness. The illness however was less of an autoimmune process perhaps than it was caused by the presence of human genome-incorporated B.t. or toxic yeasts which are now permanent fixtures in the body. A redesigned OspA-OspC linked antigen combo may overcome this process by training the immune system to recognize just a leptospiral/fungal agent instead of the body's tissues and any genetically-embedded B.t. toxins that may be present.[2-5]

It is interesting to read patents by Lyme notable Dr. Raymond J. Dattwyler; and also the other patent inventions referenced in each application. Several Dattwyler patents discuss recombinant constructs of *Borrelia burgdorferi*, and also those for the *Borrelia afzelii* group. Some patents refer to an older patent which describes how recombinant antibodies will not bind with those that are not "Bb." According to one patent:[6-10]

> "It does not bind to antigens produced by related spirochetes such as other species of *Borrelia*, and *Leptospira interrogans*."

If leptospires are part of an aggregate mutant Bb, then the antibodies will bind only to the Bb aggregate, and not to other native, unmutated leptospirea spirochetes according to scientists such as Dr. Dattwyler. It is also interesting to read how patents never use the word "leptonema" but instead carefully select the word "anti-OspC" antibodies or "OspC" instead of "leptonema" protein. Either that is because a leptonema is not part of the Bb organism, or because it most assuredly is, and the patent holders know it. If the latter is the case, then we may rightly ask why they or their esteemed colleagues have not spoken up about the leptospires (leptonema) before in relation to Lyme disease.[6-10]

The Fungi of Bb: Although each of the *Borrelia burgdorferi* sensu lato groups produce similar infections, individual strains are uniquely different. The differences between each may lie within the combination of pathogens that define the group and individual strain types. Strains vary by region because of the combination of insecticidal tools and pollutants that exist in the environment. I believe that the precise combination of microbes and engineered toxins determines the final outcome and strength of a particular Bb strain.

This is probably why symptoms vary widely between patients and can manifest as a mild skin infection, a fatigue syndrome, an arthritis; to more severe neurologic forms, or an encephalitis, meningitis, or "polio"-like illness. Keep in mind there are additional factors which comprise the Bb spirochete including engineered "natural" toxins; and animal and plant co-infections. Bb also requires two hosts in order to form a complete infection, including an insect and animal or human. Any interruption in the transmission cycle disrupts the aggregation/reassortment phase, and the result will be a transmitted infection, but not necessarily one that is a full-blown Bb spirochete, but a Lyme-like illness.

Let's examine some of the fungi that were applied in the environments where Bb-harboring insects are found. The entomopathogenic fungi include but are not necessarily limited to *Beauveria, Aspergillus, Paecilomyces, Coelomomyces, Verticillium, Entomophthora,* and *Metarhizium* species. Remember natural and recombinant fungi and *molds* parasitize insects as part of mixed infections. Fungi and molds may bind with the microbes of insecticides where they may be transmitted by insect or arthropod vectors to human hosts.

The most globally deployed agricultural fungi are *Beauveria bassiana* and *Metarhizium anisopliae. Beauveria bassiana* is perhaps the earliest fungi used as a biocide against inects in 1835. It is also a natural fungal infection of insects including silkworms and beetles. We know that in 1863 Bassi suggested the use of sprayable liquid insecticides made from dead larvae under techniques that caught on in Europe by 1873. The first human ECM rash illnesses were described just two years later in 1875. These could have been caused by the early applied fertilizers and sprayable liquid insecticides.

Borrelia afzelii strains may contain the fungi of insects (and) the early sprayed insecticides (*Beauveria bassiana*). This same fungus was applied in the US beginning in 1867, but it didn't take off in the US which explains why no ECM rash patients emerged in the states at the time. When *Beauveria bassiana* was used in later decades in the US, it was used as a stand-alone fungi. Therefore it lacked the other important ingredients found in the European sprays including the liquified insect viruses and bacteriae.

Since *Borrelia afzelii* strains are found mainly in Europe and Asia, we can see which fungi most likely affect people with these strains. The viruses and bacteria that were part of the sprayable insecticides were probably those that caused the "blue" disease of Japanese beetles and the caterpillar "wilt" diseases of silkworms. I propose that the agent of "blue" disease (*Coxiella popilliae*) could be a mutated rickettsia (bacteria) Q fever; a Japanese beetle virus (i.e. "Pj"); and a fungus such as *Beauveria bassiana* in conjunction with the soil bacterium *Bacillus thuringiensis* (B.t.). Remember that B.t. is found naturally in these insects.

Since *Metarhizium anisopliae* fungi were applied as insecticides beginning in 1878, it is our next likely candidate for the *Borrelia garinii* strains found in Europe and the Far East (Russia, Asia). We also find evidence of *Borrelia garinii* in Africa in the 20th century because metarhizium strains were deployed agriculturally in that region of the world. There are HIV/AIDS epidemics around the world; but we find them concentrated in Africa, Russia, and the US. There may be a connection between HIV/AIDS; the use of this green muscardine fungus; and the gemini viruses (i.e. cassava latent virus) of certain tuber crops like cassava that are important food and industrial staples (i.e. starch, propellants).

Borrelia garinii strains are found in the US, Europe, Asia, and Africa. *B. garinii* strains may include the bacteria, viruses, and fungi naturally found in Asian beetles and silkworms. Remember that reoviruses and related viruses play a role in infections. They are able to infect bacteria and fungi when in contact with same. Reovirus-infected fungi may be the deciding factor which separates the Bb groups. In the US the most commonly applied agricultural fungi are probably the *Beauveria bassiana* and *Coelomomyces.* The latter is naturally found in mosquitoes, and was used as an agricultural tool to combat them.[13-15]

Reoviruses may also explain why there is a fourth group, *Borrelia japonica* that is not considered to be a group that causes human Lyme disease. Perhaps the agent simply lacks an important fungal-virus ingredient which makes an aggregate particularly pathogenic. Or perhaps it lacks a leptonema component. At any rate it is clear that the *B. japonica* group strains are *incomplete* agents in the sense that with the addition of a few microbes, they would produce a bona fide Bb spirochete.

The soil bacilli which act as bacteriophages (i.e. *B. popilliae, B. lentimorbus, B. sphaericus, B. thuringiensis* etc.) in the region where a Bb strain emerges is an additional factor which determines Bb strain types. The various rickettsiae and individual viruses found in a given region will further define individual strains. The adaptation between insect host and its co-infections are contributing factors to strain types that evolve, and depend on interfering viruses and other components of mixed infections.

Soil bacteriophages or virophages which infect bacteria or viruses may also cause Lyme-like infections that are not considered to be "true" Lyme disease. I am speaking of the very Lyme-like STARI infection found in the southern US. This infection likely includes similar elements to those found in the Bb spirochete, but some of its ingredients are different. It may for example include the fungus *Coccidioides immitus* instead of an agriculturally applied fungus. Its virus component is also slightly different since we know about the lone star virus and its very own satellite virus. It is possible that a fire ant virus is part of the STARI complex.

The difference in the spirochetal component between a STARI and a Bb spirochete, may be that STARI spirochetes are *unmutated* relapsing fevers, while Bb spirochetes are *mutated* leptonema which contain only *a few* relapsing fever genes.[13-15]

Bb strains also seem to incorporate reoviruses or a degraded form of same (i.e. flavivirus). This may include a borrelina virus that was released beginning in 1951 in the US; or another region after that period. Since the US obtained its sample stocks from Sweden, it is probable these viruses were first released in Europe. It could likewise include a powassan, eyach, west nile, EEE or other degraded form or related virus. The "classic" ECM rash illnesses of Europe probably emerged from natural recombinant events from the early sprayable fungal insecticides made from dead insects that harbored these kinds of viruses. Otherwise latent insect viruses could simply have been brought to life by the early applied sprays and the application of superphosphate fertilizers.[13-15]

In American Lyme patients we find a mixture of all three *Borrelia burgdorferi* sensu lato groups. The most common is the *B. burgdorferi* sensu stricto strains; followed by *B. garinii* (mainly in the northeast); and last *B. afzelii* in extremely few case numbers which are mostly anecdotal. We might examine the kinds of fungi that have been applied, and that are found naturally for clues to the fungal components of any given Bb strains.

Early USDA imports of coccinellid and vedalia beetles from Australia occurred during the late 1880s. Those beetles probably imported the fungi *Coccidiodes immitus* and which became endemic to the American southwest and California by the mid-1940s when the earliest spiroplasmas arrived. Remember this was when the triple superphosphates and chemical herbicides and pesticides were deployed agriculturally. By the way *Sporotrichum globuliferum* is a known fungal agent for the alfalfa weevil and also chinch bugs like those used in 1867 during the early days of biological controls in the midwest. Perhaps this fungus, first identified in Salt Lake City, Utah in 1914, is present in some western and midwestern Bb strains such as the Bb 25015 strain discussed in the Q&A section. In countries such as Australia, the predominant fungal strains found in Bb patients may include *Coccidioides immitus,* and a common insect virus called *Bergoldia virulenta*.[16]

I have already proposed that the viruses from the *Borrelia afzelii* group probably came from the Japanese beetles or the silkworms of the Far East. A similar contribution could have been made to *Borrelia burgdorferi* sensu stricto and *B. garinii* strains found in the US, since there was a large silk industry in the northeast; and gypsy moths and Japanese beetles were highly prevalent in the east and midwest. The pests of the great plains and the Pacific coasts (i.e. citrus) and other areas may help decide what kind of insect viruse(s) are at the core of the Bb strains in those regions. This probably also explains why there are more cases of *B. garinii* in the northeast than elsewhere in the US – because this is where Japanese beetles, gypsy moths, silkworms, and brown-tailed moths proliferated. In the south we find the lone star virus and a relapsing fever agent that causes STARI infections. In neighboring Ontario, the development of the Powassan virus that dove down into New York and its apparent affinity for mining regions is one example of the kinds of viruses that can develop in industrial areas.

Another fungi to be found in some Bb strains could include the rice blast or wheat stem rust spores. Remember the latter was studied for its ability to bioremediate herbicides. After the ban on biological weapons, the US was left with a stockpile of rice blast fungus. Perhaps it was reengineered into an agricultural insecticide. Remember we saw a recent grant award to study OspA proteins in rice, a cereal crop. This could loosely describe a Bb pathogen that contains an outer surface protein "A" that belongs to a rice blast fungus.

Fungal agents applied agriculturally, or molds found in any part of the world could contribute to an aggregate Bb spirochete. The *Borrelia burgdorferi* sensu stricto strains probably include the bacteria and viruses of the imported beetles commonly seen on citrus groves. They may as well contain the agents of gypsy and other moths that have decimated crops and forests in many parts of the world; or pathogens from the early parasitoid wasps, flies, and other insects released in the states. Of course in any Bb group we may include mixed infections from other agriculturally important pests, such as cockchafers, army worms, bollworms, cutworms; and the blood-feeding ticks, mites, mosquitoes, and other insects and arthropods. Many of these infections are present because they were first engineered into industrial and agricultural insecticides or biocides.

We find important fungal toxins on moldy corn (i.e. *Beauveria bassiana*, or *Trichothecium roseum* which produces roseotoxin B). We also know there are other entomopathogenic fungi that are naturally found in the bodies of insects (i.e. *Aspergillus, Paecilomyces, Coelomomyces*), so we may expect over time to see new groups of *Borrelia burgdorferi* sensu lato emerge. Scientists have already acknowledged these expectations. Is this because they know the true origins of Bb and its connections to applied insecticides and the recombinant and natural fungi and molds?[17]

Rickettsial agents and viruses are another part of the equation of a Bb aggregate. The difference between Bb strains may also be determined by the various rickettsial species involved. However rickettsial infections may simply "come along for the ride" so to speak as insect-borne mixed infections. They might not reassort but may be phagocytized by soil bacteria and become accidental passengers in the journey from insect gut to animal or human host.

An assortment of rickettsial infections may be found in Lyme patients. These vary between regions of the world, as do viruses.

In Europe we find Mediterranean spotted fever; and Russian Spring-Summer encephalitis, or Eyach viruses for example. In the states we find Rocky Mountain spotted fever, Q fever, Brucellosis; or Powassan and West Nile viruses. Additional bacteria that may become part of a mixed infection including the relapsing haverhill or rat-bite fevers from the eastern US or Europe. Tickborne encephalitis viruses vary depending on region, and so do other agents. Regardless of the variability of the strains, the basic structure of the Bb spirochete is similar across the groups. We should also assume that the various B.t. biocides used around the world are based upon standardized formulas. This may be why we see fifteen original Bb strains identified by a Dattwyler/Luft/Gomes-Solecki patent for a Lyme vaccine and diagnostic test; and we have noticed there were fifteen original B.t. insecticidal formulas.[18]

The possible ingredients of an aggregate Bb spirochete contribute to its complex genome. However the different ingredients determine the virility of the individual strains. Furthermore co-infections which are dumped into the insect gut through the degrading action of B.t. pesticides will complicate the individual's infectious disease complex. For the most part, here are the hypothetical ingredients as a model for how Bb agents are formed. Ingredients will vary but will probably follow a standard formula to make an aggregate, infectious spirochete that causes Lyme, Morgellon's, or other Lyme-like infections.

A.) An engineered insecticide used for industry or agriculture as a biocide (i.e. anti-bacterial or insecticide)

Engineered baculovirus + B.t. bacteriophage + Cry toxins + yeast from the fermentation process

Add in engineered "natural" spider, scorpion, mite, fungal toxins and insect genes. These formulas may include *Agrobacterium tumefaciens, Pseudomonas aeruginosa,* other bacteria; and viruses such as *Autographa californica, Sindbis, Semliki Forest, Trichoplusia ni, Heliothis zea,* mosaic viruses, and others which work together to greatly increase toxic kill times.

B.) A mutated leptospira spirochete that becomes polluted by industrial, chemical, and/or nuclear wastes

Leptonema = plant spirillum mutant (see C) or leptospirillum + bacterionema infected with gammaproteobacteria and a pathogenic or saprotrophic leptospira such as *Leptospira interrogans* (or genes from a recombinant *Leptospira meyeri*).

C.) There is a spiroplasma component that is probably part fungal, part plant spirillum that mutated from agricultural or industrial chemicals and their activity upon plant/soil or water-borne spirochetes.

D.) There is an insect virus component to the Bb aggregate, which could include any *poxvirus* or an insect iridopox (iridescent) virus such as "Pj" virus from Japanese beetles or silkworms. Pj virus is a member of the reovirus family. The reoviruses include the cypoviruses (CPVs) of insects (i.e. borrelina viruses). These may be present simply because they infect insects, or because they were picked up by a vector from recombinant insecticides that were applied agriculturally and industrially. The biocides engineer poxviruses, baculoviruses, herpesviruses, and reoviruses right into their formulas; and these may help to reactivate latent viruses not only in insects, but also in animals and humans.

Other gene insertions complicate Bb's basic structure, and enlarge its genome. These genes may be derived from natural sources or from recombinant insecticidal formulas. It is not difficult to imagine that the majority of "ingredients" of Bb strains are in fact derived from recombinant insecticides or wastewater pollutants. While many of these agents are available in the environment, they are more highly prevalent because of the global use of applied insecticides. This makes them readily available ingredients for a complicated Bb organism. In a Bb aggregate we are also likely to find multiple lab-designed recombinant genes.

E.) Taq polymerase or similar enzyme genes from any extremophile, either wild or recombinant in origin may be part of the Bb organism. This seems particularly evident when we find genes that seem to be derived from blue-green algae in Bb strains, and we know these genes are used in the laboratory to engineer GM plants and insecticides.

F.) *Chromobacterium violaceum* is an example of a managanese-dependent intracellular proteobacterium from a marine environment. Some kind of manganese-dependent organism has probably contributed its genes to the Bb organism because Bb has replaced all of its enzymes with those which utilize manganese. This is a process that occurs in only a few bacterial species. We need to identify the species which utilize manganese to get a good idea of the origin of Bb manganese enzyme genes.

G.) Insect co-infections: These are released from intracellular spaces when B.t. enters an insect gut and degrades the gut tissues. These will vary by region and insect host, and are numerous – far more than the few commonly cited co-infections ehrlichiosis, bartonella, or babesia. Additional infections that are microsporidian/protozoan in nature (i.e. nosema, wolbachia, theleria, ips, etc.) are also likely. Nematodes are also deployed in the insecticides and they carry their own co-infections including wolbachia, an agent known to manipulate host genes including sex ratios. It is possible that nematodes will come along for the ride as a co-infection in most Lyme patients, and so will their symbiont infections.

The Origins of Bb: It appears that multiple factors collided with insect pathogens and the wastewaters and soils polluted by industrial and agricultural products. In earlier centuries, this process naturally caused insect epidemics to arise; followed by animal and human epidemics. Once these toxic ingredients blended with the wastes of the textile, agricultural, mining, tanning, glassmaking, plastics, and other industries, Lyme and Morgellon's could be found. We also saw a disease emerge during the mid-1800s in the silkworm population once stronger phosphate fertilizers and fungi were deployed as sprayable insecticides.

Agricultural insecticides forced latent insect infections to reactivate and to cause diseases in pest populations. As time passed and agricultural and industrial processes evolved, the beginnings of ECM rash illnesses emerged in Europe. We began to see similar effects from the ingredients deployed agriculturally and industrially when biological controls came to America. Insects, animals, and people began to to get sick with novel infections. The modern era brought with it new chemical fertilizers and insecticides; and a parallel course of emerging infections. The epidemics in insect and animal populations were analyzed and tracked by public health experts before surfacing in the human population. While "everybody" tracked epidemics, very little was revealed to the public about their probable origins. Instead, vaccines were promoted as solutions to infectious disease while the offending products and their pollutants may have continued to perpetuate animal and human diseases over decades.

The development of modern Lyme disease that I discuss in my books has been interesting to analyze in relation to outbreaks of various human diseases (i.e. yellow fever, Spanish influenza, Kaposi's sarcoma, HIV/AIDS), and the history of various industries. We can see what appear to be intrinsic connections between infectious diseases, phosphates and fertilizers; and industrial processes (i.e. mining, chemicals, metals, plastics, agriculture, textiles, nuclear sciences). We can understand how infectious microbes make their way from industries, agriculture, and pharmaceutical laboratories into soils and watersheds. There they are free to reassort under direction of highly mutagenic chemicals and microbial formulas, especially in polluted soils and wastewaters where the chemistry is markedly skewed.

When imported insects and industry came to the US, they transported fungi, microsporidiae, bacteria, viruses, nematodes, and parasites culled from their environment. This further exacerbated the range of newly introduced foreign pathogens from the Old World into the New. The tools of agriculture and industry (especially surfactants, acids, and other chemical wastes) over time contributed to disease outbreaks that emerged. If we look carefully we can see that infectious disease experts have for a long time been acutely aware of the relationships between the diseases they study and the industrial contributors to same, although these connections are rarely publicly acknowledged.

It is not a stretch of the imagination to imagine how natural microbes will intermingle with the well-meaning efforts of those who desire better crop yields, or who work to keep animals and humans free of pest insects and their associated pathogens. While there may be additional infective agents which arrived as remnants of military experiments into weapons of biological warfare, the truth seems to be that most of the factors which created the Lyme disease organism were in place long before modern human warfare exploits were undertaken.

That is not to say that some microbial biowarfare remnants have not contributed to infectious animal or human diseases. They may have, and we may find evidence of this in animal surveys around areas contaminated from past experiments. So too is the possibility that chemicals have caused the mutation of many forms of bacteria; nonetheleast of which are part and parcel to the Bb organism (i.e. spiroplasmas). As we track the history of the Lyme disease organism from its humble origins, the savvy observer will likely find that the path to modern Lyme disease or *Borrelia burgdorferi* sensu lato, is one that involved a very different set of "biowarfare" weapons. Those chemical and microbial tools have long been pointed at pests of military, medical, veterinary, industrial, and agricultural industrial importance.

When we observe those whose eyes and talents are focused on tracking emerging diseases in the environment, in animals, and finally humans; and compare scientific interests in agriculture, wastewaters, and the chemicals and microbes found within, we find there are many truths to the story in these pages that have never been publicly revealed to an audible degree. When we carefully follow the timeline of events which involved multiple industries, we continually find connections that are impossible to ignore. The truth about Lyme disease therefore probably lies somewhere in between what we have been told, and the ideas presented here.

In my opinion the agent of Lyme disease that we are familiar with today, was an evolutionary process that took place under direction of several important factors. Agricultural and industrial pollutants combined and mutated resident microbes which became polluted and infected with these agents. It is also apparent that those who hold patent interests which seek Bb spirochetes and many other important agents may have understood the origins of Bb in relation to their own products or processes decades ago. The original ECM disease of Europe was the first evidence that mutagenic chemicals and microbes were causing human disease. Since mankind did not heed the warnings a century ago, the result over time has been the creation of the superbugs *Borrelia burgdorferi* sensu lato that we find today.

Another problem to address has to do with the earliest vaccines. According to the historical literature it is clear that the earliest vaccines were contaminated with "adventitious agents." It is also evident that this contamination problem continues today. The very first attempts at vaccine production were undertaken slightly before the Pasteur Institute in Paris, France was founded in 1887. Louis Pasteur, the father of fermentation and pasteurization, saved the silk industry with his research from 1865-1870, and invested his time in vaccines and other important studies. Although vaccines, their cells, and their cell lines have improved over time; even today patent texts describe the contaminants that are still found in modern vaccines. Unfortunately some contaminants *cannot be removed* because they are inherently part of the insect and animal products used to create vaccines. As genetic engineering techniques for agriculture, industries, and medicine continue to evolve, the human species is left vulnerable to these formulas that are both unpredictable and uncontrollable.

At some point we should expect to see a biological conflict of interest in one or more populations. We have seen these described in patents as "accidents" or "illegitimate" recombinant events. The reason that Bb has become far more virulent over time from its early days as a rash-producing illness, is likely because of the increased virulence of the agricultural weapons of biowarfare; and the chemical, microbial, and nuclear pollutants that have made their way into soils and waters over decades. What we have put into our environment, we have put into ourselves – beginning with the earliest days of industry. With the modernization of societies, we have seen a parallel progression of infectious diseases. The more sophisticated the tools, the more complex the illnesses to which we have been exposed; and the story of infectious diseases may be as simple as that.

With respect to Morgellon's disease (or "Lyme-plus"), we have already decided there is an additional group of co-factors involved. These may include silk-producing mites that have incorporated the genes of silkworms, spiders, or natural or synthetic fibers (i.e. GM crops), or those found in wastewaters. These mites may include the demodex normally found on the human body or the mite passengers of vectoring insects. Nematodes and collembola and their co-infections may also be part of the Morgellon's skin manifestations. These passengers ride on the backs of blood-feeding ticks or mites, and dislodge during the feeding process to contaminate the victim's skin. Silk-producing mites are known to have incorporated artificial genes into their genome, and such genes may be capable of generating the multi-colored "hairs" or "fibers" found in skin lesions of infected patients.

The color scheme of the fibers or hairs may be driven by human hair genes, or by the bacteriae that infect silkworms or mites which are taken up by microbes once degraded in the environment. Expressed in the human body, these genes may allow bacteriae to produce the colors seen in the Morgellon's "hairs." We may also ask if such hairs may be produced in part from toxic plastics or synthetic fibers that are stored inside the human body but which are extracted by *remediative bacteria.* These bacteria may have genes that are able to break down the toxins in the human body, and express them under instructions from recombinant genes that are also part of the infectious organisms.

The bacterial portion of Morgellon's infections may represent a manifestation of a "failed" recombinant formula in the sense that it duplicates in humans what was designed to occur in the insect or plant body. The ulcerative sores could be evidence of a B.t. agent that is fermented in the human gut to produce an anthrax-like cutaneous infection. We have also seen that fusobacteria are sought by an Amoco patent, and these may cause the ulcerative lesions seen in Morgellon's. The expression of peculiar fibers in human hair follicles is evidence that a natural or engineered formula may be wrongly expressed by human skin cells (follicles) or by the bacteria that infect them.

However Bb spirochetes come about, whether through the application of mining chemicals which encourage acid-tolerant spirochetes to thrive in those areas, or from highly polluted wastewater flows from sewage treatment, industrial ponds, nuclear reactor wastes, or otherwise contaminated waters; leptonemas will form and complicate insect-borne infections. The chemicals used in many industries, the radioactive elements that are found in our highly polluted environment; and the recombinant cocktails of applied insecticides and vaccine formulas are the final catalysts that actively drive the mutation of microbes and the new diseases of our day.

What additional factors may have influenced the decisions made at the Dearborn conference? Leptospirosis was on the rise during the 1940s in humans and animals. Scientists would have had their attentions on this growing infectious disease. They would have attempted animal vaccines, and possibly human Syphilis vaccines since treponemes are distantly related to them. Contaminated or failing animal vaccines or insecticides if discovered, could have necessitated a medical conference such as Dearborn. The most important topics of discussion at the Dearborn conference were an infection that was being transmitted by insects and arthropods to cause human "Lyme" disease, and the surveillance and detection of same.

We also know that during the 1920s and 1930s, rat-bite fever was introduced in five "controlled" epidemics in an attempt to treat Syphilis. What this means to us today is difficult to ascertain, however we can see an important connection between the Tuskegee experiments that were underway from 1932 until they were exposed in 1972; the scientific investigations into rat-bite fever and Syphilis; and their attempts to use *Spirillum* and *Streptobacillus moniliformis* to "cure" Syphilis.

Scientists were already aware of "slime fever" spirochetes during the early part of the 20th century and were actively studying them because Japanese scientists were doing the same. Were the covert Tuskegee studies really aimed at studying the effects of biowarfare agents the Japanese already had in their possession? Was a diagnosis of "Syphilis" used to describe a mutant Syphilis/ slime fever or rat-bite fever spirochete? If we find a Lyme disease spirochete today that also involves similar components, this would undoubtedly raise suspicions of early "biowarfare" weapons – at least until we remember that these agents have been ubiquitous to the global environment for centuries.

They were present as individual infections decades before they were experimented with as biowarfare tools or for Syphilis studies of the mid-20th century. Some people will ask if this is true, then why did Lyme disease become a problem only from the 1960s forward? The answers are clear that what we think of as "Lyme disease" involves multiple pathogens. These were clearly a growing problem in animal and human populations prior to the sixties, although they were not publicly acknowledged as a human concern until then. Some Lyme-like illnesses emerged a century and a half ago, and again during the 20th century with the application of important chemicals and recombinant microbes. The difference between the classic Lyme and modern Lyme disease therefore may be the menu of infectious microbes that comprise an aggregate spirochete.

We can reasonably address the possible animal vaccine component to the story. We may find evidence from early patents that there were scientific interests in fabricating meaningful animal leptospirosis vaccines. For example a 1971 patent assigned to Johnson & Johnson of New Brunswick, New Jersey describes a culture medium that was designed to produce high yields of leptospires. The patent is intended to produce vaccines. It could also be used to produce large numbers of leptospires for insecticides.[19]

The year 1971 was a period whereby a large consortium of academic institutions were collaborating on the creation of a Syphilis vaccine. These exploits may have included studies of the Tuskegee sort, or those which involved a slime fever or rat-bite fever spirochete masquerading as Syphilis. If we study research grant abstracts from this period, it seems as if everyone's attentions were turned toward creating a Syphilis vaccine. The real intent could have been to create a slime fever/rat-bite fever-like vaccine that today might address an infection called "Lyme." The patent text is highly revealing and indicates that while the invention was designed for vaccines; instead of "Syphilis," it describes "leptospirosis" as a pathogen of dogs and cattle. Slime fever and rat-bite fever spirochetes are animal pathogens, and so are the spirochetes of Lyme disease that would be announced only a few years later, and which would also seem to include the leptospires.[19]

The patent also describes the use of the chemical Tweens, which as we have learned are an important vaccine component that helps aggregate bacteria and promotes their growth. The threat of leptospirosis infections was a well-known problem by the 1970s, so it is clear that scientists were more than aware of the ubiquitous presence and the pathogenic nature of these spirochetes. We just don't know for certain whether "leptospirosis" vaccines were inclusive of pathogenic slime fever or rat-bite fever leptospires, or of the mutated leptonema that would also be found in at least one Lyme patient a decade later.[19]

Was the scientific community really interested in and working to create Syphilis vaccines? Or were their attentions turned toward attempting to solve the problem of contaminated animal vaccines, or animal infections that by 1971 were already known to infect people in the US Midwest and the northeast? Were the leptonema agents expected to cause a global human epidemic that would soon emerge? We know that researchers often substitute one term for another to conceal the true nature of their inventions and studies (i.e. use the name of one arbovirus in place of another), it is reasonable to guess that in the case of Syphilis, scientists may have really been studying leptospirosis, slime fever, an "escaped" rat-bite fever, or in more specific terms, the leptonema that were already being detected in animals.

The discovery that there were contaminated insect cell lines could have been a catalyst to establish the kinds of surveillance and diagnostic criteria such as emerged following the 1994 Dearborn conference. If we go back to the early days of poultry vaccines, we find that leptospirosis infections also affect turkeys and chickens. These are important food animals, and the latter's eggs are used to create vaccine cell lines for animals and humans. We also learned that sterile water used in the laboratory to create vaccines and other products is commonly contaminated with leptospires that scientists felt were *unimportant* as possible disease agents.

We know that the CDC was tracking the emergence of several odd leptospira strains; in particular soon after the mutated leptonema emerged in Romania in 1953. After that time public health experts were checking water and fauna samples for evidence of similar mutated leptonema in the United States. Some new leptonema strains were found during the 1960s in the midwest and in Georgia near a CDC laboratory. We can guess that when human Lyme disease emerged over the next decade, scientists were trying to ascertain how these mutants came about. Scientists even considered whether they had come from research laboratory wastewaters. When we look to the 1960s we find Dr. Burgdorfer and others investigating many pathogens that infect livestock, and their relationship to chicken embryos like those used to make vaccines. Scientists also studied the ability of livestock ticks to transmit infections including to humans. It seems clear that before the identification of the Lyme disease agent that one part of the "Bb" equation was intently studied by CDC and NIH scientists.

When the cluster of juvenile arthritis cases emerged in Connecticut, we saw a Rheumatologist and CDC-EIS employee on task every step of the way from disease origin to the politics of the infection today. He and his colleagues were the first to identify a novel mutated leptonema spirochete from a Lyme patient's ECM rash. However the discovery would only be quietly published several years later, shortly before the Dearborn conference where he would make recommendations for Lyme disease surveillance and testing. Those criteria would affect an upcoming Lyme vaccine for which Dr. Steere would also be lead investigator. However the Steere et al. team's discovery never became part of the Dearborn conference, or public discussions of Lyme disease.

The Dearborn conference occurred immediately after new insect cell lines were fabricated to replace older cell lines that mysteriously and suddenly disappeared. Could contaminated cell lines have led to the deer, cattle, and human AIDS-like or prion diseases? The missing lines which were used to create insecticides and animal vaccines were admittedly contaminated with important agents. Immediately after the new cell lines were created and their patents filed, the Dearborn conference produced highly restrictive criteria which eliminated two of the most important diagnostic bands for the Lyme disease organism. If the hypotheses in this book are accurate, these bands became unnecessary because they interfered with an upcoming Lyme vaccine. They were also probably unnecessary to detect an aggregate Bb spirochete since the remaining probes could theoretically do the job. The remaining bands would look for a few key pieces of an aggregate spirochete and also evidence of how the body responds to the presence of same. Unfortunately this setup was very limited in terms of which strains could be detected. Either those who established the criteria underestimated the number of Bb strains that would emerge, or they were more concerned with the potential success of the upcoming Lyme disease vaccine to fully optimize the test criteria defined at Dearborn.

Immediately following the Dearborn conference, we saw many agriculturally related patents filed which involve the microbial pesticide *Bacillus thuringiensis* (B.t.). Dr. Allen Steere has acknowledged receiving at least one grant from Novartis, a company that patented multiple B.t. formulas in the days following the Dearborn conference. Were these new B.t. formulas designed to replace older formulas that were found to have contributed to the formation of Bb organisms and other diseases due to cell line contaminants? Why were new insect cell lines and new B.t. insecticides formulated on and around the Dearborn conference? Around the same time that Dr. Barbara Johnson organized the Dearborn event, we find several key Johnson patents that seemed to have been designed to "fix" a problem that occurred in wastewaters by organisms that can cause infectious diseases including Lyme. Why were new chaperonin patents filed at this time? Were each of these events mere coincidences, or an indication that there was a globally-important public health problem that needed to be "controlled" by public health officials?

The chaperonin patents seem to provide a "solution" to preventing at least one aspect of Lyme disease. They seem to describe an agent that can be added to wastewaters, lakes, ponds, or even vaccines to circumvent a problem caused by animal vaccines or environmental wastes. And we also see key representatives at the Dearborn conference including from universities with important ties to agriculture, military, and/or nuclear waste disposal; and from industries which include manufacturers of important chemicals including polymers. For example, a representative was listed in the Dearborn conference booklet from the Alfred I. du Pont Institute Research Department (Wilmington, DE).

The Bb agent requires at least two hosts to become an aggregate organism. It is obvious that there may be a leptonema component to Lyme disease infections which involve a tick bite and an ECM rash. It is less clear whether a leptonema is required in other diseases that resemble Lyme. For example some people who have Lyme-like illnesses but where an ECM rash or other symptoms are absent; may have only one half of a Bb aggregate equation, such as no leptonema component. We know that the Bb spirochete is not cultured from the environment as a whole organism.

This supports the idea that part of the Bb aggregate can lead to other infectious disease states. Such an illness may be the Lyme-like chronic fatigue syndrome, or fibromyalgia. Chronic fatigue and fibromyalgia patients may be infected with Bb spirochetes. Or they may lack the spirochete but retain the "something else" including a combination of microbes and persisting pollutants derived from their environment, from vectoring insects or from contaminated foods. Combined with a leptonema they make up an infectious Lyme disease or Morgellon's organism, while without the spirochete but with the individual agents they remain infectious and may produce symptoms similar to Lyme.

It is clear that Bb spirochetes emerged as aggregate pathogens. They clearly involve an insect and an animal host, but it is doubtful whether the animal or human host makes a difference except to add co-infections. While contaminated animal vaccines may contribute to a mutated leptonema, a similar problem may occur in vaccinated humans who have covert leptospirosis and other latent infections that may reactivate and reassort their genes upon introduction of recombinant insecticides.

In the 1980s when pregnant with my first child, I swam in the polluted Kankakee River (southern Illinois). The park was downstream of the Braidwood nuclear plant, although I did not know it at the time. I could have very easily picked up a contaminated leptonema infection which would have been transmitted to each of my unborn children after this time.

I think about how many people are exposed to polluted waters of rivers or lakes, such as when I swam regularly in Lake Michigan during the 1980s. This is just one lake that is widely known to be contaminated with many chemicals including persisting pollutants. A publication long ago carried an announcement that Lansing, Michigan was building a "mammoth" plant for "the government's war needs." The plant was to manufacture the toxic picric acid. What was manufactured by industry often ended up in wastewaters including Lake Michigan over the last century. Many chemicals found in the environment as pollutants are also found in vaccines; and may contribute to the mutation and infection of organisms. The same issues that arise during the manufacture of animal vaccines (i.e. contaminants); and their chemicals (i.e. Triton-X, Tweens) are found in human vaccines.[20]

What mutates in vaccinated animals may be used as a model to understand what happens in vaccinated humans who harbor latent or low-level active infections when exposed to infected vectoring insects or arthropods. What appears in the external environment sets the stage for highly virulent pathogens that are transmissible to humans in any number of ways. Some of these routes include ingesting contaminated foods and animal products, or exposures to vectoring insects which first get their infections from the chemicals, and natural and recombinant microbes found in their environment.[20]

A main consideration with recombinant techniques and the reassortment of microbes, is that complex mixed infections now appear in microbes, plants, and animals. Microbes are commonly infected with more than one pathogen which may be either complimentary or antagonistic to the microbe. Interfering viruses prevent the more severe symptoms of some plant, animal, or human diseases. But the reassortment of genes that naturally occurs has been heightened by the large assortment of recombinant constructs that have been applied to the environment as biocides. The problem with blending nature with manmade recombinant constructs is that genes can reassort. Gene reassortments are known and acknowledged as "accidents" of genetic engineering. This problem frequently occurs with geminiviruses, where new viruses are created by those which love to reassort. The attachment of viruses to other viruses including those of recombinant constructs is a problem that scientists attempt to avoid, but which appears to be unavoidable in nature. Recombinant formulas become "heavy" with things that were not intended to be part of the recombinant formula, and this may cause constructs to fail, to release their components, and to form new infectious pathogens. There is simply no way to predict what nature may create once recombinant formulas are released into the environment; and this may be the fundamental flaw in genetic engineering techniques that cannot be overcome.[21,22]

In ticks viral attachment to the gut membrane is important and can be found within the cytoplasm (cell interior) of the symbiont microbes that live inside the ticks. When the symbionts are disturbed by gut-damaging biocides, the contents of the cells are dumped into the midgut where they are regurgitated during blood meals. Reoviruses will also infect insect (or avian) offspring in utero by way of infected egg yolks. This is key to remember in the case of infected poultry embryos that are used for vaccines. Some reoviruses only last a few generations, while others (i.e. rice stripe disease) have persisted through twenty generations of insects without a loss of virulence. This speaks to the existence of generational viruses and retroviruses.[23-25]

A problem with mixed infections in insects is that microbes often become polymorphic. This means they mutate into different types of the same microbe. Transgenic plants may extend the kinds of new mutant microbes that can be found and transmitted by insect vectors. Another consequence of these mixed pathogen interactions is viral resurfacing. This is the incorporation of one viral genome into another viral genome through mutation. Alterations in the virus capsid genes may extend the host range for mutant viruses and other infections, depending upon whether the viruses can attach to the gut cells or the microbes found in the guts of insects, animals, or humans. Each of these factors are exploited in the creation of insecticides to specifically cause diseases in insect populations. The result of those designs may also adversely affect non-targeted species including humans. Scientists have also used nematodes as virus vectors. This is problematic because even their eggs are known to contain viruses which are acquired from animals, for example from swine with influenza. However nematodes are more commonly known to transmit plant viruses.[23,24,26]

The reactivation of latent viruses by insect poxviruses, and the possibility of cancers are also an aspect of the story. Remember that latent (dormant) poxviruses can be reactivated during a mixed infection in the presence of another live poxvirus. This can occur even if the two strains of poxvirus are different (i.e. insect poxvirus and human vaccinia virus). This can occur because the live virus contributes valuable genes to the dead virus. The application of insect poxviruses in biocides purposely reactivates latent viruses in pest insect populations. With the use of these insecticides, we find that they may also force animal (i.e. rickettsialpox in pheasants, horses), and human epidemics (i.e. rickettsialpox, polio, Lyme, Morgellon's). Since insecticides are based on insect poxviruses and they have additional microbes added to the formulas, the virulence of the mixed infections is significantly increased. The patent says:

> "The virus yield from cells infected with inactivated virus of one strain and active virus of another strain contains infectious particles of both strains, and also, if the viruses are sufficiently closely related, recombinants. Inactivation by heat, therefore, does not inactivate the [DNA] of the virus particles, since all known genetic markers are preserved."

Again this means that the reactivating virus provides essential genes that are lacking in the dead or latent virus. Therefore a new insect-borne infection from an insecticide can reactivate the remnants of an inactive infection (i.e. from past natural infection); or perhaps even the live or dead recombinant vaccine virus particles that are found in animal and human bodies.[27]

Remember also that poxviruses infect humans including variola, monkeypox, smallpox, cowpox, and vaccinia. Variola and vaccinia have been used within human vaccines for generations. Of the animal poxviruses we find fowlpox, swinepox, sheep pox, and a few others. Sheep pox for example may cause a human vaccine virus to reactivate during *Borrelia garinii* infections, or it may simply reassort to cause an anthrax-like infection that is then transmissible by insects. The insect entomopoxviruses include Type A: *Melolontha melolontha* entomopoxvirus of the European cockchafer beetle (May bug); Type B *Amsacta moorei* entomopoxvirus (gypsy moth); an NPV found in mosquitoes, flies, midges, grasshoppers, and locusts; and Type C *Chironomus luridus* entomopoxvirus of the Israeli benthic midge.[28-31]

Cytoplasmicpolyhedrosis viruses, also called cypoviruses or CPVs, are the reovirus/poxviruses, and so are the insect iridescent viruses of silkworms, gypsy moths, and other insects. The CPVs were applied in the environment as insecticidal helpers beginning in the 1950s. Poxviruses were probably causing animal and human infections long before the 1950s with the earliest applications of B.t., *B. popilliae, B. lentimorbus,* and other insecticides, but their increased presence may have caused animal and human outbreaks.

If the accidental activation of vaccine viruses in animals and humans is driving many of the disease epidemics of today, this could mean that insecticides and vaccines create *biological conflicts of interest* in non-targeted species. It could also imply that genetic engineering is highly flawed, ever since the earliest vaccines developed from the 1800s forward. Human infections occur by entirely natural forces. However they may be far more easily accomplished with the addition of chemical and microbial formulas, toxic chemical pollutants, and recombinant vaccines when these components collide (i.e. insect bite).

It may also mean that there is no way to avoid this reactivation problem; at least not yet. Scientists may be working to devise a way to circumvent certain problems that seem to have caused infectious diseases. In the meantime such scenarios if proven to exist, could and would absolutely drive the silencing of epidemics, research scientists, and some physicians. We can see how this might occur with an illness such as Lyme disease, which can produce very polio-like symptoms. While Lyme disease may be "curable" in its earliest stages, once it disseminates into the body, the illness becomes harder to eradicate. Furthermore, once a former vaccine virus reactivates into a disease state, it may be difficult or impossible to "turn off" the viral aspects of what becomes a complex multi-system disease. Viral reactivation complicates infections with antibiotic-resistant organisms, and may even contribute to their persistence. The continued ingestion of insecticide-tainted foods and other products (i.e. antibiotics, tobacco) contributes to ongoing disease states that may continue to reassort gut bacteria, toxic molds, or yeasts in the presence of mutagenic chemicals and recombinant microbes that constantly enter the body. Therefore eliminating all sources of chemical toxins (i.e. fluorides, chlorides, metals), recombinant microbes, drugs, and eating an organic diet that is as free of B.t. insecticides as possible is key to reducing the overall toxin burdens the immune system has to fight each day while combatting infectious disease agents.[32]

Picric acid, amines, fluorides, chlorides, radioactive elements, Tweens, anilines, acetates, lacquers, detergents, and other chemicals are the key to the mutation of microbes that cause Lyme disease. When mutated leptospires and their passenger co-infections are not killed during acute infection, they persist in the body, and may be detected by newly emerging laboratory tests. These tests are not yet recognized by public health experts or their organizations, but are known by Lyme patients and their physicians. It should make no difference what kind of test is used to detect an infectious organism.

The pathogenicity of the leptospiral component of Lyme disease is increased by the presence of a spiroplasma, an extremophile, viruses, and other agents that due to antibiotic resistance and other tolerances, are left untouched by short-term therapies. The spiroplasma and the extremophile components of a Bb aggregate may prove to be the toughest part of the Bb spirochetes. We know that spiroplasmas are found in the bodies of ticks, and also that extremophile bacteriae are found where ticks venture. These highly pollution-friendly microbes thrive equally well in the toxic environment, as they do in the gut of insects, animals, or humans.

The spiroplasma affinity for brain and nervous system tissues allows a reasonable explanation for virulent disease states including ALS and prion diseases. The differences between disease course may be determined by the kinds of extremophile bacteria or viruses present. We know that insecticides have been engineered using any of the components discussed herein. So we may understand why they are found in the vectors which bite us; and why they are found in the brains of deceased patients upon autopsy who suffer from diseases such as ALS, prion disease, or Lyme.

The reoviruses share similar characteristics with the wound-tumor virus (WTV) of plants, *phytoreovirus*. Scientists suspected in 1965 that the reoviruses may be oncogenic or cancer-causing agents. A 1965 study funded under an NIAID grant was undertaken by scientists at the University of California-Berkeley, the California State Department of Public Health, and the Naval Biological Laboratory. The paper reveals that reoviruses associate with the chromosomes in the cell nucleus of infected host cells. This means that reoviruses will incorporate into the cellular DNA of plants, invertebrates, or higher animals. This incorporation may make them become latent *retroviruses*. At least one reovirus was isolated from Burkitt's lymphoma cells. This also suggests that reoviruses which bind with insect, arthropod, animal, or human genes (i.e. poultry) create *genetic viral infections* (retroviruses) which may be passed *generationally* to offspring. In the case of chickens, such retroviruses have been found to retain reverse transcription (RT) activity, and may be passed through eggs and embryos like those used to fabricate animal and human vaccines or insect cell lines for industrial and agricultural insecticides.[33-35]

The question is whether such retroviruses may be reactivated by wild or recombinant viruses which provide the right genetic materials to reactivate these latent viruses. Such viruses may come from pharmaceuticals, from genetically manipulated insects that are released as "population replacers," from animal or human vaccines, or from the agricultural and industrial biocides that are widely used around the globe.

I suspect that the answer to this question is a firm "yes." I also suspect that if this is true, then it could become one of the best kept secrets of the biotech industry because it would negatively impact everything from insecticides and GM crops to bioremediation tools and vaccines or other human biologicals.[33-35]

The *Namalwa* cell line that was created and used to produce *Interferon,* was established from a B-cell lymphoma tumor obtained from a patient who had an Epstein Barr virus-caused Burkitt's lymphoma. These cells are also used to make *baculovirus expression vectors*, and they may be grown in *nude* mice (mice that lack specific genes). If grown in the lab before making cell lines, they may first be passaged through mice and then chicken embryos, where they may become contaminated with animal retroviruses, rodent leptospires, leptonema, and other agents. This would make them inherent to cell lines used for insecticides or vaccines. These cells are known to produce a variety of novel gene reassortments, some of which have not been clearly identified.Others sound like *prion* disease agents since they secrete low levels of IgM antibodies and other proteins, including those that may be excreted by phages. They may be used to grow *E. coli* or *Saccharomyces cerevisiae* (yeast) such as that used to ferment global B.t. insecticides.[36,48]

We may wonder whether reoviruses are found associating with all Burkitt's lymphoma tumors, or whether they act as virophages which infect EBV and other large viruses in the same way that cypoviruses may do in the environment. We may rightfully be concerned if reoviruses, poxviruses, baculoviruses, and others which have been used agriculturally and which may contaminate vaccines (or cell lines), may be helping to increase cancer epidemics and infectious diseases worldwide. Retroviruses and other latent infections are by design, desired to reactivate and to kill insects. Unfortunately nature plays by her own rules, and the latent infections of higher animals may also be reactivated through exposures to recombinant formulas. These include highly toxic formulas that although designed to force insect epizootics and to remediate chemical and organic pollutants, instead appear to be targeting the animal and human populations.[36]

If insect and animal cell lines were found to be contaminated with prion and other disease-causing agents, such information probably would never be revealed to the public for fear of liability, public panic, loss of genetic tools, and other issues. Instead we may expect that new cell lines might be quietly created, as well as new insecticides and animal vaccines. At least around the time period of the Dearborn conference, we saw each of these items suddenly redesigned, although we cannot assume it was for the stated hypothesis. However insect cell lines were suddenly declared "contaminated" or "destroyed" and new livestock vaccines were made. We also saw the emergence of livestock, wild deer, and human prion and immunodeficiency diseases in the latter half of the 20th century; and the detection of spiroplasmas or other agents in the brain tissues of deceased patients. Therefore we may suspect that any human infections which might be associated with failed vaccine or insecticide cell lines and with livestock or deer might transmit prion agents or other infections which could drive the silencing of human epidemics in perpetuity.

What else do we need to know? One of the more disturbing aspects of this story is that the combination of insecticides which include B.t., yeasts, toxins, fungi, and viruses; is that not only are new and improved insecticides being designed, some of the insect viruses that have long been used, and which occur naturally, may leave *no evidence of infection* that is detectable by current laboratory tests. For example we know that the borrelina viruses have been used extensively as insecticidal enhancers. The polyhedrosis viruses that cause natural insect diseases and which were used as insecticides typically create what are called *inclusion bodies* or crystals which can be detected in the scientific laboratory. However there is a group of insect viruses which cause insect diseases and in which *no visible pathological inclusion body of any kind is produced.* This group of *stealth viruses* is named *Bergoldia Steinhaus,* after the University of California scientist Edward A. Steinhaus who discovered them.

These viruses are granulosis viruses (GVs), and are slowly progressing infections which *cannot be seen under an electron microscope*. However infected cells may reveal inclusion bodies that are irregularly shaped and which originate in the cytoplasm of the cell. GVs cause a kind of *wilt disease* in caterpillar larvae. There is a wilt disease called *Paillotella* that is seen in cabbage white butterflies in Europe, and which has been reported in France. This may be the "unseen" GVs which infected silkworm larvae centuries ago, and the same viruses that infect many kinds of larvae today.[38-44]

The *Bergoldia* group of GVs were discussed at the fifth international congress for microbiology in Rio de Janeiro in 1950. It is currently believed that one of the "undetectable" GVs of silkworms, when combined with the bacterium *Bacillus bombycis,* also called *Cubonianus,* which is a disease of *mulberry trees and grapevines*, gives rise to the true "*flacherie*" disease that has been seen within silkworm populations. When this same GV is accompanied by *Streptococcus bombycis,* the result is the silkworm disease "*gattine.*" [38-44]

There is an important bacteria-virus link that is exploited by current microbial insecticides, and these viruses are the latent viruses that are sought by scientists who design insecticides. The only way to prove the existence of these "unseen" GV viruses is by their infectivity, where they produce symptoms in infected insects. This means also that if the viruses are able to infect animals and humans, that *they will also remain undetectable.* The only practical way of determining their presence is by culturing cells or by symptom presentation. This tells us that the very real and important chronic infections that are found in humans today *may be undetectable by laboratory tests of any kind.* Scientists are aware that honey bees are also affected by these same pathogens, which likewise produces no evidence of infection. It may be some time before science catches up with the idea that these viruses may be contributing to "chronic" infections of our day, including quite possibly Lyme disease, Morgellon's, Chronic Fatigue, Fibromyalgia, MS, ALS, and other neurologic and/or brain-affecting diseases.[38-44]

Perhaps these viruses are what Dr. Maurice Hilleman was referring to when he cautioned us years ago to "detect the undetectable viruses." This group of insect viruses has been known to exist since at least 1949. One example of this group is *Bergoldia virulenta*, which causes a virulent infection in the cabbage white butterfly (*Pieris rapae*), an *Australian* native, and a species that has been used as a sentinel species in the US to gauge the effectiveness of the applied microbial insecticides. This butterfly is highly prevalent in North America and is a particular pest of rapeseed (canola) crops.[38-44]

The presence of "undetectable" viruses in the human body is quite disconcerting, especially when patients complain they are "still" sick and laboratory tests yield no discernable infections. If scientists cannot "see" these infections under electron microscopy, and they cannot be detected using any laboratory tests; then they may be entirely missed and dismissed. Their presence is nearly impossible to detect during the fabrication of cell lines, recombinant insecticides, or genetically modified food crops.

While the presence of these viruses has been known since at least the late 1940s, their "undetectable" nature makes these viruses the *perfect stealth organisms for biological warfare of any kind*, be it an insecticide or something far more imaginative. They also provide a practical and very real explanation as to why some patients do not improve even after long-term antibiotics, if these infections are part of an illness complex, such as that brought about by an aggregate spirochete named *Borrelia burgdorferi.* They also explain the sudden emergence of anti-retroviral agents and pharmaceuticals meant to "fix" gene folding problems from viruses and retroviruses that have become in a word, reactivated.

The unstable nature of arboviruses that have been used in genetically engineered chimera is troubling as well when we understand that some recombinant constructs can and probably have already failed. This may have occurred upon exposure to viruses from insect vectors that were exposed to recombinant insecticides and polluted microbes. The literature shows that attempts to correct this problem have already been made. Patents lend clues to this process and also to the idea that some recombinant constructs can cause *molecular mimicry* because they resemble proteins found in the human body. Molecular mimicry is a problem that occurred with the first generation Lyme vaccine, and which led to a treatment-resistant form of arthritis in some vaccine recipients.

A 1995 patent assigned to the University of North Carolina at Chapel Hill describes a method to keep a live Venezuelan equine encephalitis virus from spreading in a vaccine using an inhibiting compound. This virus is used instead of its parent virus sindbis, to create genetic constructs for vaccines, because of problems caused by sindbis virus in earlier formulas. The patent text reveals there may indeed have been a problem with the sindbis (SIN) model alphavirus in genetic chimera, of which scientists had awareness:[45]

> "Venezuelan equine encephalitis virus...Insofar as applicant is aware, *a problem with the Sindbis vector is that the heterologous insert is unstable therein and is 'kicked out' of the vector,* with the practical limit for stable inserts being about 1 kb."

Another patent addresses molecular mimicry:[46]

> "...the prior art is deficient in the lack of effective means of inhibiting the spread of certain viruses...[it] is also *deficient in the lack of effective means to ensure the non-infectivity of viruses used as vaccines*. The present invention fulfills these longstanding needs and desires in the art."

The latter patent appears to state that the prior art was ineffective at inhibiting the spread of a recombinant alphavirus such as, but not necessarily limited to sindbis from genetically engineered vaccines. It may also be stating that prior recombinant vaccines or insecticides that used sindbis or its relatives could not ensure that the viruses did not remain infective, stable, or that they would not be kicked out of the recombinant chimera to cause disease in vaccinated animals or humans.

The term "longstanding needs" is not a good indicator either if sindbis and other viruses used in recombinant formulas of all kinds from vaccines and human biologicals to biological controls were not properly stabilized, and effectively neutralized all these years. The sindbis or other vaccine viruses may be able to reactivate and cause human diseases with symptoms which mimic polio-like diseases from Lyme to chronic fatigue, fibromyalgia, Rheumatoid Arthritis, Multiple Sclerosis, and others with "no known cause." Indeed it is the reactivation of latent viruses and bacterial recombinations that may be at the heart of the silencing of human epidemics including Lyme disease; and also the thrust forward for new recombinant vaccine formulas. The underlying problem of course may be that the recombinant tools of genetic engineering which we were warned about decades ago, might be highly dangerous and unpredictable – warnings which were temporarily heeded, but in the long term perhaps largely dismissed.

If telling the truth about what is applied to the environment and within our bodies, and the relationships these applications may have had to modern disease epidemics does not get the world's attention, then I do not know what will. I do know that from where I sit observing the evolution of recombinant tools that are globally applied, and the pollutants which abound from many important industries; that these "tools" seem to be making a very different impact upon the world than what was intended as a result of their deployment. We are now better informed about some of the chemicals and microbes that appear in the environment as pollutants. Although it is tempting to target a single chemical or mutagenic agent, the truth is that there are likely to be several chemicals and radioactive wastes that are part of the microbial mutation process, at least when we discuss natural recombinant events. However there are very clear genetically engineered formulas that if sought may be detectable in organisms that are causing specific human diseases. The explanations for how they managed to infect humans will be left up to those who designed the recombinant formulas. However we may certainly narrow down the path from laboratory tool to disease state; as well as determine which industries may be contributors to infective agents the likes of *Borrelia burgdorferi*.

Among the highly mutagenic chemicals found in the environment are the organofluoride and organochloride compounds, and the surfactants. Other important factors include picric acid, azo and aniline dyes, amines, Tweens, chromium, uranium, thorium, dioxins, and other persisting pollutants. Quite frankly whatever we put into the environment will make its way into our bodies. The results of living in a toxic environment will never be compatible with maintaining optimum health regardless of what any manufacturers or "safety" scientists may say about industrial products and processes.

While the evidence appears convincing that insect biowarfare has been targeting far more than its intended insect populations, my hope is that long overdue admissions will be forthcoming while new tools will be created to correct what may prove in the long run to be accidents of genetic engineering. While this may not be good news for industries or for the scientists of same, it may be the breath of fresh air that is needed for ill patients who suffer from many diseases. I sincerely doubt that recombinant accidents were ever intentional if and when they occurred. But I do believe that there may have been a lack of foresight, and possibly also an irresponsible misuse of technologies that were applied long before they were able to be proven "safe." Sometimes even when found to be flawed and to contain risks, recombinant tools were used anyway. Unfortunately it is obvious that these risks may have been both grossly underestimated, and largely realized.

I also feel that the equally irresponsible disposal of important industrial wastes which has been undertaken over a century and a half by many industries has been a key contributing factor to the development of important human diseases. Some public health experts may have long known about some of the connections described in my books, but have said very little to the public. I also believe that the imperfect science of genetic engineering produces ongoing problems which will continue; and that those who regulate industrial and academic "products" including genetic tools have failed in their responsibility to protect the environment and the species that inhabit same. I feel also that the ability to patent living and synthetic organisms that are based on the genes of living organisms, should be immediately reconsidered or even rescinded.

If we do not change current academic and industrial trends, then the human race may soon end up as extinct as the insects we set out to exterminate a century and a half ago. We must accept the idea that genetic engineering tools and industrial wastes of yesterday and today have caused or contributed to some of the most important diseases we have faced. If we fail to correct our former mistakes, then the end result may be a world full of insects – and one devoid of humans brought about by "yet another method of massive killing of large populations." This is precisely why the techniques of insect biowarfare and nuclear energy were to be undertaken under great urgency and secrecy at the start of the War Research Service – because they were felt at the beginning to be entirely likely to cause massive human epidemics.[47]

The reason why the development of tools for insect biowarfare was to remain a closely guarded secret seems obvious. If the techniques deployed are not fool-proof; if they lead to genetic engineering "accidents;" if they reactivate latent infections in animals or humans; and if new human disease epidemics arise because of their use, then such tools will have to be scrapped for being "junk science" – but only if such flaws exist and the public and regulators become aware of same. If the modern tools of potentially flawed design are what the world depends upon to protect it from insects of medical, military, veterinary, industrial, and agricultural importance; then evidence of adverse events could remain hidden for as long as these highly profitable global tools are considered to be useful and important. The discovery of recombinant "accidents" would therefore allow the quiet replacement of flawed tools with better tools to avoid similar mistakes. The problem comes only from the idea that if such accidents are leading to human diseases, that these diseases and their patients sadly are rarely, if ever acknowledged.

If these tools are not flawed; do not cause human diseases; and this entire book has been a fantastic portrayal of an imaginery world, then consider this book merely a novel of dire warning. Therefore there should be no problems and no kept secrets, as secrets have a way of being revealed over time. However if the technologies *are* as flawed as they appear to be, and as described by so many sworn patents, then there are huge biotech secrets that have been waiting decades to be told. I for one hope that this book holds truths which will be proven to be valuable clues to the paradigms of denial that certain diseases currently share. I also pray that the adage will prove applicable to the present silence that surrounds infectious diseases of our day when I tell you that *the truth shall set us free.* ❑

Afterword: About "Evidence-Based" Medicine

"Evidence-based medicine" while perhaps useful in days long past, seems wholly impractical in this new era of recombinant genetics and rapid microbial change. Unfortunately it also appears to have very little practicality within a clinical setting. This is especially obvious with the continued laboratory and natural production of novel recombinant organisms which change classification over time. Nomenclature appears largely based on who discovers an organism; what kind of vector transmits it; how intimately and often the organism is studied; and how many different ways it mutates in the environment or within its hosts.

Further complicating the situation is the invention of recombinant "natural" microbes and toxins; new organisms that never before existed, and those that have long been present but which remain elusive to diagnostic tests and laboratory microscopes. Following the old order of establishing medical guidelines and treatment options based on "evidence-based" laboratory studies of individual organisms is no longer feasible or even remotely appropriate. Rather the new recombinant aggregate organisms in multiply co-infected people demand flexibility in the lab, in the clinical setting, and in the formation of medical treatment and insurance guidelines. This is because genetic mutations occur naturally, even once inside the host animal or human – far away from the laboratory scientist's ability to duplicate or define these processes.

Now that we are aware that there are insect viruses that cannot even be seen under electron microscopy, we know that such infections will not only be impossible to quantify by laboratory tests, but they will remain difficult to prove for insurance or disability purposes, even when they are clearly present by the manifestation of symptoms. This will further blur the lines between "allowable" insurance coverages and the establishment of accurate diagnoses, and may demand the formation of a new category of environmental illnesses based solely on symptom presentations. This has already begun, but the bulk of the "unknown" illnesses are unfortunately being relegated to a new category of "mental" illnesses.

Natural recombinations make established standards difficult if not impossible to follow since humans and their microbial infections can and do vary greatly across regional or continental areas. Multiply infected patients require combined antibiotics and other treatments to remediate highly complex diseases, toxic chemical pollutants, and their deleterious and often systemic effects upon the human body over a lifetime of exposures. Recombinant organisms will likely display characteristics of each of their individual components and therefore should herald a more liberal approach to treatment therapies. This should force all to stop thinking in terms of black and white, but rather in shades of grey and every color in between. Patients are multiply infected with many pathogens from a variety of sources and their collective effects upon the human body contribute to the development of complex diseases which cannot easily be defined within the pages of an insurance handbook of "allowable" coverages. As the world of recombinant microbes expands, so too must the clinical practitioner's repertoire of knowledge about infectious diseases, and the willingness of legislators to force insurance companies to accept and pay for the diseases caused by these tools.

The accessibility of meaningful diagnostic tools and treatments geared toward patients must expand and should never be limited or obscured by industrial or academic research interests or opinions. What becomes available for use in the laboratory should also be developed for commercial use as a mandate under federal grant award contracts. Scientists whom endow or merely study organisms with the ability to cross species barriers have no business setting rigid, "evidence-based" diagnostic and treatment guidelines or testing standards when microorganisms are far more flexible and unpredictable than the scientists who study them – scientists whose interests may conflict when hired by industries with important ties to such organisms. Public health officials must be made aware of, and accept that clinical physicians require a greater arsenal of antibiotics and other therapies. They must be allowed to prescribe therapies for longer durations to accommodate the complex microbes being released into the environment; and that are likely leading to infectious diseases which affect global populations.

In the physician's office, diagnoses are supposed to be based upon symptoms and clinical findings. The decision to diagnose and to treat any illness has always been, and should remain sacred and private between patient and physician. What purpose does the government have in the examining room unless perhaps there are industrial secrets that are supposed to remain hidden? Patients and physicians should be allowed individually to decide their medical care without threat of interference by medical boards or public health experts who enforce restrictive disease definitions or standardized diagnostic tests. Perhaps the invisible arm of government in our clinics is a reflection of protecting flawed industrial products and profits. If there are hidden motivations behind the implementation of government-sponsored "health" care, we may guess that these might include protecting the formerly transparent arm of industry and academic science that already has, and will continue *unchecked* to intrude into every aspect of our lives. It is quite simply time to accept and to acknowledge that patients are ill; and that they want, need, and deserve to be provided with adequate, accessible, and affordable tools to diagnose and treat their illnesses. Anything less than this is irresponsible, inhumane, and absolutely unacceptable. ❑

References

Introduction

A Moving Target

1.) US Army. Summaries for US Army Lyme Disease Risk Assessments, 1996 Nov 1. Doherty AJ. Major, USAF, Retired. FOIA request. Report No. 16-44-0578-88.
2.) Novel diagnostic test to detect *Borrelia burgdorferi* in patient sera. Advanced Laboratory Services. http://advanced-lab.com. Blood samples from the author were sent during the summer and fall of 2011 during the development phase of the new Lyme diagnostic test.
3.) Kramer JP. Parasites in Laboratory Colonies of Mosquitos. WHO Bulletin. 1964;31:475-478.
4.) Christophers Sir S. Rickard. *Aëdes Aegypti* (L.) The Yellow Fever Mosquito. Its Life History, Bionomics and Structure. 1960 Cambridge University Press. (d) Parasites. p. 63-68.
5.) Noguchi Hideyo, Kaliski David J. The Spirochetal Flora of the Normal Female Genetalia. JEM. 1918 Jun:559-561. From the Rockefeller Institute for Medical Research Laboratories.
6.) US Patent 4,721,617. Johnson. Vaccine against Lyme disease. Filed 8/14/86 published 1/26/88. Assignee: Regents of the University of Minnesota (Minneapolis, MN).

Chapter One: Don't Ask, Don't Tell Policies of Biowarfare

What We "Know" About Lyme

1.) Town of Guilford, Connecticut. Natural Resource Inventory and Assessment. 2005 Jan. [bulletin] [web page]
2.) Johnson Russell C. (ed.). In The Biology of Parasitic Spirochetes. Academic Press. New York 1976:101.
3.) Masuzawa T, Suzuki H, Kawabata H, et al. Identification of Spirochetes Isolated from Wild Rodents in Japan as Borrelia japonica. J Clin Microbiol. 1995 May;33(5):1392-1394.
4.) Fukunaga M, Takahashi Y, Tsuruta Y, et al. Genetic and Phenotypic Analysis of Borrelia miyamotoi sp. nov., Isolated from Ixoded Tick Ixodes persulcatus, the Vector for Lyme Disease in Japan. Inter J System Bacteriol. 1995 Oct;45(4):804-810.
5.) Kaya G, Berset M, Prins C, et al. Chronic Borreliosis Presenting with Morphea- and Lichen sclerosus et atrophicus-Like Cutaneous Lesions. A Case Report. Dermatol 2001;202(4):373-375.
6.) Aberer E, Duray Paul H. Morphology of Borrelia burgdorferi: Structural Patterns of Cultured Borreliae in Relation to Staining Methods. 1991 Apr;29(4):764-772.
7.) CDC. Lyme Disease Data. (web page) www.cdc.gov.
8.) Montgomery RR, Nathanson MH, Malawista SE. The fate of Borrelia burgdorferi, the agent for Lyme disease, in mouse macrophages. Destruction, survival, recovery. J Immunol. 1993 Feb 1;150(3):909-915.
9.) Steere AC, Taylor E, Wilson ML, Levine JF, Spielman A. Longitudinal assessment of the clinical and epidemiological features of Lyme disease in a defined population. J Infect Dis. 1986 Aug;154(2):295-300.
10.) Dr. Rudolph Scrimenti, phone interview with the author, November 10, 2011.
11.) Scrimenti RJ. Erythema chronicum migrans. Arch Dermatol. 1970 Jul;102(1):104-105.
12.) Brock Thomas D. (ed.) from the University of WI. Microorganisms From Smallpox to Lyme Disease. Readings from Scientific American. 1990 W.H. Freeman and Company, New York. From the chapter: Lyme Disease by Gail S. Habicht, Gregory Beck and Jorge L. Benach. Page 28-37.
13.) Micrographs from my office visit 10-27-11 where my blood was viewed using live blood microscopy; and in vitro darkfield microscopy, PCR, and by DNA sequencing of new diagnostic tests in development at Advanced Laboratory Services, Sharon Hill PA. Samples sent for culture July-November 2011. Press Release issued in September, 2011.
14.) UniProt Consortium Taxonomy Browser. 2002-2010. Species group Borrelia burgdorferi group. www.uniprot.org
15.) Casjens Sherwood. Borrelia Genomes in the Year 2000. J Mol Microbiol. Biotechnol. 2000;2(4):401-410.
16.) Burgdorfer Willy. The Possible Role of Ticks as Vectors of Leptospirae. I. Transmission of Leptospira pomona by the Argasid Tick, Ornithodoros turicata, and the Persistance of This Organism in Its Tissues. Exper Parasitol. 1956;V:571-579.

The Hallmark Infection

1.) Jenner W. The Medical Times and Gazette. Clinical Lectures on Diseases of the Skin. Chapter on Roseola. 1857 Jan – June. Vol. 14 (old series Vol. 35). Begins page 181. Published by John Churchill, London, England.
2.) Ramos A, Ballenilla F, Martin P. Uncommon epiloptogenic lesions affecting the temporal lobe. Semin Ultrasound CT MR. 2008 Feb;29(1):47-59.
3.) Lundberg P, Ramakrishna C, Brown J, et al. The immune response to herpes simplex virus type 1 infection in susceptible mice is a major cause of central nervous system pathology resulting in fatal encephalitis. J Virol. 2008 Jul;82(14):7078-88. Epub 2008 May 14.
4.) Auyeung P, Dunn A. Atypical case of Herpes simplex encephalitis. Intern Med J. 2008 Apr;38(4):294-5.
5.) Itzhaki RF, Cosby SL, Wozniak MA. Herpes simplex virus type 1 and Alzheimer's disease: the autophagy connection. J Neurovirol. 2008 Jan;14(1):1-4.
6.) US Patent 5,244,802. Rangan. Regeneration of cotton. Filed 3/29/91 published 9/14/93. Assignee: Phytogen (Pasadena, CA).]

The Dearborn Conference

1.) Steere AC, Matawista SE, Hardin JA, et al. Erythema chronicum migrans and Lyme arthritis: the enlarging clinical spectrum. Ann Intern Med 1977;86:685-98.
2.) Grant 5R03TW000514-03. Lyme Borreliosis in Russia. Steere, Allen C. Grant award to New England Medical Center Hospitals, Boston, MA. Fiscal year 1997. Project start: 9/30/95 ended 9/29/99. ICD: Fogarty International Center.
3.) Proceedings of the Second National Conference on Serologic Diagnosis of Lyme Disease. 1994 Oct. 27-29, Dearborn, MI. 106pages. Sponsors: Assoc. of State and Territorial Public Health Laboratory Directors, US CDC and Prevention, MI Dept. of Health. Co-sponsors: USFDA, NIH, Council of State and Territorial Epidemiologists and National Committee for Clinical Laboratory Standards.
4.) Transcripts of the US Dept. of Health and Human Services FDA Center for Biologics Evaluation and Research Vaccines and Related Biological Products Advisory Committee Meeting. 1998 May 26. At the Versailles Rooms I and II, Holiday Inn, 8120 Wisconsin Ave., Bethesda, Maryland. 364 pages.
5.) Original PLA #97-1052. Statistical Review and Evaluation. Sponsor: SKB. Product: Lyme Disease vaccine (Lymerix). From Pamela R. Getson, PhD through Peter A. Lachenbruch, PhD, Branch Chief, Biostatistics, DBE. Report. FDA [web page]
6.) Complete Review Comments and Questions to SKB for the Lyme Disease Vaccine PLA. Sponsor: SmithKline Beecham (SKB) Pharmaceuticals. Vaccine: LYMErix (OspA Lyme Disease Vaccine): PLA 97-1052. Review date July 7, 1998. From FDA [web page]
7.) Letter and report from the US Dept. of Health and Human Services of the FDA. 1998 Dec 21. Letter concerns licensing of LYMErix vaccine with comments noting that the manufacturer agreed to submit a completed study report concerning the cellular immunity study described in the document titled "Report on Cellular Immunity to Outer-surface Protein A (OspA) in a Subset of Subjects in the SmithKline Beecham Lyme Disease Vaccine Trial #008,"submitted on Jun 23, 1998 (pp. 90-109) to the manufacturer's vaccine license application.

Guidelines for a Silent Epidemic

1.) D. Scott Samuels, Justin D. Radolf (eds.). Preface: Borrelia: Molecular Biology, Host Interaction and Pathogenesis. 2010 March. Horizon Press.
2.) US Patent application 20090060932. Dattwyler et al. Filed 3/9/06published 3/5/09. Groups of Borrelia Burgdorferi and Borrelia Afzelii That Cause Lyme Disease in Humans. Inventors: Raymond Dattwyler, Gerald Seinost, Daniel Dykhuizen, Benjamin Luft, Maria Gomes-Solecki. Assignee: Research Foundation of the State University of New York (Stony Brook) and Brook Biotechnologies, Inc. (Stony Brook, NY).
3.) US Patent 5,582,829. Alliger, et al. Sonicated borrelia burgdorferi vaccine. Filed July 28, 1992, published 12/10/96. Assignee: Rx Technologies, Inc. (Garden City, NY).
4.) IRS Tax return form 990 Kaiser Foundation Health Plan Inc. Oakland, CA. 2006.
5.) IRS Tax return form 990 Kaiser Foundation Health Plan of Ohio 2003.
6.) Press Release. Richard Blumenthal. Office of the Attorney General of Connecticut. 2008 May 1.

Biowarfare in History

1.) Smadel, Joseph E., Army Medical Department Research and Graduate School, Washington, DC. Laboratory Diagnosis of Viral and Rickettsial Diseases, A Reappraisal after Ten Years. Symposium on Viral and Rickettsial Diseases. Presented at the Golden Jubilee Meeting of the Society of American Bacteriologists at Baltimore, MD. May 15, 1950.
2.) CDC. Centers for Disease Control and Prevention. Emergency Preparedness and Response.
3.) Reimer LG. Q fever. Clin Microbiol Rev 1993 Jul;6(3):193-198
4.) Stoenner HG, Lackman DB, Benson WW, et al. The Role of Dairy Cattle in the Epidemiology of Q Fever in Idaho. J Infect Dis 1961 Jul-Aug;109(1):90-97.
5.) Brock TD. Microorganisms From Smallpox to Lyme Disease. Scientific American. W.H. Freeman and Company. 1990. p. 28-37.
6.) Endicott Stephen, Hagerman Edward. The United States and Biological Warfare, Secrets from the Early Cold War and Korea. Indiana University Press 1998.
7.) Katz SL, Gershon AA, Hotez PJ. Krugman's Infectious Diseases of Children, 10th Edition, 1998 Mosby-Year Book, Inc.
8.) Langer Elinor, Listowel Judith. Chemical and Biological Warfare. Survival. 1967 Apr;9(4):128-135.
9.) The Wednesday Report. Canada's Aerospace & Defence Weekly. Weapons of Mass Destruction (Chem/Bio).
10.) Turner MD. Project Whitecoat. 1970. Spectrum.
11.) Langhoff PJ. God Science: The Secret World of Rampant Genetics, Hidden Illness, and Biotech Profiteering. 2010 Allegory Press LLC, Hustisford, WI
12.) Technical Report: DDC AD408401. February 3-4, 1960. Conference on Biological Control of Insects of Medical Importance. American Institute of Biological Sciences (Washington, DC). 148 pages. Unclassified documents retrieved from the public domain. Dr. Steinhaus speaking, page 123.
13.) Harry S. Truman Library & Museum. The War Relocation Authority & the incarceration of Japanese-Americans during World War II. 1942 Chronology.
14.) US Congress Appropriations Committee Hearing, Research, Development, Testing, and Evaluation of Synthetic Biological Agents. (Subcommittee on DOD, HB15090). Published by the US Government Printing Office. Reposted on the Internet by the Phil Fam Committee 22 June 1998.
15.) Nixon Ends Biological Weapons Program. American Experience web site. wwpbs.org
16.) Homeland Security Digital Library. www.hsdl.org Chemical Warfare Agent Experiments Among U.S. Service Members
17.) Welsome Eileen. The Plutonium Files: America's secret medical experiments in the Cold War NEJM. 1999 Dec 16;341:1941-1942.
18.) Plutonium Files: How the US Secretly Fed Radioactivity to Thousands of Americans. 2004 May 5. Democracy Now! [web site]
19.) Krueger Joline Gutierrez. Eileen Welsome, Albuquerque Tribune made history with "The Plutonium Experiment." The Times of the Tribune. 2008 Feb 22. [monograph]

Ethics Violations Become Public Knowledge

1.) US Patent 6,492,113. Vojdani. Detection of Mycoplasma genus and species in patients with chronic fatigue syndrome and fibromyalgia. Filed 4/1/99 published 12/10/02. Assignee: Immunosciences Lab, Inc., Calif. Corporation (Beverly Hills, CA).
2.) US Patent 6,815,161. Vojdani. Detection of Mycoplasma in patients with chronic fatigue syndrome and related disorders. Filed 4/1/99 published 11/9/04. Assignee; Immunosciences Lab, Inc. (Beverly Hills, CA).
3.) Nicolson Garth L, Nicolson Nancy L. Project Day Lily, An American Biological Warfare Tragedy. 2006 Xlibris Corp.
4.) US Patent 5,242,820. Lo. Pathogenic mycoplasma. Filed 6/6/91, issued 9/7/93. Assignee: American Registry of Pathology (Washington, DC)
5.) Drury Tom. How Iraq built its weapons programs. 2003 Mar 16. St. Petersburg Times.
6.) US Food and Drug Administration. Pyridostigmine Bromide Information Page.
7.) J. Stryker Meyer. Executive order gives DOD power to use investigational drugs on military. [monograph]
8.) Jonathan D. Moreno. Is there an ethicist in the house?: on the cutting edge of bioethics. 2005 Indiana Press.
9.) US Patent 5,672,485. Foster, et al. Immortalized cell lines for viral growth. Filed 8/13/96. Assignee: Regents of the University of Minnesota (Minneapolis, MN)
10.) NOVA Online. Global Guide to Bioweapons. www.pbs.org
11.) BBC News. Analysis: Threat from disease weapons. 2001 Nov 1. [monograph on the Internet]
12.) Money, Nicholas P. Triumph of the Fungi. Chapter 8: Blights, Rusts, and Rots Never Sleep: Forestry and Agriculture, Biological Warfare, and the Global Impact of Fungal Disease. 2006 Sept:137-197. Oxford Scholarship Online Monographs.
13.) Madden LV, Wheelis M. The Threat of Plant Pathogens as Weapons Against US Crops. Ann Rev. Phytopathol. 2003 Sept;41:155-176.
14.) Langer Elinor, Listowel Judith. Chemical and Biological Warfare. Survival. 1967 Apr;9(4):128-135.
15.) Choffnes Eileen. Germs on the loose. Bioweapons tests tainted sites around the globe. Will the mess ever be cleaned up? Bulletin of Atomic Scientists. 2001 Mar-Apr;57(2):57-61.
16.) Joshua Lederberg (ed.). Biological weapons: limiting the threat. 2001. Belfer Center for Schience and International Affairs. John F. Kennedy School of Government Harvard University. Chapter 6, p. 99.
17.) The National Security Archive. Stimson. Biological and Chemical Weapons. History of the US Offensive Biological Warfare Program (1941-1973). [web site]
18.) Anonymous. The Bacteriological Weapon. Bulgarian V. anniya, 1959;9(3):20-21. Translated by Claudius F. Mayer, N.D., July 1959, Washington. From: Army Biological Labs, Frederick MD report AD0845947, July 1959.
19.) USDA Agricultural Research Center. Wheat stem rust. [web site] www.ars.usda.gov
20.) Los Angeles Times. Kaplan Karen. A 'time bomb' for world wheat crop. 2009 Jun 14.
21.) Monsanto. Monsanto Invests in Wheat through WestBred Acquisition. www.monsanto.com
22.) CNS. James Martin Center for Nonproliferation Studies. Monterey Institute of International Studies. Agricultural Biowarfare: State Programs to Develop Offensive Capabilities
23.) Alibek Ken, Handelman Stephen. Biohazard: The Soviet Union's Agricultural Biological Weapons. 1999 Random House, NY.
24.) Line Roland F, Peet Clyde E, Kingsolver Charles H. Stem Rust Infection and Development in Artificially Inoculated Fields of Wheat at Hays, Kansas, and its Effect on Yield, 1960 to 1965. Corporate Author: Fort Detrick Frederick MD. Report date 1968Aug. 10 pages. Report #AD0843597. Project #DA-1-B-522301-A-061.
25.) SeedQuest News section. Dangerous wheat disease jumps Red Sea – Devastating fungal pathogen spreads from eastern Africa to Yemen, following path scientists predicted. 2007 Jan 16.
26.) Suryanarayanan S, McConnell WB. The Metabolism of Perlargonate-1-C14 by Wheat Stem Rust Uredospores. 1964 May 8. 1 page [abstract] AD0456244. Corp. author: National Research Council of Canada Saskatoon (Saskatchewan) Prairie Regional Lab.
27.) US Patent Application 20100130561. Andersch, Wolfram, et al. Controlling Pests by Combining Insecticides and Transgenic Plants by Applying Directly to Leaves and Roots. Andersch; Wolfram; et al. Filed 4/14/08 published 5/27/10. Assignee: Bayer Cropscience AG. (Monheim, DE).
28.) Technical Report: DDC AD408401. Conference on Biological Control of Insects of Medical Importance. American Institute of Biological Sciences (Washington, DC). 148 pages. Date stamped June 28, 1961 Naval Medical Field Research Laboratory, Camp LeJeune, North Carolina. (DDC) July 16, 1963. Unclassified documents retrieved from the public domain.
29.) Serratia marcescens. Schenectady County Community College. www.sunysccc.edu
30.) USDA. Beltsville, MD. News and Reviews. Biological Control at National Entomology Society Meetings. Presentation at the 1995 National Meeting of the Entomological Society of America in Las Vegas. [newsletter]. Farrar R. Strain of *Serratia marcescens* with high virulence when fed to corn earworm larvae.
31.) US Patent 7,763,465. Abad, et al. Unique novel Bacillus thuringiensis gene with lepidopteran activity. Filed 3/12/09 Assignee: Pioneer Hi-Bred International, Inc. (Johnston, IA).
32.) US Patent 3,888,887. Jirkovsky. Derivatives of 3-amino-2-halo-2-cyclohexen-1-one. Filed 5/6/74. Assignee: American Home Products Corporation (New York, NY).
33) US Patent 4,223,007. Spence, et al. Microbial insecticide. Filed 4/27/79. Assignee: Battelle Development Corporation (Columbus, OH).
34.) US Patent 3,073,749. Megna. Preparation of Microbial Insecticide. Filed 6/9/59. Issue date: 1/15/63. Assignee: Bioferm Corp., Wasco, CA.
35.) US Patent 2,776,926 Sharpe E. et al. Preparation of Alpha-Ketoglutaric Acid by Serratia Marcescens. Assignee: US Secretary of Agriculture. Filed 8/4/55. (granted under Title 35, U.S. Code [1952], sec. 266).
36.) Stojek Nimfa Maria, Dutkiewicz Jacek. Studies on the Occurrence of Gram-Negative Bacteria in ticks: Ixodes Ricinus as a potential vector of Pasteurella. Ann Agric Environ Med (AAEM) 2004;11:319-322.
37.) Duncan JT. On a bactericidal principle present in the alimentary canal of insects and arachnids. Parasitol. 1926;18:238-252
38.) Tanada, Yoshinori and Kaya, Harry K. Insect pathology. University of California. Academic Press, Inc. 1993.
39.) Radnedge L, Agron PG, Hill KK, et al. Genome Differences That Distinguish Bacillus anthracis from Bacillus cereus and Bacillus thuringiensis. Appl Environ Microbiol. 2003

May;69(5):2755-2764.
40.) Helgason E, Okstad OA, Caugant DA, et al. Bacillus anthracis, Bacillus cereus, and Bacillus thuringiensis – one species on the basis of genetic evidence. Appl Environ Microbiol. 2000;66:2627-2630.
41.) Bell JF, Moore GJ, Raymond GH, Tibbs CE. Characteristics of Rabies in Bats in Montana. AJPH. 1962 Aug;52(8):1293-1301.
42.) Bell, J. Frederick; Burgdorfer, Willy; and Moore, G. John. The Behavior of Rabies Virus in Ticks. J Infect Dis 1957;100:278-283, 1957. And Bell JF, Burgdorfer W, Moore GJ. The Behavior of Rabies Virus in Ticks.
43.) California Jail to Test Ray Gun on Prisoners. Article on Internet. Accessed Oct 26, 2011.

The "Secret" History of Lyme Disease

1.) Russel Darrell A, Williams Gerald G. History of Chemical Fertilizer Development. Soil Sci Soc Am J. 1977;41:260-265.
2.) Searls James P. Potash. US Geological Survey report. 9pages. [web page]
3.) Anonymous. The Phosphate Industry of the United States. A public domain reprinting of the Sixty Special Report of the Commissioner of Labor. Carroll D. Wright. Washington Government Printing Office. 1893.
4.) Smith DR, Moore, Jr. PA, Griffis CL, et al. Effects of Alum and Aluminum Chloride on Phosphorus Runoff from Swine Manure. J Environ Quality. 2001;30:992-998.
5.) University of South Florida. Florida Institute of Phosphate Research. Phosphate Primer. Discovery of Phosphate in Florida. [web site]
6.) Phosphorus. Chemistry Explained. Foundations and Applications. [web site]
7.) The New York Times. Mining Phosphate Rock. Regulating South Carolina's Great Industry. 1891 Jan. 29. Article dated Jan. 28, Charleston, S.C.
8.) US Marines. Marine Corp. News. (Report of five studies including natural resources in the Kazakstan, Kyrgystan, Tajikistan, Turkmenistan and Uzbekistan regions).
9.) Lowenstein TK, Spencer RJ, Pengxi Z. Origin of Ancient Potash Evaporites: Clues from the Modem Nonmarine Qaidam Basin of Western China. Science 1989 Sep. 8;245(4922):1090-1092
10.) Bloch David. Saltpeter. www.salt.org.il/frame_saltpet.html
11.) US Patent X1. Samuel Hopkins. Filed 1/31/1790. Handwritten patent for "in the making of Pot ash and Pearl ash by a new apparatus and process." Signed by George Washington in the City of New York, with attorney Edm. Randolph Attorney General of the United States.
12.) Cohen Y, Kirchmann H, Enfält P. Management of Phosphorus Resources. Historical Perspective, Principal Problems and Sustainable Solutions. Integr Waste Manag. (date unknown) Vol II:247-268.
13.) FIPR. Florida Institute of Phosphate Research. Phosphate Primer. [web site]
14.) Connett Michael. The Phosphate Fertilizer Industry: An Environmental Overview. Fluoride Action Network. [web site]
15.) Bellis Mary. Charles Martin Hall (1863-1914) – Aluminum. Hall's patent was US patent #400,666.
16.) State Symbols USA. Arkansas State Rock. [web site]
17.) Bush William V, and White Bekki. State of Arkansas. Arkansas Geological Survey. History of Bauxite in Arkansas. AGES Brochure Series 3. 2007.
18.) US Geological Survey. The Mineral Industry of North Carolina. 2003, 8 pages. Report prepared under a memorandum of understanding between the US Geological Survey and the North Carolina Geological Survey for collecting information on all nonfuel minerals.
19.) US Geological Survey. The Mineral Industry of North Carolina. 2003, 8 pages. Report prepared under a memorandum of understanding between the US Geological Survey and the North Carolina Geological Survey for collecting information on all nonfuel minerals.
20.) Cooper Jr WJ. The Conservative Regime. South Carolina, 1877-1890. 2005. John Hopkins Press
21.) Phosphate Primer. History of Phosphate Fertilizer Production. USF Polytechnic. FIPR Institute. 2010.
22.) EPA. 8.5.2 Triple Superphosphates. Inorganic Chemical Industry. 1997 July, reformatted 1/95.
23.) Wiley-VCH (ed.) Ullmann's Agrochemicals, Vol. 1. Verlag GmbH & Co. KGaA. 2007.
24.) Superior Minerals. www.superiorminerals.co.nz/phosphorus.htm
25.) Samish M, Rehacek J. Pathogens and Predators of Ticks and Their Potential in Biological Control. Annu Rev Entomol. 1999;44:149-82.
26.) The New York Times. Wasps Enlisted to Fight Ticks That Spread Lyme Disease. 1990 Mar 6. [monograph on the Internet].
27.) Roxburgh AC. Annual Centrifugal Erythema ("Erythème Annulaire Centrifuge," Darier, 1916. In: Section of Dermatology. 1931 June 18. Proc R. Soc Med. 1931 Oct;24(12):1645-1646.
28.) Stanek Gerold. Behandlung der Lyme-Borreliose. [Treatment of Lyme Borreliosis]. [Article in German]. Antibiotika Monitor. 2009May 6.
29.) Edlow Jonathan A. Bull's-eye: unraveling the medical mystery of Lyme disease. 2003 Yale University Press. pp.55-60.
30.) University of California San Diego. Bacillus thuringiensis. History of Bt. [web page]
31.) Ninfa M. Rosas-García. Biopesticide Production from Bacillus thuringiensis: An Environmentally Friendly Alternative. Recent Patents on Biotechnology. 2009;3:28-36.
32.) A. Béchamp. La maladie microzymateuse des vers à soie et les granulations moléculaires. Comptes rendus de l'Académie des sciences. 1868;67:443. [publication in french]. Reference from Wikipedia on Flacherie
33.) Gutiérrez Yezid. Diagnostic pathology of parasitic infections with clinical correlations. 2000 Oxford University Press, Inc. New York. p. 34-36.
34.) Silk in America. The Story of Silk and Cheney Silk. 1916.
35.) Walton Perry. The story of textiles: a bird's-eye view of the history of the beginning and the growth of the industry by which mankind is clothed. Compiled and written for John S. Lawrence. 1912 Boston MA.
36.) Brockett LP. The Silk Industry in America. A History: Prepared for the Centennial Exposition. 1876. George F. Nesbitt & Co. Printers NY.
37.) Harper's new monthly magazine. Alden, Henry Mills (ed). 1885 June-Nov;71.
38.) Timelines – History of Vaccines. College of Philadelphia.
39.) Duffy John. *Epidemics in Colonial America.* Baton Rouge. 1953. Louisiana State University Press.
40.) Godwin E. The US GenWeb Project. Lackawanna County News. Excerpts from the Scranton Times. The Silk Industry in Scranton. An illustrated description of the Sauquoit, Harvey's and Meadow-brook silk mills. 1893 Dec 8. The Scranton Republican, page 8.
41.) Hoffecker, Carol. Familiar Relations. The du Ponts & the University of Delaware (Newark, NJ). Monograph on the Internet
42.) Reading 1: Working "In the Silk" Paterson New Jersey. [web page]
43.) ParkNet National Park Service. Paterson, New Jersey: America's Silk City. [web site]
44.) Breed RS, Philip CB, Nellis L, Couch JN, Cleveland EMD, Seeliger H, Morse EV, Clark FE, Starr MP, Pittman M. Symposium on Taxonomy. 1955. 270-274. The symposium was presented before the 55th General Meeting of the Society of American Bacteriologists at New York on May 12, 1955.
45.) Samish M, Rehacek J. Pathogens and Predators of Ticks and Their Potential in Biological Control. Annu Rev Entomol. 1999;44:149-82.
46.) The New York Times. Wasps Enlisted to Fight Ticks That Spread Lyme Disease. 1990 Mar 6. [monograph on the Internet].
47.) Roxburgh AC. Annual Centrifugal Erythema (Erythème Annulaire Centrifuge, Darier, 1916. In: Section of Dermatology. 1931 June 18. Proc R. Soc Med. 1931 Oct;24(12):1645-1646.
48.) Stanek Gerold. Behandlung der Lyme-Borreliose. [Treatment of Lyme Borreliosis]. [Article in German]. Antibiotika Monitor. 2009 May 6.
49.) Edlow Jonathan A. Bull's-eye: unraveling the medical mystery of Lyme disease. 2003Yale University Press. pp. 55-60.
50.) Abridged agriculture records. Volume I. Domestic Animals and Dairying. New York State College of Agriculture at Cornell University, Ithaca NY. Agricultural Service Company 1912, Washington, DC.
51.) Godwin E. The US GenWeb Project. Lackawanna County News. Excerpts from the Scranton Times. The Silk Industry in Scranton. An illustrated description of the Sauquoit, Harvey's and Meadow-brook silk mills. 1893 Dec 8. The Scranton Republican, page 8.
52.) McBride TJ, Schneider JE, Floyd RA, Loeb LA. Mutations induced by methylene blue plus light in single-stranded M13mp2. Proc Natl Acad Sci USA. 1992 Aug 1;89(15):6866-6870.
53.) The Influenza Pandemic of 1918. [Monograph on the Internet].
54.) SR Dutky, EL Gooden. Coxiella popilliae, N. Sp., a Rickettsia Causing Blue Disease of Japanese Beetle Larvae. J Bacteriol. 1952Jun;63(6):743-750.
55.) Alfred W. Crosby, Jr. Epidemic and Peace, 1918. Greenwood Press, Westport, CT, 337 pages.

56.) Flexner Simon. Epidemic Encephalitis and Simple Herpes. J Gen Physiol. 1927:713-726.
57.) Cargill company history. www.cargill.com
58.) Hu X, Boyer GL. Siderophore-Mediated Aluminum Uptake by Bacillus megaterium ATCC 19213. Environ Microbiol. 1996 Nov;62(11):4044-4048.
59.) Mullen MD, Wolf DC, Ferris FG, et al. Bacterial Sorption of Heavy Metals. Appl Environ Microbiol. 1989 Dec;55(12):3143-3149.
60.) Artenstein AW, Opal JM, Opal SM, Tramont EC, Peter G, Russell PK. History of US Military Contributions to the Study of Vaccines against Infectious Diseases. Military Med. 2005;170(April Suppl):3-11.
61.) Roche Facets Viruses. [monograph] www.roche.com
62.) Schaechter M, Engleberg NC, DiRita VJ, Dermody T. (eds.) Schaechter's mechanisms of microbial disease. Page 324. Endogenous and Exogenous Viruses. Fourth Edition Lippencott Williams & Wilkins. 1998.
63.) Marlow Susan A, Wilson Louise E, Lawrie Alison M. et al. Assembly of Amsacta moorei entomopoxvirus spheroidin into spheroids following synthesis in insect cells using a baculovirus vector. J Gen Virol. 1998;79:623-628.
64.) Corbet SA, Danahar GW, King V, et al. Surfactant-enhanced essential oils as mosquito larvicides. Entomologia Experimentalis et Applicata. 1995;75(3):229-236.
65.) Seif Al, Husseiny IM, Soliman BA, et al. Development of Wuchereria bancrofti in Culex pipiens L. (Diptera: Culicidae) exposed in the larval instar to sublethal dosages of insecticides and one insect growth regulator and their influence on reproduction of filaria-infected mosquitoes. J Egypt Soc Parasitol. 1997 Dec;27(3):843-53.
66.) Wilkins Mira. The history of foreign investment in the United States to 1914. The Presidents and Fellows of Harvard College. 1989. p.358-360
67.) Abelshauser Werner, von Hippel Wolfgang, Johnson Jeffrey Allan, Stokes Raymond G. German Industry and Global Enterprise. BASF: The History of a Company. 2004 Cambridge University Press.
68.) BASF Aktiengesellschaft. Company History. [web page]
69.) Kliene Robert. The Management of Silkworms in China – a Translation from the Chinese of Tsou Tsu-Tang. In Sci Amer 1890 Jul-Dec;30 (Suppl. 775):12378-12381. Munn & Co. Publishers.
70.) Druding Susan C. Dye History from 2600 BC to the 20th Century.
71.) Woodruff NW, Durant JL, Donhoffner LL, et al. Human cell mutagenicityof chlorinated and unchlorinated water and the disinfection byproduct 3-chloro-4-(dichloromethyl)-5-hydroxy-2(5H)-furanone (MX). Mutat Res. 2001 Aug 22;495(1-2):157-168.
72.) Smith, Michael Stephen. The emergence of modern business enterprise in France, 1800-1930. Harvard University Press 2006. 575 pp.
73.) Smith, George Otis. US Congress. Department of the Interior. US Geological Survey. Water-Supply Papers Nos. 273-274. Congressional edition, Volume 6012. Washington Government Printing Office 1911.
74.) Daddow SE, Bannan B. Coal, iron, and oil, or, The practical American miner. A plain and popular work on Our Mines and Mineral Resources. JB Lippincott & Co. Philadelphia, PA. Pottsville, PA. 1866.
75.) First World War. Dunnite and Lyddite. www.firstworldwar.com
76.) American Heritage Dictionary. Picric Acid. [monograph]
77.) Armstrong Charles. Experience with the picric acid-alum spray in the prevention of poliomyelitis in Alabama, 1936. Am J Public Health and the Nation's Health. 1937 Feb;27(2). 9 pages.
78.) Schonberg A, Camey C, Kahl O, et al. First isolation of Borrelia burgdorferi, the agent of Lyme borreliosis, from Ixodes ricinus (Acari: Ixodidae) in Berlin (West). Mendeley. 1988;268(4):487-494.
79.) Garfield Eugene. Lyme Disease Researcher Uncovers a Case of Delayed Recognition: Arvid Afzelius and His Successors. Current Comments. #49. 1989 Dec 4;p.3-8. In Scientist: Creativity, Delayed Recognition, and other Essays, 1989;12:345.
80.) Pointe Jacques Pierre. Histoire topographique et médicale du Grand Hôtel-Dieu de Lyon, dans laquelle sont traitées. Ch. Savy Jeune (ed.) Lyon. 1842.
81.) Ackermann R, Hörstrup P, Schmidt R. Tickborne Meningopolyneuritis (Garin-Bujadoux, Bannwarth). Yale J Biol Med. 1984;57:485-490.
82.) Garin CH, Bujadoux. Paralysie par les Tiques. J Méd Lyon. 1922;71:765-767.
83.) Hellerström S. Erythema chronicum migrans Afzelii. Acta Derm Venereol (Stockholm). 1930;11:315-321.
84.) Gelbjerg-Hansen G. Erythema chronicum migrans Afzelii and meningitis after a tick bite. Acta Derm Venereol. (Stockholm). 1945;25:458-463.
85.) Afzelius-Alm. Verhandlungen der dermatologischen Gesellschaft zu Stockholm. 16 Dezember 1909. Arch Derm Syph (Berlin). 1910;101:405-407.
86.) Lipschütz B. Uber eine seltene Erythemform (Erythema chronicum migrans). Arch Derm Syph (Berlin). 1918;118:349-356.
87.) Strickland C. Note on a case of Tick Paralysis in Australia. Parasitol. 1915;VII:379.
88.) Hawden. On Tick paralysis in Sheep and man following bites of Dermacentor venustus. Parasitol. 1913;VI:283-297.
89.) Todar Ken. Bacillus anthracis and Anthrax. 2001. Todar's Online Textbook of Bacteriology.
90.) Lord JC. From Metchnikoff to Monsanto and beyond: The path of microbial control. 2005 J. Invert Path. 89:19-29.
91.) Müller-Kögler E. Insect Pathology and Microbial Control. PA van der Laan (ed.) North-Holland Publishing Company, Amsterdam. Pp. 339-353.
92.) US EPA. 2000 Aug. Report. Potassium Dichromate listing for background document for the inorganic chemical listing determination.
93.) Roto P, Sainio H, Reunala T, Laippala P. Addition of ferrous sulfate to cement and risk of dermatitis among construction workers. Contact Dermatitis. 1996 Jan;34(1):43-50.
94.) Tan S, Nixon R. Allergic contact dermatitis caused by chromium in a mobile phone. Contact Dermatitis. 2011 Oct;65(4):246-247.
95.) Gao X, He RX, Yan SG, Wu LD. Dermatitis associated with chromium following total knee arthroplasty. J Arthroplasty. 2011 Jun;26(4):665.
96.) Darling MI, Horn HM, McCormack SK, Schofield OM. Sole Dermatitis in Children: Patch Testing Revisited. Pedia Derma. 2011 Aug 19.
97.) Ahmad MK, Syma S, Mahmood R. Cr(VI) induces Lipid Peroxidation, Protein Oxidation and Alters the Activities of Antioxidant Enzymes in Human Erythrocytes. Biol Trace Elem Res. 2011 Jun 17.
98.) Bate G. A survey of recent advances in magnetic recording materials. IEEE Transactions on Magnetics. 1978;14(4):136-142.
99.) The Nobel Prize in Physiology or Medicine 1908 Ilya Mechnikov, Paul Ehrlich. Biography. www.nobelprize.org/nobel_prizes/medicine/laureates/1908/mechnikov-bio.html
100.) Lord JC. From Metchnikoff to Monsanto and beyond: The path of microbial control. 2005J. Invert Path. 89:19-29.
101.) Pasteur, Compt. Rend. 1961; and Revue Scientifique, 1883.
102.) US Environmental Protection Agency (EPA). Pesticides: Regulating Pesticides. Metarhizium anisopliae strain F52(029056) Biopesticide Fact Sheet. [web site]. www.epa.gov
103.) Import Risk Analysis Secretariat. Plant Biosecurity, Biosecurity Australia (was Plant Quarantine Policy Branch of the Australian Quarantine and Inspection Service). Viruses, Phytoplasmas and Spiroplasmas of Clonal Grasses and Their Diagnosis. Consultancy Report 2000 Dec. Chapter title: Maize rough dwarf fijivirus, p. 90.
104.) Par JM Dory, Chastel C, Couatarmanach A, et al. Question Étiologiques et Épidémiologiques Posées par L'érythème chronique migrant et la maladie de Lyme. A propos de 4 observations réalisées au centre hospitalier regional de Rennes. [Article in French]. Bull. Soc. Path. Exot. 1985;78(3):512-525.
105.) Geison Gerald L. Pasteur's Work On Rabies: Reexamining the Ethical Issues. The Hastings Center Report 1978 Apr;8(2):26-33.
106.) Carpentier S, Moilleron R, Beltran C, et al. Quality of dredged material in the river Seine basin (France). II. Micropollutants. Sci Total Environ. 2002 Nov 1;299(1-3):57-72.
107.) France in the Age of Les Misérables. The Sewers of Paris: A Brief History. [web site]
108.) Institut Pasteur web site. Louis Pasteur and Rabies vaccination. www.pasteur.fr
109.) The Journal of the American Medical Association. 1910 Oct 1;LV(14)
110.) Crop Protection Compendium. Botrytis bassiana Balsamo. Common name: white muscardine fungus. Web page.
111.) Johnson GW, Hogg R. The Journal of Horticulture, Cottage Gardener, Country Gentleman, Bee-Keeper, and Poultry Chronicle Journal of Horticulture, 1868 Jul 30; Vol. XL, pp. 87-88. London
112.) A Brief History of Polio. From Ancient Egypt to the 20th Century. [web site] www.columbia.edu
113.) Pessarakli M. Handbook of turfgrass management and physiology. 2008 CRC Press. Boca Raton, FL.
114.) Clausen CP. Scarabaeidae. In Introduced Parasites and Predators of Arthropod Pests and Weeds: A World Review. Clausen CG (Ed.) USDA Agriculture Handbook. 1978;480:277.
115.) Godfrey KE. Tiphia wasps. In Japanese beetle white grubs and other beetle pests of turf. In Classical Biological Control in the Southern United States. Habeck DH, Bennett FD, Frank JH. (eds.). Southern Coop. Ser Bull. 1990;355:143.
116.) White R.T. Effect of Milky Disease on Tiphia Parasites of Japanese Beetle Larvae. 1943 Sept.;51(3):213-218.

117.) Tiffany Elberton J, Martorana Nancy F. Leptospirosis in New York City. A serological survey. Am J Epidemiol. 1942;36:195-204.
118.) US Patent 4,859,377. Shasha, et al. Starch encapsulation of entomopathogens. Filed 7/10/87, issued 8/22/89. Assignee: The United States of America, as represented by the Secretary of [?] (Washington DC).
119.) Dubois Normand R, Lewis Franklin B. What is Bacillus Thuringiensis. Report presented at the annual conference of the International Society of Arboriculture in Hartford, Connecticut, August 1980. 8 pages.
120.) Metalnikov S, Corine V. On the infection of the gypsy moth and other insects with Bacterium thuringiensis. A preliminary report. Inter Corn Borer Invest Sec. Repts. 1929;2:60-61.
121.) Brindley TA, Dicke FF. Significant Developments in European Corn Borer Research. Agricultural Research Serv., Corn Borer Investigations, USDA, Ankey IA, and IA State University of Science and Technology, Ames, IA.
122.) And Stadelmann R. Ein Beitrag zum Krankheitsbild des Erythema chronicum Lipschutz. Inaugural dissertation, Marburg, 1934.
123.) Scrimenti RJ, Scrimenti M. Lyme disease redux: the legacy of Sven Hellerstrom. WI Med Journal 1993 Jan;92(1):20-21.
124.) Burges HD, Hussey NW. Microbial Control of Insects and Mites. 1971 Academic Press Inc. London, New York.
125.) Briggs John D. Mass Propagation of Bacteria Pathogenic for Insects. WHO Bulletin. 1964;31:495-497.
126.) Hatfield Laura. Bad year for anthrax outbreaks in US livestock. CIDRAP. [web page]
127.) Aitken LD (ed). Diseases of Sheep. Fourth Edition. 2000 Blackwell Science, UK.
128.) Stöcker Friedrich W. (ed). Concise Encyclopedia Biology (ABC Biologie). 1995Spektrum Akademischer Verlag GmbH (Germany). Translated and revised by Scott Thomas A, PhD. Great Britain.
129.) BBC News. Britain's 'Anthrax Island'. 2001 Jul 25. News blog.
130.) Mustard Disaster at Bari. Force Health Protection and Readiness. Chemical-Biological Warfare Exposures. [web page]
131.) Blister Agent: Sulfur Mustard (H,HD,HS). 2005. [web page]
132.) Olson Kyle B. Aum Shinrikyo: Once and Future Threat? CDC. Emerging Infectious Diseases. 1999 Jul-Aug;5(4):491-602.
133.) Carroll MC. Lab 257. The disturbing story of the government's secret germ laboratory. 2005. Harper paperback.
134.) Scannell's New Jersey's First Citizen's and State Guide. Vol. II. 1919-1920. John James Scannell (ed.) J.J. Scannell, Paterson, New Jersey. 1920. p.
519. 135.) Lockyer Sir Norman (ed). Nature. 1897 May-Oct;1435(56):16.
136.) The Rabbits of Australia. The New York Times. 1888 Mar 11.
137.) Wilkinson W Camac. (Chaiman of Executive Committee of Rabbit Commission, Manchester Square, London). Brit Med J. 1890 Mar 22. p. 693.
138.) Pound CJ. The Destruction of Rabbits by means of the Microbes of Chicken-Cholera. In The agricultural gazette of New South Wales. New South Wales Dept. of Agriculture. 1897 Jan-Dec;8.
139.) The Spectator. A Weekly Review of Politics, Literature, Theology, and Arts. 1887 Vol. 60. John Campbell, London.
140.) AH Benson. Fruits of Queensland, Australia. Department of Agriculture and Stock, Brisbane. 1908.
141.) Magraw Roger. France, 1815-1914: the bourgeois century. 1983 Oxford University Press, New York. p.112
142.) Debré Patrice. (Translated by Elborg Forster). Louis Pasteur. 1994 Flammarion. The Johns Hopkins University Press. Baltimore, MD. p. 475
143.) Dowling Edward. Australia and America in 1892. A Contrast. New South Wales Commissioners for the World's Columbian Exposition, Chicago. 1893. 193 pages.
144.) Pratt EE. US Deparment of Commerce. Bureau of Foreign and Domestic Commerice. Commercial Organizations of the United States. Government Printing Office, Washington, DC. Revised to July 1, 1917. 1181 pages.
145.) Lawrenz M, Mitchell HH, Ruth WA. A comparison of the toxicity of fluorine in the form of cryolite administered in water and in food. J Nutrition 1939 Mar:127-141.

Chapter Two: Weapons of Mass (Pest) Destruction

Weapons of Mass Pest Destruction

1.) Technical Report: DDC AD408401. Conference on Biological Control of Insects of Medical Importance. American Institute of Biological Sciences (Washington, DC). 148 pages. Unclassified documents retrieved from the public domain. Dr. Steinhaus speaking, page 123.
2.) Helgason E, Okstad OA, Caugant DA, et al. Bacillus anthracis, Bacillus cereus, and Bacillus thuringiensis – one species on the basis of genetic evidence. Appl Environ Microbiol. 2000;66:2627-2630.
3.) W. Kenneth Hoover. The Biological Control of Detrimental Insects. 1933 Oct;4(3):75-89.
4.) US Patent 3,337,395. Robert Z. Page (Springfied, VA). Termite Control by Induced Epizootics of Entomophagous Microorganisms. Filed 11/27/63, published 8/22/67.
5.) DeBach P, Rosen D. Biological control by natural enemies. Cambridge University Press 1974, 1991. pp. 136
6.) Lord JC. From Metchnikoff to Monsanto and beyond: The path of microbial control. 2005 J. Invert Path. 89:19-29.
7.) Technical Report: DDC AD408401. February 3-4, 1960. Conference on Biological Control of Insects of Medical Importance. American Institute of Biological Sciences (Washington, DC). 148 pages. Unclassified documents retrieved from the public domain. Dr. Steinhaus speaking, page 123.
8.) Helgason E, Okstad OA, Caugant DA, et al. Bacillus anthracis, Bacillus cereus, and Bacillus thuringiensis – one species on the basis of genetic evidence. Appl Environ Microbiol. 2000;66:2627-2630.
9.) Bolckmans Karel JF. (R. Albajes, M. Lodovic Gullino, JC van Lenteren and Y. Elad editors). Developments in Plant Pathology (series). Integrated Pest and Disease Management in Greenhouse Crops. 2000 Vol. 14, p. 310-318. Springer Netherlands.
10.) Burgess HD, Hussey NW. Microbial Control of Insects and Mites. 1971 Academic Press (London).

Fungal Feasts for Insect Pests

1.) Lord JC. From Metchnikoff to Monsanto and beyond: The path of microbial control. 2005 J. Invert Path. 89:19-29.
2.) US Environmental Protection Agency (EPA). Pesticides: Regulating Pesticides. Metarhizium anisopliae strain F52(029056) Biopesticide Fact Sheet. [web site]
3.) DeBach Paul, Rosen David. Biological control by natural enemies. Cambridge University Press 1974, 1991;pp.124.
4.) Müller-Kögler E. Insect Pathology and Microbial Control. (P.A. van der Laan, ed.), North-Holland Publishing Company, Amsterdam. Pp. 339-353.
5.) Klein. Micro-organisms and Disease. 1885.
6.) Newman, Barclay Moon. Japan's Secret Weapon. (Peter Greenleaf ed.) Current Publishing Co. 1944.
7.) Burgess HD, Hussey NW. Microbial Control of Insects and Mites. 1971 Academic Press Inc. London. p. 175-179.
8.) Schole EJ, Knols BGJ, Samson RA, Takken W. Entomopathogenic fungi for mosquito control: A review. J Insect Sc. 2004;4:1-24.
9.) Technical Report: DDC AD408401. Conference on Biological Control of Insects of Medical Importance. American Institute of Biological Sciences (Washington, DC). 148 pages. Unclassified documents retrieved from the public domain.
10.) Barci LAG. 1997. Biological control of the cattle tick Boophilus microplus (Acari, Ixodidae) in Brazil. Arq. Inst. Biol. 64:95–101.
11.) Cherepanova NP. Fungi which are found on ticks. Bot. Z. Mosk. 1964;49:696–99.
12.) W. Kenneth Hoover. The Biological Control of Detrimental Insects. 1933 Oct;4(3):75-89.
13.) US Patent 3,337,395. Page. Termite Control by Induced Epizootics of Entomophagous Microorganisms. Filed 12/27/63 published 8/22/67. No Assignee listed. Inventor: Robert Z. Page (Springfield, VA)
14.) US Patent 4,956,343. Dowd, et al. Control of insects by Roseotoxin B. Filed 5/2/88 published 9/11/90. Assignee: The United States of America as represented by the Secretary of (Washington, DC). [Agriculture]
15.) Burges HD, Hussey NW. Microbial Control of Insects and Mites. 1971 Academic Press Inc. London. p. 127.
16.) Nome C, Magalhães PC, Oliveira E, et al. Differences in intracellular localization of corn stunt spiroplasmas in magnesium treated maize. Biocell (Mendoza) 2009;33(2):133-136.
17.) Schole EJ, Knols BGJ, Samson RA, Takken W. Entomopathogenic fungi for mosquito control: A review. J Insect Sc. 2004;4:1-24.
18.) Hamm JJ, Styer EL, Lewis WJ. Comparative virogenesis of filamentous virus and polydnavirus in the female reproductive tract of Cotesia marginiventris (Hymenoptera: Braconidae). J Invert Path. 1990;55:357-374.
19.) Pirali-Kheirabadi K, Haddadzadeh H, Razzaghi-Abyaneh M, et al. Biological control of Rhipicephalus (Boophilus) annulatus by different strains of Metarhizium anisopliae, Beauveria bassiana and Lecanicillium psalliotae fungi. Parasitol Res. 2007;100:1297-1302.

20.) US Patent 2,933,504. Klopping. Derivatives of Polyakloxycarbonylimine. Filed 8/10/59, Published 4/19/60. Assignee: E.I. du Pont de Nemours and Company, Wilmington, DE.
21.) US Patent 2,933,502Klopping et al. Benzimidazole Derivatives. Filed 2/12/58 Published 4/19/60. Assignees: E.I. du Pont de Nemours and Co. (DE)
22.) US Patent 3,541,213Klopping et al. Fungicidal and Mite Ovicidal Substituted 2-Aminobenzimidazoles. Filed 4/11/67 Published 11/17/70. Assignee: E.I. du Pont de Nemours and Company, Wilmington, DE.
23.) Vaeck M, Reynaerts A, Höeft H, et al. Transgenic plants protected from insect attack. Nature. 1987;328:33-37.
24.) Barton KA, Whiteley HR, Yang NS. Bacillus thuringiensis delta-endotoxins expressed in transgenic Nicotiana tabacum provides resistance to lepidopteran insects. Plant Physiol. 1987;85:1103-1109.
25.) Frazzon APG, Vaz Jr. IdS, Masuda A, et al. In vitro assessment of Metarhizium anisopliae isolates to control the cattle tick Boophilus microplus. Vet Parasitol. 2000 Dec 20;94(1-2):117-125.
26.) Kurtti Timothy J, Keyhani Nemat O. Intracellular infection of tick cell lines by entomopathogenic fungus Metarhizium anisopliae. Microbiol. 2008;154:1700-1709.
27.) Benjamin MA, Zhioua E, Ostfeld RS. Laboratory and field evaluation of the entomopathogenic fungus Metarhizium anisopliae (Deuteromycetes) for controlling questing adult Ixodes scapularis (Acari: Ixodidae). J Med Entomol. 2002;39:723-728.
28.) Bittencourt VR. Trials to control South American ticks with entomopathogenic fungi. Ann NY Acad Sci. 2000;916:555-558.
29.) Fernandes EK, da Costa GL, de Souza EJ, et al. Beauveria bassiana isolated from engorged females and tested against eggs and larvae of Boophilus microplus (Acari: Ixodidae). J Basic Microbiol. 2003;43:393-398.
30.) Kaaya GP. Laboratory and field evaluation of entomogenous fungi for tick control. Ann NY Acad Sci. 2000;916:559-564.
31.) Kirkland BH, Cho EM, Keyhani NO. Differential susceptibility of Amblyomma maculaturm and Amblyomma americanum (Acari: Ixodidea) to the entomopathogenic fungi Beauveria bassiana and Metarhizium anisopliae. Biol Control. 2004;31:414-421.
32.) Kirkland BH, Westwood GS, Keyhani NO. Pathogenicity of entomopathogenic fungi Beauveria bassiana and Metarhizium anoisopliae to Ixodidae tick species Dermacentor variabilis, Rhipicephalus sanguineus, and Ixodes scapularis. J Med Entomol. 2004;41:705-711.
33.) Kirkland BH, Eisa A, Keyhani NO. Oxalic acid as a fungal acaracidal virulence factor. J Med Entomol. 2005;42:346-351.
34.) Maranga RO, Hassanali A, Kaaya GP, Mueke JM. Performance of a prototype baited-trap in attracting and infecting the tick Amblyomma variegatum (Acari: Ixodidae) in field experiments. Exp Appl Acarol. 2006;38:211-218.

Invasion of the Gypsys

1.) DeBach P, Rosen D. Biological control by natural enemies. Cambridge University Press 1974, 1991. pp. 150-154
2.) Reading 1: Working "In the Silk" Paterson New Jersey. [web page]
3.) Scrimenti RJ. Erythema chronicum migrans. Arch Dermatol. 1970 Jul;102(1):104-105.
4.) ParkNet National Park Service. Paterson, New Jersey: America's Silk City. [web page]
5.) Breed RS, Philip CB, Nellis L, Couch JN, Cleveland EMD, Seeliger H, Morse EV, Clark FE, Starr MP, Pittman M. Symposium on Taxonomy. 1955. 270-274. The symposium was presented before the 55th General Meeting of the Society of American Bacteriologists at New York on May 12, 1955.
6.) Gerardi MH, Grimm JK. The History, Biology, Damage, and Control of the Gypsy Moth. 1979 Associated University Presses, Inc., Cranbury, New Jersey.
7.) Rutgers School of Environmental and Biological Sciences. Department of Entomology. Gypsy Moth. [web page]
8.) MCClung RM. Gypsy Moth Its History in America. 1974 William Morrow and Company.
9.) Gerardi MH, Grimm JK. The History, Biology, Damage, and Control of the Gypsy Moth. 1979 Associated University Presses, Inc., Cranbury, New Jersey.
10.) Jones CG, Ostfeld RS, Richard MP, Schauber EM, Wolff JO. Chain reactions linking acorns to gypsy moth outbreaks and Lyme disease risk. Science 1998;279(5353):1023-1026.
11.) W. Kenneth Hoover. The Biological Control of Detrimental Insects. 1933 Oct;4(3):75-89.
12.) Webber RT, Schaffner JV. Host Relations of Compsilura concinnata Meigen, An Important Tachinid Parasite of the Gipsy Moth and Brown-Tail Moth. USDA Bulletin #1363, Washington, DC. 1926.
13.) Schaffner JV, Griswold CL. Macro-lepidoptera and their Parasites reared from field collections in the Northeastern part of the United States. USDA Publication #188, Washington, DC. 1934.
14.) Culver JJ. A study of Comsilura concinnata, an imported tachinid parasite of the gipsy moth and brown-tail moth. USDA Bulletin #766. Washington, DC. 1919.
15.) Boettner GH, Elkinton JS, Boettner CJ. Effects of a biological control introduction on three nontarget native species of Saturniid moths. Conserv Biol. 2000;14:1798-1806.
16.) Mahr, Susan. Know Your Friends. Ground Beetles. Midwest Biological Control News. University of WI Madison. 2001 [monograph]
17.) Munson Steve. Asian Gypsy Moth (AGM) Mission Trip Report. USDA Forest Service, R-4FHP. [monograph]
18.) DeBach P, Rosen D. Biological control by natural enemies. Cambridge University Press 1974, 1991. pp. 124-125
19.) USDA Departmental Regulation Number 5600-001. OPI: Forest Pest Management S&PF, Forest Service. 1990 June 1.
20.) Hamilton RA. Increase in Moth Eggs Seen in Fairfield County. New York Times Article on the Internet. 1988 Feb 14.
21.) Leonard David E. Recent Developments in Ecology and Control of the Gypsy Moth. 1974Jan. Ann Rev Entomol. 19:197-229.
22.) Rippere KE, Tran MT, Yousten AA, Hilu KH, Klein MG. Bacillus popilliae and Bacillus lentimorbus, bacteria causing milky disease in Japanese beetles and related scarab larvae. Inter J Syst Bacteriol. 1998;48:395-402.
23.) Todar Kenneth. Todar's Online Textbook of Bacteriology. The Genus Bacillus [web page]
24.) Dettori G, Grillo R, Cattani P, et al. Comparative study of the enzyme activities of Borrelia burgdorferi and other non-intestinal and intestinal spirochaetes. New Microbiol. 1995 Jan;18(1):13-26.
25.) Glaser RW. The cultivation of a nematode parasite of an insect. Science 1931;73:614-615.
26.) Knapp R, Caasey TM. Thermal ecology, behavior and growth of gypsy moth and eastern tent caterpillars. Biol. 1986;67:598-608.
27.) US Patent 3,950,225. Skole, et al. Filed 10/15/74, issued 4/13/76. Medium, component thereof and process employing same for the production of microbial insecticides, such as Bacillus popilliae spores and the like, for the control of Japanese beetles and other insects. Assignee: Amstar Corporation (New York, NY).
28.) US Patent 3,616,250. Hrubant et al. Preferential enzymatic lysis of vegetative cells in presence of sporulated Bacterial Cells. Filed 10/22/68, issued 10/26/71.
29.) US Patent 3,616,250. Hrubant, et al. Preferential Enzymatic lysis of vegetative cells in presence of sporulated bacterial cells. Filed 10/22/68, published 10/26/71. Inventors: Hrubant GR, Rhodes RA, (Peoria, IL). No assignee listed.
30.) Clausen CP. Biological Antagonists in the future of Insect Control. Agricul Food Chem. 1954 Jan 6;2(1):12-18.
31.) USDA. Agricultural Research Service. Research Project: Biologically-Based Technologies for Management of Crop Insect Pests in Local and Areawide Programs. Location: Insect Behavior and Biocontrol Research Unit. 2002 Annual Report.
32.) US Patent 3,616,250. Hrubant, et al. Preferential Enzymatic lysis of vegetative cells in presence of sporulated bacterial cells. Filed 10/22/68, published 10/26/71. Inventors: Hrubant GR, Rhodes RA, (Peoria, IL). No assignee listed.

Wasps as Insect Controls

1.) Samish M, Rehacek J. Pathogens and Predators of Ticks and Their Potential in Biological Control. Annu Rev Entomol. 1999;44:149-82.
2.) The New York Times. Wasps Enlisted to Fight Ticks That Spread Lyme Disease. 1990 Mar 6. [monograph on the Internet].
3.) Roxburgh AC. Annual Centrifugal Erythema (Erythème Annulaire Centrifuge, Darier, 1916. In: Section of Dermatology. 1931 June 18. Proc R. Soc Med. 1931 Oct;24(12):1645-1646.
4.) Stanek Gerold. Behandlung der Lyme-Borreliose. [Treatment of Lyme Borreliosis]. [Article in German]. Antibiotika Monitor. 2009 May 6.
5.) Edlow Jonathan A. Bull's-eye: unraveling the medical mystery of Lyme disease. 2003 Yale University Press. pp.55-60.
6.) Technical Report: DDC AD408401. Conference on Biological Control of Insects of Medical Importance. American Institute of Biological Sciences (Washington, DC). 148 pages. Date stamped June 28, 1961 Naval Medical Field Research Laboratory, Camp LeJeune, North Carolina. (DDC) July 16, 1963. Unclassified documents from the public domain.
7.) Crookshank Edgar M. Manual of Bacteriology, Third Edition. JH Vail & Co, Astor Place, NY. 1890.
8.) World Health Organization Bulletin. IX. Ticks and Mites – Acarina. 1. Parasites of Ticks. 1964;31(1):80-84.
9.) Barci LAG. 1997. Biological control of the cattle tick Boophilus microplus (Acari, Ixodidae) in Brazil. Arq. Inst. Biol. 64:95–101.
10.) Cherepanova NP. Fungi which are found on ticks. Bot. Z. Mosk. 1964;49:696–99.

11.) Renjie Hu, KE Hyland, HJ Oliver Jr. A review on the use of Ixophagus wasps (Hymenoptera: Encyrtidae) as natural enemies for the control of ticks (Acari: Ixodidae). System Appl Acarol Soc. 1998;3:19-28.
12.) Cole MM. 1965. Biological control of ticks by the use of hymenopterous parasites — a review. World Health Organization. Publ. WHO/ebl /4365:1–12.
13.) Volkov VI. 1969. Ecology of Ixodidae and eradication of tick encephalitis. PhD thesis. Voronez Univ., Russia. 29 pages.

Japanese Beetles

1.) A Brief History of Polio. From Ancient Egypt to the 20th Century. [web page]
2.) Pessarakli M. Handbook of turfgrass management and physiology. 2008 CRC Press. Boca Raton, FL.
3.) Clausen CP. Scarabaeidae. In Introduced Parasites and Predators of Arthropod Pests and Weeds: A World Review. Clausen CG (Ed.) USDA Agriculture Handbook. 1978;480:277.
4.) Godfrey KE. Tiphia wasps. In Japanese beetle white grubs and other beetle pests of turf. In Classical Biological Control in the Southern United States. Habeck DH, Bennett FD, Frank JH. (eds.). Southern Coop. Ser Bull. 1990;355:143.
5.) White R.T. Effect of Milky Disease on Tiphia Parasites of Japanese Beetle Larvae. 1943 Sept.;51(3):213-218.
6.) Pessarakli Mohammad (ed). Handbook of Turfgrass Management and Physiology. 2007. CRC Press. Pages 288-289.
7.) Fitzgerald TD. The Tent Caterpillars. 1995. Cornell University Press.
8.) Martignoni ME, Iwai PJ, Breillatt JP. Heterogeneous buoyant density in batches of viral nuclopolyhedra. J Invertebr Pathol. 1971 Sept;18(2):219-26.
9.) Steinhaus EA, Thompson CG. Preliminary field tests using a polyhedrosis virus to control the alfalfa caterpillar. J Econ Entomol. 1949 Apr;42(2):301-5.
10.) Reading 1: Working "In the Silk" Paterson New Jersey. [web page]
11.) Dyck VA, Hendrichs J, Robinson AS. Sterile Insect Technique. Chap. 5.2 Environment and the Sterile Insect Technique. IAEA. Springer. Dordrecht. 2005;pp. 499-524.
12.) Brookhaven National Laboratory. History. The Founding of Brookhaven, a Laboratory for Peacetime Research. [web page]
13.) Steinkraus KH, Tashiro H. Milky Disease Bacteria. Appl Microbiol. 1967 Mar;15(2):325-333.
14.) Gerardi MH, Grimm JK. The History, Biology, Damage, and Control of the Gypsy Moth. 1979 Associated University Presses, Inc., Cranbury, New Jersey.
15.) Steinkraus KH. Tashiro H. Production of Milky-Disease Spores (Bacillus popilliae Dutky and Bacillus lentimorbus Dutky) on Artificial Media. Science 1955 Jun 17;121(3155):873-874.
16.) Magnoler A. Susceptibility of Gypsy Moth Larvae to Lymantria spp. Nuclear- and Cytoplasmic-polyhedrosis Viruses. Entomophaga. 1970;15(4):407-412.
17.) Leonard David E. Recent Developments in Ecology and Control of the Gypsy Moth. 1974 Jan. Ann Rev Entomol. 19:197-229.
18.) Rhodes RA, Sharpe ES, Hall HH, Jackson RW. Characteristics of the Vegetative Growth of Bacillus popilliae. Appl Microbiol. 1966 Mar;14(2):189-195.
19.) Rutgers School of Environmental and Biological Sciences. Department of Entomology. Gypsy Moth. [web page]
20.) MCClung RM. Gypsy Moth Its History in America. 1974 William Morrow and Company.
21.) Gerardi MH, Grimm JK. The History, Biology, Damage, and Control of the Gypsy Moth. 1979 Associated University Presses, Inc., Cranbury, New Jersey.
22.) Steere AC, Taylor E, Wilson ML, Levine JF, Spielman A. Longitudinal assessment of the clinical and epidemiological features of Lyme disease in a defined population. J Infect Dis. 1986 Aug;154(2):295-300.
23.) Spielman A, Wilson ML, Levine JF, Piesman J. Ecology of Ixodes Dammini-Borne Human Babesiosis and Lyme Disease. Ann Rev Entomol. 1984 Jan;30:439-460.
24.) Jaenson TGT. The epidemiology of lyme borreliosis. Parasit Today. 1991;7(2):39-45.]
25.) White R.T. Effect of Milky Disease on Tiphia Parasites of Japanese Beetle Larvae. 1943 Sept.;51(3):213-218.
26.) Steinhaus EA. Nomenclature and classification of insect viruses. Bact Revs. 1949;13:203-223.
27.) Kaya, H. K., M. G. Klein, et al. Impact of Bacillus popilliae, Rickettsia popilliae, and entomopathogenic nematodes on a population of the scarabaeid Cyclocephala hirta. Biocontrol Science & Technology 3. 1993:443-453.
28.) Dutky SR, Gooden EL. Coxiella Popilliae, n. sp., a Rickettsia Causing Blue Disease of Japanese Beetle Larvae. Am Soc Microbiol. J Bacteriol. 1952;63:743-750.
29.) Noguchi Hideyo. Cultivation of Rickettsia-Like Microorganisms from the Rocky Mountain Spotted Fever Tick, Dermacentor Andersoni. J Exp Med. 1926 Mar 31;43(4):515-532.
30.) Dutky SR, Gooden EL. Coxiella Popilliae, n. sp., A Rickettsia causing Blue Disease of Japanese Beetle Larvae. Am Soc Microbiol. 1951 Nov 9;63:743-750.
31.) Macfarlane GT, Herbert RA. Nitrate Dissimilation by Vibrio spp. Isolated From Estuarine Sediments. J Gen Microbiol. 1982;128:2463-2468.
32.) Fritz Industries. Autotrophic vs. Heterotrophic Bacteria. www.bioconlabs.com/autoheterobac.html
33.) Bynum Jim. Heterotrophic Bacteria in sewage sludge biosolids, reclaimed water & drinking water. [web page]
34.) Nitrate Reducers. Heterotrophic Metabolism. [web page]
35.) Arivudainambi S, Selvanarayanan V, Vikash A. Enhancing the efficacy and persistency of Spodoptera litura (Fab.) nuclear polyhedrosis virus using UV irradiation protectants. Indian J Exper Biol. 2000;38(11):1175-1176.
36.) Smith KM. Viruses. The Syndics of the Cambridge University, London 1962.
37.) Rhodes RA, Sharpe ES, Hall HH, Jackson RW. Characteristics of the Vegetative Growth of Bacillus popilliae. Appl Microbiol. 1966 Mar;14(2):189-195.
38.) Gerardi MH, Grimm JK. The History, Biology, Damage, and Control of the Gypsy Moth. 1979 Associated University Presses, Inc., Cranbury, New Jersey.

Mosquito Manipulations

1.) Technical Report: DDC AD408401. Conference on Biological Control of Insects of Medical Importance. American Institute of Biological Sciences (Washington, DC). 148 pages. Unclassified documents retrieved from the public domain.
2.) Grant 1P01AI016289-01 *Arthropod-borne Diseases and Their Control.* University of Maryland, Baltimore. Fiscal year 1980. Richard H. Baker. Project start: 6/1/80, ended 5/31/85. NIAID.
3.) Grant 1P01AI016289-01. *Arthropod-borne Diseases and Their Control.* Fiscal year 1980. Project start date 6/1/80, ended 5/31/85. NIAID. University of Maryland (Baltimore). Granted to Richard H. Baker.
4.) Grant 5R07AI010049-15. International Center for Medical Research. University of Maryland Baltimore. Fiscal year 1974. Project start: 6/1/70 ended 5/31/75. NIAID.
5.) Grant 5R01AI007807-08. Genetic Studies on the Control of Arbovirus Vectors. University of Maryland Baltimore. Fiscal year 1974. Project start: 5/1/73, ended 4/30/75. NIAID.
6.) Grant 1R01AI032730-01. FLP-Mediated Recombination in the Mosquito Aedes Aegypti. University of California Irvine. Fiscal Year 1992. Project start: 5/1/92, ended 4/30/96. NIAID.
7.) Grant 1R01AI044238-01. Hermes and Mariner Transformation of Aedes Aegypti. Fiscal Year 1999. Project Start: 12/1/98, ended 11/30/03. NIAID.
8.) Flanders Stanley E, Bay Ernest C. Standardization of Mass Rearing Procedures for Entomophaga. WHO Bulletin. 1964;31:505-507.
9.) Filipponi A. The Feasibility of Mass Producing Macrochelid Mites for Field Trials against Houseflies. WHO Bulletin 1964;31:499-501.
10.) McLintock J. The Laboratory Cultivation of Culiseta. WHO Bulletin. 1964;31:459-460.
11.) Martínez-Palacios A. Maineance of Aedes aegypti in the Insectary in Mexico City. WHO Bulletin. 1964;341:461-462.
12.) Briggs John D. Mass Propagation of Bacteria Pathogenic for Insects. WHO Bulletin 1964;31:495-497.
13.) Weiser J. Parasitology of Blackflies. WHO Bulletin. 1964;31:483-485.
14.) Kramer JP. Parasites in Laboratory Colonies of Mosquitos. WHO Bulletin. 1964;31:475-478.
15.) Craig Jr. George B. Applications of Genetic Technology to Mosquito Rearing. WHO Bulletin 1964;31:469-473.
16.) US Patent 5,891,431. Palli, et al. Transgenic virus. Filed 1/22/97published 4/6/99. Assignee: Her Majesty the Queen in right of Canada, as represented by the Minister (Ottawa, CA).
17.) O'Reilly DR, Miller LK. A baculovirus blocks insect molting by producing ecdysteroid UDP-glucosyl transferase. Science. 1989 Sept 8;245(4922):1110-1112.
18.) US Patent 6,300,488. Gage, et al. Modified lepidopteran receptors and hybrid multifunctional proteins for use in transcription and regulation of transgene expression. Filed 7/10/97 published 10/9/01. Assignee: The Salk Institute for Biological Studies (La Jolla, CA).
19.) CRISP Grant 1DP1OD003878-01. Engineering the genetics of wild mosquito populations to fight infectious disease. California Institute of Technology. Office of Sponsored Research, Mail Code 201-15. Pasadena, CA. Fiscal Year 2008. Project start: 9/30/08, end 7/31/2013. Office of the Director, National Institutes of Health.

20.) Guangpu Li, Prágai Béla M, Rice Charles M. Rescue of Sindbis Virus-Specific RNA Replication and Transcription by Using a Vaccinia Virus Recombinant. J Virol. 1991 Dec;65(12):6714-6723.
21.) Pollack Andrew. Concerns Are Raised About Genetically Engineered Mosquitoes. The New York Times Online. 2011 October 30. [web page]
22.) Lindquist AW (ed.) International Atomic Energy Agency. Insect Population Control by the Sterile-Male Technique. Comprehensive report from a panel held in Vienna, Austria, 1962 Oct 16-19. No. 21. 67 pages
23.) Joint FAO/IAEA Division of Atomic Energy in Food and Agriculture. Sterile-Male Technique for Eradication or Control of Harmful Insects. Proceedings of a Panel, Vienna, Austria. 1968 May 27-31. 149 pages.

Fire Ants and Lone Star Ticks

1.) Brinkley Charles Kevin. Economic Impact of the Red Imported Fire Ant, Solenopsis Invicta (Buren), in Texas. Texas Tech University. August, 1989 (Thesis).
2.) Bastiaan M. Drees, S. Bradleigh Vinson. Fire Ants and their Management. Texas Agricultural Extension Service. The Texas A&M University System.
3.) Sokolova YY, McNally LR, Fuxa JR, Vinson SB. Spore morphotypes of Thelohania solenopsae (microsporidia) described microscopically and confirmed by PCR of individual spores microdissected from smears by position ablative laser microbeam microscopy. Microbiol. 2004;150:1261-1270.
4.) Hajek AE, Glare TR, O'Callaghan M (eds). Use of Microbes for Control and Eradication of Invasive Arthropods (Progress in Biological Control). 2009 Springer Science and Business Media.
5.) Gutrich John J, VanGelder Ellen, Loope Lloyd. Potential economic impact of introduction and spread of the red imported fire ant, Solenopsis invicta, in Hawaii. Environ Science & Policy. 2007 Nov-Dec;10(7-8):685-696.
6.) American-Lawns. Fire ants (soil-inhabiting). [web page]
7.) USDA. Univ. of Wisconsin submitted to CRIS. Shoemaker DD. Effects of Wolbachia on Host mtDNA Evolution. [web page]
8.) Dedeine F, Ahrens ME, Calcaterra L, Shoemaker DD. Social parasitism in fire ants (Solenopsis spp.): A potential mechanism for interspecies transfer of Wolbachia. Molecular Ecology. 2005;14:1543-1548.
9.) TN Depart. Of Agriculture. Rules of Plant Industries Division. Chapter 0080-6-19 Imported Fire Ant Quarantine Table of Contents. [web page]
10.) University of Tennessee Fire Ant Management Project. [web site]
11.) APHIS. Citrus Commodity Survey Reference. Cooperative Agriculture Pest Survey. Arthropod Pests. Solenopsis invicta (Buren) [red imported fire ant]. 2005 July. [web page]
12.) Rhoades WC. A Synecological Study of the Effects of the Imported Fire Ant Eradication Program. I. Alcohol Pitfall Method of Collecting. The Florida Entomologist. 1962 Dec;45(4):161-173.
13.) Rhoades WC. A Synecological Study of the Effects of the Improted Fire Ant Eradication Program. II. Light Trap, Soil Sample, Litter Sample and Sweep Net Methods of Collecting. The Florida Entomologist. 1963 Dec;46(4):301-310.
14.) Samish M, Rehacek J. Pathogens and Predators of Ticks and Their Potential in Biological Control. Annu Rev Entomol. 1999;44:149-82.
15.) Harris WG, Burns EC. Predation on the Lone Star Tick by the Imported Fire Ant. Envir Entomol. 1972 Jun;1(3):362-365.
16.) Myers Judith H. Eradication and Pest Management. An Rev Entomol. 1998 Jan;43:471-491.
17.) Fleetwood SC, Teel PD, Thompson G. Impact of imported fire ants on lone star tick mortality in open and canopied pasture habitats of east central Texas. Southwest Entomol. 1984;9:158-62.
18.) Department of the Army. Department of Defense, United States of America. U.S. Army Environmental Hygiene Activity – Scuth Forth McPherson, Georgia 30330-5000. 1990 Apr 24-27.
19.) USDA Agricultural Research Service. Agriculture Handbook. Management of Lone Star Tick in Recreation Areas. 1989 Aug,Vol. 682, 33 pages.
20.) Schulze TL, Bowen GS, Bosler EM, et al. Amblyomma americanum: a potential vector of Lyme disease in New Jersey. Science 1984 May;224(4649):601-603.
21.) Bacon RM, Pilgard MA, Johnson BJB, Raffel SJ, Schwan TG. Glycerophosphodiester Phosphodiesterase Gene (*glpQ*) of *Borrelia lonestari* Identified as a Target for Differentiating *Borrelia* Species Associated with Hard Ticks (Acari:Ixodidae). J Clin Microbiol. 2004 May; 42(5):2326–2328.
22.) US Patent 5,932,220. Barbour, et al. Diagnostic tests for a new spirochete, Borrelia lonestari sp. Filed 5/8/95 published 8/3/99. Assignee: Board of Regents University of Texas System (Austin, TX).
23.) Varela AS, Luttrell MP, Howerth EW, Moore VA, Davidson WR, Stallknecht DE, Little SE. First culture isolation of Borrelia lonestari, putative agent of southern tick-associated rash illness. J Clin Microbiol. 2004 Mar;42(3):1163-9.
24.) USDA Agricultural Research Service. Viruses as Biocontrol Agents. New Virus. [web page]
25.) USDA Agricultural Research Service. Accomplishments. www.ars.usda.gov
26.) USDA Grain Inspection Packers and Stockyards Administration. Principle stored insects. [web page]
27.) Lord JC. Mattesia oryzaephili (Neogregarinorida: Lipotrophidae), a Pathogen of Stored-Grain Insects: Virulence, Host Ragne and Comparison with Mattesia dispora. Biocontrol Science and Technol. 2003 Sept.;13(6):589-598.
28.) USDA ARS. Biological Control of Fire Ants Using New Species of Phorid Decaptiating Flies. Project start date 10/1/07, end date 9/30/2012. [web page]
29.) USDA ARS. Biology, Genomics and Integrated Pest Management of Invasive Ants. Project# 6615-32000-044-00. Start date: 9/8/09, ends 9/7/2014. [web page]
30.) Valles Steven M, Porter Sanford D. Pseudacteon Decapitating Flies: Potential Vectors of a Fire Ant Virus? Florida Entomol. 2007 Mar;90(1):268-270.

Filariasis – Nematodes as Biological Control

1.) Glare TR, Jackson TA, et al. Occurence of Bacillus popilliae and two nematode pathogens in populations of Amphimallon solstitialis (Col.: Scarabaeidae) near Darmstadt, Germany. Entomophaga 1993;38(4):441-450.
2.) Jaroslav Weiser. Diseases of Insects of Medical Importance in Europe. WHO Bulletin. 1963;28:121-127.
3.) Society for Invertebrate Pathology. 41st Annual Meeting of the Society for Invertebrate Pathology and 9th International Conference on Bacillus thuringiensis. [web page]
4.) Platzer EG. Biological Control of Mosquitoes with Mermithids. J Nematol. 1981 Jul;13(3):257-262.
5.) Burges HD, Hussey NW. Microbial Control of Insects and Mites. 1971 Academic Press London.
6.) Reuther Walter, Calavan E. Clair, Carman Glenn E. (ed). The Citrus Industry, Volume IV. Crop Protection. Diseases and Injuries; Viruses; Registration, Certification, Indexing; Regulatory Measures; Vertebrate Pests; Biological Control of Insects; Nematodes. Revised Edition. 1978University of California Div. of Agricultural Sciences. The Regents of the University of California.
7.) US Patent 7,396,536. Chandrashekar, et al. Parasitic helminth cuticlin proteins and uses thereof. Filed 6/9/04, published 6/8/08. Inventors: Chandrashekar R and Morales TH (Ft. Collins, CO). Assignee; Heska Corp. (Loveland, CO).
8.) Kaya Harry K. Infectivity of Neoaplectana carpocapsae and Heterorhabditis heliothidis to pupae of the parasite Apanteles militaris. J. Nematol. 1978 Jul;10(3):241-244.
9.) Smith Ray F. Considerations on the safety of certain biological agents for arthropod control. Bull Org mond. Santé. Bull. Wld Hlth Org. 1973;48:685-698. Prepared by participants in the Conference on the Safety of Biological Agents for Arthropod Control held at the Centers for Disease Control, Atlanta GA Apr. 16-19, 1973.
10.) Nematodes. Pathogenic parasites transmitted by fish and shellfish. [monograph on the Internet]
11.) Cheng TC. Larval nematodes parasitic in shellfish. Marine Fish Rev no date. Abstract.
12.) Moreno-Ancillo A. Caballero MT et al. Allergic reactions to anisakis simplex parasitizing seafood. Ann Allergy Asthma Immunol. 1997 Sep;79(3):246-50.
13.) Torres Borrego J, Martinez Cuevas JF, Tejero Garcia J. [Cross reactivity between fish and shellfish] [Article in Spanish] Allergol Immunopathol (Madr). 2003 May-Jun;31(3):146-51. [abstract]
14.) Armentia A, Martin-Gil FJ, Pascual C, et al. Anisakis simplex allergy after eating chicken meat. J Investig Allergol Clin Immunol. 2006;16(4):258-63.
15.) US Patent 5,789,194. Tripp, et al. Parasitic helminth venom allergen antigen 5-like genes and proteins. Filed 5/23/95, issued 8/4/98. Assignee: Heska Coporation (Ft. Collins, CO).
16.) Beaver Paul C, Burgdorfer Willy. A Microfilaria of Exceptional Size from the Ixodid Tick, Ixodes Dammini, from Shelter Island, New York. J Parasitol. 1984;70(6):963-966.
17.) Shukla-Dave A, Srivastava VML, Chatterjee RK. Ivermectin: Effect on sugar metabolism in Acanthocheilonema viteae, a rodent filarial parasite. Div. of Parasitology and Division of Biochemistry, Central Drug Research Institute, Lucknow, India.
18.) Koppenhöfer AM, Wilson M, Brown I, Kaya HK, Gaugler R. Biological control agents for white grubs (Coleoptera: Scarabaeidae) in anticipation of the establishment of the Japanese beetle in California. J Econ Entomol. 2000 Feb;93(1):71-80.

19.) US Patent 6,248,872. Chandrashekar et al. Parasitic nematode transglutaminase, nucleic acid molecules, and uses thereof. Filed 12/3/96. Issued 6/19/01. Assignee: Heska Corporation, Ft. Collins, CO.
20.) US Patent 6,309,644. Chandrashekar, et al. Parasitic nematode transglutaminase proteins and uses thereof. Filed 6/12/97. Issued 10/30/01. Assignee: Heska Corporation, Ft. Collins, CO and The Board of Regeants, The University of Texas System (Austin, TX).
21.) United States Patent 7,396,536 Chandrashekar, et al. Parasitic helminth cuticlin proteins and uses thereof. Filed 6/9/4, issued 6/8/8. Inventors: Chandrashekar R and Morales TH (Ft. Collins, CO). Assignee: Heska Corp. (Loveland, CO).
22.) US Patent 5,242,820. Lo. Pathogenic mycoplasma. Filed 6/6/91, issued 9/7/93. Assignee: American Registry of Pathology (Washington, DC)
23. Transglutaminase. Wikipedia. [web page]
24. Laki K, Lóránd L. On the Solubility of Fibrin Clots. Science. 1948 Sept.; 108(2802):280.
25.) US Patent 4,701,326. Nelson et al. Membrane-coated hydrogel encapsulated nematodes. Filed 5/19/86 published 10/20/87. Assignee: Plant Genetics, Inc. (Davis, CA).
26.) Renaudin J, Bodin-Ramiro C, Bové JM. Spiroplasma citri Virus SpV1-78, A Non-Lytic Rod-Shaped Virus with Single-Stranded, Circular DNA: Presence of Viral Sequences in the Spiroplasma Genome. Tenth IOCV Conference. (International Organization of Citrus Virologists) Report. Diseases Induced by Procaryotic Pathogens;2002:285-290.
27.) Sha Y, Melcher U, Davis R, et al. Resistance of Spiroplasma citri Lines to the Virus SVTS2 Is Associated with Integration of Viral DNA Sequences into Host Chromosomal and Extrachronosomal DNA. Appl Envir Microbiol. 1995 Nov;61(11):3950-3959.
28.) June-Der Lee and Chuan-Min Yen. Protease Secreted by the Infective Larvae of Angiostrongylus Cantonensis and its Role in the Penetration of Mouse Intestine. Am J Trop Med Hyg. 2005;72(6):831-836.
29.) Patterson Stark JE, Lacey LA. Susceptibility of Western Cherry Fruit Fly (Diptera: Tephritidae) to five species of entomopathogenic nematodes in laboratory studies. J Invertebr Pathol. 1999Sept;74(2):206-208 [abstract].
30.) El-Sadawy HA, El-Shazly A, El-Khateeb RMM, et al. Histopathological Studies of Hard Ticks Hyalomma dromedarii Infected of Entomopathogenic Nematodes. J Entomol. 2008;5(2):62-76.
31.) Zdene K Mrácek, Stanislav Becvái, et al. Canadian Steinernematid (Nematoda) Isolates and Their Infectivity, under Cold Conditinos, to Greater Wax Moth (Galleria mellonella) Larvae. Biol Control 1997 Feb;8(2):160-164.
32.) US Patent 4,701,326. Nelson et al. Membrane-coated hydrogel encapsulated nematodes. Filed 5/19/86, published 10/20/87. Assignee: Plant Genetics, Inc. (Davis, CA).
33.) Grant 5R01AI067434-04. Eradication of a Primary Filariasis Vector Population at an Endemic Field Site. University of Kentucky. Fiscal Year 2009. Project start: 8/15/06, end 7/31/2011. NIAID.
34.) Scott Marilyn E, Koski Kristine G. Zinc and Health: Current Status and Future Directions. Zinc Deficiency impairs immune Responses against Parasitic Nematode Infections at Intestinal and Systemic Sites. J Nutrition 2000;130:1412S-1420S.
35.) Scott ME, Koski KG. Zinc Deficiency Impairs Immune Responses against Parasitic Nematode Infections at Intestinal and Systemic Sites. Am Soc Nutr Sc. 2000;130:1412S-1420S.

Sawflies and Suspensions

1.) Bird FT, Burk JM. Artificially Disseminated Virus as a Factor Controlling the European Spruce Sawfly, Diprion hercyniae (Htg.) in the Absence of Introduced Parasites. The Canadian Entomologist. 1961;93(3):228-238.
2.) Bird FT. The Use of a Virus Disease in the Biological Control of the European Pine Sawfly, Neodiprion sertifer (Geoffr.) The Canadian Entomologist. 1953 Dec 1;85(12):437-446.
3.) McIntyre T, Dutky SR. Aerial Application of Virus for Control of a Pine Sawfly, Neodiprion prati pratti. J Econ Ent. 1961;54(4):809-810.
4.) Lewis Franklin B. (Entomologist, Forest Insect Laboratory Northeastern Forest Experiment Station Forest Service, U.S.D.A., New Haven, CT), in Forest Research Note. How to Collect and Process Small Polyhedral Viruses of Insects. Forest Service USDA, Upper Darby, PA. 1960;109:1-8.
5.) Lewis Franklin B. (Entomologist, Forest Insect Laboratory Northeastern Forest Experiment Station Forest Service, U.S.D.A., New Haven, CT), and Rollinson WB (Biological Aide); in Forest Research Note. How to Collect and Process Large Polyhedral Viruses of Insects. Forest Service USDA, Upper Darby, PA. 1962;130:1-6.
6.) Lauzon HAM, Garcia-Maruniak A, Zanotto PM de A et al. Genomic comparison of Neodiprion sertifer and Neodiprion lecontei nucleopolyhedroviruses and identification of potential hymenopteran baculovirus-specific open reading frames. J Gen Virol. 2006;87:1477-1489.
7.) St. Julian G, Bulla Jr LA, Sharpe ES, Adams GL. Bacteria, Spirochetes, and Rickettsia as Insecticides. Ann NY Acad Sci. 1973 Jun 22;217:65-75.
8.) International Bulletin of Bacteriological Nomenclature and Taxonomy. 1955 July 15;5(3):121-128. Status of the Generic Names Chlamydozoon von Prowazek and Borrelina Paillot. A Preliminary Statement. [web page]
9.) Holmes FO. Order Virales: The filterable viruses: in: Breed, RS, EGD Murray and A Parker Hitchens. Bergey's Manual of Determinative Bacteriology. 6th Edition. 1948.
10.) Holmes Kenneth M. Conservation of the generic name Borrelina and designation of the type species. Int. Bull. Bact. Nomen. Tax. 1953;3:134-137.
11.) Prowazek S von. Chlamydozoa I. Zusammenfassende Uebersicht. Arch f. Protistenkunde. 1970;10:336-358.
12.) Cowdry Edmund V. The Supravital Staining of Vaccine Bodies. J Exp Med. 1922;36:667-686. [web page]
13.) Storz Johannes, Page Leslie A. Taxonomy of the Chlamydiae: Reasons for Classifying Organisms of the Genus Chlamydia, Family Chlamydiaceae, in a Separate Order, Chlamydiales ord. nov. Internat. J System. Bacteriol. 1971 Oct;21(4):332-334.
14.) Åkerstedt J, Hofshagen M. Bacteriological Investigation of Infectious Keratoconjunctivitis in Norwegian Sheep. Acta Veter Scandin. 2004;45:19-26.
15.) Steinhaus Edward A. (University of CA Berkeley). Nomenclature and Classification of Insect Viruses. 1949;13:203-223.
16.) Turner PC, Young DC, Flanegan JB, Moyer RW. Interference with vaccinia virus growth caused by insertion of the coding sequence for poliovirus protease 2A. Virology 1989 Dec;173(20):509-521.
17.) Cornell University. Biological Control: A Guide to Natural Enemies in North America. Cotesia (=Apanteles) glomerata. (Hymenoptera: Braconidae). [web site]
18.) Benson J, Pasqualte A, Van Driesche RG, Elkinton J. Assessment of risk posed by introduced braconid wasps to Pieris virginiensis, a native woodland butterfly in New England. Biol Control. 2002. [in press at time of publication]
19.) Kolomiets NG, Stadnitskii GV, Vorontsov AI. The European Pine Sawfly: Distribution, Biology, Economic Importance, Natural Enemies and Control. [Ryzhii Sosnovyi Pilil'Shchik-Rasprostrainenie, Biologiya, vred, estestvennye vragi, mery bor'by] Nauka Publishers, Siberian Branch, Novosibirsk, 1972. [translated from Russian]. Published for the Forest Service, USDA, and NSF Washington, DC. Amerind Publishing Co., New Delhi, 1979.]
20.) Boucias Drion G, Pendland Jacquelyn C. Principles of Insect Pathology. 1998Kluwer Academic Publishers. (Netherlands).
21.) Smith Ray F. Considerations on the safety of certain biological agents for arthropod control.* Bull Org mond. Santé. Bull. Wld Hlth Org. 1973;48:685-698. *Prepared by participants in the Conference on the Safety of Biological Agents for Arthropod Control held at the Centers for Disease Control, Atlanta GA Apr. 16-19, 1973.
22.) Rollinson WD, Lewis FB, Waters WE. The Successful Use of a Nuclear-Polyhedrosis Virus against the Gypsy Moth. Notes. 1965:515-517. Forest Insect and Disease Laboratory Northeastern Forest Experiment Station Forest Service, US Department of Agriculture West Haven, CT.
23.) Hughes Kenneth. University of California. Conservation of the Generic Name Borrelina and Designation of the Type Species. International Bulletin. Request for an Opinion. File No. 53.
24.) Smirnoff WA. A staining method for differentiating spores, crystal and cell of Bacillus thuringiensis (Berliner). 1962 J Insect Path 4,384-386.192-200.
25.) Smirnoff WA, O'Connell DC. Detection of polyhedral from insect virus diseases on filter membranes. Stain Technol. 1962 Jul;37:207-10.
26.) Koyama R, Katagiri K. An Application of Nuclear and Cytoplasmic Polyhedrosis Viruses Against Lymantria fumida Butler (Lepidoptera: Lymantridae). Report translated from Japanese.
27.) US Patent 3,716,634. Insect Virus Compositions and Process. Filed 10/19/70, issued 2/13/73. Assignee: McLaughlin Gormley King Company (Minneapolis, MN).
28.) US Patent 3,541,203. Protected Virus Composition for Insect Control. Filed 5/8/69, published 11/17/70. Assignee: The National Cash Register Company, Dayton, Ohio.
29.) US Patent 2,853,797. Graham et al. Dehydration of Biological Substances. Filed 12/13/56 published 9/30/58. Assignee: United States of America as represented by the Secretary of Agriculture.
30.) US Patent 3,072,528. Kludas et al. Ingestible Dry Microorganism Preparations. Filed 7/13/57, published 6/8/63. Assignee: Med. Fabrik Chemisch-Pharmazeutischer.
31.) US Patent 3,113,066. Emond. Bacillus thuringiensis Spore Pesticide. Filed 1/3/61 published 12/3/63. Assignee: Esso Research and Engineering Company.
32.) US Patent 3,337,395. Page. Termite Control by Induced Epizootics of Entomophagous Microorganisms. Filed 12/27/63published 8/22/67. Inventor: Robert Z. Page, Springfield, VA. No assignee listed.

33.) US Patent 3,378,443. Cooper, et al. Anhydrous Liquid Suspensions of Biologics. Filed 7/29/60, published 4/16/68. Assignee: American Cyanamid Company, Stamford, Connecticut.
34.) US Patent 3,541,203. Fogle. Protected Virus Composition for Insect Control. Filed 5/8/69 published 11/17/70. Assignee: The National Cash Register Company, Dayton, OH.
35.) World Health Organization Patent #WO/2008/147879 – Automated Method and Device for DNA Sequence Determination, and Identification. Filed 5/22/08, published 12/4/08. Applicant: Ryan Golhar (US).
36.) Louda SM, Pemberton RW, Johnson MT, Follett PA. Nontarget Effects – The Achilles' Heel of Biological Control? Retrospective Analyses to Reduce Risk Associated with Biocontrol Introductions. Ann Rev Entomol. 2003;48:365-396.
37.) US Patent 3,716,634. Wells. Insect Virus Compositions and Process. Filed 10/19/70 published 2/13/73. Assignee: McLaughlin Gormley King Company (Minneapolis, MN).

The Tail of the Scorpion

1.) Schole EJ, Knols BGJ, Samson RA, Takken W. Entomopathogenic fungi for mosquito control: A review. J Insect Sc. 2004;4:1-24.
2.) Pava-Ripoll M, Posada FJ, Momen B, Wang C, St Leger R. Increased pathogenicity against coffee berry borer, Hypothenemus hampei (Coleoptera: Curculionidae) by Metarhizium anisopliae expressing the scorpion toxin (AaIT) gene. J Invertebr Pathol. 2008 Oct;99(2):220-6. Epub 2008 May 25.
3.) Pedarzani P, D'hoedt D, Doorty KB, et al. Tamapin, a Venom Peptide from the Indian Red Scorpion (Mesobuthus tumulus) that Targets Small Conductance Ca2+-activated K+ Channels and Afterhyperpolarization Currents in Central Neurons. J Biol Chem. 2002;277(48):46101-46109.772
4.) Lu D, Pava-Ripoll M, Li Z, Wang C. Insecticidal evaluation of Beauveria bassiana engineered to express a scorpion neurotoxin and a cuticle degrading protease. Appl Microbiol. Biotechnol. 2008 Dec;81(3):515-22. Epub 2008 Sept 18.
5.) Yao B, Pang Y, Fan Y, Zhao R, Yang Y, Wang T. Construction of an insecticidal baculovirus expressing insect-specific neurotoxin AaIT. Sci China C Life Sci. 1996 Apr;39(2):199-206.
6.) Castle NA, Strong PN. Identification of two toxins from scorpion (Leiurus quinquestriatus) venom which block distinct classes of calcium-activated potassium channel. FEBS Lett. 1986 Dec 1;209(1):117-21.
7.) Evans RL, Turner RJ. New insights into the upregulation and function of the salivary Na+-K+-2Cl-cotransporter. Eur J Morphol. 1998;36:142-6.
8.) Gazit E, Bach D, Kerr I, et al. The α-5 segment of Bacillus thuringiensis δ-endotoxin: in vitro activity, ion channel formation and molecular modeling. Biochem. J. 1994;304:895-902.
9.) Grove A, Tomich JM, Montal M. A molecular blueprint for the pore-forming structure of voltage-gated calcium channels. Proc Natl Acad Sci. USA Biophysics. 1991 Aug;88:6418-6422.
10.) Dee A, Belagaje RM, Ward K, Chio E, Lai MH. Expression and secretion of a functional scorpion insecticidal toxin in cultured mouse cells. Biotech (NY). 1990 Apr;8(4):339-42.
11.) Burges HD, Hussey NW. Microbial Control of Insects and Mites. 1971 Academic Press. London. p. 403.
12.) T. Yao B, Fan Y, Zeng Q, Zhao R. Insect-resistant tobacco plants expressing insect-specific neurotoxin AaIT. Chin J Biotechnol. 1996;12(2):67-72.
13.) US Patent 5,674,846. Johnson, et al. Insecticidal peptides from Sigestria sp. spider venom. Filed 9/4/96published 10/7/97. Assignee: NPS Pharmaceuticals, Inc. (Salt Lake City, UT).
14.) US Patent 6,156,539. Johnson, et al. 16KDA insecticidal toxin from bracons hebetor, nucleic acids encoding said toxin, and methods of use. Filed 2/22/99 published 12/5/00. Assignee: NPS Pharmaceuticals, Inc. (UT).
15.) US Patent 5,874,298. Johnson, et al. Insecticidal toxins from Bracon hebetor nucleic acid encoding said toxin and methods of use. Filed 2/17/95 published 2/23/99. Assignee: NPS Pharmaceuticals, Inc. (Salt Lake City, UT).
16.) US Patent 5,441,934. Krapcho, et al. Insecticidally effective peptides. Filed 12/20/93, published 8/15/95. Assignee: FMC Corporation (Philadelphia, PA).
17.) US Patent 4,879,236. Smith, et al. Method for producing a recombinant baculovirus expression vector. Filed 4/16/87 published 11/7/89. Assignee: The Texas A&M University System (College Station, TX). Original applications May 1983 and May 1984.
18.) Matsuura et al. Baculovirus expression vectors: The requirements for high level expression of proteins, including glycoproteins. J Gen Virol. 1987;68:1233-1250.
19.) Carbonell et al. Synthesis of a gene encoding an insect-specific scorpion neurotoxin and attempts to express it using baculovirus vectors. Gene 1988;73:409-418.
20.) US Patent 5,244,805. Miller. Baculovirus expression vectors. Filed 1/17/91 published 9/14/93. Assignee: University of Georgia Research Foundation, Inc. (Athens, GA).
21.) US Patent 6,673,340. Harrison, et al. Basement membrane degrading proteases as insect toxins and methods of use for same. Filed 7/12/00 published 1/6/04. Assignee: Iowa State University Research Foundation, Inc. (Ames, IA).
22.) Zlotkin E, Eitan M, Bindokas VP, et al. Functional duality and structural uniqueness of depressant insect-selective neurotoxins. Biochem 1991 May 14;30(19):4814-21.
23.) Zlotkin E, Fishman Y, Elazar M. AaIT: from neurotoxin to insecticide. Biochimie. 2000 Sep-Oct;82(9-10):869-881.
24.) Zlotkin E, Kadouri D, Gordon D, et al. An excitatory and a depressant insect toxin from scorpion venom both affect sodium conductance and possess a common binding site. Arch Biochem Biophys. 1985 Aug 1;240(2):877-887.
25.) US Patent 7,354,993. King, et al. Insecticidal polypeptides and methods of use thereof. Filed 11/4/05, Published 4/8/08.
26.) Eitan M, Fowler E, Herrmann R, et al. A scorpion venom neurotoxin paralytic to insects that affects sodium current inactivation: purification, primary structure, and mode of action. Biochem 1990 Jun 26;29(25):5941-7.
27.) Fan Y, Fang W, Guo S, et al. Increased Insect Virulence in Beauveria bassiana Strains Overexpressing an Engineered Chitinase. Amer Soc Microbiol. 2007 Jan;73(1):295-302.
28.) Fuxa JR, Richter AR, Ameen AO, Hammock BD. Vertical transmission of TnSNPV, TnCPV, AcMNPV, and possibly recombinant NPV in Trichoplusia ni. J Invertebr Pathol. 2002 Jan;79(1):44-50.
29.) Monett R, Potvin L, Baines, D et al. Interaction between Calcium Ions and Bacillus thuringiensis Toxin Activity against Sf9 Cells (Spodoptera frugiperda, Lepidoptera). Appl Environ Microbiol. 1997 Feb;63(2):440-447.
30.) Friedlander Ed. Pancreatic disease (including diabetes). [web page]
31.) de Roodt AR, Lago NR, Salomón OD, et al. A new venomous scorpion responsible for severe envenomation in Argentina: Tityus confluens. Toxicon. 2009 Jan;53(1):1-8.
32.) Koma Y, Furuno T, Hagiyama M, et al. Cell adhesion molecule 1 is a novel pancreatic-islet cell adhesion molecule that mediates nerve-islet cell interactions. Gastroenterol. 2008 May;134(5):1544-1554.
33.) Morel G. A cytoplasmic virus in the scorpion Buthus occitanus AMoreux. CR Acad Sci Hebd Seances Acad Sci D. 1975 Jun 30;280(25):2893-2894.
34.) Bartholomew C, Murphy J McGeeney K, Fitzgerald O. Pancreatic response to Tityus trinitatis venom. West Indian Med J. 1974 Mar;23(1):42-43.
35.) Reddy CR, Suvarnakumari G, Devi CS, Reddy CN. Pathology of scorpion venom poisoning. J Trop Med Hyg. 1972 May;75(5):98-100.
36.) Lamy J, Goyffon M. [Hepato-pancreas catalase from the scorpion Androctonus australis L. Kinetics of decomposition of hydrogen peroxide. Action of aminotraizole.
37.) CR Acad Sci Hebd Seances Acad Sci D. 1969 Dec 15;269(24):2449-2452. [Article in French].
38.) Petricevich VL, Reynaud E, Cruz AH, Possani LD. Macrophage activation, phagocytosis and intracellular calcium oscillations induced by scorpion toxins from Tityus serrulatus. Clin Exp Immunol. 2008 Dec;154(3):415-423
39.) US Patent 6,559,359. Laten. Plant retroviral polynucleotides and methods for use thereof. Filed 8/25/97 published 5/6/03. Assignee: Loyola University of Chicago (Chicago, IL).

Chapter Three: The Elements of Surprise Epidemics

Arboviruses and Multiple Infections

1.) Blaškovic. The Public Health Importance of Tickborne Encephalitis in Europe. World Health Organization Bulletin. 1967;36(Suppl. 1):5-13.
2.) Chumakov MP, Seitlenok NA. Tickborne Human Encephalitis in the European Part of USSR and Siberia. 1940 Sept. 20;92(2385):264-268.
3.) Casals J, Webster LT. Close Relation Between Russian Spring-Summer Encephalitis and Louping-Ill Viruses. Science 1943;97(2515):246-248.
4.) Parker RR. Public Health Report 1942;57:1963-66.
5.) Chambers TJ, Monath TP, (eds.) Chambers TJ, Maramorosch K, Monath TP, Murphy FA, Shatkin AJ. (eds.) The Flaviviruses: Pathogenesis and Immunity. Advances in Virus Research, Vol. 60. 2006 Elsevier Academic Press.
6.) Tokarz R, Jain K, Bennett A, et al. Assessment of Polymicrobial Infections in Ticks in New York State. Vector-Borne and Zoonotic Diseases. 2010;10(3). 6 pages.
7.) NI Grašcenkov. Tickborne encephalitis in the USSR. World Health Organization Bulletin. 1964;30:187-196.
8.) Vanlandingham DL, Davis BS, Lvov DK, et al. Molecular Characterization of California Serogroup Viruses Isolated in Russia. Am J Trop Med Hyg. 2002;67(3):306-309.
9.) Hoff Gerald L, Iversen John O, Yuill Thomas M, et al. Isolations of Silverwater Virus from Naturally Infected Showshoe Hares and Haemaphysalis Ticks from Alberta and

Wisconsin. Am J Trop Med Hyg. 1971;20(2):320-325.
10.) Hoff Gerald L, Yuill Thomas M, Iversen John O, Hanson Robert P. Silverwater Virus Serology in Snowshoe Hares and Other Vertebrates. Am J Trop Med Hyg. 1971;20(2):326-330.
11.) Shubladze AK, Andzhaparidze OG. [Effectiveness of a new vaccine in prevention of vernal tickborne encephalitis]. [Article in Russian]. Zh Mikrobiol Epidemiol Immunobiol. 1954 Sept;9:74-77.
12.) Miles JAR. Epidemiology of the Arthropod-borne Encephalitides. WHO Bulletin 1960;22:339-371.
13.) Warren Joel. Epidemic Encephalitis in the Far East. A Review. Am J Trop Med Hyg;1946;S-1-26(4):417-436. Div. of Virus and Rickettsial Diseases Army Medical School.
14.) Keirans JE, Lacombe EH. First records of Amblyomma americanum, Ixodes (Ixodes) dentatus, and Ixodes (Ceratixodes) uriae (Acari Ixodidae) from Maine. J Parasitol. 1998 Jun;84(3):629-631.
15.) Standard Corporation Service, Daily revised May-August, 1917. Standard Statisics Company Inc. New York. P. 234.
16.) Silber LA. Arch Sci Biol. (Moscow). 1939;56:9.
17.) Pearce JM. Baron Constantin von Economo and encephalitis lethargic. 1996;60:167.
18.) von Economo C. Encephalitis lethargica. Wien Klin Wschr. 1917;30:581-585.
19.) Duvoisin Roger C. Yahr Melvin D. Encephalitis and Parkinsonism. Arch Neurol. 1965;12(3):227-239.
20.) Whitman Loring, Wallis RC, Leventhal EA. Isolation of a California-Group Arbovirus from Aedes Abserratus (Felt and Young) in Simsbury, Connecticut. Am J Trop Med Hyg. 1968;17(3):449-450.
21.) Jennings Wm L, Lewis Arthur L, Sather Gladys E, et al. California-Encephalitis-Group Viruses in Florida Rabbits: Report of Experimental and Sentinel Studies. Am J Trop Med Hyg. 1968;17(5):781-787.
22.) Whitney Elinor, Jamnback Hugo, Means Robert G, et al. California Virus in New York State. Isolation and Characterization of California Encephalitis Virus Complex from Aedes cinereus. Am J Trop Med Hyg. 1969;18(1):123-131.
23.) Monti G, Galli M, Invernizzi F, et al. Cryoglobulinaemias: a multi-centre study of the early clinical and laboratory manifestations of primary and secondary disease. GISC. Italian Group for the Study of Cryoglobulinaemias. QJM. 1995 Feb;88(2):115-126.
24.) World Health Organization. Crimean-Congo haemorrhagic fever. [web page]
25.) Par JM Dory, Chastel C, Couatarmanach A, et al. Question Étiologiques et Épidémiologiques Posées par L'érythème chronique migrant et la maladie de Lyme. A propos de 4observations réalisées au centre hospitalier regional de Rennes. [Article in French]. Bull. Soc. Path. Exot. 1985;78(3):512-525.
26.) Chastel C, Main AJ, Couatarmanac'h A. et al. Isolation of Eyach virus (Reoviridae, Colorado tick fever group) from Ixodes ricinus and I. ventalloi ticks in France. Arch Virol. 1984;82(3-4):161-71.
27.) Shope, RE. World Reference Center for Arboviruses. 1977 Aug. Project #s: 3M161102BS01 and 3A161102B71Q.
28.) Carpentier S, Moilleron R, Beltran C, et al. Quality of dredged material in the river Seine basin (France). II. Micropollutants. Sci Total Environ. 2002Nov 1;299(1-3):57-72.
29.) Alfeev NI, YV Klimas. Experience in cultivating Ichneumon Flies, Hunterellus hookeri, obtained from United States, which destroy Ixodid ticks of Soviet fauna. Priroda, Moskva 1938;2:98-101. [NAMRU No. 3, Translation 1674from Russian]. [Abstract]
30.) Alfeev NI, YaV Klimas. On the possibility of developing Hunterellus hookeri in climatic conditions of USSR. Sovetsk. Vet. 1938;15(3):55. [NAMRU No. 3, Translation 1676 from Russian].[Abstract]
31.) Bernadskaya ZM.A case of parasitism on ixodid ticks. Trudy Uzbek. Nauch. Issled. Vet. Opyt. Sta.Narkom. USSR. 1939;2(11):28-30. [NAMRU No. 3, Translation 1686 from Russian]. [Abstract] The ichneumon parasitizing nymphal H. asiaticum [sp. Ixodes] proved to be a species that is widespread in the USA, eastern Africa, and when introduced to Leningrad area became adapted to northern condition of the USSR.
32.) Blagoveshchensky DI. Hymenopterous parasite of ticks of the family Ixodidae. Parazit. Sborn. Zool. Inst. Akad. Nauk SSSR. 1947;9:115-124. [NAMRU No. 3, Translation 1681 from Russian].
33.) Hurwitz Eugene S, Schell Wendy, Nelson Donald, et al. Surveillance for California Encephalitis Group Virus Illness in Wisconsin and Minnesota, 1978. Am J Trop Med Hyg. 1983:32(3):595-601.
34.) Huhn GD, Austin C, Langkop C, et al. The Emergence of West Nile Virus During a Large Outbreak in Illinois in 2002. Am J Trop Med Hyg. 2005;72(6):768-776.
35.) Boyd KR, Whitaker-Dowling P. Flanders virus replication and protein synthesis. Virol. 1988 Apr;163(2):349-358.
36.) Robert E. Shope, MD. Yale University. Annual Report for 1976Yale Arbovirus Research Unit, International Center for Arboviruses. WHO Collaborating Center for Arbovirus Reference and Research. Report #ADA038877. Dept of Epidemiology and Public Health, Yale School of Medicine, New Haven, CT. Controlling office: Department of the Army, US Army Medical Research and Development Command, Washington, DC. Annual Report from 7/1/75to 6/30/76. Contract or Grant No. DADA-17-72-C-2170. Report date July 1, 1976. 92 pages.
37.) Langhoff PJ, God Science: The Secret World of Rampant Genetics, Hidden Illness, and Biotech Profiteering. 2010 Allegory Press LLC, Hustisford, WI.
38.) 14. Pond WL, Ehrenkranz NJ, Danauskas JX, Davies JE. Arboviruses and Human Disease in South Florida. Am J Trop Med Hyg. 1966;18(2):205-210.
39.) Chamberlain RW, Sudia WD, Coleman PH. Isolations of an Arbovirus of the Bunyamwera Group (Tensaw Virus) from Mosquitoes in the Southeastern United States, 1960-1963. Am J Trop Med Hyg. 1969;18(1):92-97.
40.) Coleman PH. Tensaw Virus, A New Member of the Bunyamwera Arbovirus Group from the Southern United States. Am J Trop Med. 1969;18(1):81-91.
41.) Sudia WD, Coleman PH, Chamberlain RW. Experimental Vector-Host Studies with Tensaw Virus, a Newly Recognized Member of the Bunyamwera Arbovirus Group. Am J Trop Med Hyg. 1969;18(1):98-102. (Scientists were from the National Communicable Disease Center, Health Services and Mental Health Administration, US Dept. of Health, Education, and Welfare, Atlanta, Georgia.)
42.) Kokernot RH, Hayes J, Will RL, et al. Arbovirus Studies in the Ohio-Mississippi Basin, 1964-1967. II. St. Louis Encephalitis Virus. Am J Trop Med Hyg. 1969;18(5):750-761.
43.) Clifford Carleton M, Sonenshine Daniel E, Atwood Earl L, Robbins Chandler S, Hughes Lyndahl E. Tests on Ticks from Wild Birds Collected in the Eastern United States for Rickettsiae and Viruses Am J Trop Med Hyg November 1969 18:1057-1061.
44.) Kinnunen PM, Inkeroinen H, Ilander M, et al. Intracerebral Borna disease virus infection of bank voles leading to peripheral spread and reverse transcription of viral RNA. PLoS One. 2011;6(8):323622. Epub 2011 Aug 22.
45.) Fort P, Albertinni A, Van-Hua A, et al. Fossil Rhabdoviral Sequencees integrated into Arthropod Genomes: Ontogeny, Evolution, and Potential Functionality. Mol Biol Evol. 2011 Oct 14. [Epub ahead of print].
46.) Wünschmann A, Honkavuori K, Briese T, et al. Antigen tissue distribution of Avian bornavirus (ABV) in psittacine birds with natural spontaneous proventricular dilatation disease and ABV genotype 1 infection. J Vet Diagn Invest. 2011 Jul;23(4):716-26.
47.) Hori M, Tomonaga K. [Endogenous bornavirus elements in mammalian genome]. Uirusu. 2010 Dec;20(2):143-153. Review. [Article in Japanese].
48.) Rackova S, Janu L, Kabickova H. Borna disease virus (BDV) circulating immunocomplex positivity in addicted patients in the Czech Republic: a prospective cohort analysis. BMC Psychiatry. 2010 Sept 8;10:70.
49.) Belyi VA, Levine AJ, Skalka AM. Unexpected inheritance: multiple integrations of ancient bornavirus anad ebolavirus/marburgvirus sequences in vertebrate genomes. PLos Pathog. 2010 Jul 29;6(7):e1001030.
50.) Heinrich A. Adamaszek M. Anti-Borna disease virus antibody responses in psychiatric patients: long-term follow up. Psychiatry Clin Neurosci. 2010 Jun;64(3):255-261. Epub 2010 Apr 8.
51.) Reutler A, Ackermann A, Kothlow S. et al. Avian bornaviruses escape recognition by the innate immune system. Viruses. 2010 Apr;2(4):927-938.
52.) Ludwig H, Koester V, Pauli G, Rott R. The cerebrospinal fluid of rabbits infected with Borna disease virus. Arch Virol. 1977;55(3):209-223.
53.) Metzler A, Frei U, Danner K. [Virologically confirmed outbreak of Borna's disease in a Swiss herd of sheep]. Schweiz Arch Tierheilkd. 1976 Nov;118(11):483-492. [German].

Leptospires, Reoviruses, and Reassortments, Oh My

1.) Shope, RE. World Reference Center for Arboviruses. Annual Report. July 1, 1975- Jun 30, 1976. Report ADA060051. Projects # 3M161102BS01, 3A161102B71Q. Supported by the US Army Medical Research and Development Command, Fort Detrick, Frederick, MD 21701. Under Contract No. DADA 17-72-C-2170. Department of Epidemiology and Public Health, Yale University School of Medicine, New Haven, CT 06510.

2.) Chastel C, Main AJ, Couatarmanac'h A. et al. Isolation of Eyach virus (Reoviridae, Colorado tick fever group) from Ixodes ricinus and I. ventalloi ticks in France. Arch Virol. 1984;82(3-4):161-71.

3.) Chastel C, Main AJ, Couatarmanac'h A, et al. Isolation of Eyach virus (Reoviridae, Colorado tick fever group) from Ixodes ricinus and I. ventalloi ticks in France. Arch Virol. 1984;82(3-4):161-71.

4.) CDC. MedScape Today. Attoui H, Jaafar FM, de Micco P, de Lamballerie X. Coltiviruses and Seadornaviruses in North America, Europe, and Asia. Emerg Infect Dis 2005 Nov 15;11(11).

5.) Knudson DL. Genome of Colorado Tick Fever Virus. Virol. 1981;112:361-364. From Yale Arbovirus Research Unit, Yale University, New Haven, Connecticut.

6.) Hariharasubramanian V, Hadidi A, Singer B, Fraenkel-Conrat H. Possible identification of a protein in brome mosaic virus infected barley as a component of viral RNA polymerase. Virology. 1973 Jul;54(1):190-198.

7.) Shih DS, Kasberg P. Translation of brome mosaic viral ribonucleic acid in a cell-free system derived from wheat embryo. Proc Natl Acad Sci USA. 1973 Jun;70(6):1799-1803.

8.) Cooper JI. Viruses and the Environment. Second Edition. 1995 Chapman and Hall, London.

9.) Offit PA. Rotaviruses: immunologic determinants of protection against infection and disease. Adv Virus Res. 1994;44:161-202.

10.) Brakke MK. Degradation of brome mosaic and tobacco mosaic viruses in bentonite. Virology. 1971 Dec;46(3):575-585.

11.) Pfeiffer P, Dorne B. The reversible reaction of brome grass mosaic virus and its RNA with mercuric ions. Biochim Biophys Acta. 1971 Jan 28;228(2):456-470.

12.) Hamilton RI. Properties of brome mosaic virus and its related antigens. Virol. 1961 Dec;15:452-464.

13.) Herzog M, Pfeiffer P, Hirth L. Pathways of degradation of brome mosaic virus particles as influenced by their RNA content. Virol. 1976 Feb;69(2):394-407.

14.) McGirr Scott C, Endrizzi JE. The Effects of B, K10, and AR Chromosoms on the Resistance of Maize to Viral Infection. Genetics. 1978 Oct;90(2):331-338.

15.) JW Davies. The multipartite genome of brome mosaic virus: aspects of in vitro translation and RNA structure. Ann Microbiol (Paris). 1976 Jan;127A(1):131-142.

16.) RI Graham, Rao S, Possee RD, et al. Detection and characterisation of three novel species of reovirus (Reoviridae), isolated from geographically separate populations of the winter moth Operophtera brumata (Lepidoptera: Geometridae) on Orkney. J Invert Path. 2006 Feb;91(2):79-87.

17.) Lucarotti CJ, Morin B, Graham RI, Lapointe R. Production, application, and field performance of Abietiv, the balsam fir sawfly nucleopolyhedrovirus. Virologica Sinica. 2007;22(2):163-172.

18.) Graham RI, Rao S, Hails RS, et al. Sequence analysis of a reovirus isolated from the winter moth Operophtera brumata (Lepidoptera: Geometridae) and its parasitoid Phobocampe tempestiva (Hymenoptera: Ichneumonidae). Virus Res. 2008;135:42-47.

19.) Graham RI, Rao S, Possee RD, et al. Detection and characterisation of three novel species of reovirus (Reoviridae), isolated from geographically separate populations of the winter moth Operophtera brumata (Lepidoptera: Geometridae) on Orkney. J Invertebr Pathol. 2006;91:79-87.

20.) Bigot, Y., Drezen, J.M., Sizaret, P.Y., Rabouille, A., Hamelin, M.H. and Periquet, G. The genome segments of DpRV, a commensal reovirus of the wasp Diadromus pulchellus (Hymenoptera). Virology New York 1995;210 (1): 109 - 119.

21.) Borsa J, Sargent MD, Lievaart PA, Copps TP. Reovirus: Evidence for a second step in the intracellular uncoating and transcriptase activation process. Virol. 1981 May;111(1):191-200.

22.) Morgan Exeen M, Kingsbury David W. Reovirus enzymes that modify messenger RNA are inhibited by perturbation of the lambda proteins. Virol. 1981 Sept;113(2):565-572. Chapter One 797References 797

23.) Ahmed Rafi, Fields BN. Reassortment of genome segments between reovirus defective interfering particles and infectious virus: Construction of temperature-sensitive and attenuated viruses by rescue of mutations from DI particles. Virol. 1981 May;111(2):351-363.

24.) Macdonald RD, Gower DA. Genomic and phenotypic divergence among three serotypes of aquatic bunyaviruses (infectious pancreatic necrosis virus). Virol. 1981 Oct;114(1):187-195.

25.) Dies J, Miralles L, Tarrasa F, et al. Thermoluminescence Response of Calcic Bentonite Subjected to Conditions of High Nuclear Waste Underground Storage. Radiat Prot Dosimetry 2002;100(1-4):389-393.

26.) Zlobenko EP, Movchan NP, Vovk IF, et al. Studies of Clays from Deposits in Ukraine as Barrier Material for Radioactive Waste Repositories. In: Proceedings 5th International Conference on Radioactive Waste Management and Environmental Remediation. 1995;1:587-859.

27.) López-Galindo A, Hach-Alí PF, Pushkarev AV, et al. Tritium redistribution between water and clay minerals. Appl Clay Sci. 2008;39:151-159.

28.) Beaurepaire C, Chaconas G. Topology-dependent transcription in linear and circular plasmids of the segmented genome of Borrelia burgdorferi. Mol Microbiol. 2007 Jan;63(2):443-453.

29.) Pascale Bourhy, Laurence Salaün, Aurélie Lajus, et al. A Genomic Island of the Pathogen Leptospira interrogans Serovar Lai Can Excise from Its Chromosome. Infect Immun. 2007 Feb;75(2):677-683.

30.) Sherwood JL, Fulton RW. The specific involvement of coat protein in tobacco mosaic virus cross protection. Virol. 1982 May;119(1):150-158.

31.) Tyulkina LG, Mankin AS. Inhibition of ribonuclease contamination in preparations of T4RNA ligase, polynucleotide kinase, and bacterial alkaline phosphatase with bentonite. Analyt Biochem. 1984 May;138(2):285-290.

32.) Hall TC, Shih DS, Kaesberg P. Enzyme-Mediated Binding of Tyrosine to Brome-Mosaic-Virus Ribonucleic Acid. Biochem J. 1972;129:969-976.

33.) Beaurepaire C, Chaconas G. Topology-dependent transcription in linear and circular plasmids of the segmented genome of Borrelia burgdorferi. Mol Microbiol. 2007 Jan;63(2):443-453.

34.) Maan S, Maan NS, Nomikou K, et al. Complete Genome Characterisation of a Novel 26th Bluetongue Virus Serotype from Kuwait. PLOS One 2011 Oct 21;6(10). 11 pages.

35.) López DR, Miranda MA, Paredes-Esquivel C, et al. Recovery rates of bluetongue virus serotypes 1, 2, 4 and 8 Spanish strains from orally infected Culicoides imicola in South Africa. Med Vet Entomol. 2011 Nov 13. [Epub ahead of print].

36.) Cox Herald R. Bluetongue. From Viral and Rickettsial Research Section, American Cyanamid Company Research Laboratories, Pearl River, New York. Bacteriol Rev. 1954 Dec;18:239-253.

37.) Dutky SR, Gooden EL. Coxiella Popilliae, N. Sp., A Rickettsia Causing Blue Disease of Japanese Beetle Larvae. J Bacteriol.1952 Jun;63(6):743-750.

38.) Cytec. Products Overview. www.cytec.com/products/overview.htm and

39.) US Patent 8,003,675. Nagata et al. 3,4-dihalogenoisothiazole derivative, and agricultural or horticultural plant disease-controlling agent. Filed 7/6/07 published 8/23/11. Assignee: Kumiai Chemical Industry Co., Ltd. (Tokyo, JP).

40.) US Patent 6,995,185. Jansen et al. .DELTA.1-pyrrolines used as pesticides. Filed 9/10/01 published 2/7/06. Assignee: Bayer Cropscience AG (Monheim, DE).

41.) BASF. American Cyanamid acquisition by BASF closed within three months. [web page]

42.) Aftalion Fred. A History of the International Chemical Industry. 1991. Mining and Scientific Press Vol. 114. 1917 Jan-Jul. San Francisco, CA. 1070 pages.

43.) Wilson Nixon, Kale II Herbert W. Ticks Collected From Indian River County, Florida (Araci: Metastigmata: Ixodidae). The Florida Entomol. 1972 Mar;55(1):53-57.

44.) Reovirus. Lohmann Animal Health International. [web page]

45.) Lahinternational. Reovirus. [web page]

46.) Clark FD. Poultry Site. Avian Reovirus Infections. www.thepoultrysite.com/articles/96/avian-reovirus-infections.

47.) Ishii N, Isogai E, Isogai H, et al. T cell response to Borrelia garinii, Borrelia afzelii, and Borrelia japonica in various oncogenic mouse strains. Microbiol. Immunol. 1995;39(12):929-935.

48.) Le Fleche A, Postic D, Girardet K, et al. Characterization of Borrelia lusitaniae sp. nov. by 16S Ribosomal DNA Sequence Analysis. Int J Syst Bacteriol. 1997 Oct;47(4):921-925.

49.) Gouvea V, Schnitzer TJ. Pathogenicity of Avian Reoviruses: Examination of Six Isolates and a Vaccine Strain. Infect Immun. 1982;38(2):731-738.

50.) Spandidos DA, Graham AF. Physical and Chemical Characterization of an Avian Reovirus. J Virol. 1976 Sept.;19(3):968-976.

51.) Mullen Gary R, Durden Lance A. (ed.). Medical and Veterinary Entomology, Second Edition. 2009 Academic Press, an imprint of Elsevier. Burlington, MA. P. 154.

52.) US Patent 5,990,388. Roth, et al. Resistance to viruses and viroids in trasgenic plants and animals expressing dsRNA-binding protein. Filed 6/7/95 published 11/23/99. Assignee: Research Corporation Technologies, Inc. (Tucson, AZ).

53.) Wellings FM, Lewis AL, Pierce LV. Agents Encountered During Arboviral Ecological Studies: Tampa Bay Area, Florida, 1963 to 1970. Am J Trop Med Hyg. 1972;21(2):201-213.

54.) Taylor DJ, Lewis AL, Edman JD, Jennings WL. California Group Arboviruses in Florida. Host-Vector Relations. Am J Trop Med Hyg. 1971;20(1):139-145.

55.) Weidhaas DE. Mosquito Population Control Through the Use of Chemosterilants. Am J Trop Med Hyg. 1972;21(5):772-776.

56.) Weidhaas DE, Schmidt CH, Seabrook EL. Field studies on the release of sterile males for the control of Anopheles quadrimaculatus. Mosquito News. 1962;22:283-291.

57.) Morlan HB, McCray EM Jr., Kilpatrick JW. Field tests with sexually sterile males for control of Aedes aegypti. Mosquito News. 1962;22:295-300.
58.) Lofgern CS, Dame DA, Breeland SG, et al. Release of chemosterilized males for the control of Anopheles Albimanus in El Salvador. III. Field Methods and Population Control. Am J Trop Med Hyg. 1974;23(2):288-297.
59.) Breeland SG, Jeffery GM, Lofgren CS, Weidhaas DE. Release of Chemosterilized Males for the Control of Anopheles Albimanus in El Salvador. Am J Trop Med Hyg. 1974;23(2):274-281.
60.) Petersen JJ, Willis OR, Chapman HC. Release of Romanomermis culicivorax for the control of anopheles albimanus in El Salvador. I. Mass Production of the Nematode. Am J Trop Med Hyg. 1978;27(6):1265-1267.
61.) Lowe RE, Bailey DL, Dame DA, Savage KE, Kaier PE. Efficiency of Techniques for the Mass Release of Sterile Male Anopheles Albimanus Wiedemann in El Salvador. Am J Trop Med. 1980;29(4):695-703.
62.) Pond WL, Ehrenkranz NJ, Danauskas JX, Davies JE. Arboviruses and Human Disease in South Florida. Am J Trop Med Hyg. 1966;18(2):205-210.
63.) Chamberlain RW, Sudia WD, Coleman PH. Isolations of an Arbovirus of the Bunyamwera Group (Tensaw Virus) from Mosquitoes in the Southeastern United States, 1960-1963. Am J Trop Med Hyg. 1969;18(1):92-97.
64.) US Patent 3,891,756. Kasugai et al. Agricultural pesticide composition. Filed 12/26/73published 6/24/75. Assignee: Mitsubishi Chemical Industries Ltd. (Tokyo, JA).
65.) US Patent 3,716,634. Wells. Insect Virus Compositions and Process. Filed 10/19/70 published 2/13/73. Assignee: McLaughlin Gormley King Company (Minneapolis, MN).
66.) Burgdorfer W, Eklund CM. Studies of the ecology of Colorado tick fever virus in Western Montana. Am J Hyg. 1959 Mar;69(2):127-137.
67.) Kelly DC, Lescott Thelma, Ayres MD, et al. Induction of a nonoccluded baculovirus persistently infecting Heliothis zea cells by Heliothis armigera and Trichoplusia ni nuclear polyhedrosis viruses. Virol. 1981 Jul;112(1):174-189.
68.) Shope Robert E, Rozhont Edward J, Bishop David HL. Role of the middle-sized bunyavirus RNA segment in mouse virulence. Virology 1981 Oct;114(1):273-276.
69.) Beaty BJ, Rozhon EJ, ensemer P, Bishop DHL. Formation of reassortant bunyaviruses in dually infected mosquitoes. Virology. 1981 May;111(2):662-665.
70.) Trent DW, Grant JA, Vorndam AV, Monath TP. Genetic heterogeneity among Saint Louis encephalitis virus isolates of different geographic origin. 1981 Oct;114(2):319-332.
71.) Acoles Glen A, Papero Michele, Beati Lorenza, Fish Durland. A Relapsing Fever Group Spirochete Transmitted by Ixodes scapularis Ticks. Vector Borne Zoonot Dis. 2001;1(1):21-34.
72.) Ebel GD, Foppa I, Spielman A, Telford SR. A Focus of deer tick virus transmission in the northcentral United States. Emerg Infect Dis. 1999;5:570-574
73.) Telford SR 3rd, Armstrong PM, Katavolos P, Foppa I, et al. A new tickborne encephalitis-like virus infecting New England deer ticks, Ixodes dammini. Emerg Infect Dis. 1997;3:165-170.
74.) Belyaev VG. Yu I, Mirotvortsev GM et al. Contribution to zoological and parasitological characteristics of the tularemia infection areas in Primor'ye region. Mater, Nauch, Prakt. Konf. Tulyarem. Soputst. Infekts. 1965:272-273. [NAMRU No. 3, Translation 1525 from Russian]. [Abstract]
75.) Gaidamovich S Ya. Classification and identification of Arboviruses. Vestn. Akad. Med. Nauk. SSSR. 1972;27(6):25-33. [NAMRU No. 3, Translation 677 from Russian]
76.) Garfield Eugene. Lyme Disease Researcher Uncovers a Case of Delayed Recognition: Arvid Afzelius and His Successors. Current Comments. #49. 1989 Dec 4;p.3-8. In Scientist: Creativity, Delayed Recognition, and other Essays, 1989;12:345.
77.) Fitzpatrick Tony. Washington Univesrity in St. Louis, Monsanto Co., awarded patent for technology that creates disease-resistant crops. 2003 Aug 20. Washington University in St. Louis. Newsroom.
78.) Belyaev VG. Yu I, Mirotvortsev GM et al. Contribution to zoological and parasitological characteristics of the tularemia infection areas in Primor'ye region. Mater, Nauch, Prakt. Konf. Tulyarem. Soputst. Infekts. 1965:272-273. [NAMRU No. 3, Translation 1525 from Russian]. [Abstract]
79.) Gaidamovich S Ya. Classification and identification of Arboviruses. Vestn. Akad. Med. Nauk. SSSR. 1972;27(6):25-33. [NAMRU No. 3, Translation from Russian] [Abstract]
80.) Lenhoff C. Spirochetes in aetiologically obscure diseases. Acta Dermato-Venreol. 1948;28:295-324.

Wolbachia as Symbiont

1.) USDA. Univ. of Wisconsin submitted to CRIS. Shoemaker DD. Effects of Wolbachia on Host mtDNA Evolution. [web page]
2.) Bastiaan M. Drees, S. Bradleigh Vinson. Fire Ants and their Management. Texas Agricultural Extension Service. The Texas A&M University System.
3.) Dedeine F, Ahrens ME, Calcaterra L, Shoemaker DD. Social parasitism in fire ants (Solenopsis spp.): A potential mechanism for interspecies transfer of Wolbachia. Molecular Ecology. 2005;14:1543-1548.
4.) APHIS. Citrus Commodity Reference. Cooperative Agriculture Pest Survey. Arthropod Pests. Solenopsis invicta (Buren) [red imported fire ant]. 2005 July. [web page]
5.) Wikipedia. Wolbachia. [web page]
6.) Kathrin Hartelta, Rainer Oehmea, Henning Franka, Stefan O. Brockmanna, Dieter Hasslerb and Peter Kimmiga. Pathogens and symbionts in ticks: prevalence of Anaplasma phagocytophilum (Ehrlichia sp.), Wolbachia sp., Rickettsia sp., and Babesia sp. in Southern Germany International Journal of Medical Microbiology Supplements Volume 293, Supplement 37, April 2004, Pages 86-92.
7.) Williams JC, Weiss E, Dasch GA. The genera Coxiella, Wolbachia, and Rickettsiella. Naval Medical Command. Naval Medical Research Institute. Department of the Navy, Washington, DC. In: The Prokaryotes: a handbook on the biology of bacteria: ecophysiology, isolation, identification, applications. 2nd ed. Edited by A. Balows et al. NY Springer-Verlag. 1992;111:2471-2484. Document AD-A250-768.
8.) Brock TD. Microorganisms From Smallpox to Lyme Disease. Scientific American. W.H. Freeman and Company. 1990. p. 28-37.
9.) Burgdorfer W, Brinton LP, Hughes LE. Isolation and characterization of symbiotes from the Rocky Mountain wood tick, Dermacentor andersoni. J Invertebr Pathol. 1973 Nov;22(3):424-34.
10.) Hoerauf A, Rau RU, (ed.) Wolbachia: A Bug's Life in another Bug. Issues in Infectious Diseases. 2007S. Karger AG. (Switzerland) Vol. 5.
11.) Science Daily. Science News. River Blindness Caused by Bacteria, Not Worms, Suggesting Antibiotic Treatment for the Disease, Researchers Report. [Monograph on the Internet] 2002 Mar 12.
12.) Hertig M, Wolbach SB. Studies on Rickettsia-like microorganisms in insects. J Med Res. 1924;44:329-74.
13.) Yen JH, Barr AR. New hypothesis of the cause of cytoplasmic incompatibility in Culex pipiens. Nature 1971;232:657-658.
14.) New England Biolabs. Wolbachia Genome Project. Sequencing the Brugia malayi endosymbiont. [web site] 2002-2005 New England Biolabs.
15.) Zhiyong Xi, Dean Jeffry L, Khoo Cynthia, Dobson Stephen L. Generation of a novel Wolbachia infection in Aedes albopictus (Asian tiger mosquito) via embryonic microinjection. Insect Biochem Mol Biol. 2005;35:903-910.
16.) BBC News. Bug could combat dengue fever. 2009 Jan 2. [web page]
17.) McMeinman CF, Lane RV, Cass BN et al. Stable Introduction of a Life-Shortening Wolbachia Infection into the Mosquito Aedes aegypto. 2009. Science. 323:141.
18.) Sylvain Charlat, Markus Riegler, Isabelle Baures, et al. Incipient Evolution of Wolbachia Compatibility Types. Evolution. 2004;58(9):1901-1908.
19.) Hiroakinoda, Ulrike G. Munderloh, Timothy J. Kurtti. Endosymbionts of Ticks and Their Relationship to Wolbachia spp. and Tickborne Pathogens of Humans and Animals. Proceedings of the VII International Potsdam Symposium on Tickborne Diseases. Appl Environ Microbiol. 1997 Oct;63(10):3926-3932.
20.) Suitor EC Jr. Studies on the Cell Envelope of Wolbachia Persica. J Infect Dis. 1964 Apr;114:125-34.
21.) Cory J, Yunker CE, Howarth JA, Hokama Y, Hughes LE, Thomas LA, Clifford CM. Isolation of spotted fever group and Wolbachia-like agents from field-collected materials by means of plaque formation in mammalian and mosquito cells. Acta Virol. 1975 Sep;19(5):443-5.
22.) Stevens Lori, Giordano Rosanna, Fialho Roberto F. Male-Killing, Nematode Infections, Bacteriophage Infection, and Virulence of Cytoplasmic Bacteria in the Genus Wolbachia. Ann Rev Ecol System. 2001 Nov;32:519-545.
23.) Wenseleers T. Wolbachia: microbial insect symbionts and manipulators of reproduction. University of Sheffield. 2003. [slide presentation on the Internet].
24.) Stevens Lori. Male-Killing, Nematode Infections, Bacteriophage Infection, and Virulence of Cytoplasmic Bacteria in the Genus Wolbachia. Ann Rev. 2001 Nov;32:519-545.
25.) Masui S, Kuroiwa H, Sasaki T, et al. Bacteriophage WO and virus-like particles in Wolbachia, an endosymbiont of arthropods. Biochem Biophys Res Commun. 2001 May 25;283(5):1099-104.
26.) Grant 1Z01AI000062-06. Brinton, LP. Cellular and Subcellular Aspects of Vector-Pathogen Relationships. (Dr. Brinton was at the Rocky Mountain Laboratories at Hamilton, MT, although the location is not mentioned in the grant). Fiscal year 1975. No start and end date for the project. NIAID.
27.) CRISP. Grant 1Z01AI000062-06. Cellular and Subcellular Aspects of Vector-Pathogen Relationships. No school listed. Fiscal year 1975. National Institute of Allergy and Infectious Diseases.

28.) CRISP Grant 1Z01AI000062-07. Cellular and Subcellular Aspects of Vector-Pathogen Relatinoships. No school listed. Fiscal year 1977. National Institute of Allergy and Infectious Diseases.
29.) Brinton LP, Burgdorfer W. Intracellular manipulators of mite reproduction. Exp Appl. Acarol 1976;20:421–434.
30.) Burgdorfer W, Brinton LP. Intranuclear Growth of Rickettsia Canada, a Member of the Typhus Group. Infect Immun. 1970 Jul;2(1):112-114.
31.) Brinton LP, Burgdorfer W. Fine structure of Rickettsia Canada in tissues of Dermacentor andersoni Stiles. J Bacteriol. 1971 Mar;105(3):1149-59.
32.) Brinton LP, Burgdorfer W. Fine structure of normal hemocytes in Dermacentor andersoni Stiles (Acari: Ixodidae). J Parasitol. 1971 Oct;57(5):1110-27.
33.) Burgdorfer W, Brinton LP, Hughes LE. Isolation and characterization of symbiotes from the Rocky Mountain wood tick. Dermacentor andersoni. J Invertebr Pathol. 1973 Nov;22(3):424-34.
34.) Brinton LP, Burgdorfer W, Oliver JH Jr. Histology and fine structure of spermatozoa and egg passage in the female tract of Dermacentor andersoni stiles (acari-Ixodidae). Tissue Cell. 1974;6(1):109-25.
35.) Burgdorfer W, Brinton LP. Mechanisms of transovarial infection of spotted fever Rickettsiae in ticks. Ann NY Acad Sci. 1975;266:61-72.
36.) Burgdorfer W, Brinton LP), Hughes LE. Isolation and characterization of symbiotes from the Rocky Mountain wood tick, Dermacentor andersoni. J Invertebr Pathol. 1973;22:424-434.
37.) Pickens Edgar G, Gerloff Robert K, Burgdorfer Willy. Spirochete from the Rabbit Tick, Haemaphysalis leporispalustris (Packard). I. Isolation and Preliminary Characterization. J Bacteriol. 1968 Feb;95(2):291-299.
38.) Kettyls GD, Hopper JMH, Schmitt N. Serological Survey of Human Arbovirus Infections in Southeastern British Columbia. Canad Med Ass J. 1968 Sept 28;99:600-603.
39.) New Perspectives on The West. Montana. PBS. [web page]
40.) The Copper King. 125 Montana Newsmakers. Greatfalls Tribune. [web page]
41.) Wright John Burghardt. Montana places: exploring Big Sky Country. 2000 University of Minnesota Press, Minneapolis.
42.) Kettyls GD, Hopper JMH, Schmitt N. Serological Survey of Human Arbovirus Infections in Southeastern British Columbia. Canad Med Ass J. 1968 Sept 28;99:600-603.
43.) CRISP. Grant 5R22AI011847-08Cytoplasmic Incompatibility for Filariasis Control. University of California Los Angeles. Fiscal year 1975. Project began 1/6/73, ended 5/31/76. NIAID.
44.) CRISP Grant 5R29AI034355-03. Trans-Infection of Mosquitoes with Wolbachia Pipientis. Yale University. Fiscal year 1995. Project start 1/7/93, ended 6/30/98. NIAID.
45.) CRISP Grant 5R29AI034355-05. Trans-Infection of Mosquitoes with Wolbachia Pipientis. Yale University. Fiscal year 1997. Project start 1/7/93, ended 6/30/98. NIAID.
46.) Grant 1R01AI080597-01A1. Zhiyong Xi. Endosymbiont, Arbovirus & Mosquito Interactions and the Disease Control. Michigan State University. Fiscal year 2009. Project start 3/1/9, ends 2/28/14. ICD: NIAID.
47.) Grant 5R29AI034388-05. O'Neil, Scott L. Trans-Infection of Mosquitoes with Wolbachia Pipientis. Yale University. Fiscal year 1997. Project start: 7/1/93, ended 6/30/98. ICD: NIAID.
48.) Grant 5R01GM023468-30. Cline, Thomas. Regulation of Sex Specific Genes in Drosophila. University of California Berkeley. Fiscal year 2006. Project start: 1/1/77, ends 7/31/10. ICD: National Institute of General Medical Sciences.
49.) Grant 1R43AI061865-01. Carlow, Clotilde K. Development of a novel nematode/Wolbachia target. New England Biolabs, Inc. Fiscal year 2004. Project start date: 7/1/04, ended 12/31/04. NIAID.
50.) Grant 5R22AI011847-08. Barr, A Ralph. Cytoplasmic Incompatibility for Filariasis Control. University of California Los Angeles. Fiscal year 1975. Project start date 6/1/73, ends 5/31/76. NIAID.
51.) Grant 5R29AI034355-04. O'Neill Scott L. Trans-Infection of Mosquitoes with Wolbachia Pipientis. Yale University School of Public Health. Fiscal year 1996. Project start date: 7/1/93, ended 7/30/98. NIAID.
52.) CRISP Grant 5R31AI009553-03. Minority Predoctoral Fellowship Program. Melinda M. Pettigrew. Yale University. EPH (School of Public Health). Project start 10/1/97. No end date. NIAID.
53.) Niebylski ML, Peacock MG, Fischer ER, Porcella SF, Schwan TG. Characterization of an endosymbiont infecting wood ticks, Dermacentor andersoni, as a member of the genus Francisella. Appl Environ Microbiol. 1997 Oct;63(10):3933-40.
54.) Zhiyong Xi, Dean Jeffry L, Khoo Cynthia, Dobson Stephen L. Generation of a novel Wolbachia infection in Aedes albopictus (Asian tiger mosquito) via embryonic microinjection. Insect Biochem Mol Biol. 2005;35:903-910.
55.) Cheng LL, Rodas JD, Schultz KT. Et al. Potential for Evolution of California Serogroup Bunyaviruses by Genome Reassortment in Aedes Albopictus. Am J Trop Med Hyg. 1999;60(3):430-438
56.) Personal communication between the author and Marketing Director for the North Carolina Center for Reproductive Medicine. Sharon McCloud. (www.nccrm.com) October 3, 2008.
57.) North Carolina Center for Reproductive Medicine. [web page]
58.) Talbert LM, Hammond MG, Halme J, O'Rand M, Sloan C, Bailey L. In vitro fertilization at the North Carolina Memorial Hospital in Chapel Hill. NC Med J 1985 Jun;46(6):338-40.
59.) Talbert LM, Hammond MG, Halme J, O'Rand M, Fryer JG, Ekstrom RD. Semen parameters and fertilization of human oocytes in vitro: a multivariable analysis. Fertil Steril 1987 Aug;48(2):270-7.
60.) Cory J, Yunker CE, Howarth JA, et al. Isolation of spotted fever group and Wolbachia-like agents from field-collected materials by means of plaque formation in mammalian and mosquito cells. Acta Virol. 1975 Sept;19(5):443-445.
61.) Tully JG, Whitcomb RF, Rose DL, et al. Characterization and Taxonomic Status of Tick Spiroplasmas: A Review. The Yale J Biol Med. 1983;56:599-603.
62.) van Overbeek L, Gassner F, van der Plas CL, Kastelein P, Nunes-da Rocha U, Takken W. Diversity of Ixodes ricinus tick-associated bacterial communities from different forests. FEMS Microbiol Ecol. 2008 Oct;66(1):72-84.
63.) Avakyan AA, Popov VL. Rickettsiaceae and Chlamydiaceae: comparative electron microscopic studies. Acta Virol. 1984 Mar;28(2):159-173.
64.) 81. Cory J, Yunker CE, Howarth JA, et al. Isolation of spotted fever group and Wolbachia-like agents from field-collected materials by means of plaque formation in mammalian and mosquito cells. Acta Virol. 1975 Sept;19(5):443-445.
65.) Schmid George P, Steere Allen C, Kornblatt Arnold A, Kaufmann Arnold F, Moss C. Wayne, Johnson Russell C, Hovind-Hougen Kari, Brenner Don J. Newly Recognized Leptospira Series ("Leptospira inadai" serovar lyme) Isolated from Human Skin. J Clin Microbiol. 1986 Sept.;24(3):484-486.

March of the Spiroplasmas

1.) Ludwig W, Schleifer KH, Whitman WB. Revised road map to the phylum Firmicutes. In De Vos P et al (eds) Bergey's Manual of Systematic Bacteriology. Vol 3, 2nd ed. 2009 Sep 15. Springer-Vertag, New York. ISBN: 0-387-95041-9.
2.) Nienhaus F, Sikora RA. Mycoplasmas, Spiroplasmas, and Rickettsia-like Organisms as Plant Pathogens. Ann Rev Phytopathol. 1979;17:37-58.
3.) Jensen DD. A plant virus lethal to its insect vector. Virol. 1959 Jun;8(2):164-175.
4.) Phillips RN, Humphery-Smith I. The Histopathology of Experimentally Inducted Infections of Spiroplasma taiwanense (Class: Mollicutes) in Anopheles stephensi Mosquitoes. J Invert Pathol. 1995 Sept;66(2):185-195.
5.) Hackett KJ, Whitcomb RF, Tully JG, et al. Lampyridae (Coleoptera): A plethora of mollicute associations. Microb Ecol. 1992 Jun;23(2):181-193.
6.) Carle P, Laigret F, Tully JG, Bové JM. Heterogeneity of Genome Sizes within the Genus Sprioplasma. Inter J System Bacteriol. 1995 Jan;45(1):178-181.
7.) Tully JG, Rose DL, Yunker CE, et al: Helical mycoplasmas (spiroplasmas) in Ixodes ticks. Science 1982;212:1043-1045.
8.) Whitcomb RF. The Genus Spiroplasma. Ann Rev Microbiol. 1980 Oct;34:677-704.
9.) Agricultural Microbes Genome 2: First Glimpses into the Genomes of Plant-Associated Microbes. The Plant Cell. 2001 Mar;13:451-457.
10.) Nome C, Magalhães PC, Oliveira E, et al. Differences in intracellular localization of corn stunt spiroplasmas in magnesium treated maize. Biocell (Mendoza) 2009;33(2):133-136.
11.) Nejat N, Vadaalai G, Dickinson M. Spiroplasma citri: A Wide Host Range Phytopathogen. Plant Pathol Journal. 2011;10(2):46-56.
12.) Miklossy Judith, Kasas Sandor, Zurn Anne D, et al. J Neuroinflam. 2008 Sept 25;5:40.
13.) US Patent 7,432,419. Gupta. Compositions and methods for the treatment of Pierce's disease. Filed 5/14/04, published 10/7/08. Assignee: Los Alamos National Security, LLC (Los Alamos, NM)
14.) Tully et al. Helical Mycoplasmas (Spiroplasmas) from Ixodes Ticks. Science. 1981;212(4498):1043-1045.

15.) Fawcett HS, Perry JC, Johnston JC. The stubborn disease of citrus. Calif. Cirtog. 1944;29:146-147.
16.) Fawcett HS, Wallace JM. Evidence of virus nature of citrus quick decline. Calif. Citrog. 1946;32:88-89.
17.) Reuther W, Calavan EC, Carman GE (ed.) The Citrus Industry. Vol. IV Crop Protection. University of California Div. of Agricultural Sciences. 1978. Page 128.
18.) Agricultural Microbes Genome 2: First Glimpses into the Genomes of Plant-Associated Microbes. The Plant Cell. 2001 Mar;13:451-457.
19.) Williamson DL, Brink PR, Zieve GW. Spiroplasma fibrils. Isr J Med Sci. 1984 Sep;20(9):830-835.
20.) US Patent 7,405,342. Finberg. Transgenic mice expressing heterologous complement receptor type 1 (CR1) molecules on erythrocytes and uses therefor. Filed 5/10/04 published 7/29/08. Assignee: University of Massachusetts (Worcester, MA).
21.) Baar J, Shulman MJ. The Ig heavy chain switch region is a hotspot for insertion of transfected DNA. J Immunol. 1995;155:1911-1920.
22.) Ronai Diana, Berru Maribel, Shulman Marc J. Variegated Expression of the Endogenous Immunoglobulin Heavy-Chain Gene in the Absence of the Intronic Locus Control Region. Mol Cell Biol. 1999 Oct;19(10):7031-7040.
23.) US Patent 7,521,424. Rosen et al.Albumin fusion proteins. Filed 7/7/05 published 4/21/09. Assignee: Human Genome Sciences , Inc. (Rockville, MD).
24.) US Patent 3,709,782. Smith et al. Heterploid Cell Lines. Filed 10/3/69, issued 1/9/73. Assignee: Burroughs Wellcome Co., Research Triangle Park, NC.
25.) O'Leary William Michael. Practical handbook of microbiology. 1977 Condensed version of CRC handbook of microbiology. CRC Press LLC. (Boca Raton, FL). Laskin AI, Lechevalier HA (ed). 2nd ed.
26.) Barbour AG, Hayes SF. Biology of Borrelia Species. Microbiol Rev 1986 Dec;50(4):381-400
27.) Clark TB. Spiroplasma sp. a new pathogen in honey bees. J Inverteb. Pathol. 1977;29:112-113.
28.) Williamson DL, Poulson DF. Sex ratio organisms (spiroplasmas) of Drosophila. 1979 p. 175-208. In RF Whitcomb and JG Tully (ed.), The mycoplasmas, vol. 3. Academic Press, Inc. NY.
29.) Williamson DL. Whitcomb RF. Helical, wall-free prokaryotes in Drosophila, leafhoppers and plants. 1974 Colloq. INSERM 33:282-290.
30.) Stalheim Ole HV, Ritchie Alfred E. Whitcomb Robert F. Cultivation, Serology, Ultrastructure, and Virus-Like Particles of Spiroplasma 277F. Curr Micrbiol. Vol. 1. 1978:365-370.
31.) Steiner Theodor, McGarrity Gerard J, Phillips David M. Cultivation and Partial Characterization of Spiroplasmas in Cell Cultures. Infect Immun. 1982 Jan;35(1):296-304.
32.) US Patent 4,166,118. Cosgrove, et al. Use of chlorhydroxyquinolone to inhibit growth of mycoplasmas. Filed 10/2/78 published 8/28/79. Assignee: E.R. Squibb & Sons, Inc. (Princeton, NJ).
33.) Bastian Frank O, Sanders Dearl E, Forbes Will A., et al. Spiroplasma spp. from transmissible spongiform encephalopathy brains or ticks induce spongiform encephalopathy in ruminants. J Med Microbiol. 2007;56:1235-1242.
34.) Bastian FO, Purnell DM, Tully JG. Neuropathology of Spiroplasma Infection in the Rat Brain. AJP. 1984 Mar;114(3):496-514.
35.) US Patent 4,129,721. Michel, et al. A-40104antibiotics and process for production thereof. Filed 12/8/77, issued 12/12/78. Assignee: Eli Lilly and Company (Indianapolis, IN).
36.) Townsend R, Burgess J, Plaskitt KA. Morphology and ultrastructure of helical and nonhelical strains of Spiroplasma citri. J Bacteriol. 1980 Jun;142(3):973-981.
37.) Johnson Russell C. (ed.) The Biology of Parasitic Spirochetes. 1976 Academic Press, New York.
38.) CRISP. Grant 1Z01AI000062-06. Cellular and Subcellular Aspects of Vector-Pathogen Relationships. No school listed. Fiscal year 1975. National Institute of Allergy and Infectious Diseases.
39.) Bové JM. Spiroplasmas: infectious agents of plants, arthropods and vertebrates. Wien Klin Wochenschr. 1997 Aug 8;109(14-15):604-612.
40.) CRISP Grant 1Z01AI000062-07. Cellular and Subcellular Aspects of Vector-Pathogen Relatinoships. No school listed. Fiscal year 1977. National Institute of Allergy and Infectious Diseases.
41.) Williamson DL, Tully JG, Whitcomb RF. Serological Relationships of Spiroplasmas as Shown by Combined Deformation and Metabolism Inhibition Tests. Inter J System Bacteriol. 1979 Oct;29(4):345-351.
42.) Stalheim OHV, Ritchie AE, Whitcomb RF. Cultivation, serology, ultrastructure, and virus-like particles of sprioplasma 277F. Curr Microbiol. 1978 Dec;1(6):365-370. US Department of Agriculture, National Animal Disease Center (Ames, Iowa) and USDA Plant Protection Institute (Beltsville, MD).
43.) Reuther Walter, Calavan E. Clair, Carman Glenn E. (ed) The Citrus Industry. Volume IV. Diseases and Injuries; Viruses; Registration, Certification, Indexing; Regulatory Measures; Vertebrate Pests; Biological Control of Insects; Nematodes. University of California Div. of Agriculture and Natural Resources. 1978 The Regents of the University of California.
44.) Christiansen Claus, Freundt EA, Maramorosch K. Identity of cactus and lettuce spiroplasmas with Spiroplasma citri as determined by DNA-DNA hybridization. Curr Micrbiol. 1980 Nov;4(6):353-356.
45.) Babbar OP, Shukla US, Agnihotri VP, Singh K. Appearance of transmissible disease syndrome in maize (Zea mays L.) plants infected with avian mycoplasma. Curr Sci. 1973;42:190-92.
46.) USDA. Agricultural Research Service. National Program 303: Plant Diseases FY 2004 Annual Report. [web page]
47.) Lee RF, Raju BC, Nyland G. Phytotoxin(s) produced by the Pierce's disease organism grown in culture. Phytopathol News. 1978;12:216 [abstract].
48.) Hopkins DL. Diseases caused by leafhopper-borne, Rickettsia-like bacteria. Ann Rev Phytopathol. 1977;15:277-94.
49.) Tully JG, Rose DL, Yunker CE, Cory J, Whitcomb RF, Williamson DL. Helical mycoplasmas (spiroplasmas) from Ixodes ticks. Science. 1981 May 29;212(4498):1043-5.
50.) Agricultural Microbes Genome 2: First Glimpses into the Genomes of Plant-Associated Microbes. The Plant Cell. 2001 Mar;13:451-457.
51.) Moreira LM, DeSouza RF, Digiampietri LA, et al. Comparative Analyses of Xanthomonas and Xylella Complete Genomes. J Integrat Biol. 2005 Spring;9(1):43-76.
52.) Los Alamos National Security. Wikipedia.
53.) US Patent 7,432,419Gupta. Compositions and methods for the treatment of Pierce's disease. Assignee Los Alamos National Security, LLC (Los Alamos, MN). Filed 5/14/04, published 10/7/08.
54.) Kamoun Sophien, Hogenhout Saskia A. Agricultural Microbes Genome 2: First Glimpses into the Genomes of Plant-Associated Microbes. Amer Soc Plant Biologists. The Plant Cell. 2001 Mar;13:451-457.
55.) Garcia R, Gusmani L, Murgia R, et al. Elastase is the only Human Neutrophil Granule Protein that alone is Responsible for In Vitro killing of Borrelia burgdorferi. Infect Immun. 1998;66:1408-1412.
56.) Montgomery RR, Lusitani D, de Boisfleury Chevance A, Malawista SE. Human Phagocytic Cells in the Early Innate Immune Response to Borrelia burgdorferi. J Infect Dis. 2002;185:1773-9.
57.) Campanelli D, Detmers PA, Nathan CF, Gabay JE. Azurocidin and a homologous serine protease from neutrophils. Differential antimicrobial and proteolytic properties. J Clin Invest. 1990 May;85(3):904-915.
58.) Tully JG, Whitcomb RF, Rose DL, Williamson DL, Bové JM. Characterization and taxonomic status of tick spiroplasmas: a review. Yale J Biol Med. 1983 Sep-Dec;56(5-6):599-603.
59.) Henning K, Greiner-Fischer S, Hotel H, Ebsen M, Theegarten D. Isolation of Sprioplasma sp. from an Ixodes tick. Int J Med Microbiol. 2006 May;296Suppl. 40:157-61. Epub 2006 Mar 9.
60.) Halos L, Mavris M, Vourc G, et al. Broad-range PCR-TTGE for the first-line detection of bacterial pathogen DNA in ticks. Vet Res. 2006;37:245-253.
61.) Tully JG, DL Rose, CE Yunker, J Cory, RF Whitcomb, DL Williamson. 1981. Helical mycoplasmas (spiroplasmas) from Ixodes ticks. Science 1981;212(4498):1043-1045.
62.) Mouchès C, Candresse T, Barroso G, Saillard C, Wroblewski H, Bové JM. Gene for Spiralin, the Major Membrane Protein of the Helical Mollicute Spiroplasma citri: Cloning and Expression in Escherichia coli. J Bacteriol. 1985 Dec;164(3):1094-1099.
63.) Wise KS. Adaptative surface variation. Trends Microbiol. 1993;1:59-63.
64.) Watson HL, Zheng X, Cassell GH. Structural variations and phenotypic switching of mycoplasmal antigens. Clin Infect Dis. 1993;17:S183-S186.
65.) MacDonald AB. The Molecular Link Between Alzheimer's Disease and Borrelia. [Internet podcast].
66.) Comer John B. Genesis of Jamaican Bauxite. Economic Geology. 1974 Dec;69(8):1251-1264.
67.) Compton SR, Riley LK. Detection of infectious agents in laboratory rodents: traditional and molecular techniques. Comparative Med. 2001;51:113-119.
68.) Lipson SM, Stotzky G. Effect of proteins on reovirus adsorption to clay minerals. Appl. Environ. Microbiol. 1984 Sept;48(3):525-530.
69.) Proceedings of the Second National Conference on Serologic Diagnosis of Lyme Disease. 1994 Oct. 27-29, Dearborn, MI. 106 pages. Sponsors: Assoc. of State and Territorial Public Health Laboratory Directors, US CDC and Prevention, MI Dept. of Health. Co-sponsors: USFDA, NIH, Council of State and Territorial Epidemiologists and National Committee for Clinical Laboratory Standards.

70.) MacDonald AB. Alzheimer's neuroborreliosis with trans-synaptic spread of infection and neurofibrillary tangles derived from intraneuronal spirochetes. Med Hypotheses. 2007;68(4):822-825. [Epub 2006 Oct. 20]
71.) Duret S, Berho N, Danet JL et al. Spiralin Is Not Essential for Helicity, Motility, or Pathogenicity but Is Required for Efficient Transmission of Spiroplasma citri by Its Leafhopper Vector Circulifer haematoceps. Appl Envir Microbiol. 2003 Oct;69(10):6225-6234
72.) Tilly K, Krum J, Bestor A, et al. Borrelia burgdorferi OspC Protein Required Exclusively in a Crucial Early Stage of Mammalian Infection. Infec Immun. 2006 June;74(6):3554-3564.
73.) Neelakanta G, Li X, Pal U, Liu X, Beck DS, DePonte K, Fish D, Kantor FS, Fikrig E. Outer Surface Protein B Is Critical for Borrelia burgdorferi Adherence and Survival within Ixodes Ticks. PLOS Pathogens. 2007 Mar;3(3). 11 pgs.]
74.) Johnson Norman. Evolution in Action: A New Mutualism. Watching the Detectives Blog.
75.) Yong Ed. Friendly bacteria protect flies from sterilising worms. Discover. 2010 Jul 9. [web page]
76.) Jaenike J, Stahlhut JK, Boelio LM, Unckless RL. Association between Wolbachia and Spiroplasma within Drosophila neotestacea: an emerging symbiotic mutualism? Mol Ecol. 2010 Jan;19(2):414-425.]
77.) Keim Brandon. Parasite-Busting Bugs Throw Fruit Fly Evolution in Overdrive. Wired Science. 2010 Jul 8. (internet monograph).
78.) McKeever S, Gorman GW, Chapman JF et al. Incidence of Leptospirosis in Wild Mammals from Southwestern Georgia, with a Report of New Hosts for Six Serotypes of Leptospires. CDC, Bureau of State Services, Public Health Service, US Dept. of Health, Education and Welfare, Atlanta, Georgia and Emory University Field Station, Newton, GA. Am J Trop Med Hyg. 1958;7(6):646-655.
79.) Wiki: Eugene Odum. [web page]
80.) Cole RM, Tully JG, Popkin TJ, Bové JM. Morphology, Ultrastructure, and Bacteriophage Infection of the Helical Mycoplasma-Like Organism (Spiroplasma citri gen. nov., sp. nov.) Cultured from "Stubborn" Disease of Citris. J Bacteriol. 1973 July;115(1):367-386
81.) Hackett KJ, Henegar RB, Whitcomb RF, et al. Distribution and biological control significance of Colorado potato beetle spiroplasmas in North America. Biol Control. 1992 Aug;2(3):218-225.
82.) Clark TB, Whitcomb RF. Pathogenicity of mollicutes for insects: possible use in biological control. Ann Microbiol (Paris). 1984 Jan-Feb;135A(1):141-150.
83.) Humphery-Smith I, Grulet O, LeGoff F, Robaux P, Chastel C. [Basic research on the use of mosquito spiroplasmas in the control of the major tropical diseases transmitted by mosquitoes]. [Article in French]. [abstract] Bull Soc Pathol Exot. 1991;84(5Pt 5):693-696.
84.) Clark TB, Whitcomb RF, Tully JG. Spiroplasmas from Coleopterous Insects: New Ecological Dimensions. Microb Ecol. 1982;8:401-409.

A Fungal Spiroplasma is Born

1.) W. Kenneth Hoover. The Biological Control of Detrimental Insects. 1933 Oct;4(3):75-89.
2.) US Patent 3,337,395. Robert Z. Page (Springfied, VA). Termite Control by Induced Epizootics of Entomophagous Microorganisms. Filed 11/27/63, published 8/22/67.
3.) DeBach P, Rosen D. Biological control by natural enemies. Cambridge University Press 1974, 1991. pp. 136
4.) Castleberry MW, Converse JI, Sinski JT, Lowe EP, Pakes SP. Coccidioidomycosis: Studies of Canine Vaccination and Therapy. University of Chicago. J Infect Dis. 1965 Feb;115:41-48.
5.) Converse John Lay, Fakes Steven P., Snyder Ernest Manford, Castleberry Merida William. Experimental Primary Cutaneous Coccidioidomycosis in the Monkey. AD288870. Tech. Manuscript 22. US Army Biological Laboratories, Fort Detrick. 1962 Nov. The report was presented at the 7th annual meeting of the VA-Armed Forces Coccidioidomycosis Study Group, Los Angeles, CA November 1962. The work was conducted under project 4B11-02-066, Bacterial and Fungal Agent Research, Task -02, Bacterial and Fungal Laboratory Research.
6.) Smith CE, Pappagiania D, Saito M. The Public Health Significance of Coccidioidomycosis. Public Health Service Publication. 1957;575:3-9.
7.) Colwell Ja. Remission in disseminated coccidiodomycosis produced by amphotericin B. Ann Intern Med 1959 Apr;50(4):1028-1035.
8.) Gephardt MC, Hanlon TJ. Treatment of disseminated coccidiomycosis with stilbamidine (case history). J Okla State Med Assoc. 1954 Mar;47(3):55-58.
9.) Comparative Pathogenesis of Canine and Simian Coccidioidomycosis. 1963 March. US Army Biological Laboratories, Fort Detrick. Technical Manual 41. AD 401301. Presented at the 7th annual meeting of the VA-Armed Forces Coccidioidomycosis Study Group, Los Angeles, CA, 1962 November.
10.) Rixford E, Gilchrist TC. Two Cases of Protozoan (Coccidioidal) Infection of the Skin and Other Organs. Johns Hopkins Hospital. Report 1. 1896. pages 209-265.
11.) Posodas A. Psorospuniose Infectant Generalise. Rev. Chir. Paris. 1900;20:277-282.
12.) Kisielswicz Josef et al. Case of Coccidioidomycosis of the Lungs. Prlski Tygodnik Lekarski (Polish Medical Weekly) 1968;23(2) 760-762. Department of the Army. Fort Detrick, MD. AD854029. Translation no. 2434 dated May 1969.
13.) Reuther Walter, Calavan E. Clair, Carman Glenn E. (eds.) The Citrus Industry, Volume IV. Diseases and Injuries: viruses; Registration, Certification, Indexing; Regulatory Measures; Vertebrate Pests; Biological Control of Insects; Nematodes. Revised Edition. 1978. University of California Division of Agricultural Sciences. The Regents of the University of Califonia.
14.) Contemporary State of Experimental Investigations on the Specific Prophylaxis of Coccidiodomycosis (Review). Translated text of poor quality. 1968 November. Translation No. 2360, document AD680493. Department of the Army, Fort Detrick, Frederick, Maryland.
15.) APHIS National Select Agents Registry. HHS Select Agents and Toxins. Coccidioides posadasii / Coccidioides immitis. [web page]
16.) Green Deborah R, Koenig Gina, Fisher Matthew C, Taylor John W. Soil Isolation and Molecular Identification of Coccidioides immitis. Mycologia. 2000 May-June;92(3):406-410.
17.) Micorbiology and Immunology on-line. University of South Carolina School of Medicine. C. coccidioidomycosis (Coccidioides immitis). [web page]
18.) Bordeaux Mixture now on the Chem One Copper Sulfate Crystals Pesticide Label. Approval pending in California. [web page]
19.) Langhoff PJ. God Science: The Secret World of Rampant Genetics, Hidden Illness, and Biotech Profiteering. 2010 Allegory press LLC. Hustisford, WI.
20.) US Patent 3,699,223. Bergy et al. Enhygrofungin and Process for Preparing the Same. Filed 6/13/69 published 10/17/72. Assignee: The Upjohn Company (Kalamazoo, MI).
21.) US Patent 3,709,782. Smith et al. Heterpoloid Cell Lines. Filed 10/3/69, issued 1/9/73. Assignee: Burroughs Wellcome Co., Research Triangle Park, NC.
22.) O'Leary William Michael. Practical handbook of microbiology. 1977Condensed version of CRC handbook of microbiology. CRC Press LLC. (Boca Raton, FL). Laskin AI, Lechevalier HA (ed). 2nd ed.
23.) Barbour AG, Hayes SF. Biology of Borrelia Species. Microbiol Rev 1986 Dec;50(4):381-400
24.) Clark TB. Spiroplasma sp. a new pathogen in honey bees. J Inverteb. Pathol. 1977;29:112-113.
25.) Williamson DL, Poulson DF. Sex ratio organisms (spiroplasmas) of Drosophila. 1979 p. 175-208. In RF Whitcomb and JG Tully (ed.), The mycoplasmas, vol. 3. Academic Press, Inc. NY.
26.) Williamson DL. Whitcomb RF. Helical, wall-free prokaryotes in Drosophila, leafhoppers and plants. 1974 Colloq. INSERM 33:282-290.
27.) Stalheim Ole HV, Ritchie Alfred E. Whitcomb Robert F. Cultivation, Serology, Ultrastructure, and Virus-Like Particles of Spiroplasma 277F. Curr Micrbiol. Vol. 1. 1978:365-370.
28.) Steiner Theodor, McGarrity Gerard J, Phillips David M. Cultivation and Partial Characterization of Spiroplasmas in Cell Cultures. Infect Immun. 1982 Jan;35(1):296-304.
29.) US Patent 4,166,118. Cosgrove, et al. Use of chlorhydroxyquinolone to inhibit growth of mycoplasmas. Filed 10/2/78 published 8/28/79. Assignee: E.R. Squibb & Sons, Inc. (Princeton, NJ).
30.) Bastian Frank O, Sanders Dearl E, Forbes Will A., et al. Spiroplasma spp. from transmissible spongiform encephalopathy brains or ticks induce spongiform encephalopathy in ruminants. J Med Microbiol. 2007;56:1235-1242.
31.) Bastian FO, Purnell DM, Tully JG. Neuropathology of Spiroplasma Infection in the Rat Brain. AJP. 1984 Mar;114(3):496-514.
32.) US Patent 4,129,721. Michel, et al. A-40104antibiotics and process for production thereof. Filed 12/8/77, issued 12/12/78. Assignee: Eli Lilly and Company (Indianapolis, IN).
33.) St George TD, Standfast HA, Cybinski DH, et al. Peaton virus: a new Simbu group Arbovirus isolated from cattle and Culicoides brevitarsis in Australia. Aust J Biol. Sci. 1980 May;33(2):235-43.
34.) Hardy JL, Lyness RN, Rush WA. Experimental Vector and Wildlife Host Ranges of Buttonwillow Virus in Kern County, California. Am J Trop Med Hyg. 1972;21(1):100-109. School of Public Health, University of California, Berkeley, California 94720.
35.) Hardy JL, Scrivani RP, Lyness RN, et al. Ecologic Studies on Buttonwillow Virus in Kern County, California, 1961-1968. Am J Trop Med Hyg. 1970;19(3):552-563.
36.) Reeves WC, Scrivani RP, Hardy JL, et al. Buttonwillow Virus, a New Arbovirus Isolated from Mammals and Culicoides Midges in Kern County, California. Am J Trop Med Hyg. 1970;19(3):544-551.

37.) Gerone PJ, Couch RB, Keefer GV, et al. Assessment of Experimental and Natural Viral Aerosols. Bacteriol. Rev. 1966 Sept;30(3):576-584.
38.) A Brief History of Polio. From Ancient Egypt to the 20th Century. [web site]
39.) Goodwin Ronald H, Filshie Barry K. Morphology and development of entomopoxviruses from two Australian scarab beetle larvae (Coleoptera: Scarabaeidae). J Invert Pathol. 1975Jan;25(1):35-46.
40.) Scotti PD, Dearing Sally, Mossop DW. Flock house virus: A Nodavirus isolated from Costelytra zealandica (White) (Coleoptera: Scarabaeida). Arch Virol. 1983 Sept;75(3):181-189.
41.) Dasgupta R, Cheng LL, Bartholomay LC, Christensen BM. Flock house virus replicates and expresses green fluorescent protein in mosquitoes. J Gen Virol. 2003;84:1789-1797.
42.) Burges HD, Hussey NW. Microbial Control of Insects and Mites. 1971 Academic Press Inc. London. p. 105-118.
43.) Hirschmann Jan V. The Early History of Coccidioidomycosis: 1892-1945. Clin Infect Dis. 2007;44:1202-1207.
44.) Reuther W, Calavan EC, Carman GE. The Citrus Industry Vol. IV. Diseases and Injuries, Viruses Registration, Certification, Indexing, Regulatory Measures, Vertebrate Pests, Biological Control of Insects; Nematodes. Revised Edition. Div. of Agriculture and Natural Resources. 1978. University of California Div. of Agricultural Sciences.
45.) Suryanarayanan S, McConnell WB. The Metabolism of Perlargonate-1-C14by Wheat Stem Rust Uredospores. 1964 May 8. 1 page [abstract] AD0456244. Corp. author: National Research Council of Canada Saskatoon (Saskatchewan) Prairie Regional Lab.
46.) US Patent Application 20100130561. Andersch, Wolfram, et al. Controlling Pests by Combining Insecticides and Transgenic Plants by Applying Directly to Leaves and Roots. Andersch; Wolfram; et al. Filed 4/14/08 published 5/27/10. Assignee: Bayer Cropscience AG. (Monheim, DE).
47.) Line Roland F, Peet Clyde E, Kingsolver Charles H. Stem Rust Infection and Development in Artificially Inoculated Fields of Wheat at Hays, Kansas, and its Effect on Yield, 1960 to 1965. Corporate Author: Fort Detrick Frederick MD. Report date 1968Aug. 10 pages. Report #AD0843597. Project #DA-1-B-522301-A-061.
48.) Bové JM, Mouches C, Carle-Junca P. et al. Spiroplasmas of Group I: The Spiroplasma citri Cluster. Yale J Biol Med. 1983;56:573-582.
49.) Murray Polly. The Widening Circle. A Lyme Disease Pioneer Tells Her Story. 1996. St. Martin's Press, NY.
50.) Tully JG, Whitcomb RF, Bové JM et al. Plant mycoplasmas: serological relation between agents associated with citrus stubborn and corn stunt diseases. Science 1973;182:827-829.
51.) Clark HF, Rorke LB. Spiroplasmas of tick origin and their pathogenicity. In The Mycoplasmas, Volume 3. Plant and Insect Mycoplasmas. Whitcomb RF, Tully JG (ed.) New York, Academic Press. 1979:155-174.
52.) Zeigel RF, Clark HF. Electron microscopy of the suckling mouse cataract agent, a noncultivable animal pathogen possibly related to mycoplasma. Infect Immun. 1974;9:430-443.
53.) Junca P, Saillard C, Tully JG et al. Caractérisation de spirooplasmes isolés d'insectes et de fleurs de France continentale, de Course et du Maroc. Proposition pour une classification des spiroplasmes. CR Acad Sci (Paris) 1980;Ser D 290:1209-1212.
54.) Tully Joseph G, Rose David L, Yunker Conrad E, et al. Helical Mycoplasmas (Spiroplasmas) from Ixodes Ticks. Science 1981;212(4498):1043-1045.
55.) Grant 1Z01AI000062-06. Cellular and Subcellular Aspects of Vector-Pathogen Relationships. No school listed. Fiscal year 1975. National Institute of Allergy and Infectious Diseases (NIAID).
56.) Grant 1Z01AI000062-07. Cellular and Subcellular Aspects of Vector-Pathogen Relationships. No school listed. Fiscal year 1977. NIAID.
57.) Reimer LG. Q fever. Clin Microbiol Rev 1993 Jul;6(3):193-198 And Tylewska-Wierzbanowska S, Kruszewska D, Chmielewski T, et al. [Ticks as a reservoir of Borrelia burgdorferi and Coxiella burnetii on Polish terrain]. Przegl Epidemiol. 1996;50(3):245-251. Article in Polish
58.) Cherry CB, Bartlett AG. The Diagnosis of Acute Coccidioides immitis Infections. Bulletin US Army M Dept. 6. 1946 Feb;5:190-193.
59.) Rifkin Feldman D.J. II, Hawes LJ, Gordon LE. Coexisting Tuberculosis and Coccidioidomycosis. Arch Int Mod. 1947 Apr;79:381-390.
60.) Smith CE, Saito MT, Beard RR, Rosenberger HG, Whiting EG. Histoplasmin Sensitivity and Coccidioidal Infection. 1. Occurrence of Cross-Reactions. Am J Pub Health. 1949 Jun;39(722-736).
61.) Castleberry MW, Converse JI, Sinski JT, Lowe EP, Pakes SP. Coccidioidomycosis: Studies of Canine Vaccination and Therapy. University of Chicago. J Infect Dis. 1965 Feb;115:41-48.
62.) Converse John Lay, Fakes Steven P., Snyder Ernest Manford, Castleberry Merida William. Experimental Primary Cutaneous Coccidioidomycosis in the Monkey. AD288870. Tech. Manuscript 22. US Army Biological Laboratories, Fort Detrick. 1962 Nov. The report was presented at the 7th annual meeting of the VA-Armed Forces Coccidioidomycosis Study Group, Los Angeles, CA November 1962. The work was conducted under project 4B11-02-066, Bacterial and Fungal Agent Research, Task -02, Bacterial and Fungal Laboratory Research.
63.) Smith CE, Pappagiania D, Saito M. The Public Health Significance of Coccidioidomycosis. Public Health Service Publication. 1957;575:3-9.
64.) Colwell Ja. Remission in disseminated coccidiodomycosis produced by amphotericin B. Ann Intern Med 1959 Apr;50(4):1028-1035.
65.) Gephardt MC, Hanlon TJ. Treatment of disseminated coccidiomycosis with stilbamidine (case history). J Okla State Med Assoc. 1954 Mar;47(3):55-58.
66.) Comparative Pathogenesis of Canine and Simian Coccidioidomycosis. 1963March. US Army Biological Laboratories, Fort Detrick. Technical Manual 41. AD 401301. Presented at the 7th annual meeting of the VA-Armed Forces Coccidioidomycosis Study Group, Los Angeles, CA, 1962 November.
67.) Rixford E, Gilchrist TC. Two Cases of Protozoan (Coccidioidal) Infection of the Skin and Other Organs. Johns Hopkins Hospital. Report 1. 1896. pages 209-265.
68.) Posodas A. Psorospuniose Infectant Generalise. Rev. Chir. Paris. 1900;20:277-282.
69.) Kisielswicz Josef et al. Case of Coccidioidomycosis of the Lungs. Prlski Tygodnik Lekarski (Polish Medical Weekly) 1968;23(2):760-762. Department of the Army. Fort Detrick, MD. AD854029. Translation no. 2434 dated May 1969.
70.) Reuther Walter, Calavan E. Clair, Carman Glenn E. (eds.) The Citrus Industry, Volume IV. Diseases and Injuries: viruses; Registration, Certification, Indexing; Regulatory Measures; Vertebrate Pests; Biological Control of Insects; Nematodes. Revised Edition. 1978. University of California Division of Agricultural Sciences. The Regents of the University of California.
71.) Contemporary State of Experimental Investigations on the Specific Prophylaxis of Coccidiodomycosis (Review). Translated text of poor quality. 1968November. Translation No. 2360, document AD680493. Department of the Army, Fort Detrick, Frederick, Maryland.
72.) Garrity, George M, Brenner Don J, Krieg Noel R, Staley James T. (eds.) Bergey's Manual of Systematic Bacteriology, Volume Two: The Proteobacteria, Part C: The Alpha-, Beta-, Delta-, and Epsilonproteobacteria. 2005 Springer, New York, New York.
73.) Langer Elinor, Listowell Judith. Chemical and Biological Warfare. Survival. 1967 Apr;9(4):128-135.
74.) US Patent 3,699,223. Bergy et al. Enhygrofungin and Process for Preparing the Same. Filed 6/13/69 published 10/17/72. Assignee: The Upjohn Company (Kalamazoo, MI).

Spirochetes and Yellows Diseases

1.) Ritambhara T, Girjesh K. Genetic loss through heavy metal induced chromosomal stickiness in Grass pea. Caryologia. 2010;63(3):223-228.
2.) US Patent 3,674,866. Fritz Lindner et al. Moenomycin and process for producing same. Filed 9/1/64, issued 7/4/72. Assignee: Farbwerke Moechst Aktiengesellschaft vormals Meister Lucius & Bruning, Frankfurt/Main, Germany. (BASF)
3.) Cassity TR, Kolodziej BJ. Role of the capsule produced by Bacillus megaterium ATCC 19213in the accumulation of metallic cations. Microbios. 1984;41(160):117-25.
4.) Gong CS, Chen LF, Flickinger MC, et al. Production of ethanol from D-xylose by using D-xylose isomerase and yeasts. Appl Environ Microbiol. 1981;41:430-436.
5.) Wang PY, Shopis C, Schneider H. Fermentation of a pentose by yeasts. Biochem Biophys Res Commun. 1980;94:248-254.
6.) Lin-Chang Chiang, Humg-Yu Hsiao, Pear P. Ueng, George T. Tsao. Enzymatic and Microbial Preparation of D-Xylulose from D-Xylose. Appl Environ Microbiol. 1981 Jul;42(1):66-69.
7.) Cassity TR, Kolodziej BJ. Rose of the capsule produced by Bacillus megaterium ATCC 19213in the accumulation of metallic cations. Microbios 1984;41(160):117-25.
8.) H. Naik, L. Owings, D. Soybel. Tapping the zinc sink: Mitochondrial regulation of intracellular Zn2+ loading. J Amer Coll Surg. 2006;203(3):S11-S12.
9.) Kartha KK, Gamborg OL, Constabel F, Shyluk JP. Regeneration of Cassava Plants from Apical Meristems. Corp. Author: National Research Council of Canada Saskatoon (Saskatchewan) Prairie Regional Lab. Assession No. AD0781056. Report Date: Sept. 4, 1973. 8 pages. Report #NRC13475.
10.) Lister RM. [Mechanical transmission of cassava brown streak virus.] Nature. 1959 Jun 6;183(4675):1588-1589.
11.) Grant 1U01TW001021-01. Ecologically Guided Bioprospecting in Panama. Smithsonian Institution, Arlington, VA. 1998. Project start: 9/30/98, ended 9/29/03. ICD: Fogarty International Center.
12.) Grant 3U01TW001021-01S1. Ecologically Guided Bioprospecting in Panama. Smithsonian Institution, Arlington, VA. 1998. Project start: 9/30/98, ended 9/29/03. ICD: Fogarty International Center.
13.) Grant 5U01TW001021-02. Ecologically Guided Bioprospecting in Panama. Institution: Smithsonian Institution, Arlington, VA. Fiscal year 1999. Project start date: 9/30/98, ended 9/29/03. ICD: Fogarty International Center.

14.) Grant 5U01TW001021-03. Ecologically Guided Bioprospecting in Panama. Institution: Smithsonian Institution, Arlington, VA. Fiscal year 2000. Project start date: 9/30/98, ended 9/29/03. ICD: Fogarty International Center.

15.) Grant 5U01TW001021-04. Ecologically Guided Bioprospecting in Panama. Institution: Smithsonian Institution, Arlington, VA. Fiscal year 2001. Project start date: 9/30/98, ended 9/29/03. ICD: Fogarty International Center.

16.) Grant 5U01TW001021-05. Ecologically Guided Bioprospecting in Panama. Institution: Smithsonian Institution, Arlington, VA. Fiscal year 2002. Project start date: 9/30/98, ended 9/29/03. ICD: Fogarty International Center.

17.) Carabali A, Bellotti AC, Montoya-Lerma J, Fregene M. Resistance to the Whitefly, Aleurotrachelus socialis, in Wild Populations of Cassava, Manihot Tristis. J Insect Sci. 2010;10:170.

18.) Capinera John L (ed.) Encyclopedia of entomology, 2nd Edition. 2008 Springer Science + Business Media B.V.

19.) Golden Harvest Organics. Soil Amendment and Nutrient Deficiency Chart. [web page]

20.) Osunlaja SO. Effect of organic soil amendments on the incidence of brown spot disease in maize caused by Physoderma maydis J Basic Microbiol. 2007 Jan 10;29(8):501-505.

21.) Bonanomi G, Antignani V, Capodilupo M, Scala F. Identifying the characteristics of organic soil amendments that suppress soilborne plant diseases. Soil Biol Biochem. 2010 Feb;42(2):136-144.

22.) Gordon AS, Howell LD, Harwood V. Responses of diverse heterotrophic bacteria to elevated copper concentations. Can J Microbiol. 1994 May;40(5):408-411. (From Old Dominion University, Norfolk, VA).

23.) Starr TJ, Jones ME. The Effect of Copper on the Growth of Bacteria Isolated from Marine Environments. US Fish and Wildlife Service, Gulf Fishery Investigations, Galveston, TX. 1957;2(1):36

24.) Kartha KK, Gamborg OL, Constabel F, Shyluk JP. Regeneration of Cassava Plants from Apical Meristems. Corp. Author: National Research Council of Canada Saskatoon (Saskatchewan) Prairie Regional Lab. Assession No. AD0781056. Report Date: Sept. 4, 1973. 8 pages. Report #NRC13475.

25.) Lister RM. [Mechanical transmission of cassava brown streak virus.] Nature. 1959Jun 6;183(4675):1588-1589.

26.) Grant 1U01TW001021-01. Ecologically Guided Bioprospecting in Panama. Smithsonian Institution, Arlington, VA. 1998. Project start: 9/30/98, ended 9/29/03. ICD: Fogarty International Center.

27.) Grant 3U01TW001021-01S1. Ecologically Guided Bioprospecting in Panama. Smithsonian Institution, Arlington, VA. 1998. Project start: 9/30/98, ended 9/29/03. ICD: Fogarty International Center.

28.) Grant 5U01TW001021-02. Ecologically Guided Bioprospecting in Panama. Institution: Smithsonian Institution, Arlington, VA. Fiscal year 1999. Project start date: 9/30/98, ended 9/29/03. ICD: Fogarty International Center.

29.) Grant 5U01TW001021-03. Ecologically Guided Bioprospecting in Panama. Institution: Smithsonian Institution, Arlington, VA. Fiscal year 2000. Project start date: 9/30/98, ended 9/29/03. ICD: Fogarty International Center.

30.) Grant 5U01TW001021-04. Ecologically Guided Bioprospecting in Panama. Institution: Smithsonian Institution, Arlington, VA. Fiscal year 2001. Project start date: 9/30/98, ended 9/29/03. ICD: Fogarty International Center.

31.) Grant 5U01TW001021-05. Ecologically Guided Bioprospecting in Panama. Institution: Smithsonian Institution, Arlington, VA. Fiscal year 2002. Project start date: 9/30/98, ended 9/29/03. ICD: Fogarty International Center.

32.) Carabali A, Bellotti AC, Montoya-Lerma J, Fregene M. Resistance to the Whitefly, Aleurotrachelus socialis, in Wild Populations of Cassava, Manihot Tristis. J Insect Sci. 2010;10:170.

33.) Capinera John L (ed.) Encyclopedia of entomology, 2nd Edition. 2008 Springer Science + Business Media B.V.

34.) International Bulletin of Bacteriological Nomenclature and Taxonomy. 1955 July 15;5(3):121-128. Status of the Generic Names Chlamydozoon von Prowazek andBorrelina Paillot. A Preliminary Statement. [web page]

35.) Prowazek S von. Chlamydozoa I. Zusammenfassende Uebersicht. Arch f. Protistenkunde. 1970;10:336-358.

36.) Steinhaus Edward A. (University of CA Berkeley). Nomenclature and Classification of Insect Viruses. 1949;13:203-223.

37.) Babu KR, Ramakrishna S, Reddy YHK, et al. Metabolic alterations and molecular mechanism in silkworm larvae during viral infection: A Review. African J Biotechnol. 2009 Mar;8(6):899-907.

38.) Knight V, Gerone PJ, Griffith WR, et al. Studies in Volunteers with Respiratory Viral Agents: Small Particle Aerosol; Heterotypic Protection; Viral Chemotherapy; Bovine Reovirus in Man. Am Rev Respir Dis. 1963 Sept;88:SUPPL 135-147.

39.) Sinha RC, Chemistry and Biology Research Institute, Agriculture Canada, Ottawa, Ontario, Canada. The Aster Yellows Controversy: Current Status. Yale J Biol Med. 1983;56:737-743.

40.) Robert E. Shope, MD. Yale University. Annual Report for 1976Yale Arbovirus Research Unit, International Center for Arboviruses. WHO Collaborating Center for Arbovirus Reference and Research. Report #ADA038877. Dept of Epidemiology and Public Health, Yale School of Medicine, New Haven, CT. Controlling office: Department of the Army, US Army Medical Research and Development Command, Washington, DC. Annual Report from 7/1/75 to 6/30/76. Contract or Grant No. DADA-17-72-C-2170. Report date July 1, 1976. 92 pages.

41.) Monti G, Galli M, Invernizzi F, et al. Cryoglobulinaemias: a multi-centre study of the early clinical and laboratory manifestations of primary and secondary disease. GISC. Italian Group for the Study of Cryoglobulinaemias. QJM. 1995 Feb;88(2):115-126.

42.) Davis LE, Beckham JD, Tyler KL. North American encephalitic arboviruses. Neurol Clin. 2008 Aug;26(3):727. 26 pages.

43.) Gilmour Marion H, Howell Jr. Arden, Bibby Basil G. The Classification of Organisms Termed Leptotrochia (Leptothrix) Buccalis. I. Review of the Literature and Proposed Separation into Leptotrichia buccalis Trevisan, 1879 and Bacterionema Gen. Nov., B. matruchotii (Mendel, 1919) Comb. Nov. 1961;Vol. 25:131-141.

44.) Batrakov SG. Specific Lipids of Mycobacteria and Related Organisms. 1985 Mar;21(3):137.

45.) Shaw Cheng-Mei, Alvord JR Ellsworth C, Kies Marian W. Straight Chain Hydrocarbons as Substitutes for the Oil in Freund's Adjuvants in the Production of Experimental "Allergic" Encephalomyelitis in the Guinea Pig. J Immunol. 1964;92:24-27.

46.) Kuroda Y, Nacionales DC, Akaogi J, Reevees WH, Satoh M. Autoimmunity induced by adjuvant hydrocarbon oil components of vaccine. Biomed Pharmacother. 2004;48:325-337.

47.) Idodo-Umeh G, Ogbeibu AE. Bioaccumulation of the heavy metals in cassava tubers and plantain fruits grown in soils impacted with petroleum and non-petroleum activities. Res. J. Environm Sc. 2010;4:33-41.

48.) Cannon GW, Openshaw S, Clayton F, et al. Adjuvant arthritis in rats: susceptibility to arthritis induced by Mycobacterium butyricum and Mycobacterium tuberculosis. Transplantation Proceedings. 1999 May;31(3):1590-1591.

49.) EMD4Biosciences USA. 344289 Freund's Complete Adjuvant, Modified, Mycobacterium butyricum. [web page]

50.) Carreiro MM, Laux DC, Nelson DR. Characterization of the Heat Shock Response and Identification of Heat Shock Protein Antigens of Borrelia burgdorferi. Infect and Immun. 1990 Jul;58(7):2186-2191.

51.) Tawadros Marianne. Borrelia burgdorferi. From the Wadsworth Center, NY State Dept. of Health Student presentation. MCB 233Pathogenic Microbiology, University of Connecticut-Department of Molecular and Cell Biology.

52.) Aberer E, Duray Paul H. Morphology of Borrelia burgdorferi: Structural Patterns of Cultured Borreliae in Relation to Staining Methods. 1991 Apr;29(4):764-772.

53.) Anecdotal statements from a male patient diagnosed with Rheumatoid Arthritis when discussing his past military medical test results pertaining to Syphilis. Personal communication to the author.

54.) Brinton LP, Burgdorfer W. Cellular and Subcellular Organization of the 277F Agent, a Spiroplasma from the Rabbit Tick Haemaphysalis leporispalustris (Acari: Ixodidae). Int J Syst Bacteriol. 1976;26:554-560.

55.) Stalheim Ole HV, Ritchie Alfred E. Whitcomb Robert F. Cultivation, Serology, Ultrastructure, and Virus-Like Particles of Spiroplasma 277F. Curr Micrbiol. Vol. 1. 1978:365-370.

56.) Tully Joseph G, Whitcomb Robert F, Rose David L, et al. Characterization and Taxonomic Status of Tick Spiroplasmas: A Review. The Yale Journal of Biology and Medicine. 1983;56:599-603.

57.) Williamson DL, Tully JG, Whitcomb RF: Serological relationships of spiroplasmas as shown by combined deformation and metabolism inhibition tests. Int J Syst Bacteriol. 1979;29:345-351.

58.) Stalheim OHV, Richie AE, Whitcomb RF: Cultivation, serology, ultrastructure, and virus-like particles of spiroplasma 277F. Curr Microbiol 1978;1:365-370.

59.) Junca P, Saillard C, Tully J et al: Caracterisation de spiroplasmes isoles d'insectes et de fleurs de France conttinentale, de Course et du Maroc. Proposition pour une classification

des spiroplasmes. C R Acad Sci (Paris) 1980;290:1209-1212.
60.) Likins RC, McClure FJ, Steere AC. Urinary excretion of fluoride following defluoridation of a water supply. Public Health Rep. 1956 Mar;71(3):217-20.
61.) Sivakumar K. Actinomycetes. Report for Centre of Advanced Study in Marine Biology. Annamalai University. No date. P. 197-204. [web page]

Q Fever – Spiroplasma Connection

1.) Williams JC, Thompson HA, (eds). Q Fever: The biology of Coxiella burnetii. 1991 CRC Press, Boca Raton, FL
2.) Tylewska-Wierzbanowska S, Kruszewska D, Chmielewski T, et al. [Ticks as a reservoir of Borrelia burgdorferi and Coxiella burnetii on Polish terrain]. Przegl Epidemiol. 1996;50(3):245-251. [Article in Polish]
3.) Burgdorfer Willy, Pickens Edgar G. A Technique Employing Embryonated Chicken Eggs for the Infection of Argasid Ticks with Coxiella burnetti, Bacterium tularense, Leptospira icterohaemorrhagiae, and Western Equine Encephalitis Virus. 1954 Jan-Feb;94(1):84-89
4.) Parker RR, Pickens EG, Lackman DB, et al. Isolation and Characterization of Rocky Mountain Spotted Fever Rickettsiae from the Rabbit Tick Haemaphysalis leporis-palustris Packard. Public Health Reports. 1951 Apr 13;66(15)
5.) Luoto L, Casey ML, Pickens EG. Q Fever Sudies in Montana. Detection of Asymptomatic Infection Among Residents of Infected Dairy Premises. Am J Epidemiol. 1965 May;81:356-369
6.) Burgdorfer W, Pickens EG, Newhouse VF, Lackman DB. Isolation of Coxiella burnetii from rodents in western Montana. J Infect Dis. 1963 Mar-Apr;112:181-186
7.) Luoto L, Pickens EG. A resume of recent research seeking to define the Q fever problem. Am J Hyg. 1961 Jul;74:43-49.
8.) Nienhaus F, Sikora RA. Mycoplasmas, Spiroplasmas, and Rickettsia-like Organisms as Plant Pathogens. Ann Rev Phytopathol. 1979;17:37-58
9.) Henning K, Greiner-Fischer S, Hotel H, Ebsen M, Theegarten D. Isolation of Spiroplasma sp. from an Ixodes tick. Int J Med Microbiol. 2006 May;296 Suppl. 40:157-61. Epub 2006 Mar 9.
10.) Swiss Institute of Bioinformatics. HAMAP: Borrelia burgdorferi (strain ZS7) complete proteome. General Information. [web page]
11.) Pickens Edgar G, Gerloff Robert K, Burgdorfer Willy. Spirochete from the Rabbit Tick, Haemaphysalis leporispalustris (Packard). I. Isolation and Preliminary Characterization. J Bacteriol. 1968 Feb;95(2):291-299
12.) Clark TB. Spiroplasma sp. a new pathogen in honey bees. J Inverteb. Pathol. 1977;29:112-113
13.) Lackman DB, Bell EJ, Bell JF, Pickens EG. Intradermal Sensitivity Testing in Man with a Purified Vaccine for Q Fever. AJPH, 1962 Jan;52(1)86-93
14.) Luoto L. The Epidemiology of Q Fever in the United States. AJPH 1959 Mar;49:334-338
15.) Stoenner HG, Lackman DB, Benson WW, et al. The Role of Dairy Cattle in the Epidemiology of Q Fever in Idaho. J Infect Dis. 1961 Jul-Aug.;109:90-97
16.) Stoenner HG, Lackman DB. The Biologic Properties of Coxiella burnetii Isolated from Rodents Collected in Utah. Am J Hyg. 1960 Jan;71:45-51
17.) McDade, JE. Historical Aspects of Q Fever. In Marrie, Thomas J. Q Fever, Volume I: The Disease. CRC Press. 1990.
18.) Tully JG, Whitcomb RF, Rose DL, Williamson DL, Bové JM. Characterization and taxonomic status of tick spiroplasmas: a review. Yale J Biol Med. 1983 Sep-Dec;56(5-6):599-603
19.) Halos L, Mavris M, Vourc G, et al. Broad-range PCR-TTGE for the first-line detection of bacterial pathogen DNA in ticks. Vet Res. 2006;37:245-253
20.) Tully JG, DL Rose, CE Yunker, J Cory, RF Whitcomb, DL Williamson. 1981. Helical mycoplasmas (spiroplasmas) from Ixodes ticks. Science 1981;212(4498):1043-1045
21.) RD Andrews, JR Reilly, DH Ferris, LE Hanson. Leptospiral Agglutinins in Sera from Southern Illinois Herpetofauna. College of Vet. Med. Univ. of IL Urbana, IL. Bulletin Wildlife Dis Assoc. 1965 Oct;1:55-59
22.) Hovind-Hougen Kari. Leptospiraceae, a new family to include Leptospira Noguchi 1917and Leptonema gen. nov. Int. J Syst. Bacteriol. 1979;29:245-251
23.) Clark HF, Rorke LB. Spiroplasmas of tick origin and their pathogenicity. In The Mycoplasmas, Volume 3. Plant and Insect Mycoplasmas. Whitcomb RF, Tully JG (ed.) New York, Academic Press. 1979:155-174
24.) Zeigel RF, Clark HF. Electron microscopy of the suckling mouse cataract agent, a noncultivable animal pathogen possibly related to mycoplasma. Infect Immun. 1974;9:430-443
25.) Junca P, Saillard C, Tully JG et al. Caractérisation de spirooplasmes isolés d'insectes et de fleurs de France continentale, de Course et du Maroc. Proposition pour une classification des spiroplasmes. CR Acad Sci (Paris) 1980;Ser D 290:1209-1212
26.) Whitcomb Robert F. The Bioloogy of Spiroplasmas. Ann Rev Entomol. 1981;26:397-425
27.) Clark HF. Suckling mouse cataract agent. J Infect Dis. 1964;114:476-487
28.) Tully Joseph G, Rose David L, Yunker Conrad E, et al. Helical Mycoplasmas (Spiroplasmas) from Ixodes Ticks. Science 1981;212(4498):1043-1045
29.) Tully JG, Whitcomb RF, Rose DL, et al. Yale 1983: Three serologically distinct groups of spiroplasmas have been recovered from ticks. Yale J Biol Med. 1983 Sept-Dec;603.
30.) Tully JG, Whitcomb RF, Rose DL, et al. Characterization and Taxonomic Status of Tick Spiroplasmas: A Review. The Yale J Biol. Med. 1983;56:599-603
31.) Megraud F, Gamon LB, McGarrity GJ. Characterization of Spiroplasma mirum (Suckling Mouse Cataract Agent) in a Rabbit Lens Cell Culture. Infect Immun. 1983 Dec;42(3):1168-1175
32.) Tully JG, Rose DL, Yunker CE, et al. Spiroplasma ixodetis sp. nov., a New Species from Ixodes pacificus Ticks Collected in Oregon. Inter J System Bacteriol. 1995 Jan;45(1):23-28
33.) Tenckhoff B, Kölmel HW, Wolf V, Lange R. Production and characterization of a polyclonal antiserum against Spiroplasma mirum (ATCC 29335). Zentralbl Bakteriol. 1994 Jan;280(3):409-415
34.) Stanek G, Laber G, Hirschl A. Survival of spiroplasma on different carriers and resistance against three disinfectants. Proceedings of the 3rd International Organ. Mycoplasm. Custer, South Dakota, 1980 Sept. Abstract 107.
35.) Tully JG, Rose DL, Yunker CE, et al. Spiroplasma ixodetis sp. nov.,, a New Species from Ixodes pacificus Ticks Collected in Oregon. Inter J System Bacteriol. 1995 Jan;45(1):23-28
36.) Proceedings of the Second National Conference on Serologic Diagnosis of Lyme Disease. 1994 Oct. 27-29, Dearborn, MI. 106pages. Sponsors: Assoc. of State and Territorial Public Health Laboratory Directors, US CDC and Prevention, MI Dept. of Health. Co-sponsors: USFDA, NIH, Council of State and Territorial Epidemiologists and National Committee for Clinical Laboratory Standards.
37.) Alfred I. duPont Testamentary Trust. [web page]
38.) Williamson DL, Whitcomb RF, Tully JG, et al. Revised group classification of the genus Spiroplasma. Inter J Bacteriol. 1998;48:1-12
39.) Steere Allen C, Broderick Thomas F, Malawista Stephen E. Erythema Chronicum Migrans and Lyme Arthritis: Epidemiologic Evidence for a Tick Vector. Am J Epidemiol. 1978;108(4):312-321
40.) Reik Louis, Steere Allen C, Bartenhagen Nicholas H, Shope Robert E, Malawista Stephen E. Neurologic Abnormalities of Lyme Disease. Medicine. 1979;58(4):281-294
41.) Steere AC, Hardin JA, Malawista SE. Lyme arthritis: serum cryoprecipitates associated with skin and joint lesion. Arthritis Rheum. 1977;20:136
42.) Steere AC, Hardin JA, Malawista SE. Erythema chronicum migtans and Lyme arthritis: serum cryoimmunoglobulins and clinical activity of skin and joints. Science 1977;196:1121-1122

Mollicutes and Swine Diseases

1.) Bazovská S, Hovind-Hougen K, Rudiová A, Kmety E. Leptospira sp. Strain Dimbovitza, First Isolate in Europe with Characteristics of the Proposed Genus Leptonema. Inter J System Bacteriol. 1983 Apr.;33(2):325-328. (Institut of Epidem, Med Faculty of Komensky Univ, Bratislava, Czechoslovakia, and Dept of Biophysics, Statens Seruminstitut, Copenhagen, Denmark).
2.) Petrina Ecaterina. Corn and the Development of Agricultural Science in Romania, 1864-1939. Agricult. History. 1995 Winter;69(1):54-78. Published by Agricultural History Society.
3.) Michael LG. Agricultural Survey of Europe: The Danube Basin, Part 2: Romania, Bulgaria and Yugoslavia. USDA Technical Bulletin No. 126. 1929 Oct:6-81.
4.) Hovind-Hougen Kari. Leptospiraceae, a new family to include Leptospira Noguchi 1917and Leptonema gen. nov. Int. J Syst. Bacteriol. 1979;29:245-251.
5.) Lewis FR. How to Collect and Process Small Polyhedral Viruses of Insects. Northeast Forest Experiment Station. Forest Research Notes. No. 109. 1960. 8 pages. By the Forest Insect Laboratory Northeastern Forest Experiment Station Forest Service, USDA New Haven, CT.
6.) Rollinson WD, Lewis FB. How to Collect and Process Large Polyhedral Viruses of Insects. In Forest Research Notes. Forest Service, USDA, Upper Darby, PA. 1962 No. 130, 6 pages. By the Forest Insect Laboratory Northeastern Forest Experiment Station Forest Service, USDA New Haven,CT.
7.) Rollinson WD, Lewis FB, Waters WE. The Successful Use of a Nuclear-Polyhedrosis Virus against the Gypsy Moth. Notes. 1965. Forest Insect and Disease Laboratory

Northeastern Forest Experiment Station Forest Service, US Department of Agriculture, West Haven, Connecticut.
8.) Volkin Elliot, Astrachan L. Phosphorus incorporation in Escherichia coli ribonucleic acid after infection with bacteriophage T2 Virology. 1956 Apr;2(2):149-161.
9.) Ritchie AE, Ellinghausen HC. In Proc. Electron-Microscopy Soc Amer. J Marceaux (ed.), Baton Rouge, LA. Claiton. 1969:228-229.
10.) Sefer M. Growth and multiplication specific serum inhibition test applied to acvicola leptospira, p. 77-83. In Sefer M (ed.), Leptospirosis, leptospira and other spirocheta. Cantacuzino Institute, Bucharest, Hungary. 1975.
11.) Tripathy DN, Hanson LE. Studies of Leptospira illini strain 3055: immunologic and serologic determinations. Am J Vet Res. 1973;34:563-565.
12.) Becker Klaus. Health Effects of High Radon Environments in Central Europe: Another Test for the LNT Hypothesis? Nonlinear Biol Toxicol Med. 2003;1(1):3-35.
13.) Hanford Cultural Resources Program, US Department of Energy. Hanford Site Historic District: History of the Plutonium Production Facilities, 1943-1990. 2002. Battelle Press. Columbus, OH. p.1.22-1.27.
14.) Findlay John, Hevly Bruce. Nuclear Technologies and Nuclear Communities: A History of Hanford and the Tri-Cities, 1943-1993. Seattle, WA: Hanford History Project, Center for the Study of the Pacific Northwest, University of Washington. 1995:p. 50.
15.) Wiki: Savannah River Site. Wapedia. http://wapedia.mobi
16.) Federation of American Scientists. Special Weapons Primer. Heavy Water. Weapons of Mass Destruction. [web site] 1998 Oct. 21.
17.) SRNL. Savannah River National Laboratory. [web site] Last updated 2010 June 25
18.) Phillips RW, Wiegel J, Berry, CJ, et al. Kineococcus radiotolerans sp. nov., a radiation-resistant, Gram-positive bacterium. Inter J System Evol Microbiol. 2002;52:93-938.
19.) Field Paul E, Shaffer James H. The solubilities of hydrogen fluoride and deuterium fluoride in molten fluorides. J Phys Chem. 1967;71(10):3218-3222.
20.) Johnson MW, Sándor E, Arzi E. The Crystal Structure of Deuterium Fluoride. Acta Cryst. 1975;B3:1998-2003.
21.) McLain SE, Benmore CJ, Siewenie JE, Molaison JJ, Turner JF. On the variation of the structure of liquid deuterium fluoride with temperature. J Chem Phys. 2004 Oct 1;121(13):6448-6455.
22.) Giovanni Rosalie. The Effects of Deuterium Oxide on Certain Microorganisms. Annals NY Acad Sci. 1960 Nov;84:16:644-647.
23.) RD Andrews, JR Reilly, DH Ferris, LE Hanson. Leptospiral Agglutinins in Sera from Southern Illinois Herpetofauna. College of Vet. Med. Univ. of IL Urbana, IL. Bulletin Wildlife Dis Assoc. 1965 Oct;1:55-59.
24.) Odum Eugene, Odum Howard T. Fundamentals of Ecology. 1953 First Edition. Reprinted 1971 Philadelphia: Saunders.
25.) McKeever S, Gorman GW, Chapman JF, Galton MM, Powers DK. Incidence of Leptospirosis in Wild Mammals from Southwestern Georgia, with a Report of New Hosts for Six Serotypes of Leptospires. (CDC, Bureau of State Services, Public Health Service, US Department of Health, Education, and Welfare, Atlanta, GA and Emory University Field Station, Newton, GA). Am J Trop Med Hyg. 1958:646-655.
26.) Johnson Russell C. (ed.). University of Minnesota, Minneapolis. The Biology of Parasitic Spirochetes. 1976 Academic Press, New York. Chapter 3. Morphology of Leptospires. p.19-37.
27.) Charon NW, Johnson RC, Muschel LH. Antileptospiral Activity in Lower-Vertebrate Sera. Infect and Immun. 1975 Dec;12(6):1386-1391. (University of MN).
28.) Robinson FR. Pathogenesis of a Mycoplasm Infection in Swine. 1966Feb. AD066711. Air Force Report AMRL-TR-66-14. Final report 1962-1964. [abstract] 70 pages.
29.) Ennis RS, Dalgard D, Willerson JT et al. Mycoplasma Hyorhinis Swine Arthritis. II. Morphologic Features. Arthrit Rheum. 2005 Nov 22;14(2):202-211.
30.) Kawashima K, Yamada S, Kobayashi H, Narita M. Detection of procine reproductive and respiratory syndrome virus and Mycoplasma hyorhinis antigens in pulmonary lesions of pigs suffering from respiratory distress. J Compar Pathol. 1996Apr;114(3):315-323.
31.) Fraser KB, Shirodaria PV, Haire M, Middleton D. Mycoplasmas in cell cultures from rheumatoid synovial membranes. J Hyg Camb. 1971;69:17-25.
32.) Reed Sylvia E. The Interaction of Mycoplasmas and Influenza Viruses in Trachael Organ Cultures. J Infect Dis. 1971 Jul;124(1):18-25.
33.) Jansson E, Backman A, Hakkarainen K, et al. Mycoplasmas and arthritis. Z Rheumatol. 1983Nov-Dec;42(6):315-319.
34.) 36. Duncan JR, Ross RF. Fine Structure of the Synovial Membrane in Mycoplasma hyorhinis Arthritis in Swine. Am J Pathol. 1969 Oct;57(1):171-186.
35.) Fraser CM, Casjens S, Huang WM, et al. Genomic sequence of a Lyme disease spirochaete, Borrelia burgdorferi. Nature 1997 Dec 11;390:580-592.
36.) Noguchi Hideyo. Morphological Characteristics and Nomenclature of Leptospira (Spirochaeta) Icterohaemorrhagiae (Inada and Ito). J Exp Med. 1918;27:575-598.
37.) Studies from the Rockefeller Institute for Medical Reesarch Reprints. Volume XXXIV. 1920. The Rockefeller Institute for Medical Research. Waverly Press, Baltimore. 607 pages.
38.) Otteraaen Andrew. The Spirochete of Infectious Jaundice (Spirocheta icterohemorrhagiae, Inada; Leptospira, Noguchi) in House Rats in Chicago. J Infect Dis. 1919;24(5):485-488.

Chapter Four: What We Are Told (or Not) Matters

Secrets of the Agricultural Biocides

1.) Steinkraus KH. Tashiro H. Production of Milky-Disease Spores (Bacillus popilliae Dutky and Bacillus lentimorbus Dutky) on Artificial Media. Science 1955 Jun 17;121(3155):873-874.
2.) Rhodes RA, Sharpe ES, Hall HH, Jackson RW. Characteristics of the Vegetative Growth of Bacillus popilliae. Appl Microbiol. 1966 Mar;14(2):189-195.
3.) Hamilton RA. Increase in Moth Eggs Seen in Fairfield County. New York Times Article on the Internet. 1988 Feb 14. [web page]
4.) University of California San Diego. Bacillus thuringiensis. History of Bt. [web page]
5.) Ninfa M. Rosas-García. Biopesticide Production from Bacillus thuringiensis: An Environmentally Friendly Alternative. Recent Patents on Biotechnology. 2009;3:28-36.
6.) Technical Report: DDC AD408401. Conference on Biological Control of Insects of Medical Importance. American Institute of Biological Sciences (Washington, DC). 148 pages.
7.) Steinhaus EA, Thompson CG. Preliminary field tests using a polyhedrosis virus to control the alfalfa caterpillar. J Econ Entomol. 1949 Apr;42(2):301-5.
8.) Koppenhöfer AM, Wilson M, Brown I, Kaya HK, Gaugler R. Biological control agents for white grubs (Coleoptera: Scarabaeidae) in anticipation of the establishment of the Japanese beetle in California. J Econ Entomol. 2000 Feb;93(1):71-80.
9.) US Patent 3,950,225. Skole, et al. Filed 10/15/74, issued 4/13/76. Medium, component thereof and process employing same for the production of microbial insecticides, such as Bacillus popilliae spores and the like, for the control of Japanese beetles and other insects. Assignee: Amstar Corporation (New York, NY).
10.) Grant St. Julian, Lee A. Bulla Jr., Eugene S. Sharpe, Gordon L. Adams. Bacteria, Spirochetes, and Rickettsia as Insecticides. Ann NY Acad Sci. 1973 Jun 22;217:65-75.
11.) Technical Report: DDC AD408401. Conference on Biological Control of Insects of Medical Importance. American Institute of Biological Sciences (Washington, DC). 148 pages.
12.) Burges HD, Hussey NW. Microbial Control of Insects and Mites. 1971 Academic Press Inc. London, New York.
13.) Hernandez Eric, Ramisse Francoise, Ducoureau Jean-Pierre, et al. Bacillus thuringiensis subsp. Konkukian (Serotype H34) Superinfection: Case Report and Experimental Evidence of Pathogenicity in Immunosuppressed Mice. J Clin Microbiol. 1998 Jul;36(7):2138-2139.
14.) US Patent 4,859,377. Shasha, et al. Starch encapsulation of entomopathogens. Filed 7/10/87, issued 8/22/89. Assignee: The United States of America, as represented by the Secretary of [Agriculture] (Washington DC).
15.) Technical Report: DDC AD408401. Conference on Biological Control of Insects of Medical Importance. American Institute of Biological Sciences (Washington, DC). 148 pages.
16.) Joklik WK, Abel Pamela, Holmes IH. Reactivation of Poxviruses by a Non-Genetic Mechanism. Nature 1960 Jun 18;186(4729):992-993.
17.) Cooper JL. Viruses and the Environment. Second Edition. Chapman & Hall. 1995 Cambridge, Great Britain.
18.) Brindley TA, Dicke FF. Significant Developments in European Corn Borer Research. Ann Rev Entomol. 1963;8:155-176.
19.) Vossbrinck CR, Andreadis TG. Thephylogenetic position of Ovavesicula popilliae (Microsporisia) and its relationship to Antonospora and Paranosema based on small subunit rDNA analysis. J Invert Path. 2007;96:270-273.
20.) Weiser J, Holuša J, Žižka Z. Larssoniella duplicati n. sp. (Microsporidia, Unikaryonidae), a newly described pathogen infecting the double-spined spruce bark beetle, Ips duplicatus (Coleoptera, Scolytidae) in the Czech Republic. J Pest Sci. 2006;79(3):127-135.
21.) US Patent 4,282,238. Goetz, et al. Insecticidal process. Filed 7/26/79 published 8/4/81. Assignee: BASF Aktiengesellschaft (DE)
22.) US Patent 2,404,300. Kyrides. Substituted Imidazoles. Filed 3/22/44 published 7/16/46. Assignee: Monsanto Chemical Company, St. Louis, Missouri.
23.) World Federation for Culture Collections. WFCC-MIRCEN World Data Centre for Microorganisms. [web page]
24.) Krieg A. In vitro determination of Bacillus thuringiensis, Bacillus cereus, and related bacilli. J Invert Path. 1969;15:313-320.
25.) US Patent 4,609,550. Fitz-James. Bacillus ereus subspecies israelensis. Filed 1/20/83, issued 9/2/86. Assignee: The University of Western Ontario, Health Sciences Centre (London, CA).
26.) US Patent 3,271,243. Cords et al. Stable Concentrated Bacterial Insecticide Suspensions. Filed 3/13/63, issued 9/6/66. Assignee: International Minerals & Chemical Corporation,

a corporation of New York.
27.) Yelton David B, Thorne Curtis B. Transduction in Bacillus cereus by Each of Two Bacteriophages. J Bacteriol. 1970 May;102(2):573-579. Phages referenced in the document are CP-51 and CP-53.
28.) USDA Agricultural Research Service. Handbook. The Genus Bacillus. 1973;427. 283 pages.
29.) World Federation for Culture Collections. WFCC-MIRCEN World Data Centre for Microorganisms. [web page]
30.) Pan SC, Bonanno S, Wagman GH. Efficient Utilization of Fatty Oils as Energy Source in Penicillin Fermentation. Appl Environ Microbiol. 1959;7:176-180.
31.) Mycologia 1955;47:429-493), Accession numbers ATCC 11710, IFO 9250, QM 6890.
32.) Riegel Emil Raymond, Kent James Albert. (eds). 2003 Kluwer Academic / Plenum Publishers, NY. Riegel's handbook of industrial chemistry. Tenth Edition. P. 1023
33.) Novak RO, Backus MP. A New Species of Mycotypha with a Zygosporic Stage. Mycol Soc Amer. 1963:790.
34.) US Patent 7,605,248. Dattwyler, et al. Recombinant constructs of Borrelia burgdorferi. Filed 9/26/06, published 10/20/09. Inventors: Dattwyler Raymond J, Gomes-Solecki Maria JC, Luft Benjamin
35.) Toxic Plume from the town of Brookhaven Landfill. Long Island. News12 Exclusive Report. Karen Hassen. 2009 April 17
36.) Adams J, Cowgill M, Moskowitz P. (Brookhaven Natl Lab) and Rokhvarger A. (Nucon Systems Inc.). Effect of Radiation on Spinel Ceramics for Permanent Containers for Nuclear Waste Transportation and Storage. BNL-67518 Informal Report. 9 pages. A continuation of the series of presentations on the "ceramic container" project made at the Waste Manaegment Technology Section of the American Ceramic Society Annual Meetings of 1995, 1998, and 1999.
37.) GE document: Amersham Biosciences. Preparation and separation of Borrelia burgdorferi plasmid DNA. Report. 3 pages. [web page]
38.) Manieri DA, Truran WH. The Industrial Atom. Radioactive Waste Disposal at Knolls Atomic Power Laboratory. TID-8017 March 1958 Monograph. 22 pages. Technical Information Service Atomic Energy Commission, Washington, DC.
39.) Dykhuizen Daniel E, Polin David S, Dunn John J, Wilske Bettina, Preac-Mursic Vera, Dattwyler Raymond J, Luft Benjamin J. Borrelia burgdorferi is clonal: Implications for taxonomy and vaccine development. Proc Natl Acad Sci. 1993 Nov;90:10163-10167. The paper was written in collaboration with scientists from SUNY, Brookhaven National Laboratory and University of Munich, Germany.
40.) Eilenberg J, Enkegaard An, Vestergaard S, Jensen B. Boicontrol of Pests on Plant Crops in Denmark: Present Status and future Potential. Biocntrl Sci Tech. 2000;10:703-716.
41.) Frederiksen K, Rosenquist H, Jørgensen K, Wilcks A. Occurrence of Natural Bacillus thuringiensis Contaminants and Residues of Bacillus thuringiensis-Based Insecticides on Fresh Fruits and Vegetables. Appl Environ Microbiol. 2006;72(5):3435-3440.
42.) Sullivan DJ Jr. et al. A complete set of human telomeric probes and their clinical application. National Institutes of Health and Institute of Molecular Medicine collaboration. Nat Genet 1996;14:86-89.
43.) US Geological Survey. USGS Studies in Long Island Sound: Geology, Contaminants, and Environmental Issues. [web page]
44.) US Patent 3,616,250. Hrubant, et al. Preferential Enzymatic Lysis of Vegetative Cells in Presence of Sporulated Bacterial Cells. Filed 10/22/68 published 10/26/71.
45.) Orlando Sentinel. Nuclear Laboratory Cited for Pollution Violations. Press Release 1998 March 10. [web page]
46.) Sherwood Jeff. Brookhaven Science Associates Cited for Failure to Follow Safety Rules. Press Release No. R-99-084. 1999 Apr 19. [web page]
47.) US Department of Energy Briefs. News You Can Use. DOE Cites Brookhaven, Los Alamos National Labs for Safety Violations. Press Release. 1997 January 8. [web page]
48.) Federal Contractor Misconduct Database. Brookhaven Science Associates, LLC. [web page]
49.) Yamamoto M, Magara J, Takagi S, et al. Activity of agricultural chemicals to modify mitomycin C induced growth inhibition of Bacillus subtilis in the rec assay. Tohoku J Exp Med. 1988 Aug;155(4):385-386.
50.) Damgaard PH, Hansen BM, Pedersen JC, Eilenberg J. Natural occurrence of Bacillus thuringiensis on cabbage foliage and in insects associated with cabbage crops. J Appl Microbiol. 1997;82:253-258.
51.) Jensen Wayne I, Owen Cora R, Jellison William L. Yersinia philomiragia sp. n., a New Member of the Pasteurella Group of Bacteria, Naturally Pathogenic for the Muskrat Ondatra zibethica). J Bacteriol. 1969:100(3):1237-1241.
52.) Davis R.E. 1978. Spiroplasma associated with flowers of the tulip tree (Liriodendron tulipifera L.). Can J Microbiol. 24(8):954-959.
53.) Orent Wendy. Plague: The Mysterious Past and Terrifying Future of the World's Most Dangerous Disease. 2004 New York: Free Press. p. 135-136.
54.) Ed Regis. The Biology of Doom. The History of America's Secret Germ Warfare Project. 1999 Henry Holt and Company, New York.
55.) US Congress Appropriations Committee Hearing, Research, Development, Testing, and Evaluation of Synthetic Biological Agents. Published by the U.S. Government Printing Office. Reposted on the Internet by the PhilFam Committee 22 June 1998.
56.) US Patent 3,073,749 Megna. Preparation of Microbial Insecticide. Filed 6/9/59, issued 1/15/63. Assignee: Bioferm Corporation, Wasco, CA.
57.) Chemical Heritage Foundation. Award for Supporting Industries. Past Recipients of the Richard J. Bolte, Sr. Award for Supporting Industries. Jerry M. Sudarsky, 2008.
58.) US Patent 6,886,784. Howe. High Pressure Spray System. Filed 10/20/03 published 5/3/05. No Assignee listed.
59.) US Patent 5,747,416. McArdle. Herbicidal and insecticidal protein-polysaccharide delivery compositions and methods for controlling plant and insect populations. Field 8/16/96 published 5/5/98.
60.) US Patent 4,694,013. Lahm. Insecticidal and acaricidal phenoxypyrdinyl esters and intermediates. Filed 9/26/86 published 9/15/87. Assignee: E.I. Du Pont de Nemours and Company (Wilmington, DE).
61.) US Patent 3,113,066. Emond. Bacillus thuringiensis spore pesticide. Filed 1/3/61, published 12/3/63. Inventor: Robert E. Emond, Mooretown, Ontario, Canada, assignor to Esso Research and Engineering Company.
62.) BH Weil, I Kirshenbaum, SB Sweetser. Information Operations at Esso Research and Engineering Company. J Chem Doc. 1969;9(4):207-212.
63.) Rohm and Haas. Committed to Sustainable Development. [web page]
64.) US Patent 3,087,865. Process for Making Pesticidal Compositions. Assignees: Rohm & Haas Company, Philadelphia, PA. Filed 5/2/61, patented 4/30/63.
65.) US Patent 3,911,110. Smirnoff. Insecticidal compositions. Filed 12/22/72, published 10/7/75. Assignee: Canadian Patents and Development Limited (Ottawa, CA).
66.) US Patent 4,626,508. Steinkraus. Method for extending the viability of virulent Bacillus popilliae. Assignee: Cornell Research Foundation, Inc. (Ithaca, NY).
67.) Burges HD, Hussey NW. Microbial Control of Insects and Mites. 1971 Academic Press Inc. London, New York.
68.) Krieg A, Schmidt L. NachrBl. Dt. PflSchutzdienst. Braunschw. 1962;14:177-182.
69.) Weiser Jaroslav. Diseases of Insects of Medical Importance in Europe. World Health Organization Bulletin. 1963;28:121-127.
70.) Ghelardi E, Celandroni F, Salvetti S, et al. Requirement of flhA for Swarming Differentiation, Flagellin Export, and Secretion of Virulence-Associated Proteins in Bacillus thuringiensis. J Bacteriol. 2002 Dec;184(23):6424-6433.
71.) Hernandez Eric, Ramisse Francoise, Ducoureau Jean-Pierre, et al. Bacillus thuringiensis subsp. Konkukian (Serotype H34) Superinfection: Case Report and Experimental Evidence of Pathogenicity in Immunosuppressed Mice. J Clin Microbiol. 1998 Jul;36(7):2138-2139.
72.) US Patent 5,874,289 Liu, et al. Bacillus thuringiensis mutants which produce high yields of crystal delta-endotoxin. Filed 8/28/97, issued 2/23/99. Assignee: Abbott Laboratories (Abbott Park, IL).
73.) Lewis Franklin B. (Entomologist, Forest Insect Laboratory Northeastern Forest Experiment Station Forest Service, USDA, New Haven, CT), in Forest Research Note. How to Collect and Process Small Polyhedral Viruses of Insects. Forest Service USDA, Upper Darby, PA. 1960;109:1-8.
74.) Lewis Franklin B. (Entomologist, Forest Insect Laboratory Northeastern Forest Experiment Station Forest Service, U.S.D.A., New Haven, CT), and Rollinson WB (Biological Aide); in Forest Research Note. How to Collect and Process Large Polyhedral Viruses of Insects. Forest Service USDA, Upper Darby, PA. 1962;130:1-6.
75.) Maramorosch Karl. Advances in Virus Research. Vol. 22. 1978 Academic Press, Inc., London.
76.) Brown Dennis T, Waite Marilynn RF, Pfefferkorn Elmer R. Morphology and Morphogenesis of Sindbis Virus as Seen with Freeze-Etching Techniques. J Virol. 1972 Sept;10(3):524-536.
77.) Woods DR, Bevan EA. Studies on the nature of the killer factor produced by Saccharomyces cerevisiae. J Gen Microbiol. 1968 Apr;51(1):115-26.
78.) Fink GR, Styles CA. Curing of a killer factor in Saccharomyces cerevisiae. Proc Natl Acad Sci. 1972 Oct;69(10):2846-9.
79.) Steinhaus Edward A. Nomenclature and Classification of Insect Viruses. Bact Rev. 13(1949):203-223.
80.) Kropinski AM, Ghiorse WC, Greenberg EP. The intracellular polyglucose storage granules of Spirochaeta aurantia. Arch Microbiol. 1988;150(3):289-295. The paper was written by scientists from Queen's Unviersity, Ontario, Canada; and Cornell University, Ithaca, NY.
81.) Adler Ben, Faine Solly. Leptospira. 2010 Mar 15. Epub. Copley and Wilson's Microbiology and Microbial Infections. [web page]

82.) US Patent 6,130,074. Brennan. Recombinant insect virus with reduced capacity for host-to-host transmission in the environment and methods to produce said virus. Filed 5/28/93, issued 10/10/00. Assignee: American Cyanamid Company Five Giralda Farms (Madison, NJ).
83.) Frederiksen K, Rosenquist H, Jørgensen K, Wilcks A. Occurrence of Natural Bacillus thuringiensis Contaminants and Residues of Bacillus thuringiensis-Based Insecticides on Fresh Fruits and Vegetables. Appl Environ Microbiol. 2006;72(5):3435-3440.
84.) Damgaard PH, Hansen BM, Pedersen JC, Eilenberg J. Natural occurrence of Bacillus thuringiensis on cabbage foliage and in insects associated with cabbage crops. J Appl Microbiol. 1997;82:253-258.
85.) Lemke Paul A, Nash Claude H. Fungal Viruses. Bacteriol. Rev. 1974;38(1):29-56.
86.) Nuclear Energy in Denmark. World Nuclear Association. [web page]
87.) Nuclear Legislation in OECD Countries. Regulatory and Institutional Framework for Nuclear Activities Denmark. 2007 Report. 16 pages. [web page]
88.) Wilske B, Preac-Mursic V, Göbel UF, et al. An OspA Serotyping System for Borrelia burgdorferi Based on Reactivity with Monoclonal Antibodies and OspA Sequence Analysis. J Clin Microbiol. 1993 Feb;31(2):340-350.
89.) NCME. Network for Continuing Medical Education. Lyme Disease and Concomitant Tickborne Infections. [videotape, 3hrs.] 1997 June 27. Narrator: Dr. Benjamin Luft State University of New York at Stony Brook.
90.) Okubo Masayoshi (ed.) Polymer Particles. Springer Berlin Heidelberg, NY. P. 331,332.
91.) Thomas John A, Colby Howard D. (eds.) Endocrine toxicology. Second Edition. Target Organ Toxicology Series. Hayes AW, Thomas JA, Gardner DE (series eds.) Taylor & Francis, 1997. Washington DC.
92.) Graham EE, Mitchell RF, Reagel PF, et al. Treating Panel Traps with a Fluoropolymer Enhances their Efficiency in Capturing Cerambycid Beetles. J Econ Entomol. 2010;103(3):641-647.
93.) Ministry of the Environment, Climate Protection and the Energy Sector Baden-Württemberg. In Germany. [web page]
94.) Chang SC, Wei YH, Wei DL, et al. Factors affecting the production of eremofortin C and PR toxin in Penicillium roqueforti. Appl Environ Microbiol. 1991 Sep;57(9):2581-2585.
95.) Food and Drug Administration (FDA). Food. Chapter 13: Clostridium botulinum Toxin Formation (A Biological Hazard) – 3rd Edition. Fish and Fisheries Products Hazards and Controls Guidance. 2001 Jun. Monograph. [web page]
96.) ATCC. Strain 19113 – Listeria monocytogenes (Murray et al.) Pirie Isolation: Human Denmark. [web page]
97.) The EcoTipping Points Project. [web page]
98.) Plastipedia.co.uk A History of Plastics. The Shape of Plastics (1962) [web page]
99.) Cowen DV. Flowering Trees and Shrubs in India, Sixth Edition. Bombay. 1984. Thacker and Co. Ltd. And Nair KSS (ed). Insect Pests and Diseases in Indonesian Forests. Center for International Forestry Research 2000. SMT Grafika Desa Putera, Indonesia. 95 pages. [web page]
100.) How to Manage Pests. Pests in Gardens and Landscapes. Acacia. University of California Agriculture & Natural Resources. [web page]
101.) Niimura Noriyasu, Miyakoshi Tetsuo. Characterization of Natural Resin Films and Identification of Ancient Coating. J Mass Spectrom Soc Jpn. 2003;51:440.
102.) Brunello Franco, Neri Pozza (ed.). The Art of Dyeing in the History of mankind. 1973 Sept. Translated by Bernard Hickey. Vicenza, Italy.
103.) Wang Zhongshu. Han Civilization. Translated by KC Chang et al. Yale University Press. New Haven and London. 1982.
104.) US Patent 5,686,267. Simon et al. Nucleic acid molecule encoding antigen associate with Lyme disease. Filed 3/20/95 published 11/11/97. Assignee: Max-Planck-Gesellschaft zur Forderung der Wissenscaften E.V. (Gottingen, DE) and Deutsches Krebsforschun Zentrum Stiftung des Offentlichen Rechts (Heidelberg, DE).
105.) Max-Planck-Institut Für Kernphysik in Heidelberg [web page]
106.) US Patent 5,434,077. Simon, et al. Borrelia burgdorferi strain 257. Filed 5/27/93 published 7/18/95. Assignee: Max-Planck-Gesellschaft zur Forderung der Wissenschaften e.V. (Gottingen, DE) and Deutsches Krebsforschungszentrum Stiftung des Offentlichen Rechts (Heildelberg, DE).
107.) US Patent 5,178,859. Simon, et al. Vaccine against Lyme disease. Filed 9/19/90 published 1/12/93. Assignee: Max-Planck-Gesellschaft zur Forderung der Wissenschaften e.V. (Gottingen, DE) and Deutsche Krebsforschungszentrum Stiftung des offentlichen rechts (Heidelberg, DE).
108.) US Patent 5,780,030. Simon et al. Passive vaccine against Lyme disease. Filed 3/20/95 published 7/14/98. Assignee: Max-Planck-Gesellschaft zur Forderung der Wissenschaften e.V. (Gottingen, DE) and Deutsches Krebsforschun Zentrum Stiftung des Offentlichen Rechts (Heidelberg, DE) Invencotrs from Heidelberg, and Freiburg, Germany.
109.) US Patent 5,856,447. Simon, et al. Hybridomas producing antibodies specific for lyme disease antigens OspA and OspB. Filed 2/23/98 published 1/5/99. Assignee: Max-Planck-Gesellschaft zur Forderung der Wissenschaften (Heidelberg, DE). Inventors from Heidelberg and Freibrug.
110.) US Patent 5,942,236. Lobet et al. Osp A proteins of Borrelia burgdorferi subgroups, encoding genes and vaccines. Filed 5/16/95 published 8/24/99. Assignee: SmithKline Beecham Biologicals (GB) and Max-Planck-Gesellschaft zur Forderung der Wissenschafter e.V. (DE) and Deutsches krebsforschungszentrum Stiftung des offentlichen Rechts (DE). Inventors from Heidelberg and Frieburg.
111.) US Patent 6,676,942. Lobet et al. Osp A proteins of Borrelia burdorferi subgroups, encoding genes and vaccines. Filed 4/1/99 published 1/13/04. Assignee: SmithKline Beecham Biologicals (s.a.) (Rixensart, BE) and Max-Planck-Gesellschaft zur Forderung der Wissenschaften e.V. (Frieburg, DE) and Deutsches Krebs Forschungszentrum Stiftung des Offentlichen Rechts (Heidelberg, DE). Inventors from Heidelberg and Freiburg.
112.) Syngenta's corn amylase – Enogen Technology – the breakthrough biotechnology corn trait for ethanol production. What if corn already knew its destiny? Biofuels Digest. [monograph] (Syngenta is a Monsanto owned company).
113.) Innovating Corn Hybrid Technology. More About Enogen. [web page]
114.) Enogen Press Release. USDA Approves Enogen™ Trait – Syngenta's Corn Amylase. 2011 Feb 11.
115.) DuPont Washington Works. [web page]
115a.) DuPont Reports First-Phase Results of Health Study Examining PFOA Exposure. 2005 Jan 11. [web page]
116.) Rockwood LP. Sporotrichum globuliferum Spegazzini, A Natural Enemy of the Alfalfa Weevil. J Econ Entomol. 1916 Oct;9:493.
117.) Finney Dee. Yucca Mountain Nuclear Waste Dump. The Road to Disaster. Monograph. And Sussex Alan. The Road to Yucca Mountain: Nuclear Waste and Terrorism. 2003 February. Excerpted.
118.) Citizen Alert. Yucca Mountain Story. 2002 Apr. [web page]
119.) Lankat-Buttgereit B, Göke R, Fehmann HC, et al. Molecular cloning of a cDNA encoding for the GLP-1 receptor expressed in rat lung. Exp Clin Endocrinol. 1994;102(4);341-347. (This came from the Clinical Research Unit for Gastrointestinal Endocrinology at the University of Marburg, Germany.)
120.) Norway Rat. The Mammals of Texas. [web page]
120a.) Mourad S, Friedman L. Pathogenicity of Candida. J Bacteriol 1961;81(5):550-556.
121.) Lebech AM, Hansen K, Wilske B, Theisen M. Taxonomic classification of 29 Borrelia burgdorferi strains isolated from patients with Lyme borreliosis: a comparison of five different phenotypic and genotypic typing schemes. Med Microbiol Immunol. 1994;183:325-341.
122.) Rosenthal Elisabeth. Europe Finds Clean Energy in Trash, but U.S. Lags. The New York Times. 2010 Apr 12. [web page]
123.) Vancha AR, Govindaraju S, Parsa KV, et al. Use of polyethyleneimine polymer in cell culture as attachment factor and lipofection enhancer. BMC Biotechnol. 2004 Oct 15;4:23.
124.) Greene LA, Tischler AS. Establishment of a noradrenergic clonal lnie of rat adrenal pheochromocytoma cells which respond to nerve growth factor. Proc Natl Acad Sci USA. 1976 Jul;73(7):2424-2428.
125.) Graham FL, Siley J, Russell WC, Nairn R. Characteristics of a human cell line transformed by DNA from human adenovirus type 5. J Gen Virol. 1977 Jul;36(1):59-74
126.) Ohta H, Tsuchihara K, Mitsumasu K, et al. Comparative pharmacology of two D1-like dopamine receptors cloned from the silkworm Bombyx mori. Insect Biochem Mol Biol. 2009 May-Jun;39(5-6):342-347.
127.) Narahashi T, Carter DB, Frey J, et al. Sodium channels and GABAA receptor-channel complex as targets of environmental toxicants. Toxicol Lett. 1995 Dec;82-83:239-245. Review.
128.) Seo BB, Matsuno-Yagi A, Yagi T. Modulation of oxidative phosphorylation of human kidney 293 cells by transfection with the internal rotenone-insensitive NADH-quinone oxidoreductase (NDI1) gene of Saccharomyces cerevisiae. Biochim. Biophys Acta. 1999 May 26;1414(1):56-65.
129.) US Patent 6,670,127. Evans. Method for assembly of a polynucleotide encoding a target polypeptide. Filed 8/2/01 published 12/30/03. Assignee: Egea Biosciences, Inc. (San Diego, CA).

130.) US Patent 6,310,034. Woychik, et al. Agouti polypeptide compositions. Filed 3/3/98 published 10/30/01. Assignee: UT-Battelle, LLC (Oak Ridge, TN).
131.) US Patent 4,736,866. Leder et al. Transgenic non-human mammals. Filed 6/22/94 published 4/12/88. Assignee: President and Fellows of Harvard College (Cambridge, MA).
131.) US Patent 5,175,385. Wagner et al. Virus-resistant transgenic mice. Filed 9/3/87 published 12/29/92. Assignee: Ohio University/Edison Animal Biotechnology Center (Athens, OH).
133.) Wu A-J, Dean DH. Functional significance of loops in the receptor binding domain of Bacillus thuringiensis CryIIIA.delta.-endotoxin. J Mol Biol. 1996;255:628-640.
134.) Fagone P, Shedlock DJ, Bao H, et al. Molecular adjuvant HMGB1 enhances anti-influenza immunity during DNA vaccination. Gene Ther. 2011 Nov;18(11):1070-1077.
135.) Firth AE, Atkins JF. Evidence for a novel coding sequence overlapping the 5'-terminal ~90 codons of the Gill-associated and Yellow head okavirus envelope glycoprotein gene. Virol J. 2009;6:222. 5 pages.
136.) Jonsson M, Noppa L, Barbour AG, Bergström. Heterogeneity of outer membrane proteins in Borrelia burgdorferi: comparison of osp operons of three isolates of different geographic origins. Infect Immun. 1992;60(5):1845-1853.
137.) AgroAtlas. Interactive Agricultural Ecological Atlas of Russia and Neighboring Countries. Economic Plants and their Diseases, Pests and Weeds. [web page]
138.) Sickles GM, Mutterer M, Feorino P, Plager H. Recently classified types of Coxsackie virus, group A; behavior in tissue culture. Proc Soc Exp Biol Med. 1955 Nov;90(2):529-531.
139.) Contreras G, Barnett VH, Melnick JL. Identification of Coxsackie viruses by immunological methods and their classification into 16 antigenically distinct types. J Immunol. 1952 Oct;69(4):395-414.
140.) Gear JH. Poliomyelitis. Papers and Discussions presented at the Second International Poliomyelitis Conference. Philadelphia, PA. Lippincott; 1952.
141.) Piczak CV et al. A hepatitis virus complicating studies with mouse leukemia. J Natl Cancer Inst. 1961;27:29-51.
142.) Russia nuclear factories. globalsecurity. [web page]
143.) Russial nuclear storage. globalsecurity. [web page]
144.) GE document: Amersham Biosciences. Preparation and separation of Borrelia burgdorferi plasmid DNA. Report. 3 pages. [web page]
145.) Gamaleya Scientific Research Institute of Epidemiology and Microbiology. [web site]
146.) Firth AE, Atkins JF. A case for a CUG-initiated coding sequence overlapping torovirus ORF Ia and encoding a novel 30 kDa product. 2009;6:136. 6 pages.
147.) Firth AE, Atkins JF. Anaysis of the coding potential of the partially overlapping 3' ORF in segment 5 of the plant fijiviruses. Virol J. 2009;6:32. 5 pages.
148.) BR Petrobras. [web site]
149.) Petrobas.us What we do. [web page]
150.) Jauris-Heipke S, Liegl G, Preac-Mursic V, et al. Molecular Analysis of Genes Encoding Outer Surface Protein C (OspC) of Borrelia burgdorferi Sensu Lato: Relationship to ospA Genotype and Evidence of Lateral Gene Exchange of OspC. J Clin Microbiol. 1995 Jul;33(7):1860-1866.
151.) EMBL-EBI gene database. Nucleotide sequence / EMBL Release (normal divisions) X83554. Borrelia bavariensis OspC gene strain PTrob. [web page]
152.) Margos G, Vollmer SA, Cornet M, et al. A New Borrelia Species Defined by Multilocus Sequence Analysis of Housekeeping Genes. Appl Environ Microbiol. 2009 Aug;75(16):5410-5416.
153.) US Patent 6,248,562. Dunn et al. Chimeric proteins comprising borrelia polypeptides and uses therefor. Filed 4/29/94 published 6/19/01. Assignee: Research Foundation State University of New York (Stony Brook, NY). And Brookhaven Science Associates (Upton, NY). Inventors: Lyme notables John J. Dunn (Bellport, NY), and Benjamin J.Luft (Port Jefferson, NY).
154.) Byrd Davis Mary. Nuclear France: Materials and sites. [web page]
155.) Jonsson M, Noppa L, Barbour A, Bergström S. Heterogeneity of outer membrane proteins in Borrelia burgdorferi: comparison of osp operons of three isolates of different geographic origins. Infect Immun. 1992 May;60(5):1845-1853.
156.) Samuels DS, Marconi RT, Garon CF. Variation in size of the ospA-containing linear plasmid, but not the linear chromosome, among the three Borrelia species associated with Lyme disease. J Gen Microbiol. 1993;139:2445-2449.
157.) Play Golf America. [web page]
158) Luft BJ, Pawagi S, Jiang W, Fiseene S, Gorevic PD, Dunn J. Analysis and expression of the Borrelia burgdorferi P/Gau fla gene: identification of heterogeneity with the B31 strain. FEMS Microbiol. Lett. 1992 May;1(72):63-67.
159.) Bosanac I, Takayuki M, Mikoshiba K, Ikura M. Structural insights into the regulatory mechanism of IP_3. Biochimica et Biophysica Acta. 2004;1742(1):89-102.
160.) Stutzmann GE. Calcium Dysregulation, IP3 Signaling, and Alzheimer's Disease. Neuroscientist. 2005;11(2):110-115.
161.) Galione A, Patel S, Churchill GC. NAADP-induced calcium release in sea urchin eggs. Biol Cell. 2000;92:197-204.
162.) US Patent 7,777,097. Glazebrook et al. Plant disease resistance genes. Filed 6/21/02 published 8/17/10. Assignee: Syngenta Participations AG (Basel, CH). Inventors from Research Triangle Park, North Carolina and from San Diego, La Jolla, and Del Mar, California; and Toronto, Canada.
163.) Plastipedia.co.uk A History of Plastics. The Shape of Plastics (1962) [web page]
164.) Wierschke SC, Shoemaker JR, Haaland PD, et al. Electronic structure and properties of strained polymers: 2. Rigid-rod PBI, PBO and PBZT. Polymer 1992;33(16):3357-3368
165.) Leclerc, Mario. Polyfluorenes: Twenty Years of Progress. J Polym Sci. Part A: Polym. Chem 2001;39:2867-2873. And Bioportal. PKO. [web page]
166.) Cruel Oil Report Exposes Palm Oil's Impact on Health & Environment. Center for Science in the Public Interest. 2005 Jun 2. [web page]
167.) ATCC 58768 Mycotypha indica Kirk et Benny. Isolation: soil, India. [web page]
168.) Benny GL, et al. Observations on Thamnidiaceae (Mucorales). III. Mycotyphaceae fam. nov. and a re-evaluation of Mycotypha sensu Benny & Bemjamin illustrated by two new species. Mycotaxon 22: 119-148, 1985.
169.) ATCC 96974. Saccharomyces paradoxis Bachinskaya, teleomorph. Isolation exudate of Quercus sp., Yalta, Ukraine. [web page]
170.) Naumov GI, Naumova ES, Sniegowski PD. Differentiation of European and Far East Asian populations of Saccharomyces paradoxus by allozyme anaylsis. Int J Syst Bacteriol. 1997 Apr;47(2):341-344.
171.) Naumov ES, Naumov GI, Molina EI. Genetic variation among European stranis of Saccharomyces paradoxus: results from DNA fingerprinting. Syst Appl Microbiol. 2000 Apr;23(1):86-92.
172.) Chatonnet Pascal, Fleury Antoine Boutou Stéphane. Identification of a New Sources of Contamination of Quercus sp. Oak Wood by 2,4,6,-Trichloroanisole and Its Impact on the Contamination of Barrel-Aged Wines. J Agric. Food Chem. 2010;58(19):10528-10538.
173.) Zygomycetes. Mycotypha. Mycotypha Fenner, 1932. [web site]
174.) Delgado-Àvila AE, Urdaneta LM, García y Albino U, et al. Mycotypha indica P.M. Kirk & Benny, in turkey dung, a new record for Venezuela. Multiciencias. 2007;7(2):176-180.
175.) ATCC. Francisella philomiragia (Jensen et al.) Hollis et al. deposited as Yersinia Philomiragia.Isolated from a dying muskratm Brigham City, Utah. ATCC.org
176.) ATCC MGC-25015. Human kidney hypernephroma cell line. [web page]
177.) ATCC 82636. Human fetal brain female 17-18 weeks DNA sample. [web page]
178.) Schutzer SE, Fraser-Liggett CM, Casjens SR, Qui W-G, Dunn JJ, Mongodin EF, Luft BJ. Whole-genome sequences of thirteen isolates of Borrelia burgdorferi. J Bacteriol. 2011;193:1018-1020.
179.) Brookhaven History. The Cosmotron. [web page]
180.) Johnson LJ, Koufopanou V, Goddard MR, et al. Population genetics of the wild yeast Saccharomyces paradoxus. Genetics. 2004 Jan;166(1):43-52.
181.) ATCC 20047 Aspergillus flavus. [web page]
182.) ATCC 56496 Kluyveromyces lactis. [web page]
183.) ATCC MGC-6488 [web page]
184.) ATCC 51383 Borrelia garinii Baranton et al. Isolation: tick, Ixodes ricinus, France. [web page]
185.) Fukunaga M, Koreki Y. A Phylogenic Analysis of Borrelia burgorferi Sensu Lato Isolates Associated with Lyme Disease in Japan by Flagellin Gene Sequence Determination. Inter J Syst Bacteriol. 1996 Apr;46(2):416-421.
186.) US patent 3,620,923. Laboureur, et al. Urate Oxidase and Process for the Production Thereof. Filed 3/25/68 published 11/16/71. Assignee: Societe D'Etudes et D'Applications Biochimiques. [French]. This invention is for a new enzyme or urate oxidase enzyme that promotes oxidation of uric acid to allantoin under fermentation in a medium that has been seeded with bacteria, fungi or yeasts. The patent describes methods to treat gout, rheumatism, urinary calculi and tissue changes in the cardiovascular system.
187.) US Patent 3,431,176. Fukumoto et al. Preparation of Uricase. Filed 1/17/67, published 3/4/69. Assignee: Toyo Boseki Kabushiki Kaisha, Osaka, Japan.
188.) US Patent 3,475,276. Kano. Method of Producing Uricase from Yeast. Filed 7/26/66 published 10/28/69. Assignee: Ono Pharmaceutical Co., Ltd.

189.) Shehata ET, et al. Yeasts isolated from Drosophila and their suspected feeding places in southern and central California. Mycologia 1955;47:799-811.
190.) Chen XJ, et al. A gene-cloning system for Kluyveromyces lactis and isolation of a chromosomal gene required for killer toxin production. J. Basic Microbiol. 1988;28:211-220.
191.) Chen XJ, Wésolowski-Louvel M, Tanguy-Rougeau C, et al. A gene-cloning system for Kluyveromyces lactis and isolation of a chromosomal gene required for killer toxin production. J Basic Microbiol. 1988;28(4):211-220.
192.) US Patent 4,054,515. Sawyer Jr. Water purification methods. Filed 11/28/75 published 10/18/77. Assignee: International Telephone and Telegraph Corporation (Nutley, NJ) (This is AT&T).
193.) US Patent 5,162,331. Staub et al. Aspernomine, an antiinsectan metabolie. Filed 7/19/91 published 11/10/92. Assignee: The United States of America as represented by the Secretary of [Agriculture] (Washington, DC); the University of Iowa Research Foundation (Iowa City, IA); and the Biotechnology Research and Development Corporation (Peoria, IL).
194.) Kurztman et al. Aspergillus nomius, A New Aflatoxin-Producing Species Related to Aspergillus flavus and Aspergillus tamarii. Antonie Van Leeuwenhoek. 1987;53:147-158.
195.) Gloer et al. Nominine: A New Insecticidal Indole Diterpene from the Sclerotia of Aspergillus nomius J Org Chem. 1989;54:2530-2532.
196.) US Patent 5,017,598. Dowd, et al. Nominine, an insecticidal fungal metabolite. Filed 5/17/89 published 5/21/91. Assignee: The United States of America, as represented by the Secretary of [Agriculture] (Washington, DC); and the University of Iowa Research Foundation (Iowa City, IA).
197.) US Patent 5,801,153. Badaway. Method of enhancing the antimicrobial properties of antibacterial antibiotics to massively control and prevent bacterial, fungal, and viral diseases in plants. Filed 2/20/96, published 9/1/98.
199.) Broadbent L. In: International Atomic Energy Agency. Isotopes and radiation in plant pathology. 1966. 8 pages.
199.) Rexrode Charles O, Brown Daniel. USDA Forest Service. Forest Insect & Disease Leaflet. Oak Wilt. [web page]
200.) French DW, Stienstra WC. Oak wilt. University of Minnesota Agricultural Extension Service. Minneapolis, MN. 1980. Folder 310:11.

B.t. is Widely Deployed

1.) US Recall News. USDA. History of the US Department of Agriculture USDA. 2008 Jun 9. [web page]
2.) USDA National Agricultural Library. History, Art and Biography. USDA History. [web site]
3.) Sinclair Upton. The Jungle. New American Library of World Literature, Inc., New York. 1960.
4.) USDA Agricultural Research Service. [web page]
5.) USDA to Open New Lab and Large Animal Facilities in Iowa. The Facilities are Part of a $460-million modernization effort. 2006Jul 26. [news article]
6.) News Brief. U.S. Expert Said Behind Anthrax Mail. 2001 Nov. 29. Discoverynews.com [web page]
7.) Reuters. Group Says U.S. Exeprt Believed Behind Anthrax Attacks. 2001 Nov 28. [web site]
8.) Weiss Rick, Warrick Joby. Army Working on Weapons-Grade Anthrax. 2001 Dec 13. The Washington Post. [web page]
9.) Foster Don. The Message in the Antrax. UCLA Dept. of Epidemiology School of Public Health. In: Vanity Fair, pp. 180-200, Oct. 2003.
10.) Madsen Wayne. Fort Detrick Scientist "Commits Suicide" as Anthrax investigation closes in. Global Research.ca [web page]
11.) The Palm Beach Post. Opinion. Settle the anthrax lawsuit: Government has made Maureen Stevens' case. 2010 Feb. 25. [web page]
11a.) Greenwald Glenn. Serious doubt cast on FBI's anthrax case against Bruce Ivins. 2011 Feb 16. Salon. Topic FBI.
12.) US Recall News. USDA. History of the US Department of Agriculture USDA. 2008 Jun 9. [web site]
13.) USDA National Agricultural Library. History, Art and Biography. USDA History. [web site]
14.) Sinclair Upton. The Jungle. New American Library of World Literature, Inc., New York. 1960.
15.) USDA Agricultural Research Service. [web site].
16.) USDA to Open New Lab and Large Animal Facilities in Iowa. The Facilities are Part of a $460-million modernization effort. 2006 Jul 26. [news article]
17.) Partridge SM. I. General description and application to the qualitative analysis of sugars in apple juice, egg white, and foetal blood of sheep. Biochem J. 1948;42:238-250.
18.) Frederiksen K, Rosenquist H, Jørgensen K, Wilcks A. Occurrence of Natural Bacillus thuringiensis Contaminants and Residues of Bacillus thuringiensis-Based Insecticides on Fresh Fruits and Vegetables. Appl Environ Microbiol. 2006;72(5):3435-3440.
19.) Damgaard PH, Hansen BM, Pedersen JC, Eilenberg J. Natural occurrence of Bacillus thuringiensis on cabbage foliage and in insects associated with cabbage crops. J Appl Microbiol. 1997;82:253-258.
20.) US Patent 4,713,241. Wakisaka, et al. Bacterial insecticide and production thereof. Filed 10/15/84 published 12/15/87. Assignee: Shionogi & Co., Ltd. (Osaka, JP).
21.) US Patent 4,713,241. Wakisaka, et al. Bacterial insecticide and production thereof. Filed 10/15/84 published 12/15/87. Assignee: Shionogi & Co., Ltd. (Osaka, JP).
22.) US Patent 4,277,564. Johnson. Preparing entomocidal products with oligosporogenic mutants of bacillus thuringiensis. Filed 1/9/80 published 7/7/81. Assignee: The United States of America as represented by the Secretary of [Agriculture] (Washington, DC). This patent applies to NRRL B-4453, B-4454, B-4455, B-4456, B4457, B4458.
23.) US Patent 3,758,383 Shieh et al. Production of Exotoxin of Bacillus thuringiensis. Filed 6/1/71, published 9/11/73. Assignee: International Minerals & Chemical Corporation, Libertyville, IL. and Nishiitsutsufi Uwo et al. J Invert Path. 1975;25:355-361.
24.) Yousten AA. Can J Microbiol. 1978;24:492-494.
25.) US Patent 4,133,716. Zamola et al. Method for the biosynthesis of a microbial insecticide. Filed 11/22/76 published 1/9/79. Assignee: CRC Compagnia Ricerca Chimca, S.A. (Chiasso, CH).
26.) US Patent 3,073,749. Megna. Preparation of Microbial Insecticide. Filed 6/9/59 published 1/15/63. Assignee: Bioferm Corporation, Wasco, CA.
27.) US Patent 3,086,922. Mechalas BJ. Method for the Production of Microbial Insecticides. Filed 10/13/61 published 4/23/63. Assignee: Nutrilite Products Inc., Buena Park, CA.
28.) US Patent 3,087,865. Drake, et al. Process for Making Pesticidal Compositions. Filed 5/2/61 published 4/30/63. Assignee: Rohm & Haas Company, Philadelphia, PA.
29.) Krieg A, Schmidt L. NachrBl. Dt. PflSchutzdienst. Braunschw. 1962;14:177-182.
30.) Alibek Ken, Handelman Stephen. Biohazard: The Soviet Union's Agricultural Biological Weapons. 1999 Random House, NY.
31.) Briggs John D. Mass Propagation of Bacteria Pathogenic for Insects. WHO Bulletin. 1964;31:495-497.
32.) US Patent 3,073,749. Megna. Preparation of Microbial Insecticide. Filed 6/9/59 published 1/15/63. Assignee: Bioferm Corporation, Wasco, CA.
33.) US Patent 3,086,922. Mechalas BJ. Method for the Production of Microbial Insecticides. Filed 10/13/61 published 4/23/63. Assignee: Nutrilite Products Inc., Buena Park, CA.
34.) US Patent 3,087,865. Drake, et al. Process for Making Pesticidal Compositions. Filed 5/2/61 published 4/30/63. Assignee: Rohm & Haas Company, Philadelphia, PA.
35.) US Patent 3,920,812. Mann. Method for controlling tobacco mosaic virus disease. Filed 6/4/73 published 11/18/75. Assignee: Research Corporation (New York, NY).
36.) US Patent 3,819,829. Mann. Method for Controlling Fungal Diseases of Plants. Filed 3/4/71 published 6/25/74. Assignee: Research Corporation of New York, NY.
37.) US Patent 3,617,448. Mann. Antibiotic and Methods of Producing and Using it. Filed 10/3/67 published 11/2/71. Assignee: Research Corporation (New York, NY).
38.) Hernandez Eric, Ramisse Francoise, Ducoureau Jean-Pierre, et al. Bacillus thuringiensis subsp. Konkukian (Serotype H34) Superinfection: Case Report and Experimental Evidence of Pathogenicity in Immunosuppressed Mice. J Clin Microbiol. 1998 Jul;36(7):2138-2139.
39.) US Patent 5,874,289 Liu, et al. Bacillus thuringiensis mutants which produce high yields of crystal delta-endotoxin. Filed 8/28/97, issued 2/23/99. Assignee: Abbott Laboratories (Abbott Park, IL).
40.) Lewis Franklin B. (Entomologist, Forest Insect Laboratory Northeastern Forest Experiment Station Forest Service, USDA, New Haven, CT), in Forest Research Note. How to Collect and Process Small Polyhedral Viruses of Insects. Forest Service USDA, Upper Darby, PA. 1960;109:1-8.
41.) Lewis Franklin B. (Entomologist, Forest Insect Laboratory Northeastern Forest Experiment Station Forest Service, U.S.D.A., New Haven, CT), and Rollinson WB (Biological Aide); in Forest Research Note. How to Collect and Process Large Polyhedral Viruses of Insects. Forest Service USDA, Upper Darby, PA. 1962;130:1-6.
42.) EPA. Pesticides: Regulating Pesticides. Food Quality Protection Act (FQPA) of 1996. [web site]
43.) Society for Invertebrate Pathology. 41st Annual Meeting of the Society for Invertebrate Pathology and 9th International Conference on Bacillus thuringiensis. [web site]
44.) MR Spivey Fox, GM Briggs. Salt Mixtures for Purified-Type Diets. III. An Improved Salt Mixture for Chicks. J Nutrition. 1960;72:243-250.
45.) Food Chemical News Inc. Dow Chemical Invented Bacillus thuringiensis Cry1F, a federal court has determined. Pest and Toxic Chem News. 204;32(44):14.
46.) Ravichandra NG. Plant Nematology. IK International Publishing House Pvt. Ltd. 2008
47.) Sayre RM. Biocontrol: Bacillus penetrans and Related Parasites of Nematodes. J Nematol. 1980 Oct;12(4):260-270.
48.) Dube B, Smart GC. Biological Control of Meloidogyne incognita by Paecilomyces lilacinus and Pasteuria penetrans. J Nematol. 1987 Apr;19(2):222-227.
49.) Starr MP, Sayre RM. Pasteuria thornei sp. nov. and Pasteuria penetrans sensu stricto emend., mycelial and endospore-forming pacteria parasitic, respectively, on plant-parasitic

nematodes of the genera Pratylenchus and Meloidogyne. Ann Inst Pasteur Microbiol. 1988 Jan-Feb;139(1):11-31.
50.) R.E.D. Facts. Bacillus thuringiensis. EPA-738-F-98-001. March 1998. United States Environmental Protection Agency. Prevention, Pesticides and Toxic Substances (7511W).
51.) EPA. Pesticides: Regulating Pesticides. Food Quality Protection Act (FQPA) of 1996. [web site]
52.) Jing-Wen Z, Ya-Fei C, Zheng-Hong X, Chen YZN. Production of thuringiensin by fed-batch culture of Bacillus thuringiensis subsp. Darmstadiensis 032with an improved pH-control glucose feeding strategy. Process Biochem. 2007 Jan;42(1):52-56.
53.) Tsai SF, Liu BL, Liao JW, et al. Pulmonary toxicity of thuringiensin administered intratracheally in Sprague-Dawley rats. Toxicology. 2003 Apr 22;186(3):205-216.
54.) Transcripts of the US Dept. of Health and Human Services FDA Center for Biologics Evaluation and Research Vaccines and Related Biological Products Advisory Committee Meeting. 1998 May 26. At the Versailles Rooms I and II, Holiday Inn, 8120 Wisconsin Ave., Bethesda, Maryland. 364 pages.
55.) Wormser GP, Dattwyler RJ, Shapiro ED, et al. The Clinical Assessment, Treatment, and Prevention of Lyme Disease, Human Granulocytic Anaplasmosis, and Babesiosis: Clinical Practice Guidelines by the Infectious Diseases Society of America. Clinical Infectious Diseases. 2006;43:1089-1134.
56.) Blumenthal, Richard. Office of the Attorney General. The State of Connecticut. Connecticut Attorney General's Office Press Release. Attorney General's Investigation Reveals Flawed Lyme Disease Guideline Process, IDSA Agrees To Reassess Guidelines, Install Independent Arbiter. 2008 May 1.
57.) US Patent 6,221,363. Livey et al. Vaccine for the prevention of Lyme disease. Filed 6/25/92 published 4/24/01. Assignee: Baxter Aktiengesellschaft (Vienna, AT).
58.) NCME. Network for Continuing Medical Education. Lyme Disease and Concomitant Tickborne Infections. [videotape, 3hrs.] 1997 June 27. Narrator: Dr. Benjamin Luft State University of New York at Stony Brook.
59.) The Power of SUNY BIO. Fact Sheet. [web page]
60.) Bacillus thuringiensis. History of Bt. University of California San Diego. [web site]
61.) Pharmacia Tax Information Statement. 2002 Aug 13 [web page]
62.) Monsanto. Monsanto to Purchase Chesterfield Village Research Center From Pfizer. 2009Nov 9. [web site]
63.) Charoo NA, Rahman Z, Repka MA, Murthy SN. Electroporation: An Avenue for Transdermal Drug Delivery. Curr Drug Deliv. 2010 Feb 17. [Epub ahead of print]
64.) Ball C, Thomson KR, Kavnoudias H. Irreversible Electroporation: A New Challenge in "Out of Operating Theatre" Anesthesia. Anesth Analg. 2010 Feb 8.
65.) Hussain SM, Hess KL, Gearhart JM, et al. In vitro toxicity of nanoparticles in BRL 3A rat liver cells. Toxicol in Vitro. 2005 Oct;19(7):975-983.
66.) H. Naik, L. Owings, D. Soybel. Tapping the zinc sink: Mitochondrial regulation of intracellular Zn2+ loading. J Amer Coll Surg. 2006;203(3):S11-S12.
67.) Science News. Science Daily. New Nanoparticle Vaccine is Both More Effective and Less Expensive. 2007Sept 20. [Press release on the Internet]
68.) US Patent 7,285,289. Nagy, et al. Nanoparticle vaccines. Filed 4/4/03 published 10/23/07. No assignee listed. Inventors from Bozeman, MT and New Orleans, LA.
69.) Weiss Rick. EPA to Regulate Nanoproducts Sold As Germ-Killing. The Washington Post. [news article].
70.) Turpen Thomas H. Tobacco Mosaic Virus and the Virescence of Biotechnology. In: Philosophical Transactions: Biological Sciences. 1999 Mar 29;354(1383):665-673.
71.) Jaan Suurkula. Genetically Engineered Crops – A Threat to Soil Fertility? [monograph on the Internet].
72.) Jaan Suurkula. Genetically Engineered Crops – A Threat to Soil Fertility? [monograph on the Internet].
73.) Wertz SK. Maize: The Native North American's Legacy of Cultural Diversity and Biodiversity. J Agricul and Environ Ethics. 2005 Apr;18(2):131-156.
74.) US Patent 5,366,892. Foncerrada et al. Gene encoding a coleopteran-active toxin. Filed 1/2/92, published 11/22/94. Assignee: Mycogen Corporation (San Diego, CA).
75.) US Patent 5,747,450. Ohba, et al. Microorganism and insecticide. Filed 7/8/94, published 5/5/98. Assignee: Kubota Corporation (Ibaraki, JP).
76.) US Patent 5,723,756. Peferoen et al. Bacillus thuringiensis strains and their genes encoding insecticidal toxins. Filed 5/18/95, published 3/3/98. Assignee: Plant Genetic Systems, N.C. (Ghent, BE).
77.) US Patent 5,593,881.Thompson, et al. Bacillus thuringiensis dela-endotoxin. Filed 5/6/94, published 1/14/97. Assignee: Mycogen Corporation (San Diego, CA).
78.) US Patent 7,666,644. Castle et al. Glyphosate-N-acetyltransferase (GAT) genes. Filed 12/19/06, published 2/23/10. Assignee: Verdia, Inc. (Rewood City, CA); E.I. du Pont de Nemours & Company (Wilmington, DE); Pioneer Hi-Bred International, Inc. (Des Moines, IA).
79.) Anneclaire J. DeRoos, Aaron Blair, Jennifer A. Rusiecki, et al. Cancer Incidence among Glyphosate-Exposed Pesticide Applicators in the Agricultural Health Study. Environ Health Perspect. 2005 Jan;113(1):49-54.
80.) Andre Leu. Glyphosate: A review of its health and environmental effects. A report on the Organic Federation of Australia web site. 2002 Nov 7.
81.) Hiroyasu Kitashiba, Erina Kitazawa, Sachie Kishitani, Kinya Toriyama. Partial male serility in transgenic tobacco carrying an antisense gene for alternative oxidase under the control of a tapetum-specific promoter. Mol Breed. 1999 Oct;5(3):209-218.
82.) Wisconsin Farmers and Agri-Business Call for Glyphosate (Roundup) Stewardship. UW Extension report. 2 pages, undated, promoted by WI Corn Growers Assoc., WI Soybean Assoc., Prof. Dairy Producers of WI; UW Extension Team Grain; WI Potato and Vegetable Growers Assoc.; WI Assoc. of Prof. Crop Consultants; WI Fertilizer and Chemical Assoc.; and the UW-Madison Weed Scientists.
83.) European Commission Research. Risk assessment with genetically engineered woody plants expressing virus coat protein gene. [web site]
84.) Safety of Genetically Engineered Foods: Approaches to Assessing Unintended Health Effects. The Committee on Identifying and Assessing Unintended Effects of Genetically Engineered Foods on Human Health, the Board on Life Sciences, the Food and Nutrition Board, the Board on Agriculture and Natural Resources and the Institute of Medicine and National Research Council of the National Academies. The National Academies Press. 2004. Washington, DC. 256 pages.
85.) Mae-Wan Ho. Genetically Engineered Foods: The Hazards are Inherent in the Technology. Third World Network. Earth Summit Plus 5 Briefing No. 7. [monograph]
86.) Capdevila JA, Bisbe V, Gasser I, et al. [Enterobacter amnigenus. An unusual human pathogen]. [Article in Spanish]. Enferm Infecc Microbiol. Clin. 1998 Oct;16(8):364-366.
87.) The Institute of Science in Society. Ban GMOs Now Report. April 6, 2008. [web site]
88.) Smith Jeffrey M. The Health Dangers of Genetically Engineered Foods and the Cover-up. YouTube video.
89.) Smith Jeffrey M. The GMO Trilogy. Why Genetically Modified Organisms threaten your health, the environment and future generations. 3DVD set. www.seedsofdeception.com
90.) Kavitha Kurungati. Mass Protests against GM Crops in India. India-wide coalition against GM Brinjal in the wake of toxic GM cotton. Institute of Science in Society. [web site] Apr 30, 2008.
91.) Agrifood Awareness Australia. State governments and GM crops. Issue Paper 5. 4 pages. [monograph on the Internet]
92.) Mercer Chris. EU backs Poland's GM crop ban. 2006 May 10. Food navigator.com [web page]
93.) Ministry for the Environment. Genetically modified medicines and food. [web site] 2010.
94.) Thorsten Severin, Michael Hogan; James Jukwey (ed). Germany to ban cultivation of GMO maize-Minister. 2009 Apr 14. Reuters News. [monograph on the Internet]
95.) AusSMC. Australian Science Media Centre. Rapid Roundup: SA Government extends moratorium on genetically modified food crops – experts respond. 2008 Feb 8. Updated 2008Feb 11. [web site]39. Institute of Science in Society. [web site] Field Testing Genetically Engineered Eucalyptus: Environment Assessment Still Inadequate. ISIS Press Release. 8/2/10. [web page]
96.) Boucias Drion G, Pendland Jacquelyn C. Principles of Insect Pathology. 1998 Kluwer Academic Publishers. (Netherlands).
97.) Lewis Franklin B. (Entomologist, Forest Insect Laboratory Northeastern Forest Experiment Station Forest Service, USDA, New Haven, CT), in Forest Research Note. How to Collect and Process Small Polyhedral Viruses of Insects. Forest Service USDA, Upper Darby, PA. 1960;109:1-8.
98.) Lewis Franklin B. (Entomologist, Forest Insect Laboratory Northeastern Forest Experiment Station Forest Service, U.S.D.A., New Haven, CT), and Rollinson WB (Biological Aide); in Forest Research Note. How to Collect and Process Large Polyhedral Viruses of Insects. Forest Service USDA, Upper Darby, PA. 1962;130:1-6.
99.) Rollinson WD, Lewis FB, Waters WE. The Successful Use of a Nuclear-Polyhedrosis Virus against the Gypsy Moth. Notes. 1965. Forest Insect and Disease Laboratory Northeastern Forest Experiment Station Forest Service, US Department of Agriculture, West Haven, Connecticut.
100.) Bird FT. The Use of a Virus Disease in the Biological Control of the European Pine Sawfly, Neodiprion sertifer (Geoffr.) The Canadian Entomologist. 1953 Dec 1;85(12):437-446.

Brucellosis

1.) Starr MP, Sayre RM. Pasteuria thornei sp. nov. and Pasteuria penetrans sensu stricto emend., mycelial and endospore-forming pacteria parasitic, respectively, on plant-parasitic nematodes of the genera Pratylenchus and Meloidogyne. Ann Inst Pasteur Microbiol. 1988 Jan-Feb;139(1):11-31.
2.) Montie TC, Doyle-Huntzinger D, Craven RC, Holder IA. Loss of Virulence Associated with Absence of Flagellum in an Isogenic Mutant of Pseudomonas aeruginosa in the Burned-Mouse Model. Infect and Immun. 1982 Dec;38(3):1296-1298.
3.) US Patent 5,436,000. Barbour, et al. Flagella-less borrelia. Filed 1/11/91, published 7/25/95. Assignee: University of Texas System (Austin, TX). Inventors: Alan G. Barbour, Virgilio Bundoc.

4.) US Patent 5,585,102. Barbour, et al., Flagella-less borrelia. Filed 9/20/93, published 12/17/96. Assignee: Board of Regents, The University of Texas System (Austin, TX). Inventors: Alan G. Barbour, Virgilio G. Bundoc, Adriadna Sadziene.
5.) Johnson RC, Burgdorfer W, Lane RS, Barbour AG, Hayes SF, Hyde FW. Borrelia coriaceae sp. nov.: Putative Agent of Epizootic Bovine Abortion. Inter J Syst Evol Microbiol. 1987 Jan;37(1):72-74.
6.) Transcripts of the US Dept. of Health and Human Services FDA Center for Biologics Evaluation and Research Vaccines and Related Biological Products Advisory Committee Meeting. 1998 May 26. At the Versailles Rooms I and II, Holiday Inn, 8120 Wisconsin Ave., Bethesda, Maryland. 364 pages.
7.) Wormser GP, Dattwyler RJ, Shapiro ED, et al. The Clinical Assessment, Treatment, and Prevention of Lyme Disease, Human Granulocytic Anaplasmosis, and Babesiosis: Clinical Practice Guidelines by the Infectious Diseases Society of America. Clinical Infectious Diseases. 2006;43:1089-1134.
8.) Pharmacia Tax Information Statement. 2002 Aug 13. [web page]
9.) Monsanto. Monsanto to Purchase Chesterfield Village Research Center From Pfizer. 2009Nov 9. [web site]
10.) Charoo NA, Rahman Z, Repka MA, Murthy SN. Electroporation: An Avenue for Transdermal Drug Delivery. Curr Drug Deliv. 2010 Feb 17. [Epub ahead of print]
11.) Ball C, Thomson KR, Kavnoudias H. Irreversible Electroporation: A New Challenge in "Out of Operating Theatre" Anesthesia. Anesth Analg. 2010 Feb 8.
12.) US Patent 3,674,866. Fritz Lindner et al. Moenomycin and process for producing same. Filed 9/1/64, issued 7/4/72. Assignee: Farbwerke Moechst Aktiengesellschaft vormals Meister Lucius & Bruning, Frankfurt/Main, Germany. (BASF)
13.) Microbwiki. Brucella abortus. [web page]
14.) Taylor JG, Li X, Oberthür M, Zhu W, Kahne DE. The Total Synthesis of Moenomycin A. J Am Chem Soc. 2006Nov 29;128(47):15084-15085.
15.) Nicolson GL, Gan R, Haier J. Evidence for Brucella spp. and Mycoplasma spp. Co-Infections in Blood of Chronic Fatigue Syndrome Patients. J Chron Fat Syn. 2005;12(2):5-17.
16.) Blumenthal, Richard. Office of the Attorney General. The State of Connecticut. Connecticut Attorney General's Office Press Release. Attorney General's Investigation Reveals Flawed Lyme Disease Guideline Process, IDSA Agrees To Reassess Guidelines, Install Independent Arbiter. 2008 May 1.
17.) Hendson M, Lane RS. Genetic Characteristics of Borrelia coriaceae Isolates from Soft Tick Ornithodoros coriaceus (Acari: Argasidae). J Clin Microbiol 2000 Jul;38(7):2678-2682.
18.) US Patent 5,582,829. Alliger, et al. Sonicated borrelia burgdorferi vaccine. Filed July 28, 1992, published 12/10/96. Assignee: Rx Technologies, Inc. (Garden City, NY).
19.) Tsai SF, Liu BL, Liao JW, et al. Pulmonary toxicity of thuringiensin administered intratracheally in Sprague-Dawley rats. Toxicology. 2003Apr 22;186(3):205-216.
20.) US Patent 6,221,363. Livey et al. Vaccine for the prevention of Lyme disease. Filed 6/25/92 published 4/24/01. Assignee: Baxter Aktiengesellschaft (Vienna, AT).
21.) NCME. Network for Continuing Medical Education. Lyme Disease and Concomitant Tickborne Infections. [videotape, 3hrs.] 1997 June 27. Narrator: Dr. Benjamin Luft State University of New York at Stony Brook.
22.) The Power of SUNY BIO. Fact Sheet. [web page]
23.) Bacillus thuringiensis. History of Bt. University of California San Diego. [web site].
24.) Hussain SM, Hess KL, Gearhart JM, et al. In vitro toxicity of nanoparticles in BRL 3A rat liver cells. Toxicol in Vitro. 2005 Oct;19(7):975-983.
25.) H. Naik, L. Owings, D. Soybel. Tapping the zinc sink: Mitochondrial regulation of intracellular Zn2+ loading. J Amer Coll Surg. 2006;203(3):S11-S12.
26.) Science News. Science Daily. New Nanoparticle Vaccine is Both More Effective and Less Expensive. 2007Sept 20. [Press release on the Internet]
27.) US Patent 7,285,289. Nagy, et al. Nanoparticle vaccines. Filed 4/4/03 published 10/23/07. No assignee listed. Inventors from Bozeman, MT and New Orleans, LA.
28.) Weiss Rick. EPA to Regulate Nanoproducts Sold As Germ-Killing. The Washington Post. [news article].
29.) Turpen Thomas H. Tobacco Mosaic Virus and the Virescence of Biotechnology. In: Philosophical Transactions: Biological Sciences. 1999 Mar 29;354(1383):665-673.
30.) Jaan Suurkula. Genetically Engineered Crops – A Threat to Soil Fertility? [monograph on the Internet].
31.) Wertz SK. Maize: The Native North American's Legacy of Cultural Diversity and Biodiversity. J Agricul and Environ Ethics. 2005 Apr;18(2):131-156.
32.) US Patent 5,366,892. Foncerrada et al. Gene encoding a coleopteran-active toxin. Filed 1/2/92, published 11/22/94. Assignee: Mycogen Corporation (San Diego, CA).
33.) US Patent 5,747,450. Ohba, et al. Microorganism and insecticide. Filed 7/8/94, published 5/5/98. Assignee: Kubota Corporation (Ibaraki, JP).
34.) US Patent 5,723,756. Peferoen et al. Bacillus thuringiensis strains and their genes encoding insecticidal toxins. Filed 5/18/95, published 3/3/98. Assignee: Plant Genetic Systems, N.C. (Ghent, BE).
35.) US Patent 5,593,881.Thompson, et al. Bacillus thuringiensis dela-endotoxin. Filed 5/6/94, published 1/14/97. Assignee: Mycogen Corporation (San Diego, CA).
36.) US Patent 7,666,644. Castle et al. Glyphosate-N-acetyltransferase (GAT) genes. Filed 12/19/06, published 2/23/10. Assignee: Verdia, Inc. (Rewood City, CA); E.I. du Pont de Nemours & Company (Wilmington, DE); Pioneer Hi-Bred International, Inc. (Des Moines, IA).
37.) Anneclaire J. DeRoos, Aaron Blair, Jennifer A. Rusiecki, et al. Cancer Incidence among Glyphosate-Exposed Pesticide Applicators in the Agricultural Health Study. Environ Health Perspect. 2005 Jan;113(1):49-54.
38.) Andre Leu. Glyphosate: A review of its health and environmental effects. A report on the Organic Federation of Australia web site. 2002 Nov 7.
39.) Hiroyasu Kitashiba, Erina Kitazawa, Sachie Kishitani, Kinya Toriyama. Partial male serility in transgenic tobacco carrying an antisense gene for alternative oxidase under the control of a tapetum-specific promoter. Mol Breed. 1999 Oct;5(3):209-218.
40.) Wisconsin Farmers and Agri-Business Call for Glyphosate (Roundup) Stewardship. UW Extension report. 2 pages, undated, promoted by WI Corn Growers Assoc., WI Soybean Assoc., Prof. Dairy Producers of WI; UW Extension Team Grain; WI Potato and Vegetable Growers Assoc.; WI Assoc. of Prof. Crop Consultants; WI Fertilizer and Chemical Assoc.; and the UW-Madison Weed Scientists.
41.) European Commission Research. Risk assessment with genetically engineered woody plants expressing virus coat protein gene. [web site]
42.) Safety of Genetically Engineered Foods: Approaches to Assessing Unintended Health Effects. The Committee on Identifying and Assessing Unintended Effects of Genetically Engineered Foods on Human Health, the Board on Life Sciences, the Food and Nutrition Board, the Board on Agriculture and Natural Resources and the Institute of Medicine and National Research Council of the National Academies. The National Academies Press. 2004. Washington, DC. 256 pages.
43.) Mae-Wan Ho. Genetically Engineered Foods: The Hazards are Inherent in the Technology. Third World Network. Earth Summit Plus 5 Briefing No. 7. [monograph on the Internet]
44.) Capdevila JA, Bisbe V, Gasser I, et al. [Enterobacter amnigenus. An unusual human pathogen]. [Article in Spanish]. Enferm Infecc Microbiol. Clin. 1998 Oct;16(8):364-366.
45.) The Institute of Science in Society. Ban GMOs Now Report. April 6, 2008. [web site]
46.) Smith Jeffrey M. The Health Dangers of Genetically Engineered Foods and the Cover-up. YouTube video.
47.) Smith Jeffrey M. The GMO Trilogy. Why Genetically Modified Organisms threaten your health, the environment and future generations. 3DVD set. www.seedsofdeception.com
48.) Kavitha Kurungati. Mass Protests against GM Crops in India. India-wide coalition against GM Brinjal in the wake of toxic GM cotton. Institute of Science in Society. [web site] Apr 30, 2008.
49.) Agrifood Awareness Australia. State governments and GM crops. Issue Paper 5. 4 pages. [monograph on the Internet]
50.) Mercer Chris. EU backs Poland's GM crop ban. 2006 May 10. Food navigator.com [web page]
51.) Ministry for the Environment. Genetically modified medicines and food. [web site] 2010.
52.) Thorsten Severin, Michael Hogan; James Jukwey (ed). Germany to ban cultivation of GMO maize-Minister. 2009 Apr 14. Reuters News. [monograph on the Internet]
53.) AusSMC. Australian Science Media Centre. Rapid Roundup: SA Government extends moratorium on genetically modified food crops – experts respond. 2008 Feb 8. Updated 2008 Feb 11. [web site]
54.) Institute of Science in Society. [web site] Field Testing Genetically Engineered Eucalyptus: Environment Assessment Still Inadequate. ISIS Press Release. 8/2/10. [web page]
55.) EPA. Pesticides: Regulating Peticides. Food Quality Protection Act (FQPA) of 1996. [web page]
56.) US Patent 5,436,000. Barbour (Alan) et al. Flagella-less borrelia. Filed 1/11/91 published 7/25/95. Assignee: University of Texas System (Austin, TX).
57.) US Patent 6,077,515. Barbour, et al. Flagella-less borrelia. Filed 8/13/96 published 6/20/00. Assignee: The University of Texas System, Board of Regents (Austin, TX).

Pleuropneumonias and Animal Feeds

1.) Records of the Bureau of Animal Industry. Record Group 17 1864-1962. National Archives. [web page]
2.) Garfield Eugene. Current Comments. Lyme Disease Research Uncovers a Case of Delayed Recognition: Arvid Afzelius and His Successors. Essays of an Information Scientist: Creativity, Delayed Recognition, and Other Essays, Vol:12, p.345, 1989. Current Contents, #49, p.3-8, December 4, 1989.
3.) Noguchi Hideyo. Etiology of Yellow Fever. VIII. Presence of a Leptospira in Wild Animals in Guayaquil and its Relation to Leptospira Icterohemorrhagie and Leptospira Icteroides. 1919 May. Report from Labs at Rockefeller Institute for Medical Research. Pp. 95-107.

4.) Rice CM, Lenches EM, Eddy SR, et al. Nucleotide sequence of yellow fever virus: implications for flavivirus gene expression and evolution. Science 1985 Aug;229(4715):726-733.
5.) Clark Harold W. Lecture I: Mycoplasmas Properties and their Role in Autoimmune Diseases. San Marcos University College of Veterinarian Medicine Lima, Peru Lectures. 1999 Aug. 22 pages.
6.) Weisburg WG, Tully JG, Rose DL, et al. A Phylogenetic Analysis of the Mycoplasmas: Basis for Their Classification. J Bacteriol. 1989 Dec;171(12):6455-6467.
7.) Rink L, Nicklas W, Alvarez-Ossorio L, et al. Differential induction of tumor necrosis factor alpha in murine and human leukocytes by Mycoplasma arthriditis-derived superantigen. Infec Immun. 1994;62(2):462-467.
8.) Tully Joseph G, Rose David L, Yunker Conrad E, et al. Spiroplasma ixodetis sp. nov., a New Species from Ixodes pacificus Ticks Collected in Oregon. Inter J Syst Bacteriol. 1995 Jan;45(1):23-28.
9.) Tully JG, Rose DL, Yunker CE, et al. Helical mycoplasmas (spiroplasmas) from Ixodes ticks. Science 1981 May 29;212(4498):1043-1045.
10.) Weisburg WG, Tully JG, Rose DL, et al. A phylogenetic analysis of the mycoplasmas: basis for their classification. J Bacteriol. 1989 Dec.;171(12):6455-6467.
11.) US Patent 5,242,820. Lo. Pathogenic mycoplasma. Filed 6/6/91 published 9/7/93. Assignee: American Registry of Pathology (Washington, DC).
12.) US Patent 3,485,721. Woodhour et al. Process for Growing Mycoplasma Pneumonial Organisms. Filed 2/12/65 published 12/23/69. Assignee: Meck & Co., Rahway, NJ. And US Patent 3,627,874. Vella et al. Vaccine Preparation. Filed 7/16/69, published 12/14/71. Assignee: Merck & Co., Inc. (Rahway, NJ).
13.) Low Iolanda E, Eaton Monroe D. Replication of Mycoplasma pneumonia in Broth Culture. J Bacteriol. 1965 Mar;89(3):725-728.
14.) Rodwell AW, Rodwell ES. The breakdown of carbohydrates by Asterococcus mycoides, the organism of bovine pleuropneumonia. Australian J Biol Sci. 1954;7:18-30.
15.) North Dakota State University. News Archive. Use Care When Adding Monensin. 2005Feb. 17. [web site].
16.) Hutjens Michael F. Managing Monensin. 2007 Sept 1. (Extension Dairy Specialist University of Illinois, Urbana). [monograph on the Internet]
17.) Kabel Marcus. USDA revokes OK for Tyson chicken labels. [Monograph on the Internet] 2007 Nov 20.
18.) US Patent 6,682,762. Register. Poultry and livestock feed additive. Filed 10/9/01, published 1/27/04. Assignee: Heart-O-Dixie Animal Nutrition, LLC (Montgomery, AL).
19.) Houlihan Adam J, Russell James B. The susceptibility of ionophore-resistant Clostridium aminophilum F to other antibiotics. J Antimicrob Chemo. 2003;52:623-628.
20.) USDA Agricultural Research Service. Two Strategies for Protecting Poultry from Coccidia. [web site]
21.) Schneider Keith. AIDS-Like virus is Found at High Rate in US Cattle. The New York Times. 1991 June 1.
22.) Langhoff PJ. God Science: The Secret World of Rampant Genetics, Hidden Illness, and Biotech Profiteering. Allegory Press LLC. 2010. 825 pages. Bovine Immunodeficiency virus, page 657.
23.) Harris Jr. Emmett D, Genung WG, Haines CE. Cattle Grub Control with Bayer 21/199 in the Everglades. The Florida Entomologist. 1959;42(4):155-157.
24.) The Cass City Chronicle. New Material For Insect Pest Control. Bayer 21/199Added to Approved Pesticides. 1958 Oct 16, Cass City, Michigan. [Newspaper Article]
25.) Marquardt WC, Lovelace SA, Fritts DH. Spray treatment of calves with Bayer 21/199 for control of cattle grubs and lice in Montana. J Am Vet Med Assoc. 1960 Nov 15;137:589-594.
26.) Raun ES, Herrick JB. Feedlot tests of the efficacy of Dow ET-57(trolene) for control of cattle grubs. J Am Vet Med Assoc. 1957 Nov 1;131(9):421-423.
27.) Wilson HG, LaBrecque GC. Tests with Larvicides for the Control of House Flies in Poultry Houses. The Florida Entomologist. 1960 Mar;43(1):19-21.
28.) Bailey Donald L, Meifert DW, Bishop PM. Control of House Flies in Poultry Houses with Larvicides. The Florida Entomologist. 1968 Jun;51(2):107-111.
29.) Kane PF, Cohen CJ, Betker WR, MacDougall D. Insecticide Assay, Assay of Co-Ral in Technical Material and Formulated Products. J Agric. Food Chem. 1960;8(1):26-29.
30.) Tietz Jeff. Pork's Dirty Secret: The nation's top hog producer is also one of America's worst polluters. 2009May 4. Global Research.ca Centre for Research on Globalization. From Rolling Stone.com 2006 Dec 14.
31.) Faine Solomon. Leptospira and Leptospirosis. CRC Press, Inc. Boca Raton, FL.
32.) Schraufnagel FH. Disposal of Indusrial Wastes by Irrigation. Public Health Reports. 1959 Feb;74(2):133-140.
33.) Eldridge EF. Industrial Wastes. Recent Trade Waste Disposal Methods. Sewage Works Journal. 1941 Jan;13(1):105-114. Presented at the First Annual Convention of the Sewage Works Federation, Chicago, IL 1940 Oct 5.
34.) Subcommittee on Underutilized Resources and Animal Feedstuffs, Committee on Animal Nutrition, National Reserach Council. Underutilized Resources as Animal Feedstuffs. National Academy of Sciences, Washington, DC. 1983. 253 pages.
35.) EPA. Pesticides: Regulating Pesticides. Food Quality Protection Act (FQPA) of 1996. [web site]
36.) Society for Invertebrate Pathology. 41st Annual Meeting of the Society for Invertebrate Pathology and 9th International Conference on Bacillus thuringiensis. [web site]
37.) MR Spivey Fox, GM Briggs. Salt Mixtures for Purified-Type Diets. III. An Improved Salt Mixture for Chicks. J Nutrition. 1960;72:243-250.
38.) US Patent 3,949,079. Brandl, et al. Antibiotic derivatives. Filed 8/14/67, issued 4/6/76. Assignee: Biochemie Ges.m.b.H. (Vienna, OE).
39.) US Patent 2,903,356. Lampen et al. Animal growth stimulation compositions. Filed 7/22/57. Assignee: Olin Mathieson Chemical Corporation, New York.
40.) Swiss Institute of Bioinformatics. HAMAP: Borrelia burgdorferi (strain ZS7) complete proteome. Generl Information. [web page]
41.) Pickens Edgar G, Gerloff Robert K, Burgdorfer Willy. Spirochete from the Rabbit Tick, Haemaphysalis leporispalustris (Packard). I. Isolation and Preliminary Characterization. J Bacteriol. 1968Feb;95(2):291-299.
42.) Houlihan Adam J, Russell James B. The susceptibility of ionophore-resistant Clostridium aminophilum F to other antibiotics. J Antimicrob Chemo. 2003;52:623-628.
43.) USDA Agricultural Research Service. Two Strategies for Protecting Poultry from Coccidia. [web site] www.ars.usda.gov
44.) Mac Kenzie William R, Hoxie Neil J, Proctor Mary E, Blair Kathleen A, Peterson Dan E, Kazmierczak James J, Addiss David G, Fox Kim R, Rose Joan B, Davis Jeffrey P. A Massive Outbreak in Milwaukee of Cryptosporidium Infection Transmitted through the Public Water Supply. 1994 Jul 21;331(3):161-167.
45.) Mather RE, Pratt AD, Holdaway CW. Fused Tricalcium Phosphate as a Low-Fluorine Phosphorus Supplement for Dairy Cattle. J Dairy Science 1949;32:228-236.
46.) Morris Hanson. Diseases of Feedlot Cattle. Canadian J Compar. Med. 1958 Dec;22(12):433-436.
47.) Shah PK. Rendering Plants. Recycling of Dead Animals and Slaughterhouse Wastes. [web page]
48.) Loehr RC. Effluent quality from anaerobic lagoons treating feedlot wastes. J Water Poll Control Fed. 1967 Mar;39(3):384-391.
49.) Mahloch JL, McGriff EC Jr. Agricultural wastes. J Water Pollut Control Fed. 1974Jun;46(6):1280-1283.
50.) Wheeler RP. Waste disposal and agriculture. Treatment and disposal of farm wastes. R Soc Health J. 1979 Aug;99(4):143-151.
51.) Schraufnagel FH. Disposal of Indusrial Wastes by Irrigation. Public Health Reports. 1959Feb;74(2):133-140.
52.) Eldridge EF. Industrial Wastes. Recent Trade Waste Disposal Methods. Sewage Works Journal. 1941 Jan;13(1):105-114. Presented at the First Annual Convention of the Sewage Works Federation, Chicago, IL 1940 Oct 5.
53.) Ryan William A. Industrial Wastes. Effect of Cannery Wastes on Operation of Sewage Treatment Plants. Sewage Works Journal 1940 Jan ;12(1):99-105. Presented at the Fall Meeting of the New York State Sewage Works Association, Olean. 1939 Oct 7.
54.) Neubert AM, Graham DW, Henry JL, et al. Sugar Recovery, Recovery of Sugars from Pear-Canning Waste. J Agric. Food Chem. 1954 Jan;2(1):30-36.
55.) Murphy Homer S, Hepler JM, Eldridge EF. Water pollution control: cannery wastes: a compilation covering activities, experimental work and cooperative investigations as conducted by the Department of Conservation, the Department of Health and the Michigan Canners' Association. Michigan Dept. of Conservation, Michigan Dept. of Health, Michigan Canners Assoc. 1927 Apr 1. 18 pages. Available from the EPA National Library Network.
56.) Warrick Louis F. Methods of treating cannery waste a summary of cooperative work conducted in Wisconsin by the Wisconsin State Board of Health and the National Canners Association. 1939. 91 pages. Available from the EPA National Library Network.
57.) Environmental Protection Agency EPA National Library Network. Canneries Waste Disposal. 24 reports.
58.) Law James P, Thomas RE, Myers Leon H. Water Pollution Control Research Series. Nutrient removal from cannery wastes by spray irrigation of grassland. 1969. US Federal Water Pollution Control Administration, Washington, DC.
59.) Cornell, Howeland, Hayes, Merryfield. Seafood cannery waste study: Phase I. 1971 National Cannery Association, Seattle, Washington. Vol. 48.
60.) Marine Studies of San Pedro Bay, California. Part 16. Alan Hancock Foundation, Harbors Environmental Projects and the Office of Sea Grant Programs, Institute of Marine and Coastal Studies, University of Southern California. 1979, 579 pages. A report for the City of Los Angeles, Dept. of Public Works, Bureau of Engineering, for the Terminal Island Treatment Plant and the Environmental Protection Agency, Report to Congress on seafood waste effluents, for the Tuna Research Foundation.
61.) Green Giant Company. Pilot plant installation for fungal treatment of vegetable canning wastes. 1971, Washington. 77 pages. Corporate Author US EPA. Part of the Water pollution control research series. Available from the EPA National Library Network.
62.) Morris Hanson. Diseases of Feedlot Cattle. Canadian J Compar. Med. 1958 Dec;22(12):433-436.

63.) US Patent 2,980,586. Norden et al. Method of Producing Swine Erysipelas Vaccine. Filed 6/9/58 published 4/18/61. Assignee: Norden Laboratories, Inc. (Lincoln, NE).
64.) Pierson RE. Polyarthritis in Colorado feedlot lambs. J Am Vet Med Assoc.1967 Jun 15;150(12):1487-1492.
65.) Cutlip RC, Smith PC, Page LA. Chlamydial polyarthritis of lambs: a review. J Am Vet Med Assoc. 1972 Dec 1;161(11):1213-1216.
66.) Hopkins JB, Stephenson EH, Storz J, Pierson RE. Conjunctivitis associated with chlamydial polyarthritis in lambs. J Am Vet Med Assoc. 1973 Nov 15;163(10):1157-1160.
67.) Technical Report: DDC AD408401. Conference on Biological Control of Insects of Medical Importance. American Institute of Biological Sciences (Washington, DC). 148pages. Date stamped June 28, 1961 Naval Medical Field Research Laboratory, Camp LeJeune, North Carolina. (DDC) July 16, 1963. Unclassified documents from the public domain.
68.) Serratia marcescens. Schenectady County Community College. [web page]
69.) USDA. Beltsville, MD. News and Reviews. Biological Control at National Entomology Society Meetings. Presentation at the 1995 National Meeting of the Entomological Society of America in Las Vegas. [newsletter]. Farrar R. Strain of Serratia marcescens with high virulence when fed to corn earworm larvae.
70.) US Patent 3,087,865. Drake et al. Process for Making Pesticidal Compositions. Filed 5/2/61, published 4/30/63. Assignee: Rohm & Haas Company, Philadelphia, PA.
71.) US Patent 4,016,265 Inoue, et al. Synergistic insecticidal compositions containing .beta.-exotoxin. Filed 11/8/71, published 4/5/77. Assignee: Sandoz, Inc. (E. Hanover, NJ).
72.) US Patent 4,888,276. Shelburne. Method and composition for the diagnosis of Lyme disease. Filed 6/26/86 published 12/19/89. Assignee: Minnesota Mining and Manufacturing Company (St. Paul, MN).
73.) News: Evaluation of Surfactants in Fertilizers Calm Enthusiastic Claims. J Agric Food Chem. 1954 Sept;2(20):1015-1016.
74.) US Patent 3,681,441. Robertson. Filed 4/13/70 published 8/1/72. Quaternary Fluorinated Ammonium Salts. Assignee: Minnesota Mining and Manufacturing Company (Saint Paul, MN).
75.) Freedman Alix M. 'Impact Booster' Tobacco Firm Shows How Ammonia Spurs Delivery of Nicotine. 1995 Dec 28. The Pulitzer Prizes. [web site]
76.) US Patent 3,615,654. Ayukawa et al. Method of treating microbial cells. Filed 5/17/68 published 10/26/71. Assignee: CPC International Inc.
77.) Brock TD. Microorganisms From Smallpox to Lyme Disease. Scientific American. W.H. Freeman and Company. 1990. p. 28-37.
78.) Dhillon AS, Winterfield RW, Thacker HL. Quaternary Ammonium Compounds Toxicity in Chickens. Avian Dis. 1982 Oct-Dec;26(4):928-931.
79.) Quaternary ammonium compound toxicity in broiler chickens. Nova Scotia. Cross Canada Disease Report. Can Vet J. 1996 Aug;37:482.
80.) General Farm Biosecurity. The University of Vermont. [web page]
81.) Marriott NG, Gravani RB. Principles of food sanitation. Fifth Edition. 2006 Springer Science+Business Media Inc. and Cleaning and Disinfecting. 2005 Jan. [web page]
82.) Jeffrey JS. Sanitation-Disinfection Basics. Poultry Fact Sheet #27. Cooperative Extension. University of California. 1997.
83.) Lacy MP, French JD. Effective Broiler House Clean Out and Disinfection Techniques. The University of Georgia College of Agricultural & Environmental Sciences Cooperative Extension Service. [web page]
84.) US Patent 3,571,844. Stiles. Poultry Conveyor System. Filed 6/4/68 published 3/23/71. Assignee: The University of Connecticut (Storrs, CT).
85.) ATCC 33825. Spiroplasma monobiae Whitcomb et al. Isolation: vespid wasp hemolymph, Monobia quadridens, Maryland. [web page]
86.) US Patent 5,296,371. Razin, et al. DNA encoding spiroplasma sp. dna methylase. Filed 10/4/91 published 3/22/94. Assignee: Yissum Research Development Company of the Hebrew University of Jerusalem, an Israeli Corp.
87.) US Patent 4,886,750 Bertola et al. Process for the preparation of a pharmaceutically active compound in a sterospecific form of the formula. Filed 1/6/87 published 12/12/89. Assignee: Gist-Brocades N.V (Delft, NL) and Shell Internationale Research Mattschappij B.V. (The Haag, NL).
88.) US Patent 4,565,782. Bewick. Process for producing optically active aryloxypropionic acids and derivatives thereof useful as herbicides. Filed 7/26/84 published 1/21/86. Assignee: Imperial Chemical Industries PLC (London, GB2).
89.) Lock EA, Gyte A, Sturgess NC, et al. 2-Halopropionic acid-induced cerebellar granule cell necrosis in rat: in vivo and in vitro studies. From Syngenta Central Toxicology Laboratory, Macclesfield, Cheshire, UK. Neurotoxicol. 2001 Jun;22(3):363-374.
90.) US Patent 4,601,987. Klibanov, et al. Enzymatic production of optical isomers of 2-halopropionic acids. Filed 2/27/85 published 7/22/86. Assignee: Massachusetts Institute of Technology (Cambridge, MA).
91.) Kricheldorf Hans R. Handbook of Polymer Synthesis Part A. 1992. Marcel Dekker Inc., New York.
92.) Schubert EF. Doping with II-V Semiconductors. Section 5-Doping with elemental sources. P. 165-207. AT&T Bell Laboratories, New Jersey Cambridge University Press 1993.
93.) Park JH, Cho YW, Kwon IC, et al. Assessment of PEO/PTMO multiblock copolymer/segmented polyurethane blends as coating materials for urinary catheters: in vitro bacterial adhesion and encrustation behavior. Biomaterials. 2002 Oct;23919):3991-4000.
94.) Anderson JP, Cappello J, Martin DC. Morphology and primary crystal structure of a silk-like protein polymer synthesized by genetically engineered Escherichia coli bacteria. Biopolymers. 1994 Aug;34(8):1049-1058.
95.) Anthierens T, Ragaert P, Verbrugghe S, et al. Use of endospore-forming bacteria as an active oxygen scavenger in plastic packaging materials. Innovative Food Science and Emerging Technologies.2011;12:594–599
96.) US Patent 5,232,850. Casida, Jr. Predatory Pseudomonas strain as a control of bacterial and fungal plant pathogens. Filed 7/19/91 published 8/3/93. Assignee: The Penn State Research Foundation (University Park, PA).
97.) Domb AJ, Kost J, Wiseman DM. (eds). Handbook of biodegradable polymers. 1997 Harwood Academic publishers. Overseas Publishers Association (OPA). Amsterdam B.V., The Netherlands.
98.) US Patent 4,503,155. Miller et al. Multifunctional, cloning vectors for use in Streptomyces, Bacillus, and E. coli. Filed 2/1/82 published 3/5/85. Assignee: Eli Lilly and Company (Indianapolis, IN).
99.) US Patent 4,918,006. Ellar et al. Gene coding for insecticidal crystal protein. Filed 2/3/86 published 4/17/90. Assignee: E.I. Du Pont de Nemours and Company (Wilmington, DE).
100.) US Patent application 20050070486. Wieland-Berghausen SC, et al. Microspherules containing a pleuromutilin derivative. Filed 11/27/07 published 3/31/05. Assignee: Novartis.
101.) US Patent 3,978,228. Yoshinaga et al. Method for killing noxious fungi in plants using dihalo sulfonates. Filed 3/24/75 published 8/31/76. Assignee: Kumiai Chemical Industry Co., Ltd. (Tokyo, JA).

Minerals and Reoviruses

1.) Lottes Jordan J. UM earth materials. Malachite. [web page]
2.) Kirk, Charles T. Conditions of Mineralization in the Copper Veins at Butte, Montana. Economic Geology VII(1912): 35-82.
3.) WHO. Evaluation of certain veterinary drug residues in food. Technical Report Series 954. Seventieth report of the Joint FAO/WHO Expert Committee on Food Additives. 2009. 144 pages. [web page]
4.) Fuchs T, Huber H, Teiner K, et al. Metallosphaera prunae, sp nov, a novel metal-mobilizing, thermoacideophilic archaeum, isolated from a uranium mine in Germany. Systematic and Applied Microbiology 1996;18(4):560-566
5.) Nordén B, Tjerneld F, Palm E. Linear dichroism studies of binding site structures in solution. Complexes between DNA and basic arylmethane dyes. Biophys Chem. 1978;8:1-15
6.) Bhasikuttan AC, Mohanty J, Pal H. Interation of malachite green with guanine-rich single-stranded DNA: Preferential binding to a G-quadruplex. Agnew. Chem Int Ed Engl. 2007;46:9305-9307.
7.) The Salmon Farm Monitor. www.salmonfarmmonitor.org/intlnewsseptember2003.shtml
8.) Tamez-Guerra P, McGuire MR, Medrano-Roldan HM et al. Sprayable Granule Formulations for Bacillus thuringiensis. J Econ Entomol. 1996 Dec;89(6):1414-1430.
9.) Comer John B. Genesis of Jamaican Bauxite. Economic Geology. 1974 Dec;69(8):1251-1264.
10.) Lipson Steven M, Stotzky G. Effect of Proteins on Reovirus Adsorption to Clay Minerals. Appl Environ Microbiol. 1984 Sept;48(3):525-530.
11.) Lipson SM, Stotzky G. Effect of bacteria on the inactivation and adsorption on clay minerals of reovirus. Can J Microbiol. 1985 Aug;31(8):730-5.
12.) Zoologix. Molecular diagnostic testing for animals. Rodent and rabbit assay data sheet. Reovirus type 3 (REO3). [web site]
13.) Compton SR, Riley LK. Detection of infectious agents in laboratory rodents: traditional and molecular techniques. Comparative Med. 2001;51:113-119.
14.) Lipson SM, Stotzky G. Effect of proteins on reovirus adsorption to clay minerals. Appl. Environ. Microbiol. 1984 Sept;48(3):525-530.
15.) Friesen PD, Miller LK. Insect viruses. In: Knipe DM, Howley PM, Griffin DE, Lamb RA, Marin MA, Roizman B, Straus SE (Eds.). Fund Virol. Lippincott Williams and Wilkins, Philadelphia, pp. 446-456.
16.) Krywienczyk J, Bergold GH. Serological relationships of viruses from some lepidopterous and hymenopterous insects. Virology. 1960 Mar;10(3):308-315.

17.) Shope RE. World Reference Center for Arboviruses. Yale University New Haven Conn. School of Medicine. 1981 Jul 1-Dec 31. Published 1982Jan. 121 pages. Accession #ADA153831. Contract #DAMD17-81-C-1121 and DADA17-72-C-2170.
18.) Shope RE. World Reference Center for Arboviruses. Yale University New Haven Conn. School of Medicine. 1983 Jan. 89 pages. #ADA181440. Contract# DAMD17-81-C-1121. Annual Progress report 1982Jan 1-Dec 31.
19.) CDC. Robert Ellis Shope In Memoriuam. Emerg Infect Dis 2004 Apr;10(4):762-765.
20.) Meshik, A. P. (November 2005). The workings of an ancient nuclear reactor. Scientific American. [web page]
21.) Gauthier-Lafaye F, Holliger P, Blanc PL. Natural fission reactors in the Franceville Basin, Gabon: a review of the conditions and results of a "critical event" in a geologic system. Geochimica et Cosmochimica Acta 1996;60(25):4831–4852.
22.) Karam A. The Natural Nuclear Reactor at Oklo: a Comparison with Modern Nuclear Reactors. Report. [web page]
23.) Lottes Jordan J. UM earth materials. Malachite. [web page]
24.) Import Risk Analysis Secretariat. Plant Biosecurity, Biosecurity Australia (formerly Plant Quarantine Policy Branch of the Australian Quarantine and Inspection Service). Viruses, Phytoplasmas and Spiroplasmas of Clonal Grasses and Their Diagnosis. Consultancy Report 2000 Dec. Chapter title: Maize rough dwarf fijivirus, p. 90.
25.) Geison Gerald L. Pasteur's Work On Rabies: Reexamining the Ethical Issues. The Hastings Center Report 1978 Apr;8(2):26-33.
26.) Carpentier S, Moilleron R, Beltran C, et al. Quality of dredged material in the river Seine basin (France). II. Micropollutants. Sci Total Environ. 2002 Nov 1;299(1-3):57-72.
27.) Andrews Richard David. Leptospiral Flora of Aquatic Turtles in Illinois. University of IL, PhD thesis. 1966. 158 pages.
28.) Shope, RE. World Reference Center for Arboviruses. Annual Report. July 1, 1975- Jun 30, 1976. Report ADA060051. Projects # 3M161102BS01, 3A161102B71Q. Supported by the US Army Medical Research and Development Command, Fort Detrick, Frederick, MD 21701. Under Contract No. DADA 17-72-C-2170. Department of Epidemiology and Public Health, Yale University School of Medicine, New Haven, CT 06510.
29.) Chastel C, Main AJ, Couatarmanac'h A. et al. Isolation of Eyach virus (Reoviridae, Colorado tick fever group) from Ixodes ricinus and I. ventalloi ticks in France. Arch Virol. 1984;82(3-4):161-71.
30.) Chastel C, Main AJ, Couatarmanac'h A, et al. Isolation of Eyach virus (Reoviridae, Colorado tick fever group) from Ixodes ricinus and I. ventalloi ticks in France. Arch Virol. 1984;82(3-4):161-71.
31.) US Patent 6,500,617. Stemmer, et al. Optimization of pest resistance genes using DNA shuffling. Filed 4/22/99 published 12/31/02. Assignee: Maxygen, Inc. (Redwood City, CA).
32.) Federici Brian A, Vlak Just M. Hamm John J. Comparative Study of virion structure, protein composition and genomic DNA of three ascovirus isolates. J Gen Virol. 1990;71:1661-1668.
33.) Knudson DL. Genome of Colorado Tick Fever Virus. Virol. 1981;112:361-364. From Yale Arbovirus Research Unit, Yale University, New Haven, Connecticut.
34.) Mullen Gary R, Durden Lance A. (ed.). Medical and Veterinary Entomology, Second Edition. 2009Academic Press, an imprint of Elsevier. Burlington, MA. P. 154.
35.) Hu R, Hyland KE, Oliver JH. A review on the use of Ixodiphagus wasps (Hymenoptera: Encyrtidae) as natural enemies for the control of ticks (Acari: Ixodidae). 1998. Systematic Applied Acarology. 3:19-28.
36.) Hu R, Hyland KE. Human babesiosis in the United States: a review with emphasis on its tick vectors. Systematic & Applied Acaraology. 1997;2:3-16.
37.) Hu R, Hyland KE, Mather TN. Occurrence and distribution in Rhode Island of Hunterellus hookeri (Hymenoptera: Encyrtidae), a wasp parasitoid of Ixodes dammini. J Med Entomol. 1993;30:277-280.
38.) Knipling EF, Steelman CD. Feasibility of Controlling Ixodes scapularis Ticks (Acari: Ixodidae), the Vector of Lyme Disease, by Parasitoid Augmentation. 2000. J Med Entomol. 37(5):645-652.
39.) US Patent 5,643,576. Johnston, et al. Method of inducing an immune response with a live Venezuelan Equine Encephalitis virus expressing a heterologous immunogen. Filed 5/19/95 published 7/1/97. Assignee: The University of North Carolina at Chapel Hill (Chapel Hill, NC).
40.) US Patent 4,447,537. Yunker et al. Tick cell lines. Filed 1/22/81 published 5/8/84. Assignee: The United States of Americas as represented by the Department of Health (Washington, DC).
41.) US Patent 4,497,793. Cummins. Method of regulating appetite and efficiency of food utilization employing interferon. Filed 12/13/82 published 2/5/87. Assignee: The Texas A&M University System (College Station, TX).
42.) US Patent 3,699,222. Isaacs et al. Production of Viral Interfering Substances. Filed 8/5/68 published 10/17/72. Assignee: National Research Development Corporation (London, EN).
43.) US Patent 3,144,390. Burke. Process for the purification of interferon. Filed 6/21/61 published 8/11/64. Assignee: National Research Development Corporation (London, EN).
44.) US Patent 3,265,581. Fantes et al. Process of purifying interferon with alumino-silicate adsorbants. Filed 8/2/63 published 8/9/66. Assignee: Glaxo Laboratories Limited, (Greenford, EN).
45.) US Patent 3,385,757. Finter. Quantitative hemadsorption assay technique for the estimation of interferon. Filed 11/14/63 published 5/28/68. Assignee: Imperial Chemical Industries Limited (London, EN).
46.) US Patent 3,414,651. Fantes. Purification of interferon-containing material. Filed 12/10/63published 12/3/68. Assignee: Glaxo Laboratories Limited (Greenford, EN).
47.) US Patent 3,548,053. Joshi. Interferon Production. Filed 9/7/65 published 12/15/70. Assignee: Frank W. Horner Limited, Mount Royal, Quebec, Canada.
48.) Ensign-Bickford Industries, Inc. About us. [web page] www.ensign-bickfordcompany.com/about.html
49.) EBA&D. Ensign-Bickford Aerospace & Defense Company. [web site]
50.) The Lewiston Daily News. Sunday August 16, 1984. Three killed in Connecticut explosives blast.
51.) Connecticut Siting Council. Docket No. 203. New England Site Management Application for a Certificate of Environmental Compatibility and Public Need for the construction, maintenance, and operation of a cellular telecommunications facility located on Grist Mill Road, known as the Powder Forest, Simsbury, Connecticut. [web site]
52.) Global InfoMine. Dyno Nobel Inc. Dyno Nobel Acquired by Incitec Pivot Still Delivering Groundbreaking Performance. [web site]
53.) EPA Great Lakes Contaminated Sediments. Contaminated Sediments Program. Sediment Remediation. [web site]
54.) Whitman Loring, Wallis RC, Leventhal EA. Isolation of a California-Group Arbovirus from Aedes Abserratus (Felt and Young) in Simsbury, Connecticut. Am J Trop Med Hyg. 1968;17(3):449-450.
55.) Corporate Watch. Syngenta. 2002 Nov. [web page]
56.) Munderloh UG, Liu Y, Wang M, Chen C, Kurtti TJ. Establishment, maintenance and description of cell lines from the tick Ixodes scapularis. J Parasitol. 1994;80(4):533-543.
57.) Cargill Timeline 1865-Present. [web page]
58.) Johnson Russell C. (ed.) The Biology of Parasitic Spirochetes. 1976 Academic Press. New York.
59.) Begum F, Wisseman Jr. CL, Casals J. Tickborne Viruses of West Pakistan: II. Hazara Virus, a new agent isolated from Ixodes Redikorzevi ticks from the Kaghan Valley, W. Pakistan. Am J Epidem 1970;92(3):192-194. The research was carried out under the auspices of the US Armed Forces Epidemiological Board's Commission on Rickettsial Diseases under contract DA-49-193-MD2277. Collaborators belonged to the US Army Medical Research and Development Command and were working together under an NIH grant (TW00142), and with additional support (in the case of YARU), from the Rockefeller Foundation.
60.) No. 211 Hazara (HAZ) Strain: JC 280. Am J Trop Med Hyg. 1970;19(6):1095-1096.
61.) Washington University in St. Louis and AstraZeneca announce Alzheimer's research collaboration. 2008 April 17. Press release AstraZeneca [web page]

It's Elementary Dear Watsons

1.) National Parks Conservation Association. Yellowstone National Park. [web page]
2.) Brock TD, Brock ML, Bott TL, Edwards MR. Microbial Life at 90C: The Sulfur Bacteria of Boulder Spring. J Bacteriol. 1971 Jul;107(1):303-314.
3.) Mindat.org the mineral and locality database. Mineral database search engine. [web page]
4.) 65.) Stieff LR, Stern TW, Sherwood AM. Preliminary Description of Coffinite - A New Uranium Mineral. Science. 1955;121:608-609.
5.) 66.) Hoekstra HR, Fuchs LH. Synthesis of Coffinite-UsiO4. Science 1956;123:105. And CaseWestern Reserve University. Case Institute of Technology. [web page]
6.) Gregg EC. A Flux-Forced Field-Biased Betatron. Rev Sci Instrum 1951;22(176). 7 pages.
7.) Waloschek Pedro. Box 12: Betatrons and Industry. [web page]
8.) Hempstead C, Worthington WE (eds). Encyclopedia of 20th century technology. Vol. 2, M-Z Index 2005 Routledge, NY p. 529
9.) Kathren RL, Gough JB, Benefiel GT. (eds). The Plutonium Story, the Journals of Professor Glenn T. Seaborg. 1939-1946. Battelle Press, columbus, OH. 1994.

10.) Jacobson Leon O. From Atom to Eve. Perspectives in Biology and Medicine. 1981 Winter;24(2). 23 pages
11.) Adams JASA, Richardson KA. Thorium, uranium and zirconium concentrations in bauxite. Econom Geol.1960 Dec;55(8):1653-1675.
12.) Fischer-Brandies E, Pratzel H, Wendt T. [Radioactive burden resulting from zirconia implants]. Dtsch Zahnarzti A. 1991 Oct;46(10):688-690. [Article in German.]
13.) Argonne National Laboratory. Zirconium Human Health Fact Sheet 2005 August. 2 pages.
14.) US Patent 4,732,859. Hershberger et al. Method to protect bacteria form natural bacteriophage. Filed 9/5/84 published 3/22/88. Assignee: Eli Lilly & Co. (Indianapolis, IN).
15.) Joint FAO/IAEA Division of Nuclear Techniques in Food and Agriculture. Agrochemicals and environmental concerns. P. 32, In Nuclear Strategies in Food and Agriculture. 25 Years of Progress. 1964-1989. Vienna, Austria.
16.) US Patent 4,609,550. Fitz-James. Bacillus cereus subspecies israelensis. Filed 1/20/83 published 9/2/86. Assignee: The University of Western Ontario, Health Sciences Centre (London, CA).
17.) EPA. History of the Clean Water Act. www.epa.gov/lawsregs/laws/cwahistory.html and Khater AE. Uranium and trace elements in phosphate fertilizers-Saudi Arabia. Health Phys. 2012 Jan;102(1):63-70.
18.) FAO Plant Production and Protection Paper #165. Pesticide residues in food – Evaluations 2000. Part I Residues. Food and Agriculture Organization of the United Nations (FAO). Joint Meeting of the FAO Panel of Experts on Pesticide Residues in Food and the Environment and the WHO Core Assessment Group. Geneva, Switzerland, 2000 Sep 20-29.
19.) Boukhalfa H, Icopini GA, Reilly SD, Neu MP. Plutonium (IV) Reduction by the Metal-Reducing Bacteria Geobacter metallireducens GS15 and Shewanella oneidensis MR1. Appl Environ Microbiol. 2007 Sep;73(1):5897-5903.
20.) Icopini GA, Boukhalfa H, Neu P. Biological reduction of Np(V) and Np(V) citrate by metal-reducing bacteria. Environ Sci Technol. 2007 Apr 15;41(8):2764-2769.
21.) Francis AJ, Dodge CJ. Bioreduction of uranium (VI) complexed with citric acid by Clostridia affects its structure and solubility. Environ Sci Technol. 2008 Nov 15;42922):8277-8282.
22.) Updegraff DM, Wren GB. The Release of Oil from Petroleum-Bearing Materials by Sulfate-Reducing Bactreia. 1954 May 17. Report from the Field Research Laboratories, Magnolia Petroleum Company, Dallas, Texas. 14 pages.
23.) Stacy Adrian. Deinococcus-Thermus: Adaptations to "nearly out of this world" environments. 2004 Tree of Life Project. [web page]
24.) Brock TD, Brock ML, Bott TL, et al. Microbial Life at 90 C: the Sulfur Bacteria of Boulder Spring. J Bacteriol. 1971 Jul;107(1):303-314.
25.) Co-Ordinated Research Project on Validation and Application of Plants as Biomonitors of Trace Element Atmospheric Pollution, Analysed by Nuclear and Related Techniques. Report on the First Research Co-ordination Meeting (RCM) Vienna, Austria, 1998 Sept 28-Oct 1. 171 pages. Report No. NAHRES-45.
26.) International Symposium on Induced Mutations in Plants. IAEA/FAO. Report on abstracts for the use of nuclear radiation to improve crop plants. 2008 August 12-15, Vienna, Austria. 207 pages.
27.) Allen David, Glover, Sam. Site Profiles for Atomic Weapons Employers that Worked Uranium and Thorium Metals – Appendix BB. General Steel Industries. 2007 Jun 25. 12 page report. Appendix to Battelle-TBD-6000 describing the use of the TBD for claims at General Steel Industries.
28.) US Patent 5,466,577. Weisburg. Nucleic acid probes for the detection of Lyme disease spirochetes. Filed 10/27/93, published 11/14/95. Inventor: William G. Weisburg (Milford, MA); Assignee: Amoco Corp.
29.) US Patent 4,888,276. Shelburne. Method and composition for the diagnosis of Lyme disease. Filed 6/26/86 published 12/19/89. Assignee: Minnesota Mining and Manufacturing Company (St. Paul, MN).
30.) US Patent 3,607,235. Duncan et al. Rapid bacteriological metal extraction method. Filed 2/23/68 published 9/21/71. Assignee: British Columbia Research Council (Vancouver, British Columbia, CA).
31.) Hernandez G, Fardeau ML, Cayol JL, et al. Clostridium thiosulfatireducens sp. nov., a proteolytic, thiosulfate- and sulfur-reducing bacterium isolated from an upflow anaerobic sludge blanket (UASB) reactor. IJSEM 2002 Sept;52(5):1461-1468.
32.) Ravot G, Ollivier B, Magot M, et al. Thiosulfate Reduction, an Important Physiological Feature Shared by Members of the Order Thermotogales. Appl Environ Microbiol. 1995 May;61(5):2053-2055.
33.) Miranda-Tello E, Fardeau ML, Thomas P, et al. Petrotoga mexicana sp. nov., a novel thermophilic, anaerobic and xylanolytic bacterium isolated from an oil-producing well in the Gulf of Mexico. Int J Syst Evol Microbiol. 2004 Jan;54(Pt 1):169-174.
34.) ATCC 644090. Deinococcus radiodurans clone from Thiobacillus ferrooxidans. [web page]
35.) ATCC 643058. Deinococcus radiodurans clone from Thiobacillus ferrooxidans. [web page]
36.) ATCC 653025. Deinococcus radiodurans clone from Thiobacillus ferrooxidans. [web page]
37.) White O, et al. Genome sequence of the radioresistant bacterium Deinococcus radiodurans R1. Science 1999;286:1571-1577.
38.) US Patent 2,829,964. Zimmerley et al. Cyclic leaching process employing iron oxidizing bacteria. Filed 10/24/55 published 4/8/58. Assignee: Kennecott Copper Corporation, Salt Lake City, Utah.
39.) US Patent 2,134,679. Allen. Process for treating biologic material. Filed 10/17/35 published 11/1/38. Assignee: Health Research Foundation Inc., Boston, MA.
40.) US Patent 3,894,770. Huff et al. Wellbore oxidation of lixiviants. Filed 6/12/74 published 7/15/75. Assignee: Kennecott Copper Corporation (New York, NY).
41.) Strongin DR, Moore JF, Ruckman MW. Synchrotron radiation assisted deposition of aluminum oxide from condensed layers of trimethylaluminum and water at 78K. Appl Phys Ltrs. 1992;61(6):729-731.
42.) Shenkenberg DL. Taking Semiconductor Manufacturing to the extreme. Photonics Spectra. [web page]
43.) Science Daily. First Beam for Large Hadron Collider, World's Mightiest Particle Accelerator. 2008 Sept. 10. [web page]
44.) Bocchi S, Malgioglio A. Azolla-Anabaena as a biofertilizer for Rice Paddy Fields in the Po Valley, a Temperate Rice Area in Northern Italy. Inter J Agronomy. 2010. ID#152158. 5 pages
45.) Washington State Department of Health. Cyanobacterial Toxins and Symptoms. [web page]
46.) Stacy Adrian. Deinococcus-Thermus: Adaptations to "nearly out of this world" environments. [web page]
47.) US Patent 4,782,022 Puhler, et al. Nigtrogen fixation regulator genes. Filed 5/22/85 published 11/1/88. Assignee: Lubrizol Genetics, Inc. (Wickliffe, OH).
48.) Halperin JJ, Kaplan GP, Brazinsky S, et al. Immunologic reactivity against Borrelia burgdorferi in patients with motor neuron disease. Arch Neurol 1990 May;47(5):586-594.
49.) US Patent 3,271,243. Cords et al. Stable concentrated bacterial insecticide suspensions. Filed 3/13/63 published 9/6/66. Assignee: International Materials and Chemical Corp. New York.
50.) US Patent 5,516,693 Vaeck, et al. Hybrid gene incorporating a DNA fragment containing a gene coding for an insecticidal protein, plasmids, transformed cyanobacteria expressing such protein and method for use as a biocontrol agent. Filed 3/4/87 published 5/14/96. Assignee: Board of Trustees operating Michigan State University (East Lansing, MI).
51.) US Patent 5,516,674. Roe et al. Insecticide resistance associated cytochrome 450. Filed 8/30/94 published 5/14/96. Assignee: North Carolina University (Raleigh, NC).
52.) US Patent 6,020,491. Wonley et al. Monomeric and polymeric cyclic amine and N-halamine compounds. Filed 7/7/98 published 2/1/00. Assignee: Auburn University, AL.
53.) Methylobacterium bacteremia in AIDS. Clin Microbiol. 1998;4:112-113.
54.) Lai CC, Cheng A, Liu WL, et al. Infections Caused by Unusual Methylobacterium Species. J Clin Microbiol. 2011 Sep;49(9):3329-3331.
55.) Curran Chris. University of Cincinnati Bio-Medicine monograph. [web page]
56.) Induced mutations and in vitro culture techniques for improving crop plant resistance to diseases. Report No. IAEA-TECDOC-728. Proceedings of a final Research Co-ordination Meeting organized by the Joint FAO/IAEA Division of Nuclear Techniques in Food and Agriculture and held in Grünbach, Germany. 1991 Oct 7-11. 97 pages.
57.) Printed in Vienna, Austria. And Whitcomb RF, Tully JG, McCawley P, Rose DL. Application of the Growth Inhibition Test to Spiroplasma Taxonomy. Inter J Sys Bacteriol. 1982 Oct;32(4):387-394.
58.) Mouches C, Bové JM. A Plasmid from S. citri Strain M14 Hybridizes with Extrachromosomal DNAs from Other Spiroplasmas, Including Corn Stunt Spiroplasma E275, Tick Spiroplasma 277F, and Coco Spiroplasma N525. Yale J Biol Med. 1983;56:723-727.
59.) US Patent 4,076,981. Sparks et al. Position sensitive area detector for use with X-ray diffractometer or X-ray camera Filed 7/29/75 published 2/28/78. Assignee: Syntex (USA) Inc. (Palo Alto, CA).
60.) US Patent 4,910,758. Herrick. X-ray diffraction method for generating mineralogy record of whole core. Filed 8/9/88 published 3/20/90. Assignee: Amoco Corporation (Chicago, IL).
61.) US Patent 4,710,946. Hinch et al. Method and apparatus for X-ray video fluoroscopic analysis of rock samples. Filed 8/6/85 published 12/1/87. Assignee: Amoco Corporation (Chicago, IL).

62.) US Patent 587,883. E. Thomson. Device for examining jewels by roentgen rays. Filed 9/4/1896, published 8/10/1897. Assignee: General Electric Company, New York.
63.) US Patent 2,476,150. Koppius. X-ray Diffraction Apparatus. Filed 2/12/47 published 7/12/49. Assignee: Philips Laboratories, Inc., Irvington on Hudson, New York.
64.) US Patent 4,715,053. Comstock, et al. Method for monitoring the crystallographic texture of metallic tubes by use of X-ray diffraction. Filed 1/25/85 published 12/2/87. Assignee: Westinghouse Electric Corp. (Pittsburgh, PA).
65.) Bolsunovsky A, Muratova E, Sukovaty A, Kornilova M. The effect of radionuclide and heavy metal contamination on the Yenisei River on cytogenetics of aquatic plant Elodea canadensis. Radioprotection. 2009;44(5):83-88.
66.) Closed Nuclear Cities Partnership. CNCP UK-Russia. Zheleznogorsk. Introduction to the Mining and Chemical Combine Industry Today. [web page]
67.) Digges Charles. Russia and America OK Deal to Shut Down Plutonium Reactors. Bellona. 2003 Mar 17. [web page]
68.) Sukovaty A, Bolsunovsky A. Exposure dose rates to aquatic organisms of the Yenisei River. In: Per Strand, Torun Jolle and Ase Sane (Eds.). Environmental Radioactivity in the Arctic & Antarctic. Norwegian Radiation Protection Authority. Norway. 2002:337-339.
69.) Danilyan VA, Vysotsky VL, Katkova MN, Kreyshev II. Dose rates to aquatic organisms and residents in the vicinity of running the ships equipped with nuclear power plants. Atomnaya energiya (Atomic Energy). 2002;92:158-168. [Article in Russian].
70.) Sazykina TG, Kryshev II. Assessment of the impact of radioactive substances on marine biota of North European waters (Report of Working Subgroup D. Marina II Project.) Commission of the European Communities Report. C6496/TR004. 2002 Aug;3. 106 pages.

The Fluoride Whitewash

1.) Provin TL, Pitt JL. Phosphorus Too Much and Plants May Suffer. Texas Cooperative Extension, Texas A&M University System. Report L-5241 6-02.
2.) Tennessee Valley Authority. From the New Deal to a New Century. [web site]
3.) FC Frary to L Branting. The ALCOA papers. 1930 Dec. 9.
4.) Cox GJ, Dodds ML, Wigman HB, Murphy FJ. The effects of high doses of aluminum and iron on phosphorus metabolism. J Biol Chem. 1931;92(XI)
5.) Health Effects: Fluoride & the Kidneys. [web page]
6.) Russel Darrell A, Williams Gerald G. History of Chemical Fertilizer Development. Soil Sci Soc Am J. 1977;41:260-265.
7.) Searls James P. Potash. US Geological Survey report. 9pages. [web page]
8.) Anonymous. The Phosphate Industry of the United States. A public domain reprinting of the Sixty Special Report of the Commissioner of Labor. Carroll D. Wright. Washington Government Printing Office. 1893.
9.) Smith DR, Moore, Jr. PA, Griffis CL, et al. Effects of Alum and Aluminum Chloride on Phosphorus Runoff from Swine Manure. J Environ Quality. 2001;30:992-998.
10.) University of South Florida. Florida Institute of Phosphate Research. Phosphate Primer. Discovery of Phosphate in Florida. [web site]
11.) Phosphorus. Chemistry Explained. Foundations and Applications. [web site]
12.) The New York Times. Mining Phosphate Rock. Regulating South Carolina's Great Industry. 1891 Jan. 29. Article dated Jan. 28, Charleston, S.C.
13.) US Marines. Marine Corp. News. (Report of five studies including natural resources in the Kazakstan, Kyrgystan, Tajikistan, Turkmenistan and Uzbekistan regions). [web page]
14.) Sobolev Dmitiri, Begonia Maria FT. Effects of Heavy Metal Contamination upon Soil Microbes: Lead-induced Changes in General and Denitrifying Microbial Communities as Evidenced by Molecular Markers. Int J Environ Res Public Health. 2008;5(5):450-456.
15.) Russel Darrell A, Williams Gerald G. History of Chemical Fertilizer Development. Soil Sci Soc Am J. 1977;41:260-265.
16.) Church RJ. Chemistry and processing of urea. In Vincent Sauchelli (ed.) Fertilizer nitrogen. Reinhold Publ Corp. 1964 New York.
17.) Hargrove T. TVA fertilizer technology used worldwide - but few new products since 1970s. [monograph]
18.) Tennessee Valley Authority Act. 40 pages. [web page]
19.) Betts Kellyn S. Perfluoroalkyl acids: what is the evidence telling us? Environ Hlth Perspect. 2007 May;115(5):A250-6.
20.) Bush William V, and White Bekki. State of Arkansas. Arkansas Geological Survey. History of Bauxite in Arkansas. AGES Brochure Series 3. 2007.
21.) Kelshall Gaylord TM. The U-boat war in the Caribbean. Originally published in 1988by Paria Publishing Co., Ltd. Port-of-Spain, Trinidad and Tobago. 1994 The United States Naval Institute, Anapolis, Maryland.
22.) US Patent 3,620,785. Root et al. Alum Containing Aluminous Cements. Filed 6/20/70 published 11/16/71. Assignee: The Dow Chemical Company, Midland, MI.
23.) Craig Klauber, Markus Gräfe, Greg Power. Australian Government. CSIRO. National Research Flagships Light Metals. Review of Bauxite Reside "Re-use" Options. 2009 May. Document No. DMR-3609. Project ATF-06-3: "Management of Bauxite Residues," Department of Resources, Energy and Tourism (DRET).
24.) US Patent 4,251,255. Wagner, et al. Agrochemical agents and their use. Filed 2/12/79, published 2/17/81. Assignee: Bayer Aktiengesellschaft (Leverkusen, DE).
25.) US Patent 3,864,138. Uchikawa, et al. Process for regulating setting time of hydraulic cement. Filed 5/15/72, published 2/4/75. Assignee: Onoda Cement Company, Limited (Onoda-shi, Yamaguchi, JA).
26.) US Patent 4,155,774. Randolph. Process for controlling the rate of growth of particulate masses. Filed 8/9/77, published 5/22/79. Inventors: Ellwood A. Randolph (Baton Rouge, LA).
27.) US Geological Survey. The Mineral Industry of North Carolina. 2003, 8 pages. Report prepared under a memorandum of understanding between the US Geological Survey and the North Carolina Geological Survey for collecting information on all nonfuel minerals.
28.) Shupe JL. Fluorine toxicosis and industry. Am Ind Hyg Assoc J. 1977;31:240-247.
29.) FIPR. Florida Institute of Phosphate Research. Phosphate Primer. [web site]
30.) Phosphorus. Chemistry Explained. Foundations and Applications. [web site]
31.) The New York Times. Mining Phosphate Rock. Regulating South Carolina's Great Industry. 1891 Jan. 29. Article dated Jan. 28, Charleston, S.C.
32.) Chernoff CB, Orris GJ. Data Set of World Phosphate Mines, Deposits, and Occurrences – Part A. Geologic Data. USGS. 2002Open File Report 02-156-A. 352 pages.
33.) Appel Adrianne. Florida Counties Try to Contain Phosphate Mines. The New York Times. 2007 Aug 4. [news article]
34.) Mather RE, Pratt AD, Holdaway CW. Fused Tricalcium Phosphate as a Low-Fluorine Phosphorus Supplement for Dairy Cattle. J Dairy Science 1949;32:228-236.
35.) Tennessee Valley Authority. From the New Deal to a New Century. [web site]
36.) US Marines. Marine Corp. News. (Report of five studies including natural resources in the Kazakstan, Kyrgystan, Tajikistan, Turkmenistan and Uzbekistan regions). [web page]
37.) State Symbols USA. Arkansas State Rock. [web site]
38.) US Geological Survey. The Mineral Industry of North Carolina. 2003, 8pages. Report prepared under a memorandum of understanding between the US Geological Survey and the North Carolina Geological Survey for collecting information on all nonfuel minerals.
39.) Shupe JL. Fluorine toxicosis and industry. Am Ind Hyg Assoc J. 1977;31:240-247.
40.) Connett Michael. The Phosphate Fertilizer Industry: An Environmental Overview. Fluoride Action Network. [web site]
41.) FC Frary to L Branting. The ALCOA papers. 1930 Dec. 9.
42.) Cox GJ, Dodds ML, Wigman HB, Murphy FJ. The effects of high doses of aluminum and iron on phosphorus metabolism. J Biol Chem. 1931;92(XI)
43.) RC Cross to HM Laudemann. The ALCOA papers. 1931 Jan. 12.
44.) In: The Australian Fluoridation News Aqua Pura. 1966Jan; 3(8). Address by FB Exner, M.D., to the Western Conference of National Food Associations, Salt Lake City, Utah. 1961 Oct. 27.
45.) Health Effects: Fluoride & the Kidneys. [web page]
46.) CDC. Achievements in Public Health, 1900-1999: Fluoridation of Drinking Water to Prevent Dental Caries. MMWR Weekly. 1999 Oct. 22;48(41):933-940.
47.) Meiers Peter. A new water supply for Oakley, Idaho. [web page]
48.) Kempf Grover A, McKay Frederick S. Mottled Enamel in a Segregated Population. Public Health Reports. 1930 Nov 28;45(48):2923-2977.
49.) Eager JM. Denti di Chiaie (Chiaie teeth). Naples, Italy. 1901 Oct 7.p. 2576-2577In: Public Health Reports of the US. 1901 November 1. 64 pages.
50.) McKay Frederick S. The Present Status of the Investigation of the Cause, and of the Geographic Distribution, of Mottled Enamel, Including a Complete Bibliography on Mottled Enamel. J Dental Res. 2930;10(5):561-568.
51.) Waldbott George L. Fluoridation: The Great Dilemma. 1978. Coronado Press. Inc. Lawrence, Kansas.
52.) CDC. Achievements in Public Health, 1900-1999: Fluoridation of Drinking Water to Prevent Dental Caries. MMWR Weekly. 1999Oct 22;48(41):933-940.
53.) US Patent 2,013,034. Sugar Acylation. Gerald J. Cox et al. Filed 6/22/32 published 9/3/35. Assignee: Niacet Chemicals Corporation, New York.

54.) US Patent 2,029,412. Manufacture of Esters of Levulinic Acid. Gerald J. Cox et al. Filed 12/19/34published 2/4/36. Assignee Niacet Chemicals Corporation, NY.
55.) US Patent 2,033,909. Manufacture of Calcium Levulinate. Gerald J. Cox et al. Filed 12/19/34published 3/17/36. Assignee: Niacet Chemicals Corporation, New York.
56.) Cox Gerald J. System of Study of Experimental Dental Caries as Related to Nutrition. In: Gies William J. International Association for Dental Research: Proceedings of the Fifteenth General Meeting. J Dent Res 1937;16:289-365. Held at the Lord Baltimore Hotel, Baltimore, Maryland March 13-14, 1937.
57.) Sugar Consumption, Supply and Demand. J Am Med Assoc. 1930;94(22):1763.
58.) Schmitz Mark. The Transformation of the Southern Cane Sugar Sector: 1860-1930. Agricul History. Vol. 53, No. 1. Southern Agriculture Since the Civil War: A Symposium (Jan 1979). Pp. 270-285.
59.) Science: Chemists at Washington. 1933 April 10. TIME article [web page]
60.) Hodge HHC, Luce-Clausen EM, Brown EF. J Nutrition. 1939;17:333.
61.) McClendon JF, Foster WC. Effect of Dietary Fluorine in Delaying Dental Caries. J Dent Res. 1942;21:139-143.
62.) US Patent 2,181,003. Salzberg Harold K. Filed 1/11/38, published 11/21/39. Assignee: The Borden Company, New York, NY.
63.) Armstrong WD, Brekhus PJ. Chemical Constitution of Enamel and Dentin: I. Principal Components. J Biol. Chem. 1937;120:677-687.
64.) Armstrong WD, Brekhus PJ. Possible Relationship Between the Fluorine Content of Enamel and Resistance to Dental Caries. J Dent Res. 1938;18:393-399.
65.) Cox Gerald J, Matuschak MC, Dixon SF, Dodds ML, Walker WE. Experimental Dental Caries: IV. Fluorine and Its Relation to Dental Caries. J Dent Res. 1939;18:481-490.
66.) Armstrong WD. Proceedings of the American Society of Biological Chemists. Thirty-first annual Meeting. J Biol Chem. 1937 119:v.
67.) Armstrong WD. Fluorine Content of Enamel and Dentin of Sound and Carious Teeth. Proceedings of the American Society of Biological Chemists. Thirty-first annual Meeting. J Biol. Chem. 1937;120:iii-cvii. Page vi.
68.) Perry Mabel W., Armstrong WD. On the Manner of Acquisition of Fluorine by Mature Teeth. J Nutrition. 1940;35-44.
69.) Anderson Jr., Oscar E. The Pure-Food Issue: A Republican Dilemma, 1906-1912. The American Historical Review. 1956 Apr;51(3):550-573.
70.) Krook L, Maylin GA. Industrial fluoride pollution. Chronic fluoride poisoning in Cornwall Island cattle. Cornell Vet. 1979 Apr;69 Suppl 8:suppl 1-70.
71.) Crissman JW, Maylin GA, Krook L. New York State and US Federal fluoride pollution standards do not protect cattle health. Cornell Vet. 1980 Apr;70(2):183-192.
72.) Eckerlin RH, Maylin GA, Krook L. Milk production of cows fed fluoride contaminated commercial feed. Cornell Vet. 1986 Oct;76(4):403-414.
73.) Bunce HW. Fluoride in air, grass, and cattle. J Dairy Sci. 1985 Jul;68(7):1706-1711.
74.) Labreche Julianne. An Island Unfit for Man or Beast. Macleans Magazine 1979 July 30. On: Fluoride Action Network web site. [web page]
75.) Clark DC. Appropriate uses of fluorides for children: guidelines from the Canadian Workshop on the Evaluation of Current Recommendations Concerning Fluorides. CMAJ. 1993 Dec 15;149(12):1787-1793.
76.) Bélanger LF, Visek WJ, Lotz WE, Comar CL. Rachitomimetic Effects of Fluoride Feeding on the Skeletal Tissues of Growing Pigs. Am J Pathol. 1958 Feb;34(1):25-35.
77.) Ashe WF. Acute Effects of Air Pollution in Donora, Pennsylvania, Air Pollution: Proc. of the U.S. Tech. Conf. on Air Pollution, Sponsored by the Interdepartmental Comm. on Air Pollution. Louis McCabe, Chairman. 1952 McGraw-Hill, NY. pp. 455-461.
78.) NIH. A Short History of the National Institutes of Health. [web site]
79.) Centers for Disease Control. Chronic Disease Prevention and Health Prevention. Oral Health.
80.) Lennon MA. One in a million: the first community trial of water fluoridation. WHO Bulletin. 2006 Sept;84(9):759-760.
81.) Rakita Philip E. Dentifrice Fluoride. Products of Chemistry. J Chem Ed 4 page report. No date.
82.) Yiamouyiannis John. Fluoride: The Aging Factor 2nd Edition. 1986 Health Action Press. [web page]
83.) Department of Health and Human Services, Food and Drug Administration. Center for Drug Evaluation and Research. Joint Meeting of the CDER Psychopharmacologic Drugs Advisory Committee and the FDA Pediatric Advisory Committee. Monday September 13, 2004, Bethesda, Maryland. [web page]
84.) Lezoualc'h F, Sparapani M, Behl C. N-acetyl-serotonin (normelatonin) and melatonin protect neurons against oxidative challenges and suppress the activity of the transcription factor NF-kB. J Pineal Res. 1998;24:168-178. [web page]
85.) International Plant Nutrition Institute. Triple Superphosphates. Norcross, GA. [web page]
86.) Fluorspar data sheet. [web page]
87.) Exner Frederick B. Economic Motives Behind Fluoridation. 1961. In Aqua Pura, 1966 Jan.
88.) Miller RF, Phillips PH. The metabolism of fluorine in the bones of the fluoride-poisoned rat. J Nutr. 1953 Oct;51(2):273-281.
89.) Peters JH. Therapy of acute fluoride poisoning. Am J Med Sci. 1948Sep;216(3):278-285.
90.) Freedman AM, Himwich HE. The effect of size, sex and pregnancy on the lethality of diisopropyl fluorophosphate. Fed Proc. 1948 Mar;7(1 Pt1):36.
91.) Welsome Eileen. The Plutonium Files: America's secret medical experiments in the Cold War NEJM. 1999Dec 16;341:1941-1942.
92.) Plutonium Files: How the US Secretly Fed Radioactivity to Thousands of Americans. 2004May 5. Democracy Now! [web site]
93.) Krueger Joline Gutierrez. Eileen Welsome, Albuquerque Tribune made history with "The Plutonium Experiment." The Times of the Tribune. 2008 Feb 22. [monograph]
94.) US Dept. of Energy. Office of History & Heritage Resources. The Manhattan Project. [web site]
95.) Political Friendster. Connection between Project F – Fluoride. [web site]
96.) Yant WP. Toxicity of Organic Fluorides. Am J Public Health Nations Health. 1933 Sept;23(9):930-934.
97.) Winter JH. Chronic fluorine intoxication: effect on bones and teeth. Vet Med. 1946 Nov;41(11):408.
98.) Charnot A. [Fluoreses: darmous, calcium fluoride poisoning in North Africa.] Sem Hop. 1952 Dec 22;28(94):3827-3831. Undetermined language.
99.) [No authors listed] Relation of malnutrition to fluoride toxicity. Nutr Rev. 1952 Aug;10(8):227-229.
100.) Miller RF, Phillips PH. The metabolism of fluorine in the bones of the fluoride-poisoned rat. J Nutr. 1953 Oct;51(2):273-281.
101.) Kauffman Joel M.Water Fluoridation: a Review of Recent Reesarch and Actions. J Amer Phys Surg. 2005 Summer;10(2):38-44.
102.) Likins RC, Scow RO, Zipkin I, Steere AC. Deposition and retention of fluoride and radiocalcium in the growing rat. Am J Physiol. 1959 Jul;197(1):75-80. No abstract.
103.) CDC. Achievements in Public Health, 1900-1999: Fluoridation of Drinking Water to Prevent Dental Caries. MMWR Weekly. 1999 Oct 22;48(41):933-940.
104.) Air and Water News Report. (no author listed) Fluoridated Water Supply Argument Rages in Wisconsin. 2009 Mar 19. [monograph]
105.) Brooker Kevin. Calgary. Hydrofluorosilicic acid: Toxic. Industrial. Waste. Calgary Herald. 2009Mar 30. On: Fluoride Action Network Internet news site.
106.) Slate, Robert. Fluoride Action Network. Fluoridated Connecticut experiencing Oral Health Crisis. New Haven Register 2005 May.
107.) Zipkin I, Likins RC, McClure FJ, Steere AC. Urinary fluoride levels associated with use of fluoridated waters. Public Health Report. 1956 Aug;71(8):767-772.
108.) Likins RC, McClure FJ, Steere AC. Urinary excretion of fluoride following defluoridation of a water supply. Public Health Report 1956 Mar;71(3):217-220.
109.) Van der Hoeven JS, Franken HCM. Effect of Fluoride on Growth and Acid Production by Streptococcus mutans in Dental Plaque. Infect Immun. 1984;45(2):356-359.
110.)Kester Dana R. Fluoride chlorinity ratio of sea water between the Grand Banks and the Mid-Atlantic Ridge. Deep Sea Res and Oceanograph Abstr. 1971 Nov;18(11):1123-1126. Report No. AD0723237. Fluoride Analysis in the Northwest Atlantic Ocean. Contract No. N00014-68-A-0215-0003. Technical report. DTIC and NTIS Defense Technical Information Center Report. Ft. Belvoir, VA.
111.) Quin LD, Quin GS. Screening for carbon-bound phosphorus in marine animals by high-resolution 31P-NMR spectroscopy: coastal and hydrothermal vent invertebrates. Comp Biochem Physiol B Biochem Mol Biol. 2001 Jan;128(1):173-185.
112.) Karl Heinz Wilm. www.ourfood.com slide presentation. WHO Guidelines for Recreational Water Environments. Slide 64 of 73.
113.) Tinanoff Norman, Camosci David. The Effect of a Low Fluoride Delviery System on Bacterial Metabolism, Bacterial Attachment and Caries. Corp. Author: Connecticut Univ. Health Center, Farmington. Report #ADA077569. Dated Sept. 1979, 103 pages. Contract #DAMD17-78-C-8066. Annual report Sept. 1, 1978-Sept. 30, 1979. Project #3S161102BS06.
114.) Rubel and Hager Inc. Tucson, AZ (Corporate authors). The Removal of Fluoride from Concentrated Fluoride Wastewater: A Literature Search. Report ADA956510. Dated June 29, 1979. 28 pages. Contract No. DAAA05-79-C-0006. Report No. XARMA. Report identifiers: U/A Reports, Defluoridation, Rocky Mountain Arsenal, Adams County (Colorado).
115.) In Depth: Fluoroquinolones: Unnecessary Risks. Keep Antibiotics Working.com. Chicago, IL. 2004 [web site]
116.) FDA. Human Health Impact of Fluoroquinolone Resistant Camplyobacter Attributed to the Consumption of Chicken. FDA Center for Veterinary Medicine. 2000 Oct 18. 109 page report.
117.) FDA. Fluoroquinolone Antimicrobial Drugs. 7/8/2008. [web site] Information for Healthcare Professionals: Fluoroquinolone Antimicrobial Drugs [ciprofloxacin (marketed

as Cipro and generic ciprofloxacin), ciprofloxacine extended-release (marketed as Cipro XR and Proquin XR), gemifloxacin (marketed as Factive), levofloxacin (marketed as Levaquin), moxifloxacin (marketed as Avelox), norfloxacin (marketed as Noroxin), and ofloxacin (marketed as Floxin)].
118.) Herrlin K, Segerdahl M, Gustafsson LL, Kalso E. Methadone, ciprofloxacin, and adverse drug reactions. Lancet 2000;356(9247):2069-2070.
119.) Tsutsui T, Suzuki N, Ohmori M, Maizumi H. Cytotoxicity, chromosome aberrations and unscheduled DNA synthesis in cultured human diploid fibroblasts induced by sodium fluoride. Mutation Res. 1984;139:193-198.
120.) Tsutsui T, Ide K, Maizumi H. Induction of unscheduled DNA synthesis in cultured human diploid fibroblasts by sodium fluoride. Mutation Res. 1984;140:43-48.
121.) Tsutsui T, Suzuki N, Ohmori M. Sodium fluoride-induced morphological and neoplastic transformation, chromosome aberrations, sister chromatid exchanges, and unscheduled DNA synthesis in cultured Syrian hamster embryo cells. Cancer Res. 1984;44:938-941.
122.) Ong SH. Utilisation of Radioisotopes and Irradiation in Crop Protection Research. June 8-11, 1981. Seminar on nuclear techniques in agriculture and environment. Kuala Lumpur, Malaysia.
123.) Tejada AW, Calumpang SMF, Magallona ED. National Crop Protection Center, University of the Philippines, College, Laguna, Philippines. 1992 p. 11-16.
124.) International Atomic Energy Agency. Progress in Peaceful Applications of Nuclear Energy During the Year 1967/68. Statements by Member States. Printed in Austria January 1969. 60 page report.
125.) Merck's 1907 Index. Third Edition. An Encyclopedia for the Chemist Pharmacist and Physician. Merck & Co., New York. p. 67.
126.) Heidelberger C, Chaudhuri NK, Danneberg P, et al. Fluorinated Pyrimidines, A New Class of Tumour-Inhibitory Compounds, Nature. 1957 Mar 30;179:663-666.
127.) Cohen Seymour. 50 years ago in cell biology. A virologist recalls his work on cell growth inhibition. The Scientist. 2008 Jan 30.
128.) Wyatt GR, Cohen SS. The bases of the nucleic acids of some bacterial and animal viruses: the occurrence of 5-hydroxymethylcytosine. Biochemical J. 1953;55:774-782.
129.) Barner Hazel D, Cohen Seymour S. The Induction of Thymine Synthesis by T2Infection of a Thymine Requiring Mutant of Escherichia Coli. J Bacteriol. 1954 Jul;68(1):80-88.
130.) Flaks JG, Cohen SS. The enzymic synthesis of 5-hydroxymethyl-deoxycytidylic acid. Biochim. Biophys. Acta 1957;25:667-668.
131.) Heidelberger C, Chaudhuri NK, Danneberg P, et al. Fluorinated Pyrimidines, a New Class of Tumor-Inhibitory Compounds. Nature 1957 Mar 30;179:663-666.
132.) Cohen SS et al. The mode of action of 5-fluorouracil and its derivatives. PNAS. 1958;44:1004-1012.
133.) Nimmo Kurt. Story on Mystery Substance Distracts from Fact Fluoride is a Deadly Killer. 2010 Mar 13.
134.) When Workers Blow Whistle on Federal Waste, Fraud. US News and World Report. 1977 Dec. 19, p. 55.
135.) Sesikeran B, Rao SH, Krishnamurthi D, et al. Studies on Sural Nerve Biopsies in Endemic Skeletal Fluorosis. Fluoride. 1994;27(4):189-193.
136.) Laboratory test results of a Lyme patient from Ireland who gave kind permission to the author to reprint.
137.) Christopher Bryson. The Fluoride Deception. 2004 A Seven Stories Press First Edition, New York, NY.
138.) Spittle Bruce. Fluoride Fatigue. Fluoride Poisoning: is fluoride in your drinking water – and from other sources – making you sick? 4th edition. 2007 Paua Press, Dunedin, New Zealand.
139.) Gupta SK, Seth AK, Gupta A, Gavane AG. Transplacental passage of Fluorides in Cord Blood. J Ped. 1993 Jul:137-141.
140.) Mullenix PJ, Denbesten PK, Schunior A, Kernan WJ. Neurotoxicity of sodium fluoride in rats. Neurotoxicology and Teratology. 1995;17(2):169-177.
141.) Waldbott GL. Acute Fluoride Intoxication. Acta Med Scand. 1963;174(Suppl. 400).
142.) Waldbott GL. Chronic Fluorine Intoxication from Drinking Water. Int Arch Allergy Appl Immunol. 1955;7:70-74.
143.) Petraborg HT, Chronic Fluoride Intoxication form Drinking Water. Fluoride. 1974;7:47-52.
144.) Faccini JM. Fluoride-induced Hyperplasia of the Parathyroid Glands. Proc Roy Soc Med. 1969;62:241.
145.) Waldbott GL. Tetaniform Convulsions Precipitated by Fluoridated Drinking Water. Confin. Neurol. 1957;17:339-347.
146.) International Society for Fluoride Research. Neurotoxicity of Fluoride. 1996;29(2):57-58. Editorial. [web page]
147.) Subcommittee on Health Effects of Ingested Fluoride. Committee on Toxicology, Board on Environmental Studies and Toxicology, Commission on Life Sciences, National Research Council. Health Effects of Ingested Fluoride. National Academy Press, Washington, DC. 1993.
148.) Hileman B. Fluoridation of water.Questions about health risks and benefits remain after more than 40 years. Chem Eng News.1988 Aug 1:26-42.
149.) Singh A, et al. Endemic fluorosis. Epidemiological, clinical and biochemical study of chronic fluoride intoxication in Punjab. Medicine. 1963;42:229-246.
150.) Waldbott GL, Burgstahler AW, McKinney HL. Fluoridation: The Great Dilemma. 1978. Coronado Press, Inc. Lawrence, Kansas.
151.) Lünemann JD, Gelderblom H, Sospedra M, et al. Cerebrospinal Fluid-Infiltrating CD4+ T Cells Recognize Borrelia burgdorferi Lysine-Enriched Protein Domains and Central Nervous System Autoantigens in Early Lyme Encephalitis. Infect Immun. 2007 Jan;75(1):243-251.
152.) CNPase Antibody. [web page]
153.) Rapaport Y.I: Les opacifications du cristallin mongolism et cataracte sénile (Donnés statistiques récentes). Rev Anthropol (Paris). 1957;2(3):133-135. [Article in French]
154.) Rapaport I. Contribution à l'étude étiologique du mongolisme. Rôdes inhibiteurs enzymatiques. Encephalie. 1957;46:468-481. [Article in French].
155.) Rapaport I. Oligophrénie mongolienne et ectodermoses congénitales. Ann Dermatol. Syphiligr. 1960;87:263-278.
156.) Rapaport I. Oligophrénie mongolienne et caries dentaires. Rev Stomatol. 1963;64:207-218.

Chapter Five: Paving Roads with Unknown Intentions

International Interests and the OPs

1.) Van Atta D. With Honor Melvin Laird in War, Peace and Politics. 2008 Univ WI Press.
2.) Melvin R. Laird. Health Care and Education Legacy. [web site]
3.) Burges HD, Hussey NW. Microbial Control of Insects and Mites. 1971 Academic Press, London.
4.) Steinhaus EA. The Microbial Flora of the Rocky Mountain Wood Tick, Dermacentor Andersoni Stiles. US Public Health Service, Rocky Mt. Laboratory, Hamilton, MT. 1942 J Bacteriol. Jan. 8;44(4):397-404.
5.) Muangman D, Frothingham TE, Spielman A. Presence of Sindbis Virus in Anal Discharge of Infected Aedes Aegypti. Am J Trop Med Hyg. 1969;18(3):401-410.
6.) Weiss E, Myers WF, Suitor EC Jr, Neptune EM Jr. Respiration of a Rickettsialike Microorganism, Wolbachia persica. J Infect. Dis. 1962 Mar-Apr;110:115-64.
7.) Steinhaus EA, Thompson CG. Preliminary field tests using a polyhedrosis virus to control the alfalfa caterpillar. J Econ Entomol. 1949 Apr;42(2):301-5.
8.) Technical Report: DDC AD408401. Conference on Biological Control of Insects of Medical Importance. American Institute of Biological Sciences (Washington, DC). 1960 Nov 1. Date stamped June 28, 1961, Camp LeJeune, NC. 148 pages. Convened at Armed Forces Institute of Pathology, Washington, DC, Feb. 3-4, 1960.
9.) Steinhaus EA. The Microbial Flora of the Rocky Mountain Wood Tick, Dermacentor Andersoni Stiles. US Public Health Service, Rocky Mt. Laboratory, Hamilton, MT. 1942 J Bacteriol. Jan. 8;44(4):397-404.
10.) Muangman D, Frothingham TE, Spielman A. Presence of Sindbis Virus in Anal Discharge of Infected Aedes Aegypti. Am J Trop Med Hyg. 1969;18(3):401-410.
11.) Weiss E, Myers WF, Suitor EC Jr, Neptune EM Jr. Respiration of a Rickettsialike Microorganism, Wolbachia persica. J Infect. Dis. 1962 Mar-Apr;110:115-64.
12.) Steinhaus EA, Thompson CG. Preliminary field tests using a polyhedrosis virus to control the alfalfa caterpillar. J Econ Entomol. 1949 Apr;42(2):301-5
13.) US Patent 3,639,578 Batzer. Virus Insecticide. Filed 2/18/70 published 2/1/72. Assignee: International Minerals & Chemicals Corporation.
14.) Barboza David. Cargill and IMC Global to Combine Fertilizer Units. The New York Times. 2004 Jan 28. [monograph on the Internet].
15.) A Summary of Cargill's History. 3 pages. [web page]
16.) Broehl Jr. Wayne G. Cargill. Trading the World's Grain. 1992 University Press of New England.
17.) Tinoco-Ojanguren R, Halperin DC. Poverty, production, and health: inhibition of erythrocyte cholinesterase via occupational exposure to organophosphate insecticides in Chiapas, Mexico. Arch Environ Health. 1998 Jan-Feb;53(1):29-35.
18.) Sulak O, Altuntas I, et al. Nephrotoxicity in rats induced by organophosphate insecticide methidathion and ameliorating effects of vitamins E and C. Pest Biochem Phys. 2005 Sep;83(1):21-28.
19.) Extoxnet. Oregon State University. Toxicology Information Briefs. Cholinesterase Inhibition. 1993 Sep. [web page]
20.) Marnett LJ. Lipid peroxidation-DNA damage by malondialdehyde. Mutat Res. 1999 Mar 8;424(1-2):83-95.
21.) Daily News. Beyond Pesticides. National Coalition Against the Misuse of Pesticides. Study Links Organophosphate Insecticide Used on Corn With ADHD. 2007 Jan 5. [monograph on the Internet]
22.) Chávez J, Seguar P, et al. Paradoxical effect of salbutamol in a model of acute organophosphates intoxication in guinea pigs: role of substance P release. Am J Physiol Lung

Cell Mol Physiol. 2007;292:L915-L923. First published 2006 Dec 8;doi:10.1152/ajplung.00253.2005.
23.) Fryer AD, Lein PJ, Howard AS, et al. Mechanisms of organophosphate insecticide-induced airway hyperreactivity. Am J Physiol Lung Cell Mol Physiol. 2004;286:L963-L969.
24.) US Patent 3,281,376. Proops. Epoxide Compositions Containing a Catalytic Amount of a Stannic Organophosphate. Filed 12/29/61 published 10/25/66. Assignee: Union Carbide Corporation a corporation of NY.
25.) US Patent 3,542,688. Crowley. Flocculant Consisting of the Condensation Product of a Polyhalogenated Organophosphate and a Polyamine. Filed 4/18/68 published 11/24/70. Assignee: Amicon Corporation, Wakefield, MA.
26.) US Patent 3,697,645. Meier, et al. Purification of antibodies. Filed 4/28/71 published 10/10/72. Assignee: The United States of America as represented by the Secretary of the Army
27.) US International Trade Commission Rulings and Harmonized Tariff Schedule. NY F83625. 2000 Apr 13. Letter to Scott A. Cohn Esq., Arent Fox Kintner Plotkin & Kahn, New York, NY on behalf of client Monsanto; from Robert B. Swierupski.
28.) Babu KR, Ramakrishna S, Reddy YHK, et al. Metabolic alterations and molecular mechanism in silkworm larvae during viral infection: A review. African J Biotechnol. 2009 Mar 20;8(6):899-907.
29.) Indian Museum, India. Department of Agriculture. Indian museum notes, 1889-1891. Vols. 1-3. P. 41.
30.) Andrianantoandro et al. Synthetic biology: new engineering rules for an emerging discipline . Mol Syst Biol. 2006;2:1-14.
31.) Isaac Freeda, Weyant Rob. National Select Agent Workshop. Select Agent Program Workshop Series. [slide presentation on the Internet] sponsored by the CDC, USDA, APHIS. Meeting date August 12, 2009, meeting held at the CDC's Roybal Campus, Auditorium A, 1600 Clifton Road, Atlanta GA according to a federal register posting from May 22, 2009. Fed. Register Vol. 74 No. 98 p. 23991. Docket No. APHIS-2009-0029 Multi-Agency Informational Meeting Concerning Compliance with the Federal Select Agent Program; Public Meeting.
32.) National Institutes of Health and the Department of Health and Human Services. National Science Advisory Board for Biosecurity. Addressing Biosecurity Concerns Related to the Synthesis of Select Agents. 2006 December. Report length 20 pages.
33.) Federal Register Notice. 2007 Oct 31;72(210):61661. Department of Health and Human Services National Institutes of Health Office of Biotechnology Activities; Recombinant DNA Research: Action Under the NIH Guidelines for Research Involving Recombinant DNA Molecules (NIH Guidelines).
34.) Federal Register Notice. 2009 Sept. 22;74(182):48275. Department of Health and Human Services. National Institutes of Health Office of Biotechnology Activities; Recombinant DNA Research: Actions Under the NIH Guidelines for Research Involving Recombinant DNA Molecules (NIH Guidelines). Action: Notice of Changes to the NIH Guidelines.
35.) Calmes Jackie, McNeil Jr. Donald G. H1N1 Widespread in 46States as Vaccines Lag. The New York Times. 2009 Oct 25.
36.) US FDA. News Release: 2009 Sept. 15. FDA Approves Vaccines for 2009 H1N1 Influenza Virus Approval Provides Important Tool to Fight Pandemic.
37.) Zhdanov VM. Recent Experience with Antiviral Vaccines. Ann Rev Microbiol. 1961 Oct;15:297-322.
38.) Parker RR. Public Health Report 1942;57:1963-66.
39.) Beckwith JR. Gene Expression in Bacteria and Some Concerns About the Misuse of Science. Bacter Rev 1970 Sept;34(3):222-227.
40.) Oshinsky DM. Polio. An American Story. 2005 Oxford University Press, New York, NY.

Chemicals and Mutated Microbes

1.) Siddharth Y. Srivastava and Aravinda M. de Silva. Characterization of Borrelia burgdorferi Aggregates. Vector-Borne Zoonotic Diseases. Jun 2009;9(3):323-329. Department of Microbiology and Immunology, University of North Carolina, Chapel Hill, North Carolina.
2.) US Patent 3,816,261. Torney. Culture Medium for Lertospira [sic] Organisms. Filed 4/1/71 published 6/11/74. Assignee: Johnson & Johnson (New Brunswick, NJ).3. Darzins Egons. Bacteriology of Tuberculosis. 1958University of Minnesota. North Central Publishing Company, St. Paul. P.239
4.) Buck John D, Cleverdon Robert C. The Effect of Tween 80 on the Enumeration of Marine Bacteria by the spread and pour plate methods. Dept. of Bacteriology, University of Connecticut.
5.) US Department of Labor. Hexavalent Chromium. OSHA web site. [web page]
6.) Vasilatos Ch, Megremi I, Economou-Eliopoulos M, Mitsis I. Hexavalent chromium and other toxic metals in groundwaters of the Asopos Valley (Attica), Greece. SEGH. Athens, Hellas 31st March-2nd April 2008.
7.) San Joaquin Valley Unified Air Pollution Control District. RULE 7012 – Hexavalent Chromium – Cooling Towers. Adopted 5/15/91 amended 12/17/92. [1 page report on California EPA Air Resources Board web site]
8.) Shaffer Matthew. Waste Lands: The Threat of Toxic Fertilizer. 2001 May 3. CALPIRG Charitable Trust. The State PIRGs. (California Public Interest Research Group Charitable Trust) Report. 31 pages. [web page]
9.) National Research Council US Committee on Biologic Effects of Atmospheric Pollutants. Div. of Medical Sciences. Medical and Biologic Effects of Environmental Pollutants. Chromium. National Academy of Sciences, Washington, DC. 1974.
10.) Grubinger VP, Gutenmann WH, Doss GJ, et al. Chromium in Swiss chard grown in soil amended with tannery meal fertilizer. Chemosphere. 1994 Feb;28(4):717-720.
11.) EPA. Background Report on Fertilizer Use, Contaminants and Regulations. Report No. 747-R-98-003. 1999 January. Washington, DC. 395 pages. [web page]
12.) The Journal of the Society of Chemical Industry. Society of Chemical Industry (Great Britain). 1891. Volume X. 1143 pages.
13.) Haynes WM. (ed) Handbook of Chemistry and Physics. Chromium. 92nd Edition. 2011-2012. CRC Press.
14.) Hingston J et al. Leaching of chromated copper arsenate wood preservatives: a review. Environmental Pollution 2001;111(1):53–66.
15.) Weckhuysen BM Schoonheydt RA. Olefin polymerization over supported chromium oxide catalyst. Catalysis Today. 1999 Jun 30;51(2):215-221.
16.) The School of Engineering and Applied Sciences at the University at Buffalo, State University of New York (SUNY). High-Density Polyethylene. Fact Sheet. [web page]
17.) Report: Hexavalent Chromium Used As Fertilizer. www.youtube.com/watch?v=PvpzcapmTUI. Grubinger VP, Gutenmann WH, Doss GJ, et al. Chromium in Swiss chard grown on soil amended with tannery meal fertilizer. Chemosphere 1994 Feb;28(4):717-720.
18.) Megharaj M, Avudainayagam S, Naidu R. Toxicity of hexavalent chromium and its reduction by bacteria isolated from soil contaminated with tannery waste. Curr Microbiol. 2003 Jul;47(1):51-54.
19.) Larkin EP, Tierney JT, Sullivan R. Persistence of virus on sewage-irrigated vegetables. J Environ Eng Div Am Soc Civ Eng. 1976;102:29-35.
20.) Edwards, Joseph. Coating and Surface Treatment Systems for Metals. Finishing Publications Ltd. and ASM International. 1997:214–217.
21.) Ragheb M. Uranium Resources in Phosphate Rocks. Report 2010 Jan 23. [web page]
22.) Wang LK, Shammas NK, Hung YT. (eds). Waste Treatment in the Metal Manufacturing, Forming, Coating, and Finishing Industries. CRC Press. 2009 Boca Raton, FL.
23.) Zelman Joanna. Hexavalent Chromium: Tap Water Industry Knew About Brockovich Chemical For Years, Reports EWG. Huff Post. 2011 Apr 4. [web page]
24.) US Dept. of Labor. OSHA Occupational Safety & Health Administration. Hexavalent Chromium. [web page]
25.) Independent Environmental Technical Evaluation Group (IETEG). Guertin J, Jacobs JA, Avakian CP (eds.) Chromium (VI) Handbook. 2005 CRC Press.
26.) Salunkhe PB, Dhakephalkar PK, Paknikar KM. Bioremediation of Cr(VI) in soil microcosms. Biotechnol Ltrs. 1998;20(8):749-751.
27.) Yao J, Wang Y, Djah A, et al. Microcalorimetric study the toxic effect of hexavalent chromium on microbial activity of Wuhan brown sandy soil: an in vitro approach. Ecotoxicol Environ Saf. 2008 Feb;69(2):289-295.
28.) Lupescu A, Jilani K, Zelenak C, et al. Hexavalent chromium-indued erythrocyte membrane phospholipid assymmetry. Biometals. 2011 Nov 13.
29.) al-Shawi AW, Dahl R. Determination of total chromium in phosphate rocks by ion chromatography. J Chromatogr A. 1999 Jul 30;850(1-2):137-141.
30.) Anderson Jamie. BP to persist with Corexit 9500 dispersant. The Money Times. 2010 May 23. [web page]
31.) Lustgarten Abrahm Chemicals Meant to Break up BP Oil Spill Present New Environmental Concerns. 2010 Apr 30. ProPublica. [web page]
32.) Townsend R, Burgess J, Plaskitt KA. Morphology and ultrastructure of helical and nonhelical strains of Spiroplasma citri. J Bacteriol. 1980 Jun;142(3):973-981.
33.) Aufderheide Jeffry John. Vaccine Ingredients: Non-Ionic Surfactants (Tween 80, Triton X-100, Nonoxynol-9. 2011 Aug 32. [web page]
34.) Sun W, Xie C, Wang H, Hu Y. Specific role of polysorbate 80 coating on targeting of nanoparticles to the brain. Biomaterials 2004 Jul;25(15):3065-3071.
35.) Garcia-Garcia E, Andrieux K, Gil S, Couvreur P. Colloidal carriers and blood-brain barrier (BBB) translocation: a way to deliver drugs to the brain? Int J Pharm 2005 Jul 25;298(2):274-292.
36.) Ogita K, Yoneda Y. Disclosure by triton X-100 of NMDA-sensitive [3H] glutamate binding sites in brain synaptic membranes. Biochem Biophys Res Commun. 1988 Jun 16;153(2):510-517.

37.) Stutzenberger FJ. Interference of the detergent Tween 80 in protein assays. Anal Biochem. 1992 Dec;207(2):249-254.
38.) Gajdová M, Jakubovsky J, Války J. Delayed effects of neonatal exposure to Tween 80 on female reproductive organs in rats. Food chem. Toxicol. 1993 Mar;31(3):183-190.
39.) Vasilatos Ch, Megremi I, Economou-Eliopoulos M, Mitsis I. Hexavalent chromium and other toxic metals in groundwaters of the Asopos Valley (Attica), Greece. SEGH. Athens, Hellas 31st March-2nd April 2008.
40.) Buck John D, Cleverdon Robert C. The Effect of Tween 80 on the Enumeration of Marine Bacteria by the Spread and Pour Plate Methods. Dept of Bacteriology, University of CT. Amer Soc Linnology and Oceanography. 1961;6(1):42-44.
41.) Feng J, Zeng Y, Ma C, et al. The Surfactant Tween 80 Enhances Biodesulfurization. Appl Environ Microbiol. 2006 Nov;72(11):7390-7393.
42.) US Patent 4,223,007. Spence, et al. Microbial insecticide. Filed 4/27/79, issued 9/16/80. Assignee: Battelle Development Corporation (Columbus, OH).
43.) Battelle. The Business of Innovation. [web page]
44.) Battelle. Working with Battelle. Battelle/DOE Use Permit for the Pacific Northwest Laboratory. Permit #DE-GM05-00RL01831. [web page] Accessed 2007 Jun 16.
45.) Burgess HD, Hussey NW. Microbial Control of Insects and Mites. 1971 Academic Press Inc. London.
46.) US Patent 4,859,377. Shasha, et al. Starch encapsulation of entomopathogens. Issued 8/22/89, Filed 7/10/87. Assignee: The United States of America, as represented by the Secretary of (Washington, DC).
47.) US Patent 7,605,248. Dattwyler, et al. Recombinant constructs of Borrelia burgdorferi. Filed 9/26/06, published 10/20/09. Inventors: Dattwyler Raymond J, Gomes-Solecki Maria JC, Luft Benjamin J, Dunn John J. Assignee: Research Foundation of the State University of New York (SUNY) and Brookhaven Sciences Associates, LLC (Upton, NY).
48.) Alibek Ken, Handelman Stephen. Biohazard: The Soviet Union's Agricultural Biological Weapons. 1999 Random House, NY.
49.) Madsen Wayne. Fort Detrick Scientist "Commits Suicide" as Anthrax investigation closes in. Global Research.ca [web page]
50.) National Toxicology Program [NTP] (1990). Toxicology and Carcinogenesis Studies of Sodium Fluoride in F344/N Rats and B6C3f1 Mice. Technical report Series No. 393. NIH Publ. No 91-2848. National Institute of Environmental Health Sciences, Research Triangle Park, N.C.
51.) Likins RC, Scow RO, Zipkin I, Steere AC. Deposition and retention of fluoride and radiocalcium in the growing rat. Am J Physiol. 1959 Jul;197(1):75-80. No abstract.
52.) Sajjadi B, Moraveji MK, Davarnejad R. Investigation of Surfactant Effect on the Operational Characteristics of a Packed Bed Internal Loop Airlift Reactor. World Appl Sc J. 2010;11(8):1004-1014.
53.) Kumar AG, Venkatesan R, Kirubagaran R, et al. Effects of nonionic surfactant on hydrolysis and fermentation of protein rich tannery solid waste. Earth and Environ Sc. 19(5):739-748.
54.) Merchuk JC, Gluz M. Bioreactors, Air-Lift Reactors. Encyclopedia of Bioprocess Technology: Fermentation, Biocatalysis and Bioseparation. John Wiley & Sons, Inc. (Eds.);1999:320.
55.) Dionex. Determination of an Anionic Fluorochemical Surfactant (FC-95) in a Steel Bath. Application Update Note 119. Dionex Corporation. Sunnyvale, California.
56.) Elewady GY, El-Said IA, Fouda AS. Anion Surfactants as Corrosion Inhibitors for Aluminum Dissolution in HCl Solutions. Int J Electrochem Sci. 2008;3:177-190.
57.) Karlin Y, Gorbachev D, Volkov A, Barinov A. Advantageous Technology for Treatment of Laundry Waters. International Atomic Energy Agency. Document IAEA-SM-357/59. [web page]
58.) US Patent 7,179,448. Dattwyler et al. Recombinant constructs of Borrelia burgdorferi. Filed 8/3/05 published 2/20/07. Assignees: Research Foundation of the State of New York (Stony Brook) and Brookhaven Science Associates, LLC (Upton, NY).
59.) Brookhaven Science Associates. Laboratory Administration. [web page]. Accessed 2007 Apr 16.
60.) Battelle. The Business of Innovation. [web page] Accessed 2007 Apr 16.
61.) Proceedings from the United States of America, Department of Health and Human Services, Food and Drug Administration, Center for Bioloics Evaluation and Research, Vaccines and Related Biological Products Advisory Committee Meeting, Bethesda, MD. 1998 May 26.
62.) IDSA. Practice Guidelines for the Treatment of Lyme Disease. CID 2000;31 (Suppl. 1). [web page] Accessed 2007 June 5.
63.) Wormser GP, Dattwyler RJ, Shapiro ED, et al. The Clinical Assessment, Treatment, and Prevention of Lyme Disease, Human Granulocytic Anaplasmosis, and Babesiosis: Clinical Practice Guidelines by the Infectious Diseases Society of America. Clinical Infectious Diseases. 2006;43:1089-1134.
64.) Blumenthal, Richard. Office of the Attorney General. The State of Connecticut. Connecticut Attorney General's Office Press Release. Attorney General's Investigation Reveals Flawed Lyme Disease Guideline Process, IDSA Agrees To Reassess Guidelines, Install Independent Arbiter. 2008 May 1. [web page]
65.) US Patent 2,681,878 Kauppi. Insect Repellent Compositions. Filed 9/4/51 published 6/22/54. Assignee: Dow Corning Corporation, Midland, Michigan
66.) US Patent 2,163,104 Salxberg. Chemical Compounds. Filed 12/17/36, published 6/20/39. Assignee: E.I. du Pont de Nemours & Company, Wilmington, DE
67.) US Patent 4,062,948. Vos et al. Dihydromocimycin antibiotics. Filed 9/11/75 published 12/13/77. Assignee: Gist-Brocades N.V. (Delft, NL)
68.) Forge F et al. Mad Cow Disease and Canada's Cattle Industry. Parliament of Canada. 2005 Jul 12. Online document. [web page]
69.) Eugene Franz Roeber, Howard Coon Parmelee (eds). Chemical & metallurgical engineering. 1917 Jul 1-Dec 15;XVII. McGraw-Hill Publishing Company, Inc. And Standard Corporation Service, Daily revised May-August, 1917. Standard Statisics Company Inc. New York. P. 147
70.) Dubos René J, Davis Bernard D. Factors affecting the growth of tubercle bacilli in liquid media. J Exp Med 1946;83:409-423.
71.) Lederberg, Joshua. Letter to Atlas Powder Company. 1946Nov 18. Profiles in Science National Library of Medicine. [web page]
72.) Condayan Chris. 1946 Joshua Lederberg and Edward L. Tatum. History of Microbiology 1930s-1940. Microbe World [web site]
73.) Warwick K. The Joshua Lederberg Papers: Profiles in Science, National Library of Medicine. 2001 Fall;24(4):978-982.
74.) Lederberg Joshua, Tatum EL. Gene recombination in E. coli. Nature. 1946 Oct 19;158:558.
75.) Maloney SE, Maule A, Smith ARW. Microbial Transformation of the Pyrethroid Insecticides: Permethrin, Deltamethrin, Fastac, Fenvalerate, and Fluvalinate. Appl Environ Microbiol. 1988 Nov;54(11):2874-2876.
76.) Vreysen MJB. Prospects for area-wide integration control of tsetse flies (Diptera: Glossinidae) and trypanosomosis in sub-Saharan Africa. Rev. Soc. Entomol. Argent. 2006 Jan/Jul. Vol 65(1-2).
77.) Navokov VA, Sadovnikov AI, Uspenskii IV. Using a helicopter for dusting forest sources of tickborne encephalitis. Foreign Technology Division Wright-Patterson Air Force Base, Ohio. [web site] 1970 Feb 20.
78.) Bastiaensen, Kouagou, Gnofam, Batawui, Napala, Hendrickx. 2004. [Acquisition of a new tsetse fly control technique by farmers of the north of Togo: socio-economic aspects.] [Article in French] Bulletin of Animal Health and Production in Africa, 52(3): 142–158.
79.) US Patent 3,671,635. Chemosterilant Compositions for Flies and Method of Use. Inventor: Philip C. Hamm, Assignee: Monsanto Company, St. Louis, MO. Filed May 27, 1970, issued June 20, 1972.
80.) US Patent 5,367,983. Pound et al. Device and method for its use as an aid in control of ticks and other ectoparasites on wildlife. Filed 8/11/93 published 11/29/94. Assignee: The United States of America as represented by the Secretary of [Agriculture] (Washington DC).
81.) CDC. Surveillance for Acute Pesticide-Related Illness During the Medfly Eradication Program—Florida, 1998. MMWR Weekly 1999 Nov 12;48(44):1015-1018,1027.
82.) Navy and Marine Corps. Pre-Service Test of the U.S. Army Ultra Low Volume Arial Spray System for Rotary Wing Aircraft. Naval Medical Field Research Lab Camp LeJeune, NC. 1971 Aug. Vol. XXI, No. 19. Project #: M4305.
83.) Kokernot RH, Calisher CH, Stannard LJ, Hayes J. Arb ovirus Studies in the Ohio-Mississippi Basin, 1964-1967. J Trop Med Hyg. 1969;18(5):789-795.
84.) Information from Kokernot RH. Lone Star (LS) Strain: TMA 1381. No. 239. Am J Trop Med Hyg. 1970;19(6):1151-1152.
85.) EPA. Technology Transfer Network. Air Toxics Web Site. Methyl Ethyl Ketone (2-Butanone). Hazard Summary. 1992 Apr, Revised 2000 Jan.
86.) Anigstein L, Anigstein D. A review of the evidence in retrospect for a rickettsial etiology in Bullis fever. Texas Rep Biol Med. 1975;33:201-211.
87.) Neelakanta G, Sultana H, Fush D, Anderson JF, Fikrig E. Anaplasma phagocytophilum induces Ixodes scapularis ticks to express an antifreeze glycoprotein gene that enhances their survival in the cold. J Clin Invest. 2010 Sept;120(9):3179-3190.
88.) Lee RE, Baust JG. Cold-hardiness in the Antarctic tick, Ixodes uriae. Physiol Zool. 1987;60(4):499-506.
89.) Graham LA, Liou YC, Walker VK, Davis PL. Hyperactive antifreeze protein from beetles. Nature. 1997;388(6644):727-728.
90.) Gaskin DJH, Starck K, Vulfson EN. Identification of inorganic crystal-specific sequences using phage display combinatorial library of short peptides: A feasibility study. Biotech Ltrs. :22(15):1211-1216.
91.) Johnson Russell C, Harris Virginia G. Differentiation of Pathogenic and Saprophytic Leptospires. I. Growth at Low Temperatures. J Bacteriol. 1967 Jul;94(1):27-31.
92.) Renaudin J, Pascarel MC, Bové MJ. Spiroplasma virus 4: nucleotide sequence of the viral DNA, regulatory signals, and proposed genome organization. J Bacteriol. 1987

Nov;169(11):4950-4961.

93.) Ellinghausen HC Jr, Painter GM. Growth, Survival, Antigenic Stability, and Virulence of Leptospira Interrogans Serotype Canicola. National Animal Disease Center, North Central Region, Agricultural Research Service, USDA, Ames, IA. J Med Microbiol. 1976;9:29-37.

94.) Tumilowicz Joseph J, Alexander Aaron D, Stafford Keith. On the Contamination of Leptospira Biflexa. In Vitro. 1974;10(3&4):238-242.

95.) Brendle JJ, Alexander AD. Contamination of Bacteriological Media by Leptospira biflexa. Appl Microbiol. 1974 Sept;28(3):505-506. (From Div. of Veterinary Medicine, Walter Reed Army Medical Center, Washington, DC).

96.) Sally Jo Rubin, Sidney Perlman, Herman C. Ellinghausen Jr. Isolation of Leptospira biflexa from Commercially Prepared Deionized Water Labeled "Sterile for Tissue Culture." J Clin Microbiol. 1980 Jul;12(1):121-123. (From St. Francis Hospital and Medical Center, Hartford, CT and National Animal Disease Laboratory, Ames, Iowa.)

97.) Hovind-Hougen K, Høybe G. Urinary excretion of an unidentified treponeme in a case of leptospirosis. Zentralbl Bakteriol A. 1981 Feb;248(4):532-40.

98.) Brendle JJ, Alexander AD. Contamination of Bacteriological Media by Leptospira biflexa. Appl Microbiol. 1974 Sept.;28(3):505-506.

99.) Faine Solomon. Leptospira and Leptospirosis. 1993 CRC Press, Inc. Boca Raton, FL.

100.) Segers RPAM. The molecular analysis of sphingomyelinase genes of Leptospiraceae. Doctoral thesis. Rijksuniversiteit te Utrecht, Netherlands. 1991 p. 147.

101.) Fikrig E, Narasimhan S, Neelakanta G, et al. Toll-Like Receptors 1 and 2 Heterodimers Alter Borrelia burgdorferi Gene Expression in Mice and Ticks. J Infect Dis. 2009 Oct 15;200(8):1331-1340.

102.) Rozen P, Zonis J, Yekutiel P, Gilat T. Crohn's disease in the Jewish population of Tel-Aviv-Yafo. Epidemiologic and clinical aspects. Gastroenterology 1979 Jan;76(1):25-30.

103.) Kelly TE, Chase GA, Kaback MM, et al. Tay-Sachs Disease: High Gene Frequency in a Non-Jewish Population. Am J Hum Genet. 1975;27:287-291.

104.) Wikipedia. Sphingomyelin phosphodiesterase. http://en.wikipedia.org

105.) Wikipedia. Ceramide. http:/en.wikipedia.org

106.) Grant 7R01HL064735-02. The Role of Plasma Sphingomyelin in Atherosclerosis. Project start 2/3/01 ended 1/31/05. SUNY Downstate Medical Center, Brooklyn, NY. Department Anatomy and Cell Biology. National Heart, Lung, and Blood Institute.

107.) Ozbayraktar FB, Ulgen KO. Molecular facets of sphingolipids: mediators of diseases. Biotechnol. J. 2009 Jul;4(7):1028-1041.

108.) Ng CG, Griffin DE. Acid Sphingomyelinase Deficiency Increases Susceptibility to Fatal Alphavirus Encephalomyelitis. J Virol. 2006 Nov;80(22):10989-10999.

109.) Faine Solomon. Leptospira and Leptospirosis. 1994. CRC Press Inc., Boca Raton, FL. p. 78.

110.) Kasarov LB, Addamiano L. Metabolism of the lipoproteins of serum by leptospires: degradation of the triglycerides. J Med Microbiol. 1969;2:165-168.

111.) Groman Neal B, Bobb Dolores. The inhibition of adsorption of Cornybacterium diphtheria phage by Tween 80. Virol. 1955 Sept;1(3):313-323.

112.) Ouyang Z, He M, Oman T, et al. A manganese transporter, BB0219 (BmtA), is required for virulence by the Lyme disease spirochete, Borrelia burgdorferi. Proc Natl Acad Sci USA. 2009 Mar 3;106(9):3449-3454. Epub 2009 Feb 13.

113.) Posey JE, Gherardini FC. Lack of a role for iron in the Lyme disease pathogen. Science 2000 Jun 2;288(5471):1651-1653.

114.) Sueyoshi N, Kita K, Okino N, et al. Molecular cloning and expression of Mn(2+)-dependent sphingomyelinase/hemolysin of an aquatic bacterium, Pseudomonas sp. strain TK4. J Bacteriol. 2002 Jan;184(2):540-546.

115.) Smith MCM, Socket RE (eds.) Methods in Microbiology. Volume 29. Genetic methods for diverse prokaryotes. 1999. Academic Press, London, UK and San Diego, CA. P. 218.

116.) US Patent 7,220,385. Blecka et al. System and method for multi-analyte detection. Filed 7/19/04 published 5/22/07. Assignee: Bio-Rad Laboratories, Inc. (Hercules, CA).

117.) US Patent 7,955,555. Blecka et al. System and method for multi-analyte detection. Filed 4/6/07 published 7/7/11. Assignee: Bio-Rad Laboratories, Inc. (Hercules, CA).

118.) US Patent 8,012,768. Jafari, et al. System and method for multi-analyte detection. Filed 5/1/07 published 9/6/11. Assignee: Bio-Rad Laboratories, Inc. (Hercules, CA).

119.) Willman David. Selling the threat of bioterrorism. 2007 Jul 1. The Los Angeles Times. [monograph]. http://articles.latimes.com/2007/jul/01/nation/na-alibek1. 6 pages.

120.) Bio-rad [web page]

Herbicides and Amines to an End

1.) Friesen PD, Miller LK. Insect viruses. In: Knipe DM, Howley PM, Griffin DE, Lamb RA, Marin MA, Roizman B, Straus SE (Eds.). Fund Virol. Lippincott Williams and Wilkins, Philadelphia, pp. 446-456.

2.) Krywienczyk J, Bergold GH. Serological relationships of viruses from some lepidopterous and hymenopterous insects. Virology. 1960 Mar;10(3):308-315.

3.) TIME.com. Panic over Paraquat. [monograph on the Internet] 1978 May 1.

4.) Revkin AC. Paraquat: A potent weed killer is killing people. Science Digest 1983;91(6):36-38.

5.) Chlorfluazuron. Class action in Australia against ICI over residues in meat. Food Safety and Hygiene Bulletin. [web page]

6.) US Patent 3,615,654. Ayukawa et al. Filed 5/17/68 published 10/26/71. Assignee: CPC International Inc.

7.) Brock TD. Microorganisms From Smallpox to Lyme Disease. Scientific American. W.H. Freeman and Company. 1990. p. 28-37.

8.) US Patent 4,888,276. Shelburne. Method and composition for the diagnosis of Lyme disease. Filed 6/26/86 published 12/19/89. Assignee: Minnesota Mining and Manufacturing Company (St. Paul, MN).

9.) News: Evaluation of Surfactants in Fertilizers Calm Enthusiastic Claims. J Agric Food Chem. 1954 Sept;2(20):1015-1016.

10.) US Patent 3,681,441. Robertson. Filed 4/13/70 published 8/1/72. Quaternary Fluorinated Ammonium Salts. Assignee: Minnesota Mining and Manufacturing Company (Saint Paul, MN).

11.) Freedman Alix M. 'Impact Booster' Tobacco Firm Shows How Ammonia Spurs Delivery of Nicotine. 1995 Dec 28. The Pulitzer Prizes. [web site]

12.) Landrigan PJ, Powell KE, et al. Paraquat and Marijuana: Epidemiologic Risk Assessment. AJPH 1983 Jul;73(7):784-788.

13.) Mulroy MF, Bernards CM, McDonald SB, Salinas FV.; Gravlee Glenn P. (ed.) A Practical Approach to Regional Anesthesia. Fourth Edition. 2009 Lippincott Williams & Wilkins. Philadelphia, PA

14.) Reigart JR, Roberts JR. Recognition and Management of Pesticide Poisonings. US EPA. 1999 report.

15.) Montgomery MR. Interaction of paraquat with the pulmonary microsomal fatty acid desaturase system. Toxicol App Pharma 1976 Jun;36(3):543-554.

16.) Khazaeli AA, Nuzhdin SV, Curtsinger JW. Genetic variation for life span, resistance to paraquat, and spontaneous activity in unselected populations of Drosophila melanogaster: Implications for transgenic rescue of life span. Mech Ageing Devel 2007 Sept;128(9):486-493.

17.) Sohal RS, Mockett RJ, Orr WC. Mechanisms of aging: an appraisal of the oxidative stress hypothesis. Free Radic Biol Med 2002 Sept 1;33(5):575-586 Review.

18.) McClure Carol D, Schiller Neal L. Effects of Pseudomonas aeruginosa rhamnolipids on human monocyte-derived macrophages. J Leuk Biol. 1992 Feb;51:97-102.

19.) Laurence Zulianello, Coralie Canard, Thilo Köhler, et al. Rhamnolipids Are Virulence Factors That Promote Early Infiltration of Primary Human Airway Epithelia by Pseudomonas aeruginosa. Infect and Immun. 2006 Jun;74(6):3134-3147.

20.) Boles BR, Thoendel M, Singh PK. Rhamnolipids mediate detachment of Pseudomonas aeruginosa from biofilms. Mol Microbiol. 2005 Sept;47(5):1210-1223. [abstract]

21.) Aberer E, Duray Paul H. Morphology of Borrelia burgdorferi: Structural Patterns of Cultured Borreliae in Relation to Staining Methods. 1991 Apr;29(4):764-772.

22.) Steere AC, Tenney JH, Mackel DC, Snyder MJ, Polakavetz S, Dunne ME, Dixon R. Pseudomonas species bacteremia caused by contaminated normal human serum albumin. J Infect Dis. 1977 May;135(5):729-35.

23.) Lohmann CP, Winkler von Mohrenfels C, Gabler B, et al. [Polymerase chain reaction (PCR) for microbiological diagnosis in refractory infectious keratitis: a clinical study in 16 patients]. Klin Monbl Augenheilkd. 2000 Jul;217(1):37-42. [Article in German] [abstract]

24.) Rogers SA, Bero JD, Melander C. Chemical synthesis and biological screening of 2-aminoimidazole-based bacterial and fungal antibiofilm agents. Chembiochem. 2010 Feb 15;11(3):396-410. Chemistry, North Carolina State University, 2620 Yarborough Drive, Raleigh, NC.

25.) Imhoff, Johannes F, Petri Ralf, Süling Jörg. Reclassification of species of the spiral-shaped phototrophic purple non-sulfur bacteria of the α-Proteobacteria: description of the new genera Phaeospirillum gen. nov., Rhodovibrio gen. nov., Rhodothalassium gen. nov. and Roseospira gen. nov. as well as transfer of Rhodospirillum fulvum to Phaeospirillum fulvum comb. nov., of Rhodospirillum molischianum to Phaeospirillum molischianum comb. nov., of Rhodospirillum salinarum to Rhodovibrio salinarum comb. nov., of Rhodospirllum sodomense to Rhodovibrio sodomensis comb. nov., of Rhodospirillum salexigens to Rhodothalassium salexigens comb. nov. and of Rhodospirillum mediosalinum to Roseospira mediosalina comb. no. Int J Syst Bacteriol. 1998;48(3):793-798.

26.) Evers D, Weckesser J, Drews G. Protein on the Cell Surface of the Moderately Halophilic Phototrophic Bacterium Rhodospirillum salexigens. J Bacteriol. 1984 Oct;160(1):107-111.

27.) Harrison JJ, Turner RJ, Joo DA, et al. Copper and Quaternary Ammonium Cations Exert Synergistic Bactericidal and Antibiofilm Activity against Pseudomonas aeruginosa. Antimicrob Chemo. 2008 Aug;52(8):2870-2881.

28.) Wang EW, Agostini G, Olomu O, Runco D, Jung JY, Chole RA. Gentian violet and ferric ammonium citrate disrupt Pseudomonas aeruginosa biofilms. Laryngoscope. 2008 Nov;118(11):2050-2060. [abstract]
29.) Juergensen, L., J. Busnarda, P.-Y. Caux, and R. A. Kent. 2000. Fate, behaviour, and aquatic toxicity of the fungicide DDAC in the Canadian environment. Environ. Toxicol. 15:174–200.
30.) Littlefield NA, Gaylor DW, Blackwell BN, Allen RR. Chronic toxicity/carcinogenicity studies of gentian violet in Fischer 344 rats: two-generation exposure. Food Chem Toxicol. 1989 Apr;27(4):239-247.
31.) Littlefield NA, Blackwell BN, Hewitt CC, Gaylor DW. Chronic toxicity and carcinogenicity studies of gentian violet in mice. Fundam Appl Toxicol. 1985 Oct;5(5):902-912.
32.) Conn HJ. An Investigation of American Gentian Violets Report of Committee on Bacteriological Technic. J Bacteriol. 1922;7(5):529-537. Pepling M, Howard PH, Durkin PR. Use and Assessment of Markers Used with Herbicides. Submitted to the Animal and Plant Health Inspection Service (APHIS) Policy and Program Development, Environmental Analysis and Documentation. USDA. Riverdale, MD. Submitted by Syracuse Environmental Research Associates, Inc. Fayetteville, NY. Document SERA TR 96-21-07-03b. 1997 Dec 21. 47 pages.
33.) Morena CX, Moy F, Daniels TJ, et al. Molecular analysis of microbial communities identified in different developmental stages of Ixodes scapularis ticks from Westchester and Dutchess Counties, New York. Environ Microbiol. 2006 May;8(5):761-772.786
34.) Seal Taghavi, Fegan Hayward & Fegan. Determination of Ralstonia (Pseudomas) solanacearum rDNA subgroups by PCR tests. Plant Pathol. 2002 Jan;48(1):115-120.
35.) Holness H, Stone WR. The Separation of Quaternary Halides by Paper Chromatography. Analyst. 1958;83:71-75.

Chasing Rainbows

1.) Galston Arthur. An Accidental Plant Biologist. Plant Psysiol. Am Soc Plant Physiol. 2002Mar;128:786-787.
2.) Young Alan L. The History, Use, Disposition and Environmental Fate of Agent Orange. 2009Springer Science + Business Media, LLC. New York. ISBN: 978-0-387-87486-9.
3.) Young AL. TCDD Biomonitoring and Exposure to Agent Orange: Still the Gold Standard. Env Sci Pollut Res. 2004;11(3):143-146.
4.) Palmer MG. The Legacy of Agent Orange: Empirical Evidence from Central Vietnam. Soc Sci & Med. 2004;60:1061-1070.
5.) IOM. The Institute of Medicine. Improving the Presumptive Disability Decision-Making Process for Veterans. The Institute of Medicine, The National Academies Press, Washington, DC. 2008. 813 pages. ISBN: 978-0-309-10730-3
6.) Pearce Jeremy. Arthur Galston, Agent Orange Researcher, Is Dead at 88. The New York Times. 2008 June 23.
7.) Mockett RJ, Radyuk SN, et al. Phenotypic effects of familial amyotrophic lateral sclerosis mutant Sod alleles in transgenic Drosophila. PNAS 2003Jan 7;100(2):301-306.
8.) Fluoride in Drinking Water. A Scientific Review of EPA's Standards. 2006. National Academy of Sciences. Committee on Fluoride in Drinking Water. Board on Environmental Studies and Toxicology, Division on Earth and Life Studies. National Research Council of the National Academies. The National Academies Press, Washington, DC. 531 pages.
9.) Sokoloff L. Cerebral circulatory and metabolic changes associated with aging. Res Publ Assoc Res Nerv Ment Dis. 1966;41:237-254.
10.) Jacqmin H, Comenges D, Letenneur L, et al. Components of drinking water and risk of cognitive impairment in the elderly. Am J Epidemiol. 1994;139(1):48-57.
11.) Mouchès C, Candresse T, Barroso G, Saillard C, Wroblewski H, Bové JM. Gene for Spiralin, the Major Membrane Protein of the Helical Mollicute Spiroplasma citri: Cloning and Expression in Escherichia coli. J Bacteriol. 1985 Dec;164(3):1094-1099.
12.) Wise KS. Adaptative surface variation. Trends Microbiol. 1993;1:59-63.
13.) Watson HL, Zheng X, Cassell GH. Structural variations and phenotypic switching of mycoplasmal antigens. Clin Infect Dis. 1993;17:S183-S186.
14.) MacDonald AB. The Molecular Link Between Alzheimer's Disease and Borrelia. [Internet podcast].
15.) MacDonald AB. Alzheimer's neuroborreliosis with trans-synaptic spread of infection and neurofibrillary tangles derived from intraneuronal spirochetes. Med Hypotheses. 2007;68(4):822-825. [Epub 2006 Oct. 20.

Persisting Pollutants

1.) Dinman Bertram D. Aluminum Smelting and Refining. [monograph on the Internet].
2.) Bowell RJ, Williams KP, Connelly RJ, Sadler PJK, Dodds JE. Containment of Metalliferous Wastes. Chemical containment of mine waste. Geological Society, London, Special Publications. 1999;157:213-240.
3.) Yamashita N, Kannan K, Taniyasu S, et al. A global survey of perfluorinated acids in oceans.
4.) Assessment of PFOA in the drinking water of the German Hochsauerlandkreis. Drinking Water Commission (Trinkwasserkommission) of the German Ministry of Health at the Federal Environment Agency. 8 pages.
5.) Kudo N, Kawashima Y. Toxicity and toxicokinetics of perfluorooctanoic acid in humans and animals. J. Toxicol. Sci. 2003 May;28(2): 49–57.
6.) Strategic Challenges for the Bush Administration. Perspectives from the Institute for National Strategic Studies. 2001. National Defense University Press, Washington, DC. 76 page report.
7.) Schultz MM, Higgins CP, Huset CA, et al. Fluorochemical mass flows in a municipal wastewater treatment facility. Environ Sci Technol. 2006 Dec;40(23):7350-7357.
8.) Betts Kellyn. PFOS and PFOA in Humans: New Study Links Prenatal Exposure to Lower Birth Weight. Environ Health Perspect. 2007 Nov;115(11):A550-1.
9.) Hood Ernie. Alternative Mechanism for PFOA?: Trout Studies Shed Light on Liver Effects. Environ. Health Perspect. 2008 Aug;116(8): A351.
10.) Cookson, Clive. Researchers link synthetic chemicals to infertility. Financial Times. 2009 Jan 29. [web page]
11.) Meersman, Tom. Study: Death rate up for 3M workers exposed to PFOA. Star Tribune. 2008 Mar 5. [web page]
12.) Eder, Andrew DuPont plant linked to cancer. The News Journal. Delawareonline. 2008 Jun
13.) Betts Kellyn. PFOS and PFOA in Humans. New Study Links Prenatal Exposure to Lower Birth Weight. Environ. Health Perspect. 2007 Nov;115(111):A550.
14.) Eder Andrew. The News Journal. Delawareonline. DuPont plant linked to cancer. Company to look into high W.Va. rates; other plants blacked out in report. [monograph].
15.) Rutherford Tony. DuPont Sued for Toxic Pollution of Ohio River. Little Hocking Water Association Asserts Teflon Chemicals Harmful for 2,000 Years. HuntingtonNews.net 2009 Dec. 8.
16.) Anke Schaefer, Barbara Booth, Naomi Lubick, Kellyn S. Betts. Perfluorinated surfactants contaminate German waters – Mislabeled waste in fertilizer leads to a water scandal. Environ. Sci. Technol. ACS Publications. 2006 Dec 1;40(23):7108–14.
17.) Fluoropolymers: Dependable. Essential. Safe. 2008. SPI The plastics industry trade association. [web site]
18.) Dupont. Products & Services [web site].
19.) Giesy JP, Jones PD, Newsted JL, Kannan K. Perfluorinated Compounds: An Overview of Environmental and Analytical Issues. Slide presentation on the Internet. Michigan State University Zoology Dept. & National Food Safety and Toxicology Center. [web page]
20.) US Patent 5,516,674. Roe et al. Insecticide resistance associated cytochrome 450. Filed 8/30/94 published 5/14/96. Assignee: North Carolina State University (Raleigh, NC).
21.) Hougham Gareth. Topics in Applied Chemistry. Fluoropolymers: Synthesis. 16.2.1 Containerization of Crop Protection Channels. Hougham G, Cassidy PE, Johns K, Davidson T. (eds.) 1999 Kluwer Academic/Plenum Publishes, New York. P. 242.
22.) Carstens P, De Beer J, Le roux J. New Surface-fluorinated Products. Fluoropolymers 1: Synthesis. Topics in Applied Chemistry. 2002;II:241-259.
23.) Weber Marcus O, Schilo Diederich. Fluoropolymers 1: Synthesis. Hougham et al. (eds.) Plenum Press, New York. 1999. Series editors: Kartritzky AR (Univ. Florida) and Sabongi GJ. (3M Company, St. Paul, MN).
24.) Kansas Department of Wildlife and Parks. Fish Hatcheries. [web site]
25.) Seepage Control Inc. Sealing Lakes & Ponds with ESS-13…Empty or Full! [web site]
26.) US Patent 3,772,893. Soil Sealing Method. Filed 6/7/72, published 11/20/73. Assignee: The Dow Chemical Company (Midland, MI).
27.) US Patent 3,016,713. Deming. Method of Treating Soil with Aqueous Slurry of Lattice Clay and Anionic Polyelectrolyte. Filed 5/15/57, published 1/16/62. Assignee: The Monsanto Chemical Company, St. Louis, MO.
28.) Arneson, Gerald J. (November 1961). Toxicity of Teflon Dispersing Agents. DuPont Polychemicals Department, Research & Development Division, Experimental Station. [web page]
29.) Clapp R, Hoppin P, Jagai J, Donahue S. Case Studies in Science Policy: Perfluorooctanoic Acid. Project on Scientific Knowledge and Public Policy (SKAPP). [web page]
30.) Ward, Jr., Ken. DuPont finds high C8in Chinese workers. The Charleston Gazette. 2008 Nov 7. [web page]
31.) 2010/15PFOA Stewardship Program; PFOA and Fluorinated Telomers. US Environmental Protection Agency.
32.) Michael Janofsky. DuPont to Pay $16.5Million for Unreported Risks. The New York Times. 2005 Dec 15. [web page]

33.) MN Department of Health. News Release. 2007Mar 1. Health officials issue new health guidelines for PFOA, PFOS; reiterate protective advice on PFBA. [monograph].
34.) US EPA v. E.I. du Pont de Nemours and Company, Wilmington, DE, Washington Works Facility, WV. Complaint and Notice of Opportunity for Hearing. Docket No. TSCA-HQ-2005-5001. Date stamped 2004Dec. 6. 14 pages.
35.) Lien Dennis. 3M releases findings on PFCs. Some fish taken from river near plant have high levels of industrial chemicals that were once dumped in river. Pioneer Press. 2006 Mar 11. [web page]
36.) Skutlarek D, Exner M, Färber H. Perfluorinated surfactants in surface and drinking waters. Environ. Sci. Pollut. Res. Int. 2006 Sept.;13(5):299-307.
37.) Parsons John R, Sáez Monica, Dolfing Jan, de Voogt Pim. Biodegradation of Perfluorinated Compounds. Reviews of Environmental Contamination and Toxicology. Vol. 196. Springer New York. 2009.
38.) US Patent 4,888,276. Shelburne. Method and composition for the diagnosis of Lyme disease. Filed 6/26/86 published 12/19/89. Assignee: Minnesota Mining and Manufacturing Company (St. Paul, MN).
39.) US Patent 3,016,713. Deming. Method of Treating Soil with Aqueous Slurry of Lattice Clay and Anionic Polyelectrolyte. Filed 5/15/57, published 1/16/62. Assignee: The Monsanto Chemical Company, St. Louis, MO.
40.) Zambrana MC, Beklemisheva AA, Bryksin AV, et al. Borrelia burgdorferi binds to, invades, and colonizes native type 1 collagen lattices. Infect immun. 2004Jun;72(6):3138-3146.
41.) Domb AJ, Kumar N. (eds.) Biodegradable Polymers in Clinical Use and Clinical Development. 2011 John Wiley & Sons, Inc Hoboken, New Jersey.
42.) Beck Gregory, Benach Jorge L, Habicht Gail S. Isolation, preliminary chemical characterization, and biological activity of Borrelia burgdorferi peptidoglycan. Biochem and Biophys Res Comm. 1990 Feb 28;167(1):89-95.
43.) Shamsi SA, Igbal R, Akbay C. Glycine-based polymeric surfactants with varied polar head group: II. Chemical sensitivity in micellar eletrokinetic chromatography using linear solvation energy relationships. Electrophoresis. 2005 Nov;26(21):4138-4152.
44.) Delton Cables. Fluoropolymer Insulated wire and cables for high temperature application. ISO 9001,2000. Specification sheet. [web page]
45.) AGC Chemicals. Fluon. Fuoropolymer website. [web page]
46.) EPA. Love Canal. Press Releases and Articles. [web page]
47.) Leistner Marilyn. The Times Beach Story. (former mayor of Times Beach, Missouri). Mongraph. Synthesis/Regeneration. 1995 Summer (7-8). [web page]
48.) Proceedings of the Third Annual Hazardous Materials Management Conference & Exhibition. Philadelphia, PA. June 4-6, 1985.
49.) EPA (Environmental Protection Agency). An inventory of sources and environmental releases of dioxin-like compounds in the United States for the years 1987, 1995, and 2000. (2006) National Center for Environmental Assessment, Washington, DC; EPA/600/P-03/002F. [web page]
50.) Health Effects Dioxins [web page]
51.) Meij R, Winkel H te. Health aspects of coal fly ash. [web page]
52.) McGavran MH. Easterday BC. U.S. Army Biological Laboratories, Fort Detrick, Maryland. Technical Manuscript 34. (work originally submitted under manuscript #5033). Rift Valley Fever Virus Hepatitis. Light and Electron Microscopic Studies in the Mouse. 1963 Jun. Document# AD410394. Project 4B11-02-068.
53.) Chulov Martin. Iraq littered with high levels of nuclear and dioxin contamination, study finds. 2010 Jan 22. The guardian. [web page]
54.) The Alliance for a Clean Environment. ACE. The Toxic Triangle – A Major Factor in Shocking Childhood Cancer Rates for the Greater Pottstown Area. [web page]
55.) EPA. Technology Transfer Network. Air Toxics Web Site. Methyl Ethyl Ketone (2-Butanone). Hazard Summary. 1992 Apr, Revised 2000 Jan.
56.) Anigstein L, Anigstein D. A review of the evidence in retrospect for a rickettsial etiology in Bullis fever. Texas Rep Biol Med. 1975;33:201-211.
57.) Perkins John H. Reshaping Technology in Wartime: The Effect of Military Goals on Entomological Research and Insect-Control Practices. Technol Culture. 1978Apr;19(2):169-186.
58.) Huxsoll David L, Hildebrandt Paul K, Nims Robert M, Amyx Herbert T, Ferguson James A. Epizootiology of Tropical Canine Pancytopenia. Proceed Ann Conf. J Wildlife Dis. 1970;6:220-225.
59.) Anderson Burt E, Greene Craig E, Jones Dana C, Dawson Jacqueline E. Ehrlichia ewingii sp. nov., the Etiologic Agent of Canine Granulocytic Ehrlichiosis. Inter J Syst Bacteriol. 1992Apr;42(2):299-302.
60.) Schecter A, Cramer P, Boggess K, et al. Intake of Dioxins and Related Compounds from Food in the US Population. J Toxicol Environ Health. 2001;63:1-18 (Part A).
61.) Rogowski David, Yake Bill. Addendum to Final Report: Screening Survey for Metals and Dioxins in Fertilizer Products and Soils in Washington State. Dioxins in Washington State Agricultural Soils. 1999 Nov. Ecology Publication No. 99-333. 64 pages.
62.) Bowhay Dennis, and the Interagency Fertilizer Testing Workgroup. Screening Survey for Metals in Fertilizers and Industrial By-Product Fertilizers in Washington State. 1997 Dec. Ecology Publication No. 97-341. 85 pages.
63.) Rogowski David, Golding Steven, et al. Final Report Screening Survey for Metals and Dioxins in Fertilizer Products and Soils in Washington State. 1999 Apr. Ecology Publication No. 99-309. Washington State Dept. of Ecology, Olympia, WA. 177 pages.
64.) Alcock RE, Behnisch PA, Jones KC, Hagenmaier H. Dioxin-like PCBs in food. Their significance to human TEQ exposures. Organohalogen Compounds. 1998;38:89-92.
65.) Gladen B, Schecter A, Päpke O, et al. Polychlorinated dibenzy-p-dioxins, polychlorinated dibenzofurans, and coplanar polychlorinated biphenyls in breast milk from two cities in Ukraine. J Toxicol Environ Health. 1999;58:119-127.
66.) Kociba R. Rodent bioassays for assessing chronic toxicity and carcinogenic potential of TCDD. In Banury Report 35: Biological basis for risk assessment of dioxins and related compound. Gallo MA, Scheuplein RJ, van der Heijden KA (eds). Cold Spring Harbor, NY; Cold Spring Harbor Laboratory Press. p. 3-11.
67.) Masuda Y, Schecter AJ, Päpke O. Concentration of PCBs, PCDFs and PCDDs in the blood of Yusho patients and their toxic equivalent contributions. Organohalogen Compounds 1996;30:146-149.
68.) Hou DX, Kunitake T, Kusuda J, Fujii M. Primary culture of chicken hepatocytes as an in vitro model for determining the influence of dioxins. Biosci Biotechnol Biochem. 2001 Jan;65(1):218-221.
69.) Cohen-Barnhouse AM, Zwiernik MJ, Link JE, et al. Sensitivity of Japanese quail (Coturnix japonica), Common pheasant (Phasianus colchicus), and White Leghorn chicken (Gallus gallus domesticus) embryos to in ovo exposure to TCDD, PeCDF, and TCDF. Toxicol Sci. 2011 Jan;119(1):93-103.
70.) Kijlstra A, Traag WA, Hoodenboom LA. Effect of flock size on dioxin levels in eggs from chickens kept outside. Poult Sci 2007 Sep;86(9):2042-2048.
71.) Felsheim RF, Chávez AS, Palmer GH, et al. Transformation of Anaplasma marginale. Vet Parasitol. 2010 Feb 10;167(2-4):167-174.
72.) Hourrigan JL. Safe use of pesticides on livestock. J Am Vet Med Assoc. 1970 Dec 1;157(11):1818-1827.
73.) US Patent 7,192,905. Li et al. Organophosphate insecticide synergists for fly and tick control. Filed 6/20/03, published 3/20/07. Assignee: The United States as represented by the Secretary of Agriculture. (Washington, DC).
74.) Maamun JM, Suleman MA, Akinyi M, et al. Prevalence of Babesia microti in free-ranging baboons and African green monkeys. J Parasitol. 2011 Feb;97(1):63-67.
75.) US Patent 4,073,932. Beriger. Method of controlling insects using 1,3-dioxin-4-ones. Filed 1/10/77 published 2/14/78. Assignee: Ciba-Geigy Corporation (Ardsley, NY).
76.) US Patent 3,351,485. Langner. Stabilization and Preservation of Wood. Filed 3/6/64 published 11/7/67. Assignee: Dow Chemical Company, Midland, MI.
77.) US Patent 3,723,468. Blumenfeld et al. Ketonitriles and Methods for their Production. Filed 1/28/70 published 3/27/73. Assignee: Dynamit Nobel AG (Troisdorf, DT).
78.) US Patent 3,169,879. Wahl et al. Plasticized Plastic Compositions. Filed 11/15/60 published 2/16/65. Assignee: Agfa Aktiengesellschaft, Leverkusen, Germany.
79.) US Patent 4,123,551. Beriger. 2,2-Disubstituted-phenylcarbamoyl-6-hydroxy-m-dioxin-4-one derivatives havingn insecticidal properties. Filed 1/10/77 published 10/31/78. Assignee: Ciba-Geigy Corporation (Ardsley, NY).
80.) US Patent 4,725,306. Ueda et al. Pyridinecarboxamide plant growth inhibitors. Filed 10/21/85 published 2/16/88. Assignee: Daicel Chemical Industries Inc. (Osaka, JP).
81.) US Patent 3,816,268. Watson et al. Stabilized Distillation of Pentachlorophenol. Filed 4/20/73 published 6/11/74. Assignee: The Dow Chemical Company (Midland, MI).
82.) US Patent 3,646,225. Morrison. Treatment of Pentachlorophenol. Filed 7/24/67 published 2/29/72. Assignee: The Dow Chemical Company, Midland MI.
83.) US Patent 1,919,298. Lehmann et al. Filed 5/15/29, published 7/25/33. Disinfectant. Assignee: Winthrop Chemical Company, Inc. of New York, NY.
84.) US Patent 2,435,676. Fitzgerald, et al. Herbicide. Filed 5/31/44 published 2/10/48. Assignee: The Dow Chemical Company, Midland, MI.
85.) US Patent 2,780,546. Moyle et al. Production of Preserved Alkaline Paper. Filed 8/26/55 published 2/5/57. Assignee: The Dow Chemical Company, Midland, MI.
86.) US Patent 2,993,934. Rosen. Derivatives of Pentachlorophenol. Filed 8/8/56 published 7/25/61. Assignee: Diamond Alkali Company, Cleveland, OH.
87.) US Patent 3,408,323. Hackney. Insect Resistance Thermoplastic Compositions. Filed 5/13/65 published 10/29/68. Assignee: Union Carbide Australia Limited.

Mustard Wastes Do Catch Up

1.) Mustard Disaster at Bari. Force Health Protection and Readiness. Chemical-Biological Warfare Exposures. [web page]
2.) Blister Agent: Sulfur Mustard (H,HD,HS). 2005. [web page]
3.) Olson Kyle B. Aum Shinrikyo: Once and Future Threat? CDC. Emerging Infectious Diseases. 1999 Jul-Aug;5(4):491-602.
4.) Global Security.org. Operation CHASE. [web site]
5.) Borg James. Tending the Dragon's Fire: Shall We Bake, Steam or Baste our Obsolete Chemical Weapons? [web site]
6.) Watson AP, Griffin GD. Toxicity of vesicant agents scheduled for destruction by the Chemical Stockpile Disposal Program. Environ Health Perspect. 1992 Nov;98:259-280. Review.
7.) Chemical Warfare Primer. Minnesota Poison Control System. [web site]
8.) Ashby J, Tinwell H, Callander RD, Clare N. Genetic activity of the human carcinogen sulphur mustard towards Salmonella and the mouse bone marrow. Mutat Res. 1991 May;257(3):307-311.
9.) Goldman M, Dacre JC. Lewisite: its chemistry, toxicology, and biological effects. Rev Environ Contam Toxicol. 1989;110:75-115. Review.
10.) Robertson Campbell, Lipton Eric. BP is Criticized Over Oil Spill, but U.S. Missed Chances to Act. 2010 Apr 30. The New York Times. [web page]
11.) These are the chemicals of warfare. Daily Press. [web site] Mustard Gas. Newport News VA, Daily Press 2010.
12.) Bull John MR. Decades of Dumping Chemical Arms Leave a Risky Legacy. Part I. The Deadliness Below. 2005 Oct. 30. The Daily Press.
13.) Dumping was carried out on a global scale. The Daily Press. [web site] The Daily Press.
14.) Gibson PD, Brink RA, Stahmann MA. The mutagenic action of mustard gas on zea mays. J Hered. 1950 Sep;41(9):232-238. No abstract.
15.) Tuomi J, Rantamäki LK, Tanskanen R, Junttila J. Characterization of Finnish Borrelia burgdorferi Sensu Lato Isolates by Sodium Dodecyl Sulfate-Polyacrylamide Gel Electrophoresis and with Monoclonal Antibodies. J Clin Microbiol. 1995 Aug;33(8):1989-1996.
16.) Sanderson Hans, Fauser Patrik, Thomsen Marianne. Environmental Hazards of Sea-Dumped Chemical Weapons. Environmental Science and Technology. [web site]
17.) Runner Philippa. EU mulls Baltic Sea strategy. 2009 May 2. Euobserver.com [web site]
18.) Hawley Charles. Europe's Underwater Chemical Dump. Tons of Mercury Found in the Baltic Sea. 2006 Aug 30. [Monograph on the Internet]
19.) Missiaen T, Feller P. Geophysical investigations of a chemical munition dumpsite in the Baltic Sea. 2008 May 27-29. [monograph]
20.) Surveying Ships Sunk Off North Carolina in World War II. 2009 Aug 13. ScienceDaily. [web page]

Borrelia Mining

1.) Anke Schaefer, Barbara Booth, Naomi Lubick, Kellyn S. Betts. Perfluorinated surfactants contaminate German waters – Mislabeled waste in fertilizer leads to a water scandal. Environ. Sci. Technol. ACS Publications. 2006 Dec 1;40(23):7108–14.
2.) Skutlarek D, Exner M, Färber H. Perfluorinated surfactants in surface and drinking waters. Environ. Sci. Pollut. Res. Int. 2006 Sept.;13(5):299-307.
3.) Parsons John R, Sáez Monica, Dolfing Jan, de Voogt Pim. Biodegradation of Perfluorinated Compounds. Reviews of Environmental Contamination and Toxicology. Vol. 196. Springer New York. 2009.
4.) US Patent 4,888,276. Shelburne. Method and composition for the diagnosis of Lyme disease. Filed 6/26/86 published 12/19/89. Assignee: Minnesota Mining and Manufacturing Company (St. Paul, MN).
5.) Bush William V, and White Bekki. State of Arkansas. Arkansas Geological Survey. History of Bauxite in Arkansas. AGES Brochure Series 3. 2007.
6.) Bauxite and Alumina. Mineral Commodity Summaries. 1996 January. [web page]
7.) Kelshall Gaylord TM. The U-boat war in the Caribbean. Originally published in 1988 by Paria Publishing Co., Ltd. Port-of-Spain, Trinidad and Tobago. 1994 The United States Naval Institute, Anapolis, Maryland.
8.) US Patent 3,620,785. Root et al. Alum Containing Aluminous Cements. Filed 6/20/70 published 11/16/71. Assignee: The Dow Chemical Company, Midland, MI.
9.) US Patent 4,888,276. Shelburne. Method and composition for the diagnosis of Lyme disease. Filed 6/26/86, published 12/19/89. Assignee: Minnesota Mining and Manufacturing Company (St. Paul, MN)
10.) US Patent 4,765,982. Ronning, et al. Insect control device. Filed 7/9/87published 8/23/88. Assignee: Minnesota Mining and Manufacturing Company (St. Paul, MN).
11.) US Patent 4,888,276. Shelburne. Method and composition for the diagnosis of Lyme disease. Filed 6/26/86, published 12/19/89.
12.) 3M At a Glance. [web page].
13.) 3M. 100 A century of innovation. [online brochure].
14.) US Patent 4,888,276. Shelburne. Method and composition for the diagnosis of Lyme disease. Filed 6/26/86, published 12/19/89. Assignee: Minnesota Mining and Manufacturing Company (St. Paul, MN)
15.) Rule NG, Hickinbottom WJ. Alkylation of the Aromatic Nucleus. Part IV. Phenanthrene. J Chem Soc. 1959;2517-2520.
16.) Brown ER, Hazdra JJ, Keith L, et al. Frequency of Fish Tumors Found in a Polluted Watershed as Compared to Nonpolluted Canadian Waters. Cancer Res. 1973 Feb;33(2):189-198.
17.) US Patent 4,888,276. Shelburne. Method and composition for the diagnosis of Lyme disease. Filed 6/26/86, published 12/19/89. Assignee: Minnesota Mining and Manufacturing Company (St. Paul, MN)
18.) ATCC. HB-10878 Cell hybridoma: VIII C3.78(IVI #10256).
19.) Andersch I, Pianka S, Fritze D, Claus D. Description of Bacillus laevolacticus (ex Nakayama and Yanoski 1967) sp. nov., nom. rev. Inter J System Bacter. 1994 Oct;44(4):659-664.
20.) US Patent 4,683,132. Ronning, et al. Compositions, devices, and methods for extended control of insect activity. Filed 4/30/82 published 7/28/87. Assignee: Minnesota Mining and Manufacturing Company (St. Paul, MN).
21.) Cytec History. A Timeline of History. [web site]
22.) CYTEC. Company Overview. [web site]
23.) Wilkins Mira. The history of foreign investment in the United States to 1914. The Presidents and Fellows of Harvard College. 1989. P. 359.
24.) Schweber Nate. Costly groundwater cleanup needed at Home Depot site. Herald News. 2004 Aug. 3. [web page]
25.) Scannell's New Jersey's First Citizen's and State Guide. Vol. II. 1919-1920. John James Scannell (ed.) J.J. Scannell, Paterson, New Jersey. 1920. p. 519.
26.) Kaiser Aluminum & Chemical Corporation – CLU Profile. [web site]
27.) Gilford Steve. The Rediscovery of Contractors General Hospital – Birthplace of Kaiser Permanente. The Permanente Journal. 2006 Summer;10(2):57-60.
28.) NowPublic. "Worms-Under-Skin" Disease Puzzles Scientists. 2008 May 16. [monograph on the Internet]
29.) CDC. Press Briefing Transcripts. CDC to Launch Study on Unexplained Illness. 2008 Jan 16.
30.) Giesy JP, Kannan K. Global distribution of Perfluorooctane Sulfonate and Related Perfluorinated Compounds in Wildlife. Env. Sci. Technol. 2001;34:1339-1342.
31.) Kannan K, et al. Perfluorooctane Sulfonate and Related Fluorinated Organic Chemicals in Marine mammals. Environ Sci Technol. 2001;35:1593-1598.
32.) Kannan K, et al. Concentrations of Perfluorinated Acids in Livers of Birds from Japan and Korea. Chemosphere 2002;49:225-231.
33.) The History Channel. The Crumbling of America DVD. 100 minutes.
34.) Achorn PJ, Haseltine WG, Miller JK. Physicochmical Properties of Mono- and Diisocyanates. J Chem Eng Data. 1986;31(4):385-387.
35.) US Patent 5,677,053. Moriga et al. Acrylic plastisol adhesion structure. Filed 6/28/96 published 10/14/97. Assignee: Toyo Seikan Kaisha, Ltd. (Tokoyo, JP).

Something in the Water

1.) CDC. Achievements in Public Health, 1900-1999: Fluoridation of Drinking Water to Prevent Dental Caries. MMWR Weekly. 1999 Oct 22;48(41):933-940.
2.) Air and Water News Report. (no author listed) Fluoridated Water Supply Argument Rages in Wisconsin. 2009 Mar 19. [monograph] www.airandaqua.com
3.) Brooker Kevin. Calgary. Hydrofluorosilicic acid: Toxic. Industrial. Waste. Calgary Herald. 2009Mar 30. On: Fluoride Action Network Internet news site. http://www2.fluoridealert.org
4.) Slate, Robert. Fluoride Action Network. Fluoridated Connecticut experiencing Oral Health Crisis. New Haven Register 2005 May.
5.) Likins RC, Scow RO, Zipkin I, Steere AC. Deposition and retention of fluoride and radiocalcium in the growing rat. Am J Physiol. 1959 Jul;197(1):75-80. No abstract.
6.) Zipkin I, Likins RC, McClure FJ, Steere AC. Urinary fluoride levels associated with use of fluoridated waters. Public Health Report. 1956 Aug;71(8):767-772.
7.) Likins RC, McClure FJ, Steere AC. Urinary excretion of fluoride following defluoridation of a water supply. Public Health Report 1956 Mar;71(3):217-220.

8.) Van der Hoeven JS, Franken HCM. Effect of Fluoride on Growth and Acid Production by Streptococcus mutans in Dental Plaque. Infect Immun. 1984;45(2):356-359.
9.) Kester Dana R. Fluoride chlorinity ratio of sea water between the Grand Banks and the Mid-Atlantic Ridge. Deep Sea Res and Oceanograph Abstr. 1971 Nov;18(11):1123-1126. Report No. AD0723237. Fluoride Analysis in the Northwest Atlantic Ocean. Contract No. N00014-68-A-0215-0003. Technical report. DTIC and NTIS Defense Technical Information Center Report. Ft. Belvoir, VA.
10.) Quin LD, Quin GS. Screening for carbon-bound phosphorus in marine animals by high-resolution 31P-NMR spectroscopy: coastal and hydrothermal vent invertebrates. Comp Biochem Physiol B Biochem Mol Biol. 2001 Jan;128(1):173-185.
11.) NowPublic. "Worms-Under-Skin" Disease Puzzles Scientists. 2008 May 16. [monograph on the Internet]
12.) CDC. Press Briefing Transcripts. CDC to Launch Study on Unexplained Illness. 2008 Jan 16.
13.) Giesy JP, Kannan K. Global distribution of Perfluorooctane Sulfonate and Related Perfluorinated Compounds in Wildlife. Env. Sci. Technol. 2001;34:1339-1342.
14.) Kannan K, et al. Perfluorooctane Sulfonate and Related Fluorinated Organic Chemicals in Marine mammals. Environ Sci Technol. 2001;35:1593-1598.
15.) Kannan K, et al. Concentrations of Perfluorinated Acids in Livers of Birds from Japan and Korea. Chemosphere 2002;49:225-231.
16.) The History Channel. The Crumbling of America DVD. 100 minutes.
17.) Annual report of the Board of Regents of the Smithsonian Institution. Ancient Aboriginal Trade in Northern America. Copper. 42nd Congress, 3rd Session. House of Representatives. Mis. Doc. No. 107. The operations, expenditures, and condition of the institution for the year 1872. Government printing office, Washington, DC, 1873. page 350.
18.) Rail Chester D. Groundwater Contamination. Management, Containment, Risk Assessment & Legal Issues. Vol. 2. 2000 Technomic Publishing, Inc. Lancaster, PA
19.) Godínez Carlos, Zelaya de Romillo Blanca, et al. Antibodies against Leptopira interrogans in California Sea Lion Pups from Gulf of California. J Wildlife Dis. 1999;35(1):108-111.
20.) Iversen JG. Isolation of Leptospira Pomona from naturally infected California sea lion, Sonoma County, California. J Wildlife Dis. 1971;7:195-197.
21.) Smith AW, Brown RJ, Skilling DE, DeLong RL. Leptospira Pomona and reproductive failure in California sea lions. J Amer Vet Med Assoc. 1974;166:996-997.
22.) Stell Susan M, Hopkins Evelyn H, Buell Gary R. Hippe Daniel J. US Geological Survey. Use and Occurrence of Pesticides in the Apalachicola-Chattahoochee-Flint River Basin, Georgia, Alabama, and Florida, 1960-91. Open File Report 95-739. 72 pages.
23.) Stockholm Convention on persistent organic pollutants (POPs). [web site]
24.) US Patent 5,622,822. Ekeze, et al. Methods for capture and selective release of nucleic acids using polyethyleneimine and an anionic phosphate ester surfactant and amplification of same. Filed 9/13/94, published 4/22/97. Assignee: Johnson & Johnson Clinical Diagnostics, Inc. (Rochester, NY).
25.) Hock Winand K. (Penn State University, Extension Pesticide Specialist). Sevin (Carbaryl): A Controversial Insecticide. [monograph on the Internet].
26.) Delaplane Keith S. (ed). 1991 Georgia Pest Control Handbook, Athens, GA. The University of Georgia College of Agriculture Cooperative Extension Service Special Bulletin No. 28, 440 pages.
27.) Carson R. Silent Spring. 1962 Houghton Mifflin Company. The Riverside Press, Cambridge.
28.) Hanford Cultural Resources Program, US Department of Energy. Hanford Site Historic District: History of the Plutonium Production Facilities, 1943-1990. 2002. Battelle Press. Columbus, OH. p.1.22-1.27. ISBN 1-57477-133-7.
29.) Findlay John, Hevly Bruce. Nuclear Technologies and Nuclear Communities: A History of Hanford and the Tri-Cities, 1943-1993. Seattle, WA: Hanford History Project, Center for the Study of the Pacific Northwest, University of Washington. 1995:p. 50.
30.) Wiki: Savannah River Site. Wapedia.
31.) Savannah River Remediation. [web page]
31a.) US Department of Energy Press Release. 2008 Dec 8. DOE Selects Savannah River Remediation, LLC for Liquid Waste Contract at Savannah River Site. [web page]
32.) EPA. United States Environmental Protection Agency. Summary of the Clean Water Act. 33 U.S.C.§1251 et seq. (1972). [web page]
33.) EPA Environmental Fact Sheet. Low-Level Mixed Waste Conditionally Exempt from Hazardous Waste Regulations. EPA530-F01-008 May 2001. [web page]
34.) ScienceBlog. Researchers use transgenic trees to help clean up toxic waste site. 2003 Sept 11. [web page]
35.) Hanford Cultural Resources Program, US Department of Energy. Hanford Site Historic District: History of the Plutonium Production Facilities, 1943-1990. 2002. Battelle Press. Columbus, OH. p.1.22-1.27. ISBN 1-57477-133-7.
36.) Findlay John, Hevly Bruce. Nuclear Technologies and Nuclear Communities: A History of Hanford and the Tri-Cities, 1943-1993. Seattle, WA: Hanford History Project, Center for the Study of the Pacific Northwest, University of Washington. 1995:p. 50.
37.) Wiki: Savannah River Site. Wapedia.
38.) National Nuclear Security Administration. New Tritium Source On Line at DOE's Savannah River Site. 2007 Feb 27 press release. [web page]
39.) Meyer Bob. Professional Reactor Operator Society. New Tritium Source On Line at DOE's Savannah River Site. 2007 Feb 28. Press release
40.) About the Savannah River Site. SRS online document. [web page]
41.) Energy News Staff. MOX plant using weapons-grade plutonium being built at S. Carolina site with ominous looking reactors – located on top of region's most dangerous fault line. Press release. 2011 Sept 13. [web page]
42.) Fantle Will. Plutonium Pancakes. The Progressive. From: Project Censored. EPA Plans to Disburse Toxic/Radioactive Wastes into Denver's Sewage System. [web page]
43.) Hansen Brian. Colorado Ready to Spread Plutonium-laden Sewage on Family Farms. 2000 Feb 19.
44.) Rail Chester D. Groundwater Management, Containment, Risk Assessment & Legal Issues. Vol. 2. 2009 CRC Press.
45.) Reilly Maureen. Sludge Watch Colorado-Plutonium compost and sewage sludge. [web page]
46.) Fantle Will. Plutonium Pancakes controversy over Colorado plan to sewage sludge that may be radioactive as fertilizer. 2000 May.
47.) Lawrence Livermore National Security LLC. [web page]
48.) Lawrence Livermore National Laboratory. About LLNL. [web page]
49.) Joint Genomic Institute http://genome.jgi.doe.gov and pop-up 7/28/10 4086848.fsa, (19 major contigs, trimmed) [web page]
50.) Bonch-Osmolovskaya EA, Sokolova TG, Kostrinkina NA, Zavarzin GA. Desulfurella acetivorans gen. nov. and sp. nov. – a new thermophilic sulfur-reducing eubacterium. Arch Microbiol. 1990;153(2):151-155.
51.) Pankratov TA, Dedysh SN. Granulicella paludicola gen. nov. sp. nov., Granulicella pectinivorans sp. nov., Granulicella aggregans sp. nov. and Granulicella rosea sp. nov., acidophilic, polymer-degrading acidobacteria from Sphagnum beat bogs. IJSEM 2010 Dec;2951-2959.
52.) Agency for Toxic Substances and Discharge Registry. ATSDR Public Health Assessment for Lawrence Livermore National Laboratory Site 300 (USDOE). Report. 2005 Jan 20. [web page]
52a.) DOE Joint Genome Institute JGI. Web site. [web page]
53.) Colorado Department of Public Health and Environment. Plutonium. Technical Topics papers. Rocky Flats Public Exposure Studies. [web page]
54.) Vartabedian Ralph, Times Staff Writer. Safety issues probed at Texas Nuclear Plant. 2006 Dec 13. [web page]
55.) B&W Panex. [web page]
56.) Military Munitions Response Program. Site Inspection, Camp Bullis, Texas. Texas Commission on Environmental Quality. Letter to Colonel Garry Atkins, Fort Sam Houston, dated 2005 Aug 29. Topic Approval: Final RCRA Facility Assessment Report. [web page]
57.) Goddard J. Bug Vectors. The Mystery of Bullis Fever: What Can We Learn from an Outbreak 57Years Ago? US Air Force publication USAFAM-89-2. 2000. Infect Med 17(1):24-26. SCP Communications.
58.) Anigstein L, Anigstein D. A review of the evidence in retrospect for a rickettsial etiology in Bullis fever. Texas Rep Biol Med. 1975;33:201-211.
59.) Los Alamos National Security. Wikipedia.
60.) US Army corps of engineers. Dredging and bauxite and cleanup of solid wastes T. Neil McLellan, Robert J. Hopman. Hartman Consulting Corporation. Innovations in Dredging Technology: Equipment, Operations, and Management. US Army Corps of Engineers. ERDC TR-DOER-5 April 2000. Report. 136 pages. Approved for public release, distribution unlimited.
61.) US Patent 6,017,734. Summers, et al. Unique nucleotide and amino acid sequence and uses thereof. Filed 1/30/97published 1/25/00. Assignee: The Texas A&M University System (College Station, TX).
62.) Cregg JM, Vedvick TS, Raschke WC. Recent advances in the expression of foreign genes in Pichia pastoris. Bio/Technol. 1993;11:905-910.
63.) US Patent 5,891,431. Palli et al. Transgenic Virus. Filed 1/22/97, published 4/6/99. Assignee: Her Majesty the Queen in the right of Canada, as represented by the Minister of Natural Resources, Ottawa, Canada.

64.) Wang CH, Chou CM, Liu HC, et al. Continuous Cell Line from Pupal Ovary of Perina nuda (Lpidoptera: Lymantriidae) That Is Permissive to Nuclear Polyhedrosis Virus from P. nuda. J Invert Path. 1996;67(3):199-204.
65.) US Patent 4,870,023. Fraser, et al. Recombinant baculovirus occlusion bodies in vaccines and biological insecticides. Filed 2/8/88 published 9/26/89. Assignee: American Biogenetic Sciences, Inc. (Copiague, NY).
66.) Updegraff DM, Wren GB. The Release of Oil from Petroleum-Bearing Materials by Sulfate-Reducing Bacteria. Appl Environ Microbiol. 1954;2(6):309-321.
67.) US Patent 2,413,278. ZoBell. Bacteriological Process for Treatment of Fluid-Bearing Earth Formations. Filed /17/44 published 12/24/46. Assignee: American Petroleum Institute, New York, NY.
68.) US Patent 2,641,564. ZoBell. Process of Removing Sulfur from Petroleum Hydrocarbons and Apparatus. Filed 3/31/48 published 6/9/53. Assignee: Texaco Development Corporation, New York, NY.
69.) US Patent 2,641,566. ZoBell. Recovery of Hydrocarbons. Filed 5/15/48published 6/9/53. Assignee: Texaco Development Corporation, New York, NY.
70.) US Patent 2,742,398. ZoBell. Method of Removing Deposits of Wax and Like Materials. Filed 6/9/51 published 4/17/56. Assignee: Texaco Development Corporation, New York, NY.
71.) US Army corps of engineers. Dredging and bauxite and cleanup of solid wastes T. Neil McLellan, Robert J. Hopman. Hartman Consulting Corporation. Innovations in Dredging Technology: Equipment, Operations, and Management. US Army Corps of Engineers. ERDC TR-DOER-5 April 2000. Report. 136 pages.
72.) Tschirley FH. Defoliation in Vietnam. Science 1969;163:779-786.
73.) Hakim Joy. War, Peace, and All That Jazz. 1918-1945A History of US. Revised Third Edition. 2007 Oxford University Press.
74.) Project AGILE. Quarterly Report. Apr 1-June 30. Battelle Memorial Institute, Columbus, OH. Dated 1963 Jul 15. AD0338491. 212 pages.
75.) US Army corps of engineers. Dredging and bauxite and cleanup of solid wastes T. Neil McLellan, Robert J. Hopman. Hartman Consulting Corporation. Innovations in Dredging Technology: Equipment, Operations, and Management. US Army Corps of Engineers. ERDC TR-DOER-5 April 2000. Report. 136 pages.
76.) US Patent 5,246,844. Norris, et al. Virulence associated proteins in Borrelia burgdorferi (BB). Filed 10/22/91, published 9/21/93. Assignee: Board of Regents, The University of Texas System (Austin, TX).
77.) US Patent 6,153,194. Skare, et al. Borrelia burgdorferi outer membrane proteins. Filed 10/29/98, published 11/28/00. Assignee: The Regents of the University of California (Oakland, CA). Inventors from CA, MA, TX, NY.
78.) US Patent 6,316,005. Korshus, et al. Borrelia burgdorferi bacterin. Filed 1/21/97, published 11/13/01. Assignee: Solvay Animal Health, Inc. (Mendota Heights, MN).
79.) US Patent 5,985,595. Krider, et al. Early detection of Borrelia infection. Filed 6/6/96, published 11/16/99. Assignee: The University of Connecticut (Storrs, CT).
80.) US Patent 5,585,102. Barbour, et al. Flagella-less borrelia. Assignee: University of Texas System (Austin, TX).
81.) US Patent 5,436,000. Barbour, et al. Flagella-less borrelia. Assignee: University of Texas System (Austin, TX).
82.) US Patent 5,403,718. Dorward, et al. Methods and antibodies for the immune capture and detection of Borrelia burgdorferi. Filed 8/11/92, published 4/4/95. Inventors all from Hamilton, MT. Assignee not listed.
83.) US Patent 5,217,872. Dorward, et al. Method for detection of Borrelia burgdorferi antigens. Filed 2/27/90, published 6/8/93. Inventors all from Hamilton, MT. Assignee: The United States of America as represented by the Department of Health (Washington, DC).
84.) US Patent 6,204,018. Bergstrom, et al. 66kDa antigen from Borrelia. Filed 6/12/97, published 3/20/01. Inventors: Sven Bergstrom (Umea, SE), Alan George Barbour (Irvine, CA). Assignee: Symbicom Aktiebolag (Umea, SE).
85.) US Patent 4,721,617. Johnson. Vaccine against Lyme disease. Filed 8/14/86, published 1/26/88. Inventor: Russell C. Johnson (St. Paul, MN). Assignee: Regents of the University of Minnesota (Minneapolis, MN).
86.) US Patent 5,554,371. Caputa, et al. Recombinant vaccine against Lyme disease. Assignee: Regents of the University of Minnesota (Minneapolis, MN).
87.) US Patent 6,183,986. Bergstrom, et al. OspA DNA and lyme disease vaccine. Inventors: Sven Bergstrom (Umea, SE); Alan G. Barbour (San Antonio, TX); Louis A. Magnarelli (Durham, CT). Assignee: Symbicom Aktiebolag (Umea, SE).
88.) Schultz MM, Higgins CP, Huset CA, et al. Fluorochemical mass flows in a municipal wastewater treatment facility. Environ Sci Technol. 2006Dec;40(23):7350-7357.
89.) US Patent 6,312,915. Nelson, et al. Tick (Ixodes scapularis) vector saliva-induced Lyme disease spirochete (Borrelia burgdorferi) antigens as vaccine candidates. Filed 1/29/97, published 11/6/01. Inventors from RI and MD; Assignee: The Board of Governors for Higher Education, State of Rhode Island (Providence, RI) and Providence Plantations (Providence, RI). [These two are commonly referred to as the state of Rhode Island].
90.) US Patent 7,582,304. Dattwyler, et al. Groups of Borrelia burgdorferi and Borrelia afzelli that cause Lyme Disease in humans. Inventors: Raymond J. Dattwyler (Setauket, NY); Gerald Seinost (Graz, AU); Daniel Dykhuizen (St. James, NY); Benjamin.
91.) B&W the Babcock & wilcox company. About B&W. [web page]
92.) Inglenook Ad. Inglenook Vineyards, Nappa Valley, California. 10 Questions that wine experts ask each other. New York Magazine. 1974 Feb 11.
93.) Eldridge George Washington. Martha's Vineyard. Its History and Advantages as a Health and Summer Resort. 1889 EL Freeman & Sons. Providence, Rhode Island. 1889.
94.) Code of Federal Regulations. Title 27. Alcohol, Tobacco Products and Firearms. Tax and Trade Bureau, Treasury. Parts 1 to 39. Revised 2011 Apr 1. p. 159.
95.) Cavalloro R. Integrated Pest Control in Viticulture. Commission of the European Communities. Proceedings of a meeting of the EC Expert's Group/Portoferraio. 1985. A.A. Balkema Publishers, Brookfield, Vt. Sept 26-28. p. 188
96.) Downing RS, Moilliet TK. Comparisons between an Exotic and an Endemic Phytoseiid Mite Predator (Acarina: Phytoseiidae) in British Columbia. The Canadian Entomologist. 1974;106(7):773-776.
97.) Crookes William. The Chemical News and Journal of Physical Science. Vol. 29. 1874. Henry Gillman, Boy Court, Ludgate Hill, E.C. London. 512 pages.
98.) Moisse Katie. Morgellons: Mysterious Skin Disease Under Microscope. ABC News. 2012 January 25.

Chapter Six: Tracking Insects and Epidemics

Mites and Rickettsialpox

1.)Steinhaus, Edward Arthur. Catalog of Bacteria Associated Extracellularly with Insects and Ticks. Burgess publishing. Minneapolis, MN. 1942.
2.) Baker Edward William, Evans TM, Gould DJ, Hull WB, Keegan HL. A Manual of Parasitic Mites of medical or economic importance. A Technical Publication of the National Pest Control Association, Inc. New York 1956. p. 18.
3.) Kaya, H. K., M. G. Klein, et al. Impact of Bacillus popilliae, Rickettsia popilliae, and entomopathogenic nematodes on a population of the scarabaeid Cyclocephala hirta. Biocontrol Science & Technology 3.1993:443-453.
4.) Dutky SR, Gooden EL. Coxiella Popilliae, n. sp., a Rickettsia Causing Blue Disease of Japanese Beetle Larvae. Am Soc Microbiol. J Bacteriol. 1952;63:743-750.
5.) Huebner RJ, Stamps P, Armstrong C. Rickettsialpox. A newly recognized rickettsial disease. 1. isolation of the etiological agent. Public Health Report. 1946;61:1605.
6.) Henn T, Weinzierl R, Koehler PG. Beneficial Insects and Mites. Report of University of Florida IFAS Extension Doc# ENY-276(IN078) that was originally published as Circular 1298 by the Office of Agricultural Entomology, University of Illinois at Urbana-Champaign). 1995 Jul.
7.) Baker Edward W (Bur of Entomol and Plant Quarantine, Ag Res Admin USDA), Wharton GW (Dep Zool, Duke Univ, Durham, SC) An introduction to acarology. 1952. Marine Biology Laboratory Library, Woods Hole, Massachusetts.The Macmillan Company, New York. [web page]
8.) Raoult Didier, Parola Philippe (eds.). Rickettsial diseases. 2007. Informa Healthcare. Pages 68-72.
9.) Symposium on Viral and Rickettsial Diseases. Presented at the Golden Jubilee Meeting of the Society of American Bacteriologists at Baltimore, MD. 1950 May 15. Joseph E. Smadel was convenor and editor of the papers presented. Paper discussed was titled Newer Knowledge of the Older Rickettsial Diseases.
10.) Baker EW (USDA Agricultural Research Service), Evans TM (Walter Reed Army Institute of Research), Gould DJ (Walter Reed), Hull WB (US Naval Medical Research Institute), Keegan HL (406th Medical General Laboratory, US Army Far East). A Manual of Parasitic Mites of Medical or Economic Importance. 1956. A technical publication of the National Pest Control Association, Inc. New York, p. 18.
11.) Raoult Didier, Parola Philippe (eds.). Rickettsial diseases. 2007. Informa Healthcare. Pages 68-72.
12.) University of California, San Francisco. Environmental Health and Safety/Biosafety. Lymphyocytic Choriomeningitis Virus Exposure/Injury Response Protocol Sheet. [Safety Data Sheet] [web page]
13.) Krinsky WL. Does epizootic lymphocytic choriomeningitis prime the pump for epidemic rickettsialpox? Ev Infect Dis. 1983;5:1118-1119.
14.) White RT Effect of Milky Disease on Tiphia Parasites of Japanese Beetle Larvae. 1943 Sept.;51(3):213-218.

15.) Steinhaus EA. Nomenclature and classification of insect viruses. Bact Revs. 1949;13:203-223.
16.) Yamataka S, Hayashi R. Electron microscopic studies on the mitochondria and intramitochondrial microorganisms of Halteria gele:ana. J Electron Microsc. (Tokyo) 1970;19:50-62.
17.) Beninati T, Lo N, Sacchi L, et al. A novel alpha-proteobacterium resides in the mitochondria of ovarian cells of the tick Ixodes ricinus. Appl Environ Microbiol 2004;70:2596-2602.
18.) Parola P, Cornet JP, Sanogo YO. Et al. Detection of Ehrlichia spp., Anaplasma spp., Rickettsia spp., and other eubacteria in ticks from the Thai-Mayanmar border and Vietnam. J Clin Microbiol 2003;41:1600-1608
19.) Bhat HR, Naik SV. Transmission of Kyasanur forest disease virus by Haemaphysalis wellingtoni Nuttall and Warburton, 1907 (Acarina : Ixodidae). Indian J Med Res. 1978 May;67(5):697-703.
20.) Bourtzis Kostas, Miller Thomas A. (eds.) Insect symbiosis, volume 2. 2006 Taylor & Francis Group, CRC Press, Boca Raton, FL.
21.) Brinton LP, Oliver JH Jr., Fine structure of oogonial and oocyte development in Dermacentor andersoni Stiles (Acari: Ixodidae). J parasitol. 1971;57:720-747.
22.) Burgdorfer W, Hayes SF, Mavros AJ. Nonpathogenic rickettsiae in Dermacentor andersoni: a limiting factor for the distribution of Rickettsia rickettsii. In Rickettsiae and Rickettsial Diseases W. Burgdorfer and R.L. Anacker (Eds.). 1981:585-594. Academic Press, New York.
23.) Magnarelli LA, Anderson JF, Philip RN, Burgdorfer W, Casper EA. Endemicity of spotted fever group rickettsiae in Connecticut. Am J Trop med Hyg. 1981 May;30(3):715-721.
24.) Magnarelli LA, Anderson JF, Burgdorfer W. Rocky mountain spotted fever in Connecticut: human cases, spotted-fever group rickettsiae in ticks, and antibodies in mammals. Am J Epidemiol. 1979 Aug;110(2):148-155.
25.) US Patent 6,183,986 Bergstrom, et al. OspA DNA and Lyme disease vaccine. Filed 6/6/95, published 2/6/01. Assignee: Symbicom Aktiebolag (Umea, SE). Inventors: Sven Bergstrom (Umea), Alan G. Barbour (San Antonio, TX), Louis A. Magnarelli (Durham, CT).
26.) State of Connecticut. The Connecticut Agricultural Experiment Station. [web site]
27.) US Patent 5,523,089Bergstrom, et al. Borrelia antigen. Filed 6/22/93, issued 6/4/96. Assignee: Symbicom Aktiebolag (SE). Inventors: Sven Bergstrom (Umea, SE); Alan G. Barbour (San Antonio, TX), Louis A. Magnarelli (Durham, CT).
28.) Windhover Information Inc. Healthcare business intelligence. [web page]
29.) US Patent 5,582,990. Bergstrom, et al. DNA encoding borrelia burgdorferi OspA and a method for diagnosing borrelia burgdorferi infection. Filed 10/3/94, issued 12/10/96. Assignee: Symbicom Aktiebolag (SE).
30.) US Patent 6,083,722. Bergstrom, et al. Borrelia antigen. Filed 6/6/95, issued 7/4/00. Assignee: Symbicom AB. Inventors: Sven Bergstrom; Alan G. Barbour; Louis A. Magnarelli.
31.) US Patent 6,183,986. Bergstrom, et al. OspA DNA and lyme disease vaccine. Filed 6/6/95, issued 2/6/01. Assignee: Symbicom Aktiebolag (Umea, SE). Inventors: Sven Bergstrom; Alan G. Barbour; Louis A. Magnarelli.
32.) US Patent 6,203,798. Bergstrom, et al. Borrelia antigen. Filed 6/6/95, issued 3/20/01. Assignee: Symbicom Aktiebolag (Umea, SE). Inventors: Sven Bergstrom; Alan G. Barbour; Louis A. Magnarelli.
33.) US Patent 6,183,986. Bergstrom, et al. OspA DNA and lyme disease vaccine. Filed 6/6/95, issued 2/6/01. Assignee: Symbicom Aktiebolag (Umea, SE). Inventors: Sven Bergstrom; Alan G. Barbour; Louis A. Magnarelli.

The Emergence of Ehrlichiosis

1.) Goddard J. Bug Vectors. The Mystery of Bullis Fever: What Can We Learn from an Outbreak 57Years Ago? US Air Force publication USAFAM-89-2. 2000. Infect Med 17(1):24-26. SCP Communications.
2.) Anigstein L, Anigstein D. A review of the evidence in retrospect for a rickettsial etiology in Bullis fever. Texas Rep Biol Med 1975;33:201-211.
3.) USDA. DDT and Other Insecticides and Repellents Developed for the Armed Forces. Laboratory of the Bureau of Entomology and Plant Quarantine. August 1946, Washington, DC. 71 pgs.
4.) Michelbacher AE, Middlekauff WW. New Insecticides. Effectiveness and limitations of chlorinated hydrocarbon insecticides not yet fully determined. California Agriculture 1949 June
5.) Smith MS. Persistence of D.D.T. and Benzene Hexachloride in Soils. Ann Appl Biol. 1948 Dec;35(4):494-504.
6.) US Patent 2,329,074. Müller. Devitalizing Composition of Matter. Filed 3/7/40, published 9/7/43. Assignee: J.R. Geigy A.G., Basel, Switzerland.
7.) Livesay HR, Pollard M. Serological Studies of Bullis Fever. Am J Trop Med Sep 1944;s1-24:281-284.
8.) Livesay HR, Pollard M. Laboratory Report on a Clinical Syndrome Referred to as "Bullis Fever." From the Eighth Service Command Laboratory, United States Army. Am J Trop Med. Sep 1943;s1-23:475-479.
9.) Savage, Charlie. Ex-C.I.A. Agent Goes Public With Story of Mistreatment on the Job. The New York Times. 2011 Feb. 10.
10.) Texas State Historical Association. Camp Stanley. [web site] www.tshaonline.org
11.) Perkins John H. Reshaping Technology in Wartime: The Effect of Military Goals on Entomological Research and Insect-Control Practices. Technol Culture. 1978 Apr;19(2):169-186.
12.) Leon Springs Military Reservation. Texas State Historical Association. [web page]
13.) Department of the Army. Department of Defense, United States of America. U.S. Army Environmental Hygiene Activity – South Forth McPherson, Georgia 30330-5000. 1990 Apr 24-27.
14.) USDA Agricultural Research Service. Agriculture Handbook. Management of Lone Star Tick in Recreation Areas. 1989 Aug;Vol. 682, 33 pages.
15.) Schulze TL, Bowen GS, Bosler EM, et al. Amblyomma americanum: a potential vector of Lyme disease in New Jersey. Science 1984 May;224(4649):601-603.
16.) Bacon RM, Pilgard MA, Johnson BJB, Raffel SJ, Schwan TG. Glycerophosphodiester Phosphodiesterase Gene (*glpQ*) of *Borrelia lonestari* Identified as a Target for Differentiating *Borrelia* Species Associated with Hard Ticks (Acari:Ixodidae). J Clin Microbiol. 2004May; 42(5): 2326–2328.
17.) Barbour, et al. Diagnostic tests for a new spirochete, Borrelia lonestari sp. Nov. Patent #5,932,220 1999 Aug 3.
18.) Varela AS, Luttrell MP, Howerth EW, Moore VA, Davidson WR, Stallknecht DE, Little SE. First culture isolation of Borrelia lonestari, putative agent of southern tick-associated rash illness. J Clin Microbiol. 2004 Mar;42(3):1163-9.
19.) Thermo Scientific Nalgene. Phthalates as Endocrine Disrupters. [web page]

So-Called "Polio"

1.) Gerardi MH, Grimm JK. The History, Biology, Damage, and Control of the Gypsy Moth. 1979 Associated University Presses, Inc., Cranbury, New Jersey.
2.) Rutgers School of Environmental and Biological Sciences. Department of Entomology. Gypsy Moth. [web page]
3.) MCClung RM. Gypsy Moth Its History in America. 1974William Morrow and Company.
4.) Gerardi MH, Grimm JK. The History, Biology, Damage, and Control of the Gypsy Moth. 1979Associated University Presses, Inc., Cranbury, New Jersey.
5.) Jones CG, Ostfeld RS, Richard MP, Schauber EM, Wolff JO. Chain reactions linking acorns to gypsy moth outbreaks and Lyme disease risk. Science 1998;279(5353):1023-1026.
6.) McClanahan HM. A Brief Report of the Nebraska Epidemic of Poliomyelitis. The Journal of the American Medical Association. 1910 Oct 1;LV(14)
7.) Haeber Jonathan. Processing Sugar from Beets in the Early 1900s. [web page]
8.) University of Nebraska-Lincoln. CropWatch: Sugarbeets. History of beets in Nebraska. [web page]
9.) Lange W. Harry. Insect Pests of Sugar Beets. Ann Rev Entomol. 1982;32:341-360.
10.) Watson AP, Griffin GD. Toxicity of vesicant agents scheduled for destruction by the Chemical Stockpile Disposal Program. Environ Health Perspect. 1992 Nov;98:259-280. Review.
11.) American President: A Reference Resource. Henry L. Stimson (1940-1945): Secretary of War. Miller Center, Univeristy of VA (web site) [web page]
12.) Brock TD. Microorganisms From Smallpox to Lyme Disease. Scientific American. W.H. Freeman and Company. 1990. p. 28-37.
13.) Technical Report: DDC AD408401. February 3-4, 1960. Conference on Biological Control of Insects of Medical Importance. American Institute of Biological Sciences (Washington, DC). 148pages. Unclassified documents retrieved from the public domain. Dr. Steinhaus speaking, page 123.
14.) Smadel, Joseph E., Army Medical Department Research and Graduate School, Washington, DC. Laboratory Diagnosis of Viral and Rickettsial Diseases, A Reappraisal after Ten Years. Symposium on Viral and Rickettsial Diseases. Presented at the Golden Jubilee Meeting of the Society of American Bacteriologists at Baltimore, MD. May 15,1950.
15.) Schaal E, Kleinsorgen A. [Oral transmission of the Q-fever agent (Coxiella burnetti) by infected milk]. Dtsch Tierarztl Wochenschr. 1973 Sep 1;80(17):394-9. (Article in German)

16.) Luoto L, Casey ML, Pickens EG. Q Fever Studies in Montana. Detection of Asymptomatic Infection Among Residents of Infected Dairy Premises. Am J Epidemiol. 1965 May;81:356-69.
17.) Stoenner HG, Lackman DB, Benson WW, et al. The Role of Dairy Cattle in the Epidemiology of Q Fever in Idaho. J Infect Dis 1961 Jul-Aug;109(1):90-97.
18.) Eklund CM, Bell EJ, Gerloff RK. Poliomyelitis in Idaho after use of live virus vaccine. Public Health Reports. 1958 Jul;73:637-647.
19.) Eklund CM, Hadlow WJ, Pickens EG, Gerloff RK. Detecting Poliovirus in Vaccine Lots Used in Idaho in 1955. Public Health Reports. 1959 Jan;74(1):60-68.
20.) Luoto Lauri, Pickens Edgar G. Tissue Cultures of KB Epithelial Cells for Poliomyelitis Virus Tests. 1958 Public Health Reports. Jun;73(6):541-544.

Lone Star Virus and Asian Outbreaks

1.) Navy and Marine Corps. Pre-Service Test of the U.S. Army Ultra Low Volume Arial Spray System for Rotary Wing Aircraft. Naval Medical Field Research Lab Camp LeJeune, NC. 1971 Aug. Vol. XXI, No. 19. Project #: M4305.
2.) Kokernot RH, Calisher CH, Stannard LJ, Hayes J. Arb ovirus Studies in the Ohio-Mississippi Basin, 1964-1967. J Trop Med Hyg. 1969;18(5):789-795.
3.) Information from Kokernot RH. Lone Star (LS) Strain: TMA 1381. No. 239. Am J Trop Med Hyg. 1970;19(6):1151-1152.
4.) US Patent 5,932,220. Barbour, et al. Diagnostic tests for a new spirochete, Borrelia lonestari sp. nov. Filed 5/8/95 published 8/3/99. Assignee: Board of Regents University of Texas System (Austin, TX).
5.) US Patent 5,279,938. Rosa. Sensitive diagnostic test for Lyme disease. Filed 5/18/92, published 1/18/94. Assignee: The United States of America as represented by the Department of Health (Washington, DC).
6.) US Patent 5,283,175. Weaver, et al. Genus-specific oligomers of Borrelia and methods of using same. Filed 4/15/91 published 2/1/94. Assignee: The Research Foundation of State University of New York (Albany,NY).
7.) US Patent 5,618,533. Flavell, et al. Flagellin-based polypeptides for the diagnosis of Lyme disease. Filed 12/10/93 published 4/8/97. Assignee: Yale University (New Haven, CT).
8.) History of the UT System. The University of Texas System. [web page]
9.) Rich SM, Armstrong PM, Smith RD, Telford III SR. Lone Star Tick-Infecting Borreliae are most closely related to the Agent of Bovine Borreliosis. J Clin Micribiol. 2001 Feb;39(2):494-497.
10.) Anigstein L, Anigstein D. A review of the evidence in retrospect for a rickettsial etiology in Bullis fever. Texas Rep Biol Med. 1975;33:201-211.
11.) Anigstein L, Anigstein D. A review of the evidence in retrospect for a rickettsial etiology in Bullis fever. Texas Rep Biol Med. 1975;33:201-211.
12.) Perkins John H. Reshaping Technology in Wartime: The Effect of Military Goals on Entomological Research and Insect-Control Practices. Technol Culture. 1978Apr;19(2):169-186.
13.) Huxsoll David L, Hildebrandt Paul K, Nims Robert M, Amyx Herbert T, Ferguson James A. Epizootiology of Tropical Canine Pancytopenia. Proceed Ann Conf. J Wildlife Dis. 1970;6:220-225.
14.) US Army Medical Research Institute of Infectious Diseases, Fort Detrick, Maryland. 1981 October. Annual Report October 1, 1981 to September 30, 1982. Report # RCS-MEDDH-288(R1). 177 pages. Unclassified document in the public domain.
15.) Progress Report. Microbiology Branch Office of Naval Research, Department of the US Navy, Washington, DC. 1968 January. ONR Report ACR-141. 153 pages. Unclassified document in the public domain.
16.) Wedum Arnold G., Safety Director. Cml C Biological Laboratories. AD310671. Special Report. No. 185. Safety Division Chemical Corps Biological Laboratories. Safety Program at Camp Detrick. 1944 to 1953. 1979 July 235 pages.
17.) US Patent 5,413,931. Dawson, et al. Ehrlichia species from a patient suffering from ehrlichiosis. Filed 11/5/93published 5/9/96. Assignee: United States of America (Washington, DC).
18.) Ristic, in Microbiology 1986, L. Leive (ed). American Society for Microbiology, Washington, DC. 1986pp. 182-187.
19.) Hooda PS, Edwards AC, Anderson HA, Miller A. A review of water quality concerns in livestock farming areas. Sc Tot Environ. 2000 Apr 24;250(1-3):143-167.
20.) van der Ploeg RR, Ringe H, Machulla G, Hermsmeyer D. Postwar Nitrogen Use Efficiency in West German Agriculture and Groundwater Quality. J Envir Qual. 1996 Mar 18;26(5):1203-1212.
21.) How Britain sprayed Malaya with dioxin. New Scientist 1984 January 19. No. 1393.
22.) Westing AH (ed). Herbicides in War. The Long-Term Ecological and Human Consequences. 1984. Taylor and Francis, London.
23.) Tschirley FH. Defoliation in Vietnam. Science 1969;163:779-786.
24.) Hakim Joy. War, Peace, and All That Jazz. 1918-1945A History of US. Revised Third Edition. 2007Oxford University Press.
25.) Project AGILE. Quarterly Report. Apr 1-June 30. Battelle Memorial Institute, Columbus, OH. Dated 1963Jul 15. AD0338491. 212 pages
26.) Mac Vean DW. That New Dog Disease. Malaysian Kennel Review. 1968;66.
27.) Seamer J, Snape T. Tropical Canine Pancytopenia and Ehrlichia canis infection. Vet Rec. 1970;86:375.
28.) Spence JB, Giam CH, Theis JH. A New Canine Disease Syndrome. Vet Rec. 1967;81:328-329.
29.) Shirlaw JF. On the Relationship Between 'Lahore Canine Fever' and 'Tick Fever' of Dogs due to P. gibsoni Infection, with Observations on their Pathology and Haemocytology. Ind J Vet Sci. 1938;8:293-316.
30.) Galston Arthur. An Accidental Plant Biologist. Plant Psysiol. Am Soc Plant Physiol. 2002Mar;128:786-787.
31.) Young Alan L. The History, Use, Disposition and Environmental Fate of Agent Orange. 2009Springer Science + Business Media, LLC. New York. ISBN: 978-0-387-87486-9.
32.) Young AL. TCDD Biomonitoring and Exposure to Agent Orange: Still the Gold Standard. Env Sci Pollut Res. 2004;11(3):143-146.
33.) Palmer MG. The Legacy of Agent Orange: Empirical Evidence from Central Vietnam. Soc Sci & Med. 2004;60:1061-1070.

Agricultural Agents and Encephalitis Outbreaks

1.) W. Kenneth Hoover. The Biological Control of Detrimental Insects. 1933 Oct;4(3):75-89.
2.) Webber RT, Schaffner JV. Host Relations of Compsilura concinnata Meigen, An Important Tachinid Parasite of the Gipsy Moth and Brown-Tail Moth. USDA Bulletin #1363, Washington, DC. 1926.
3.) Schaffner JV, Griswold CL. Macro-lepidoptera and their Parasites reared from field collections in the Northeastern part of the United States. USDA Publication #188, Washington, DC. 1934.
4.) Culver JJ. A study of Comsilura concinnata, an imported tachinid parasite of the gipsy moth and brown-tail moth. USDA Bulletin #766. Washington, DC. 1919.
5.) Glaser RW. The cultivation of a nematode parasite of an insect. Science 1931;73:614-615.
6.) US Patent 2,293,890. Process for Propagating Bacteria. Samson R. Dutky. Filed 3/15/40 published 8/25/42. Assignee: Claude R. Wickard as Secretary of Agriculture of the United States of America and his successors in office.
7.) Bryant ES, Anderson CRm, van der Heide L. Case Report: An Epizootic of Eastern Equine Encephalomyelitis in Connecticut. Avian Dis. 1973 Oct-Dec;17(4):861-867.
8.) Luginbuhl Roy E, Satriano Salvatore F, Helmboldt Charles F, Lamson Arroll L, Jungherr Erwin L. Investigation of Eastern Equine Encephalomyelitis. II. Outbreaks in Connecitcut Pheasants. Am J Epidemiol. 1957;67:4-9.
9.) DeGraaf Richard M. Breeding Birds and Gypsy Moth Defoliation: Short Term Responses of Species and Guilds. Wildlife Soc. Bulletin. 1987Summer;15(2):217-221.
10.) Hayes RO, Daniels JB, Maxfield HK, Wheeler RE. Field and Laboratory Studies on Eastern Encephalitis in Warm- and Cold-Blooded Vertebrates. Am J Trop Med Hyg. 1964 Jul;13:595-606.
11.) Moro VC, Chauve C, Zenner L. Vectorial Role of Some Dermanyssoid Mites (Acari, Mesostigmata, ermanyssoidea). Parasite 2005;12:99-109.
12.) USDA. Natural Resources Conservation Service. Ring-neck Pheasant (Phasianus colchicus). 1999Octo. Fish and Wildlife Habitat Management Leaflet.
13.) Technical Report: DDC AD408401. Conference on Biological Control of Insects of Medical Importance. American Institute of Biological Sciences (Washington, DC). 148 pages. Unclassified documents retrieved from the public domain.
14.) Grant 1P01AI016289-01 *Arthropod-borne Diseases and Their Control.* University of Maryland, Baltimore. Fiscal year 1980. Richard H. Baker. Project start: 6/1/80, ended 5/31/85. NIAID.
15.) Grant 5R07AI010049-15. International Center for Medical Research. University of Maryland Baltimore. Fiscal year 1974. Project start: 6/1/70 ended 5/31/75. NIAID.
16.) Grant 5R01AI007807-08. Genetic Studies on the Control of Arbovirus Vectors. University of Maryland Baltimore. Fiscal year 1974. Project start: 5/1/73, ended 4/30/75. NIAID.
17.) Raoult Didier, Parola Philippe (eds.). Rickettsial diseases. 2007. Informa Healthcare. Pages 68-72.
18.) University of California, San Francisco. Environmental Health and Safety/Biosafety. Lymphyocytic Choriomeningitis Virus Exposure/Injury Response Protocol Sheet.

19.) Krinsky WL. Does epizootic lymphocytic choriomeningitis prime the pump for epidemic rickettsialpox? Ev Infect Dis. 1983;5:1118-1119.
20.) Kaya, H. K., M. G. Klein, et al. Impact of Bacillus popilliae, Rickettsia popilliae, and entomopathogenic nematodes on a population of the scarabaeid Cyclocephala hirta. Biocontrol Science & Technology 3. 1993:443-453.
21.) Dutky SR, Gooden EL. Coxiella Popilliae, n. sp., a Rickettsia Causing Blue Disease of Japanese Beetle Larvae. Am Soc Microbiol. J Bacteriol. 1952;63:743-750.
22.) Huebner RJ, Stamps P, Armstrong C. Rickettsialpox. A newly recognized rickettsial disease. 1. isolation of the etiological agent. Public Health Report. 1946;61:1605.
23.) Henn T, Weinzierl R, Koehler PG. Beneficial Insects and Mites. Report of University of Florida IFAS Extension Doc# ENY-276 (IN078) that was originally published as Circular 1298 by the Office of Agricultural Entomology, University of Illinois at Urbana-Champaign). 1995 Jul.
24.) Fuller Henry S. Studies of Rickettsialpox III. Life Cycle of the Mite Vector, Allodermanyssus Sanguineus. Am J Hyg. 1954;59:236-289.
25.) Fuller HS, Murray ES, Ayres JC, Snyder JC, Potash L. Studies of rickettsialpox. I. Recovery of the causative agent from house mice in Boston, Massachusetts. Amer J Hyg. 1951;54:82-100.
26.) Rindge ME. Connecticut has first rickettsialpox outbreak. Conn Health Bull. 1952;66:73-75.
27.) La Boccetta AC, Israel HL, Perri AM, Siegel MM. Rickettsialpox. Report of four apparent cases in Pennsylvania. Amer J Med. 1952;13:413-422.
28.) Raoult Didier, Parola Philippe (eds.). Rickettsial diseases. 2007. Informa Healthcare. Pages 68-72.
29.) Arzeena Hamir. The story of two mites. [web page]
30.) Tvedten Stephen. History of Pest Management. History of the Development of Organophosphate Poisons. [web page]
31.) Bourtzis K, Miller TA. (eds). Insect Symbiosis Vol. 2. CRC Press 2006 Boca Raton, FL.

An Outbreak in the Pacific

1.) Burgess HD, Hussey NW. Microbial Control of Insects and Mites. 1971 Academic Press (London).
2.) Tupanceska Daniela, Zaid Ali, Rulli Nestor E. et al. Ross River Virus: An Arthritogenic Alphavirus of Significant Importance in the Asia Pacific. Lal SK (ed): Emerging Viral Diseases of Southeast Asia. Issues Infect Dis. Basel, Karger. 2007;4:94-111.
3.) Sol M. Cancel Tirado, Kyoung-Jin Yoon. Antibody-Dependent Enhancement of Virus Infection and Disease. Viral Immunol. 2003Apr;16(1):69-86.
4.) Laird M, Colless DH. Experiments towards the biological control of mosquitoes in theTokelau Islands. First Report, Aug-Oct 1958. WHO. Mimeogr. 1959. 39 pages (Restricted).
5.) Technical Report: DDC AD408401. Conference on Biological Control of Insects of Medical Importance. American Institute of Biological Sciences (Washington, DC). 1960 Nov 1. Date stamped Jun 28, 1961, Camp LeJeune, NC. 148pages. Convened at Armed Forces Institute of Pathology, Washington, DC, Feb. 3-4, 1960. Unclassified documents retrieved from the public domain.
6.) Aaskov JG, Mataika JU, Lawrence GW, et al. An Epidemic of Ross River Virus Infection in Fiju, 1979. Am J Trop Med Hyg. 1981;30(5):1053-1059.
7.) Fraser JRE, Rowley MJ, Tait B. Collagen antibodies in Ross River virus disease (epidemic polyarthritis). Rheumatol Inter. 1987 Dec;7(6):267-269.
8.) Smith Ray F. Considerations on the safety of certain biological agents for arthropod control.* Bull Org mond. Santé. Bull. Wld Hlth Org. 1973;48:685-698. *Prepared by participants in the Conference on the Safety of Biological Agents for Arthropod Control held at the Centers for Disease Control, Atlanta GA Apr. 16-19, 1973.
9.) Sharma A, Jaimungal S, Basdeo-Maharaj K, et al. Erythema Migrans-like Illness among Caribbean Islanders. Emerg Infect Dis. 2010 Oct;16(10):1615-1617
10.) Adams Mike. Natural News. America's farmlands to be carpet-bombed with Vietnam-era Agent Orange chemical if Dow petition approved. 2011 Dec 27. [web page]

Seven: The Origin of a Human Epidemic?

1.) Ninfa M. Rosas-García. Biopesticide Production from Bacillus thuringiensis: An Environmentally Friendly Alternative. Recent Patents on Biotechnology. 2009;3:28-36.
2.) Koppenhöfer AM, Wilson M, Brown I, Kaya HK, Gaugler R. Biological control agents for white grubs (Coleoptera: Scarabaeidae) in anticipation of the establishment of the Japanese beetle in California. J Econ Entomol. 2000 Feb;93(1):71-80.
3.) US Patent 3,950,225. Skole, et al. Filed 10/15/74, issued 4/13/76. Medium, component thereof and process employing same for the production of microbial insecticides, such as Bacillus popilliae spores and the like, for the control of Japanese beetles and other insects. Assignee: Amstar Corporation (New York, NY).
4.) Steinhaus EA, Thompson CG. Preliminary field tests using a polyhedrosis virus to control the alfalfa caterpillar. J Econ Entomol. 1949 Apr;42(2):301-5.
5.) Heimpel AM, Hrubant GG. Medical Examination of Humans Exposed to Bacillus popilliae japonica During Production of Commercial Milky Disease Spore Dust. Environ. Entomol. 1973Oct.;2(5):793-795.
6.) Masuzawwa T, Suzuki H, Kawabata H, et al. Identification of Spirochetes Isolated from Wild Rodent in Japan as Borrelia japonica. J Clin Microbiol. 1995 May;33(5):1392-1394.
7.) Fraser CM, Casjens S, Huang WM, et al. Genomic sequence of a Lyme disease spirochaete, Borrelia burgdorferi. Nature 1997 Dec 11;390:580-586.
8.) Aberer E, Duray Paul H. Morphology of Borrelia burgdorferi: Structural Patterns of Cultured Borreliae in Relation to Staining Methods. 1991 Apr;29(4):764-772.
9.) Skare JT, Mirzabekov TA, Shang ES et al. The Oms66(p66) protein is a Borrelia burgdorferi porin. In-fect Immun 1997;65:3654-3661.
10.) Skare JT, Shang ES, Foley DM et al. Virulent strain associated outer membrane proteins of Borrelia burg-dorferi. J Clin Invest 1995;96:2380-2392.
11.) Skare JT, Champion CI, Mirzabekov TA et al. Porin activity of the native and recombinant outer membrane protein Oms28of Borrelia burgdorferi. J Bacteriol 1996;178:4909-4918.
12.) Shang E S, Skare JT, Exner MM, et al. Isolation and characteriza-tion of the outer membrane of Borrelia hermsii. Infect Immun 1998;66:1082-1091.
13.) Thein M, Bunikis I, Denker K et al. Oms38is the first identified pore-forming protein in the outer membrane of relapsing fever spirochetes. J Bacteriol 2008;190:7035-7042.
14.) Pascale Bourhy, Laurence Salaün, Aurélie Lajus, et al. A Genomic Island of the Pathogen Leptospira interrogans Serovar Lai Can Excise from Its Chromosome. Infect Immun. 2007 Feb;75(2):677-683.
15.) Hinnebusch J, Barbour AG. Linear- and circular-plasmid copy numbers in Borrelia burgdorferi. J Bateriol. 1992 Aug;174(16):5251-5257
16.) Melcher U, Sha Y, Ye F, Fletcher J. Mechanisms of spiroplasma genome variation associated with SpV1-like viral DNA inferred from sequence comparisons. Microb Comp Genomics. 1999;4(1):29-46.
17.) Lee HY, Krell PJ. Generation and analysis of defective genomes of Autographa californica nuclear polyhedrosis virus. J Virol. 1992 Jul;66(7):4339-4347.
18.) Diego Cadavid and Alan G. Barbour . Neuroborreliosis during Relapsing Fever: Review of the Clinical Manifestations, Pathology, and Treatment of Infections in Humans and Experimental Animals. Clin Infect Dis. 1998;26(1): 151-164.
19.) Nordstrand Annika, Bunikis Ignas, Larsson Christer, et al. Tickborne Relapsing Fever Diagnosis Obscured by Malaria, Togo. Emerg Infect Dis. 2007 Jan;13(1):117-123.

Novel Spirochetes Emerge

1.) Bazovská S, Hovind-Hougen K, Rudiová A, Kmety E. Leptospira sp. Strain Dimbovitza, First Isolate in Europe with Characteristics of the Proposed Genus Leptonema. Inter J System Bacteriol. 1983 Apr.;33(2):325-328. (Institut of Epidem, Med Faculty of Komensky Univ, Bratislava, Czechoslovakia, and Dept of Biophysics, Statens Seruminstitut, Copenhagen, Denmark).
2.) Petrina Ecaterina. Corn and the Development of Agricultural Science in Romania, 1864-1939. Agricult. History. 1995 Winter;69(1):54-78. Published by Agricultural History Society.
3.) Michael LG. Agricultural Survey of Europe: The Danube Basin, Part 2: Romania, Bulgaria and Yugoslavia. USDA Technical Bulletin No. 126. 1929 Oct:6-81.
4.) Hovind-Hougen Kari. Leptospiraceae, a new family to include Leptospira Noguchi 1917and Leptonema gen. nov. Int. J Syst. Bacteriol. 1979;29:245-251.
5.) Lewis FR. How to Collect and Process Small Polyhedral Viruses of Insects. Northeast Forest Experiment Station. Forest Research Notes. No. 109. 1960. 8 pages. By the Forest Insect Laboratory Northeastern Forest Experiment Station Forest Service, USDA New Haven, CT.
6.) Rollinson WD, Lewis FB. How to Collect and Process Large Polyhedral Viruses of Insects. In Forest Research Notes. Forest Service, USDA, Upper Darby, PA. 1962No. 130, 6 pages. By the Forest Insect Laboratory Northeastern Forest Experiment Station Forest Service, USDA New Haven,CT.
7.) Rollinson WD, Lewis FB, Waters WE. The Successful Use of a Nuclear-Polyhedrosis Virus against the Gypsy Moth. Notes. 1965. Forest Insect and Disease Laboratory Northeastern Forest Experiment Station Forest Service, US Department of Agriculture, West Haven, Connecticut.
8. Volkin Elliot, Astrachan L. Phosphorus incorporation in Escherichia coli ribonucleic acid after infection with bacteriophage T2. Virology. 1956 Apr;2(2):149-161.
9.) Schippers A, Hallmann R, Wentzien S, Sand W. Microbial Diversity in Uranium Mine Waste Heaps. Appl Environ Microbiol. 1995 Aug;61(8):2930-2935.
10.) Canchaya C, Proux C, Fournous G, et al. Prophage genomics. Microbiol Mol Biol Rev. 2003 Jun;67(2):238-276.
11.) Becker Klaus. Health Effects of High Radon Environments in Central Europe: Another Test for the LNT Hypothesis? Nonlinear Biol Toxicol Med. 2003;1(1):3-35.

12.) Nuclear Weapons Production Processes and History. 20 pages. [web page]
13.) Bellows Alan. Undark and the Radium Girls. [monograph] 2006 Dec. [web page]

Animal Trapping in Georgia

1.) Hanford Cultural Resources Program, US Department of Energy. Hanford Site Historic District: History of the Plutonium Production Facilities, 1943-1990. 2002. Battelle Press. Columbus, OH. p.1.22-1.27. ISBN 1-57477-133-7.
2.) Findlay John, Hevly Bruce. Nuclear Technologies and Nuclear Communities: A History of Hanford and the Tri-Cities, 1943-1993. Seattle, WA: Hanford History Project, Center for the Study of the Pacific Northwest, University of Washington. 1995:p. 50.
3.) Wiki: Savannah River Site. Wapedia.
4.) Federation of American Scientists. Special Weapons Primer. Heavy Water. Weapons of Mass Destruction. [web site] 1998Oct. 21.
5.) SRNL. Savannah River National Laboratory. [web site] Last updated 2010 June 25
6.) Phillips RW, Wiegel J, Berry, CJ, et al. Kineococcus radiotolerans sp. nov., a radiation-resistant, Gram-positive bacterium. Inter J System Evol Microbiol. 2002;52:93-938.
7.) Field Paul E, Shaffer James H. The solubilities of hydrogen fluoride and deuterium fluoride in molten fluorides. J Phys Chem. 1967;71(10):3218-3222.
8.) Johnson MW, Sándor E, Arzi E. The Crystal Structure of Deuterium Fluoride. Acta Cryst. 1975;B3:1998-2003.
9.) McLain SE, Benmore CJ, Siewenie JE, Molaison JJ, Turner JF. On the variation of the structure of liquid deuterium fluoride with temperature. J Chem Phys. 2004Oct 1;121(13):6448-6455.
10.) Giovanni Rosalie. The Effects of Deuterium Oxide on Certain Microorganisms. Annals NY Acad Sci. 1960 Nov;84:16:644-647.
11.) Lawrie JM, Downard JS, Whiteley HR. Bacillus subtilis bacteriophages SP82, SPO1, and phie: a comparison of DNAs and of peptides synthesized during infection. J Virol. 1978 Sept.;27(3):725-737.
12.) Stewart CR, Casjens SR, Cresawn SG, et al. The genome of Bacillus subtilis bacteriophage SPO1. J Mol Biol. 2009 Apr 24;388(1):48-70. Epub 2009 Mar 10.
13.) Strömsten NJ, Benson SD, Burnett RM, et al. The Bacillus thuringiensis linear double-stranded DNA phage Bam35, which is highly similar to the Bacillus cereus linear plasmid pBClin15, has a prophage state. J Bacteriol. 2003 Dec;185(23):6985-9.
14.) Hardies Stephen C, Thomas Julie A, Serwer Philip. Comparative genomics of Bacillus thuringiensis phage 0305phi8-36: defining patterns of descent in a novel ancient phage lineage. Virol. Journal. 2007Oct 5;4:97.
15.) UniProt Taxonomy. Species Bacillus thuringiensis phage MZTP02.
16.) Barbour AG, Hayes SF. Biology of Borrelia Species. Microbiol Rev 1986 Dec;50(4):381-400.
17.)Ferdows MS, Barbour AG. Megabase-sized linear DNA in the bacterium Borrelia burgdorferi, the Lyme disease agent. Proc Natl Acad Sci USA. 1989 Aug;86(15):5969-73.
18.) University of Massachusetts Amherst, MA. NIH Grant #5R01AI008248-07. Physiology and morphology of anaerobic spirochetes. Fiscal year 1974. Project began 1972, ended 1974.
19.) Jurkevitch E, Minz D, Ramati B, Barel G. Prey Range Characterization, Ribotyping, and Diversity of Soil and Rhizosphere Bdellovibrio spp. Isolated on Phytopathogenic Bacteria. Appl Environ Microbiol 2000 Jun;66(6):2365-2371.
20.) Grant #5R01AI008715-02. Studies on Bdellovibrio, a Parasite of Bacteria. Abram D. University of Pittsburgh (PA). Fiscal year 1974. Project start: 9/1/72, ended 8/31/74. NIAID.
21.) RD Andrews, JR Reilly, DH Ferris, LE Hanson. Leptospiral Agglutinins in Sera from Southern Illinois Herpetofauna. College of Vet, Med. Univ. of IL Urbana, IL. Bulletin Wildlife Dis Assoc. 1965 Oct;1:55-59.
22.) McKeever S, Gorman GW, Chapman JF et al. Incidence of Leptospirosis in Wild Mammals from Southwestern Georgia, with a Report of New Hosts for Six Serotypes of Leptospires. CDC, Bureau of State Services, Public Health Service, US Dept. of Health, Education and Welfare, Atlanta, Georgia and Emory University Field Station, Newton, GA. Am J Trop Med Hyg. 1958;7(6):646-655.
23.) Wiki: Eugene Odum. http://wapedia.mobi
24.) Odum Eugene, Odum Howard T. Fundamentals of Ecology. 1953First Edition. Reprinted 1971 Philadelphia: Saunders.
25.) McKeever S, Gorman GW, Chapman JF, Galton MM, Powers DK. Incidence of Leptospirosis in Wild Mammals from Southwestern Georgia, with a Report of New Hosts for Six Serotypes of Leptospires. (CDC, Bureau of State Services, Public Health Service, US Department of Health, Education, and Welfare, Atlanta, GA and Emory University Field Station, Newton, GA). Am J Trop Med Hyg. 1958:646-655.
26.) Sweeten JM, Wolfe ML. The Expanding Dairy Industry: Impact on Ground Water Quality and Quantity with Emphasis on Waste
27.) Management System Evaluation for Open Lot Dairies. Texas Water Resources Institute. Texas A&M University. TR-155 August 1993. Project No. 06 (Sept. 1, 1988 – Aug. 31, 1991. Grant #14-0800001-G1592.
28.) Freedman KA, Klein JW, Crosson CE. Beta-cyclodextrins enhance bioavailability of pilocarpine. Curr Eye Res. 1993 Jul;12(7):641-647.
29.) van der Veen BA, Uitedehaag JC, Pennings D, et al. Rational design of cyclodextrin glycosyltransferase from Bacillus circulans strain 251 to increase alpha-cyclodextrin production. J Mol Biol. 2000 Mar 3;296(4):1027-1038.
30.) Zhuang M, Oltean DI, Gómez I, et al. Heliothis virescens and Manduca sexta lipid rafts are involved in Cry1A toxin binding to the midgut epithelium and subsequent pore formation. J Biol Chem. 2002 Apr 19;277(16):13863-13872.

Bull-Turtle Studies

1.) Johnson Russell C. (ed.). University of Minnesota, Minneapolis. The Biology of Parasitic Spirochetes. 1976Academic Press, New York. Chapter 3. Morphology of Leptospires. p.19-37.
2.) Charon NW, Johnson RC, Muschel LH. Antileptospiral Activity in Lower-Vertebrate Sera. Infect and Immun. 1975 Dec;12(6):1386-1391. (University of MN).
13.) US Energy Information Administration. Independent Statistics and Analysis. Clinton Nuclear Power Plant, Illinois. www.eia.doe.gov
14.) Chicago Radiological Society. A division of the Illinois Radiological Society. History: Radiology in Illinois by Franklin Alcorn, MD. www.chi-rad-soc.org
15.) Physics Illinois. University of Illinois at Urbana-Champaign. [web page]
16.) Babudieri B. Systematics of a Leptospira strain isolated from frog. Experentia. 1972;28:1252-1253.
17.) Johnson RC, Rogers P. Differentiation of pathogenic and saprophytic leptospires with 8-azaguanine. J Bacteriol. 1964;88:1618-1623.
18.) Andrews Richard David. Leptospiral Flora of Aquatic Turtles in Illinois. 1966. University of Illinois. PhD thesis. 158 pages.
19.) Miller MM. Fluorspar. US Geological Survey, Mineral Commodity Summaries, January 2007. Information sheet. [web page]
20.) US Mine Rescue Association. 2012 Jan 3. Historical Data on Mine Disasters in the US. [web page]
21.) Renner R. The long and short of perfluorinated replacements. Environ Sci Technol. 2006 Jan 1;40(1):12-13.
22.) Thomas Gary. Prairie State Deer. [web site] www.lib.niu.edu
23.) HA Surface (ed). The Zoological bulletin of the Division of Zoology of the…Pennsylvania Department of Agriculture, Division of Zoology. 1908 May;6(1):189.
24.) Ritchie AE, Ellinghausen HC. Bacteriophage-like entities associated with a leptospire. 1969. In J. Arcenaux (ed.), Proceedings of the Electron-Microscopy Society of America. Claitor's Publishing Div., Baton Rouge. P. 228-229.
25.) Hude FW, Johnson RC. Genetic relationship of Lyme disease spirochetes to Borrelia, Treponema, and Leptospira. J Clin Microbiol. 1984;20:151-154.
26.) Schmid GP, Steigerwalt AG, Johnson SE, Barbour AG, Steere AC, Robinson IM, Brenner DJ. DNA characterization of the spirochete that causes Lyme disease. J Clin Microbiol. 1984;20:155-158.
27.) Johnson Russell C, Schmid George P, Hyde Fred W, et al. Borrelia burgdorferi sp. nov.: Etiologic Agent of Lyme Disease. Inter J Syst Bacteriol. 1984 Oct;34(4):496-497.
28.) Dahlkamp Franz J. Uranium deposits of the World, USA and Latin America. Volume 1. 2010 Springer-Verlag Berlin Heidelberg.
29.) Tripathy DN, Hanson LE. Colonial and morphologic variations of Leptospira illini strain 3055. Am J Vet Res. 1972;33:1723-1727.
30.) Tripathy DN, Hanson LE. Studies of Leptospira illini, strain 3055: pathogenicity for different animals. Am J Vet Res. 1973;34:557-562.
31.) Johnson Russell C, Schmid George P, Hyde Fred W, Steigerwalt AG, Brenner Don J. Borrelia burgdorferi sp. nov.: Etiologic Agent of Lyme Disease. Inter J System Bacteriol. 1984 Oct;34(4):496-497.
32.) Blanc G, Mailloux M, Kolochine-Erber B, Ascione L. Enquete epidemioloque sur de leptospires au Maroc. Bull. Soc. Path. Exot. 1971;54:761-776.
33.) Kolochine-Erber B, Mailloux M. Quelque differences entre leptospires pathogens et leptospires saprophytes.Biol Med. 1963;52:496-504. [Article in French]
34.) Kinyon JM, Harris DL. Treponema innocens, a New Species of Intestinal Bacteria, and Emended Description of the Type Strain of Treponema hyodysenteriae Harris et al. Inter

J System Bacteriol. 1979 Apr;29(2):102-109.
35.) Coram NJ, Rawlings DE. Molecular Relationship between Two Groups of the Genus Leptospirillum and the Finding that Leptospirillum ferriphilum sp. nov. Dominates South African Commercial Biooxidation Tanks that Operate at 40°C. Appl Environ Microbiol. 2002 Feb;68(2):838-845.
36.) Schrenk MO, Edwards KJ, Goodman RM, et al. Distribution of thiobacillus ferrooxidans and leptospirillum ferrooxidans: implications for generation of acid mine drainage. Science. 1998 Mar 6;279(5356):1519-1522.
37.) Hovind-Hougen Kari. Leptospiraceae, a new family to include Leptospira Noguchi 1917 and Leptonema gen. nov. Int. J Syst. Bacteriol. 1979;29:245-251.
38.) DePamphilis ML, Adler J. Fine structure and isolation of the hook-basal body complex of flagella from Escherichia coli and Bacillus subtilis. J. Bacteriol. 1971;105:384-395. (This was written in 1970 by scientists at the Dept of Biochem and Genetics Univ. of WI Madison)
39.) Barbour Alan G, Hayes Stanley F. Biology of Borrelia Species. Microbiol Rev. 1986 Dec;50(4):381-400.
40.) Motaleb MA, Corum L, Bono JL. Et al. Borrelia burgdorferi periplasmic flagella have both skeletal and motility functions. PNAS. 2000 Sept. 26;97(2):10899-10904.
41.) Goldstein Stuart F, Charon Nyles W, Kreiling Jill A. Borrelia burgdorferi swims with a planar waveform similar to that of eukaryotic flagella. Proc Natl Acad. Sci. USA. 1994 Apr;91:343-3437. (These scientists were from the University of MN [St. Paul], and West Virginia University).
42.) Tawadros Marianne. Borrelia burgdorferi. From the Wadsworth Center, NY State Dept. of Health Student presentation. MCB 233Pathogenic Microbiology, University of Connecticut-Department of Molecular and Cell Biology.
43.) Johnson Russell C. (ed.). University of Minnesota, Minneapolis. The Biology of Parasitic Spirochetes. 1976Academic Press, New York. Chapter 3. Morphology of Leptospires.
44.) Aberer E, Duray Paul H. Morphology of Borrelia burgdorferi: Structural Patterns of Cultured Borreliae in Relation to Staining Methods. 1991 Apr;29(4):764-772.
45.) Johnson RC, Schmid GP, Hyde FW, et al. Borrelia burgdorferi sp. nov.: Etiological Agent of Lyme Disease. Inter J Syst Bacteriol. 1984 Oct;34(4):496-497.
46.) Brinkley BR, Fuller EM, Highfield DP. Cytoplasmic microtubules in normal and transformed cells in culture: analysis by tubulin antibody immunofluorescence. PNAS 1975 Dec 1;72(12):4981-4985.
47.) Bazovská S, Hovind-Hougen K, Rudiová A, Kmety E. Leptospira sp. Strain Dimbovitza, First Isolate in Europe with Characteristics of the Proposed Genus Leptonema. Inter J Syst Bacteriol. 1983;3(2):325-328.
48.) Anecdotal statements from a male patient diagnosed with Rheumatoid Arthritis when discussing his past military medical test results pertaining to Syphilis. Personal communication to the author.
49.) Iridoviruses. [web site] University of Otago, Dunedin, New Zealand. 1998.
50.) Weiser J. Recent Advances in Insect Pathology. 1970 Jan.;15:245-256. From the laboratory of insect pathology, Institute of Entomology, Academy of Sciences, Praha, Czechoslovakia.
51.) Tidona CA, Schnitzler P, Kehm R, Darai G. Is the major capsid protein of iridoviruses a suitable target for the study of viral evolution? Virus Genes. 1998;16(1):59-66. From the Institut für Medizinische Virologie, Universität Heidelberg, Federal Republic of Germany.
52.) Dixon LK, Abrams CC, Bowick G, Goatley LC, Kay-Jackson PC, Chapman D, Liverani E, Nix R, Silk R, Zhang F. African swine fever virus proteins involved in evading host defence systems. Vet Immunol Immunopathol. 2004Aug;100(3-4):117-34.
53.) US Patent 4,211,711. Witkowski, et al. Treatment of human viral diseases with 1-B-D-ribofuranosyl-1,2,4-triazole-3-carboxamide. Filed 2/13/78, published 7/8/80. No assignee listed. Inventors from Morris Township, NJ and Provo, UT.
54.) Leonard David E. Recent Developments in Ecology and Control of the Gypsy Moth. 1974Jan. Ann Rev Entomol. 19:197-229.
55.) Rippere KE, Tran MT, Yousten AA, Hilu KH, Klein MG. Bacillus popilliae and Bacillus lentimorbus, bacteria causing milky disease in Japanese beetles and related scarab larvae. Inter J Syst Bacteriol. 1998;48:395-402.
56.) Todar Kenneth. Todar's Online Textbook of Bacteriology. The Genus Bacillus [web site]
57.) Dettori G, Grillo R, Cattani P, et al. Comparative study of the enzyme activities of Borrelia burgdorferi and other non-intestinal and intestinal spirochaetes. New Microbiol. 1995Jan;18(1):13-26.
58.) Glaser RW. The cultivation of a nematode parasite of an insect. Science 1931;73:614-615.
59.) US Patent 2,293,890. Process for Propagating Bacteria. Samson R. Dutky. Filed 3/15/40 published 8/25/42. Assignee: Claude R. Wickard as Secretary of Agriculture of the United States of America and his successors in office.
60.) Tilly Kit. Independence of Bateriophage N15 Lytic and Linear Plasmid Replication from the Heat Shock Proteins DnaJ, DnaK, and GrpE. J Bacteriol. 1991 Oct;173(20):6639-6642
61.) US Patent 6,670,127. Evans. Method for assembly of a polynucleotide encoding a target polypeptide. Filed 8/2/01 published 12/30/03. Assignee: Egea Biosciences, Inc. (San Diego, CA).
62.) Brezhak JA, Canale-Parola E. Spirochaeta aurantia, a Pigmented, Facultatively Anaerobic Spirochete. J Bacteriol. 1969;97(1):386-395
63.) Cox CD, Stover RC, Treick RW. Serological Studies on Hemolytic Antigen from Leptospira. Exper Biol Med. 1958 Jun;98(2):265-269
64.) Shi W, Yang Z, Geng Y, et al. Chemotaxes in Borrelia burgdorferi. J Bacteriol. 1998 Jan;180(2):231-235.]
65.) DN Tripathy, LE Hanson. Leptospires from Water Sources at Dixon Springs Agricultural Center. J Wildlife Dis. 1973 Jul;9:209-212.
66.) St. Julian G, Bulla Jr. LA, Sharpe ES, Adams GL. Bacteria, Spirochetes, and Rickettsia as Insecticides. 1973Jun 22;217:65-75.
67.) RD Andrews, JR Reilly, DH Ferris, LE Hanson. Leptospiral Agglutinins in Sera from Southern Illinois Herpetofauna. College of Vet. Med. Univ. of IL Urbana, IL. Bulletin Wildlife Dis Assoc. 1965 Oct;1:55-59.
68.) Wier Andrew, Ashen Jon, Margulis Lynn. Canaleparolina darwiniensis, gen. nov., sp. nov., and other pillotinaceous spirochetes frominsects. Intern Microbiol. 2000;3:213-223.
69.) University of Illinois at Urbana-Champaign. Animal Sciences Laboratory. [web site]
70.) Lane Robert S. Susceptibility of the Western Fence Lizard (Sceloporus Occidentalis) to the Lyme Borreliosis Spirochete (Borrelia burgdorferi). Am J Trop Med Hyg. 1990;42(1):75-82.
71.) Shenberg EA, Friedlander A, Torten M, Ben-Efraim S. Leptospiral agglutinating factor in turtles. Further studies on fractioned sera. Isr J Med. Sci. 1970;6:408-412.
72.) Van der Hoeden J. Agglutination of leptospires in sera of fresh water turtles. Antonie van Leeuwenhoek J. Microbiol. Serol. 1968;34:458-464.
73.) Glosser JW, Sulzer CR, Eberhardt M, Winkler W. Cultural and serologic evidence of Leptospira interrogans serotype tarassovi infection in turtles. J Wild Dis. 1974;10:429-435.
80.) Combiesco D, Sturdza N, Radu I. et al. Recherches concernant les sources d'infection dans les leptospiroses. Arch Roumaines Path Exper et Microbiol. 1959;18:361-372. [Article in French]
81.) Van Der Hoeden J, Szenberg E, Evenchik Z. Leptospira-agglutinating factors in turtle sera. Nature 1961;190:95-96.
82.) Blanc G, Mailloux M, Kolochine-Erber B, Ascione L. Enquete epidemioloque sur de leptospires au Maroc. Bull. Soc. Path. Exot. 1971;54:761-776.
83.) Tripathy DN, Hanson LE. Leptospires from Water Sources at Dixon Springs Agricultural Center. J Wildlife Dis. 1973Jul;9:209-212.
84.) Morbidity and Mortality Weekly Reports. Centers for Disease Control, Atlanta, Georgia, 30333, USA. 1973;22(6):48-49.
85.) Morbidity and Mortality Weekly Reports. Centers for Disease Control, Atlanta, Georgia, 30333, USA. 1973;22(6):48-49.
86.) Noguchi Hideyo. Cultivation of Treponema Calligyrum (New Species) from Condylomata of Man. J. Exp Med. 1913;17(1):89-100.
87.) Listgarten Max A, Lewis DW. The distribution of spirochetes in the lesion of acute necrotizing ulcerative gingivitis. An electron microscopic and statistical survey. J Periodontol. 1967;38:379-386. (University of PA)
88.) Aberer E, Duray Paul H. Morphology of Borrelia burgdorferi: Structural Patterns of Cultured Borreliae in Relation to Staining Methods. 1991 Apr;29(4):764-772.
89.) Albrecht SL, Okon Y, Burris RH. Effects of Light and Temperature on the Association between Zea mays and Spirillum lipoferum. Plant Physiol. 1977;60:528-531.
90.) Hovind-Hougen K, Høybe G. Urinary excretion of an unidentified treponeme in a case of leptospirosis. Zentralbl Bakteriol A. 1981 Feb;248(4):532-40.
91.) Brendle JJ, Alexander AD. Contamination of Bacteriological Media by Leptospira biflexa. Appl Microbiol. 1974Sept.;28(3):505-506.
92.) Faine Solomon. Leptospira and Leptospirosis. 1993 CRC Press, Inc. Boca Raton, FL.
93.) Segers RPAM. The molecular analysis of sphingomyelinase genes of Leptospiraceae. Doctoral thesis. Rijksuniversiteit te Utrecht, Netherlands. 1991 p. 147.
94.) Bazovská S, Hovind-Hougen K, Rudiová A, Kmety E. Leptospira sp. Strain Dimbovitza, First Isolate in Europe with Characteristics of the Proposed Genus Leptonema. Inter J Syst Bacteriol. 1983 Apr;33(2):325-328.
95.) Hude FW, Johnson RC. Genetic relationship of Lyme disease spirochetes to Borrelia, Treponema, and Leptospira. J Clin Microbiol. 1984;20:151-154.
96.) Hovind-Hougen Kari. Leptospiraceae, a New Family to Include Leptospira Noguchi 1917and Leptonema gen. nov. Inter J Syst Bacteriol. 1979 Jul;29(3):245-251.

97.) Wier A, Ashen J, Margulis L. Canaleparolina darwiniensis, gen. nov., sp. nov., and other pillotinaceous spirochetes from insects. Int Microbiol. 2000 Dec;3(4):213-223.
98.) Hovind-Hougen Kari. Leptospiraceae, a new family to include Leptospira Noguchi 1917and Leptonema gen. nov. Int. J Syst. Bacteriol. 1979;29:245-251.
99.) Wiki: Savannah River Site. Wapedia. http://wapedia.mobi
100.) Bazovská S, Hovind-Hougen K, Rudiová A, Kmety E. Leptospira sp. Strain Dimbovitza, First Isolate in Europe with Characteristics of the Proposed Genus Leptonema. Inter J Syst Bacteriol. 1983Apr;33(2):325-328.
101.) Hude FW, Johnson RC. Genetic relationship of Lyme disease spirochetes to Borrelia, Treponema, and Leptospira. J Clin Microbiol. 1984;20:151-154.
102.) US Patent 5,466,577. Weisburg. Nucleic acid probes for the detection of Lyme disease spirochetes. Filed 10/27/93, published 11/14/95. Inventor: William G. Weisburg (Milford, MA); Assignee: Amoco Corp.
103.) LeFebvre RB, Perng GC, Johnson RC. Characterization of Borrelia burgdorferi Isolates by Restriction Endonuclease Analysis and DNA Hybridization. J Clin Microbiol.1989 Apr;27(4):636-639.
104.) US Patent 5,698,394. Duhamel, et al. Nucleotide sequences and methods for detection of Serpulina hyodysenteriae. Filed 6/1/94, published 12/16/97. Assignee: Board of Regents of the University of Nebraska. Notice how this patent was filed just 4months before the Lyme disease Dearborn, MI conference to standardize its laboratory testing.
105.) US Patent 5,869,630. Duhamel, et al. Nucleotide sequences for detection of serpulina hyodysenteriae. Filed 10/8/96, published 2/9/99. Assignee: Board of Regents, University of Nebraska Lincoln (Lincoln, NE).
106.) US Patent 6,068,843. Duhamel, et al. Nucleotide sequences and methods for detection of Serpulina hyodysenteriae. Filed 10/2/97, published 5/30/00. Assignee: Board of Regents University of Nebraska (Lincoln, NE).
107.) LeFebvre RB, Perng GC, Johnson RC. Characterization of Borrelia burgdorferi Isolates by Restriction Endonuclease Analysis and DNA Hybridization. J Clin Microbiol.1989 Apr;27(4):636-639.
108.) US Patent 5,837,263. Haake, et a. Leptospira membrane proteins. Filed 5/19/95, published 11/17/98. Assignee: The Regents of the University of California (Oakland, CA).
109.) Glosser JW, Sulzer CR, Eberhardt M, Winkler W. Cultural and serologic evidence of Leptospira interrogans serotype tarassovi infection in turtles. J Wild Dis. 1974;10:429-435.
110.) RD Andrews, JR Reilly, DH Ferris, LE Hanson. Leptospiral Agglutinins in Sera from Southern Illinois Herpetofauna. College of Vet. Med. Univ. of IL Urbana, IL. Bulletin Wildlife Dis Assoc. 1965 Oct;1:55-59.
111.) Tripathy DN, Hanson LE. Leptospires from Water Sources at Dixon Springs Agricultural Center. J Wildlife Dis. 1973 Jul;9:209-212.
112.) Glosser JW, Sulzer CR, Eberhardt M, Winkler W. Cultural and serologic evidence of Leptospira interrogans serotype tarassovi infection in turtles. J Wild Dis. 1974;10:429-435.
113.) News China View. Health. Report on China origin of swine flu "groundless": agriculture ministry. 2009 Apr 29. [news report on the Internet]
114.) The Pig Site Pig Health. [web site] Sheffield, England. www.thepigsite.com
115.) Haughey Jim, Simonson Ken, Baker Kermit. Reed Construction Data 2010 Market Insights Webcast Series. Economic Recovery: Under Construction. CDC Directors Emergency Ops Ctr Bldg A. [monograph]
116.) Johnson Russell C. (ed.). University of Minnesota, Minneapolis. The Biology of Parasitic Spirochetes. 1976 Academic Press, New York. Chapter 3. Morphology of Leptospires. p.19-37.
117.) Haines FJ, Griffiths CM, Possee RD, Hawes CR. King LA. Involvement of lipid rafts and cellular actin in AcMNPV GP64 distribution and virus budding. Virol Sinica. 2009Aug;24(4):333-349.
118.) Johnson RC, Rogers P. Differentiation of pathogenic and saprophytic leptospires with 8-azaguanine. J Bacteriol. 1964;88:1618-1623.
119.) Faine Solomon. Leptospira and Leptospirosis. CRC Press, Inc. Boca Raton, FL.
120.) Kasarov LB, Addamiano L. Metabolism of the lipoproteins of serum by leptospires: degradation of the triglycerides. J Med Microbiol. 1969;2:165-168.
121.) Johnson RC, Harris VG. Purine analogue sensitivity and lipase activity of leptospires. Appl. Microbiol. 1968;16:1584-1590.
122.) Yasuda PH, Steigerwalt AG, Sulzer KR, et al. Deoxyribonucleic acid relatedness between serogroups and serovars in the family Leptospiraceae with proposals for seven new Leptospira species. Int J Syst Bacteriol. 1987;37:407-415.
123.) Johnson Russell C. (ed.). University of Minnesota, Minneapolis. The Biology of Parasitic Spirochetes. 1976 A cademic Press, New York. Chapter 3. Morphology of Leptospires. p.19-37.
124.) Sommer Patricia, Bormann Christiane, Götz Friedrich. Genetic and Biochemical Characterization of a New Extracellular Lipase from Streptomyces cinnamomeus. Appl Environ Microbiol. 1997 Sept;:63(9):3553-3560.
125.) US Patent 3,626,060. Grier. Filed 1/12/70, published 12/7/71. Agricultural Compositions and Process for Utilizing Same. Assignee: Merck & Co.,Inc. (Rahway, NJ)
126.) Schmid George P, Steere Allen C, Kornblatt Arnold N, Kaufmann Arnold F, Moss C. Wayne, Johnson Russell C, Hovind-Hougen Kari, Brenner Don J. Newly Recognized Leptospira Species ("Leptospira inadai" serovar lyme) Isolated from Human Skin. J Clin Microbiol. 1986 Sept.;24(3):484-486.
127.) US Patent 4,703,010. Yunker et al. Electrolytic bioreactor assembly and method. Filed 5/2/86 published 10/27/87. Assignee: The Board of Regents for the University of Oklahoma.
128.) US Patent 4,888,293. Hackl et al. Adapting bacteria to low pH and high arsenic concentration for use in oxidizing sulfide ores. Filed 7/10/87 published 12/19/89. Assignee: Giant Bay Biotech Inc. (Burnaby, CA).
129.) US Patent 3,607,235. Duncan et al. Rapid Bacteriological Metal Extraction Method. Filed 2/23/68 published 9/21/71. Assignee: British Columbia Research Council (Vancouver, British Columbia, CA).
130.) US Patent 3,266,889. Duncan et al. Method of Extracting Metals from Sulfide Ores Using Bacteria and an Accelerating Agent. Filed 4/7/64 published 8/16/66. Assignee: British Columbia Research Council, Vancouver, British Columbia, Canada.
131.) US Patent 2,829,964. Zimmerley et al. Cyclic Leaching Process Employing Iron Oxidizing Bacteria. Filed 10/24/55 published 4/8/58. Assignee: Kennecott Copper Corporation, Salt Lake City, Utah.
132.) US Patent 3,218,252. Glover et al. Process for the Bacteriological Oxidation of Ferrous Salts in Acidic Solution. Filed 8/27/63 published 11/16/65. Assignee: Coal Industry (Patents) Limited, Grosevenor Place, London, England.
133.) US Patent 3,305,353. Duncan te al. Filed 3/30/64 published 2/21/67. Accelerated Microbiological Ore Extraction Process. Assignee: British Columbia Research Council, Vancounver, British Columbia, Canada.
134.) US Patent 3,347,661. Mayling. Cyclic Leaching Process Employing Iron Oxidizing Bacteria. Filed 2/15/65 published 10/17/67. Assignee: Bio Metals Corporation Ltd., Vancouver British Columbia, Canada.
135.) US Patent 3,856,913. McElroy et al. Copper Extraction by Rapid Bacteriological Process. Filed 9/21/72 published 12/24/74. Assignee: British Columbia Research Council (Vancouver, British Columbia, Canada).
136.) US Patent 3,260,593. Zimmerley et al. Process for Leaching Copper from Low-grade Copper-bearing Ore Materials. Filed 9/12/62 published 7/12/66. Assignee: Kennecott Copper Corporation, New York.
137.) US Patent 3,679,397. O'Connor et al. Bacterial Leaching Process. Filed 12/29/69 published 7/25/72. Assignee: Teh Regents, New Mexico Institution of Mining and Technology, Socorro, New Mexico.
138.) US Patent 3,433,629. Imai et al. Process of Recovering Manganese from Manganese Ores. Filed 1/30/65 published 3/18/69. Assignee: Tomoji Murata, Akashi-shi, Japan.
139.) US Patent 3,455,679. Mayling. Bacterial Leaching of Ores with an Alkaline Matrix. Filed 2/28/67 published 2/1/67. Assignee: Roan Selection Limited, Vancouver, British Columbia, Canada.
140.) US Patent 3,894,770. Huff et al. Wellbore oxidation of lixiviants. Filed 6/12/74 published 7/15/75. Assignee: Kennecott Copper Corporation. (New York, NY).
141.) US Patent 3,278,233. Hurd et al. In Situ Leaching of Subterranean Deposits. Filed 3/27/64 published 10/11/66. Assignee: Mobil Oil Corporation, New York.
142.) Adachi K, Suzuki I. Purification and properties of glutamate synthase from Thiobacillus thioparus. J Bacteriol. 1977;129:1173-1182.
143.) Hallbeck L, Pedersen K. Autotrophic and mixotrophic growth of Gallionella ferruginea. J Gen Microbiol. 1991;137:2657-2661.
144.) Mondani L, Benzerara K, Carrière M et al. Influence of uranium on bacterial communities: a comparison of natural uranium-rich soils with controls. PloS One. 2011;6(10): e25771. Epub 2001 Oct 5.
145.) Emerson D, Rentz JA, Lilburn TG, et al. A Novel Lineage of Proteobacteria Involved in Formation of Marine Fe-Oxidizing Microbial Mat Communities. PLoS One. 2007 Aug 1;2(7):e667.
146.) Reddy KR, DeLaune RD. Biogeochemistry of Wetlands Science and Applications. 2008 CRC Press. Boca Raton, FL.

Rocky Mountain Leptospires

1.) Rentko VT, Ross LA. Canine Leptospirosis. In: Bonagura JD (ed.), Kirk's Current Veterinary Therapy XI. W.B. Saunders, Philadelphia. 1992. pp. 260-263.

2.) US Patent 6,852,322Nascimento, et al. Surface proteins of Leptospira. Filed 2/28/03 published 2/8/05. Assignee: Fundacao de Amparo a Pesquisa do Estado de Sao Paolo (Sao Paulo, BR).

3.) Yager Robert H, Gochenour Jr. William S. Leptospirosis in North America. Veterinary Div. Walter Reed Army Medical Center, Washington, DC. Am J Trop Med Hyg. 1952;1(3):457-461.

4.) Merck. Chloramphenicol. [web page]

5.) Little RB, Beck JD. McCahon JV. An outbreak of bovine leptospirosis in Pennsylvania. Vet Med. 1950;45:104-110.

6.) Reinhard KR, Tierney WF, Roberts SJ. A study of two enzootic occurrences of bovine leptospirosis. Cornell Vet. 1950;40:148-164.

7.) Meyer K.F, Stewart B, Stewart-Anderson Eddie B. Canicola fever, a professional hazard, JAVMA 1938;93:332-333.

8.) Abdulla Pk, Karstad L. Experimental infections with Leptospira Pomona in snakes and turtles. Zoonoses Res. 1962 Dec 31;1:295-306.

9.) Takeuchi Akio, Zeller Jack A. Ultrastructural Identification of Spirochetes and Flagellated Microbes at the Brush Border of the Large Intestinal Epithelium of the Rhesus Monkey. Infect and Immun. 1972Dec;6(6):1008-1018.

10.) Reilly JR, Muraschi TF, Dean DJ. Experimental Leptospira Pomona infection in white-tailed deer. Odocoileus virginafanus, and in cattle. J Am Vet Med Assoc. 1962 Jan 1;140:53-7.

11.) Maramorosch Karl. Do Developmental Stages Occur in the Reproductive Cycle of Aster-Yellows Virus? Cold Spring Harbor Symposia on Quantitative Biology. 1953;18:51-54.

12.) CDC. MMWR Update: Leptospirosis and Unexplained Acute Febrile Illness Among Athletes Participating in Triathlons – Illinois and Wisconsin. 1998;47(32):676.

13.) Friedland JS, Warrell DA. The Jarisch-Herxheimer reaction in leptospirosis: possible pathogenesis and review. Rev Infect Dis 1991;13:207-10.

14.) Guo BP, Brown EL, Dorward DW, et al. Decorin-binding adhesions from Borrelia burgdorferi. Mol Microbiol. 1998 Nov;30(4):711-723.

15.) Taylor Kathleen A, Barbour Alan G, Thomas Denee. Pulsed-Field Gel Electrophoretic Analysis of Leptospiral DNA. Infect Immun. 1991 Jan;59(1):323-329.

16.) Baril C, Saint-Girons I. FEMS Microbiol. Lett. 1990;71:95.

17.) Schutzer Steven E. Lyme Disease: Molecular and Immunologic Approaches. 1992 Cold Spring Harbor Laboratory Press. New York.

18.) Haake DA, Chao G, Zuerner RL, et al. The Leptospiral Major Outer Membrane Protein LipL32Is a Lipoprotein Expressed during Mammalian Infection. Infect Immun. 2000;68:2276-2285.

19.) Haake DA et al. Molecular cloning and sequence analysis of the gene encoding OmpL1, a transmembrane outer membrane protein of pathogenic Leptospira spp. J. Bacteriol. 1993 Jul;175:4225-4234.

20.) Haake DA, Chao G, Zuerner RL, et al. The leptospiral major outer surface protein, LipL32, is a lipoprotein expressed during mammalian infection. Infect. Immun. 2000;68:2276-2285.

21.) Haake DA, Martinich C, Summers TA et al. Characterization of leptospiral outer membrane lipoprotein LipL36: Downregulation associatd with late-log-phase growth and mammalian infection. Infect. Immun. 1998;66:1579-1587.

22.) Haake DA, Mazel MK, McCoy AM, et al. Leptospiral outer membrane proteins OmpL1 and LipL41 exhibit synergistic immunoprotetion. Infect. Immun. 1999;67:6572-6582.

23.) Shang ES, Exner MM, Summers TA, et al. The rare outer membrane protein, OmpL1, of pathogenic Leptospira species is a heat-modifiable porin. Infect. Immun. 1995 Aug;63:3174-3181.

24.) Masuzawa T, Nakamura R, Shimizu T, Yanagihara Y. Biological activities and endotoxic activities of protective antigens (PAgs) of Leptospira interrogans. Zentralbl. Bakteriol. 1990;274:109–117.

25.) US Patent 5,989,547. Haake. Leptospiral outer membrane proteins. Filed 1/21/97 published 11/23/99. Assignee: University of California (Los Angeles, CA).

26.) US Patent 5,837,263. Haake, et al. Leptospira membrane proteins. Filed 5/19/95 published 11/17/98. Assignee: The Regents of the University of California (Oakland, CA).

27.) Radolf, et al. Characterization of Outer Membranes Isolated from Borrelia burgdorferi, the Lyme Disease Spirochete. Infect Immun. 1995;63:2154-2163.

28.) Skare, et al. Virulent Strain Associated Outer Membrane Proteins of Borrelia burgdorferi. J Clin Invest. 1995;96:2380-2392.

29.) Jackson LA, Kaufmann AF, Adams WG, et al. Outbreak of leptospirosis associated with swimming. Pediatr Infect Dis J 1993;12:48-54.

30.) Johnson Russell C. The Spirochetes. Ann Rev Microbiol. 1977;31:89-106.

31.) Johnson Russell C, Harris Virginia G. Differentiation of Pathogenic and Saprophytic Leptospires. J Bacteriol. 1967 Jul;94(1):27-31.

32.) Cinco M, Banfi E, Panfili E. Heterogeneity of lipopolysaccharide banding patterns in Leptospira spp. J. Gen. Microbiol 1986;132:1135–1138.

33.) Bigler Bill, Conti Lisa. Florida Department of Health, Bureau of Epidemiology. [web page]

34.) Vieira Monica L, Pimenta Daniel C, de Morais Zenaide M. et al. Proteome Analysis of Leptospira interrogans Virulent Strain. Microbiol J. 2009;3:69-74.

35.) Krøjgaard LH, Villumsen S, Markussen MD, Jensen JS, Leirs H, Heiberg AC. High prevalence of Leptospira spp. in sewer rats (Rattus norvegicus). Epidemiol Infect. 2009 Nov;137(11):1586-92. Epub 2009 Apr 27.

36.) Dorjee S, Heuer C, Jackson R, et al. Are white-spot lesions in kidneys in sheep associated with leptospirosis? NZ Vet J 2009Feb;57(1):28-33.

37.) Tilly K, Krum JG, Bestor A, et al. Borrelia burgdorferi OspC Protein Required Exclusively in a Crucial Early Stage of Mammalian Infection. Infect Immun. June 2006;74(6):3554-3564.

38.) Utpal P, Xiaofeng Y, Manchuan C, Bockenstedt LK, Anderson JF, Flavell RA, Norgard MV, Fikrig E. OspC facilitates Borrelia burgdorferi invasion of Ixodes scapularis salivary glands. J Clin Invest 2004;113(2):220-230.

39.) Doungchawee G, Kositanont U, Niwetpathomwat A, et al. Early Diagnosis of Leptospirosis by Immunoglobulin M Immunoblot Testing. 2008 Mar;15(3):492-498.

40.) US Patent 7,635,480. Andre-Fontaine et al. Peptides for Preventing, Diagnosing and Treating Animal and/or Human Leptospirosis. Filed 10/24/03, published 12/22/09. Assignee: Virbac S.A. (France).

41.) Johnson Russell C. (ed.). In The Biology of Parasitic Spirochetes. Academic Press.New York 1976:101.

42.) WHO. Technical Report Series No. 380. Current Problems in Leptospirosis Research. 1967.

43.) Rodríguez de Córdoba S, Esparza-Gordillo J, Goicoechea de Jorge E, Lopez-Trascasa M, Sánchez-Corral P. The human complement factor H: functional roles, genetic variations and disease associations. Mol. Immunol. 2004Jun;41(4):355-367.

43.) Nally JE, Chow E, Fishbein MC, Blanco DR, Lovett MA. Changes in lipopolysaccharide O antigen distinguish acute versus chronic Leptospira interrogans infections. Infect. Immun. 2005;73(6):3251–60.

44.) Vinh TU, Shi MH, Adler B, Faine S. Characterization and taxonomic significance of lipopolysaccharides of Leptospira interrogans serovar hardjo. J. Gen. Microbiol 1989;135:2663–2673.

45.) Johnson Russell C, Harris Virginia G. Differentiation of Pathogenic and Saprophytic Leptospires. J Bacteriol. 1967 Jul;94(1):27-31.

46.) PATRIC: Pathosystems Resource Integration Center. Bacteria>Spirochaetes>Borrelia burgdorferi N40:Phylogeny. [web page]

47.) Willy Burgdorfer, Edgar G. Pickens. A Technique Employing Embryonated Chicken Eggs for the Infection of Argasid Ticks with Coxiella burnetti, Bacterium tularense, Leptospira icterohaemorrhagiae, and Western Equine Encephalitis Virus. 1954 Jan-Feb;94(1):84-89.

48.) Willy Burgdorfer. The Possible Role of Ticks as Vectors of Leptospirae. I. Transmission of Leptospira Pomona by the Argasid Tick, Ornithodoros turicata, and the Persistance of This Organism in Its Tissues. Exper. Parasitol. 1956:571-579.

49.) Burgdorfer Willy. The Possible Role of Ticks as Vectors of Leptospirae. I. Transmission of Leptospira pomona by the Argasid Tick, Ornithodoros turicata, and the Persistance of This Organism in Its Tissues. Exper Parasitol. 1956;V:571-579.

50.) Burgdorfer Willy. The Possible Role of Ticks as Vectors of Leptospirae. II. Infection of the Ixoid Ticks, Dermacentor andersoni and Amblyomma maculatum, with Leptospira pomona. Exper Parasitol. 1959;8:502-508.

51.) Burgdorfer W, Pickens EG. A technique employing embryonated chicken eggs for the infection of argasid ticks with Coxiella burnetti, Bacterium tularense, Leptospira ictero-haemorrhagiae, and western equine encephalitis virus. J Infect. Dis. 1954;94:84-89.

52.) Burgdorfer Willy, Lackman David. Identification of the Virus of Colorado Tick Fever in Mouse Tissues by Means of Fluorescent Antibodies. J Bacteriol. 1960 Jul;80:131-6. Received for publication 12/7/59.

54.) J Frederick Bell, Willy Burgdorfer, G John Moore. The Behavior of Rabies Virus in Ticks. J Infect Dis. 1957May-June;100(3):278-283.

55.) Mackintosh C, Haigh JC, Griffin F. Bacterial diseases of farmed deer and bison. Rev Sci Tech Off Int Epiz. 2002;21(2):249-263.

56.) Stuart RD. The Occurrence of Weil's Disease among Miners in the West of Scotland. J Hygiene. 1939 May;39(3):316-323.
57.) Inada R, Ido Y, Hoke R, Kaneko R, Ito H. The Etiology, mode of infection and specific therapy of Weil's Disease. J Exper Med. 1916;23:377.
58.) Rentschler Harey C, Nagy Rudolph, Mouromseff Galina. Bactericidal Effect of Ultraviolet Radiation. J Bacteriol. 1941 Jun;41(6):745-774. From the Research Department, Westinghouse Lamp Division, Bloomfield, New Jersey.
59.) Burgdorfer Willy. The Possible Role of Ticks as Vectors of Leptospirae. I. Transmission of Leptospira Pomona by Argasid Tick, Ornithodoros turicata, and the Persistance of This Organism in Its Tissues. Exp Parasitol. 1956;V:571-579.
60.) Burgdorfer Willy. The Possible Role of Ticks as Vectors of Leptospirae. I. Transmission of Leptospira pomona by the Argasid Tick, Ornithodoros turicata, and the Persistance of This Organism in Its Tissues. Exper Parasitol. 1956;V:571-579.
61.) Burgdorfer Willy. The Possible Role of Ticks as Vectors of Leptospirae. II. Infection of the Ixoid Ticks, Dermacentor andersoni and Amblyomma maculatum, with Leptospira pomona. Exper Parasitol. 1959;8:502-508.
62.) Burgdorfer W, Pickens EG. A technique employing embryonated chicken eggs for the infection of argasid ticks with Coxiella burnetti, Bacterium tularense, Leptospira ictero-haemorrhagiae, and western equine encephalitis virus. J Infect. Dis. 1954;94:84-89.
63.) Burgdorfer Willy, Lackman David. Identification of the Virus of Colorado Tick Fever in Mouse Tissues by Means of Fluorescent Antibodies. J Bacteriol. 1960 Jul;80:131-6. Received for publication 12/7/59.
64.) Willy Burgdorfer. Artificial Feeding of Ixodid Ticks for Studies on the Transmission of Disease Agents. J Infect Dis. 1957 Jun;100(3):212-214.
65.) J Frederick Bell, Willy Burgdorfer, G. John Moore. The Behavior of Rabies Virus in Ticks. J Infect Dis. 1957 May-Jun;100(3):278-283.
66.) US Patent 2,293,890. Process for Propagating Bacteria. Samson R. Dutky. Filed 3/15/40 published 8/25/42. Assignee: Claude R. Wickard as Secretary of Agriculture of the United States of America and his successors in office.
67.) Likar M, Kmet J. Virus Meningo-encephalitis in Slovenia. WHO Bulletin. 1956;15:275-279.
68.) Belyaev VG. Yu I, Mirotvortsev GM et al. Contribution to zoological and parasitological characteristics of the tularemia infection areas in Primor'ye region. Mater, Nauch, Prakt. Konf. Tulyarem. Soputst. Infekts. 1965:272-273. [NAMRU No. 3, Translation from Russian]. [Abstract]
69.) Gaidamovich S Ya. Classification and identification of Arboviruses. Vestn. Akad. Med. Nauk. SSSR. 1972;27(6):25-33. [NAMRU No. 3, Translation 677 from Russian]
70.) Missouri Digital Heritage. Photographic print. Titled: Sarah A. Luse and A.K. Shubladze, 1957. May 29, 2004. Housed in the Bernard Becker Medical Library, Washington University School of Medicine.
71.) Shubladze AK, Dick GWA. Russian Vaccine for Multiple Sclerosis. Correspondence, British Medical Journal. 1958 Jul 26; page 245.
72.) Belyaev VG. Yu I, Mirotvortsev GM et al. Contribution to zoological and parasitological characteristics of the tularemia infection areas in Primor'ye region. Mater, Nauch, Prakt. Konf. Tulyarem. Soputst. Infekts. 1965:272-273. [NAMRU No. 3, Translation 1525 from Russian]. [Abstract]
73.) Kolonin GV. Effect of industrial activity on ixodid tick numbers and distribution in Primor'ye region. Zool. Zh. 1981;60(3):363-370. NAMRU No. 3. Translation 1691 from Russian.
74.) Williams RE, Casals J, Moussa MI, Hoogstraal H. Royal Farm Virus: A New Tickborne Group B Agent Related to RSSE Complex. Am J Trop Med Hyg. 1972;21(5):582-586.
75.) Miles JAR. Epidemiology of the Arthropod-borne Encephalitides. WHO Bulletin. 1960;22:339-371.
76.) Missouri Digital Heritage. Photographic print. Titled: Sarah A. Luse and A.K. Shubladze, 1957. May 29, 2004. Housed in the Bernard Becker Medical Library, Washington University School of Medicine. 10. Shubladze AK, Dick GWA. Russian Vaccine for Multiple Sclerosis. Correspondence, British Medical Journal. 1958 Jul 26; page 245.
77.) Fitzpatrick Tony. Washington Univesrity in St. Louis, Monsanto Co., awarded patent for technology that creates disease-resistant crops. 2003 Aug 20. Washington University in St. Louis. Newsroom.
78.) US Patent 6,608,241. Beachy et al. Protection of plants against viral infection. Filed 10/9/86, published 8/19/03. Assignee: Monsanto Technology LLC (St. Louis, MO) and Washington University (St. Louis, MO).
79.) US Patent 4,966,852. Wun, et al. DNA Clone of human tissue factor inhibitor. Filed 11/23/87, published 10/30/90. Assignee: Monsanto Company (St. Louis, MO) and Washington University (St. Louis, MO).
80.) McKeever S, Gorman GW, Chapman JF, Galton MM, Powers DK. Incidence of Leptospirosis in Wild Mammals from Southwestern Georgia, with a Report of New Hosts for Six Serotypes of Leptospires. (CDC, Bureau of State Services, Public Health Service, US Department of Health, Education, and Welfare, Atlanta, GA and Emory University Field Station, Newton, GA). Am J Trop Med Hyg. 1958:646-655.
81.) Williams RE, Casals J, Moussa MI, Hoogstraal H. Royal Farm Virus: A New Tickborne Group B Agent Related to RSSE Complex. Am J Trop Med Hyg. 1972;21(5):582-586.
82.) Alfred I. duPont Testamentary Trust. [web site] www.alfrediduponttrust.org
83.) Washington University in St. Louis and AstraZeneca announce Alzheimer's research collaboration. 2008April 17. Press release AstraZeneca web site.
84.) Miles JAR. Epidemiology of the Arthropod-borne Encephalitides. WHO Bulletin. 1960;22:339-371.
85.) Schmid George P, Steere Allen C, Kornblatt Arnold N, Kaufmann Arnold F, Moss C. Wayne, Johnson Russell C, Hovind-Hougen Kari, Brenner Don J. Newly Recognized Leptospira Species ("Leptospira inadai" serovar lyme) Isolated from Human Skin. J Clin Microbiol. 1986 Sept.;24(3):484-486.
86.) Coleman James L, Benach Jorge L. Identification and Characterization of an Endoflagellar Antigen of Borrelia burgdorferi. J Clin Invest. 1989 Jul;84:322-330.
87.) Luft Benjamin J, Jiang Wei, Munoz Priscilla, Dattwyler Raymond J, Gorevic Peter D. Biochemical and Immunological Characterization of the Surface Proteins of Borrelia burgdorferi. Infec Immun. 1989 Nov;57(11):3637-3645.

Spiroplasma 277F

1.) Pickens Edgar G, Gerloff Robert K, Burgdorfer Willy. Spirochete from the Rabbit Tick, Haemaphysalis leporispalustris (Packard). I. Isolation and Preliminary Characterization. J Bacteriol. 1968 Feb;95(2):291-299.
2.) O'Leary William Michael. Practical handbook of microbiology. 1977 Condensed version of CRC handbook of microbiology. CRC Press LLC. (Boca Raton, FL). Laskin AI, Lechevalier HA (ed). 2nd ed.
3.) Grant 1Z01AI000062-06. Cellular and Subcellular Aspects of Vector-Pathogen Relationships. No school listed. Fiscal year 1975. National Institute of Allergy and Infectious Diseases. (NIAID)
4.) Grant 1Z01AI000062-07. Cellular and Subcellular Aspects of Vector-Pathogen Relationships. No school listed. Fiscal year 1977. NIAID.
5.) Williamson DL, Tully JG, Whitcomb RF. Serological Relationships of Spiroplasmas as Shown by Combined Deformation and Metabolism Inhibition Tests. Inter J System Bacteriol. 1979 Oct;29(4):345-351.
6.) Stalheim OHV, Ritchie AE, Whitcomb RF. Cultivation, serology, ultrastructure, and virus-like particles of spiroplasma 277F. Curr Microbiol. 1978Dec;1(6):365-370. US Department of Agriculture, National Animal Disease Center (Ames, Iowa) and USDA Plant Protection Institute (Beltsville, MD).
7.) Reuther Walter, Calavan E. Clair, Carman Glenn E. (ed) The Citrus Industry. Volume IV. Diseases and Injuries; Viruses; Registration, Certification, Indexing; Regulatory Measures; Vertebrate Pests; Biological Control of Insects; Nematodes. University of California Div. of Agriculture and Natural Resources. 1978 The Regents of the University of California.
8.) Fletcher J, Schultz GA, Davis RE, Eastmann CE, Goodman RM. Brittle root disease of horseradish: evidence for an etiological role of Spiroplasma citri. Phytopathol. 1981;71:1073-1080.
9.) Tully JG, Rose DL, Yunker CE, Cory J, Whitcomb RF, Williamson DL. Helical mycoplasmas (spiroplasmas) from Ixodes ticks. Science. 1981 May 29;212(4498):1043-5.
10.) Tully JG, Whitcomb RF, Rose DL, Williamson DL, Bové JM. Characterization and taxonomic status of tick spiroplasmas: a review. Yale J Biol Med. 1983 Sep-Dec;56(5-6):599-603.
11.) Henning K, Greiner-Fischer S, Hotel H, Ebsen M, Theegarten D. Isolation of Sprioplasma sp. from an Ixodes tick. Int J Med Microbiol. 2006 May;296 Suppl. 40:157-61. Epub 2006 Mar 9.
12.) US Patent 5,296,371. Razin et al. DNA encoding spiroplasma sp. dna methylase. Filed 10/4/91, published 3/22/94. Assignee not listed. Inventors from Jerusalem, Illinois.,11d
13.) Barbour AG, Hayes SF. Biology of Borrelia Species. Microbiol Rev 1986 Dec;50(4):381-400
14.) Merck. Chloramphenicol. [web page]
15.) Stalheim Ole HV, Ritchie Alfred E. Whitcomb Robert F. Cultivation, Serology, Ultrastructure, and Virus-Like Particles of Spiroplasma 277F. Curr Micrbiol. Vol. 1. 1978:365-370.
16.) Steiner Theodor, McGarrity Gerard J, Phillips David M. Cultivation and Partial Characterization of Spiroplasmas in Cell Cultures. Infect Immun. 1982 Jan;35(1):296-304.

17.) Pickens EG, Gerloff RK, Burgdorfer W. Spirochete from the rabbit tick Haemphysalis leporispalustris (Packard). J Bacteriol. 1968;95:291-299.
18.) Poulson DF, Sakaguchi B. Nature of the "sex-ratio" agent in Drosophila. Science 1961;133:1489-1490.
19.) Stalheim OHV1, Ritchie AE1, Whitcomb RF2. Cultivation, serology, ultrastructure, and virus-like particles of spiroplasma 277F. 1USDA National Animal Disease Center (Ames, IA); 2USDA Plant Protection Institute, Agricultural Research Science and Education Administration (Beltsville, MD). Current Microbiol. 1978 Dec.;1(6):365-370.
20.) Steiner Theodor, McGarrity Gerard J, Phillips David M. Cultivation and Partial Characterization of Spiroplasmas in Cell Cultures. Infect and Immun. 1982 Jan;35(1):296-304.
21.) Tsai JH, Miller JW. Corn Stunt Spiroplasma. Plant Pathol Circular No. 373. 1995 Sept/Oct. FL Dept of Agriculture & Consumer Services, Division of Plant Industry.
22.) CABI and EPPO for the EU under Contract 90/399003. Data Sheets on Quarantine Pests. Spiroplasma citri. [web page]
23.) Brinton LP, Burgdorfer W. Cellular and subcellular organization of the 277F agent: A spiroplasma from the rabbit tick. Haemaphysalis leporispalustris (Acari: Ixodidae). Inter J Syst Bacteriol. 1976;26:554-560.
24.) Tully JC. The Emmy Klieneberger-Nobel Award Lecture. Reflections on Recovery of Some Fastidious Mollicutes with Implications of the Changing Host Patterns of These Organisms. The Yale J Biol Med. 1983;56:799-813.
25.) Tully JG. Laboratory diagnosis of Mycoplasma pneumonia infections. Isr J Med Sci. 1981 Jul;17(7):644-647.
26.) Brown MB, Brown DR, Klein PA, et al. Mycoplasma agassizii sp. nov., isolated from the upper respiratory tract of the desert tortoise (Gopherus agassizii) and the gopher tortoise (Gopherus polyphemus). Inter J System Evol Microbiol. 2001;51:413-418.
27.) Brown DR, Merritt JL, Jacobson ER, et al. Mycoplasma testudineum sp. nov., from a desert tortoise (Gopherus agassizii) with upper respiratory tract disease. Inter J System Evol Microbiol. 2004;54:1527-1529.

Will the Real Bb Stand Up?

1.) WHO. Technical Report Series No. 380. Current Problems in Leptospirosis Research. Report of a WHO Expert Group. 1967.
2.) Gonder, R., Spironemacea (Spirochaeten), in yon Prowazek, S., Handbuch der pathogenen Protozoen, Leipsic, Liefg. 6, 1914, 671. And
3.) Noguchi H. The spirochetal Flora of the Normal Male Genitalia. J Exp Med. 1918 Jun 1;27(6):667-678.
4.) Meleney HE. Relapse Phenomena of Spironema Recurrentis. J Exp Med. 1928 Jun 30;48(1):65-82. And Berks G, Goodwin LG. Terramycin and Spironema duttoni Infections. Nature 1951 Mar 17;167(4246):447-448.
5.) Berks G, Goodwin LG. Terramycin and Spironema duttoni Infections. Nature 1951 Mar 17;167(4246):447-448.]
6.) Emerson, Charles Phillip. Clinical diagnosis: a textbook of clinical microscopy and clinical chemistry for medical students, laboratory workers, and practitioners of medicine. 4th Edition. 1913 JB Lippencott Co.
7.) Bai Xiaodong. Insect transmitted plant pathogenic mollicutes, Spiroplasma kunkelii and aster yellows witches' broom phytoplasma: from structural genomics to functional genomics. Vii, 232 p. [web page]
8.) Schmid George P, Steere Allen C, Kornblatt Arnold N, Kaufmann Arnold F, Moss C. Wayne, Johnson Russell C, Hovind-Hougen Kari, Brenner Don J. Newly Recognized Leptospira Species ("Leptospira inadai" serovar lyme) Isolated from Human Skin. J Clin Microbiol. 1986 Sept.;24(3):484-486.
9.) Evans Alfred S, Brachman Philip S. (eds.) Bacterial infections of humans: epidemiology and control. Third edition. 1998 Kluwer Academic/Plenum Publishers, NY.
10.) Barbour AG. Isolation and cultivation of Lyme disease spirochetes. Yale J Biol Med. 1984 Jul-Aug;57(4):521-5.
11.) Burgdorfer Willy, Barbour Alan G., Hayes Stanley F., Benach Jorge L., Grunwaldt Edgar, Davis Jeffrey P. Lyme Disease – A Tick-borne Spirocheosis? Science 1982Jun;216(18):1317-1319. Drs. Burgdorfer and Barbour were at the Rocky Mt. Lab in Hamilton, MT; Dr. Benach was at State University of New York (SUNY) Stony Brook; Dr. Grunwaldt was at Shelter Island, NY; Dr. Davis was at the Dept. of Health and Social Services, Madison, WI and is now a WI State Epidemiologist.
12.) The Encyclopaedia britannica. Eleventh Edition. Volume XX. 1910-1911. The Encyclopaedia Britannica Company, 1911, New York. Parasitic diseases. Page 770-792.
13.) Jones KL, Glickstein LJ, Damle N, Sikand VK, McHugh G, Steere AC. Borrelia burgdorferi genetic markers and disseminated disease in patients with early Lyme disease. J Clin Microbiol. 2006 Dec;44(12):4407-4413.
14.) Private conversation between the author and a producer of the Lyme disease documentary film *Under Our Skin,* September 2009.
15.) Wormser GP, Dattwyler RJ, Shapiro ED, et al. The Clinical Assessment, Treatment, and Prevention of Lyme Disease, Human Granulocytic Anaplasmosis, and Babesiosis: Clinical Practice Guidelines by the Infectious Diseases Society of America. Clinical Infectious Diseases. 2006;43:1089-1134.
16.) Blumenthal, Richard. Office of the Attorney General. The State of Connecticut. Connecticut Attorney General's Office Press Release. Attorney General's Investigation Reveals Flawed Lyme Disease Guideline Process, IDSA Agrees To Reassess Guidelines, Install Independent Arbiter. 2008 May 1. [web page]
17.) Grant 5R03TW000514-03. Lyme Borreliosis in Russia. Steere, Allen C. Grant award to New England Medical Center Hospitals, Boston, MA. Fiscal year 1997. Project start: 9/30/95ended 9/29/99. ICD: Fogarty International Center.
18.) Proceedings of the Second National Conference on Serologic Diagnosis of Lyme Disease. 1994Oct. 27-29, Dearborn, MI. 106pages. Sponsors: Assoc. of State and Territorial Public Health Laboratory Directors, US CDC and Prevention, MI Dept. of Health. Co-sponsors: USFDA, NIH, Council of State and Territorial Epidemiologists and National Committee for Clinical Laboratory Standards.
19.) Schmid GP, Steigerwalt AG, Johnson SE, Barbour AG, Steere AC, Robinson IM, Brenner DJ. DNA characterization of the spirochete that causes Lyme disease. J Clin Microbiol. 1984;20:155-158.
20.) Johnson Russell C, Schmid George P, Hyde Fred W, et al. Borrelia burgdorferi sp. nov.: Etiologic Agent of Lyme Disease. Inter J Syst Bacteriol. 1984 Oct;34(4):496-497.
21.) Steere AC, Grodzicki RL, Kornblatt AN, Kraft JE, Barbour AG, Burgdorfer W, Schmid GP, Johnson E, Malawista SE. The spirochetal Etiology of Lyme disease. N Engl J Med. 1983;308:733-740.
22.) Pershina MIu, Shaginian IA, Anan'ina IuV, Prozorovskiĭ SV. [Analysis of genomic polymorphism in leptospira by polymerase chain reaction with random primers] [Article in Russian]. Mol Gen Mikrobiol Virusol. 1998;(1):29-32.
23.) Woo TH, Patel BK, Smythe LD, et al. Identification of Leptospira inadai by continuous monitoring of fluorescence during rapid cycle PCR. Syst Appl Microbiol. 1998Mar;21(1):89-96. [abstract]
24.) Brenner DJ, Kaufmann AF, Sulzer KR, et al. Further determination of DNA relatedness between serogroups and serovars in the family Leptospiraceae with a proposal for Leptospira alexanderi sp. nov. and four new Leptospira genomospecies. Inter J Syst Bacteriol. 1999;49:839-858.
25.) Esser RP, El-Gholl NE. Harposporium, a fungus that parasitizes and kills nematodes utilizing conidia swallowed by or sticking to its prey. Nematol Circular No. 200. 1992Jul-Aug. FL Department of Agriculture & Consumer Services Div. of Plant Industry. 6 pages.
26.) Adler Ben, Faine Solly. Leptospira. 2010 Mar 15. Epub. Copley and Wilson's Microbiology and Microbial Infections. [web page]
27.) Hovind-Hougen K, Ellis W, Birch-Andersen A. Leptospira parva sp. npv.: some morphological and biological characters. Zentralbl Bakteriol Mikrobiol Hyg A. 1981 Sep;250(3):343-354.
28.) Levett PN, Morey RE, Galloway R, Steigerwalt AG, Ellis WA. Reclassification of Leptospira parva Hovind-Hougen et al. 1982as Turneriella parva gen. nov., comb. Nov. Int J Syst Evol Microbiol. 2005 Jul;55(Pt 4):1497-1499.
29.) Burgdorfer Willy. Discovery of the Lyme Disease Spirochete and Its Relation to Tick Vectors. Yale J Biology and Medicine. 1984;57:515-520.
30.) Yasuda PH et al. Deoxyribonucleic acid relatedness between serogroups and serovars in the family leptospiraceae with proposals for seven new leptospira species. Int J Syst Bacteriol. 1987;37:407-415.
31.) US Patent 5,945,586. Steiger et al. Soybean variety 93B01. Filed 2/13/98 published 8/31/99. Assignee: Pioneer Hi-Bred International, Inc. (Des Moines, IA).
32.) Plant & Soil Sciences Library. Gene Expression Part 1: Reading Genes to Make Proteins. [web page]
33.) US Patent 4,888,172. Szebenyi, et al. Pharmaceutical for treating tumors and methods for making it. Filed 9/17/85 published 12/19/89. Assignee: Alfaceu Corporation (Bloomfield, NJ).
34.) US Patent 5,659,026. Baszczynski et al. ALS3 promoter. Field 3/24/95 published 8/19/97. Assignee: Pioneer Hi-Bred International (Des Moines, IA).
35.) US Patent 4,970,224. Jacobson et al. 1-dimethylcarbamoyl-3-substituted-5-substituted-1H-1,2,4-triazzoles. Filed 4/15/88 published 11/13/90. Assignee: Rohm and Haas Company (Philadelphia, PA).
36.) US Patent 3,308,131. McKusick. Tertiary Carbamyl Triazoles. Filed 7/9/64 published 5/7/67. Assignee: E.I. du Pont de Nemours and Company.
37.) Willy Burgdorfer, Edgar G. Pickens. A Technique Employing Embryonated Chicken Eggs for the Infection of Argasid Ticks with Coxiella burnetti, Bacterium tularense, Leptospira icterohaemorrhagiae, and Western Equine Encephalitis Virus. 1954Jan-Feb;94(1):84-89.

38.) Willy Burgdorfer. The Possible Role of Ticks as Vectors of Leptospirae. I. Transmission of Leptospira Pomona by the Argasid Tick, Ornithodoros turicata, and the Persistance of This Organism in Its Tissues. Exper. Parasitol. 1956:571-579.
39.) Willy Burgdorfer. Artificial Feeding of Ixodid Ticks for Studies on the Transmission of Disease Agents. J Infect Dis. 1957 Jun;100(3):212-214.

The Secret Agent

1.) Tully JG, Whitcomb RF, Rose DL, Williamson DL, Bové JM. Characterization and taxonomic status of tick spiroplasmas: a review. Yale J Biol Med. 1983Sep-Dec;56(5-6):599-603.
2.) US Patent 5,296,371. Razin et al. DNA encoding spiroplasma sp. dna methylase. Filed 10/4/91, published 3/22/94. Assignee not listed. Inventors from Jerusalem, Illinois.
3.) Pickens Edgar G, Gerloff Robert K, Burgdorfer Willy. Spirochete from the Rabbit Tick, Haemaphysalis leporispalustris (Packard). I. Isolation and Preliminary Characterization. J Bacteriol. 1968 Feb;95(2):291-299.
4.) O'Leary William Michael. Practical handbook of microbiology. 1977 Condensed version of CRC handbook of microbiology. CRC Press LLC. (Boca Raton, FL). Laskin AI, Lechevalier HA (ed). 2nd ed.
5.) Grant 1Z01AI000062-06. Cellular and Subcellular Aspects of Vector-Pathogen Relationships. No school listed. Fiscal year 1975. National Institute of Allergy and Infectious Diseases. (NIAID)
6.) Grant 1Z01AI000062-07. Cellular and Subcellular Aspects of Vector-Pathogen Relatinoships. No school listed. Fiscal year 1977. NIAID.
7.) Williamson DL, Tully JG, Whitcomb RF. Serological Relationships of Spiroplasmas as Shown by Combined Deformation and Metabolism Inhibition Tests. Inter J System Bacteriol. 1979 Oct;29(4):345-351.
8.) Whitcomb RF, Tully JG, Clark TB, et al. Revised Serological Classification of Spiroplasmas, New Provisional Groups, and Recommendations for Serotyping of Isolates. Curr Microbiol. 1982;7:291-296.
9.) Davis RE et al. Spiroplasma floricola, a new species isolated from surfaces of flowers of the tulip tree, Liriodendron tulipifera L. Int J Syst Bacteriol. 1981;32:456-464.
10.) Whitcomb RF, Tully JG, Clark TB et al. Revised Serological Classification of Spiroplasmas, New provisional Groups, and Recommendations for Serotyping Isolates. Curr Microbiol. 1982;7:291-296.
11.) US Patent 3,837,834. Hill et al. Plant Regulator Compositions and Method. Filed 6/19/72 published 9/24/74. Assignee: FMC Corporation (New York.)
12.) FMC Corporation web site.
13.) US Patent 2,843,617. Kaufman. Dialkyl Propynyl Phosphonates. Filed 5/31/56 published 7/15/58. Assignee: Monsanto Chemical Company, St. Louis, MO.
14.) US Patent 2,882,304. Weber. Production of Organic Phosphonyl Halide. Filed 10/30/53 published 4/14/59. Assignee: M.W. Kellogg Company, Jersey City, NJ.
15.) US Patent 2,898,300. Norton et al. High Temperature Lubricating Greases. Filed 4/25/57 published 8/4/59. Assignee: Esso Research and Engineering Company, DE.
16.) US Patent 2,927,014. Goyette. Method for Killing Plants. Filed 2/14/57 published 3/1/60. Assignee: Virginia-Carolina Chemical Corporation, Richmond, VA.
17.) US Patent 3,094,405. Toy et al. Defoliant methods using thio esters of Chloromethyl Phosphonous and Chloromethyl Phosphonic Acids. Filed 2/8/61 published 6/18/63. Assignee: Stauffer Chemical Company, New York.
18.) US Patent 3,209,020. Schraeder. Thiophosphonic acid esters containing at least one S-alkyl Group. Filed 9/29/61 published 9/28/65. Assignee: Farbenfabriken Bayer Aktiengesellschaft, Leverkusen, Germany.
19.) US Patent 3,346,669. Regel. Halo-Phosphorus Compounds and Process for their preparation. Filed 4/6/64 published 10/10/67. Assignee: Chemagro Corporation, Kansas City, MO.
20.) US Patent 5,082,485. Evans. Treatment for prevention for oak wilt disease or decline. Filed 10/5/88 published 1/21/92. Assignee: David W. Evans, Kerrville, TX.

The Secret Agent

1.) Tully JG, Whitcomb RF, Rose DL, Williamson DL, Bové JM. Characterization and taxonomic status of tick spiroplasmas: a review. Yale J Biol Med. 1983Sep-Dec;56(5-6):599-603.
2.) US Patent 5,296,371. Razin et al. DNA encoding spiroplasma sp. dna methylase. Filed 10/4/91, published 3/22/94. Assignee not listed. Inventors from Jerusalem, Illinois.
3.) Pickens Edgar G, Gerloff Robert K, Burgdorfer Willy. Spirochete from the Rabbit Tick, Haemaphysalis leporispalustris (Packard). I. Isolation and Preliminary Characterization. J Bacteriol. 1968 Feb;95(2):291-299.
4.) O'Leary William Michael. Practical handbook of microbiology. 1977 Condensed version of CRC handbook of microbiology. CRC Press LLC. (Boca Raton, FL). Laskin AI, Lechevalier HA (ed). 2nd ed.
5.) Grant 1Z01AI000062-06. Cellular and Subcellular Aspects of Vector-Pathogen Relationships. No school listed. Fiscal year 1975. National Institute of Allergy and Infectious Diseases.
6.) Grant 1Z01AI000062-07. Cellular and Subcellular Aspects of Vector-Pathogen Relatinoships. No school listed. Fiscal year 1977. National Institute of Allergy and Infectious Diseases.
7.) Williamson DL, Tully JG, Whitcomb RF. Serological Relationships of Spiroplasmas as Shown by Combined Deformation and Metabolism Inhibition Tests. Inter J System Bacteriol. 1979 Oct;29(4):345-351.
8.) Whitcomb RF, Tully JG, Clark TB, et al. Revised Serological Classification of Spiroplasmas, New Provisional Groups, and Recommendations for Serotyping of Isolates. Curr Microbiol. 1982;7:291-296.
9.) Davis RE et al. Spiroplasma floricola, a new species isolated from surfaces of flowers of the tulip tree, Liriodendron tulipifera L. Int J Syst Bacteriol. 1981;32:456-464.
10.) Whitcomb RF, Tully JG, Clark TB et al. Revised Serological Classification of Spiroplasmas, New provisional Groups, and Recommendations for Serotyping Isolates. Curr Microbiol. 1982;7:291-296.
11.) US Patent 3,837,834. Hill et al. Plant Regulator Compositions and Method. Filed 6/19/72 published 9/24/74. Assignee: FMC Corporation (New York.)
12.) FMC Corporation web site. www.fmc.com/
13.) US Patent 2,843,617. Kaufman. Dialkyl Propynyl Phosphonates. Filed 5/31/56 published 7/15/58. Assignee: Monsanto Chemical Company, St. Louis, MO.
14.) US Patent 2,882,304. Weber. Production of Organic Phosphonyl Halide. Filed 10/30/53 published 4/14/59. Assignee: M.W. Kellogg Company, Jersey City, NJ.
15.) US Patent 2,898,300. Norton et al. High Temperature Lubricating Greases. Filed 4/25/57 published 8/4/59. Assignee: Esso Research and Engineering Company, DE.
16.) US Patent 2,927,014. Goyette. Method for Killing Plants. Filed 2/14/57 published 3/1/60. Assignee: Virginia-Carolina Chemical Corporation, Richmond, VA.
17.) US Patent 3,094,405. Toy et al. Defoliant methods using thio esters of Chloromethyl Phosphonous and Chloromethyl Phosphonic Acids. Filed 2/8/61 published 6/18/63. Assignee: Stauffer Chemical Company, New York.
18.) US Patent 3,209,020. Schraeder. Thiophosphonic acid esters containing at least one S-alkyl Group. Filed 9/29/61 published 9/28/65. Assignee: Farbenfabriken Bayer Aktiengesellschaft, Leverkusen, Germany.
19.) US Patent 3,346,669. Regel. Halo-Phosphorus Compounds and Process for their preparation. Filed 4/6/64 published 10/10/67. Assignee: Chemagro Corporation, Kansas City, MO.
20.) US Patent 5,082,485. Evans. Treatment for prevention for oak wilt disease or decline. Filed 10/5/88 published 1/21/92. Assignee: David W. Evans, Kerrville, TX.
21.) Indiana State Tree. [web page]
22.) Australian Government Department of Agriculture, Fisheries and Forestry. Mangoes from India. Draft Revised Import Policy. 2004 July. 250 pg. [web page]
23.) Australia's Prime Ministers. National Archives of Australia. Timeline. Robert Menzies. [web page]
24.) Benjamin Clemins Masterman Stone. Pandanus tectorius var. heronensis (H. St. John ed.) in Bot J Linn Soc. 1982;85(2):138.
25.) REG Pichi Sermolli 1 March 1991, R.W. Kiger 11 July 1991, Barbara Parris' Fern List. Taxon. 1999;48(4):788. Biographical details incl. portr. In Iridos 2005;16(2):18-19.
26.) The International Plant Names Index. Author Details. Stone, Benjamin Clemens Masterman (1933-1994). [web page]
27.) Australian Government Cocos Islands Environment and Heritage. Geography and Climate. [web page]
28.) Williamson DL, Poulson DF. Sex ratio organisms (spiroplasmas) of Drosophila. 1979p. 175-208. In RF Whitcomb and JG Tully (ed.), The mycoplasmas, vol. 3. Academic Press, Inc. NY.
29.) Williamson DL. Whitcomb RF. Helical, wall-free prokaryotes in Drosophila, leafhoppers and plants. 1974 Colloq. INSERM 33:282-290.
30.) Parthasarathy MV. Mycoplasmalike organisms associated with lethal yellowing disease of palms. Phytopathology 1974;64:667-74.
31.) Agricultural Microbes Genome 2: First Glimpses into the Genomes of Plant-Associated Microbes. The Plant Cell. 2001 Mar;13:451-457.
32.) Nuclear test, Kiritimati (Christmas) Island. Museum of New Zealand, Te Papa Tongarewa. [web page]
33.) Farmer Brian. Families fight to sue over Christmas Island nuclear weapons tests. Manchester Evening News. UK newspaper & website. 2011 Nov 15. [web page]
34.) 1957: Britain drops its first H-bomb. On this day 15 May 1957. BBC News. [web page]

35.) Johnston Martin. Genetic damage found among N-test veterans. Genetic Engineering. New Zealand Herals. 2005 Sep 23. [monograph on the internet]
36.) Hua Q, Woodroffe CD, Smithers SG, Barbetti M, Fink D. Radiocarbon in corals from the Cocos (Keeling) Islands and implications for Indian Ocean circulation. Geophys Res Ltr. 2005;32(L21602). 4 pages.
37.) Bové JM, Mouches C, Carle-Junca P. et al. Spiroplasmas of Group I: The Spiroplasma citri Cluster. Yale J Biol Med. 1983;56:573-582.
38.) Junca P, Saillard C, Tully JG et al. Caractérisation de spirooplasmes isolés d'insectes et de fleurs de France continentale, de Course et du Maroc. Proposition pour une classification des spiroplasmes. CR Acad Sci (Paris) 1980;Ser D 290:1209-1212.
39.) Whitcomb Robert F. The Bioloogy of Spiroplasmas. Ann Rev Entomol. 1981;26:397-425.
40.) Clark HF. Suckling mouse cataract agent. J Infect Dis. 1964;114:476-487.
41.) Tully Joseph G, Rose David L, Yunker Conrad E, et al. Helical Mycoplasmas (Spiroplasmas) from Ixodes Ticks. Science 1981;212(4498):1043-1045.
42.) Tuomi J, Rantamäki LK, Tanskanen R, Junttila J. Characterization of Finnish Borrelia burgdorferi Sensu Lato Isolates by Sodium Dodecyl Sulfate-Polyacrylamide Gel Electrophoresis and with Monoclonal Antibodies. J Clin Microbiol. 1995 Aug;33(8):1989-1996.
43.) Sanderson Hans, Fauser Patrik, Thomsen Marianne. Environmental Hazards of Sea-Dumped Chemical Weapons. Environmental Science and Technology. [web site]
44.) Runner Philippa. EU mulls Baltic Sea strategy. 2009 May 2. Euobserver.com [web site]
45.) Hawley Charles. Europe's Underwater Chemical Dump. Tons of Mercury Found in the Baltic Sea. 2006 Aug 30. [Monograph on the Internet]
46.) Missiaen T, Feller P. Geophysical investigations of a chemical munition dumpsite in the Baltic Sea. 2008 May 27-29. [monograph]
47.) Surveying Ships Sunk Off North Carolina in World War II. 2009 Aug 13. ScienceDaily. [web page]
48.) Tully Joseph G, Rose David L, Yunker Conrad E, et al. Helical Mycoplasmas (Spiroplasmas) from Ixodes Ticks. Science 1981;212(4498):1043-1045.
49.) Tully JG, Whitcomb RF, Rose DL, et al. Yale 1983: Three serologically distinct groups of spiroplasmas have been recovered from ticks. Yale J Biol Med. 1983Sept-Dec;603.
50.) Tully JG, Whitcomb RF, Rose DL, et al. Characterization and Taxonomic Status of Tick Spiroplasmas: A Review. The Yale J Biol. Med. 1983;56:599-603.
51.) Megraud F, Gamon LB, McGarrity GJ. Characterization of Spiroplasma mirum (Suckling Mouse Cataract Agent) in a Rabbit Lens Cell Culture. Infect Immun. 1983 Dec;42(3):1168-1175.
52.) Tully JG, Rose DL, Yunker CE, et al. Spiroplasma ixodetis sp. nov., a New Species from Ixodes pacificus Ticks Collected in Oregon. Inter J System Bacteriol. 1995 Jan;45(1):23-28.
53.) Tenckhoff B, Kölmel HW, Wolf V, Lange R. Production and characterization of a polyclonal antiserum against Spiroplasma mirum (ATCC 29335). Zentralbl Bakteriol. 1994 Jan;280(3):409-415.
54.) Stanek G, Laber G, Hirschl A. Survival of spiroplasma on different carriers and resistance against three disinfectants. Proceedings of the 3rd International Organ. Mycoplasm. Custer, South Dakota, 1980 Sept. Abstract 107.
55.) Tully JG, Rose DL, Yunker CE, et al. Spiroplasma ixodetis sp. nov.,, a New Species from Ixodes pacificus Ticks Collected in Oregon. Inter J System Bacteriol. 1995Jan;45(1):23-28.
56.) Stanek Gerold. Behandlung der Lyme-Borreliose. [Treatment of Lyme Borreliosis]. [Article in German]. Antibiotika Monitor. 2009 May 6.
57.) Proceedings of the Second National Conference on Serologic Diagnosis of Lyme Disease. 1994 Oct. 27-29, Dearborn, MI. 106pages. Sponsors: Assoc. of State and Territorial Public Health Laboratory Directors, US CDC and Prevention, MI Dept. of Health. Co-sponsors: USFDA, NIH, Council of State and Territorial Epidemiologists and National Committee for Clinical Laboratory Standards.
58.) Alfred I. duPont Testamentary Trust. [web site]
59.) Williamson DL, Whitcomb RF, Tully JG, et al. Revised group classification of the genus Spiroplasma. Inter J Bacteriol. 1998;48:1-12.
60.) Steere Allen C, Broderick Thomas F, Malawista Stephen E. Erythema Chronicum Migrans and Lyme Arthritis: Epidemiologic Evidence for a Tick Vector. Am J Epidemiol. 1978;108(4):312-321.
61.) Reik Louis, Steere Allen C, Bartenhagen Nicholas H, Shope Robert E, Malawista Stephen E. Neurologic Abnormalities of Lyme Disease. Medicine. 1979;58(4):281-294.
62.) Steere AC, Hardin JA, Malawista SE. Lyme arthritis: serum cryoprecipitates associated with skin and joint lesion. Arthritis Rheum. 1977;20:136.
63.) Steere AC, Hardin JA, Malawista SE. Erythema chronicum migtans and Lyme arthritis: serum cryoimmunoglobulins and clinical activity of skin and joints. Science 1977;196:1121-1122.
64.) Shulman S, Witebsky E. The thyroid gland as source and target in autosensitization. Ann NY Acad Sci. 1960;86:400.
65.) US Patent 5,582,829. Alliger, et al. Sonicated borrelia burgdorferi vaccine. Filed July 28, 1992, published 12/10/96. Assignee: Rx Technologies, Inc. (Garden City, NY).
66.) Shulman S, Bronson P, Clelia Riera, Brandt Eva J, Yantorno C. Studies in Cryo-Immunology. III. The Immunoglobulin Nature of the Antibody Response. Immunol. 1968;14:541-551.
67.) Sugarman Michael, Stobie Dennis G, Quismorio Francisco P, Terry Roger, Hanson Virgil. Plant Thorn Synovitis. Arthritis & Rheumat. 2005 Nov 22;20(5):1125-1128.
68.) Johnston YE, Duray PH, Steere AC, Kashgarian M, Buza J, Malawista SE, Askenase PW. Lyme arthritis. Spirochetes found in synovial microangiopathic lesions. Am J Pathol. 1985 Jan;118(1):26-34.
69.) Gérard HC, Wang Z, Wang GF, et al. Chromosomal DNA From a Variety of Bacterial Species Is Present in Synovial Tissue From Patients With Various Forms of Arthritis. Arthrit Rheum. 2001 Jul;44(7):1689-1697.
70.) Gran JT, Hjetland R, Andraessen AH. Pneumonia, myocarditis, and reactive arthritis due to Chlamydia pneumonia. Scand J Rheumatol. 1993;22:43-44.
71.) Braun J, Laitko S, Treharne J, et al. Chlamydia pneumoniae – a new causative agent of reactive arthritis and undifferentiated oligoarthritis. Ann Rheum Dis. 1994;53:100-105.
72.) Beaudreuil J, Hayem G, Meyer O, et al. Reactive arthritis ascribed to Chlamydia pneumonia. Rev Rhum Engl Ed. 1995;3:222-224.
73.) Wilkinson NZ, Kingsley GH, Sieper J, et al. Lack of correlation between the detection of Chlamydia trachomatis DNA in synovial fluid from patients with a range of rheumatic diseases and the presence of an antichlamydial immune response. Arthritis Rheum. 1998;41:845-854.
74.) Schaeverbeke T, Gilroy CB, Bebear C, et al. Mycoplasma fermentans, but not M. penetrans, detected by PCR Assays in synovium from patients with rheumatoid arthritis and other rheumatic disorders. J Clin Pathol. 1996;49:824-828.
75.) Tully Joseph G, Whitcomb Robert F, Rose David L, Williamson David L, Bové Joseph M. Characterization and Taxonomic Status of Tick Spiroplasmas: A Review. The Yale Journal of Biology and Medicine 1983;56:599-603.
76.) Grant 1Z01AI000062-06. Cellular and Subcellular Aspects of Vector-Pathogen Relationships. No school listed. Fiscal year 1975. National Institute of Allergy and Infectious Diseases (NIAID)
77.) Grant 1Z01AI000062-07. Cellular and Subcellular Aspects of Vector-Pathogen Relationships. No school listed. Fiscal year 1977. NIAID.
78.) US Patent 7,122,715. Korte et al. In vitro method to create circular molecules for use in transformations. Filed 9/20/01 published 10/17/06. Assignee: Monsanto Technology LLC (St. Louis, MO).
79.) US Patent 5,015,580. Hinchey et al. Maize cytoplasmic glutamine synthetase promoter compositions and methods for use thereof. Filed 11/20/01 published 11/21/06. Assignee: Monsanto Technology, LLC (St. Louis, MO).
80.) Tilly Kit, Lubke Lori, Rosa Patricia. Characterization of Circular Plasmid Dimers in Borrelia burgdorferi. J Bacteriol. 1998 Nov;180(21):5676-5681.

Drink To Our Health

1.) Bové JM, Mouches C, Carle-Junca P. et al. Spiroplasmas of Group I: The Spiroplasma citri Cluster. Yale J Biol Med. 1983;56:573-582.
2.) Junca P, Saillard C, Tully JG et al. Caractérisation de spirooplasmes isolés d'insectes et de fleurs de France continentale, de Course et du Maroc. Proposition pour une classification des spiroplasmes. CR Acad Sci (Paris) 1980;Ser D 290:1209-1212.
3.) Tully JG, Whitcomb RF, Bové JM et al. Plant mycoplasmas: serological relation between agents associated with citrus stubborn and corn stunt diseases. Science 1973;182:827-829.
4.) Clark HF, Rorke LB. Spiroplasmas of tick origin and their pathogenicity. In The Mycoplasmas, Volume 3. Plant and Insect Mycoplasmas. Whitcomb RF, Tully JG (ed.) New York, Academic Press. 1979:155-174.
5.) Zeigel RF, Clark HF. Electron microscopy of the suckling mouse cataract agent, a noncultivable animal pathogen possibly related to mycoplasma. Infect Immun. 1974;9:430-443.
6.) Junca P, Saillard C, Tully JG et al. Caractérisation de spirooplasmes isolés d'insectes et de fleurs de France continentale, de Course et du Maroc. Proposition pour une classification des spiroplasmes. CR Acad Sci (Paris) 1980;Ser D 290:1209-1212.
7.) Head Elizabeth. The Oleander – From Whence Came Thee. International Oleander Society. 2011 Nov 23. [web page]
8.) Oleander (Nerium Oleander) Adelfa. [web page]
9.) USDA Agricultural Research Service database. [web page]

10.) PD/GWSS Board Bulletin. Newsletter of the California Department of Food and Agriculture. 2007 Spring. [web page]
11.) Pierce's Disease. About Pierce's Disease. [web page]
12.) Foreign Agricultural Service. Horticultural & Tropical Products Division. 2002 Apr. The US Peach & Nectarine Industry Situation. [web page]
13.) South Carolina Department of Agriculture. Historical Retrospective of SC's Peach Industry. [web page]
14.) Purdue University. Purdue Fruit and Vegetable Connection. Peaches [web page]
15.) University of California Agriculture and Natural Resources. Bordeaux Mixture. [web page]
16.) The Great French Wine Blight. Wine Tidings 1986 Jul-Aug;96. The Wampum Keeper. [web page]
17.) PD/GWSS Board Bulletin. Newsletter of the California Department of Food and Agriculture. 2007 spring. [web page]
18.) Pierce's Disease. About Pierce's Disease. [web page]
19.) Tennekes Henk A. The significance of the Druckrey-Küpfmüller equation for risk assessment. The toxicity of neonicotinoid insecticides to arthropods is reinforced by exposure time. Toxicol. 2010. [web page]
20.) US Environmental Protection Agency. Pesticides: Registration Review. 2011 Feb. [web page]
21.) Syngenta. Cruiser Exploring the Thiamethoxam Vigor Effect. [web page]
22.) Los Alamos National Laboratory. [web page]
23.) Los Alamos National Security, LLC. [web page]
24.) Agricultural Microbes Genome 2: First Glimpses into the Genomes of Plant-Associated Microbes. The Plant Cell. 2001 Mar;13:451-457.
25.) Moreira LM, DeSouza RF, Digiampietri LA, et al. Comparative Analyses of Xanthomonas and Xylella Complete Genomes. J Integrat Biol. 2005 Spring;9(1):43-76.
26.) US Patent 7,432,419Gupta. Compositions and methods for the treatment of Pierce's disease. Assignee Los Alamos National Security, LLC (Los Alamos, MN). Filed 5/14/04, published 10/7/08.
27.) Kamoun Sophien, Hogenhout Saskia A. Agricultural Microbes Genome 2: First Glimpses into the Genomes of Plant-Associated Microbes. Amer Soc Plant Biologists. The Plant Cell;2001 Mar;13:451-457.
28.) Garcia R, Gusmani L, Murgia R, et al. Elastase is the only Human Neutrophil Granule Protein that alone is Responsible for In Vitro killing of Borrelia burgdorferi. Infect Immun. 1998;66:1408-1412.
29.) Ruth R. Montgomery, Denise Lusitani, Anne de Boisfleury Chevance, Stephen E. Malawista. Tick Saliva Reduces Adherence and Area of Human Neutrophils. Infect Immun. 2004 May;72(5):2989-2994.
30.) Glassy-winged Sharpshooter. Fact Sheet. [web page]
31.) Furukawa T, Sasaoka T, Hosoya Y. Effects of tetrodotoxin on the neuromuscular junction. Jpn J Physiol. 1959 Jun 25;9(2):143-152.
32.) Firth AL, Remillard CV, Platoshyn O, et al. Functional ion channels in human pulmonary artery smooth muscle cells: Voltage-dependent cation channels. Pulm Circ. 2011 Jan 1;(1):48-71.
33.) Sahraian MA, Maghzi AH, Etemadifar M, Minagar A. Dalfampridine: Review of its Efficacy in Improving Gait in Patients with Multiple Sclerosis. J Centrl Nerv Sys Dis. 2011;3:87-93.
34.) US Patent 4,950,739. Cherksey et al. Membrane calcium channels and factors and methods for blocking, isolating and purifying calcium channels. Filed 7/14/88 published 8/21/90. Assignee: New York University (New York, NY).
35.) US Patent 5,064,657. Hunter Jackson et al. Spider toxins and methods for their use as blockers of amino acid receptor function. Filed 5/11/90 published 11/12/91. Assignee: University of Utah (Salt Lake City, UT).
36.) US Patent 5,461,032. Krapcho et al. Insecticidally effective peptides. Filed 3/18/94 published 10/24/95. Assignee: FMC Corporation and NPS Pharmaceuticals Inc.

Morgellon's: Another Multi-Factored Infection

1.) Schulte, Brigid. Figments of the Imagination?" Washington Post Magazine: 2008 Jan 20;pp. W10. [web page]
2.) Morgellon's Research Foundation web site. www.morgellons.org and CDC. Unexplained Dermopathy (also called "Morgellons"). [web page]
3.) Savely VR, Stricker RB. Morgellons disease: Analysis of a population with clinically confirmed microscopic subcutaneous fibers of unknown etiology. Clin Cosmet Investig Dermatol. 2010 May 13;3:67-78.
4.) Skinner Charles E, Emmons Chester W, Tsuchiya Henry M. Henrici's Molds, Yeasts and Actinomycetes - A Handbook for Students of Bacteriology. Second Ed. John Wiley & Sons, London. 1945.
5.) NowPublic. "Worms-Under-Skin" Disease Puzzles Scientists. 2008 May 16. [monograph on the Internet]
6.) CDC. Press Briefing Transcripts. CDC to Launch Study on Unexplained Illness. 2008 Jan 16.
7.) Schoeck RJ. Sir Thomas Browne and the Republic of Letters: Introduction. Engl Lang Notes. 1982;19(4):299-312.
8.) Shaw AB. Vicary Lecture, 1977. Sir Thomas Browne: the man and the physician. Ann R Coll Surg Engl. 1978 July;60(4):336-344.
9.) Huntley Frank Livingstone. The Occasion and Date of Sir Thomas Browne's "A Letter to a Friend". Modern Philology. 1951 Feb;48(3):157-171.
10.) Allwords.com English Dictionary definitions. Morgellons. [web page]
11.) Kellett CE. Sir Thomas Browne and the Disease Called the Morgellons. Annals of Medical History. 1935;VII:467-479.
12.) Coghlan Avril. Nematode genome evolution. WormBook. *C. elegans*. 15 pages, Dublin, Ireland. [web page]
13.) Shapiro-Ilan DI, Byron GA, Gaugler R. Nematodes. (Rhabditida: Steinernematidae & Heterorhabditidae). [web page]
14.) USDA. How to Identify and Manage Pine Wilt Disease and Treat Wood Products Infested by the Pinewood Nematodes. [web page]
15.) Jaroslav Weiser. Diseases of Insects of Medical Importance in Europe. WHO Bulletin. 1963;28:121-127.
16.) Burges HD, Hussey NW. Microbial Control of Insects and Mites. 1971 Academic Press London.
17.) Reuther Walter, Calavan E. Clair, Carman Glenn E. (ed). The Citrus Industry, Volume IV. Crop Protection. Diseases and Injuries; Viruses; Registration, Certification, Indexing; Regulatory Measures; Vertebrate Pests; Biological Control of Insects; Nematodes. Revised Edition. 1978 University of California Div. of Agricultural Sciences. The Regents of the University of California.
18.) US Patent 7,396,536. Chandrashekar, et al. Parasitic helminth cuticlin proteins and uses thereof. Filed 6/9/04, published 6/8/08. Inventors: Chandrashekar R and Morales TH (Ft. Collins, CO). Assignee; Heska Corp. (Loveland, CO).
19.) Kaya Harry K. Infectivity of Neoaplectana carpocapsae and Heterorhabditis heliothidis to pupae of the parasite Apanteles militaris. J. Nematol. 1978 Jul;10(3):241-244.
20.) The Silk Industry of Lyon, A Fabric Collector's Diary. [web page]
21.) Jash Botanicals. Demodex Folliculorum – The Unseen Culprit? [web page]
22.) Amin OM. In Their Own Words. Or: Symptoms of Morgellons and Neuro-cutaneous Syndrome (Ncs) Upon First Examination at the Parasitology Center, Inc. (Pcl). Explore 2010;19(2). [web page]
23.) Johnson GW, Hogg R. The Journal of Horticulture, Cottage Gardener, Country Gentleman, Bee-Keeper, and Poultry Chronicle. Journal of Horticulture, 1868 Jul 30; Vol. XL, pp. 87-88. London.
24.) Morgellon's Disease: Mysterious Ecto-Parasites. [monograph on the Internet]
25.) US Patent 3,987,169. Maurer, et al. S-[O-alkyl-isoureido-carbonylmethyl]-(thiono) (di)thiolphosphoric(phosphonic) acid esters and ester-amides. Filed 9/18/75, issued 10/19/76. Assignee: Bayer Aktiengesellschaft (DT).
26.) Bird mite characteristics. [web page]
27.) Todar's Online Textbook of Bacteriology. Pseudomonas aeruginosa. [web page]
28.) Charles E. Holman Foundation. Morgellon's Disease Fiber Analysis. [web page]
29.) Leclercq J, lardet L, Martin F, et al. The green fluorescent protein as an efficient selection marker for Agrobacterium tumefaciens-mediated transformation in Hevea brasiliensis (Müll. Arg). Plant Cell Rep. 2010 May;29(5):513-522.
30.) Langhoff PJ. God Science: The Secret World of Rampant Genetics, Hidden Illness, and Biotech Profiteering. Allegory Press LLC. 2011. Hustisford, WI.
31.) US Patent 6,232,270. Branly et al. Agricultural compositions containing bacteria. Filed 11/29/96 published 5/15/01. Assignee: Micro Flo Company (Memphis, TN).
32.) US Patent 2,921,410 Merritt. Cotton Seed Treatment and Composition, Using Gibberellin and Fungicide. Filed 12/11/57 published 1/19/60. Assignee: Merck & Co., Inc.

Rahway, NJ.
33.) US Patent 5,171,505. Lock. Process for spinning polypeptide fibers. Filed 11/28/90 published 12/15/92. Assignee: E.I. du Pont de Nemours and Company (Wilmington, DE).
34.) US Patent R22,650. Bley. Fibroin Spinning Solutions. Filed 2/7/39 published 6/12/45. Assignee: North American Rayon Corporation, New York.
35.) Chilton MD, Drummond MH, Merio DJ, Sciaky D, Montoya AL, Gordon MP, Nester EW., Stable incorporation of plasmid DNA into higher plant cells: the molecular basis of crown gall tumorigenesis, Cell. 1977 Jun;11(2):263-71.
36.) Chan JWYF, Ramey WD, Moore LW, Bell CR. Potential of Agrobacterium tumefaciens and Octopine-Utilizing Fluorescent *Pseudomonas* Strains To Attach to Susceptible Potato Tissues. Appl Environ Microbiol. 1990 September; 56(9): 2826–2833.
37.) Dewan P, Miller J, Musters C et al. Delusional infestation with unusual pathogens: a report of three cases. Clin Exp Dermatol. 2011 Oct;36(7):745-8.
38.) US Patent 4,771,002. Gelvin. Transcription in plants and bacteria. Filed 2/24/84 published 9/13/88. Assignee: Lubrizol Genetics, Inc. (Wickliffe, OH).
39.) Hannes Melasniemi, Anne Hernesmaa. Yeast spores seem to be involved in biological phosphate removal: a microscopic in situ case study. Microbiol. 2000;146:701-707.
40.) Fan Y, Fang W, Guo S, et al. Increased Insect Virulence in Beauveria bassiana Strains Overexpressing an Engineered Chitinase. Amer Soc Microbiol. 2007Jan;73(1):295-302.
41.) Great Vista Chemicals. Chitin. [web site]. www.greatvistachemicals.com
42.) Bokura H, Kobayashi S. Chitosan decreases total cholesterol in women: a randomized, double-blind, placebo-controlled trial Eur J Clin Nutrit. 2003;57:721-725.
43.) Pierre Jollès, Muzzarelli Riccardo AA. (eds.) Chitin and Chitinases. 1999. Birkhäuser.
44.) US Patent 4,940,840. Suslow, et al. Novel chitinase-producing bacteria and plants. Filed 7/18/86 published 7/10/90. Assignee: DNA Plant Technology Corporation (Mt. Kisco, NY).
45.) Burgess HD, Hussey NW. Microbial Control of Insects and Mites. 1971 Academic Press (London).
46.) US Patent 3,890,198. Kobayashi, et al. Cell wall-lysing complex enzymes and a process for the production thereof. Filed 12/14/72 published 6/17/75. Assignee: Kumiai Chemical Industry Co., Ltd. (Tokyo, JA).
47.) US Patent 6,521,454. Becnel, et al. Baculoviruses, insecticidal compositions, and methods for control of invertebrates. Filed 6/30/99 published 2/18/03. Assignee: The United States of America, as represented by the Secretary of Agriculture (Washington, DC).
48.) US Patent 4,911,913. Hostetter, et al. Multiple embedded nuclear polyhedrosis virus from celery looper with activity against lepidoptera. Filed 3/7/89 published 3/27/90. Assignee: The United States of America as represented by the Secretary of (unmarked, probably Agriculture) (Washington, DC).
49.) US Patent 3,911,110. Smirnoff. Insecticidal compositions. Filed 12/22/72 published 10/7/75. Assignee: Canadian Patents and Development Limited (Ottawa, CA).
50.) Mah et al. A Genetic Basis for Pseudomonas aeruginosa Biofilm Antibiotic Resistance. Nature. 2003;426:306-310.
51.) Kielty CM, Baldock C, Lee D, Rock MJ, Ashworth JL, Shuttleworth CA (February 2002) Fibrillin: from microfibril assembly to biomechanical function. Philos. Trans. R. Soc. Lond., B, Biol. Sci. 2002;357(1418): 207–217.
52.) Bergey David Hendricks, Boone David R. Bergey's manual of systematic bacteriology, 2nd Edition, Volume 3. The Firmicutes. 2009
53.) Johnson GW, Hogg R. The Journal of Horticulture, Cottage Gardener, Country Gentleman, Bee-Keeper, and Poultry Chronicle. Journal of Horticulture, 1868 Jul 30; Vol. XL, pp. 87-88. London
54.) US Patent 5,171,505. Lock. Process for spinning polypeptide fibers. Filed 11/28/90 published 12/15/92. Assignee: E.I. du Pont de Nemours and Company (Wilmington, DE)
55.) US Patent 7,157,615. Karatzas et al. Production of biofilaments in transgenic animals. Filed 3/17/98 published 1/2/07. Assignee: Nexia Biotechnologies, Inc. (Montreal).
56.) Bates Daniel. Making science-fiction a reality: Bulletproof human skin made from spider silk and goat milk developed by researchers. Mailonline. 2011 Aug 16.
57.) US Patent 3,835,176. Matsuo et al. Alpha-Cyanobenzyl Cyclopropanecarboxylates. Filed 6/26/72 published 9/10/74. Assignee: Sumitomo Chemical Company, Limited (Osaka, JA).
58.) US Patent 4,053,625. Insecticides. Filed 11/24/75 published 10/11/77. Assignee: Sumitomo Chemical Company, Limited (Osaka, JA).
59.) US Patent 5,245,012. Lombari, et al. Method to achieve solubilization of spider silk proteins. Filed 9/29/92 published 9/14/93. Assignee: The United States of America as represented by the Secretary of the Army (Washington, DC).
60.) US Patent RE21,454. Bley. Fibroin Spinning Solutions. Filed 1/20/36 published 5/21/40. Assignee: North American Rayon Corporation, New York, NY.
61.) Daly R, Hearn MT. Expression of heterologous proteins in Pichia pastoris: a useful experimental tool in protein engineering and production. J Mol Recognit. 2005;18(2):119-138.
62.) Life technologies. pPICZα A, B, C. Invitrogen™ [web page]
63.) US Patent 6,268,169 Fahnestock. Recombinantly produced spider silk. Filed 6/15/94 published 7/31/01. Assignee: E. I. du Pont de Nemours and Company (Wilmington, DE).
64.) Lazaris et al. Spider Silk Fibers Spun From Soluble Recombinant Silk Produced in Mammalian Cells. Science. 2002;295:472-476.
65.) Lee et al. Virus-Based Fabrication of Micro- and Nanofibers Using Electrospinnig. Nano Letters. 2004;4(3):387-390.
66.) Kaplan. Fibrous Proteins-Silk as A Model System. Polymer Degradation and Stability. 1998;59:25-32.
67.) US Patent 6,268,169. Fahnestock. Recombinantly produced spider silk. Filed 12/11/95 published 7/31/01. Assignee: EI du Pont de Nemours and Company (Wilmington, DE).
68.) Mondal M, Trivedy K, Nirmal Kumar S. The silk proteins, sericin and fibroin in silkworm, Bombyx mori Linn., a review. Caspian J Env Sci. 2007;5:63-76 [web page]
69.) Houssay AB, Arias NH, Davison TA, Epper CE. Effects of prostaglandins upon hair growth in mice. Acta Physiol Lat Am. 1976;26(3):186-91.
70.) Johnstone MA, Albert DM. Prostaglandin-induced hair growth. Surv Ophthalmol. 2002 Aug;47 Suppl 1:S185-202.
71.) Brockett LP. The Silk Industry in America. A History: Prepared for the Centennial Exposition. 1876. George F. Nesbitt & Co. Printers NY
72.) US Patent 6,127,146. Lal, et al. Human fibrous protein. Filed 3/3/98 published 10/3/00. Assignee: Incyte Pharmaceuticals, Inc. (Palo Alto, CA).
73.) US Patent 7,041,797. Vollrath. Precursor silk feedstock for forming filaments. Filed 10/28/02 published 5/9/06. Assignee: Spin'Tec Engineering GmbH (Fellbach, DE)
74.) US Patent 4,771,002. Gelvin. Transcription in plants and bacteria. Filed 2/24/84 published 9/13/88. Assignee: Lubrizol Genetics, Inc. (Wickliffe, OH).
75.) US Patent 5,495,070. John. Genetically engineering cotton plants for altered fiber. Filed 5/18/92, published 2/27/96. Assignee: Agracetus, Inc. Middleton, WI.
76.) Firoozabady, E. et al., Transformation of Cotton (Gossypium hirsetum L.) by Agrobacterium Tumefaciens and Regeneration of Transgenic Plants. Plant Molecular Bio. 1987;10:105-116.
77.) Umbeck, P. et al., Genetically Transformed Cotton (Gossypium hirsutum L.) Plants. Bio/Technology 1987;5:3:263-266.
78.) US Patent 5,004,863. Umbeck. Genetic engineering of cotton plants and lines. Filed 12/3/86 published 4/2/91. Assignee: Agracetus (Middleton, WI).
79.) Roeske CA, Widholm JM, Ogren WL. Photosynthetic Carbon Metabolism in Photoautotrophic Cell Suspension Cultures Grown at Low and High CO2[1]. Plant Physiol. 1989;91:1512-1519.
80.) Schulte, Brigid. Figments of the Imagination?" Washington Post Magazine: 2008 Jan 20;pp. W10. [web page]
81.) Morgellon's Research Foundation web site. www.morgellons.org and CDC. Unexplained Dermopathy (also called "Morgellons"). [web page]
82.) Lacey N, Delaney S, Kavanagh K, Powell FC. Mite-related bacterial antigens stimulate inflammatory cells in rosacea. British J Dermatol. 2007 Sept;157(3):474-481.
83.) Heyndrckx M, Coorevits A, Scheldeman P. et al. Emended descriptions of Bacillus sporothermodurans and Bacillus oleronius with the inclusion of dairy farm isolates of both species. Int J Syst Evol Microbiol. 2011 Mar 11. [Epub ahead of print].

Trouble Ahead for Biocides and Animal Vaccines

1.) US Patent 3,709,782. Smith et al. Heterploid Cell Lines. Filed 10/3/69, issued 1/9/73. Assignee: Burroughs Wellcome Co., Research Triangle Park, NC.
2.) Clark TB. Spiroplasma sp. a new pathogen in honey bees. J Inverteb Pathol 1977;29:112-113.
3.) Williamson DL, Poulson DF. Sex ratio organisms (spiroplasmas) of Drosophila. 1979 p. 175-208. In RF Whitcomb and JG Tully (ed.), The mycoplasmas, vol. 3. Academic Press, Inc. NY.
4.) US Patent 4,447,537. Yunker, et al. Tick Cell Lines. Filed 1/22/81, issued 5/8/84. Assignee: The USA as represented by the Dept. of Health (Washington, DC)
5.) Varma MGR, Pudney Mary, Leake CJ. The Establishment of Three Cell Lines from the Tick Rhipicephalus appendiculatus (Acari: Ixodidae) and Their Infection with Some Arboviruses. J Med Entomol. 1975 Jan;11(6):698-706.
6.) US Patent 2,658,021. Earle. Single Tissue Cell Culturing Procedure. Filed 11/30/49 published 11/3/53. Assignee: United States of America as represented by the Administrator of the Federal Security Agency.
7.) US Patent 3,647,633. Dawson. Apparatus for the Continuous phased culturing of cells. Filed 8/16/68 published 3/7/72. Assignee: Canadian Patents and Development Limited, Ottawa, Ontario, Canada.
8.) US Patent 4,017,631. Janssen, et al. Imadazolium salts. Filed 3/1/76 published 4/12/77. Assignee: Janssen Pharmaceutica N.V. (Beerse, BE).
9.) US Patent 4,021,302. Smith et al. Cell cultures. Filed 8/20/75 published 5/3/77. Assignee: Burroughs Wellcome & Co., Inc. (Tuckahoe, NY).
10.) US Patent 4,040,905. Petricciani et al. Sub-human primate diploid cell lines as substrates for virus vaccine production. Filed 10/27/71 published 8/9/77. Assignee: The United

States Government (Washington, DC).
11.) US Patent 3,709,782. Smith et al. Heterpoloid Cell Lines. Filed 10/3/69 published 1/9/73. Assignee: Burroughs Wellcome Co., Research Triangle Park, NC.
12.) US Patent 4,447,537. Yunker, et al. Tick Cell Lines. Filed 1/22/81, issued 5/8/84. Assignee: The USA as represented by the Dept. of Health (Washington, DC).
13.) Varma MGR, Pudney Mary, Leake CJ. The Establishment of Three Cell Lines from the Tick Rhipicephalus appendiculatus (Acari: Ixodidae) and Their Infection with Some Arboviruses. J Med Entomol. 1975 Jan;11(6):698-706
14.) Presti RM, Zhao G, Beatty WL. Quaranfil,Johnston Atoll, and Lake Chad viruses are novel members of the family Orthomyxoviridae. J Virol. 2009 Nov;83(22):11599-11606.
15.) Work TH. Tick-borne Viruses. A Review of an Arthropod-borne Virus Problem of Growing Importance in the Tropics. WHO. Bulletin. 1963;29:59-74.
16.) US Patent 4,447,537. Yunker, et al. Tick Cell Lines. Filed 1/22/81, issued 5/8/84. Assignee: The USA as represented by the Dept. of Health (Washington, DC).
17.) Meyer P, Heidmann I, Niedenhof I. The use of African cassava mosaic virus as a vector system for plants. Gene. 1992 Jan 15;110(2):213-217.
18.) Eckholm Erik. French scientists report discovery of AIDS Virus in African Insects. The New York Times. 1986 Aug 27.
19.) Schneider Keith. AIDS-Like virus is Found at High Rate in US Cattle. The New York Times. 1991 June 1.
20.) Other Viruses May Activate Dormant AIDS Viruses. 1986 Dec 31.
21.) Toh H, Kikuno R, Hayashida H, et al. Close structural resemblance between putative polymerase of a Drosophila transposable genetic element 17.6 and pol gene product of Moloney murine leukaemia virus. The EMBO Journal. 1985;4(5):1267-1272.
22.) Coutts RHA, Buck KW. Cassava latent virus specific DNAs in mosaic diseased cassava of Nigerian origin. Neth J Pl Path. 1987;93:241-244.
23.) Gbadegesin MA, Wills MA, Beeching JR. Diversity of LTR-retrotransposons and Enhancer/Suppressor Mutator-like transposons in cassava (Manihot esculenta Crantz). Mol Genet Genomics. 2008Oct;280(4):305-317. Epub 2008 Jul 18.
24.) Espinoza AM, Usmany M, Pirone TP, et al. Expression of cauliflower mosaic virus ORF II in a baculovirus system. Intervirol 1992;34(1):1-12.
25.) US Patent 3,709,782. Smith et al. Heteroploid Cell Lines. Filed 10/3/69, issued 1/9/73. Assignee: Burroughs Wellcome Co., Research Triangle Park, NC.
26.) US Patent 4,447,537. Yunker, et al. Tick Cell Lines. Filed 1/22/81, issued 5/8/84. Assignee: The USA as represented by the Dept. of Health (Washington, DC).
27.) US Patent 3,709,782. Smith et al. Heterploid Cell Lines. Filed 10/3/69, issued 1/9/73. Assignee: Burroughs Wellcome Co., Research Triangle Park, NC.
28.) US Patent 3,520,972. Smith et al. Feline virus vaccines obtained by propagation and serial passage attenuation of virulent feline viruses in diploid feline embryo tissue cell serial passage subculture strains. Filed 2/14/67, published 7/21/70. Assignee: Burroughs Wellcome & Co. (USA) Inc., Tuckahoe, NY.
29.) US Patent 3,293,130. Slater et al. Panleukopenia Vaccine and Method for the Production Thereof. Filed 11/27/62, published 12/20/66. Assignee: Philips Roxane, Inc. St. Joseph MO.
30.) US Patent 3,562,387. Lauerman Jr. Mink Virus Enteritis Vaccine and Method for the Production Thereof. Filed 12/1/67, published 2/9/71. Assignee: The Mogul Corp.
31). US Patent 7,429,690. Robl, et al. Transgenic bovines having reduced prion protein production. Filed 11/10/03published 9/30/08. Assignee: Kirin Holdings Kabushiki Kaisha (Tokyo, JP).
32.) US Patent 7,405,342. Finberg. Transgenic mice expressing heterologous complement receptor type 1 (CR1) molecules on erythrocytes and uses therefor. Filed 5/10/04 published 7/29/08. Assignee: University of Massachusetts (Worcester, MA).
33.) US Patent 5,587,311 Cobon, et al. DNA encoding a cell membrane glycoprotein of a tick gut. Filed 10/19/94, published 12/24/96. Assignee: Biotechnology Australia Pty. Ltd. (Roseville, AU), and Commonwealth Scientific and Industrial Research Organization (Campbell, AU).
34.) US Patent Application 20090297560. Dattwyler et al. Oral vaccine for Borrelia. Filed 6/30/05and 8/3/09, published 12/3/09. No assignee listed, correspondence to San Francisco, CA.
35.) Sund Julian M, Niedermeier RP, Burris Robert H. NASD. National AG Safety Database. Watch Out for Silage Gas! University of Wisconsin-Extension. Fact Sheet A1871. Depart. Of Agricultural Journalism, College of Agricultural and Life Sciences, University of Wisconsin-Madison.
36.) Wormser GP, Dattwyler RJ, Shapiro ED, Halperin JJ, Steere AC, Klempner MS, Krause PJ, Bakken JS, Strle F, Stanek G, Bockenstedt L, Fish D, Dumler JS, Nadelman RB. The Clinical Assessment, Treatment, and Prevention of Lyme Disease, Human Granulocytic Anaplasmosis, and Babesiosis: Clinical Practice Guidelines by the Infectious Diseases Society of America. (IDSA Guidelines). Clin Infect Dis. 2006;43:1089-1134
37.) US Patent 7,531,180. Polo, et al. Chimeric Alphavirus replicon particles. Filed 4/22/02, published 5/12/09. Assignee: Novartis Vaccines and Diagnostics, Inc. (Emeryville, CA).
38.) Snider BB, Patricia JJ, Kates SA. Mechanism of manganese (III)-based Oxidation of ß-keto esters. Am Chem Soc. 1988 May 13;53(10:2137-2143.

When Good Ideas Turn Bad

1.) HHS-FDA Center for Biologics Evaluation and Research. Advisory Committee Meeting. International Conference on Harmonisation; Guidance on Viral Safety Evaluation of Biotechnology Products Derived From Cell Lines of Human or Animal Origin; Availability. Federal Register. 1998 Sept. 24;63(185):51074-51084.
2.) Wimmer Eckard, Hellen Christopher UT, Cao Xuemei. Genetics of Polio virus. Annu Rev Gent. 1993;27:353-436. Department of Microbiology, School of Medicine, State University of New York at Stony Brook, Stony Brook, New York.
3.) Marlow Susan A, Wilson Louise E, Lawrie Alison M. et al. Assembly of Amsacta moorei entomopoxvirus spheroidin into spheroids following synthesis in insect cells using a baculovirus vector. J Gen Virol. 1998;79:623-628.
4.) Fenner Frank, Woodroofe Gwendolyn M. The Reactivation of Poxviruses II. The Range of Reactiving Viruses. Virol. 1960;11(1):185-201.
5.) Joklik WK, Woodroofe Gwendolyn M, Holmes IH, Fenner Frank. The Reactivation of Poxviruses I. Demonstration of the phenomenon and techniques of assay. Virol. 1960;11(1):168-184.
6.) Nelson AM, Jorsburgh Jr. CR. Pathology of Emerging Infections (2). ASM Press Washington, DC. 1998. Amer Soc Micrbiol. Chapter 1, page 1. Burke, DS. Evolvability of Emerging Viruses.
7.) Burges HD, Hussey NW. Microbial Control of Insects and Mites. 1971 Academic Press. London.
8.) Pavlovsky EN, Soloviev VD. Experimental Study of the Encephalitis Virus in the Organism of the Tick, Ixodes persulcatus. Arkh Sci Biol. (USSR) [Article in Russian]. 1940;59:111-17.
9.) US Patent 2,966,443. Cox. Trivalent Poliomyelitis Live Virus Vaccine. Filed 6/22/59 published 12/27/60.
10.) US Patent 4,497,793. Cummins. Method of regulating appetite and efficiency of food utilization employing interferon. Filed 12/13/82 published 2/5/87. Assignee: The Texas A&M University System (College Station, TX).
11.) US Patent 3,699,222. Isaacs et al. Production of Viral Interfering Substances. Filed 8/5/68published 10/17/72. Assignee: National Research Development Corporation (London, EN).
12.) US Patent 3,144,390. Burke. Process for the purification of interferon. Filed 6/21/61 published 8/11/64. Assignee: National Research Development Corporation (London, EN).
13.) US Patent 3,265,581. Fantes et al. Process of purifying interferon with alumino-silicate adsorbants. Filed 8/2/63published 8/9/66. Assignee: Glaxo Laboratories Limited, (Greenford, EN).
14.) US Patent 3,385,757. Finter. Quantitative hemadsorption assay technique for the estimation of interferon. Filed 11/14/63published 5/28/68. Assignee: Imperial Chemical Industries Limited (London, EN).
15.) US Patent 3,414,651. Fantes. Purification of interferon-containing material. Filed 12/10/63published 12/3/68. Assignee: Glaxo Laboratories Limited (Greenford, EN).
16.) US Patent 3,548,053. Joshi. Interferon Production. Filed 9/7/65published 12/15/70. Assignee: Frank W. Horner Limited, Mount Royal, Quebec, Canada.
17.) US Patent 3,401,084. Rubella vaccine and its preparation. Filed 7/29/65published 9/10/68. Inventors: Eugene B. Buynak (North Wales) and Maurice R. Hilleman, (Lafayette Hill, PA). Assignee: Merck & Co., Inc. (Rahway, NJ).
18.) Horowitz, L. Merck Vaccine Chief Brings HIV/AIDS to America. [video] from the DVD In Lies We Trust, The CIA, Hollywood and Bioterrorism. Access: www.inlieswetrust.com.
19.) US Patent 3,541,202. Meyer Jr. et al. Detection of Rubella by Hemagglutination-Inhibition. Filed 6/26/67, published 1/17/70. Assignee: United States of America as represented by the Secretary of the Department of Health, Education, and Welfare.
20.) US Patent 3,544,680. Plotkin. Intranasal Immunization Agent Rubella. Filed 10/9/68 published 12/1/70. Assignee: The Wistar Institute (Philadelphia, PA).
21.) Pardigon Nathalie, Strauss James H. Cellular Proteins Bind to the 3' End of Sindbis Virus Minus-Strand RNA. J Virol. 1992 Feb;66(2):1007-1015.
22.) Parkman PD, Buescher EL, Artenstein MS, et al. Studies of Rubella. I. Properties of the Virus. J Immunol. 1964;93:595-607.
23.) US Patent 3,544,680 Plotkin Stanley A. Intranasal Immunization Against Rubella. Filed 10/9/68 issued 12/1/70. Assignee: Wistar Institute (Philadelphia, PA).
24.) US Patent 3,873,421. Chagnon. Propagation of attenuated rubella virus on turkey embryo tissue. Filed 8/13/73, issued 3/25/75.
25.) US Patent 6,982,087. Johnston et al. Vectors derived from South African Arbovirus No. 86. Filed 9/6/01, issued 1/3/06. Assignee: The University of North Carolina at Chapel Hill.
26.) Naides Stanley J. Viral arthritis including HIV. Edited by Robert T. Schoen. Current Opinion in Rheumatology. 1995 Jul 7(4):epub only.
27.) Oldstone MBA, Bokisch VA, Dixon FJ, et al. Subacute sclerosing panencephalitis: Destruction of human brain cells by antibody and complement in an autologous system. Clin

Immunol Immunopath. 1975 May;4(1):52-58.
28.) Newcastle Disease Virus (NDV). AvianBiotech
29.) Gilardi Gerald L. Glucose nonfermenting gram-negative bacteria in clinical microbiology. CRC Press. 1978.
30.) Klinger R. Untersuchungen über menschliche Aktinomykose. Zentralbl Bakteriol Parasit Infect Hyg. 1912;62:191.
31.) Osawa R, Rainey F, Fujisawa T, et al. Lonepinella koalarum gen. nov., sp. nov., a New Tannin-Protein Complex Degrading Bacterium. Syst Appl Microbiol. 1995;18(3):368-373.
32.) Foster G, Ross HM, Malnick H, et al. Phocoenobacter uteri gen. nov., sp. nov., a new member of the family of Pasteurellaceae Pohl (1979) 1981 isolated from a harbour porpoise (Phocoena phocoena). Inter J Syst Evol Microbiol. 2000;50:135-139.
33.) Casolari C, Fabio U. Isolation of Pasteurella multocida from Human Clinical Specimens: First Report in Italy. European Journal of Epidemiology. 1988 Sept;4(3):389-390.
34.) Nielsen JP Vaccination against progressive atrophic rhinitis with a recombinant "Pasteurella multocida" toxin derivative. Canadian Journal of Veterinary Research.55(2):128-138.
35.) Pasteur Louis. The Attenuation of the Causal Agent of Fowl Cholera. 1880. From Pasteur Brewing. [web page]
36.) Burmester and Witter, An Outline of the diseases of the avian leukosis complex, production research report No. 94, USDA 1966
37.) USDA Statistical Reporting Service POW 2-1, crop reporting board, Washington DC 20250.
38.) US Patent 3,548,054. Bowen. Method for improving weight gains and reducing grass lesions in chickens exposed to Marek's disease. Filed 6/6/69 published 12/15/70. Assignee: Eli Lilly and Company.
39.) Hitchner, Johnson. A Virus of Low Virulence for Immunizing Fowls Against Newcastle Disease. Vet Med. 1948;43:525-530.
40.) Hanson, Brandley. Identification of Vaccine Strains of Newcastle Disease Virus. Science. 1955;122:156-157.
41.) Churchill AE et al. Agent of Marek's Disease in Tissue Culture. Nature 1967 Jul 29;215:538-540.
42.) Churchill AE. Res. Studies on the Serological and Interferring Properties of Avian Leukosis Virus Isolated from Field Outbreaks of Disease and from Three Vaccines. Vet Sci. 1968 Jan;9(1):68-75.
43.) US Patent 3,674,861. Churchill. Live attenuated Marek's disease virus vaccine for poultry. Filed 10/31/69 published 7/4/72.
44.) US Patent 3,326,767 Holper Jacob C (Waukegan, IL) and Kiggins Edward M. (Kenosha, WI). Avian Leukosis Treatment with Inactivated Rous Sarcoma Virus. Filed 3/21/66, published 6/20/67. Assignee Abbott Laboratories, North Chicago IL.
45.) Merchant et al. Veterinary Bacteriology and Virology, 6th Ed. Published by Iowa State University Press, Ames, Iowa. 1961 pp. 766-767.
46.) Witter RL et al. Isolation from Turkeys of a Cell-Associated Herpesvirus Antigenically Related to Marek's Disease Virus. Am J Vet Res. 1970 Mar;31(3):525-538.
47.) Okazaki W et al. Protection Against Marek's Disease by Vaccination With a Herpesvirus of Turkeys. Avian Diseases 1970 May;14(2):413-428.
48.) US Patent 3,642,574. Okazaki, et al. Method for producing vaccine for immunization of Poultry against Marek's Disease. Filed 4/29/70, published 2/15/72.
49.) Miller Hatcheries. Marek's Disease in Chickens. [web page]
50.) US Patent 3,548,054. Bowen. Method for Improving Weight Gain and Reducing Gross Lesions in Chickens Exposed to Marek's Disease. Filed 6/6/69 published 12/15/70. Assignee: Eli Lilly and Company.
51.) US Patent 3,326,767. Holper. Avian Leukosis Treatment with Inactivated Rous Sarcoma Virus. Filed 3/21/66 published 6/20/67. Assignee: Abbott Laboratories, North Chicago, IL.
52.) Zavala G, Cheng S. Experimental infection with avian leukosis virus isolated from Marek's disease vaccines. Avian Dis. 2006 Jun;50(2):232-237.
53.) Scarduzio Lin. The Nestor. The Historical Society of Glastonbury. [web page]
54.) Annual Report of the Secretary of War. United States War Dept. University of California. Vol. II Part 1. 1880.
55.) Long Island Sound Dredged Materials. [web page]
56.) Ignoffo, Possibilities of Mass-Producing Insect Pathogens, Internat. Colloq. Insect Pathol. Netherlands, pp. 91-117(1967); Ignoffo, Viruses-Living Insecticides, Current Topics in Microbiology and Immunology, Vol. 42, pp. 129-167(1968)
57.) Jersey City Past and Present. Black Tom Explosion. [web site]
58.) Arbor Acres Farms Inc. [web page]
59.) Verdon R. Lyme Disease and the SS Elbrus. 2006 Elderberry Press, Oakland, Oregon.
60.) US Patent 3,326,767. Avian Leukosis Treatment with Inactivated Rous Sarcoma Virus. Filed 3/21/66 published 6/20/67. Assignee: Abbott Laboratories, North Chicago, IL.

Eight: If All Else Fails, Play the Red Herring

Even Microbes Get Sick

1.) Lakshminarayan M. Iyer, Aravind L, Koonin Eugene V. Common Origin of Four Diverse Families of Large Eukaryotic DNA Viruses. J Virol. 2001 Dec;75(23):11720-11734.
2.) Richardson Christopher D. (ed). Baculovirus Expression Protocols. Methods in Molecular Biology. 1995 Humana Press, Totowa, New Jersey. Vol. 39. p. 2.
3.) Fischer MG, Suttle CA. A Virophage at the Origin of Large DNA Transposons. Science Apr 2011 8;332(6026):231-234.
4.) D'Amico Vince. Baculoviruses (Baculoviridae). Cornell University College of Agriculture and Life Sciences Department of Entomology. [web page]
5.) Vaughn JL, Goodwin RH, Tompkins GH, McCawley P. The establishment of two cell lines from the insect Spodoptera frugiperda (Lepidoptera; Noctuidae). In Vitro. 1977 Apr;13(4):213-217.
6.) Pearson Helen. 'Virophage' suggests viruses are alive. Nature 2008 Aug 6;454(677). Published online.
7.) Fischer MG, Allen MJ, Wilson WH, Suttle CA. Giant virus with a remarkable complement of genes infects marine zooplankton. PNAS 2010 Nov 9;107(45):19508-19512.
8.) Monier A, Claverie JM, Ogata H. Taxonomic distribution of large DNA viruses in the sea. Genome Biol. 2008;9(7):R106.
9.) Suzan-Monti M, La Scola B, Raoult D. Genomic and evolutionary aspects of Mimivirus. Virus Res. 2006;117(1):145-155.
10.) Virophage, the virus eater. 2011 Mar. Virology blog [web page]
11.) d'Hérelle Félix. The bacteriophage, its rôle in immunity. Pasteur Institute. Translated to English by George H. Smith. 1922. Williams & Wilkins Co., Baltimore, MD.
12.) Whitfield JB. Parasitoids, polydnaviruses and endosymbiosis. Parasitol. Today. 1990 Dec;6(12):381-384.

Another Look at Dearborn's Elite

1.) Copy of letter that appears to have been written by Dr. Allen C. Steere at Tufts University, New England Medical Center to Dr. George Kraus, Connecticut Department of Health. July 30, 1990. Letter was provided to the author by Dr. Joseph Burrascano, Jr., of New York
2.) Copy of letter that appears to be from Dr. Allen C. Steere at Tufts University School of Medicine, New England Medical Center as Chief Rheumatology/Immunology to Dr. Kenneth B. Liegner of Armonk, NY. Dated June 14, 1990. Letter provided to the author by Dr. Joseph Burrascano, Jr., of New York
3.) Copy of from letter that appears to be from Dr. Allen C. Steere at Tufts University School of Medicine, New England Medical Center to former Lyme patients for follow-up study. Dated August 11, 1994. Provided to the author by Dr. Joseph Burrascano, Jr., of New York
4.) Proceedings of the Second National Conference on Serologic Diagnosis of Lyme Disease. 1994Oct. 27-29, Dearborn, MI. 105pages. Sponsors: Assoc. of State and Territorial Public Health Laboratory Directors, US CDC and Prevention, MI Dept. of Health. Co-sponsors: USFDA, NIH, Council of State and Territorial Epidemiologists and National Committee for Clinical Laboratory Standards.

Monoclonal Antibodies at Dearborn

1.) Proceedings of the Second National Conference on Serologic Diagnosis of Lyme Disease. 1994Oct. 27-29, Dearborn, MI. 105pages. Sponsors: Assoc. of State and Territorial Public Health Laboratory Directors, US CDC and Prevention, MI Dept. of Health. Co-sponsors: USFDA, NIH, Council of State and Territorial Epidemiologists and National Committee for Clinical Laboratory Standards.
2.) Burgdorfer Willy, Barbour Alan G., Hayes Stanley F., Benach Jorge L., Grunwaldt Edgar, Davis Jeffrey P. Lyme Disease – A Tick-borne Spirocheosis? Science 1982 Jun;216(18):1317-1319. Note: Drs. Burgdorfer and Barbour were at the Rocky Mt. Lab in Hamilton, MT; Dr. Benach was at State University of New York (SUNY) Stony Brook; Dr. Grunwaldt was at Shelter Island, NY; Dr. Davis was at the Dept. of Health and Social Services, Madison, WI and is now a WI State Epidemiologist.
3.) Magnarelli LA, Anderson JF, Johnson RC, Nadelman RB, Wormser GP. Comparison of Different Strains of Borrelia burgdorferi Sensu Lato Used as Antigens in Enzyme-Linked Immunosorbent Assays. J Clin Microbiol. 1994 May;32(5):1154-1158
4.) Fikrig E, Barthold SW, Persing DH, Sun X, Kantor FS, Flavell RA. Borrelia burgdorferi strain 25015: characterization of outer surface protein A and vaccination against infection. J Immunol. 1992;148(7):2256-2260.

5.) Luft BJ, Mudri S, Jiang W, Dattwyler RJ, et al. The 93-Kilodalton Protein of Borrelia burgdorferi: an Immunodominant Protoplasmic Cylinder Antigen. Infect and Immun. 1992 Oct;60(10):4309-4321.

6.) Volkman DJ, Luft BJ, Gorevic PD, Schultz J, Padovano L. Characterization of an immunoreactive 93-kDa core protein of Borrelia burgdorferi with a human IgG monoclonal antibody. J Immunol. 1991;9(146):3177-3182.

7.) Chiu FC, Barnes EA, Das K, et al. Characterization of a novel 66kd subunit of mammalian neurofilaments. Neuron 1989 May;2(5):1435-45.

8.) Zest for Life. [web site] Leucine amino acid information page.

9.) Sigal LH, Williams S, Soltys B, Gupta R. H9724, a monoclonal antibody to Borrelia burgdorferi's flagellin, binds to heat shock protein 60 (HSP60) within live neuroblastoma cells: a potential role for HSP60 in peptide hormone signaling and in an autoimmune pathogenesis of the neuropathy of Lyme disease. Cell Mol Neurobiol. 2001 Oct;21(5):477-95.

10.) Roessler D, Hauser U, Wilske B. Heterogenicity of BmpA (P39) among European Isolates of Borrelia burgdorferi Sensu Lato and Influence of Interspecies Variability on Serodiagnosis. J Clin Microbiol. 1997Nov;35(11):2752-2758.

11.) Reddi A H. Bone Morphogenetic Proteins: an Unconventional Approach to Isolation of First Mammalian Morphogens. Cytokine & Growth Factor Reviews. 1997;8(1):11–20.

12.) Renkema GH, Boot RG, Au FL, et al. Chitotriosidase, a chitinase, and the 39-kDa human cartilage glycoprotein, a chitin-binding lectin, are homologues of family 18glycosyl hydrolases secreted by human macrophages. Eur J Biochem. 1998Jan 15;251(1-2):504-9.

13.) Risco C, Rodríguez JR, Demkowicz W, et al. The vaccinia virus 39-kDa protein forms a stable complex with the p4a/4a major core protein early in morphogenesis. Virol. 1999 Dec 20;265(2):375-86.

14.) Alia Hussam Al-Haj, Sawada Takuo, et al. Characterization of a 39kDa capsular protein of avian Pasteurella multocida using monoclonal antibodies. Vet Microbiol. 2004;100(1-2):43-53.

15.) UniprotKB. Taxonomy browser. Insertion element IS630 uncharacterized 39kDa protein. Shigella sonnei. [web page]

16.) Yang F, Yang J. Genome dynamics and diversity of Shigella species, the etiologic agents of bacillary dysentery. Nucleic Acid Res. 2005;33(9): 6445-6458.

17.) US Patent 3,444,222. Roberts. (Decamethylenedithio)Dialanine Compounds. Filed 6/22/66 published 5/13/69. Assignee: Dow Chemical Company, Midland, MI.

18.) Barchiese F, Tortorano AM, Falconi Di Francesco L, et al. Genotypic variation and antifungal susceptibilities of Candida pelliculosa clinical isolates. J Med Microbiol. 2005 Mar;54(3):279-285.

19.) US Patent 5,665,595. Petell et al. Immunoglobulins against insect tissue. Filed 3/18/94 published 9/9/97. Assignee: DowElanco (Indianapolis, IN).

20.) US Patent 5,770,696. Warren, et al. Auxiliary proteins for enhancing the insecticidal activity of pesticidal proteins. Filed 6/6/95 published 6/23/98. Assignee: Novartis corporation.

21.) US Patent 5,840,868. Warren, et al. Pesticidal proteins and strains. Filed 6/6/95 published 11/24/98. Assignee: Novartis Finance Corporation (New York, NY).

22.) US Patent 5,942,664. Baum et al. Bacillus thuringiensis Cry1C compositions toxic to lepidopteran insects and methods for making Cry1C mutants. Filed 11/27/96 published 8/24/99. Assignee: Ecogen, Inc. (Langhorne, PA).

23.) US Patent 5,965,428. Gilmer et al. Chimeric lepidopteran-toxic crystal proteins. Filed 10/8/96 published 10/12/99. Assignee: Ecogen, Inc. (Langhorne, PA).

24.) US Patent 5,888,801. Warren et al. Pesticidal strains of bacillus. Filed 6/6/95 published 3/30/99. Assignee: Novartis Finance Corporation (New York NY).

25.) US Patent 5,470,712. Simpson et al. Antigenic proteins of Borrelia burgdorferi. Filed 2/19/93published 11/28/95. Assignee: none listed. Inventors: Warren Simpson, T.G. Schwan (Hamilton, MT).

26.) Di Zhang, Tözser Jozsef, Waugh David S. Molecular cloning, overproduction, purification and biochemical characterization of the p39nsp2protease domains encoded by three Alphaviruses. Protein expression and purification. 2009;64(1):89-97.

27.) Patent WO/2005/019414– Insecticidal Proteins Secreted from Bacillus Thuringiensis and Uses Therefor. Inter. Filing date: 6/7/04. Assignees: Monsanto Technology, LLC.

28.) Risco C, Rodríguez JR, Demkowicz W, et al. The vaccinia virus 39-kDa protein forms a stable complex with the p4a/4a major core protein early in morphogenesis. Virol. 1999Dec 20;265(2):375-86.

29.) Alia Hussam Al-Haj, Sawada Takuo, et al. Characterization of a 39kDa capsular protein of avian Pasteurella multocida using monoclonal antibodies. Vet Microbiol. 2004;100(1-2):43-53.

30.) Xu S, Zheng G, Li M, Shu B. [Direct effects of fluoride on activities of bone morphogenetic protein]. [Article in Chinese]. Zhonghua Yu Fang Yi Xue Za Zhi. 2000 Jul;34(4):215-217.

31.) Roessler D, Hauser U, Wilske B. Heterogenicity of BmpA (P39) among European Isolates of Borrelia burgdorferi Sensu Lato and Influence of Interspecies Variability on Serodiagnosis. J Clin Microbiol. 1997 Nov;35(11):2752-2758.

32.) Reddi A H. Bone Morphogenetic Proteins: an Unconventional Approach to Isolation of First Mammalian Morphogens. Cytokine & Growth Factor Reviews. 1997;8(1):11–20.

33.) Renkema GH, Boot RG, Au FL, et al. Chitotriosidase, a chitinase, and the 39-kDa human cartilage glycoprotein, a chitin-binding lectin, are homologues of family 18glycosyl hydrolases secreted by human macrophages. Eur J Biochem. 1998Jan 15;251(1-2):504-9.

34.) Risco C, Rodríguez JR, Demkowicz W, et al. The vaccinia virus 39-kDa protein forms a stable complex with the p4a/4a major core protein early in morphogenesis. Virol. 1999Dec 20;265(2):375-86.

35.) Risco C, Rodriguez JR, Demkowicz W, et al. The vaccinia virus 39-kDa protein forms a stable complex with the p4a/4a major core protein early in morphogenesis. Virol. 1999 Dec 20;254(2):375-386.

36.) Park MY, Kim YE, Seo MR, et al. Interactions among Four Proteins Encoded by the Human Cytomegalovirus UL112-113 Region Regulate Their Intranuclear Targeting and the Recruitment of UL44to Prereplication Foci. J Virol. 2006 Mar;80(6):2718-2727.

37.) US Patent 5,308,760. Brown, et al. Crystal proteins of Bacillus thuringiensis, genes encoding them, and host expressing them. Filed 2/3/92, issued 5/3/94. Assignee: Washington Research Foundation (Seattle, WA).

38.) Zepter K, Häffner A, Soohoo LF, et al. Induction of biologically active IL-1 beta-converting enzyme and mature IL-1 beta in human keratinocytes by inflammatory and immunologic stimuli. J Immunol. 1997 Dec 15;159(12):6203-8.

39.) Vertrees S, Wilson CA, Ubungen R, et al. Interleukin-1 beta regulation of islet and thyroid autoimmunity in the BB rat. J Autoimmun. 1991 Oct;4(5):717-32.

40.) Kenefick KB, Lederer JA, Schell RF, Czuprynski CJ. Borrelia burgdorferi stimulates release of interleukin-1 activity from bovine peripheral blood monocytes. Infect Immun. 1992 Sept;60(9):3630-3634.

41.) Arella M, Belloncik S, Devauchelle G. Protein synthesis in a Lymantria dispar Cell Line Infected by Cytoplasmic Polyhedrosis Virus. J Virol. 1984;52(3):1024-1027.

42.) Span Diagnostics SARL. [web site] www.spandiag.com

43.) The Center for Food Security & Public Health. Institute for International Cooperation in Animal Biologics. Lyme Disease. Lyme Borreliosis, Lyme Arthritis, Erythema Migrans with Polyarthritis. 2005 May 1. Bulletin. 5pages. [web page]

44.) Dunn MG, Ellar DJ. Identification of two sequence elements associated with the gene encoding the 24-kDa crystalline component in Bacillus thuringiensis ssp,. fukuokaensis: an example of transposable element archaeology. Plasmid. 1997;37(3):205-15.

45.) Tessier DC, Thomas DY, Laliberte F, et al. Enhanced secretion from insect cells of a foreign protein fused to the honey bee melittin signal peptide. Gene. 1991;98:177-183.

46.) Friesen PD, Miller LK. Insect viruses. In: Knipe DM, Howley PM, Griffin DE, Lamb RA, Marin MA, Roizman B, Straus SE (Eds.). Fund Virol. Lippincott Williams and Wilkins, Philadelphia, pp. 446-456.

47.) Burges HD, Hussey NW. Microbial Control of Insects and Mites. 1971 Academic Press London.

48.) Engstrom SM, Shoop E, Johnson RC. Immunoblot interpretation criteria for serodiagnosis of early Lyme disease. J Clin Microbiol 1995;33:419-22.

49.) Kenefick KB, Lederer JA, Schell RF, Czuprynski CJ. Borrelia burgdorferi stimulates release of interleukin-1 activity from bovine peripheral blood monocytes. Infect Immun. 1992 Sept;60(9):3630-3634.

50.) Dunn MG, Ellar DJ. Identification of two sequence elements associated with the gene encoding the 24-kDa crystalline component in Bacillus thuringiensis ssp,. fukuokaensis: an example of transposable element archaeology. Plasmid. 1997;37(3):205-15.

51.) Cullen Paul A. Cordwell SJ, Baluch DM, Haake DA, Adler B. Global Analysis of Outer Membrane Proteins from Leptospira interrogans Serovar Lai. Infect Immun. 2002 May;70(5):2311-2318.

52.) Templeton TJ. Borrelia Outer Membrane Surface Proteins and Transmission Through the Tick. J Exp Med. 2004Mar 1;199(5):603-606.

53.) Sigal LH, Williams S, Soltys B, Gupta R. H9724, a monoclonal antibody to Borrelia burgdorferi's flagellin, binds to heat shock protein 60 (HSP60) within live neuroblastoma cells: a potential role for HSP60 in peptide hormone signaling and in an autoimmune pathogenesis of the neuropathy of Lyme disease. Cell Mol Neurobiol. 2001 Oct;21(5):477-95.

54.) Lundstrom Kenneth*. Alphavirus Vectors: Applications for DNA Vaccine Production and Gene Expression. Intervirology 2000;43:247-257. *F. Hoffmann-La Roche, Research

Laboratories, Basel, Switzerland.
55.) Lundstrom Kenneth. Novel developments for applications of Alphavirus vectors in gene therapy. Review Article. Gen Ther Mol Biol. 2001;6:25-31.
56.) Gwag BJ, Kim EY, Ryu BR*, et al. A neuron-specific gene transfer by a recombinant defective Sindbis virus. Brain Res Mol Brain Res. 1998Dec 10;63(1):53-61. *Department of Pharmacology, Ajou University School of Medicine, Suwon, Kyungkido, South Korea.
57.) US Patent 5,523,089 Bergstrom, et al. Borrelia antigen. Filed 6/22/93, issued 6/4/96. Assignee: Symbicom Aktiebolag (SE). Inventors: Sven Bergstrom (SE), Alan G. Barbour (TX), Louis A. Magnarelli (CT).
58.) Daly R, Hearn MT. Expression of heterologous proteins in Pichia pastoris: a useful experimental tool in protein engineering and production.[J Mol Recognit. 2005;18(2):119-138.
59.) Life technologies. pPICZα A, B, C. Invitrogen™ [web page]
60.) US Patent 6,268,169 Fahnestock. Recombinantly produced spider silk. Filed 6/15/94 published 7/31/01. Assignee: E. I. du Pont de Nemours and Company (Wilmington, DE).
61.) InvivoGen. Zeocin™. [web page]
62.) Invitrogen life technologies Instruction Manual, Zeocin™. From the company's [web page]
63.) US Patent 5,162,222. Guarino, et al. Use of baculovirus early promoters for expression of foreign genes in stably transformed insect cells or recombinant baculoviruses. Filed 9/17/90, issued 11/10/92.
64.) US Patent 5,547,871. Black, et al. Heterologous signal sequences for secretion of insect controlling proteins. Filed 1/25/93, issued 8/20/96. Assignee: American Cyanamid Co. (Wayne, NJ).
65.) US Patent 5,662,897. Miller, et al. Insect viruses, sequences, insecticidal compositions and methods of use. Filed 7/27/94, issued 9/2/97. Assignee: U of GA Research Foundation (Athens, GA) and American Cyanamid Co. (Wayne, NJ).
66.) World Intellectual Property Organization International Patent (WO/1993/024145) Compositions Useful in Diagnosis and Prophylaxis of Lyme Disease. Assignees: Smithkline Beecham Corporation, Government of the United States of America represented by The Department of Health and Human Services Centers for Disease Control and Prevention; William T. Golde, John T. Roehrig, Thomas Burkot, Joseph F. Piesman, Barbara JB Johnson, Leonard W Mayer, Mark G. Keen, Ann R Hunt. Filed 5/26/93, published 9/12/93.
67.) Fischer Matthias G. Suttle Curtis A. A Virophage at the Origin of Large DNA Transposons. Science 2011 Apr 8;332(6026):231-234.
68.) US patent 5,077,214. Guarino et al. Use of baculovirus early promoters for expression of foreign genes in stably transformed insect cells. Filed 7/7/89 published 12/31/91. Assignee: The Texas A&M University System (College Station, TX).
69.) Pugachev KV, Pletnev AG. [Expression of gene codingn for the NS1 protein of the tick-borne encephalitis virus in Escherichia coli cell]. [Article in Russian]. Mol Biol (Mosk). 1990 Nov-Dec;24(6):1631-1639.

Silly Rice and the Dearborn Conference

1.) The Nature of Gibberellins. www.plant-hormones.info/gibberellins.htm and Grennan AK. Gibberellinn Metabolism Enzymes in Rice. Plant Physiol. 2006 Jun;141(2):524-526.
2.) Akai S. History of Plant Pathology in Japan. Ann Rev Phytopath. 1974 Sept;12:13-26.
3.) Munkvold Gary Ear rot and mold problems. Iowa State University. Integrated Crop Management newsletter. 2001 Oct 22.
4.) Otis JS, Ashikhmin Yl, Brown LA, Guidot DM. Effect of HIV-1-related protein expression on cardiac and skeletal muscles from transgenic rats. AIDS Res Ther. 2008 Apr 25;5:8.
5.) Newman KP, Neal MT, Roberts M, et al. The importance of lost minerals in heart failure. Cardiovasc Hematol Agents Med Chem. 2007 Oct;5(4):295-299.
6.) Burnham EL, Moss M, Ziegler TR. Myopathies in critical illness: characterization and nutritional aspects. J Nutr 2005 Jul;135(7):1818S-1823S.
7.) Foster HD. How HIV-1 causes AIDS: implications for prevention and treatment. Med Hypotheses. 2004;62(4):549-553.
8.) US Patent 2,747,334. Routien et al. Cultivation of Plant Tissue. Filed 5/20/52 published 5/29/56. Assignee: Pfizer & Co., Inc. New York, NY
9.) US Patent 5,168,059. Roberts. Micropropagation process. Filed 6/19/87, published 12/1/92. Assignee: Imperial Chemicals Industries PLC (London, GB2).
10.) US Patent 3,920,443 Drewe et al. Herbicidal compositions. Filed 3/23/73 published 11/18/75. Assignee: Imperial Chemical Industries Limited (London, EN).
11.) US Patent 2,972,528. Coles BR et al. Dipyridyl derivatives and herbicidal methods and compositions containing the same. Filed 3/25/57 published 2/21/61. Assignee: Imperial Chemical Industries Limited, London, England.
12.) US Patent 3,527,593. Coles RB et al. Herbicide-Amine Oxide Compositions and their Use. Filed 11/30/66 published 9/8/70. Assignees: Imperial Chemical Industries Limited, London, England.
13.) US Patent 3,620,711. White. Herbicidal Process and Compositions for Use Therein. Filed 7/11/68 published 11/16/71. Assignee: Imperial Chemical Industries Limited, London, GB2.
14.) Paraquat Fact Sheet. [web page]
15.) US EPA. Reregistration Eligibility Decision (RED) paraquat dichloride. 1997 Aug. EPA 738-F-96-018 Report. Prevention, Pesticides, and Toxic Substances (7508W). 267 pages. [web page]
16.) Peacock Bill. Gibberellin and Flame Seedless Grapes. Pub. TB14-00. University of California. Tulare County Cooperative Extension. Report, 2 pages. [web page]
17.) Pullman GS, Mein J, Johnson S, Yhang Y. Gibberellion inhibitors improve embryogenic tissue initiation in conifers. Plant Cell Rep. 2005 Feb;23(9):596-605.
18.) Yung KH, Mann JD. Inhibition of early steps in the gibberellin-activated synthesis of alpha-amylase. Plant Physiol. 1967 Feb;42(2):195-200.
19.) CDC. 2,4,5-Trichlorophenoxyacetic Acid. General Information. [web page]
20.) Yabuta et al. Biochemical Studies on Bakanae Fungus. Part 15, Effect of Gibberellin and Heteroauxin on Rice Seedlings (1) J Ag Chem Soc Japan. 1943;19(4):244-248.
21.) Miller. Study Seed Protectants and Peanuts. Agricul Chem. 1950 June;5(6):59,61,63,91.
22.) Kemp. Gibberellic Acid. Agricul Chem. 1957 Apr;12(4):30-31.
23.) Sigal LH, Williams S, Soltys B, Gupta R. H9724, a monoclonal antibody to Borrelia burgdorferi's flagellin, binds to heat shock protein 60 (HSP60) within live neuroblastoma cells: a potential role for HSP60 in peptide hormone signaling and in an autoimmune pathogenesis of the neuropathy of Lyme disease. Cell Mol Neurobiol. 2001 Oct;21(5):477-95.
24.) Anzola J, Luft BJ, Gorgone G, Dattwyler RJ, et al. Borrelia burgdorferi HSP70 homolog: characterization of an immunoreactive stress protein. Infect Immun. 1992 Sep;60(9):3704-3713.
25.) Penn CW, Bassford PJ, Yelton DB, Dunn J, Nelson DR, Fukunaga M, Stanek G. Genetic approaches to cell biology and metabolism of spirochetes. Res Microbiol. 1992 Jul-Aug;143(6):605-613.
26.) Ijdo JW, Zhang Y, Anderson ML, Goldberg D, Fikrig E. Heat shock protein 70 of the agent of human granulocytic ehrlichiosis binds to Borrelia burgdorferi antibodies. Clin Diagn Lab Immunol. 1998 Jan;5(1):118-120.
27.) Wong SJ, Brady GS, Dumler JS. Serological responses to Ehrlichia equi, Ehrlichia chaffeensis, and Borrelia burgdorferi in patients from New York State. J Clin Microbiol. 1997 Sep;35(9):2198-2205.
28.) Coleman JL, Benach JL. Characterization of antigenic determinants of Borrelia burgdorferi shared by other bacteria. J Infect Dis. 1992 Apr;165(4):658-666.
29.) Luft BJ, Gorevic PD, Jiang W, Munoz P, Dattwyler RJ. Immunologic and structural characterization of the dominant 66- to 73-kDa antigens of Borrelia burgdorferi. J Immunol. 1991 Apr 15;146(8):2776-2782.
30.) CDC. Notice to Readers Recommendations for Test Performance and Interpretation from the Second National Conference on Serologic Diagnosis of Lyme Disease. 1995 Aug 11;44(31):590-591.
31.) Engstrom SM, Shoop E, Johnson RC. Immunoblot interpretation criteria for serodiagnosis of early Lyme disease. J Clin Microbiol. 1995;33:419-422.
32.) Dressler F, Whelan JA, Reinhart BN, Steere AC. Western blotting in the serodiagnosis of Lyme disease. J Infect Dis. 1993;167:392-400.
33.) Giordano G, Afsharinejad Z, Guizzetti M, et al. Organophosphorus insecticides chlorpyrifos and diazinon and oxidative stress in neuronal cells in a genetic model of glutathione deficiency. Toxicol Appl Pharmacol. 2007 Mar219(2-3):181-189.
34.) Flaskos J. The developmental neurotoxicity of organophosphorus insecticides: A direct role for the oxon metabolites. Toxicol Lettr. 2011 Dec 3.
35.) Saxena R, Garg P, Jain DK. In Viro Anti-oxidant Effect of Vitamin E on Oxidative Stress induced due to pesticides in rat erythrocytes. Toxicol Int. 2011 Jan;18(1):73-76.
36.) Wu H, Zhang R, Liu J, et al. Effects of malathion and chlorpyrifos on acetylcholinesterase and antioxidant defense system in Oxya chinensis (Thunberg) (Orthoptera: Acrididae). Chemosphere 2011 Apr;83(4):599-604.
37.) Cheng MY, Hartl FU, Martin J, et al. Mitochondrial heat-shock protein hsp60 is essential for assembly of proteins imported into yeast mitochondria. Nature 1989 Feb 16;337(6208):620-625.

38.) Sigal LH, Williams S. A monoclonal antibodyto Borrelia burgdorferi flagellin modifies neuroblastoma cell neuritogenesis in vitro: a possible role for autoimmunity in Lyme disease. Infect Immun. 1997 May;65(5):1722-1728.
39.) Dai Z, Lackland H, Stein S, Li Q, Radziewicz R, Williams S, Sigal LH. Molecular mimicry in Lyme disease: monoclonal antibody H9724 to B. burgdorferi flagellin specifically detects chaperonin-HSP60. Biochim Biophys Acta. 1993 Mar 24;1181(1):97-100.
40.) Robinson A, Hudson MJ Cranage MP. (eds.) Vaccine protocols. Methods in Molecular Medicine. Second edition.
41.) 2.4 Toxicity Testing and Immunogenicity Testing. 2003 Humana Press. Totowa, New Jersey.
42.) US Patent 3,978,228. Yoshinaga, et al. Method for killing noxious fungi in plants using dihalo sulfonates. Filed 3/24/75 published 8/31/76. Assignee: Kumiai Chemical Industry Co., Ltd. (Tokoya, JA).
43.) US patent 7,005,255. Kaddurah-Daouk et al. Methods for drug discovery, disease treatment, and diagnosis using metabolomics. Filed 1/13/04 published 2/28/06. Assignee: Metabolon, Inc. (Research Triangle Park, NC) and Cornell Research Foundation, Inc. (Ithaca, NY).
44.) US Patent 7,812,219. Baum et al. Compositions and methods for control of insect infestations in plants. Filed 11/30/07 published 10/12/2010. Asignee: Monsanto Technology LLC (St. Louis, MO).
45.) US Patent 5,037,745. McAllister. Plasmid for overproduction of bacteriophage T3 RNA polymerase, transcription vectors that carry a promoter recognized by its polymerase, gene coding for T3 RNA polymerase and application of these plasmids. Filed 4/1/86 published 8/6/91. Assignee: University of Medicine and Dentistry of New Jersey (Newark, NJ).
46.) US Patent 4,349,629. Carey et al. Plamid vectors, production and use thereof. Filed 5/29/80 published 9/14/82. Assignee: G.D. Searle and Co. (Skokie, IL).
47.) US Patent 5,077,214. Guarino et al. Use of baculovirus early promoters for expression of foreign genes in stably transformed insect cells. Filed 7/7/89 published 12/31/91. Assignee: The Texas A&M University System (College Station, TX).
48.) Pugachev KV, Pletnev AG. [Expression of gene codingn for the NS1 protein of the tick-borne encephalitis virus in Escherichia coli cell]. [Article in Russian]. Mol Biol (Mosk). 1990 Nov-Dec;24(6):1631-1639.

Calling "Doctor Johnson"

1.) World Intellectual Property Organization International Patent (WO/1993/024145) Compositions Useful in Diagnosis and Prophylaxis of Lyme Disease. Assignees: Smithkline Beecham Corporation, Government of the United States of America represented by The Department of Health and Human Services Centers for Disease Control and Prevention; William T. Golde, John T. Roehrig, Thomas Burkot, Joseph F. Piesman, Barbara JB Johnson, Leonard W Mayer, Mark G. Keen, Ann R Hunt. Filed 5/26/93, published 9/12/93.
2.) US Patent Application #20090047240 (A1). Johnson Barbara J. et al. Chaperonin 10-Induced Immunomodulation. Filed in Australia 7/11/06. Published 2/19/09. Correspondence to San Francisco, CA. Assignee: CBio Limited, Queensland, AU.
3.) US Patent Application # 20070275890 (A1). Johnson Barbara Jane et al. Filed in Australia 1/16/04 under 200400190 and 2004903914. Published 11/29/07. Correspondence to Irvine, CA.
4.) US Patent Application #20090325882(A1). Johnson Barbara Jane et al. Chaperonin 10 Modulation of Toll-Like Receptor-Inducible Cytokine and Chemokine Secretion. Filed in Australia 9/3/09. Published 12/31/09. Correspondence to Irvine, CA.
5.) US Patent Application #20090305400. Naylor et al. Modified chaperonin 10. Inventors include Barbara Jane Johnson. Filed 1/16/06and 8/31/06. Published 12/10/09. Assignee: CBio Limited. Correspondence to San Francisco, CA.
6.) Broadley SA, Vanags D, Williams B, Johnson B, et al. Results of a phase IIa clinical trial of an anti-inflammatory molecule, chaperonin 10, in multiple sclerosis. Mult Scler. 2009Mar;15(3):329-336. Epub 2008Nov 27.
7.) Vanags D. et al. Therapeutic efficacy and safety of chaperonin 10 in patients with rheumatoid arthritis. A double-blind randomized trial. Lancet 2006 Sep 2;368:855-863.
8.) Teshima T, Kohda J, Kondo A, et al. Protein refolding system using holo-chaperonin from the thermophilic bacterium Thermus thermophilus. J Ferment Bioengin. 1998Jun;85(6):564-570.
9.) Teshima T, Kohda J, Kondo A, et al. Protein refolding system using holo-chaperonin from the thermophilic bacterium Thermus thermophilus. J Ferment Bioengin. 1998Jun;85(6):564-570.
10.) Suehara K, Kawamoto Y, Fujii E, et al. Biological treatment of wastewater discharged from biodiesel fuel production plant with alkali-catalyzed transesterification. J Biosc Bioengin. 2005 Oct;100(4):437-442.
11.) US Patent 5,401,631. Lane, et al. Universal eubacteria nucleic acid probes and assay methods. Filed 9/27/91, published 3/28/95. Assignee: Amoco Corporation (Naperville, IL).
12.) US Patent 4,971,151. Sheehy. Recovery of oil from oil reservoirs. Filed 3/9/89 published 11/20/90. Assignee: B.W.N. Live-Oil Pty. Ltd. (Dandenong, AU).
13.) US Patent 5,083,610. Sheehy. Recovery of oil from oil reservoirs. Filed 4/25/90 published 1/28/92. Assignee: B.W.N. Live-Oil Pty. Ltd. (Dandenong, AU).
14.) Pikuta EV, Hoover RB, Tang J. Microbial Extremophiles at the Limits of Life. Critical Rev Microbiol. 2007;33(3):183-209.
15.) US Patent 5,352,608. Kaplan, et al. Bioreduction of metal oxides and oxyanions by photosynthetic bacteria. Filed 1/13/92published 10/4/94. Assignee: The Board of Regents, The University of Texas (Austin, TX).
16.) US Patent 5,561,221. Yoshida, et al. Methods and compositions for promoting protein folding. Filed 8/3/94published 10/1/96. Assignee: Nippon Oil Company Limited (Minato-ku, JP).
17.) US Patent 5,618,711. Gelfand, et al. Recombinant expression vectors and purification methods for Thermus thermophilus DNA polymerase. Filed 2/6/ 95published 4/8/97. Assignee: Hoffmann-La Roche Inc. (Nutley, NJ).
18.) Mann Jeffrey E. Recent advances in the development of Deinococcus in bioremediation of mixed radioactive waste. MMG 445Basic Biotech. 2009;5(1):
19.) Bertin PB, Lozzi SP, Howell JK et al. The Thermophilic, Homohexameric Aminopeptidase of Borrelia burgdorferi Is a Member of the M29Family of Metallopeptidases. Infect Immun. 2005Apr;73(4):2253-2261.
20.) Sekine K, Fukii H, Abe F. Induction of apoptosis by bestatin (ubenimex) in human leukemic cell lines. Leukemia. 1999May;13(5):729-734.
21.) Stallings WC, Pattridge KA, Strong RK, Ludwig ML. The structure of manganese superoxide dismutase from Thermus thermophilus HB8at 2.4-A resolution. J Biol Chem. 1985 Dec 25;260:16424-16432.
22.) Whitehouse CA, Williams LR, Austin FE. Identification of superoxide dismutase activity in Borrelia burgdorferi. J Infect Immun. 1997Nov;65(11):4865-4868.
23.) Manganese Superoxide Dismutase (MnSOD) [web page]
24.) Fore Jr. Joe, Wiechers Ilse R, Cook-Deegan Robert. The effects of business practices,licensing, and intellectual property on development and dissemination of the polymerase chain reaction: case study. J Biomed Discov Collab. 2006;1:7. 17 pages.
25.) Ignoffo CM, Dropkin VH. Deletrious Effects of the Thermostable Toxin of Bacillus thuringiensis on Species of Soil-Inhabiting Myceliophagus, and Plant-Parasitic Nematodes. J Kansas Entomol Soc. 1977;50(3):394-398.
26.) Ahmed R, Sankar-Mistry P, Jackson S, et al. Bacillus cereus Phage Typing as an Epidemiological Tool Outbreaks of Food Poisoning. J Clin Microbiol. 1995 Mar;33(3):636-640.
27.) US Patent 5,401,631. Lane, et al. Universal eubacteria nucleic acid probes and assay methods. Filed 9/27/91, published 3/28/95. Assignee: Amoco Corporation (Naperville, IL).
28.) Rudenko N, Golovchenko M, Grubhoffer L, Oliver Jr. JH. Borrelia carolinensis sp. nov., a New (14th) Member of the Borrelia burgdorferi Sensu Lato Complex from the Southeastern Region of the United States. J Clin Microbiol. 2009 Jan;47(1):134-141.
29.) ATCC. Strain Number BAA-816Deinococcus radiodurans (ex Raj et al.) Brooks and Murray, designations: USUHS. Depositor: MJ Daley. History: MJ Daley, KW Minton, BE Mosley. BSL-1. Strain references PubMed ID: 10567266. [web page]
30.) White O, Eisen JA, Heidelberg JF, et al. Genome sequence of the radioresistant bacterium Deinococcus radiodurans R1. Science 1999Nov 19;286(5444):1571-1577.
31.) Brim H, McFarlan SC, Fredrickson JK, et al. Engineering Deinococcus radiodurans for metal remediation in radioactive mixed waste environments. Nat Biotechnol. 2000 Jan;18(1):85-90.
32.) Craig Venter on DNA and the Sea. TED Talks 2005Feb. He discusses in an 18minute segment the Sorcerer II Expedition sampling the world's ocean bacteria, gene sequencing and how D. radiodurans is the ultimate genome assembly machine. [web page]
33.) Young John D, Martel Jan. The Truth about Nanobacteria. 2010 Jan. Scientific American. [web page]
34.) Jacquot Jeremy. Concrete + Extremophile Bacteria = Walls That Repair Themselves. Discover. Blogs/Science Not fiction. 2010 Sep 3.
35.) Karl Jeff. Scientists Creating 'Extremophile' Super Bug to Make Fuel. 2010 May 18. Science and Technology. Treehugger, a Discovery Company. [web page]
36.) Carey Bjorn. Wild Things: The Most Extreme Creatures. Live Science. 2005 Feb 7. [web page]
37.) White O, Eisen JA, Heidelberg JF, et al. Genome sequence of the radioresistant bacterium Deinococcus radiodurans R1. Science 1999Nov 19;286(5444):1571-1577.
38.) Brim H, McFarlan SC, Fredrickson JK, et al. Engineering Deinococcus radiodurans for metal remediation in radioactive mixed waste environments. Nat Biotechnol. 2000

Jan;18(1):85-90.

39.) Craig Venter on DNA and the Sea. TED Talks 2005 Feb. He discusses in an 18minute segment the Sorcerer II Expedition sampling the world's ocean bacteria, gene sequencing and how D. radiodurans is the ultimate genome assembly machine. [web page]

40.) New Scientist. McDowell Natasha. Data stored in multiplying bacteria. 2003 Jan 8. [web page]

41.) US Patent 6,890,527. Thomas, et al. Methods of treatment. Filed 5/24/02 published 5/10/05. Assignee: The University of Arkansas (Fayetteville, AR).

42.) Patent application 20070122826. Glass et al. Minimal bacterial genome. Filed 5/31/07. Inventors from Maryland.

43.) Jensen JS. Mycoplasma genitalium: the aetiological agent of urethritis and other sexually transmitted diseases. J Eur Acad Dermatol. Venereol. 2004 Jan;18(1):1-11.

44.) Fraser CM, Casjens S, Huang WM, et al. Genomic sequence of a Lyme disease spirochaete, Borrelia burgdorferi. Nature 1997 Dec 11;390(6660):580-586.

45.) Johansson KE, Tully JG, et al. Mycoplasma cavipharyngis and Mycoplasma fastidiosum, the closest relatives to Eperythrozoon spp. and Haemobartonella spp. FEMS Microbiol Ltrs. 2006Jan 17;174(2):321-326.

46.) Haemobartonellosis, Haemobartonella infection. [monograph on the Internet] 2006Vetcentric.com Inc. [web page]

47.) Mann Jeffrey E. Recent advances in the development of Deinococcus in bioremediation of mixed radioactive waste. MMG 445 Basic Biotech. 2009;5(1):

48.) Bertin PB, Lozzi SP, Howell JK et al. The Thermophilic, Homohexameric Aminopeptidase of Borrelia burgdorferi Is a Member of the M29 Family of Metallopeptidases. Infect Immun. 2005Apr;73(4):2253-2261.

49.) Sekine K, Fukii H, Abe F. Induction of apoptosis by bestatin (ubenimex) in human leukemic cell lines. Leukemia. 1999 May;13(5):729-734.

50.) US Patent 5,466,577. Weisburg. Nucleic acid probes for the detection of Lyme disease spirochetes. Filed 10/27/93, published 11/14/95. Assignee: Amoco Corporation.

Another Use for Chaperonin

1.) Irani SR. Autoimmune Encephalitis – New Awareness, Challenging Questions. Discovery Medicine. Johns Hopkins. 2011 May 17. [web page]

2.) Javierre BM, Hernando H, Ballestar E. Environmental Triggers and Epigenetic Deregulation in Autoimmune Disease. 2011 Dec 26. Discovery Medicine. Johns Hopkins. [web page]

3.) US Patent 2,773,800. Powell Horace M. Rabies Vaccine Production. Filed 4/28/53, published 12/11/56. Assignee: Eli Lilly and Company, Indianapolis, IN.

4.) US Patent 2,768,114. Koprowski Hilary, et al. Rabies Vaccines and Methods of Preparing the Same. Filed 8/21/53, published 10/23/56. Assignees: The American Cyanamid Company, New York.

5.) Shaw Cheng-Mei, Alvord JR Ellsworth C, Kies Marian W. Straight Chain Hydrocarbons as Substitutes for the Oil in Freund's Adjuvants in the Production of Experimental "Allergic" Encephalomyelitis in the Guinea Pig. J Immunol. 1964;92:24-27.

6.) Kuroda Y, Nacionales DC, Akaogi J, Reevees WH, Satoh M. Autoimmunity induced by adjuvant hydrocarbon oil components of vaccine. Biomed Pharmacother. 2004;48:325-337.

7.) Waksman BH. Int Arch Allergy 1959;14(Suppl.)

8.) Waksman BH. Auto-Allergic Diseases and Their Relation to the Immediate and Delayed Types of Allergic Reactivity. Transact. College Int Allerg. 4th Symp. Rome 1959. Int Arch Allergy. 1961;18(55).

9.) US Patent 3,906,092. Hilleman, et al. Stimulation of antibody response. Filed 11/26/71 published 9/16/75. Assignee: Merck & Co., Inc. (Rahway, NJ). Inventors Hilleman Maurice R., Tytell Afred A., Woodhour Allen F.

10.) US Patent Application #20090305400. Naylor et al. Modified chaperonin 10. Inventors include Barbara Jane Johnson. Filed 1/16/06and 8/31/06. Published 12/10/09. Assignee: CBio Limited. Correspondence to San Francisco, CA.

11.) Duncan AJ, Bott CB, Terlesky KC, Love NG. Detection of GroEL in activated sludge: a model for detection of system stress. Lett Appl Microbiol. 2000 Jan;30(1):28-32.

12.) US Patent Database. Patent 4,888,276 Shelburne. Method and composition for the diagnosis of Lyme disease. 1989 Dec 19. [web page]

13.) US Patent 5,643,723. Persing, et al. Detection of a genetic locus encoding resistance to rifampin in mycobacterial cultures and in clinical specimens. Filed 5/26/94, published 7/1/97. Assignee: Roche Molecular systems, Inc. (Branchburg, NJ) and Mayo Foundation for Medical Education and Research (Rochester, MN). Inventors: David H. Persing, John J Hunt (Rochester, MN); Karen KY Young (San Ramon, CA); Teresa A. Felmlee (Oronoco, MN); Glenn D Roberts and Christian A. Whelan (Rochester, MN).

14.) Cockerill, III FR. Genetic Methods for Assessing Antimicrobial Resistance. Minireview. Antimicrobial Agents Chemo. 1999Feb;43(2):199-212.

15.) Patel R, Piper K, Cockerill III, FR, et al. The Biopesticide Paenibacillus popilliae Has a Vancomycin Resistance Gene Cluster Homologous to the Enterococcal VanA Vancomycin Resistance Gene Cluster. 2000 Antimicrob Agents Chemo. 2000 Mar;44(3):705-709.

16.) Cockerill III, Franklin R. CV. [web page]

17.) Jespersen DJ, Smith TF, Rosenblatt JE, Cockerill III, FR. Comparison of the Borrelia DotBlot G, MarDx, and VIDAS Enzyme Immunoassays for Detecting Immunoglobulin G Antibodies to Borrelia burgdorferi in Huma Serum. J Clin Microbiol. 2002Dec;40(12):4782-4784.

18.) Espy MJ, Cockerill III FR, Meyer RF, et al. Detection of smallpox virus DNA by LightCycler PCR. J Clin Microbiol. 2002 Jun;40(6):1985-1988.

19.) Ravin V, Ravin N, Casjens S, et al. Genomic sequence and analysis of the atypical temperate bacteriophage N15. J Mol. Biol. 2000;209:53-73.

20.) The Bovine Tubercle Bacillus in Joint Tuberculosis. J Bone Joint Surg Am. 1913;s2-10:465-466.

21.) Stover Kendall, Bansal Geetha P, Hanson, Mark S, Burlein Jeanne E, Palaszynski Susan R, Young James F, Koenig Scott, Young Douglas B, Sadziene Adriadna, Barbour Alan G. Protective Immunity Elicited by Recombinant Bacille Calmette-Guerin (BCG) Expressing Outer Surface Protein A (OspA) Lipoprotein: A Candidate Lyme Disease Vaccine. J Exp Med. 1993Jul;178:197-209. (The Rockefeller University Press).

22.) Krebs JR, Anderson T, Clutton-Brock WT, et al. Bovine tuberculosis in cattle and badgers: an independent scientific review. London: Ministry of Agriculture, Fisheries and Food. 1997.

23.) Rajasekaran S, Gunasekaran M, Jayakumar DD, et al. Tuberculous Cervical Lymphadenitis in HIV Positive nad Negative Patients. Ind J Tub. 2001;48:201-205.

24.) US Patent 4,743,591. Fukushima et al. Composition for animals. Filed 12/24/86 published 5/10/88. Assignee: Toyo Jozo Company (Shizuoka, JP).

25.) Kulski et al. Use of a Multiplex PCR To Detect and Identify Mycobacterium avium and M. intracellular in Blood Culture Fluids of AIDS Patients. J Clin Microbiol. 1995;33(3):668-674.

26.) Bale Kumar. Healing the Achilles Heel of Proteomics. Gen Eng Biotech News. Tech Updates 2010 Feb 1;30(3). [web page]

27.) Mac Síomóin Tomás. The gene is out of the bottle. The menace of genetic enginering. Red Banner 2000 July 7. 5 pages. [web page]

Cooking the Red Herring

1.) Feder Henry M JR., Johnson Barbara JB, O'Connell Susan, Shapiro Eugene D, Steere Allen C, Wormser Gary P, and the Ad Hoc International Lyme Disease Group*. NEJM;2007Oct 4;357:1422-1430. *The Ad Hoc Group consisted of these individuals: WA Agger (Gundersen Lutheran Medical Foundation, La Crosse, WI); H. Artsob, (National Microbiology Laboratory, Health Canada, Winnipeg, MB, Canada); P. Auwaerter, J.S. Dumler, (Johns Hopkins Medical Institutions, Baltimore); J.S. Bakken, (St. Luke's Hospital, Duluth, MN); LK Bockenstedt, J Green, (Yale University School of Medicine, New Haven, CT); RJ Dattwyler, J Munoz, RB Nadelman, I Schwartz, (New York Medical College, Valhalla); T. Draper, (Danbury Hospital, Danbury, CT); E. McSweegan, (Johns Hopkins Medical Institutions, Crofton, MD); JJ Halperin, (Atlantic Neuroscience Institute, Summit NJ and the New York University School of Medicine, New York); MS Klempner, (Boston University School of Medicine and Boston Medical Center, Boston); PJ Krause, (University of Connecticut School of Medicine and Connecticut Children's Medical Center, Farmington); P. Mead, (Centers for Disease Control and Prevention); M. Morshed, (University of British Columbia, Vancouver, Canada); R. Porwancher, (Univesrity of Medicine and Dentistry of New Jersey-Robert Wood Johnson Medical School, Piscataway); JD Radolf, (University of Connecticut Health Center, Farmington); RP Smith, Jr., (Maine Medical Center, Portland, ME); S. Sood, (Schneider Children's Hospital at North Shore, Manhasset, NY); A. Weinstein, (Washington Hospital Center and Georgetown University Medical Center, Washington, DC. SJ Wong, (Wadsworth Center, New York State Department of Health, Albany); and L. Zemel, (Connecticut Children's Medical Center, University of Connecticut, Hartford).

2.) Langhoff PJ. The Baker's Dozen & the Lunatic Fringe: Has Junk Science Shifted the Lyme Disease Paradigm? 2008Allegory Press LLC. Milwaukee, WI. ISBN:978-0-9654580-6-1

3.) US Patent 6,210,676. Callister, et al. Compositions and methods using the borreliacidal epitope(s) of borrelia burgdorferi outer surface protein C (OspC) for the diagnosis and prevention of Lyme disease. Filed 7/30/99 published 4/3/01. Assignee: Gundersen Lutheran Medical Foundation (La Crosse, WI).

4.) Cargill Timeline 1865-Present. [web page]

5.) Broehl Jr. Wayne G. Cargill. Trading the World's Grain. 1992 University Press of New England.

6.) Health Protection Agency of UK. Unorthodox Clinical and Laboratory Practices Related to Lyme borreliosis. [web page]

7.) Health Protection Agency. Report on Lyme Disease. Unorthodox and Unvalidated Laboratory Tests in the Diagnosis of Lyme Borreliosis and In Relation to Medically Unxplained Symptoms. By Professor Brian I. Duerden, Inspector of Microbiologyand Infection Control, UK Department of Health. [web page]

8.) Klempner MS, Schmid CH, Hu L et al. Intralaboratory reliability of serologic and urine testing of Lyme disease. Am J Med. 2001;110(3):217-9.
9.) Caution regarding testing for Lyme disease. MMWR 2005;54(05):125. [web page]
10.) Halperin JJ, Logigian EL, Finkel MF et al. Practice parameters for the diagnosis of nervous system Lyme borreliosis. *Neurology* 1996;46(3):619-27.
11.) Sigal LH. Anxiety and persistence of Lyme disease. Am J Med 1995;98(4A):74S-78S.
12.) Steere AC. Lyme disease. New Engl J Med 2001;345(2):115-25.
13.) Stanek G, Strle F. Lyme borreliosis. Lancet 2003;362(9396):1639-47
14.) Wormser G P, Dattwyler R J, Shapiro E D, et al. The Clinical Assessment, Treatment, and Prevention of Lyme Disease, Human Granulocytic Anaplasmosis and Babesiosis: Clinical Practice Guidelines by the Infectious Diseases Society of America. Clin Infect Dis 2006; 43: 1089-34.
15.) US Patent 7,344,720. Haensler. Vaccine composition. Filed 11/15/04published 3/18/08. Assignee: Sanofi Pasteur SA (Lyon cedex, FR).
16.) US Patent 5,618,533. Flavell, et al. Flagellin-based polypeptides for the diagnosis of Lyme disease. Filed 12/10/93 published 4/8/97. Assignee: Yale University (New Haven, CT). Inventors: Richard A. Flavell, Erol Fikrig, Robert Berland.
17.) Garfield Eugene. Lyme Disease Researcher Uncovers a Case of Delayed Recognition: Arvid Afzelius and His Successors. Current Comments. #49. 1989 Dec 4;p.3-8. In Scientist: Creativity, Delayed Recognition, and other Essays, 1989;12:345. [web page]
18.) Steere AC. Lyme disease. N Eng Med J. 1989;321(9):586-596.
19.) Barbour AG. The diagnosis of Lyme disease: rewards and perils. Ann Intern Med. 1989;110(7):501-502.
20.) US Patent 5,747,294. Flavell, et al. Compositions and methods for the prevention and diagnosis of Lyme disease. Filed 10/7/94published 5/5/98. Assignee: Yale University (New Haven, CT).
21.) Duesberg Peter H. Inventing the AIDS Virus. Regnery Publishing, Inc., Washington, DC. 1996. p. 381
22.) CDC. Guide E. Smallpox Preparation and Response Activities: Communication Plan and Activities.
23.) US Patent 6,719,983. Norris, et al. VMP-like Sequences of pathogenic Borrelia. Filed 8/16/02 published 4/13/04. Assignee: Board of Regents, The University of Texas System (Austin, TX).
24.) US Patent 5,466,577. Weisburg. Nucleic acid probes for the detection of Lyme disease. Filed 10/27/93 published 11/14/95. Assignee: Amoco Corporation.
25.) Program from Eastern Branch Entomological Society of America. 75th Annual Meeting. Entogration: Discipline Integrationin Entomology. 2004 Mar 7-9. Omni Hotel, New Haven, CT.
26.) NCME. Lyme Disease and Concomitant Tick-borne Infections. Narrator: Benjamin J. Luft, MD. #7161997 Jun 27. Video (60 Min.)
27.) US Patent 5,558,993. Champion, et al. Cloned Borrelia burgdorferi virulence protein. Filed 6/17/94published 9/24/96. Assignee: The Regents of the University of California (Oakland, CA).

Some Very Real Threats Lurk on the Horizon

1.) Finsterer J, Stölberger C, Sehnal E, Stanek G. Mild leptospirosis with three-year persistence of IgG- and IgM-antibodies, initially manifesting as carpal tunnel syndrome. J Infect 2005 Aug;51(2):E67-70.
2.) Daxboeck F, Khanakah G, Bauer C, Stadler M, Hofmann H, Stanek G. Detection of Mycoplasma pneumonia in serum specimens from patients with mycoplasma pneumonia by PCR. Int J Med Microbiol. 2005 Aug;295(4):27-85. Erratum in: Int J Med Microbiol. 2006 Feb;296(1):55.
3.) Kocianová E, Kost'anová Z, Stefanidesová K, Spitalská E, Boldis V, Hucková D, Stanek G. Serologic evidence of Anaplasma phagocytophilum infections in patients with a history of tick bite in central Slovakia. Wien Klin Wochenschr. 2008;120(13-14):427-31.
4.) Blaschitz M, Narodoslavsky-Gföller M, Kanzler M, Stanek G, Walochnik J. Babesia species occurring in Austrian Ixodes ricinus ticks. Appl Environ Microbiol. 2008Aug;74(15):4841-6. Epub 2008 Jun 6.
5.) Dietrich W, Rath M, Stanek G, et al. Multiple site sampling does not increase the sensitivity of Chlamydia trachomatis detection in infertility patients. Fertil Steril. 2010 Jan;93(1):67-71. Epub 2008 Nov 6.
6.) Health Protection Agency. Diagnosis and Treatment of Lyme Borreliosis. [UK public health web site]
7.) EUCALB. European Union Concerted Action on Lyme Borreliosis. [web site]
8.) Barbour AG. Isolation and cultivation of Lyme disease spirochetes. Yale J Biol Med. 1984Jul-Aug;57(4):521-5.
9.) Stanek G, Laber G, Hirschl A. Survival of spiroplasma on different carriers and resistance against three disinfectants. Proceedings of the 3rd International Organ. Mycoplasm. Custer, South Dakota, 1980 Sept. Abstract 107.
10.) Burgdorfer Willy, Barbour Alan G, Hayes Stanley F., Benach Jorge L, Grunwaldt Edgar, Davis Jeffrey P. Lyme Disease – A Tick-borne Spirochetosis? Science. 1982 Jun;216:1317-1319
11.) US Patent Application 20090324638. Live bacterial vaccine. Dattwyler Raymond J, et al. Filed 6/12/06, published 12/31/09. Inventors: Raymond J. Dattwyler (East Setauket, NY), Maria C. Gomes-Solecki (Memphis, TN), Jozef FML Seegers (Leiden, NL). Assignee: Biopeptides Corp., New York, NY. Note: This patent utilizes the OspA protein of Bb in combination with a lactobacillus bacterium and possibly the agent of bubonic plague – yersinia pestis in a composition intended for a live bacterial vaccine!
12.) US Patent Application 20090297560. Oral vaccine for Borrelia. Dattwyler Raymond J, et al. Filed 6/30/05, published 12/3/09. Assignee: unknown however possibly Biopeptides Corp. NY, Dattwyler/Gomes-Solecki's SUNY spin-off biotech company.
13.) US Patent Application 20090098121. Immunoglobulin Directed Biocides. Imboden et al. Filed 10/19/07, published 4/16/09. Assignee: ioGenetics, LLC, Madison, WI.
14.) US Patent application 20050086715. Xenorhabdus nematophila DNA sequences induced within insects. Goodrich-Blair et al. Filed 10/14/04, published 4/21/05. No assignees but the inventors are from Madison, WI. Xenorhabdus nematophila are gram-negative nematode-like proteobacteria that are enterobacteria (gut).
15.) Sadovi Carlos and Tribune staff. U of C researcher dies after exposure to plague bacteria. Chicago Breaking News Center. [monograph] 2009 Sept 19. [web page]
16.) US Patent 5,593,882. Cano et al. Ancient microorganisms. Filed 10/28/94, issued 1/14/97. Assignee: Ambergene Corporation (San Francisco, CA).

Arsenic and Old Lace

1.) Maheshwari Dinesh K. (ed). Bacteria in Agrobiology: Crop Ecosystems. 2011 Springer Heidelberg Dordrecht London, New York. ISBN: 978-3-642-18357-7
2.) Tatum HW, Ewing WH, Weaver RE. Miscellaneous gram-negative bacteria. p. 270-294. In Lennette EH, Spaulding EH, Truant JP. (ed.) Manual of clinical microbiology. 2nd ed. American Society for Microbiology, Washington, D.C. 1974.
3.) Appendix 6. Sampling of Plant Species Studied for Phytoremediation. LID Technical Guidance Manual for Puget Sound. 6 pages. [web page]
4.) McCutcheon SC, Schnoor JL. (eds). Phytoremediation: Transformation and Control of Contaminants. 2003. Wiley-Interscience, Inc. Hoboken, New Jersey.
5.) Olson PE, Fletcher JS. Field evaluation of mulberry root structure wtih regard to phytoremediation. Biorem J. 1999;3(1):27-33.
6.) Leigh MB. The release of phenolic compounds into the soil by root turnover of mulberry (Morus rubra L.). Masters thesis, University of Oklahoma, Norman, Oklahoma. 1997.
7.) Leigh MB, Fletcher JS, Nagle DP, et al. Vegetation and fungi at Czech PCB-contaminated sites as bioremediation candidates. In: Phytoremediation, Wetlands and Sediments. A. Leeson, EA Foote, MK Banks, V. Magar (eds). Sixth International Symposium on In Situ and On-Site Bioremediation. 2001 Jun 4-7, pages 61-68. San Diego, California. Battelle Press, Columbia, OH.
8.) Hackenthal E, Mannheim W, Hackenthal R, Becher R. [The Reduction of Perchlorate by Bacteria. I. Studies on intact cells] Biochem Pharmacol. 1964 Feb;13:195-206. Article in German.
9.) Timothy Lee Scott, Stephen Harrod Buhner. Invasive Plant Medicine: The Ecological Benefits and Healing Abilities of Invasives. Healing Arts Press. 2010.
10.) Symposium on Viral and Rickettsial Diseases. Presented at the Golden Jubilee Meeting of the Society of American Bacteriologists at Baltimore, MD. 1950 May 15. Joseph E. Smadel was convenor and editor of the papers presented. Paper discussed was titled Newer Knowledge of the Older Rickettsial Diseases.
11.) Baker EW (USDA Agricultural Research Service), Evans TM (Walter Reed Army Institute of Research), Gould DJ (Walter Reed), Hull WB (US Naval Medical Research Institute), Keegan HL (406th Medical General Laboratory, US Army Far East). A Manual of Parasitic Mites of Medical or Economic Importance. 1956. A technical publication of the National Pest Control Association, Inc. New York, p. 18.
12.) Baker Edward William, Evans TM, Gould DJ, Hull WB, Keegan HL. A Manual of Parasitic Mites of medical or economic importance. A Technical Publication of the National Pest Control Association, Inc. New York 1956. p. 18.
13.) White R.T. Effect of Milky Disease on Tiphia Parasites of Japanese Beetle Larvae. 1943Sept.;51(3):213-218.
14.) Steinhaus EA. Nomenclature and classification of insect viruses. Bact Revs. 1949;13:203-223.

15.) Kaya, H. K., M. G. Klein, et al. Impact of Bacillus popilliae, Rickettsia popilliae, and entomopathogenic nematodes on a population of the scarabaeid Cyclocephala hirta. Biocontrol Science & Technology 3.1993:443-453.

16.) Dutky SR, Gooden EL. Coxiella Popilliae, n. sp., a Rickettsia Causing Blue Disease of Japanese Beetle Larvae. Am Soc Microbiol. J Bacteriol. 1952;63:743-750.

17.) Huebner RJ, Stamps P, Armstrong C. Rickettsialpox. A newly recognized rickettsial disease. 1. isolation of the etiological agent. Public Health Report. 1946;61:1605.

18.) Campbell FL. Speed of Toxic Action of Arsenic in the Silkworm. From the Entomological Laboratory of the Bussey Institution, Harvard University, Boston. J Gen Phys. 1926:433-443.

19.) Powers EB. The goldfish (Carassius carassius) as a test animal in the study of toxicity. 1880-1949 Illinois biological monographs. Natural History Survey No. 5705. 1917;4(2). University of Illinois, Urbana-Champaign, IL.

20.) Horn MA, Drake HL, Schramm A. Nitrous Oxide Reductase Genes (nosZ) of Denitrifying Microbial Populations in Soil and the Earthworm Gut are Phylogenically Similar. Appl Environ Microbiol. 2006 Feb;72(2):1019-1026.

21.) Horn MA, Ihssen J, Matthies C, et al. Dechloromonas denitrificans sp. nov., Flavobacterium denitrificans sp. nov., Paenibacillus anaericanus sp. nov. and Paenibacillus terrae strain MH72, N2)-producing bacteria isolated from the gut of the earthworm Aporrectodea caliginosa. Inter J Syst Evol Microbiol. 2005 May;55(3):1255-1265.

22.) Park M, Lu S, Ryu SH, et al. Flavobacterium croceum sp. nov., isolated from activated sludge. Inter J Syst Evol Microbiol. 2006;56:2443-2447.

23.) Betlach MR, Tiedje JM. Kinetic Explanation for Accumulation of Nitrite, Nitric Oxide, and Nitrous Oxide During Bacterial Denitrification. Appl Environ Microbiol. 1981 Dec;42(6):1074-1084. Written by scientists from Michigan State University, and the Extraterrestrial Research Division, Ames Research Center, National Aeronautics and Space Administration, Moffett Field, CA.

24.) Ma Y, Seiler KP, Tai KF, et al. Outer surface lipioproteins of Borrelia burgdorferi stimulate nitric oxide production by the cytokine-inducible pathway. Infec Immun. 1994;62(9):3663.

25.) Holmes B. Owen RJ. Emendation of the genus Flavobacterium and the status of the genus. Developments after the 8th edition of Bergey's Manual. 1981. p. 17-26. From: H. Reichenbach and OB Weeks (ed.), The Flavobacterium-Cytophaga group. Proceedings of the International Symposium on Yellow-Pigmented Gram-Negative Bacteria of the Flavobacterium-Cytophaga Group, Braunschweig. July 8-11, 1980. Verlag Chemie, Weinheim.

26.) Woods AC, Burky EL. The Relationship of the Flavobacterium Ophthalmiae to Periodic Ophthalmia in Horses. Trans Am Opthalmol Soc. 1929;27:131-148.

27.) Twarog R, Cleverdon RC. Pigments of some flavobacteria, xanthomonads and corynebacteria. 1961;27:316-320.

28.) Owen RJ, Lapage SP. A comparison of strains of King's group IIb of Flavobacterium with Flavobacterium meningosepticum. Antonie van Leeuwenhoek J. Microbiol. Serol. 1974;40:255-264.

29.) Owen RJ, Snell JJS. Deoxyribonucleic acid reassociation in the classification of flavobacteria. J. Gen. Microbiol. 1976;93:89-102.

30.) Lavalee C, Arella M, Belloncik S, Furuichi Y. Expression of Escherichia coli of the cloned polyhedrin gene of Bombyx mori cytoplasmic polyhedrosis virus. Protein Exp Purif. 1993 Dec;4(6):570-579.

31.) Babu KR, Ramakrishna S, Reddy YHK, et al. Metabolic alterations and molecular mechanism in silkworm larvae during viral infection: A Review. African J Biotech. 2009 Mar 20;8(6):899-907.

32.) Zchori –Fein E, Perlman SJ, Kelly SE, et al. Characterization of a 'Bacteroidetes' symbiont in Encarsia wasps (Hymenoptera: Aphelinidae): proposal of 'Candidatus Cardinium hertigii'. Inter J Syst Evol Microbiol. 2004;54:961-968.

33.) Morimoto S, Kurtti TJ, Noda H. In vitro cultivation and antibiotic susceptibility of a Cytophaga-like intracellular symbiote isolated from the tick Ixodes scapularis. Curr Microbiol. 2006 Apr;52(4):324-329.

34.) Hamm JJ, Styer EL, Lewis WJ. Comparative virogenesis of filamentous virus and polydnavirus in the female reproductive tract of Cotesia marginiventris (Hymenoptera: Braconidae). J Invert Path. 1990;55:357-374.

35.) Goldstein EJC, Citron DM, Merkin TE, Pickett MJ. Recovery of an Unusual Flavobacterium Group IIb-Like Isolate from a Hand Infection following a pig bite. J Clin Microbiol. 1990 May;28(5):1079-1081.

36.) Benson MJ, Gawronski JD, Eveleigh DE, Benson DR. Intracellular Symbionts and Other Bacteria Associated with Deer Ticks (Ixodes Scapularis) from Nantucket and Wellfleet, Cape Cod, Massachusetts. Appl Environ Microbiol. 2004 Jan;70(1):616-620. This paper comes from the University of Connecticut (Storrs); and Rutgers University (New Jersey).

37.) ATCC. Database search under "flavobacterium". And Clone 39800. Bacillus thuringiensis subsp. Kurstaki de Barjac and Lemille. [web pages]

38.) Bashan Y. Interactions of Azospirillum spp. In soils: a review. Biol Fertil Soils 1999;29:246-256.

39.) Rea MC, Dobson A, O'Sullivan O, et al. Effect of broad- and narrow-spectrum antimicrobials on Clostridium difficile and microbial diversity in a model of the distal colon. PNAS 2011 Mar 15;108(Suppl. 1):4639-4644.

40.) White O, Eisen JA, Heidelberg JF, et al. Genome sequence of the radioresistant bacterium Deinococcus radiodurans R1. Science 1999 Nov 19;286(5444):1571-1577.

41.) US Patent 5,229,112. Obukowicz, et al. Combatting plant insect pests with plant-colonizing microorganisms containing the toxin gene B. thuringiensis as a chromosomal insertion. Filed 6/7/89 published 7/20/93. Assignee: Monsanto Company (St. Louis, MO).

42.) US Patent 3,763,000. Abe, et al. Enzymatic production of cephalexin. Filed 8/21/72 published 10/2/73. Assignee: Toyo Jozo Kabushiki Kaisha (Shizuoka-ken, Japan).

43.) US patent 5,229,112 Obukowicz, et al. Combatting plant insect pests with plant-colonizing microorganisms containing the toxin gene B. thuringiensis as a chromosomal insertion. Filed 6/7/89 published 7/20/93. Assignee: Monsanto Company (St. Louis, MO). Original application filed November 1985 (appl# 799369) and April 1985 (appl# 728906).

44.) US Patent 4,999,294. Looney et al. Method for producing the FokI restriction endonuclease and methylase. Filed 12/17/87 published 3/12/91. Assignee: New England Biolabs, Inc. (Beverly, MA).

45.) US patent #5,238,821. Barsomian, et al. Endo F-free PNGase. Filed 11/20/91 published 8/24/93. Assignee: Genzyme Corporation (Cambridge, MA).

46.) ATCC. Database search under "flavobacterium". [web page]

47.) ATCC. Clone 39800. Bacillus thuringiensis subsp. Kurstaki de Barjac and Lemille.

48.) Bashan Y. Interactions of Azospirillum spp. In soils: a review. Biol Fertil Soils 1999;29:246-256.

49.) Vandepitte J, Beeckmans C, Buttiaux R. [4 Cases of flavobacterium meningitis in newborns] Ann Soc Belg Med Trop. (1920). 1958 Jun 30;38(3):563-570. [Article in French].

50.) Cabrera HA, Davis GH. Epidemic meningitis of the newborn caused by flavobacteria. I. Epidemiology and bacteriology. Am J Dis Child. 1961 Mar;101:289-295.

51.) Sugathadasa AA, Arseculeratne SN. Neonatal meningitis caused by new serotype of Flavobacterium meningo-septicum. Br Med J. 1963 Jan 5;1(5322):37-38.

52.) Holmes BR. Owen J, Hollis DG. Flavobacterium spiritivorum, a new species isolated from human clinical specimens. Int J Syst Bacteriol. 1982:32157-32165.

53.) Holmes BR, Owen J, Weaver RE. Flavobacterium multivorum, a new species isolated from human clinical specimens and previously known as group IIk, biotype 2. Int J Syst Bacteriol. 1981;31:21-34.

54.) Holmes BR, Snell JSS, Lapage SP. Revised description, from clinical isolates, of Flavobacterium odoratum Stutzer and Kwaschnina 1929, and designation of the neotype strain. Int J Syst Bacteriol. 1977;27:330-336.

55.) Holmes BR, Snell JSS, Lapage SP. Revised description, from clinical strains, of Flavobacterium breve (Lustig) Bergey et al. 1923 and proposal of the neotype strain. Int. J. Syst. Bacteriol. 1978;28:201-208.

56.) Benson MJ, Gawronski JD, Eveleigh DE, Benson DR. Intracellular Symbionts and Other Bacteria Associated with Deer Ticks (Ixodes scapularis) from Nantucket and Wellfleet, Cape Cod, Massachusetts. Appl Environ Microbiol. 2004 Jan;70(1):616-620.

57.) Steere Allen C, Broderick Thomas F, Malawista Stephen E. Erythema Chronicum Migrans and Lyme Arthritis: Epidemiologic Evidence for a Tick Vector. Am J Epidemiol. 1978;108(4):312-321.

58.) Moszczynski K, Mackiewicz P, Bodyl A. Evidence for horizontal gene transfer from Bacteroidetes bacteria to dinoflagellate minicircles. Mol Biol Evol. 2011 Nov 10. [Epub ahead of print].

59.) Grimont F, Chevrier D, Grimont PA, et al.Acetylaminofluorene-labelled ribosomal RNA for use in molecular epidemiology and taxonomy. Res Microbiol. 1989 Sep;140(7):447-454.

60.) Anantharaman V, Aravind L. Application of comparative genomics in the identification and analysis of novel families of membrane-associated receptors in bacteria. BMC Genomics. 2003 Aug 12;4(1):34.

61.) Alvarez-Venegas R, Sadder M, Tikhonov A, Avramova Z. Origin of the bacterial SET domain genes: vertical or horizontal? Mol Biol Evol. 2007 Feb;24(2):482-497.

62.) Barragan VA, Mejia ME, Trávez A, et al. Interactions of leptospira with environmental bacteria from surface water. Curr Microbiol. 2011 Jun;62(6):1802-1806.

63.) Moszczynski K, Mackiewicz P, Bodyl A. Evidence for horizontal gene transfer from Bacteroidetes bacteria to dinoflagellate minicircles. Mol Biol Evol. 2011 Nov 10. [Epub

ahead of print].
64.) Grimont F, Chevrier D, Grimont PA, et al.Acetylaminofluorene-labelled ribosomal RNA for use in molecular epidemiology and taxonomy. Res Microbiol. 1989 Sep;140(7):447-454.
65.) Anantharaman V, Aravind L. Application of comparative genomics in the identification and analysis of novel families of membrane-associated receptors in bacteria. BMC Genomics. 2003 Aug 12;4(1):34.
66.) Barragan VA, Mejia ME, Trávez A, et al. Interactions of leptospira with environmental bacteria from surface water. Curr Microbiol. 2011 Jun;62(6):1802-1806.
67.) Zhong J, Jasinskas A, Barbour AG. Antibiotic treatment of the tick vector Amblyomma americanum reduced reproductive illness. PloS One. 2007 May 2;2(5):e405.
68.) Pancholi P. Kolbert CP, Mitchell PD, Reed Jr. KD, Dumler JS, Bakken JS, Telford III SR, Persing DH. Ixodes dammini as a potential vector of human granulocytic ehrlichiosis. J. Infect. Dis. 1995;172:1007-1012.
69.) Adler GH, Telford III SR, Wilson ML, Spielman A. Vegetation structure influences the burden of immature Ixodes dammini on its main host, Peromyscus leucopus. Parasitology 1992;105:105–110.
70.) Ahel I, Stathopoulos C, Ambrogelly A, et al. Cysteine Activation Is an Inherent in Vitro Property of Prolyl-tRNA Synthetases. J Biol Chem. 2002;277(38):34743-34748.
71.) Bachmann Barbara J. Studies on Cytophaga fermentans, n.sp., a Facultatively Anaerobic Lower Myxobacterium. Hopkins Marine Station, Pacific Grove, California. J Gen Microbiol. 1955;13:541-551.
72.) Clayton RA, Sutton G, Hinkle Jr PS, et al. Intraspecific Variation in Small-Subunit rRNA Sequences in GeneBank: Why Single Sequences May Not Adequately Represent Prokaryotic Taxa. Inter J Syst Bacteriol. 1995 Jul;45(3):595-599.
73.) Sundman V. The Ability of α-Conidendrin-decomposing Agrobacterium Strains to Utilize Other Lignans and Lignin-related Compounds. J Gen Microbiol. 1964;36:185-201
74.) Hendersomn EK. The metabolism of aromatic compounds related to lignin by some Hyphomycetes and yeast-like fungi of soil. J . gen. Microbiol. 1961;26:155.
75.) Ramant S, Shanmugasundaer ARM B. Metabolism of some aromatic acids by Aspergillus niger. J. Bact. 1963;84:1339.
76.) Stanierr Y, Sleeperb P, et al. The bacterial oxidation of aromatic compounds. 111. The enzymatic oxidation of catechol and protocatechuic acid to P-ketoadipic acid. J. Bact. 1950;59:137.
77.) Leopold B, Malmstromi L. Constitution of resin phenols and their biogenetic relations. Part XV. Nitrobenzene oxidation of compounds of the lignan type. Acta Chem Scand. 1951;5:936.
78.) Phillips M. The chemistry of lignin. II. Fractional extraction of lignin from corn cobs. J Am Chem Soc. 1986;50.
79.) From 8-K of Wausau-Mosinee Paper Corporation. US Securities and Exchange Commission, Washington, DC. Report dated July 6, 2005. Wausau Paper Company. 100 Paper Place, Mosinee, WI. The paper mill was located in Brokaw. [web page]
80.) Dow Wolff Cellulosics Launches Methocel™ for Flavor Emulsions. 2011 Feb 2. Dow Wolff Cellulosics. [web page]
81.) Hocking Martin B. Vanillin: Synthetic Flavoring from Spent Sulfite Liquor. University of Victoria, British Columbia, Canada. J Chem Ed. [web page]
82.) Dorey MJ. Some Properties of a Pectolytic Soil Flavobacterium. J Gen Microbiol. 1959;20:91-104.
83.) Partridge SM. Aniline hydrogen phthalate as a spraying reagent for chromatography of sugars. Nature. 1949;164:443.
84.) Pearl IA. Conidendrin from western hemlock sulfite waste liquor. J Org Chem. 1945;10:219-221.
85.) Seyferth, Dietmar. Cadet's Fuming Arsenical Liquid and the Cacodyl Compounds of Bunsen. Organometallics 2001;20(8):1488–1498.
86.) Stellman, Jeanne et al. The Extent and patterns of usage of Agent Orange and other herbicides in Vietnam. Nature. 2003 Apr 17; 422:681-687.
87.) Cevallos M. Arsenic-containing drug in chicken feed to be pulled from US. Los Angeles Times. 2011 Jun 9.
88.) 3-Nitro. Roxarsone granules. [web page]
89.) 3-Nitro (Roxarsone) and Chicken. US FDA. [web page]
90.) Kawalek JC, Carson M, Conklin S, et al. Final Report on Study 275.30. Provide data on various arsenic species present in broilers treated with roxarsone: Comparison with untreated birds. 2011 Feb 10. 39 pages. [web page]
91.) Graham N, Kanalley C. NASA Discovers New Life: Arsenic Bacteria with DNA Completely Alien to What We Know. The Huffington Post. 2010 Dec 2. [web page]
92.) Conti R, Parenti F. Rifampin Therapy for Brucellosis, Flavobacterium Meningitis, and Cutaneous Leishmaniasis. Clin Infect Dis. 1983;5(3):S600-S605.
93.) Olivares-Fuster O, Arias CR. Development and characterization of rifampicin-resistant mutants from high virulent strains of Flavobacterium columnare. J Fish Dis. 2011 May;34(5):385-394.
94.) Radeva G, Selenska-Pobell S. Bacterial diversity in water samples from uranium wastes as demonstrated by 16S rDNA and ribosomal intergenic spacer amplification retrievals. Can J Microbiol. 2005 Nov;51(11):910-923.
95.) O'Sullivan L, Weightman AJ, Fry JC. New Degenerate Cytophaga-Flexibacter-Bacteroides-Specific 16S Ribosomal DNA-Targeted Oligonucleotide Probes Reveal High Bacterial Diversity in River Taff Epilithon. Appl Environ Microbiol. 2002 Jan;68(1):201-210.
96.) Merkel BJ, Planer-Friedrich B, Wolkersdorfer C. (eds.) Uranium in the Aquatic Environment. 2002 Springer-Verlag Berlin.
97.) [Merkel BJ, Planer-Friedrich B, Wolkersdorfer C. (eds.) Uranium in the Aquatic Environment. 2002 Springer-Verlag Berlin.
98.) The Encyclopaedia britannica. Eleventh Edition. Volume XX. 1910-1911. The Encyclopaedia Britannica Company, 1911, New York. Parasitic diseases, page 776.
99.) Doukyu N, Kuwahara H, Aono R. Isolation of Paenibacillus illinoisensis that produces cyclodextrin glucanotransferase resistant to organic solvents. Biosci Biotechnol Biochem. 2003 Feb;67(2):334-340.
100.) Gordon RE, Hynes WC, Pang CHN. The genus Bacillus. Agricultural Handbook No. 427. US Department of Agriculture, Washington, D.C. 1973.
101.) Shida O, Takagi H, Kadowaki K, et al. Emended Description of Paenibacillus amylolyticus and Description of Paeniacillus illinoisensis sp. nov. and Paenibacillus chibensis sp. nov. Inter J System Bacteriol. 1997;47(2):299-306.
102.) Nakamura LK. Bacillus amylolyticus sp. nov., nom. Rev., Bacillus lautus sp. nov., nom. rev., Bacillus pabuli sp. nov., nom. rev., and Bacillus validus sp. nov., nom. rev. Inter J Syst Bacteriol. 1984 Apr;34(20:224-226.
103.) Todar Kenneth. Todar's Online Textbook of Bacteriology. The Genus Bacillus. [web page]
104.) Fukumoto J. Studies on the production of bacterial amylase. I. Isolation of bacteria secreting potent amylases and their distribution. [Article in Japanese]. J Agr. Chem Soc. Japan 1943;19:487-503.
105.) Priest FG, Goodfellow M, Shute LA, Berkeley RCW. Bacillus amyloliquefaciens sp. nov., nom. rev. Int J Syst Bacteriol. 1987;37:69-71.
106.) Dobell, C. *Antony van Leeuwenhoek and his "little animals"*. 1932
107.) Macdonald JB, Madlener EM, Socransky SS. Observations on Spirillum sputigenum and its relationship to Selenomonas species with special reference to flagellation. J Bacteriol. 1959 May;77(5):559-565.
108.) Chalcroft JP, Bullivant S, Howard BH. Ultrastructural studies on Selenomonas ruminantium from the sheep rumen. J Gen Microbiol. 1973 Nov;79(1):135-146.
109.) Macdonald JB, Madlener EM, Socransky SS. Observations on Spirillum sputigenum and its relationship to Selenomonas species with special reference to flagellation. J Bacteriol. 1959 May;77(5):559-565
110.) Horn M, Harzenetter MD, Linner T, et al. Members of the Cytophaga-Flavobacterium-Bacteroides phylum as intracellular bacteria of acanthamoebae: proposal of 'Candidatus Amoebophilus asiaticus'. Environ Microbiol. 2001 Jul;3(7):440-449.

The Iceman Cometh Bearing News of Borrelia

1.) Hall Stephen S. Iceman Unfrozen. National Geographic Magazine. 2011 November Issue.
2.) Janssens Koen HA, Grieken R. (eds). Wilson & Wilson's Comprehensive Analytical Chemistry. Non-destructive microanalysis of cultural heritage materials. Volume XLII. University of Antwerp, Belgium. 2004. Elsevier.
3.) Bellwood Peter S. The first farmers: the origins of agricultural societies. 2005 Blackwell Publishing, Australia.
4.) Bower Bruce. Serbian site may have hosted first copper makers. Finds intensify over Old world origins of metal production. 2010 Jun 25. [web page]

The Russian Model of an Agricultural Agent

1.) New York Medical College, Yale look for new tickborne disease in region. Press Release on Internet. 2011 Sept. 29. [web page]
2.) CDC. Platonov AE, Karan LA, Kolyasnikova NM, Makhneva NA, Toporkova MG, Maleev VV, Fish D, Krause PJ. Humans Infected with Relapsing Fever Spirochete Borrelia mimotoi, Russia.

3.) Bergey David Hendricks, Boone David R. Bergey's manual of systematic bacteriology, 2nd Edition, Volume 3. The Firmicutes. 2009.
4.) US Patent 5,585,102. Barbour, et al. Flagella-less borrelia. Filed 9/20/93 published 12/17/96. Assignee: Board of Regents, The University of Texas System (Austin, TX).
5.) US Patent 5,436,000. Barbour, et al. Flagella-less borrelia. Filed 1/11/91 published 7/25/95. Assignee: University of Texas System (Austin, TX).
6.) US Patent 6,077,515. Barbour et al. Flagella-less borrelia. Filed 8/13/96 published 6/20/00. Assignee: The University of Texas System, Board of Regents (Austin, TX)
7.) Ras NM, Lascola B, Postic D, et al. Phylogenesis of Relapsing Fever Borrelia spp. Inter J Syst Bacter. 1996 Oct;46(4):859-865.
8.) Fukunaga M, Takahashi Y, Tsuruta Y, et al. Genetic and Phenotypic Analysis of Borrelia miyamotoi sp. nov., Isolated from the Ixodid Tick Ixodes persulcatus, the Vector for Lyme Disease in Japan. Inter J Syst Bacteriol. 1995 Oct;45(4):804-810.
9.) Platonov AE, Karan LS, Kolyasnikova NM, Makhneva NA, Toporkova MG, Maleev VV, Fish D, Krause PJ. Humans infected with relapsing fever spirochete Borrelia miyamotoi Russia. Emerg Infect Dis. 2011 Oct;17(10):1816-1823.
10.) Richter D, Debski A, Hubalek Z, Matuschka FR. Absence of Lyme Disease Spirochetes in Larval Ixodes ricinus Ticks. Vector Borne Zoonotic Dis. 2011 Sept 16.
11.) Fomenko NV, Borgoiakov VLu, Panov VV. [Genetic features of Borrelia miyamotoi transmitted by Ixodes persulcatus]. Mol Gen Mikrobiol Virusol. 2011;(2):12-17. [Article in Russian].
12.) Richter D, Matuschka FR. Elimination of lyme disease spirochetes from ticks feeding on demostic ruminants. Appl Environ Microbiol. 2010 Nov;76(22):7650-7652. Epub 2020 Sep 24.
13.) Wilhemsson P, Fryland L, Börjesson S, et al. Prevalence and diversity of Borrelia species in ticks that have bitten humans in Sweden. J Clin Microbiol. 2010 Nov;48(11):4169-4176. Epub 2010 Dep 15. Erratum in: J Clin Microbiol. 2011 Jan;49(1):481.
14.) Barbour AG, Bunikis J, Travinsky B, Hoen AG, Diuk-Wasser MA, Fish D, Tsao JI. Niche partitioning of Borrelia burgdorferi and Borrelia miyamotoi in the same tick vector and mammalian reservoir species. Am J Trop Med Hyg 2009 Dec;81(6):1120-1131.
15.) Tokarz R, Jain K, Bennett A, et al. Assessment of polymicrobial infections in ticks in New York State. Vector Borne Zoonotic Dis. 2010 Apr;10(3):217-221.
16.) Fukunaga M, Takahashi Y, Tsuruta Y, et al. Genetic and phenotypic analysis of Borrelia miyamotoi sp. nov., isolated from the ixodid tick Ixodes persulcatus, the vector for Lyme disease in Japan. Int J Syst Bacteriol. 1995 Oct;45(4):804-810.
17.) Rich SM, Armstrong PM, Smith RD, Telford SR 3rd. Lone star tick-infecting borreliae are most closely related to the agent of bovine borreliosis. J Clin Microbiol. 2001 Feb;39(2):494-497.
18.) Richter D, Matuschka F-R. Elimination of Lyme Disease Spirochetes from Ticks feeding on Domestic Ruminants. Appl Envir Microbiol. 2010 Nov;76(22):7650-7652.
19.) Ogden NH, Margos G, Aanensen DM, et al. Investigation of Genotypes of Borrelia burgdorferi in Ixodes scapularis Ticks Collected during Surveillance in Canada. Appl Envir Microbiol. 2011 May;77(10):3244-3254.
20.) Takahashi Y, Fukunaga M. Physical Mapping of the Borrelia miyamotoi HT31 Chromosome in Comparison with That of Borrelia turicatae, an Etiologic Agent of Tickborne Relapsing Fever. Clin Diag Lab Imm. 1996 Sept;3(5):533-540.
21.) Ras NM, Lascola B, Postic D, et al. Phylogenesis of Relapsing Fever Borrelia spp. Inter J Syst Bacter. 1996 Oct;46(4):859-865.
22.) Fukunaga M, Okada K, Nakao M, et al. Phylogenetic Analysis of Borrelia Species Based on Flagellin Gene Sequences and Its Application for Molecular Typing of Lyme Disease Borreliae. Int J Syst Bacteriol. 1996 Oct;46(4):898-905
23.) Barbour Alan G, Putteet-Driver Adrienne D, Bunikis Jonas. Horizontally Acquired Genes for Purine Salvage in Borrelia spp. Causing Relapsing Fever. Infect Immun. 2005 Sept;73(9):6165-6168.
24.) CDC. Platonov AE, Karan LA, Kolyasnikova NM, Makhneva NA, Toporkova MG, Maleev VV, Fish D, Krause PJ. Humans Infected with Relapsing Fever Spirochete Borrelia mimotoi, Russia.
25.) Wisniak Jaime. Borax, Boric acid, and Boron – From exotic to commodity. Ind J Chem Technol. 2005 Jul;12:488-500.
26.) Alibek Ken, with Handelman Stephen. Biohazard. 1999 Random House.
27.) Technical Report: DDC AD408401. Conference on Biological Control of Insects of Medical Importance. American Institute of Biological Sciences (Washington, DC). 148pages. Date stamped June 28, 1961 Naval Medical Field Research Laboratory, Camp LeJeune, North Carolina. (DDC) July 16, 1963. Unclassified documents retrieved from the public domain.
28.) Radnedge L, Agron PG, Hill KK, et al. Genome Differences That Distinguish Bacillus anthracis from Bacillus cereus and Bacillus thuringiensis. Appl Environ Microbiol. 2003May;69(5):2755-2764.
29.) Helgason E, Okstad OA, Caugant DA, et al. Bacillus anthracis, Bacillus cereus, and Bacillus thuringiensis – one species on the basis of genetic evidence. Appl Environ Microbiol. 2000;66:2627-2630.
30.) Burges HD, Hussey NW. Microbial Control of Insects and Mites. 1971 Academic Press Inc. London, New York.
31.) Briggs John D. Mass Propagation of Bacteria Pathogenic for Insects. WHO Bulletin. 1964;31:495-497.
32.) Hatfield Laura. Bad year for anthrax outbreaks in US livestock. CIDRAP. [web page]
33.) Aitken LD (ed). Diseases of Sheep. Fourth Edition. 2000 Blackwell Science, UK.
34.) Stöcker Friedrich W. (ed). Concise Encyclopedia Biology (ABC Biologie). 1995 Spektrum Akademischer Verlag GmbH (Germany). Translated and revised by Scott Thomas A, PhD. Great Britain.
35.) Maramorosch Karl. Advances in Virus Research Vol. 22. 1978 Academic Press.
36.) Crookshank Edgar M. 1890. Manual of Bacteriology. Third Edition. New York J.H. Vail & Co. 3rd Edition. H.K. Lewis, London. 1890:322-335.
37.) Regis, Ed. The Biology of Doom: The History of America's Secret Germ Warfare Project. Macmillan, 2000. pp. 71-74.
38.) Siddharth Y. Srivastava and Aravinda M. de Silva. Characterization of Borrelia burgdorferi Aggregates. Vector-Borne Zoonotic Diseases. Jun 2009;9(3):323-329. Department of Microbiology and Immunology, University of North Carolina, Chapel Hill, North Carolina.
39.) Ascovirus. Viral Zone. [web page]
40.) Cheng XW, Wan XF, Xue J, Moore RC. Ascovirus and its evolution. 2007 Apr;22(2):137-147.
41.) Encyclopaedia Britannica. Facts about asfarvirus: cause of African swine fever, as discussed in African Swine Fever (ASF) (animal disease). [web page]
42.) Loh J, Zhao G, Presti RM, et al. Detection of Novel Sequences Related to African Swine Fever Virus in Human Serum and Sewage. 2009 Dec;83(24):13019-13025.
43.) Scoles GA, Papero M, Beati L, Fish D. A relapsing fever group spirochete transmitted by *Ixodes scapularis* ticks. Vector Borne Zoonotic Dis. 2001;1:21–34
44.) Barbour AG, Bunikis J, Travinsky B, Hoen AG, Diuk-Wasser MA, Fish D, Niche partitioning of *Borrelia burgdorferi* and *Borrelia miyamotoi* in the same tick vector and mammalian reservoir species. Am J Trop Med Hyg. 2009;81:1120–31.
45.) Yaroslavl Region. Engelinvest Group, Minerals and mining. [web page]
46.) Encycopledia Britannica. Torbanite. [web page]
47.) US Patent 3,620,927. Leathen. Cultivation of Micro-organisms on Hydrocarbons. Filed 6/26/69published 11/16/71. Assignee: William W. Leathen (Wexford, PA).
48.) US Patent 3,264,196. Filosa. Purification of Micro-organisms cultivated on hydrocarbon feedstock. Filed 12/16/63published 8/2/66. Assignee: The British Petroleum Company Limited of Britannic House, London, England, a British joint-stock corporation.
49.) Vossen Paul, Devarenne Alexandra Kicenik. Controlling Olive Fruit Fly at Home. University of California Cooperative Extension. 2006Jun 5. [web page]
50.) Shaw Cheng-Mei, Alvord JR Ellsworth C, Kies Marian W. Straight Chain Hydrocarbons as Substitutes for the Oil in Freund's Adjuvants in the Production of Experimental "Allergic" Encephalomyelitis in the Guinea Pig. J Immunol. 1964;92:24-27.
51.) Yaroslavl Region. Engelinvest Group, Minerals and mining. [web page]
52.) Ragheb M. Uranium Resources in Phosphate Rocks. 2010 Jan 23. Report. [web page]
53.) NIAID Grant 1R43AI082732-01. Mosquito Vector Control using BT Coupled to Seed Oil Bodies. Abdullah, Mohd Amir F, Costero Adriana. Insectigen, Inc. (awardee organization). FY2009.
54.) A Troubled Realm. Russian Agriculture's Spatial Constraints, Variance, and Prospects for Revival. Case Studies. [web site] http://www.radford.edu/~agrorus/cstudies.htm And College of Agriculture and Natural Resources, University of Maryland [web page]
55.) Mechel About Us Overview. [web page]
56.) Fomenko NV, Livanova NN, Chernousova NY. Diversity of *Borrelia burgdorferi* sensu lato in natural foci of Novosibirsk region. Int J Med Microbiol. 2008;298(suppl 1):139–48.

57.) Fukunaga M, Takahashi Y, Tsuruta Y, Matsushita O, Ralph D, McClelland M, Genetic and phenotypic analysis of *Borrelia miyamotoi* sp. nov., isolated from the ixodid tick *Ixodes persulcatus*, the vector for Lyme disease in Japan. Int J Syst Bacteriol. 1995;45:804–10.
58.) Scoles GA, Papero M, Beati L, Fish D. A relapsing fever group spirochete transmitted by *Ixodes scapularis* ticks. Vector Borne Zoonotic Dis. 2001;1:21–34.
59.) Barbour AG, Bunikis J, Travinsky B, Hoen AG, Diuk-Wasser MA, Fish D, Niche partitioning of *Borrelia burgdorferi* and *Borrelia miyamotoi* in the same tick vector and mammalian reservoir species. Am J Trop Med Hyg. 2009;81:1120–31.
60.) New York Medical College, Yale look for new tickborne disease in region. Press Release on Internet. 2011 Sept. 29. [web page]
61.) CDC. Platonov AE, Karan LS, Kolyasnikova NM, Makhneva NA, Toporkova MG, Maleev VV, Fish D, Krause PJ. Humans Infected with Relapsing Fever Spirochete Borrelia miyamotoi, Russia. 2011 Oct;17(10). [web page]
62.) McNeil Jr. Donald G. New Tickborne Disease Is Discovered. The New York Times. 2011 Sept 19. [web page]
63.) Widdel AK, Mccuiston LJ, Crans WJ, et al. Finding Needles in the Haystack: Single Copy Microsatellite Loci for Aedes Japonicus (Diptera: Culicidae). Am J Trop Med Hug. 2005;73(4):744-748.
64.) Masuzawa T, Suzuki H, Kawabata H, et al. Identification of spirochetes isolated from wild rodents in Japan as Borrelia japonica. J Clin Microbiol. 1995 May;33(5):1392-1394.
65.) Widdel AK, Mccuiston LJ, Crans WJ, et al. Finding Needles in the Haystack: Single Copy Microsatellite Loci for Aedes Japonicus (Diptera: Culicidae). Am J Trop Med Hug. 2005;73(4):744-748.
66.) Miyamoto Musashi [web page]
67.) NIAID grant 2R56AI021884-23. Larval Mosquito Feeding and Microbial Interactions. Walker Edward D. MI State University. FY2007.
68.) Nobuhiro M, Daisuke U, Takaya I, et al. Artificial Infection of Japanese Eel, Anguilla japonica, with Flavobacterium columnare. Suisan Zoshoku. 1999;47(3):431-437.
69.) Chakroun F, Urdaci MC, Faure D, et al. Ramdom Amplified Polymorphic DNA analysis provides rapid differentiation among isolates of the fish pathogen Flavobacterium psychrophilum and among Flavobacterium species. Dis Aquat Organ. 1997;31:187-196.
69.) US Patent 1,834,806. Schlack Paul. Manufacture of Artificial Threads. filed 3/1/28 published 12/1/31. Assignee: Aceta G.M.B.I. of Berlin-Lichtenberg, Germany.
70.) US Patent 1,860,473. Möhring Albert, Schultze Guido, Schlack Paul. Filed 9/21/29, published 5/31/32. Compositions consisting of woolen fibers and artificial threads. Assignee: I.G. Farbenindustrie Aktiengesellschaft, Frankfort-on-the-Main, Germany.
71.) US Patent 1,953,438. Schlack Paul. Process for Coloring Organic Products. Assignee: General Aniline Works, Inc. New York.
72.) US Patent 1,973,998. Schlack Paul. Sizing Artificial Silk. Filed 1/21/30, published 9/18/34. Assignee: Aceta G.M.B.H. Berlin-Lichtenberg, Germany.
73.) Ouyang Z, He M, Oman T, et al. A manganese transporter, BB0219 (BmtA), is required for virulence by the Lyme disease spirochete, Borrelia burgdorferi. PNAS. 20090 Mar 3;106(9):3449-3454.
74.) US Patent 11,629, July 24, 1890, 8d. W.N. Hartley, Dublin and W.F.B. Blenkinsop, London, England. Improvements in Decolourising Vegetable Oils in the Manufacture of Pale Drying Oils and Varnishes, and Apparatus therefor. P. 263. In: The Journal of the Society of Chemical Industry. 1891 March 31.
75.) Rishabh Intermediates. What is turkey Red Oil? [web page]
76.) Kinoshita S, Kageyama S, Iba, K et al. Utilization of a cyclic dimer and a linear oligomers of e-aminocaproic acid by Achromobacter guttatus. Agri Biol Chem 1975;39(6):1219-1223.
77.) Ohno S. Birth of a unique enzyme from an alternative reading frame of the preexisted, internally repetitious coding sequence. Proc Natl Acad Sci USA. 1984 Apr;81 (8): 2421–2425.
78.) Negoro S, Taniguchi T, Kanaoka M, et al. Plasmid-determined enzymatic degradation of nylon oligomers. J Bacteriol. 1983 Jul;155(1):22-31.
79.) Synthetic Yarn and Fiber Association (SYFA). Fiberworld Classroom. A service for teachrs and students. A Short History of Manufactured Fibers. [web page]
80.) NIAID grant 2R56AI021884-23. Larval Mosquito Feeding and Microbial Interactions. Walker Edward D. MI State University. FY2007.
81.) Nobuhiro M, Daisuke U, Takaya I, et al. Artificial Infection of Japanese Eel, Anguilla japonica, with Flavobacterium columnare. Suisan Zoshoku. 1999;47(3):431-437.
82.) Chakroun F, Urdaci MC, Faure D, et al. Ramdom Amplified Polymorphic DNA analysis provides rapid differentiation among isolates of the fish pathogen Flavobacterium psychrophilum and among Flavobacterium species. Dis Aquat Organ. 1997;31:187-196
83.) Neitzel DF, Johnson KA, Brogren S, Kemperman MM. First Collection Records of Aedes japonicus in Minnesota. J Am Mosq Cntrl Assoc. 2009;25(3):367-369.
84.) CDC. Information on Aedes japonicus. [monograph]. www.cdc.gov. and Widdel AK, Mccuiston LJ, Crans WJ, et al. Finding Needles in the Haystack: Single Copy Microsatellite Loci for Aedes Japonicus (Diptera: Culicidae). Am J Trop Med Hyg. 2005:744-748.
85.) US Department of Agriculture. p. Weekly newsletter, 1918 Aug 28;6:5.
86.) Vivoda Vlado. Japan's Energy Security Predicament in hte Aftermath of the Fukushima Disaster. J Energ Security. 2011 Dec 14.

The Bottom Line?

1.) Raghheb M. Uranium Resources in Phosphate Rocks. 2010. [web page]
2.) Bryan AC. IAGS. Thorium as a Secure Nuclear Fuel Alternative. Journal of Energy Security 2009 Apr. [web page]
3.) Lifton J. A report on Thorium: The newest of the technology metals. Resource Investor. 2009 Mar 18. [web page]
4.) Friedman John S. More power to thorium? Perspectives. The Bulletin of the Atomic Scientists. pps.19-20.
5.) Ragheb M. Uranium Resources in Phosphate Rocks. Report 2010 Jan 23. [web page]
6.) US Geological Survey. Thorium. Data sheet. 2009 Jan. mineral Commodity Summaries. [web page]
7.) USGS. US DOI. Hedrick James B. Thorium. 2007 Minerals Yearbook. Thorium (Advance Release). [web page]
8.) Rare Earth Elements. Minerals & Ores.
9.) Chemical & metallurgical engineering. Volume XXIV. Jan 1-June 30, 1921. McGraw-Hill Company, Inc. New York.
10.) Spear FS, Pyle JM. Apatite, monazite, and xenotime in metamorphic rocks. Dept of Earth and Environmental Sciences. Rensselaer Polytechnic Institute. Troy NY. Report 95 pgs.
11.) Bryan AC. IAGS. Thorium as a Secure Nuclear Fuel Alternative. Journal of Energy Security 2009 Apr. [web page]
12.) Castor Stephen B, Hedrick James B. Rare Earth Elements. Report 24 pages. [web page]
13.) Rothwell Richard P. The Mineral Industry, its statistics, technology and trade in the United States and Other Countries to the end of 1899. Vol. VIII. Supplement to Vols. I to VII. The Scientific Publishing Company, New York 1900. P. 430
14.) Chemical & metallurgical engineering. Volume XXIV. Jan 1-June 30, 1921. McGraw-Hill Company, Inc. New York.
15.) Goldschmidt Bertrand. Uranium's Scientific History 1789-1939. A paper that was presented at the Fourteenth International Symposium held by the Uranium Institute in London, September 1989. [web page]
16.) History of Glass Making. 2011 History.UK.com and History of French Glass Blowing and Hand Blown Glass. 2011 Aug 18. Mirakkul Glassware. [web page]
17.) Norman Remington. The Great Domaines of Burgundy: A Guide to the Finest Wine Producers of the Côte d'Or 2nd Ed. 1996. And USGS. San Francisco Bay Region Geology
18.) Geologic Hazards. About Quaternary Faults. [web page]
19.) Barchfield Jenny. Associated Press. France nuclear Site Explosion: Marcoule Waste Site Rocked by Blast. 2011 Sept 12. The Huffington Post [internet newspaper].
20.) Davis Mary Byrd. Nuclear France: materials and sites. Languedoc-Roussillon. [web page]

Nine: Now the Story is Told

Dirty Little Bacteria

1.) US Patent 7,605,248. Dattwyler, et al. Recombinant constructs of Borrelia burgdorferi. Filed 9/26/06, published 10/20/09. Inventors: Dattwyler Raymond J, Gomes-Solecki Maria JC, Luft Benjamin
2.) Miller, Victor. Institute of Medicine. National Academies. Health Effects of Project SHAD Biological Agent: Bacillus globigii. (Bacillus licheniformis; Bacillus subtilis var. niger; Bacillus atrophaeus). 2004. 52 pages. Contract # IOM-2794-04-001. [web page] Accessed 12/5/11
3.) US Department of Labor Bureau of Labor Statistics. Bulletin. No. 251. Industrial Accidents and Hygiene Series. Preventable Death in Cotton Manufacturing Industry. Arthur Reed Perry, M.D. October 1919. Government Printing Office, Washington DC. [web page]
4.) Dartmouth Toxic Metals Superfund Research Program. The Facts on Arsenic. What is Arsenic? [web page]

5.) Arima K, Beppu M. Induction and Mechanisms of Arsenite Resistance in Pseudomonas Pseudomallei. J Bacteriol. 1964 Jul;88:143-150.
6.) Beppu M, Arima K. Decreased permeability as the mechanism of arsenite resistance in pseudomonas pseudomallei. J Bacterio. 1964 Jul;88-151-157.
7.) Maschinski G. [Experimental studies on the effect of arsenic trioxide on protein catabolism and on bacteria]. Dtsch Zahnarztl Z. 1965 Mar 1;20:224-229. [Article in German].
8.) Iwainsky H, Reutgen H, Kalich R. [Studies on the endogenous metabolism of mycobacteria. 2. On the influence of enzyme inhibitors and effective antitubercular substances on 32 P-incorporation]. Z Naturforsch B. 1968 Feb;23(2):211-216. [Article in German].
9.) Rosenberg h, La Nauze JM, The Isolate of a mutant Bacillus cereus deficient in phosphate uptake. Biochim Biophys Acta. 1968 Mar 11;156(2):381-388.
10.) Kaback HR, Stadtman ER. Glycine uptake in Escherichia coli. II. Glycine uptake, exchange, and metabolism by an isolated membrane preparation. J Biol Chem. 1968 Apr 10;243(7):1390-1400.
11.) Razin S. Gottfried L, Rottem S. Amino acid transport in Mycoplasma. J Bacteriol. 1968 May;95(5):1685-1691.
12.) Adams A. Transformation and transduction of a large deletion mutation in Bacillus subtilis. Mol Gen Genet. 1972;118(4):311-320.
13.) Adams A, Oishi M. Genetic properties of arsenate sensitive mutants of Bacillus subtilis 168. Mol Gen Genet. 1972;118(4):295-310.
14.) Gentry MJ, Smith DK, Schnute SF, et al. Pseudomonas culture longevity: control by phosphate. Microbios. 1971 Dec;4(15):205-215.
15.) Smabri V, Cevenini R. Incorporation of cysteine by Borrelia burgdorferi and Borrelia hermsii. Can J Microbiol. 1992 Oct;38(10):1016-1021.
16.) Heimbuch J. Removing Arsenic from watre with ... plastic bottles and nutritional supplements?! Technol / Clean Technol. Monograph on internet. 2011 Sept 1.
17.) "Plastic bottle" solution for arsenic-contaminated water threatening 100 million people. 2011 Aug 31. Information was presented at a meeting of the American Chemical Society. ACS. Press Release. [web page] Accessed 12/6/11.
18.) Kumari B, Singh SN. Phytoremediation of metals from fly ash through bacterial augmentation. Ecotoxicology. 2011 Jan;20(1):166-176.
19.) USGS. Central Region Energy Resources Team. Fact Sheet FS-163-97 October 1997. Radioactive Elements in Coal and Fly Ash: Abundance, Forms, and Environmental Significance. And Tadmore J. Radioactivity from coal-fired power plants: A review: J Environ Radioactivity. 1986;4:177-204.
20.) Ionizing radiation exposure of the population of the United States. National Council on Radiation Protection and Measurements. 1987. Report No. 93, 87 pages.
21.) Huseyin Aytekin, Ridvan Baldik. Radioactivity of Coals and Ashes from Çatalagzi Coal-Fired Power Plant in Turkey. Rad Prot Dosim. 2011 31 May.
22.) US Environmental Protection Agency Office of Resource Conservation and Recovery Office of Solid Waste and Emergency Response. Public Hearing on EPA's Proposed Rule on Hazardous and Solid Waste Management System; Identification and Listing of Special Wastes; Disposal of Coal Combustion Residuals from Electric Utilities. Docket ID No. EPA-HQ-RCRA-2009-0640. 394 pages. 2010 Sept. 10, Pittsburgh, Pennsylvania.
23.) US EPA Office of Resource Conservation and Recovery Office of Solid Waste and Emergency Response. Public Hearing on EPA's Proposed Rule on Hazardous and Solid Waste Management System; Identification and Listing of Special Wastes; Disposal of Coal Combustion Residuals from Electric Utilities. Docket ID No. EPA-HQ-RCRA-2009-0640. 2010 Sept 8. Dallas, Texas.
24.) US EPA Office of Resource Conservation and Recovery Office of Solid Waste and Emergency Response. Public Hearing on EPA's Proposed Rule on Hazardous and Solid Waste Management System; Identification and Listing of Special Wastes; Disposal of Coal Combustion Residuals from Electric Utilities. EPA-HQ-RCRA-2009-0640. 2010 Sept 2. Denver, Colorado
25.) US EPA Office of Resource Conservation and Recovery Office of Solid Waste and Emergency Response. Public Hearing on EPA's Proposed Rule on Hazardous and Solid Waste Management System; Identification and Listing of Special Wastes; Disposal of Coal Combustion Residuals from Electric Utilities. Docket ID No. EPA-HQ-RCRA-2009-0640. 2010 Sept 14. Charlotte, NC.
26.) US EPA Office of Resource Conservation and Recovery Office of Solid Waste and Emergency Response. Public Hearing on EPA's Proposed Rule on Hazardous and Solid Waste Management System; Identification and Listing of Special Wastes; Disposal of Coal Combustion Residuals from Electric Utilities. Docket ID No. EPA-HQ-RCRA-2009-0640. 2010 Sept 16. Chicago, Illinois.
27.) US EPA. Rules and Regulations. 40 CFR Part 261. Final Regulatory Determination on Four Large-Volume Wastes From the Combustion of Coal by Electric Utility Power Plants. Federal Register 1993 Aug 9;58(151):75 pages.
28.) US EPA. Report to Congress. Wastes from the Combustion of Fossil Fuels. Vol. 2 Methods, Findings, and Recommendations. 1999 March. EPA 530-R-99-010. 231 pages EPA. And Technical Background Document on Ground Water Controls at CKD Landfills. 1998 June. Report. 199 pages.
29.) US Patent 5,436,000. Barbour, et al. Flagella-less borrelia. Filed 1/11/91, published 7/25/95. Assignee: University of Texas System (Austin, TX). Inventors: Alan G. Barbour, Virgilio Bundoc.
30.) US Patent 5,585,102. Barbour, et al., Flagella-less borrelia. Filed 9/20/93, published 12/17/96. Assignee: Board of Regents, The University of Texas System (Austin, TX). Inventors: Alan G. Barbour, Virgilio G. Bundoc, Adriadna Sadziene.
31.) Bergey David Hendricks, Boone David R. Bergey's manual of systematic bacteriology, 2nd Edition, Volume 3. The Firmicutes. 2009.

Thoughts on Bb and Lyme Disease

1.) Mattmann Lida H. Cell wall deficient forms: stealth pathogens. 3rd edition. CRC Press LLC. Boca Raton, FL
2.) Karl Heinz Wilm. www.ourfood.com slide presentation. WHO Guidelines for Recreational Water Environments. Slide 64 of 73.
3.) Tinanoff Norman, Camosci David. The Effect of a Low Fluoride Delviery System on Bacterial Metabolism, Bacterial Attachment and Caries. Corp. Author: Connecticut Univ. Health Center, Farmington. Report #ADA077569. Dated Sept. 1979, 103 pages. Contract #DAMD17-78-C-8066. Annual report Sept. 1, 1978-Sept. 30, 1979. Project #3S161102BS06.
4.) Potvin L, Laprade R, Schwartz JL. Cry1Ac, a bacillus thuringiensis toxin, triggers extracellular Ca2+ influx and Ca2+ release from intracellular stores in Cf1 cells. J Exp Biol. 1998;201:1851-1858.
5.) DelVecchio VG, Kapatral V, Redkar RJ, et al. The genome sequence of the facultative intracellular pathogen Brucella melitensis. PNAS 2002 Jan 8;99. 6 pages
6.) Monette R, Potvin L, Baines D, et al. Interaction between Calcium Ions and Bacillus thuringiensis Toxin Activity against Sf9 Cells (Spodoptera frugiperda, Lepidoptera). Appl Envir Microbiol. 1997 Feb;63(2):440-447
7.) Langhoff, PJ. God Science: The Secret World of Rampant Genetics, Hidden Illness, and Biotech Profiteering. 2010 Allegory Press, LLC. Hustisford, Wisconsin 825 pages.
8.) Thomas WE, Ellar DJ. Mechanism of action of Bacillus thuringiensis var israelensis insecticidal ß-endotoxin. FEBS Letters. 1983 Apr;154(2). 7 pages.
9.) US Congress Appropriations Committee Hearing, Research, Development, Testing, and Evaluation of Synthetic Biological Agents. (Subcommittee on DOD, HB15090). Published by the US Government Printing Office. Reposted on the Internet by the PhilFam Committee 22 June 1998.
10.) Stimson. Biological and Chemical Weapons. History of the US Offensive Biological Warfare Program (1941-1973).

The Aggregate Bb

1.) Hovind-Hougen Kari. Leptospiraceae, a new family to include Leptospira Noguchi 1917and Leptonema gen. nov. Int. J Syst. Bacteriol. 1979;29:245-251.
2.) Johnson Russell C. (ed.). In The Biology of Parasitic Spirochetes. Academic Press.New York 1976:101.
3.) Sefer M. Econological investigation on acvicola leptospira isolated in Romania, p. 49-55. In Sefer M (ed.), Leptospirosis, leptospira and other spirocheta. Cantacuzino Institute, Bucharest Hungary. 1975.
4.) Sefer M. Growth and multiplication specific serum inhibition test applied to acvicola leptospira, p. 77-83. In Sefer M (ed.), Leptospirosis, leptospira and other spirocheta. Cantacuzino Institute, Bucharest, Hungary. 1975.
5.) Bazovská S, Hovind-Hougen K, Rudiová A, Kmety E. Leptospira sp. Strain Dimbovitza, First Isolate in Europe with Characteristics of the Proposed Genus Leptonema. Inter J Syst Bacteriol. 1983Apr;33(2):325-328.
6.) Noguchi Hideyo. Cultivation of Treponema Calligyrum (New Species) from Condylomata of Man. J. Exp Med. 1913;17(1):89-100.
7.) Kurtzman RH Jr. Xylem Sap Flow as Affected by Metabolic Inhibitors. Plant Physiol. 1966;41:41-646. And Wyman JF, Guard HE, Won WD, Qay JH. Conversion of 2,4,6-trinitrophenol to a mutagen by Pseudomonas aeruginosa. Appl Environ Microbiol. 1979;37(2):222.
8.) Rebic, Ana. Biodegradation of 2,4,6-Trinitrophenol in Rhodococcus opacus and Nocardioides simplex : Developing a mutagenesis system and cloning of the nitrite eliminating enzyme. 2008 Dec 11. [web page]
9.) Whong WZ, Edwards GS. Genotoxic activity of nitroaromatic compounds and related compounds in Salmonella typhimurium. Mutat Res. 1984 Jun;136(3):209-215.
10.) Jellison WL, Eneboe PL, Parker RR, Hughes LE. Rat-bite Fever in Montana. Pub Health Rep. 1949Dec 30;64(52)1661-1665.

11.) Larson CL. Rat-bite fever in Washington, DC, due to Spirillum minus and Streptobacillus moniliforims. Pub Health Rep. 1941;56:1961-1969.
12.) Will Loren A. Rat-Bite Fever. In: Handbook of Zoonoses: Bacterial, rickettsial, chlamydial, and mycotic. Beran George W, Steele James H. (eds.) 1994 CRC Press LLC, Boca Raton, FL. ISBN: 0-8493-3205-2.
13.) CDC. MMWR Update: Leptospirosis and Unexplained Acute Febrile Illness Among Athletes Participating in Triathlons – Illinois and Wisconsin. 1998;47(32):676.
14.) Crookshank Edgar M. Manual of Bacteriology. Third Edition. J. H. Vail & Co., New York. 1890 Oct 28.
15.) Hull TG. Diseases Transmitted From Animals to Man. 3rd Ed. Thomas CC. Springfield, IL 1947.
16.) Reitzel RJ, Haim A, Prindle K. Rat-Bite Fever from Field Mouse. J Am Med Assoc. 1936;106(13):1090-1091.
17.) Jenkinson HR, Jordan CF. Case of rat-bite fever caused by bite of a wild mouse. J Iowa M. Soc. 1932;22:31-32.
18.) Skinner Charles E, Emmons Hester W, Tsuchiya Henry M. Henrici's Molds, Yeasts and Actinomycetes - a Handbook for Students of Bacteriology. Second edition. John Wiley & Sons, Inc. London. 1945.
19.) Engel A. Haverhill fever. Acta Med Scand. 1949;132:562-571.
20.) Cilento RW. Rat bite fever in New Guinea. Med J Australia. 1927 Aug:191-193.
21.) Barbour AG, Hayes SF. Biology of Borrelia Species. Microbiol Rev 1986 Dec;50(4):381-400.
22.) Francis E. Rat-bite fever and relapsing fever in the United States. Trans Assoc Am Phys. 1932;47:143-149.
23.) Simpson Walter M. Artificial Fever Therapy of Syphilis. J Am Med Assoc. 1935;105(26):2132-2140.
24.) Simpson WM, Kislig FK, Sittler EC. Ultrahigh Frequency Pyretotherapy of Neurosyphilis. A Preliminary Report. Ann Inter Med. 1933 Jul1;7(1):64-75.
25.) Short Charles L, Bauer Walter. Treatment of Rheumatoid Arthritis with Fever Induced by Diathermy. A follow-up study. J Am Med Assoc. 1935;104(24):2165-2168.
26.) Hench PS, Slocumb CH, Popp WC. Fever Therapy. Results for Gonorrheal Arthritis, Chronic Infectious (Atrophic) Arthritis, and other forms of "rheumatism". J Am Med Assoc. 1935;104(20):1779-1790.
27.) Gilbert Ruth. Report of the Diagnostic Laboratories. pp. 111-112 In Annual report. New York (State) Department of Health, New York. State of New York Forty-Second Annual Report. Year ending December 31, 1921. Volume I. By M. Lyon Company, Printers 1922.
28.) Newman Barclay Moon. Japan's Seret Weapon. Peter Greenleaf (ed.) Current Publishing Co. 1944.
29.) Inada R, Ito Y. A report of the discovery of the causal organism (a new species of spirocheta) of Weil's disease. Tokyo Ijishinshi 1908;1915:351-360.
30.) Inada R, Ido Y, Hoke R, Ito H. The Etiology, Mode of Infection and Specific Therapy of Weil's Disease. J Exper Med. 191;23(3):377.
31.) Burgdorfer W, Hayes SF, Mavros AJ. Nonpathogenic rickettsiae in Dermacentor andersoni: a limiting factor for the distribution of Rickettsia rickettsii. In Rickettsiae and Rickettsial Diseases (W. Burgdorfer and R.L. Anacker (Eds.)). 1981:585-594. Academic Press, New York.
32.) Magnarelli LA, Anderson JF, Philip RN, Burgdorfer W, Casper EA. Endemicity of spotted fever group rickettsiae in Connecticut. Am J Trop med Hyg. 1981 May;30(3):715-721.
33.) Magnarelli LA, Anderson JF, Burgdorfer W. Rocky mountain spotted fever in Connecticut: human cases, spotted-fever group rickettsiae in ticks, and antibodies in mammals. Am J Epidemiol. 1979 Aug;110(2):148-155.
34.) US Patent 6,183,986 Bergstrom, et al. OspA DNA and Lyme disease vaccine. Filed 6/6/95, published 2/6/01. Assignee: Symbicom Aktiebolag (Umea, SE). Inventors: Sven Bergstrom (Umea), Alan G. Barbour (San Antonio, TX), Louis A. Magnarelli (Durham, CT).
35.) Hayes Stanley F, Burgdorfer Willy. Reactivation of Rickettsia rickettsii in Dermacentor andersoni Ticks: an Ultrastructural Analysis. Infect Immun 1982 Aug;37(2):779-785.
36.) Cognis. Henkel & Cognis: A History of Excellence. [web page]
37.) Masuzawa T, Suzuki H, Kawabata H, et al. Identification of Spirochetes Isolated from Wild Rodents in Japan as Borrelia japonica. J Clin Microbiol. 1995 May;33(5):1392-1394.
38.) Nakao, M., and K. Miyamoto. Long-tailed shrew, Sorex unguiculatus, as a potential reservoir of the spirochetes transmitted by Ixodes ovatus in Hokkaido, Japan. Jpn J Sanit Zool. 1993;44:237–245.
39.) Sorex unguiculatus. [web page]
40.) Aksu G, Ruhi MZ, Akan H, et al. Aerobic bacterial and fungal infections in peripheral blood stem cell transplants. Bone Marrow Transplant 2001 Jan;27(2):201-205.
41.) Kudryashev M, Cyrklaff M, Baumeister W, et al. Comparative cry-electron tomography of pathogenic Lyme disease spirochetes. Mol Microbiol. 2009 Mar;71(6):1415-1434.
42.) Uchiyama T, Uchida T, Wen JW, Walker DH. Demonstration of heat-labile and heat-stable epitopes of Rickettsia japonica on ultrathin sections. Lab Invest. 1994 Sep;71(3):432-437.
43.) Silverman DJ, Wisseman CL Jr, Waddell AD, Jones M. External layers of Rickettsia prowazekii and Rickettsia rickettsii: occurrence of a slime layer. Infect Immun. 1978 Oct;22(1):233-246.
44.) Platonov AE, Karan LS, Kolyasnikova NM, Makhneva NA, Toporkova MG, Maleev VV, Fish D, Krause PJ. Human Infection with the relapsing fever spirochete Borrelia miyamotoi. Emerg Inf Dis, 2011,17:1816-1823.
45.) Masuzawa T, Suzuki H, Kawabata H, et al. Identification of spirochetes isolated from wild rodents in Japan as Borrelia japonica. J Clin Microbiol. 1995 May;33(5):1392-1394.
46.) Park William Hallock, Willaims Anna Wessels, Krumwiede Charles. Pathogenic microörganisms. A practical manual for students, physicians and health officers. 1917 Lea & Febiger, New York & Philadelphia. Sixth Edition. Pps. 513-514
47.) Kaufman J. Parasitic Infections of Domestic Animals: A Diagnostic Manual. Birkhäuser Verlag AG, Basel, Switzerland, p. 423.
48.) Pickens Edgar G, Gerloff Robert K, Burgdorfer Willy. Spirochete from the Rabbit Tick, Haemaphysalis leporispalustris (Packard). I. Isolation and Preliminary Characterization. J Bacteriol. 1968 Feb;95(2):291-299.
49.) O'Leary William Michael. Practical handbook of microbiology. 1977Condensed version of CRC handbook of microbiology. CRC Press LLC. (Boca Raton, FL). Laskin AI, Lechevalier HA (ed). 2nd ed.
50.) Tanji Y, Mizoguchi K, Akitsu T, et al. Fate of coliphage in waste water treatment process and detection of phages carrying the Shiga toxin type 2gene. Water Sci Technol. 2002;46(22-12):285-289.
51.) Gersberg Richard M, Lyon Stephen R, Brenner Robert, Elkins Bert V. Fate of Viruses in Artificial Wetlands. Appl Environ Microbiol. 1987 Apr;53(4):731-736.
52.) Schaub Stephen A, Bausum Howard T, Taylor Gordon W. Fate of Virus in Wastewater Applied to Slow-I(nfiltration Land Treatment Systems. Appl Environ Microbiol. 1982 Aug;44(2):383-394.
53.) Chauret C, Springthorpe S, Sattar S. Fate of Cryptosporidium oocysts, Giardia cysts, and microbial indicators during wastewater treatment and anaerobic sludge digestion. Can J Microbiol. 1999 Mar;45(3):257-262.
54.) Bonadonna L, Briancesco R, Cataldo C, et al. Fate of bacterial indicators, viruses and protozoan parasites in a wastewater multi-component treatment system. New Microbiol. 2002 Oct;25(4):413-420.

Bb Outer Surface Proteins

1.) Léjou JF, Diomandé I, Molas G, et al. [Human chronic gastritis associated with non-Helicobacter pylori spiral organisms (Gastrospirillum homonis). Four cases and review of the literature]. [Article in French]. Gastroenterol Clin Biol. 1990;14(11):806-810.
2.) Stevenson B, Choy HA, Pinne M, et al. Leptospira interrogans Endostatin-Like Outer Membrane Proteins Bind Host Fibronectin, Laminin and Regulators of Complement. PLOS One. 2007 November, Issue 11. 11 pages.
3.) Brissette CA, Verma A, Bowman A, et al. The Borrelia burgdorferi outer-surface protein ErpX binds mammalian laminin. Microbiol. 2009 Mar;155(Pt3):863-872.
4.) Brissette CA, Bykowski T, Cooley AE, et al. Borrelia burgdorferi RevA Antigen Binds Host Fibronectin. Infect Immun. 2009 Jul;77(7)2802-2812.
5.) Garcia RC, Murgia R, Cinco M. Complement Receptor 3 Binds the Borrelia burgdorferi Outer Surface Proteins OspA and OspB in an iC3b-Independent Manner. Infect Immun. 2005 Sept;73(9):6138-6142.
6.) US Patent 7,605,248. Dattwyler, et al. Filed 9/26/06, published 10/20/09. Recombinant constructs of Borrelia burgdorferi. Assignee: Research Foundation of the State University of New York (Stony Brook, NY).
7.) US Patent 7,179, 448. Dattwyler et al. Recombinant constructs of Borrelia burgdorferi. Filed 8/3/05, published 2/20/07. Assignee: Research Foundation of the State of New York (Stony Brook, NY).
8.) US Patent 7,060,281. Dattwyler et al. Groups of Borrelia burgdorferi and borrelia afzelii that cause lyme disease in humans. Filed 6/19/00, published 6/13/06. Assignee: Research Foundation of the State University of New York (Stony Brook, NY).
9.) US Patent 7,582,304. Dattwyler et al. Groups of Borrelia burgdorferi and Borrelia afzelii that cause Lyme disease in humans. Filed 3/9/06, published 9/1/09. Assignee: Research Foundation of the State University of New York (Stony Brook, NY).

10.) US Patent 5,217,872 Dorward, et al. Method for detection of Borrelia burgdorferi antigens. Filed 2/27/90 published 6/8/93. Assignee: The United States of America as represented by the Department of Health (Washington, DC).
11.) DeBach P., Rosen D. Biological Control by Natural Enemies. Cambridge University Press. 1974,1991, p. 124-125.
12.) Bergey David Hendricks, Boone David R. Bergey's manual of systematic bacteriology, 2nd Edition, Volume 3. The Firmicutes. 2009. Page 48.
chap 5 – mosquito release #19-21 and 5
13.) Barci LAG. 1997. Biological control of the cattle tick Boophilus microplus (Acari, Ixodidae) in Brazil. Arq. Inst.Biol. 64:95–101.
14.) Cherepanova NP. 1964. Fungi which are found on ticks. Bot. Z. Mosk. 49:696–99.
15.) W. Kenneth Hoover. The Biological Control of Detrimental Insects. 1933 Oct;4(3):75-89.
16.) Rockwood LP. Sporotrichum globuliferum Spegazzini, A Natural Enemy of the Alfalfa Weevil. J Econ Entomol. 1916 Oct;9:493.
17.) Cloyd RA. Know Your Friends. The Entomopathogenic Fungus Metarhizium anisopliae. Midwest Biological Control News. University of Illinois. [web page]
18.) US Patent 7,605,248. Dattwyler, et al. Recombinant constructs of Borrelia burgdorferi. Filed 9/26/06, published 10/20/09. Inventors: Dattwyler Raymond J, Gomes-Solecki Maria JC, Luft Benjamin
19.) US Patent 3,816,261. Torney. Culture Medium for Lertospira [sic] Organisms. Filed 4/1/71, published 6/11/74. Assignee: Johnson & Johnson (New Brunswick, NJ)
20.) Moderator Topics. (newspaper) Lansing, Michigan. 1918 Sept. 4. Volume XXXIX No. 1, Whole No. 1172, p. 91.
21.) Briddon RW, Pinner MS, Stanley J, Markham PG. Geminivirus coat protein gene replacement alters insect specificity. Virol. 1990;177:85-94.
22.) Cooper JL. Viruses and the Environment. Chapman & Hall. 2nd Edition. 1995. University Press, Cambridge, Great Britain
23.) Briddon RW, Pinner MS, Stanley J, Markham PG. Geminivirus coat protein gene replacement alters insect specificity. Virol. 1990;177:85-94.
24.) Cooper JL. Viruses and the Environment. Chapman & Hall. 2nd Edition. 1995. University Press, Cambridge, Great Britain
25.) van den Heuvel JFJM, Verbeek M, and van der Wilk F. Endosymbiotic bacteria associated with circulative transmission of potato leafroll virus by Myzus persicae. J Gen Virol. 1994;75:2559-2565.
26.) Shope RE. Epizootiology of virus diseases. Adv Vet Sci. 1955;2:1-46.
27.) Technical Report: DDC AD408401. Conference on Biological Control of Insects of Medical Importance. American Institute of Biological Sciences (Washington, DC). 148 pages.
28.) Marlow Susan A, Wilson Louise E, Lawrie Alison M. et al. Assembly of Amsacta moorei entomopoxvirus spheroidin into spheroids following synthesis in insect cells using a baculovirus vector. J Gen Virol. 1998;79:623-628.
29.) Fenner Frank, Woodroofe Gwendolyn M. The Reactivation of Poxviruses II. The Range of Reactiving Viruses. Virol. 1960;11(1):185-201.
30.) Joklik WK, Woodroofe Gwendolyn M, Holmes IH, Fenner Frank. The Reactivation of Poxviruses I. Demonstration of the phenomenon and techniques of assay. Virol. 1960;11(1):168-184.
31.)Wimmer Eckard, Hellen Christopher UT, Cao Xuemei. Genetics of Polio virus. Annu Rev Gent. 1993;27:353-436. Department of Microbiology, School of Medicine, State University of New York at Stony Brook, Stony Brook, New York.
32.) Marlow Susan A, Wilson Louise E, Lawrie Alison M. et al. Assembly of Amsacta moorei entomopoxvirus spheroidin into spheroids following synthesis in insect cells using a baculovirus vector. J Gen Virol. 1998;79:623-628.
33.) Spendlove RS, Schaffer FL. Enzymatic Enhancement of Infectivity of Reovirus. J Bacteriol. 1965 Mar;89(30):597-602.
34.) Spendlove RS, Lennette EH, John AC. The role of the mitotic apparatus in the intracellular location of reovirus antigen. J Immunol. 1963;90:554-560.
35.) Bell TM, Massie A, Ross, MGR, Williams MC. Isolation of a reovirus from a case of Burkitt's lymphoma. Brit Med J. 1964;1:1212-1213.
36.) HHS-FDA Center for Biologics Evaluation and Research. Advisory Committee Meeting. International Conference on Harmonisation; Guidance on Viral Safety Evaluation of Biotechnology Products Derived From Cell Lines of Human or Animal Origin; Availability. Federal Register. 1998Sept. 24;63(185):51074-51084.
37.) Babu KR, Ramakrishna S, Reddy YHK et al. Metabolic alterations and molecular mechanism in silkworm larvae during viral infection: A review. African J Biotech. 2009 Mar 20;8(6):899-907.
38.) Bennett AW, (ed). Journal of the Royal Microscopical Society; (Great Britain). 1898. 740 pages.
39.) Contributions from the laboratory of entomology. Harvard University. Bussey Institution of Applied Biology. Volume III. Boston. 1913-1916. 226 pages.
40.) Wilson F. The effectiveness of a granulosis virus applied to field populations of Pieris rapae (Lepidoptera). PT Bailey (ed.) Australian J Agr Res. 1960;11(4):485-497.
41.) Bailey Peter T. Pests of field crops and pastures: identification and control. 2007 Csiro Publishing, Australia.
42.) Steinhaus Edward A. Nomenclature and Classification of Insect Viruses. Bact Rev. 1949 Dec;13(4):203-223.
43.) Hughes Kenneth A. Development of the Inclusion Bodies of a Granulosis Virus. J Bacteriol. 1952 Sept;64(3):375-380
44.) Bergold GH. On the Nomenclature and Classification of Insect Viruses. 1953 Mar;56(3):495-516.
45.) US Patent 5,643,576. Johnston, et al. Method of inducing an immune response with a live Venezuelan Equine Encephalitis virus expressing a heterologous immunogen. Filed 5/19/95 published 7/1/97. Assignee: The University of North Carolina at Chapel Hill (Chapel Hill, NC).
46.) US Patent 5,532,154. Brown Dennis T. Mutated alpha virus. Filed 3/21/94, published 7/2/96. Assignee: Research Development Foundation (Carson City, NV).
47.) Smadel, Joseph E., Army Medical Department Research and Graduate School, Washington, DC. Laboratory Diagnosis of Viral and Rickettsial Diseases, A Reappraisal after Ten Years. Symposium on Viral and Rickettsial Diseases. Presented at the Golden Jubilee Meeting of the Society of American Bacteriologists at Baltimore, MD. May 15,1950.
48.) Horst Ibelgauft. COPE. Cytokines & Cells Online Pathfinder Encyclopedia. Namalwa. [web page]

Index

A

B

17259577R00221

Made in the USA
Charleston, SC
03 February 2013